Clinical Perfusion for Cardiac Surgery

Ahmed S. Awad • James DiNardo
Editors

Jiapeng Huang • Michael F. Hancock
Associate Editors

Clinical Perfusion for Cardiac Surgery

A Step-by-Step Guide to the Fundamentals

Springer

Editors
Ahmed S. Awad
Associate Professor, Department of Anesthesiology
Cooper Medical School of Rowan
University/Cooper University Health Care
Camden, NJ, USA

James DiNardo
Department of Anesthesiology
Boston Children's Hospital
Boston, MA, USA

Michael F. Hancock
Keystone Perfusion Services, P.C
Sewell, NJ, USA

Associate Editors
Jiapeng Huang
Department of Anesthesiology & Perioperative
Medicine
University of Louisville
Louisville, KY, USA

ISBN 978-3-031-91162-0 ISBN 978-3-031-91163-7 (eBook)
https://doi.org/10.1007/978-3-031-91163-7

This Springer imprint is published by the registered company Springer Nature Switzerland AG
The registered company address is: Gewerbestrasse 11, 6330 Cham, Switzerland

In Memoriam

This chapter is dedicated to Dr. David C. Wang, whose compassionate commitment to patient safety shaped Chapter 31, "Safeguards and Checklists." Though he passed away during production, his dedication to advancing safety standards will continue to inspire clinicians and safeguard patient care for generations to come.

To the loving memory of my parents, whose memory I hold dear;

To my beloved wife, Afaf, whose unwavering love, support, and friendship light my path;

And to our cherished children, Rami, Nancy, and Adam, whose patience and encouragement make all things possible.

Ahmed S. Awad

I extend my heartfelt gratitude to my wife, Morgan, and our four children for their unwavering support throughout my perfusion career. I am equally thankful to my colleagues at Cooper University Hospital and the Keystone Perfusion team for their invaluable partnership and encouragement.

Michael Hancock

I would like to thank my wife Jing Zhou, my children Emma and Justin, for their unconditional support and love. I would like to thank the BEST team of cardiac anesthesiology, cardiac surgery, cardiology, perfusion, nursing, and staff at University of Louisville Heart Hospital and Jewish Hospital.

Jiapeng Huang

I would like to thank my wife Olivia and my daughter Isabel for their unconditional love and support. I would also like to pay tribute to all my colleagues in the Heart Center at Boston Children's Hospital for their tireless devotion to the care of our patients.

Jim DiNardo

Foreword

The development of artificial heart-lung machines or cardiopulmonary bypass has allowed surgeons to operate inside the heart and create operative procedures to correct a broken heart. This technology has allowed surgeons to improve, extend, and save the lives of millions of patients afflicted with heart and large artery diseases. Cardiac surgeons were largely responsible for the development and conduction of cardiopulmonary bypass during open-heart procedures in the early days, but as it became more common and safer, highly knowledgeable and trained technical personnel took over that role. Those trained technicians became known as "perfusionists" and have become valuable members of the cardiac surgical team. Their roles have expanded from maintaining patients alive during cardiopulmonary bypass to managing and supervising patients on mechanical assist devices as simple as intra-aortic balloon pumps, to more complex ones such as extracorporeal membrane oxygenation (ECMO), ventricular assist devices, totally implantable artificial hearts, and, more recently, extracorporeal perfusion to repair and revive solid organs for transplantation.

Although cardiopulmonary bypass has become routine in cardiac operating rooms throughout the world, it remains fraught with numerous problems that continue to be slowly resolved. However, there is still much to learn, improve, and correct. In cardiopulmonary bypass as in most parts of medicine, clinical experience far exceeds the scientific basis for what we do to treat patients with various maladies. For this reason, evidence-based medicine is important in developing dynamic plans to manage patients. Dynamic because it needs frequent updates as our knowledge expands and experience increases. Cardiopulmonary bypass is no exception.

The editors of this book titled *Clinical Perfusion for Cardiac Surgery: Step-by-Step Guide to the Fundamentals* are commended for having compiled a comprehensive, pertinent, and timely compendium with topics related to cardiopulmonary bypass and mechanical circulatory support as described in 39 chapters. From basic anatomy and physiology of the heart and great vessels to the pathophysiology of cardiopulmonary bypass, the pharmacology involved in its execution, and its deleterious effect on the blood and other organs, to the management of complex clinical situations such as heart surgery in pregnancy, and advanced circulatory support, the reader will find a comprehensive textbook vital not only to perfusionists but also to cardiac anesthetists and cardiac surgeons. As often happens in textbooks with multiple authors, the contents are sometimes repetitive but always pertinent to the topic in discussion.

The reader realizes that a crucial aspect of cardiopulmonary bypass surgery is continuous communication among surgeons, anesthetists, and perfusionists and constant attention to detail to deliver a flawless outcome. It is also important to remember that for the operating team, an open-heart procedure may simply be "another day at work," but for the patient, it may be the most important day in his or her life.

This book contains the essentials on cardiopulmonary bypass, its benefits and adverse effects, and how to prevent or minimize them. It goes beyond that and offers the reader a basic understanding of how to protect the heart and other organs during cardiopulmonary bypass. It discusses in detail specialized areas such as open-heart surgery during pregnancy, fetal cardiovascular physiology, and neonate surgery. It contains a comprehensive description of the usefulness and management of intra-aortic balloon pumps, ECMO, and ventricular assist devices to support circulation. The chapters also contain a list of recommended references for additional reading. However, in highly specialized areas of cardiopulmonary bypass such as in neonates, pregnant women, and mechanical circulatory support, additional reading, updating, and training are needed.

Perfusionists, anesthetists, and cardiac surgeons will find this compendium to be an excellent source of information on the fundamentals of cardiopulmonary bypass and mechanical support of the circulation. It contains invaluable information on the science and practice of this type of life support, indispensable for the performance of open-heart operations.

Tirone E. David

Melanie Munk Chair of Cardiovascular Surgery
Peter Munk Cardiac Centre, Toronto General Hospital
Toronto, ON, Canada

Professor of Surgery, University of Toronto
Toronto, ON, Canada

Preface

Clinical Perfusion for Cardiac Surgery: A Step-by-Step Guide to the Fundamentals represents a comprehensive resource for practitioners and trainees engaged in cardiac surgery and perfusion. This book is meticulously designed to deliver practical, step-by-step guidance rooted in the fundamentals of perfusion science while also covering the complexities and specialized techniques that have evolved in the field. The purpose of this text is to serve as both an educational foundation and a detailed clinical reference, assisting perfusionists, anesthesiologists, surgeons, and other healthcare professionals involved in the intricate process of cardiopulmonary bypass (CPB) and mechanical circulatory support.

The structure of this guide, divided into 12 parts, allows for an in-depth exploration of each critical aspect of clinical perfusion. In Part I: Fundamentals of Basic Science, readers are introduced to essential cardiovascular anatomy and physiology, alongside blood physiology and pharmacology relevant to CPB. In Part II, a historical overview of CPB provides context for its evolution, highlighting how advancements in technology and technique have shaped modern perfusion practices.

Part III focuses on adult CPB, detailing physiological responses to bypass, equipment essentials, circuit assembly, and metabolic and goal-directed perfusion management strategies. The significance of monitoring is emphasized in Part IV, covering techniques for assessing perfusion adequacy and anticoagulation status during CPB. Blood management, critical to patient outcomes, is explored in Part V, addressing hematocrit and transfusion practices, anticoagulation, and conservation techniques that balance efficacy with safety.

The complexities of pediatric perfusion and congenital cardiac pathology are discussed in Part VI, while Part VII addresses clinical challenges and complications, underscoring proactive strategies for managing mechanical and emergent issues during CPB. Organ protection, a crucial consideration during bypass, is the focus of Part VIII, detailing strategies to safeguard myocardial, neurological, and renal function to support long-term patient recovery.

Safety protocols are highlighted in Part IX, featuring essential safeguards and checklists. Part X explores mechanical circulatory support options, such as Intra-Aortic Balloon Pump, Ventricular Assist Devices, and Extracorporeal Membrane Oxygenation, vital for supporting critically ill patients.

Part XI examines CPB under unique circumstances, including deep hypothermic circulatory arrest, special patient populations, distal aortic repair, and pregnancy. Part XII concludes with best practices for record-keeping, emphasizing documentation's role in patient safety and outcomes.

This book has been made possible through the collaborative expertise of leading practitioners in perfusion and cardiac surgery. Each contributor brings a wealth of knowledge and hands-on experience, ensuring that the content is both clinically relevant and reflective of current best practices. We hope this guide will serve as a valuable tool for training, a reference for seasoned professionals, and a catalyst for further innovation and research in the field of clinical perfusion.

We extend our deepest gratitude to the contributors, reviewers, and collaborators who have dedicated their time and expertise to this work. We also thank our readers, whose commitment to advancing patient care in cardiac surgery inspires us to push the boundaries of knowledge and practice in clinical perfusion.

Camden, NJ, USA — Ahmed S. Awad
Sewell, NJ, USA — Michael Hancock
Louisville, KY, USA — Jiapeng Huang
Boston, MA, USA — James DiNardo

Acknowledgments

We sincerely acknowledge all the authors and co-authors of this book, many of whom are practicing clinical perfusionists, cardiac surgeons, and cardiovascular anesthesiologists. We extend our heartfelt gratitude to the perfusion team at Cooper University Hospital, whose support was instrumental in the completion of "Clinical Perfusion for Cardiac Surgery—A Step-by-Step Guide to the Fundamentals." Although not directly involved in the authorship, their contributions were vital to this project. Special thanks to Robert Rios, Michael Campisi, Sally Fowler, Madeline Bekier, John Wallace, Yulia Fisch, and John Schultz for their unwavering assistance and expertise.

A special acknowledgment is also extended to Soojung Moon for her invaluable help in creating the complex medical illustrations. Her talent and dedication brought clarity and precision to the content of this book.

We thank you all for your invaluable support.

Contents

Part IV Monitoring During Cardiopulmonary Bypass

Part V Basics of Blood Management

Part VI Pediatrics

Part VII Clinical Problems and Complications During Cardiopulmonary Bypass

Part VIII Organ Protection During Cardiopulmonary Bypass

Part I

Fundamentals of Basic Science

Basic Cardiovascular Anatomy

1

Robert H. Anderson and Diane E. Spicer

Anatomy of the Heart

Position of the Heart in the Thorax

The heart is a cone-shaped organ with myocardial walls occupying the middle mediastinum of the thoracic cavity. Its mass is oriented such that two-thirds is usually to the left of the midline, with its long axis slanting markedly from top to bottom and right to left when viewed from the front. This discrepancy between the long axis of the heart and that of the body is significant when describing its component parts.

The heart is positioned between the lungs and rests on the top of the diaphragm's superior surface. Its apex directs downward towards the left hip, while its base aims towards the right shoulder. The apex normally is formed by the left ventricle, with the base formed by the atrial chambers and the origins of the great vessels.

The Borders and Surfaces of the Heart

The heart, being trapezoidal in shape when viewed from the front, has four borders and three surfaces. The right border is mainly formed by the right atrium, with the sloping left border formed mainly by the left ventricle, and minimally by the left atrial appendage. The lower border, which rests on the diaphragm, is formed largely by the right ventricle. The superior border is occupied largely by the intrapericardial arterial trunks as they extend into the mediastinum (Fig. 1.1).

Its surfaces are best seen when assessed along the short axis of the ventricular cone. The sternocostal surface is formed mainly by the right ventricle and the pulmonary trunk. The diaphragmatic surface is formed by the inferior surfaces of the right and left ventricles, with the posterior surface formed by the obtuse margin of the left ventricle, along with the left atrium, which has the pulmonary veins draining into its roof (Fig. 1.2).

Layers of the Heart Wall

The walls of the heart have three basic layers, with the epicardial and endocardial linings enclosing the myocardium. The myocardium is the muscle layer. The endocardium is the smooth inner endothelial lining, while the epicardium is the parietal layer of the fibrous sac known as the pericardium. Its fibrous layer is the tough sack that surrounds the heart, with its serous layers reflected on one another at the openings of the great veins and the intrapericardial arterial trunks. The fibrous layer, which can be considered to represent the cardiac seat belt, is tightly bound to the central tendon of the diaphragm. The serous layer itself has two parts. The outer parietal component lines the inner surface of the fibrous

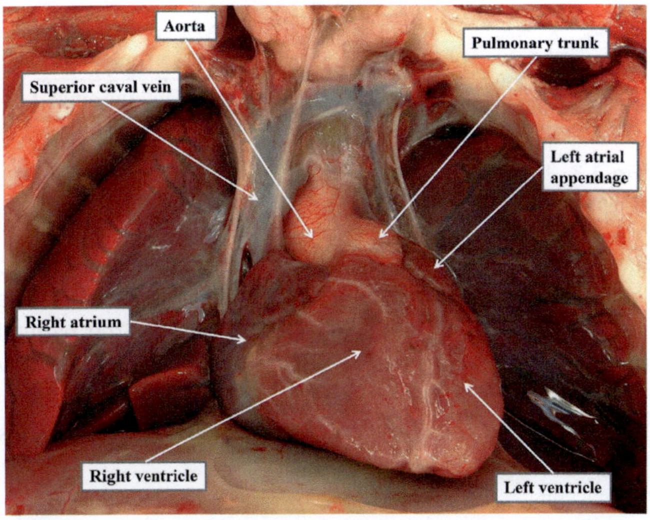

Fig. 1.1 The photograph shows the location of the heart, as seen from the front, within the mediastinum

R. H. Anderson (✉)
Newcastle University, Newcastle-upon-Tyne, UK
e-mail: sejjran@ucl.ac.uk

D. E. Spicer
Johns Hopkins All Children's Hospital, St. Petersburg, FL, USA

A. S. Awad, J. DiNardo (eds.), *Clinical Perfusion for Cardiac Surgery*, https://doi.org/10.1007/978-3-031-91163-7_1

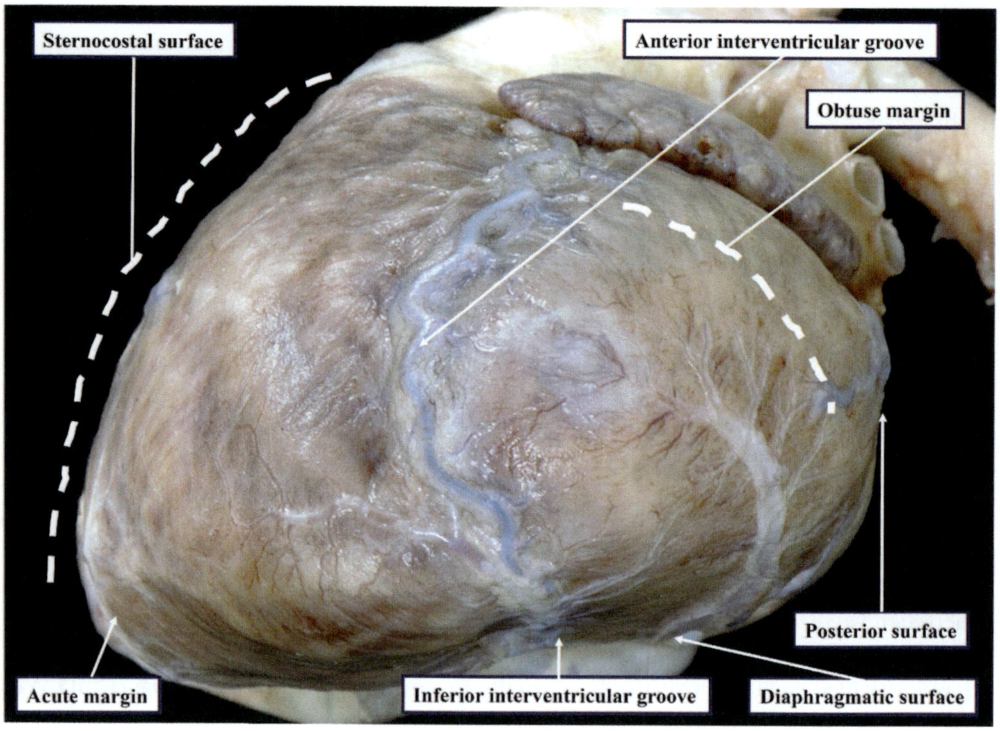

Fig. 1.2 The heart is photographed from its apex, looking towards the base, to show its surfaces. The image also shows the location of the acute and obtuse margins of the ventricular cone. The coronary arteries mark the location of the ventricular septum

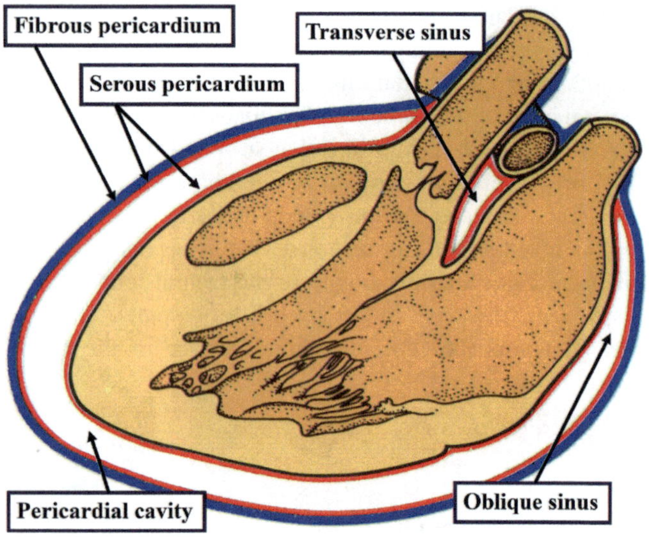

Fig. 1.3 The drawing shows the arrangement of the pericardium, along with the location of its transverse and oblique sinuses

layer. The internal layer clothes the walls of the cardiac chambers and intrapericardial vessels as the epicardium. The pericardial space is a potential space between the parietal and visceral layers of the serous pericardium. It normally contains less than 50 milliliters of serous fluid. The space has two major recesses: the transverse and oblique sinuses (Fig. 1.3).

The transverse sinus is the space between the back surfaces of the arterial trunks within the pericardium and the front walls of the atria. The oblique sinus lies posteriorly behind the left atrium, being limited by the entrances of the great veins to the right and left atrial chambers. The fibrous pericardium is supplied by several internal thoracic arteries and innervated by branches of the phrenic nerve. The visceral layer of the serous pericardium is innervated by branches of the sympathetic trunk and vagus nerves. Pain originating from the pericardium is felt as diffuse retrosternal pain, often made worse by lying down.

Chambers of the Heart

The heart functions as a dual-circuit pump. The first circuit operates at low pressure, propelling blood towards the lungs, while the second, a high-pressure system, circulates blood throughout the body. Each circuit consists of two chambers: an atrium and a ventricle. The atria are divided by the atrial septum, and the ventricular septum separates the ventricles. The left ventricle and right atrium are also separated by a small septum, the atrioventricular component of the membranous septum. The atrial chambers are then separated from the ventricles by the insulating tissues of the atrioventricular junctions. In the normal heart, there is only one myocardial connection between the atria and ventricles, the atrioventricular bundle (bundle of His).

The Right Atrium

The right atrium, when viewed from the front, occupies the right upper corner of the cardiac silhouette (Fig. 1.1). It has five anatomically distinct parts: a venous component, the vestibule, the right atrial appendage, a small part of the atrial body, and the septum (Fig. 1.4).

The venous component of the right atrium is formed by the openings of the superior and inferior caval veins and the coronary sinus. Its walls are smooth. During cardiac development, the boundaries between the venous component and the rest of the atrium are marked by the so-called venous valves. A remnant of these valves, the Eustachian valve, is usually visible at the entrance of the inferior caval vein. During fetal life, it directs oxygen-rich blood into the left atrium, bypassing the non-functioning lungs. It can persist to a greater extent in postnatal life as the Chiari network. Another remnant of the embryonic venous valves, the Thebesian valve, is usually found at the opening of the coronary sinus to inhibit blood backflow during systole. The junction of the two remnants embeds into the myocardial wall between the coronary sinus opening and the oval fossa, known as the tendon of Todaro. This serves as a crucial reference point for identifying the atrioventricular conduction axis. The vestibule refers to the smooth muscular region that converges into the leaflets of the tricuspid valve. The appendage makes up the larger part of the atrial walls. Its internal surface is marked by the pectinate muscles, with its junction with the smooth-walled atrial components demarcated by a prominent muscular band, the terminal crest or crista terminalis. The external counterpart of this crest is the terminal groove. This area is also of importance, since the cardiac pacemaker, the sinus node, lies within the groove adjacent to the opening of the superior caval vein. The septum is the partition separating the two atrial cavities. As seen from the right side, the true interatrial septum is limited to the floor of a small, oval-shaped depression known as the oval fossa, or fossa ovalis, along with an antero-inferior buttress that inserts into the insulating plane of the atrioventricular junctions. The remaining borders of the septum are formed by folds of the neighboring right and left atrial walls, which incorporate extracardiac fatty tissue. Therefore, any puncture beyond the true septum will exit outside the heart. The buttress is the true second septum, although the infolded superior rims of the fossa are often incorrectly identified as the "septum secundum." The floor of the fossa is the flap valve, which is usually, but not always, fused to the left atrial aspect of infolded rims. The lack of fusion produces persistent patency of the fossa, found in up to one-quarter of all normal individuals.

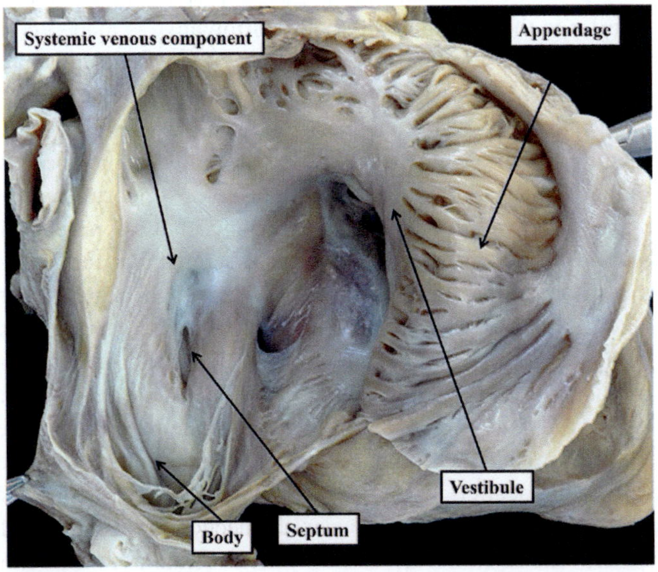

Fig. 1.4 The right atrium is opened to show its component parts. The body is the small part between the systemic venous sinus and the atrial septum

The Right Ventricle

The right ventricle is crescent-shaped, wrapping around the left ventricle to form the greater part of the ventricular mass when seen from the front. It extends from the atrioventricular to the ventriculo-arterial junctions and has three parts (Fig. 1.5).

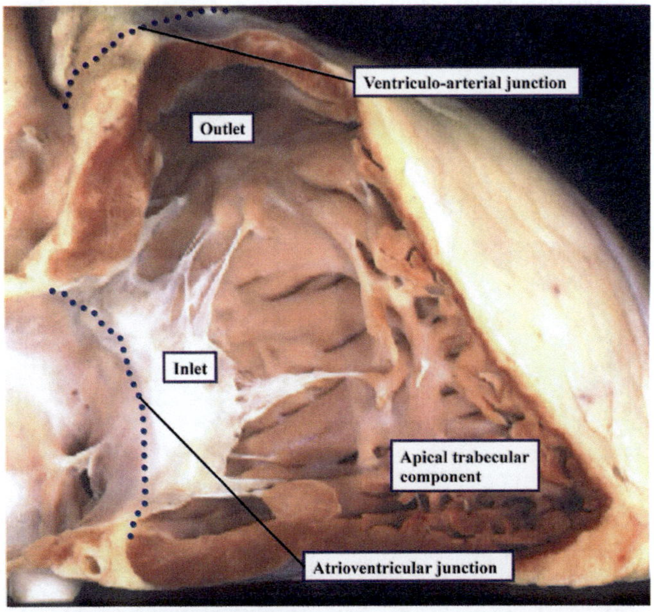

Fig. 1.5 The parietal wall of the morphologically right ventricle has been removed to show how the chamber extends from the atrioventricular to the ventriculo-arterial junctions. It has inlet, apical trabecular, and outlet components

The inlet, guarded by the tricuspid valve, extends from the atrioventricular junction to the insertions of the papillary muscles. The tricuspid valve is the largest of the four cardiac valves, with an area of 4 to 6 cm^2. It has three leaflets, which are located antero-superiorly, septally, and inferiorly when the valvar orifice is viewed in an attitudinally appropriate fashion (Fig. 1.6).

The ventricular apical component, characterized by its coarse trabeculations, extends to the ventricular apex. Among these trabeculations, the septomarginal trabeculation, also known as the septal band, is particularly prominent. This band reinforces the surface of the muscular ventricular septum. The moderator band crosses the ventricular cavity to connect with the anterior papillary muscle of the tricuspid valve and carries a significant branch of the right fascicle of the atrioventricular conduction axis. A series of septoparietal trabeculations extends from its anterior margin to the parietal wall of the ventricle. The ventricular outlet is a free-standing infundibular sleeve that supports the leaflets of the pulmonary valve. The inlet featuring the tricuspid valve and outlet featuring the pulmonic valve are separated in the roof of the ventricle by the inner heart curvature, also known as the supraventricular crest or crista supraventricularis. The pulmonary valve has three semilunar leaflets, two of which are adjacent to the aortic root. The leaflets are thin, with their semilunar hinges crossing the myocardial–arterial junction such that crescents of myocardium are incorporated within the bases of all three sinuses of the pulmonary root (Fig. 1.7).

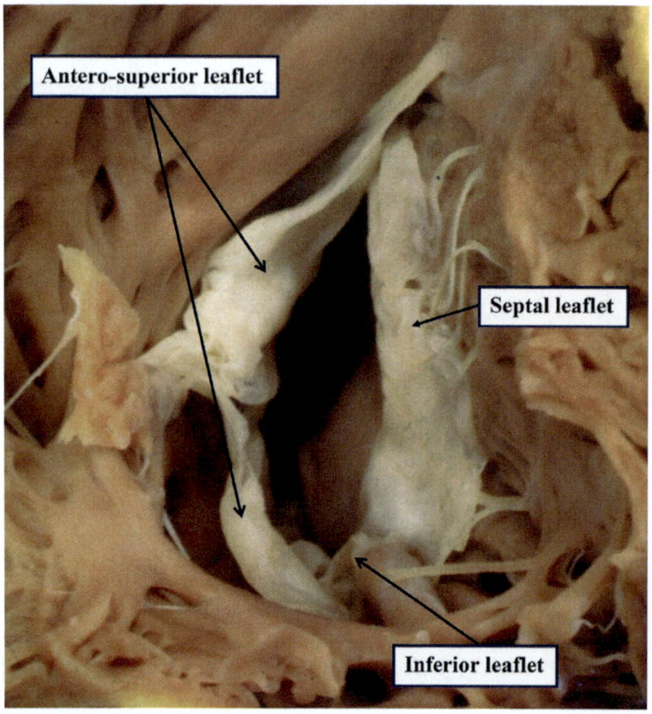

Fig. 1.6 The right atrioventricular junction is shown from the front, revealing the three leaflets of the tricuspid valve to be located antero-superiorly, septally, and inferiorly

The Left Atrium

As with its right-sided counterpart, the left atrium possesses a body, an appendage, a venous component, the vestibule, and the septum. The larger part of the body of the developing heart is committed to the left atrium. As is the case for the vestibule, which surrounds the orifice of the mitral valve, it has smooth walls. The pulmonary venous component, usually receiving a pulmonary vein at each of the corners of the atrial roof, similarly has smooth walls. The appendage of the left atrium, lined by the pectinate muscles, is limited when compared to the right atrium. It is tubular, has a narrow entrance, and is hooked, often with several constrictions along its length. The septal surface of the left atrium is formed by the flap valve of the oval foramen, with its attachments seen as horns that overlap the superior interatrial fold. The flap valve is anchored antero-inferiorly by the septal buttress, which is the true second atrial septum (Fig. 1.8).

The Left Ventricle

The left ventricle is posteriorly located within the ventricular cone, with only a small part of its leftward border projecting to make up part of the cardiac silhouette as viewed in the frontal projection (Fig. 1.1). As with its right-sided partner, it possesses an inlet, and apical component, and an outlet (Fig. 1.9).

The inlet of the ventricle is guarded by the mitral valve. Similar to the tricuspid valve, the mitral valve is made up of several parts that function in synchrony to open during diastole and close in systole. The term "annulus" is better considered as the atrioventricular junction. This junction supports the two leaflets, which are attached through tendinous cords to the paired papillary muscles, themselves supported by the ventricular walls. A malfunction of any of these parts will disturb the synchrony of the valvar apparatus thus rendering the valve incompetent. Although often described as being anterior and posterior, the leaflets are best considered as being aortic and mural, reflecting the fact that, on its ventricular aspect, the aortic leaflet is in fibrous continuity with two of the leaflets of the aortic valve. As the name suggests, the mural leaflet is hinged at the atrioventricular junction. The aortic leaflet, when viewed in its opened position, is trapezoidal. It is much broader than the mural leaflet and covers one-third of the overall valvar circumference. The mural leaflet is usually divided into three so-called scallops, although there is much individual variation, often with additional components of the skirt of valvar tissue evident at the

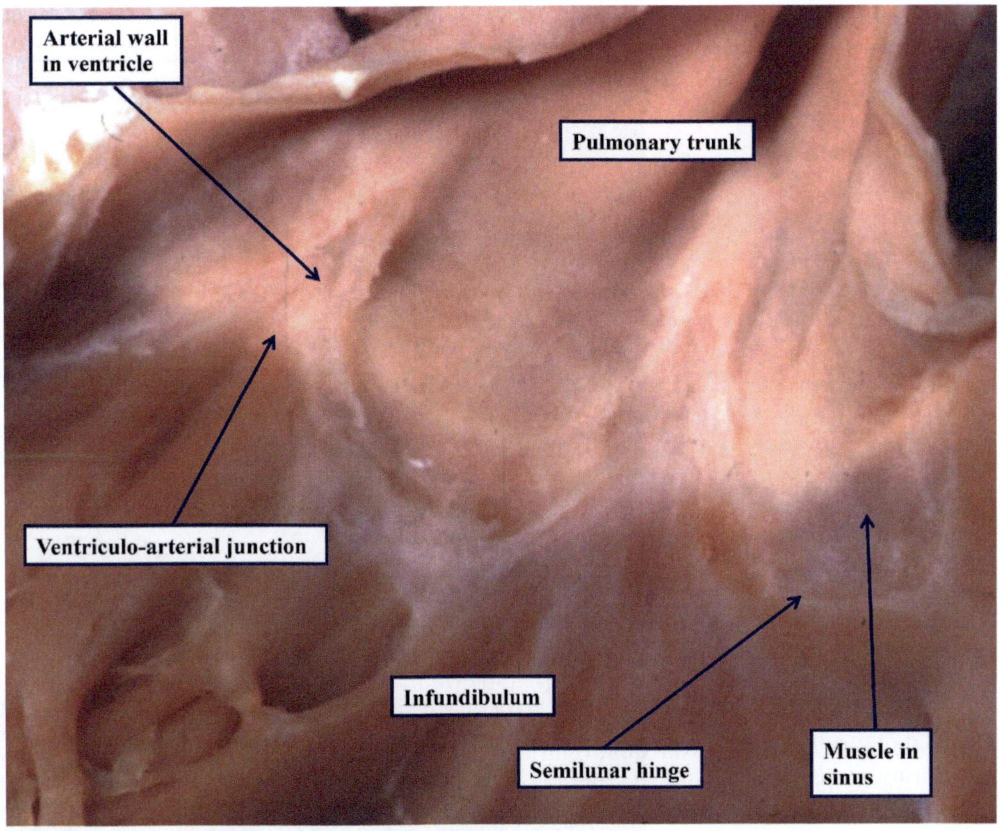

Fig. 1.7 The infundibulum of the right ventricle has been opened, and the leaflets of the pulmonary valve removed, to show how the semilunar hinges cross the junction between the myocardium of the infundibulum and the arterial wall of the pulmonary trunk

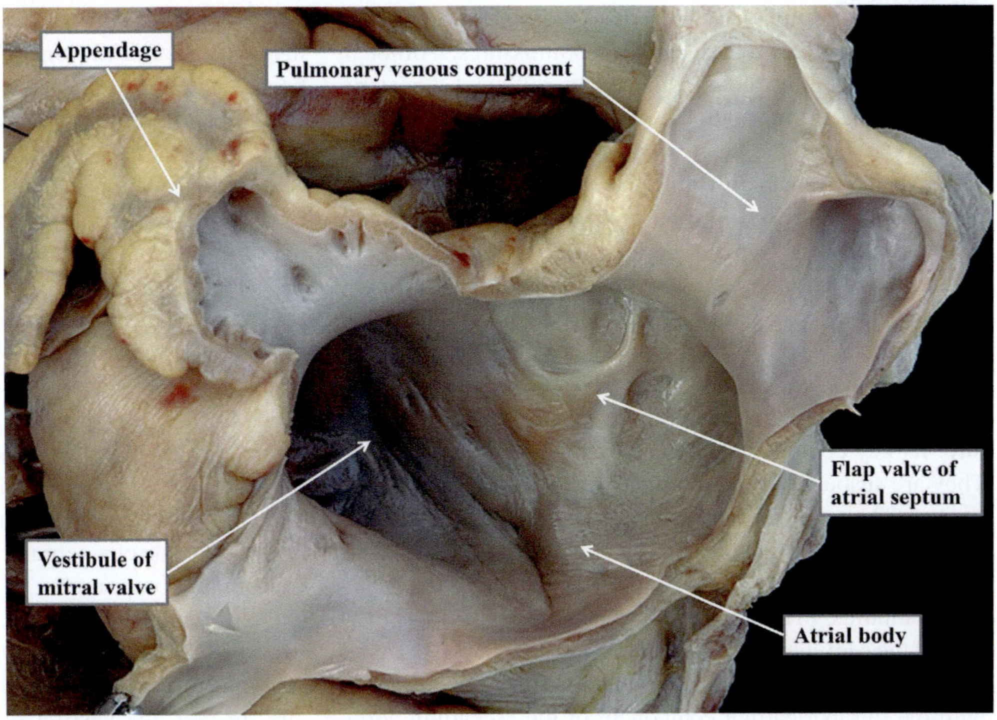

Fig. 1.8 The left atrium has been opened posteriorly and is photographed looking anteriorly to show its component parts

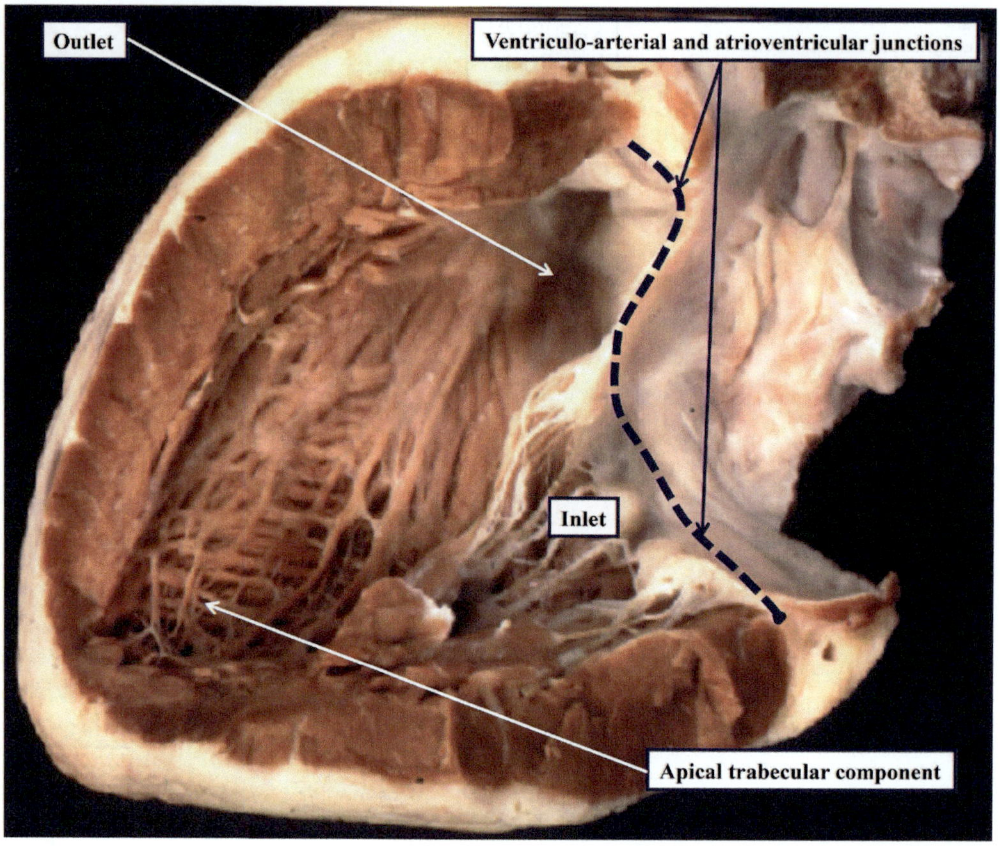

Fig. 1.9 The left ventricle has been opened to show its component parts. Unlike the right ventricle, the atrioventricular and ventriculo-arterial junctions are confluent at the ventricular base

ends of the solitary zone of apposition seen when the valve is in its closed position. It is the ends of the zone of apposition that are usually described as the commissures. Although often described as being "antero-lateral" and "postero-medial," this is a mistake, reflecting the penchant of anatomists to describe the heart as seen on its apex rather than according to its location within the body. When viewed attitudinally, the ends of the zone of apposition are positioned infero-septally and supero-laterally, mirroring the positions of the paired papillary muscles that support the tendinous cords of the leaflets (Fig. 1.10).

The apical part of the left ventricle has fine crisscrossing trabeculations, with a smooth septal surface.

The aortic root, like the mitral valve, is a complex structure. Its key components, the moving parts, are the leaflets. They are suspended in a semilunar fashion within the valvar sinuses. The nadirs of the leaflets can be joined together in a virtual fashion to provide the plane of the basal ring. This area is measured by the echocardiographer to provide the so-called annulus. In reality, it is a virtual entity. The distal margins of the semilunar leaflets come together at the sinotubular junction, which is where the aortic root becomes continuous with the intrapericardial component of the ascending aorta. When the leaflets are removed, their semilunar attachments become obvious. When assessed in three dimensions, they produce a crown-like entity, which is often described by surgeons as the valvar annulus. As was the case with the pulmonary root, the semilunar hinges of the leaflets cross the myocardial–arterial junction. Unlike the right ventricle, however, the left ventricle usually lacks a free-standing infundibular sleeve, with its leaflets in fibrous continuity at the ventricular base with the aortic leaflet of the mitral valve (Fig. 1.10). In consequence of this arrangement, myocardium is incorporated only in the bases of the two sinuses of the aortic root that give rise to the coronary arteries (Fig. 1.11).

The ventricular septum is mostly made up of the apical muscular septum. It is curved, reflecting the arrangement of the ventricular cone as seen in short axis (Fig. 1.10). A small fibrous part of the septum, located within the center of the base of the cone, is known as the membranous septum. It is crossed on its right ventricular surface by the hinge of the septal leaflet of the tricuspid valve. This divides the fibrous septum into interventricular and atrioventricular components. The part on the atrial aspect of the hinge of the septal leaflet is the only atrioventricular septal structure. It used to be thought that part of the vestibule of the right atrium was also an atrioventricular septal structure. In fact, the vestibules of the atrial chambers diverge one from the other to enclose the inferior part of the muscular ventricular septum, producing the inferior pyramidal space (Fig. 1.12).

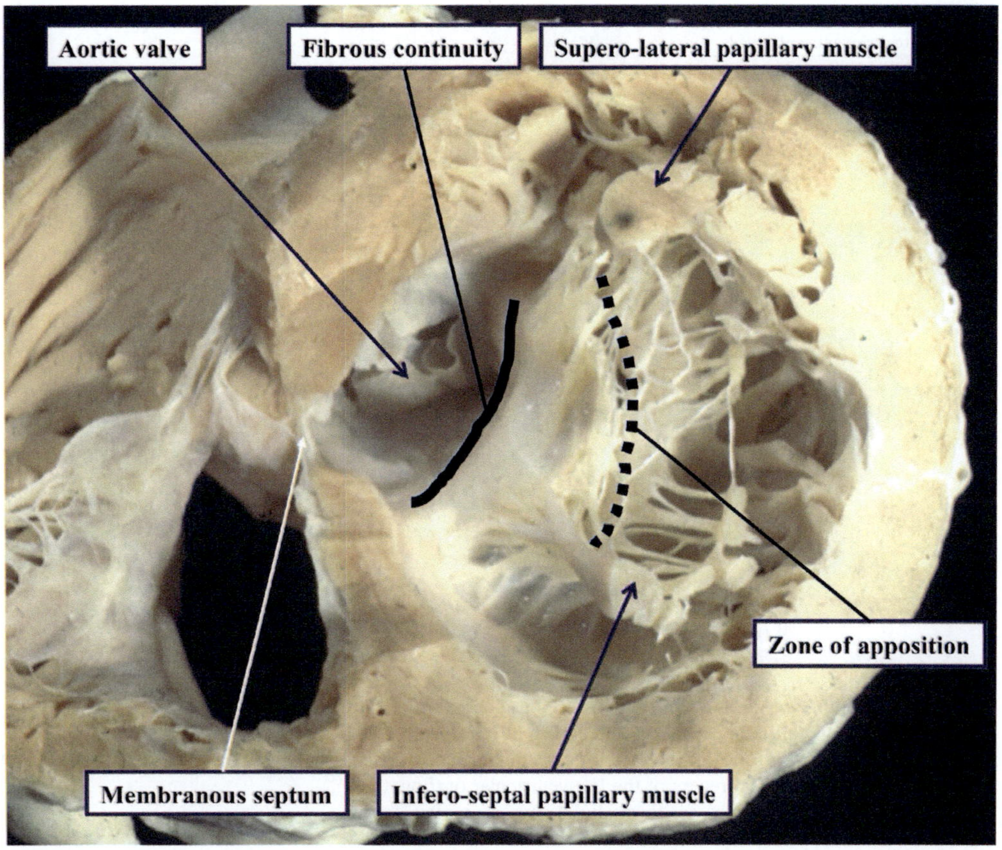

Fig. 1.10 The short axis of the ventricular cone is shown as viewed from the apex, showing the continuity between the leaflets of the aortic and mitral valves, and the location of the papillary muscles supporting the solitary zone of apposition between the leaflets of the mitral valve

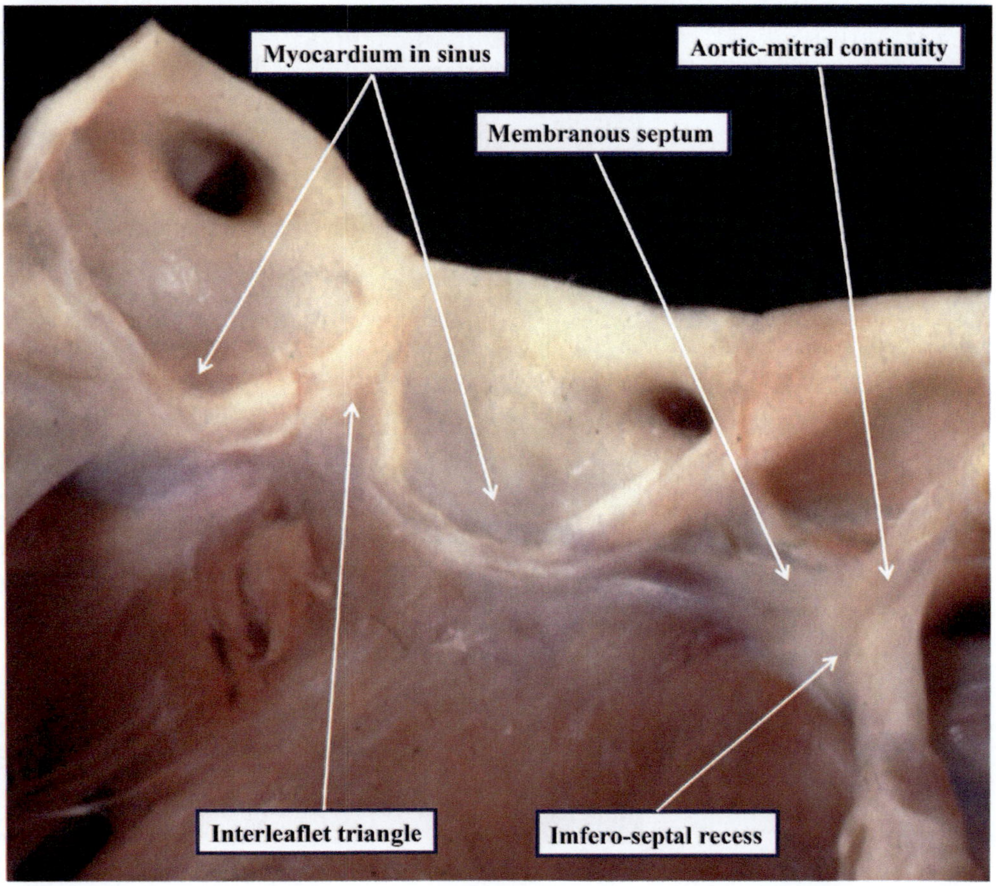

Fig. 1.11 The aortic root has been opened, and the semilunar leaflets removed, to show how the hinges cross the myocardial–arterial junction so as to incorporate myocardium at the bases of the two sinuses that give rise to the coronary arteries

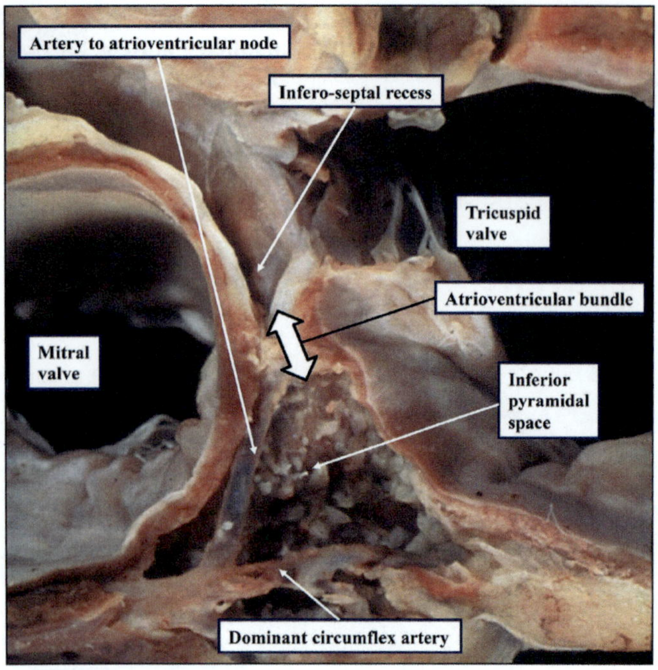

Fig. 1.12 The short axis of the ventricular cone has been dissected by removing the atrial walls and is photographed from its atrial aspect. The dissection shows how the apex of the inferior pyramidal space overlaps the apex of the infero-septal recess of the left ventricular outflow tract. The atrioventricular bundle crosses through the area of overlap. In this particular heart, the circumflex artery is dominant

Vascular Supply of the Heart

Coronary Arterial Circulation

The right and left coronary arteries provide blood supply to the heart. They arise from the sinuses of the aortic root adjacent to the pulmonary trunk, usually taking their origin just below the level of the sinutubular junction (Fig. 1.11). The right coronary artery emerges anteriorly into the right atrioventricular junction beneath the right atrial appendage. It then encircles the right atrioventricular groove as it curves around the acute margin of the ventricular cone to its diaphragmatic surface. In nine-tenths of individuals, it then gives its major branch into the inferior interventricular groove as the inferior interventricular artery. In such an arrangement, known as right coronary arterial dominance, the artery usually continues to provide branches that supply the diaphragmatic walls of the left ventricle (Fig. 1.13).

In around half of individuals, the first atrial branch of the right coronary artery supplies the sinus node. As the major stem of the artery encircles the orifice of the tricuspid valve, it gives rise to the acute marginal artery. When dominant, it also supplies the artery to the atrioventricular node.

Fig. 1.13 The right atrioventricular junction has been dissected by removing the walls of the right atrium. The dissection shows the location of the right coronary artery as seen from the atrial aspect when there is right coronary arterial dominance

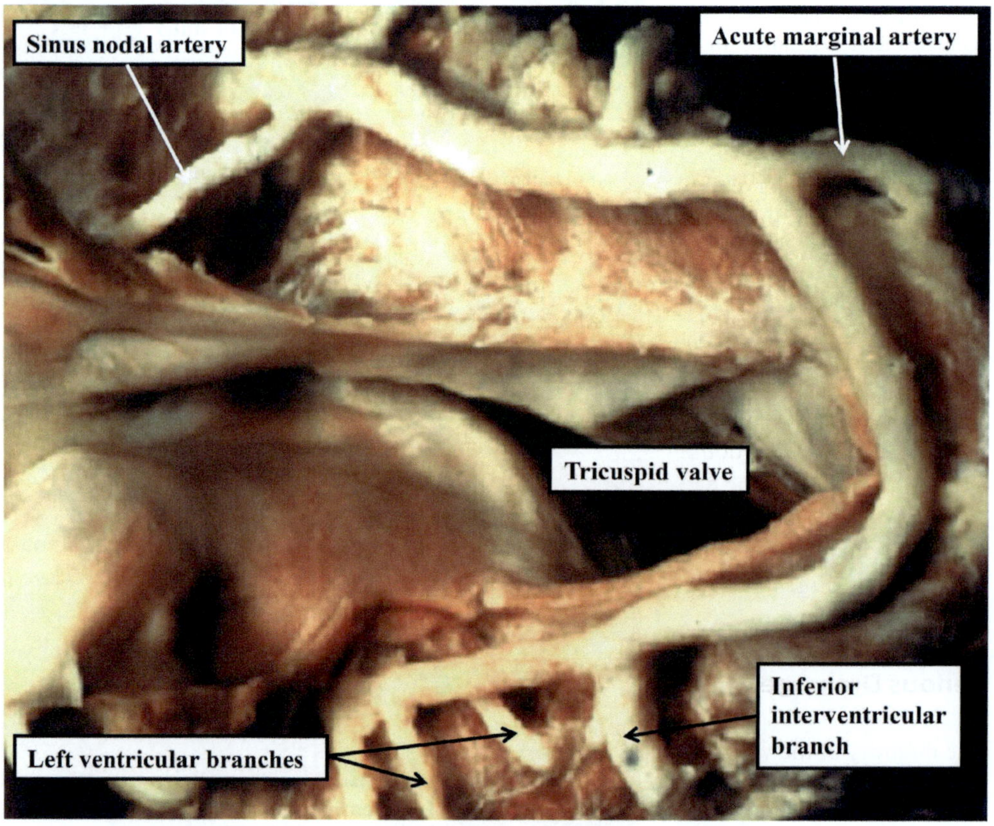

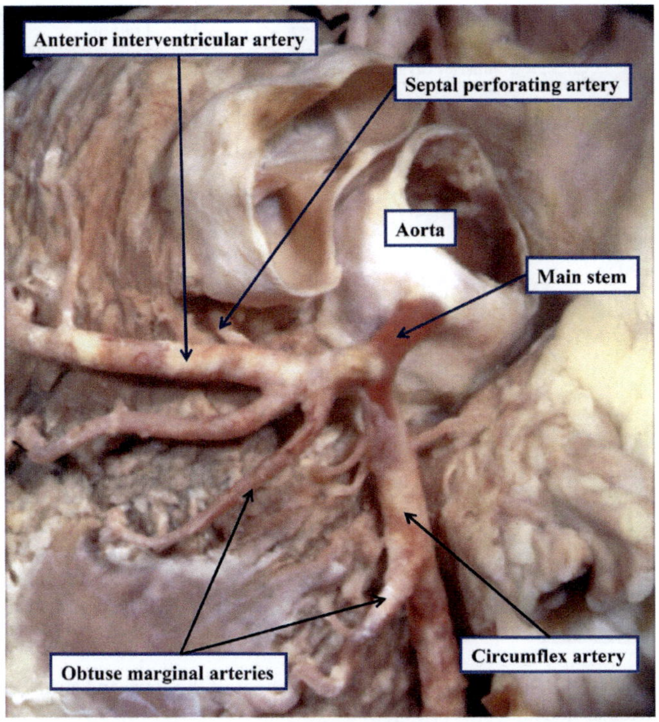

Fig. 1.14 The obtuse margin of the ventricular cone has been dissected to show the course of the main stem of the left coronary artery, which divides to become the circumflex and anterior interventricular arteries

The left coronary artery emerges from the left coronary aortic sinus. It enters the left atrioventricular groove between the pulmonary trunk and the left atrial appendage. It has a short main stem that divides into the circumflex branch, which runs in the atrioventricular groove, and the left anterior interventricular branch that runs in the anterior interventricular groove (Fig. 1.14).

The anterior interventricular artery supplies the obtuse marginal wall of the left ventricle through the diagonal branches, along with the anterior wall of the right ventricle. It supplies the anterior two-thirds of the muscular ventricular septum through septal perforating arteries. The circumflex artery also supplies branches to the obtuse margin of the left ventricle. When there is right coronary arterial dominance, the circumflex artery is relatively short. In one-tenth of normal individuals with dominance of the circumflex artery, however, it encircles the entirety of the mural part of the left atrioventricular junction. It then gives rise to the inferior interventricular artery, along with the artery to the atrioventricular node (Fig. 1.12).

Venous Drainage of the Heart

The majority of the venous drainage of the heart empties into the coronary sinus (Fig. 1.15).

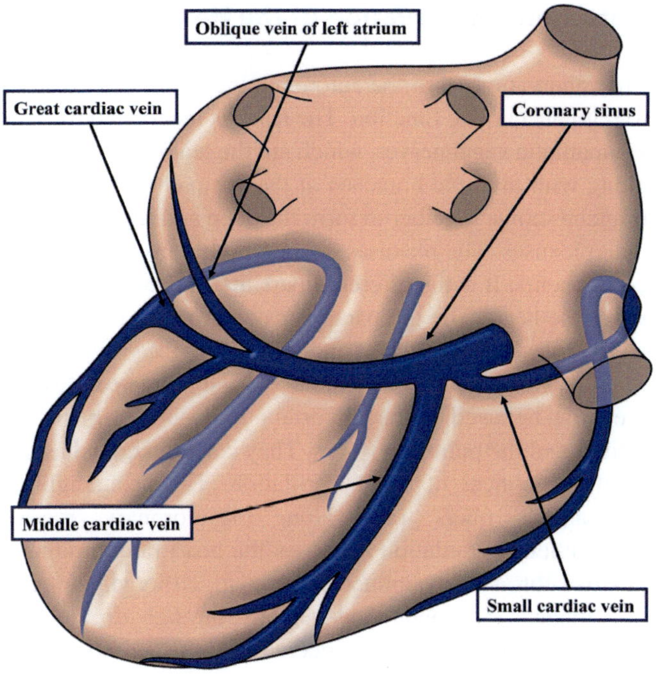

Fig. 1.15 The drawing, showing the heart as viewed from behind, illustrates the location of the veins draining into the coronary sinus

The coronary sinus, which occupies the inferior left atrioventricular groove, commences at the junction of the great cardiac vein with the oblique vein of the left atrium. It runs transversely from left to right in the left atrioventricular groove on the diaphragmatic surface of the heart, opening into the right atrium. The small, middle, and great cardiac veins all open into the coronary sinus. Thus, it receives up to five-sixths of the overall venous drainage. The great cardiac vein is the largest vein. It begins at the apex of the heart, then ascends upwards towards the ventricular base, accompanying the anterior interventricular artery. The middle cardiac vein drains most of the heart supplied by the right coronary artery. It begins at the apex, running in the inferior interventricular groove along with the inferior interventricular artery. The small cardiac vein travels in the right atrioventricular groove. It drains venous blood supplied by the marginal branches of the right coronary artery. The anterior cardiac veins, however, drain directly into the right atrial cavity. There is then a lesser network of venous drainage made up of the Thebesian veins. These small valveless vessels drain the inner layers of the myocardial walls directly into the lumens of heart chambers through openings in the endocardial surface.

Autonomic Innervation of the Heart

The innervation from the autonomic nervous system serves to regulate cardiac function. The heart is innervated by parasympathetic vagal nerves, which are the tenth cranial nerves, along with multiple branches of the sympathetic cords. The branches come together to form the deep and superficial cardiac plexuses. The plexuses contain both sensory and motor components. It is the efferent fibers that modulate the activity of the heart. The left parasympathetic vagus nerve innervates the atrioventricular node, while the right vagus innervates the sinus node. Additional ganglionated plexuses are now believed to be important in innervating the left atrium and the pulmonary vein. They can be targeted as part of the treatment of atrial fibrillation. The postganglionic sympathetic fibers travel along the coronary arteries. Sympathetic stimulation increases the heart rate, producing positive chronotropy, influences its contractility via inotropy, and impacts on conduction velocity through dromotropy. Parasympathetic stimulation decreases these activities.

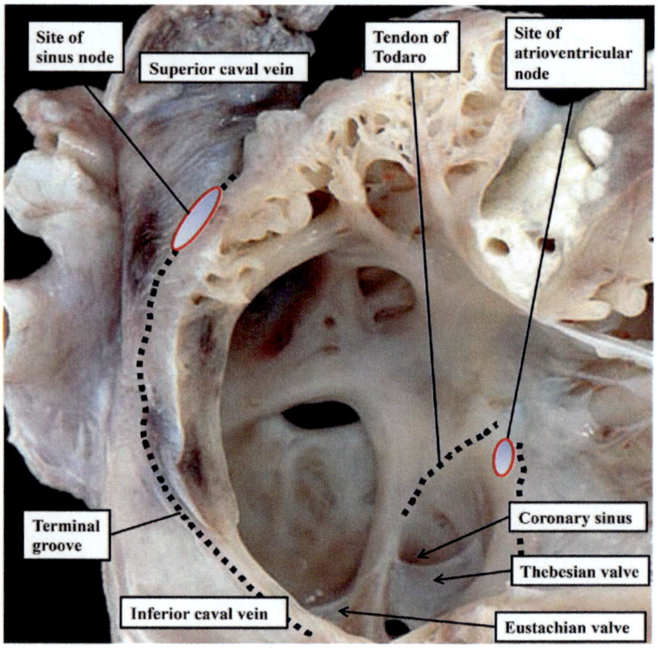

Fig. 1.16 The dissection shows the locations of the sinus and atrioventricular nodes

Anatomy of the Conduction System

The heartbeat is generated by the sinus node, a small cigar-shaped structure lying directly subepicardial within the terminal groove just below the junction of the superior caval vein with the right atrium. Along with the remainder of the so-called conduction system, which transmits the cardiac impulse to the ventricular myocardium, the cardiomyocytes making up the system are specialized, differing in this regard from the working cardiomyocytes. The nodes and conducting bundles, however, cannot be distinguished from the working myocardium simply by gross examination. Their known location (Fig. 1.16) underscores their recognition during cardiac surgical procedures, since iatrogenic damage can produce unwanted arrhythmias during cardiac surgery.

The cardiac impulse, generated by the sinus node, is conducted through the working myocardium making up the walls of the atrial chambers towards the atrioventricular junctions. The atrial myocardium is insulated from the ventricular myocardium throughout the junctions apart from at the site of penetration of the atrioventricular conduction axis. Once having been insulated, and having penetrated the plane of atrioventricular insulation, the axis becomes the non-branching bundleion, usually described as the bundle of His. It is part of the overall atrioventricular conduction axis. The atrial component of the axis is the atrioventricular node. The node is responsible for producing atrioventricular delay, permitting the atrial chambers to fill the ventricles during ventricular diastole. The node is located within the antero-inferior buttress of the atrial septum, lying at the apex of a triangle delimited by the tendon of Todaro, the septal leaflet of the tricuspid valve, and the orifice of the coronary sinus. Provided cardiac surgeons avoid the atrial vestibule making up the floor of the triangle, they will not damage the atrioventricular node. The non-branching bundle penetrates at the apex of the inferior pyramidal space, entering the infero-septal recess of the left ventricle, where it is sandwiched between the atrioventricular part of the membranous septum and the crest of the muscular ventricular septum. The axis then branches into the right and left bundle branches. These layers of specialized myocardium are insulated from the underlying septal myocardium until they reach the ventricular apexes, where they then ramify to activate the ventricular myocardium, thus ensuring that ventricular activation occurs from the apexes toward the ventricular base (Fig. 1.17).

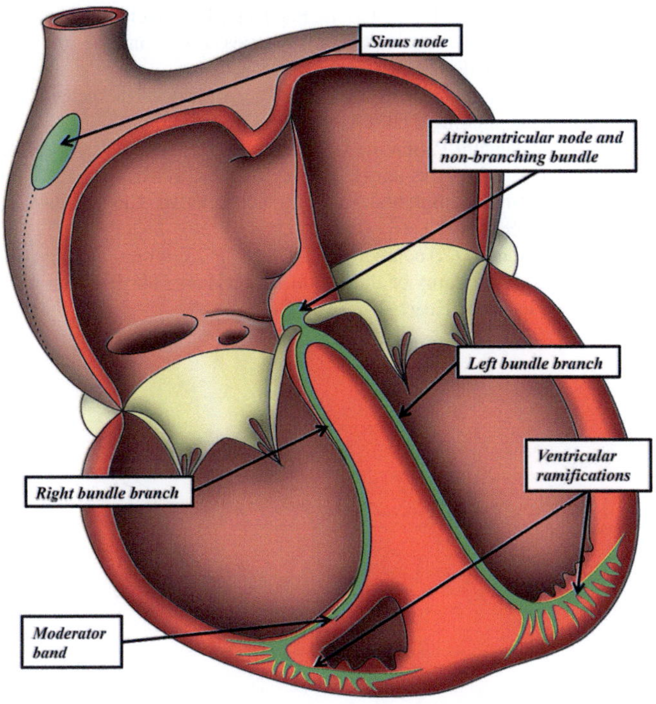

Fig. 1.17 The drawing shows the overall arrangement of the conduction system of the heart

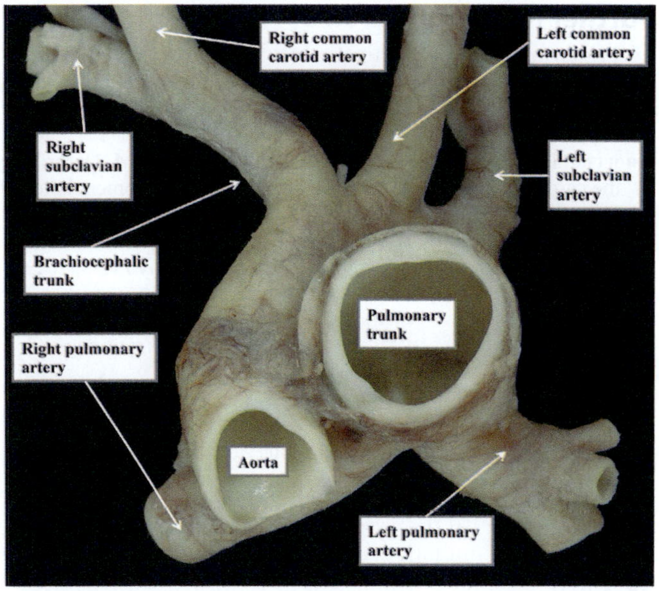

Fig. 1.18 The intrapericardial arterial trunks have been removed from the heart and photographed from the aspect of their ventricular origin, showing their major branches

Anatomy of the Great Vessels

The superior and inferior caval veins return deoxygenated blood from the body to the heart. The superior caval vein is formed by merging of the left and right brachiocephalic veins, each formed by the merger of the corresponding subclavian and jugular veins. It enters the pericardial cavity to the right side of the aorta and has only a short intrapericardial course before entering the right atrium. The inferior caval vein is formed by the merger of the common iliac veins in the pelvis. It ascends within the abdomen in the right paravertebral gutter, running to the right side of the abdominal aorta. After receiving the renal veins and hepatic veins, it passes through the central tendon of the diaphragm to drain into the right atrium.

The pulmonary trunk carries blood from the right ventricle to the lungs. It ascends from the infundibulum of the right ventricle, spiraling round the aortic root to reach the margins of the pericardial cavity where it divides into the left and right pulmonary arteries (Fig. 1.18).

The pulmonary veins, usually four in number, bring the blood back from the lungs. Each vein usually enters one of the corners of the dome of the left atrium; although, there is marked individual variation in their anatomy. The aorta carries blood from the left ventricle to the systemic circulation. It is divided into segments, with the ascending component mostly intrapericardial. After exiting the pericardium, it soon becomes the aortic arch. The arch curves upwards and backwards over the right pulmonary artery, passing along the left side of the trachea and esophagus. It supplies the brachiocephalic arteries from its superior border, with the right-sided arteries usually arising from a common brachiocephalic trunk. The left common carotid and subclavian arteries then arise separately. The arch continues as what is referred to as the isthmus. During fetal life, the arterial duct passes from the left pulmonary artery, joining the descending aorta at the distal border of the isthmus. In postnatal life, the duct usually becomes ligamentous. Distal to the union of the isthmus and the arterial ligament, the aortic arch becomes the descending thoracic aorta at the level of the body of the fourth thoracic vertebra. The thoracic aorta then enters the abdomen through the aortic opening in the diaphragm at the level of the twelfth thoracic vertebra. The aortic arch contains peripheral baroreceptors and chemoreceptors that relay blood pH and pressure information to the spinal cord medulla. The descending aorta in the thorax gives off branches to supply the intercostal, pericardial, bronchial, and mediastinal arteries. The abdominal aorta, a direct continuation of the descending aorta, gives blood to the entire abdomen, including the kidneys, foregut, midgut, and hindgut.

Acknowledgments The illustrations used by Professor Anderson and Mrs. Spicer for this chapter are all modified from previous contributions made by them. They retain the intellectual copyright in the original images from which the figures were made. They are indebted to Mrs. Gemma Price-Morgan, who produced the artwork for the drawings.

Further Reading

Anderson RH. Clinical anatomy of the aortic root. Heart. 2000;84:670–3.

Anderson RH, Razavi R, Taylor AM. Cardiac anatomy revisited. J Anat. 2004;205:159–77.

Anderson RH, Spicer DE, Hlavacek AJ, Hill A, Loukas M. Describing the cardiac components – attitudinally appropriate nomenclature. J Cardiovasc Transl Res. 2013a;6:118–23.

Anderson RH, Spicer DE, Hlavacek AL, Cook AC, Backer CL. Wilcox's surgical anatomy of the heart. Cambridge University Press; 2013b.

Anderson RH, Garbi M, Zugwitz D, Petersen SE, Nijveldt R. Anatomy of the mitral valve relative to controversies concerning the so-called annular disjunction. Heart. 2022;

Mori S, Tretter JT, Spicer DE, Bolender DL, Anderson RH. What is the real cardiac anatomy? Clin Anat. 2019;32:288–309.

Piazza N, de Jaegere P, Schultz C, Becker AE, Serruys PW, Anderson RH. Anatomy of the aortic valvar complex and its implications for transcatheter implantation of the aortic valve. Circ Cardiovasc Interv. 2008;1:74–81.

Sánchez-Quintana D, Anderson RH, Tretter JT, Cabrera JA, Sternick EB, Farré J. Anatomy of the conduction tissues 100 years on: what have we learned? Heart. 2022;108:1430–7.

Basic Cardiovascular Physiology

2

Osama M. Sayed and Irwin Gratz

Introduction

The heart is one of the most vital organs in the human body, responsible for perfusing all other organs. Composed of highly specialized cells, it employs electrical activity to generate synchronized contractions that persist throughout an individual's life. Through a complex network of blood vessels, the heart circulates blood throughout the body, both delivering essential nutrients and eliminating metabolic waste from the bodily organs. Remarkably adaptable, the heart responds to both temporary and permanent stressors, adjusting to lasting changes to meet the body's demands. However, pathological conditions may develop when the stressors' demands exceed the heart's compensatory mechanisms.

Overview of the Cardiovascular System

The cardiovascular system is responsible for maintaining the delivery of all factors necessary for metabolism to the tissues, as well as removing waste products from the tissues. It is composed of the heart, which functions as a mechanical pump, and the vasculature, which comprises the tubular system through which blood is transported. Both the heart and the vasculature respond to changes that may occur both intrinsically and extrinsically to optimize the efficiency of perfusion.

The cardiovascular system can be grouped into two major branches of circulation. The pulmonary circulation, primarily dictated by flow from the right side of the heart, is responsible for gas exchange in the lungs. Oxygen inspired from the environment diffuses into the circulation, while carbon dioxide produced from cellular metabolism diffuses out of the circulation and into the lungs. The systemic circulation, which is primarily dictated by flow from the left side of the heart, is responsible for nutrient and oxygen delivery to the organs.

The cardiac cycle consists of alternating periods of contraction (systole) and relaxation (diastole). The rhythmic contractions allow for organ perfusion, while relaxation allows for refilling of the heart with blood and perfusion of the heart itself via the coronary arteries.

All transport of blood throughout the cardiovascular system is dictated by pressure gradients from sites of high pressure to areas of low pressure. As liquids are non-compressible, contractions of smooth muscle within the vascular walls, as well as nearby skeletal muscles, result in rising pressures, which then propel the blood to the nearest site that is lower in pressure. This allows for the transport of blood both from and to the heart. As a result, the venous return should match the cardiac output in a healthy patient, usually averaging 5 liters per minute.

In the left ventricle, coronary perfusion primarily occurs during diastole, where ventricular pressure is at its lowest relative to the aortic diastolic pressure. In the right ventricle, where the pressures are lower than in the left ventricle, coronary perfusion occurs during both systole and diastole (Fig. 2.1).

Supplementary Information The online version contains supplementary material available at https://doi.org/10.1007/978-3-031-91163-7_2.

O. M. Sayed · I. Gratz (✉)
Department of Anesthesiology and Perioperative Medicine, Cooper University Hospital, Camden, NJ, USA
e-mail: sayed-osama@cooperhealth.edu; gratz-irwin@cooperhealth.edu

A. S. Awad, J. DiNardo (eds.), *Clinical Perfusion for Cardiac Surgery*, https://doi.org/10.1007/978-3-031-91163-7_2

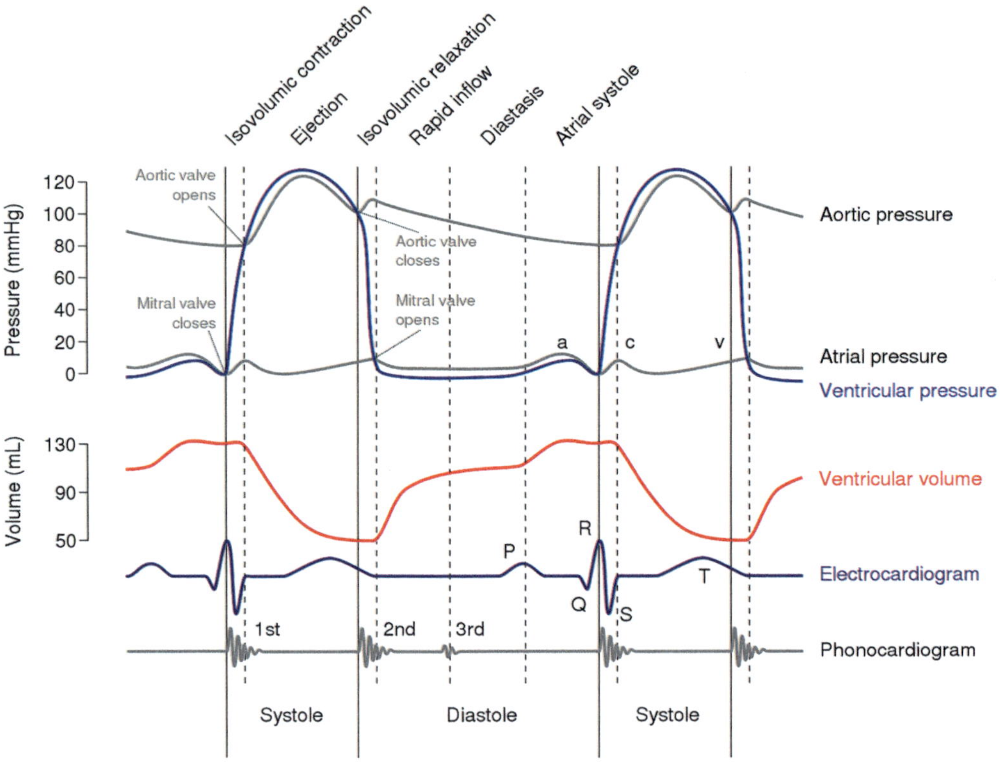

Fig. 2.1 Wiggers diagram, a comprehensive visual representation that integrates multiple cardiovascular variables into a single graph. This diagram elucidates the intricate relationship between the electrical activity of the heart, captured by the electrocardiogram (ECG), and its corresponding mechanical contractions. By examining the changes in pressure and volume at various locations within the heart, we can gain a deeper understanding of the dynamic interplay between electrical and mechanical events throughout the cardiac cycle. Specifically, the diagram illustrates how the ECG waveforms (P wave, QRS complex, T wave) correlate with changes in atrial and ventricular pressures, valve opening and closure, and the resulting changes in chamber volumes

The Arrangement of the Cardiovascular System

The Heart

The heart is divided into four chambers: two atria that act as the receiving chambers and two ventricles that serve as the primary pumping chambers. Every chamber pumps blood through a unidirectional valve. Deoxygenated blood enters the right atrium via the superior and inferior vena cava. It then flows into the right ventricle and is pumped into the pulmonary circulation, where carbon dioxide is expelled through exhalation and oxygen from inhaled air diffuses into the blood in the alveoli. Oxygenated blood returns to the heart via the pulmonary vein, entering the left atrium and then the left ventricle. Finally, the left ventricle ejects blood into the systemic circulation through the aorta, distributing it to the body's organs before it returns to the right atrium via the caval system (Fig. 2.2).

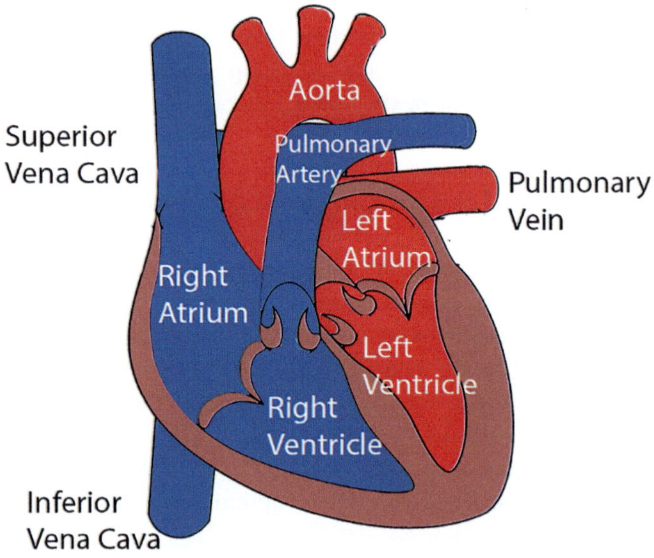

Fig. 2.2 Primary structures of the heart. This illustration, crafted by Osama M. Sayed, MD, depicts the heart's chambers and great vessels, highlighting the flow of deoxygenated blood (blue) through the right side and oxygenated blood (red) through the left

The Vascular Component

The vascular component can be characterized by the flow direction, size, and location of the vessels. Arteries are vessels that transport blood from the heart to tissues, while veins carry blood from the tissues back to the heart. The arterial system features a large muscular layer in the tunica media (the central concentric layer of the blood vessel), enabling arteries to maintain blood pressure post-ejection from the heart. With the exception of the pulmonary arteries, all arteries originate from the aorta and its branches. Arteries further divide into arterioles, which terminate in capillaries where oxygen and carbon dioxide are exchanged at the tissues, and metabolites are transported.

Although morphologically similar, arteries in pulmonary circulation exhibit several physiologic differences from arteries of the systemic circulation. One significant difference is their response to hypoxia. In systemic circulation, hypoxia induces arterial dilation in order to increase blood flow to organs, an adaptive response that enhances tissue oxygenation when oxygen levels are inadequate. This response contrasts with that of pulmonary circulation, where pulmonary arteries constrict in response to hypoxia, redirecting blood flow away from poorly oxygenated alveoli towards those with a richer oxygen supply.

The Venous System

The venous system is notable for its high degree of elasticity, which allows it to function as capacitance vessels capable of temporarily storing blood as it returns to the heart. Venous relaxation results in localized blood pooling and slows down venous return to the heart. Due to significantly lower muscle volume in vein walls compared to arteries, venous return is influenced by gravity and local muscle contractions. Venous return is greatest when venous tone is elevated, often targeted by medications such as venodilators that reduce preload by increasing venous capacitance.

The Autonomic Nervous System Role

There is a high degree of coordination between the autonomic nervous system and the cardiovascular system. Parasympathetic innervation, primarily from the vagus nerve, is concentrated at the sinoatrial (SA) node, whereas sympathetic innervation is distributed throughout the heart. At rest, the parasympathetic nervous system predominantly controls heart rate. Increases in heart rate and/or contractility, as described later in the chapter, are initially achieved by withdrawal parasympathetic dominance, followed by sympathetic activation if significant increases are required.

Vascular Responses and Baroreceptor Reflex

Changes in the vasculature prompt the heart to maintain hemodynamics and prevent rapid fluctuations. The baroreceptor reflex is a key mechanism that enables the heart to respond to swift changes in blood pressure. This reflex operates through receptors in the aortic arch and carotid sinuses, which continuously transmit neural impulses via the vagus and glossopharyngeal nerves, respectively, in response to detected pressures. A decrease in detected pressure leads to reduced neuronal firing, sensed by the solitary nucleus of the medulla oblongata, resulting in increased heart rate and systemic vascular resistance (SVR) to sustain mean arterial pressure (MAP). Conversely, an increase in pressure lowers heart rate and SVR to maintain MAP. Dysfunction of the baroreceptor, as seen in conditions like orthostatic hypotension, results in an inability to maintain MAP when rapidly standing, leading to transient cerebral hypoperfusion, dizziness, and occasionally syncope.

Cardiac Myocytes

Cardiomyocytes are specialized striated muscle cells forming the heart's musculature. A characteristic feature of cardiomyocytes is their connection with each other via gap junctions, which allow the passage of ions from cell to cell. This facilitates both the propagation of electrical signals and coordinated contraction and relaxation. The depolarization of one cardiomyocyte will result in the propagation of action potentials across surrounding cardiomyocytes, subsequently depolarizing nearby cells.

One of the most significant features of cardiomyocytes is the large concentration of mitochondria. The electrical and mechanical forces that result in synchronized cardiac contractions are energy-intensive processes. As a result of this mitochondrial density, cardiomyocytes are the most prolific utilizers of oxygen in the body.

Cardiomyocytes exhibit adaptations in response to changes in preload or afterload to maintain cardiac output. An increase in wall tension, as seen in uncontrolled chronic hypertension, may result in hypertrophy of cardiomyocytes. This occurs through an increase in the cross-sectional area of the cardiomyocyte. In response to increasing afterload, there may be an asymmetrical increase in the size of the cardiomyocytes found in the ventricle pumping against the high-pressure system. Left ventricular hypertrophy is most commonly seen in the setting of systemic hypertension, while right ventricular hypertrophy may be seen in response to pulmonary hypertension. Hypertrophy may be concentric (growing inward into the ventricular lumen) or eccentric (growing outwards with minimal changes in the luminal size).

When adapting to a chronic increase in afterload, the hypertrophy is often concentric. Hypertrophy may occur as a result of pressure overload following valvular malfunctions, such as overcoming the increased pressure gradient of a stenotic valve. Although concentric hypertrophy may decrease the space available for blood to fill during the diastole (resulting in a decrease in preload), the hypertrophied muscle allows the heart to push against the high-pressure system and indirectly maintain cardiac output by preserving ejection fraction. While this adaptive response allows the heart to compensate against rising pressures, it may become pathologic if the reductions in end-diastolic volume become significant enough such that cardiac output can no longer be maintained. Classically, this was referred to as diastolic heart failure, which is now more precisely defined as heart failure with preserved ejection fraction. Even though the percentage of blood ejected is maintained, the stroke volume is less than what is required to meet perfusion demands.

Cardiomyocytes may adapt to increase in volume by increase in length, resulting in luminal dilation. By increasing the luminal volume, the heart is able to maintain cardiac output by accommodating a larger end-diastolic volume. Although the ejection fraction (percent of blood pumped from the heart) may see a slight reduction, this is compensated for by a larger stroke volume. This may become pathologic when the stroke volume is no longer sufficient to offset the reduction in ejection fraction.

The Electrical Activity

The electrical activity of the heart involves initiation and transmission of impulses, followed by repolarization during a refractory period before the cycle repeats. All cardiac cells possess the inherent ability to generate electrical activity, known as automaticity. However, the direction and speed of electrical propagation are governed by the rates of depolarization and repolarization at each specific site within the heart. The SA node in the right atrium, possessing the fastest rate of spontaneous depolarization, serves as the heart's natural pacemaker. Electrical activity originates in the SA node and is transmitted through specialized autorhythmic cells and cardiomyocytes.

The electrical potential across the cell membrane, determined by the intracellular–extracellular gradient, is measured in millivolts (mV). Potassium ions are more abundant intracellularly, while sodium ions are predominantly extracellular. Although both sodium and potassium are positively charged ions (cations), the greater abundance of cations extracellularly creates an electrical gradient where the extracellular component is relatively more positive than the intracellular component. In the resting state, this results in a negative electrical potential within the cells, referred to as the polarized state.

Electrophysiology of the Cardiac Muscle

Like all muscle cells, cardiomyocytes rely on calcium for contraction. However, they uniquely also require calcium for electrical impulse propagation. This process begins with an electrical impulse triggering the opening of voltage-gated sodium channels, which depolarize the cardiomyocyte membrane from −96 mV to approximately +52 mV.

As with all cell membranes, the phospholipid bilayer is impermeable to most substances and ions, necessitating specialized ion channels for ions to pass into or out of the cell. Ions move along their electrochemical gradient, determined by both concentration and electrical gradient. Ion movement in this direction can occur through passive ion channels without requiring additional energy from the cell, while ion movement against this gradient necessitates energy expenditure, typically in the form of adenosine triphosphate (ATP).

The cardiomyocyte action potential (discussed later in this chapter) triggers the rapid influx of sodium ions into the cell through open channels, driven by their electrochemical gradient. This movement is driven by the electrochemical gradient for sodium, which consists of two components:

- *Chemical Gradient*: A higher concentration of sodium ions outside the cell creates a driving force for sodium to move inward.
- *Electrical Gradient*: The negative charge inside the cell attracts the positively charged sodium ions.

Together, these gradients create a strong electrochemical force that propels sodium into the cell through open channels during the action potential. As intracellular sodium concentration increases, the electrical charge within the cell becomes less negative, approaching neutrality or even a slightly positive potential. This weakening of electrical gradient, combined with the existing concentration gradient favoring potassium movement out of the cell, results in potassium efflux. This process will be explored further in the next section.

A clinical model to visualize the role of concentration and electromotive gradients can be illustrated by observing the role of potassium in cardioplegia (see Chap. 28). Normally, cardiomyocyte repolarization occurs via potassium efflux, restoring the resting membrane potential. However, a hyperkalemic cardioplegia solution, used during cardiopulmonary bypass, significantly raises extracellular potassium concentration. This not only diminishes the potassium concentration gradient but also alters the electrical gradient across the cell membrane. Consequently, potassium efflux is hindered, as more energy is required to move potassium ions against their concentration gradient, and the cell cannot fully repolarize. Instead, the resting membrane potential becomes less negative (around −50 mV instead of the usual −90 mV), making excitation less likely and effectively inducing cardiac arrest.

Action Potential in Cardiac Cells

Signals are transmitted between cells via action potentials, which are transient electrical currents that travel across the cell membranes, resulting from fluctuations in ion concentrations that affect the membrane's electrical potential. Cardiac action potentials differ from neuronal action potentials and also vary among different types of cardiac cells. Atrial, ventricular, and specialized conducting cells, for example, each exhibit distinct action potentials.

Dynamics of Action Potential in Cardiac Conduction Cells

In specialized cardiac conduction cells, the action potential begins with a gradual depolarization (**phase 4**) caused by a slow passive influx of sodium ions. Once the threshold potential is reached, voltage-gated calcium channels open, triggering a rapid depolarization phase (**phase 0**) with a steep rise in membrane potential. As the potential peaks, potassium channels open, leading to repolarization (**phase 3**) as potassium ions flow out of the cell (Fig. 2.3). The rate of this depolarization and the subsequent propagation of the action potential directly determine the heart rate. This process of pacemaker action potential occurs most rapidly in the SA node, followed by the atrioventricular (AV) node, and is slowest in the Purkinje fibers.

Autonomic Control of Heart Rate

The autonomic nervous system, composed of the sympathetic and parasympathetic branches, exerts a powerful influence on heart rate through its innervation of the SA node. It does this by modulating the activity of ion channels responsible for the SA node's action potential.

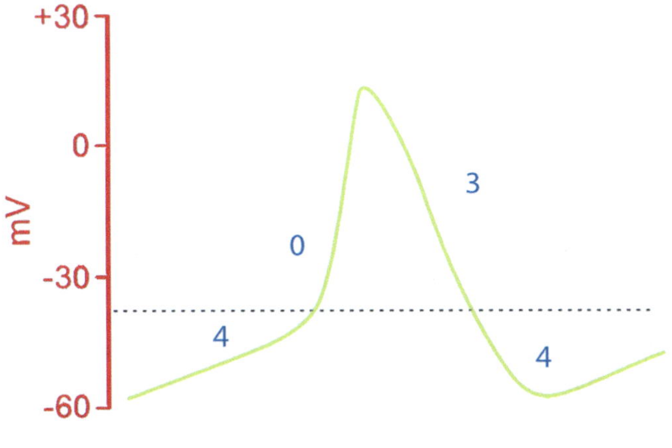

Fig. 2.3 Action potential in cardiac conduction cells. This illustration, crafted by Osama M. Sayed, MD, showcases the phases of cardiac electrical activity. Phase 4 shows gradual depolarization due to a slow influx of sodium ions. Phase 0 follows with a rapid depolarization as voltage-gated calcium channels open and membrane potential sharply increases. Phase 3 depicts repolarization with the efflux of potassium ions

Parasympathetic Stimulation: The vagus nerve releases acetylcholine, which binds to muscarinic receptors on SA node cells. This leads to increased opening of potassium channels, causing a greater efflux of potassium ions during phase 3 of the action potential. Consequently, the membrane potential becomes more negative at the start of phase 4. This hyperpolarization requires a larger influx of sodium ions to reach the threshold potential value hence prolonging phase 4 and slowing down the heart rate.

Sympathetic Stimulation: Norepinephrine released by sympathetic nerve endings binds to beta-adrenergic receptors on SA node cells. This action enhances the cellular membrane's permeability to sodium channels, allowing for a faster influx of sodium ions during phase 4. Consequently, the threshold potential is reached more quickly, resulting in a steeper phase 4 slope. This generates more action potentials in a given period, leading to an increased heart rate.

Action Potential in Cardiomyocytes

Like conduction cells, cardiomyocytes exhibit action potentials but with key differences due to unique ion channels on their membranes. In the resting phase (phase 4), potassium channels remain open, maintaining the resting membrane potential. Upon stimulation (such as activation from a conduction cell or nearby cardiomyocyte), fast sodium channels open, allowing an influx of sodium ions that lead to a rapid rise in membrane potential, causing rapid depolarization (phase 0) to its maximal point. This rise results in the closing of the sodium channels once the membrane potential becomes positive. The now positive intracellular membrane potential causes a potassium efflux along its electrical gradient, gradually lowering the potential as seen in phase 1. Unlike in conduction cells, the cardiomyocyte does not undergo rapid repolarization due to an electrical counterbalance caused by the influx of calcium ions during phase 2, which nearly matches the electrical potential lost to the simultaneous efflux of potassium ions. This calcium influx directly triggers the mechanical contraction of the cardiomyocyte (described later in this chapter). Potassium channels remain open even after the calcium channels close, allowing for the repolarization of the cell observed in phase 3. After this, cellular ion concentration gradients are restored to pre-contraction levels using active transport pumps during mechanical relaxation of the cell (Fig. 2.4).

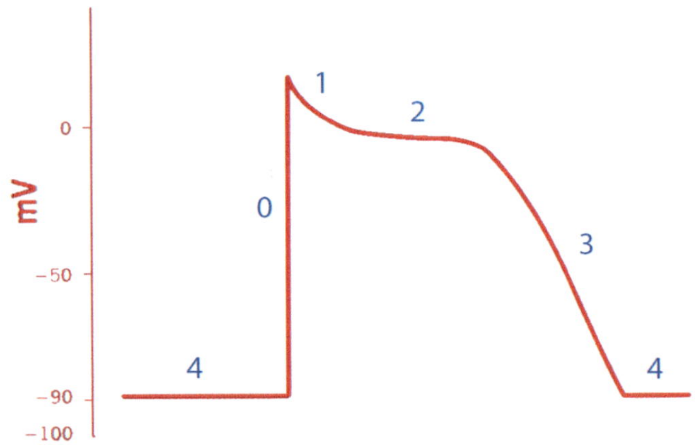

Fig. 2.4 Cardiomyocyte action potential. This illustration, crafted by Osama M. Sayed, MD, showcases the phases of cardiomyocytes action potential

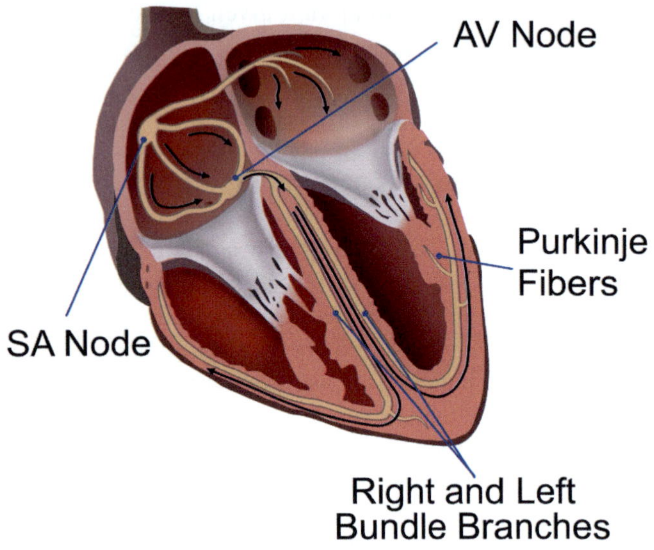

Fig. 2.5 Structures of the electrical conduction pathway. This illustration showcases the key components of the heart's electrical conduction system, including the SA node, atrioventricular AV node, bundle of His, bundle branches, and Purkinje fibers. Each element is labeled and depicted in anatomical context, illustrating the pathway through which electrical impulses travel to coordinate the heart's rhythmic contractions

The Electrical Conduction Pathway

Specialized autorhythmic cells in the heart spontaneously generate and conduct electrical activity, establishing the heart's rhythm. These cells are organized into a hierarchical system based on their anatomic location and firing rate (Fig. 2.5).

1. The SA Node: Located in the right atrium, this is the heart's primary pacemaker.

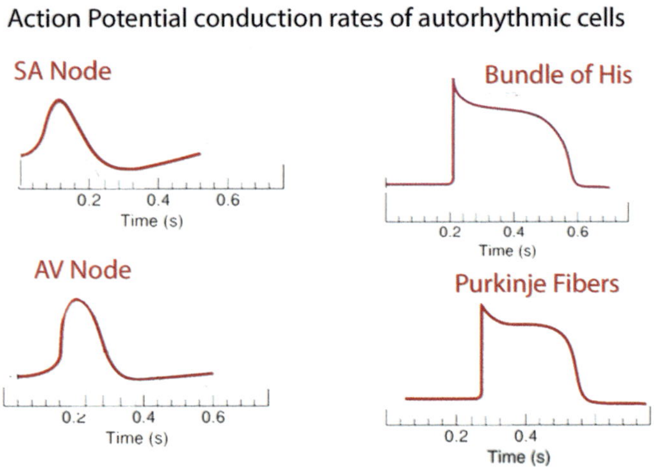

Fig. 2.6 Action potential conduction rates of autorhythmic cells. This illustration, crafted by Osama M. Sayed, MD, showcases the action potential conduction rates of autorhythmic cells across all components, including the SA node, AV node, bundle of His, and Purkinje fibers

2. The AV Node: Situated at the lower part of the right atrium, it slows conduction to allow ventricular filling.
3. Bundle of His: Divides into left and right bundles, carrying signals into the ventricles.
4. Purkinje Fibers: Distribute electrical impulses throughout the ventricles, triggering synchronized contraction.

Cardiac Autorhythmic Cells and the Pacemaker Hierarchy

The rate of action potential generation varies across different components of the cardiac conduction system, with the SA node exhibiting the fastest rate. This rate gradually slows down with each structure described above, respectively (Fig. 2.6). Although all components (SA node, AV node, bundle of His, Purkinje fibers) are capable of generating spontaneous electrical impulses (automaticity), the SA node serves as the primary pacemaker, dictating the heart rate. This hierarchy is maintained by refractory periods following each action potential, preventing downstream cells from generating their own primary action potentials prematurely.

Causes of Arrhythmias

Conduction Blockages: If there is a blockage along the conduction pathway, cells distant to the blockage will develop their own primary pacing at a slower rate than those proximal to it.

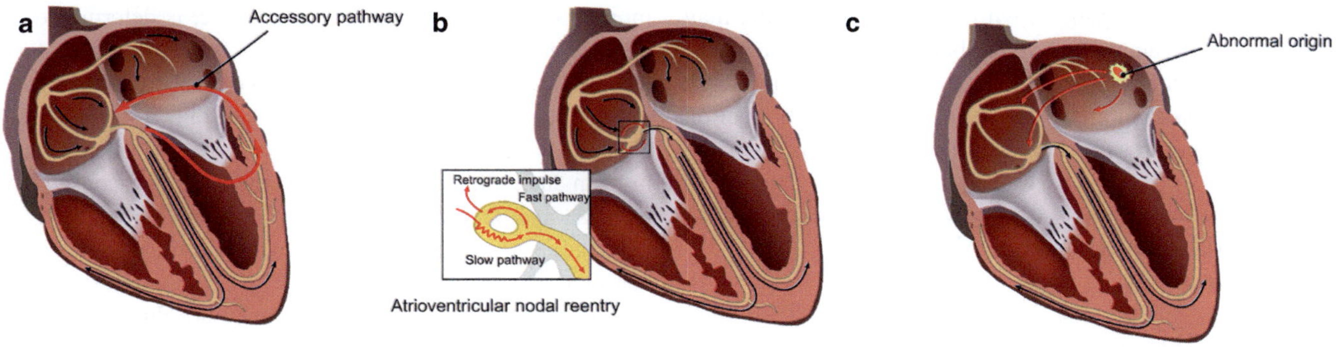

Fig. 2.7 Pathologic reentrant pathway. This illustration displays the most common types of pathologic reentrant pathways: (**a**) accessory pathway, (**b**) atrioventricular nodal reentrant tachycardia, and (**c**) abnormal foci origin

If the blockage occurs within one of the bundles of His, it results in dyssynchrony between the ventricles. Despite this dyssynchrony, most bundle branch blocks are asymptomatic due to the ventricles' intrinsic compensation capabilities. However, if there is a comorbidity that reduces the heart's ability to compensate, such as in heart failure, this lack of coordination may cause difficulty in emptying the ventricle during contraction and may exacerbate pathological conditions like heart failure.

Reentry Pathways: Alternatively, abnormal electrical connection can lead to excessively fast heart rates, which may be referred to as reentrant pathways. In these conditions, an electrical impulse may stimulate preceding nodes along the conduction pathway, resulting in a pathologically rapid heart rate (Fig. 2.7). An example of such a condition is Wolff–Parkinson–White Syndrome. Although pharmacologic management for heart rate control can be utilized for temporization, definitive treatment typically involves the ablation of the pathologic accessory pathway.

Cardiomyocytes Excitation–Contraction Coupling

The Role of Calcium

The action potential of the cardiomyocyte, as described earlier in the chapter, triggers an influx of calcium ions into the cell during phase 2. This influx activates the ryanodine receptor, which in turn releases stored calcium from the sarcoplasmic reticulum, increasing intracellular calcium levels. The presence of gap junctions facilitates the rapid propagation of excitation throughout the myocardium, leading to a unified contraction. Contraction occurs as adjacent cardiomyocytes act in response to rhythmic electrical activity.

Each cardiomyocyte contains sarcomeres, the functional units of muscle cells. The primary proteins involved in muscular contraction are actin and myosin. Under resting conditions, another protein, tropomyosin, binds to actin, blocking the myosin binding sites. Calcium triggers muscular contraction by binding to tropomyosin, inducing a conformational change that exposes the actin–myosin binding sites. Consequently, actin and myosin bind to form cross-bridges, pulling against each other to shorten the sarcomere. This coordinated shortening of sarcomeres causes the myocyte to contract, and since the signal is transmitted between adjacent myocytes, it results in a unified contraction.

This process is highly energy-intensive, requiring ATP to detach the actin–myosin bridge for relaxation or further shortening when a greater contraction is necessary. The greater the concentration of calcium, the more actin–myosin interactions occur, leading to stronger contractions. Electrical excitation primarily serves to increase intracellular calcium concentrations, which in turn primarily induce mechanical contraction.

Disruptions in Coordinated Electrical Activity and Cardiac Arrhythmias

Failure to produce coordinated electrical activity can lead to disorganized rhythms, clinically referred to as arrhythmias. The most severe form, fibrillation, involves severely disorganized electrical activity to the extent that effective contraction becomes impossible. Atrial fibrillation, a common occurrence, notably eliminates the atrial kick at the end of diastole. Its pathogenesis often involves a greater reliance on passive ventricular filling rather than on the atrial kick. Conditions that increase dependence on the atrial kick include tachycardia and diastolic filling defects. Managing atrial fibrillation typically involves reducing the heart rate to decrease reliance on the atrial kick for diastolic ventricular filling. Furthermore, patients with diastolic heart failure may experience a greater symptomatic burden if atrial fibrillation is present. Ventricular fibrillation, which is incompatible with life, causes complete failure of ventricular contraction and usually requires external electrical cardioversion.

The Cardiac Pump: Mechanics and Regulation

The passage of blood through the heart is governed by pressure gradients. At rest, most blood returns through the ventricles via passive filling during early diastole. A slight increase in ventricular volume occurs during atrial systole; as the atria contract, a rise in atrial pressure pushes additional blood through the atrioventricular valves into the relaxed ventricles. In a physiologically ideal model, all valves function as one-way valves, opening when the pressure before the valve is greater and closing when the pressure after the valve is greater.

During systole, the ventricles contract, leading to a sharp increase in pressure within these chambers in a phase known as isovolumetric contraction. This pressure rise causes the closure of the tricuspid and mitral valves to prevent backflow into the atria. When the rising ventricular pressure surpasses the pressure across the pulmonic and aortic valves, these valves open, allowing for blood ejection.

As blood is ejected into the aorta and pulmonary artery, a drop in ventricular volume leads to a reduction in pressure. This drop causes the semilunar valves to close as the pressure beyond the valve now exceeds the preceding pressure, marking the period of isovolumetric relaxation. During this phase, the ventricles have a constant volume as they continue to relax in diastole. Atrial pressure eventually rises, surpassing the pressure gradient across the mitral and tricuspid valves, which then open to allow blood refilling into the ventricles.

The Frank–Starling Law and Myocardial Contractility

The relationship between pressure and volume changes in the heart is governed by the Frank–Starling law, which underscores the heart's capacity to adjust its pumping ability based on the volume received during diastole. This law asserts that stroke volume is directly proportional to the end-diastolic volume, enabling the heart to intrinsically adjust the force of contraction in response to changes in preload. The force of contraction, and by extension, the stroke volume, is directly related to the initial length of the cardiac muscle fibers through the Frank–Starling mechanism. Preload, an indirect estimate of end-diastolic volume, is determined by the amount of blood returned to the ventricles during diastole. An increase in preload results in enhanced stretching of the cardiac muscle fibers, which, according to the Frank–Starling mechanism, leads to optimal overlap of actin and myosin filaments within the sarcomeres and a consequent increase in contraction force. In a non-pathological state, the heart adjusts its stroke volume by modifying the force of contraction in relation to preload, thus maintaining cardiac output despite fluctuations in venous return due to exercise, postural changes, or volume status.

Inotropic Therapy: Modifying Cardiac Contractility

Inotropy, the force of contraction of the heart muscle, can be either positive or negative. Positive inotropy, an increase in contractility, can be influenced both intrinsically and extrinsically through the influx of calcium ions into cardiomyocytes. Factors promoting positive inotropy include catecholamines like epinephrine and norepinephrine, released by the sympathetic nervous system bind to beta-adrenergic receptors on the heart. This triggers an intracellular cascade leading to phosphorylation of calcium channels, facilitating calcium influx. Certain drugs, such as digoxin, enhance positive inotropy indirectly by affecting the sodium–potassium pump, thereby altering transmembrane electrical potentials that result in increased calcium influx. Positive inotropic strategies may be necessary in clinical scenarios where cardiac output is insufficient, such as in heart failure.

Conversely, negative inotropy, which decreases contractility, can be achieved through factors that reduce calcium ion entry into cardiomyocytes. At rest, parasympathetic stimulation predominates, mediated by acetylcholine acting on the Muscarinic-2 (M2) receptors in the heart, which reduces intracellular cyclic-AMP and calcium influx. Activation of M2 receptor also opens potassium channels, decreasing the membrane potential and thus reducing heart rate. Negative inotropy can be induced by blocking catecholamines' actions with beta-blockers like metoprolol. Clinical indications for negative inotropy include conditions where myocardial oxygen demand exceeds supply, such as in coronary artery disease or prolonged tachyarrhythmias.

Cardiac Cycle

The cardiac cycle comprises events occurring during one heartbeat, including both contraction (systole) and relaxation (diastole) phases (Fig. 2.8).

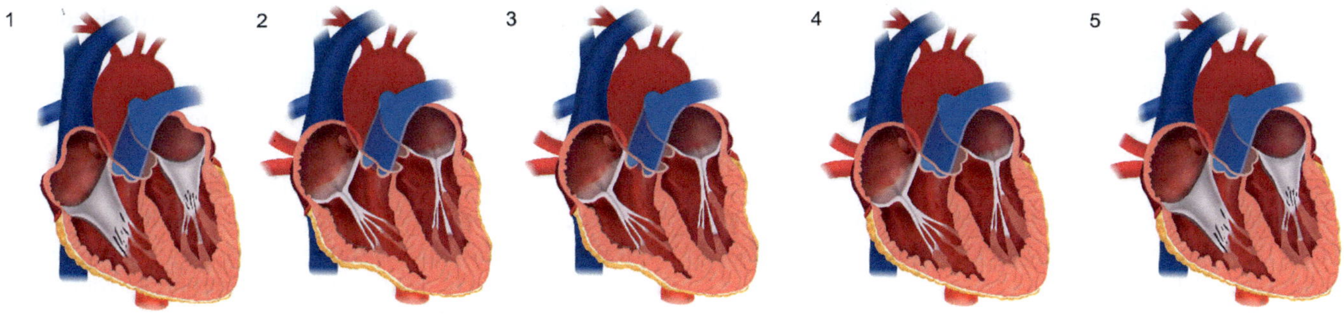

Fig. 2.8 The heart during systole and diastole. This illustration displays the actions (contract, relax, open, and close) of the different structures of the heart (atria, ventricles, atrioventricular valves, and semilunar valves) during systole and diastole

Atrial Systole

During atrial systole, which involves the contraction of the atria, an electrical impulse originating in the SA node spreads through the right atrium, stimulating the contraction of atrial cardiomyocytes. This contraction propels blood into the ventricles through the open atrioventricular valves. While most ventricular filling occurs passively before atrial contraction, the atrial kick contributes a small additional volume during rest. Following contraction, the atria enter diastole, passively filling with blood returning from the vena cava (right atrium) or pulmonary veins (left atrium).

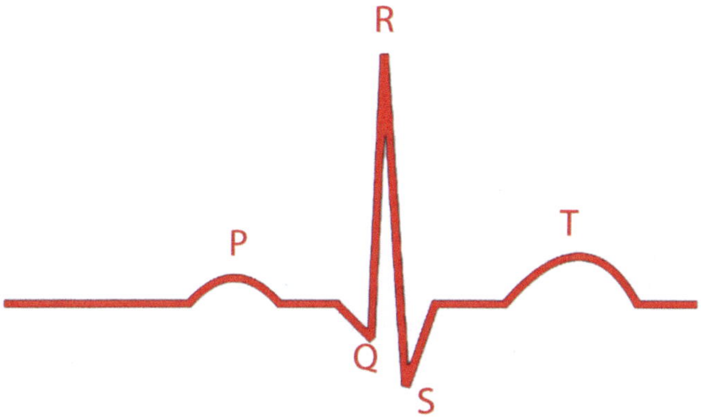

Fig. 2.9 Normal ECG waves. This illustration, crafted by Osama M. Sayed, MD, displays the normal waves found in an ECG. The P wave signifies atrial depolarization, originating from the impulse in the SA node, followed by the QRS complex, which represents ventricular depolarization. The T wave reflects ventricular repolarization, indicating the reset of ventricular cells. The PR interval measures the duration of atrial electrical activity, from the start of the P wave to the start of the QRS complex, providing insight into atrioventricular node function. Lastly, the ST-segment corresponds to the early phase of ventricular repolarization, crucial for assessing the heart's electrical recovery between beats

Ventricular Diastole

Ventricular diastole refers to the relaxation of the ventricles, creating a low-pressure environment that facilitates their filling with blood. During this phase, blood that has been accumulating in the atria during atrial systole and atrial diastole begins to flow into the ventricles, driven by the pressure gradient.

Electrocardiogram (ECG)

An ECG is a visual recording of the heart's electrical activity, obtained by placing electrodes on the body to measure the strength and direction of electrical activity. It is a valuable tool for determining heart rate, rhythm, and any deviations in the normal electrical pathway (known as the cardiac axis). A positive deflection (upward) on the ECG indicates electrical activity moving towards the electrode, while a negative deflection (downward) indicates electrical activity moving (Fig. 2.9).

The P wave represents atrial depolarization, during which the electrical impulse originates in the SA node and travels throughout the atria to the AV node. Absence of this wave suggests a failure in the SA node as the heart's natural pacemaker, indicating that heart rate regulation (chronotropy) is instead determined further down the electrical conduction pathway.

The QRS complex represents ventricular depolarization, during which the electrical impulse travels down the bundle of His and through the Purkinje fibers. The PR interval, the segment between the P and R waves, reflects the duration of atrial electrical activity prior to ventricular depolarization.

The T wave represents ventricular repolarization. A tall, peaked T wave may suggest hyperkalemia. As discussed earlier, potassium efflux during phase 2 of the cardiomyocyte action potential is crucial in maintaining the stability of the cardiac action potential.

The distance between the S and T waves, known as the ST-segment, represents the early phase of ventricular repolarization. Changes in the amplitude or morphology of the

ST-segment may be suggestive of ischemia. The location of the ischemia can often be pinpointed by identifying ST-segment elevations in the leads corresponding to the affected site and can be further supported by identifying reciprocal ST-segment depressions in the electrically opposite leads.

A traditional 12 lead ECG is composed of six limb leads (I, II, III, aVL, aVR, and aVF) and six precordial leads (V1–V6) (Table. 2.1).

The cardiac axis is a representation of the dominant locations of electrical activity in the heart. Each ECG lead can be mapped onto a hexaxial reference system (Fig. 2.10), and by measuring the amplitude of each lead, cardiac axis can be determined. This is particularly useful for identifying pathological states that may result in left or right deviation of the cardiac axis. For instance, left ventricular hypertrophy resulting from long-standing uncontrolled hypertension may lead to a left axis deviation, which can be identified using this method. Additionally, deviations in electrical activity due to

Table 2.1 Standard 12-lead ECG leads and their approximate corresponding coronary artery territories

ECG leads	Anatomical location	Coronary artery territory
II, II, AvF	Inferior wall	Right coronary artery (RCA)
I, AvL	Lateral wall	Left circumflex artery (LCx)
V1, V2	Septal wall	Proximal left anterior descending artery (LAD)
V3, V4	Anterior wall	Left anterior descending artery
V5, V6	Apex	Distal LAD artery, (and/or RCA, or LCx)

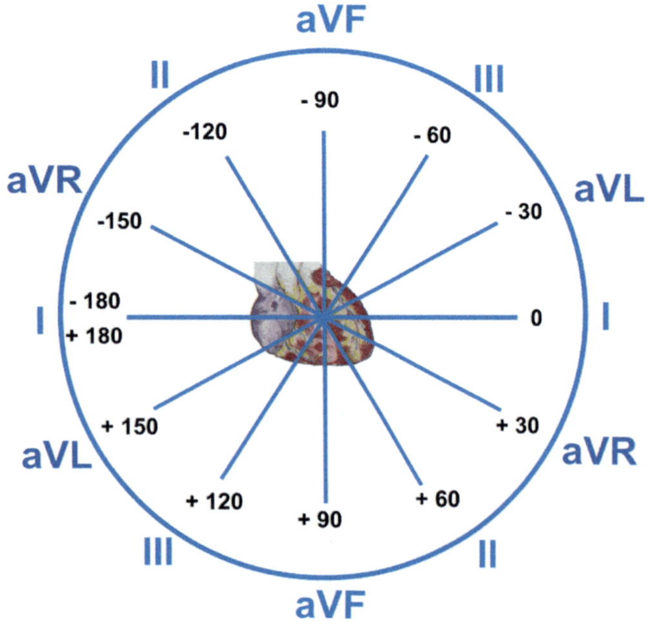

Fig. 2.10 Hexaxial reference for cardiac axis. This illustration provides a detailed view of the hexaxial reference system used to determine the cardiac axis on ECG

myocardial injury may cause deviations towards the opposing axes.

One of the most clinically significant applications of the ECG is in diagnosis of myocardial infarctions. Ventricular repolarization, denoted by the ST-segment between the S and T waves, is a critical phase. Conditions that impede ventricular repolarization can be categorized by changes in the ST-segment. Ischemic cardiomyocytes may not be able to repolarize properly, leading to an inappropriate transfer of current, which can be detected as an elevation of the ST-segment. Notably, an ST-segment elevation of greater than 0.2 mV suggests a transmural infarction, affecting the full thickness of the heart wall. However, it is crucial to recognize that not all ST-segment elevations indicate ischemia; many normal variants cause early repolarization, which may also demonstrate an elevated J-point (intersection between the QRS complex and the ST-segment) and ST-segment. Thus, the interpretation of the ECG should be contextualized within clinical symptomatology and compared to previous ECGs when available. Infarctions affecting only a portion of the wall may exhibit less pronounced ST-segment changes.

The Cardiac Output: Understanding Function and Clinical Significance

Cardiac output is a vital physiologic determinant of the heart's function, measured as the amount of blood the heart ejects per unit of time, typically expressed in liters per minute. It is calculated by multiplying the stroke volume by heart rate, and in an average adult at rest, it ranges from 4.5 to 5.5 liters per minute. In a normal heart, the cardiac output of the systemic circulation should match that of the pulmonary circulation. However, pathologic states may affect one side of the heart independently, and failure in one side can precipitate failure on the other. For example, left heart failure can lead to right heart failure due to increased hydrostatic pressure upstream. Abnormalities in cardiac output are clinically significant and can result from conditions like coronary ischemia, valvular disorders, or other cardiovascular diseases.

Measurement of Cardiac Output

Various techniques for measuring cardiac output are available, each offering different degrees of invasiveness and accuracy, depending on the monitoring modalities used.

- *Invasive Methods*: The Swan-Ganz pulmonary arterial catheter (PAC) is the gold standard for precise hemodynamic monitoring, including cardiac output measurement. However, its invasive nature limits its use to critical care settings. The PAC utilizes thermodilution, where a cold injectate is introduced into the right atrium, and the temperature change downstream is used to calculate cardiac output.

- *Fick Method*: This method indirectly calculates cardiac output by measuring oxygen consumption (the difference between inhaled and exhaled oxygen) and dividing it by the arteriovenous oxygen difference (the difference in oxygen content between arterial and venous blood). While accurate, it requires specialized equipment and is not routinely used in clinical practice.
- *Echocardiography*: This non-invasive imaging modality provides real-time visualization of the heart and can be used to estimate stroke volume. By multiplying stroke volume by heart rate, cardiac output can be calculated. Echocardiography is widely available and relatively easy to perform, making it a valuable tool for assessing cardiac function.
- *Cardiac MRI*: This non-invasive imaging technique offers detailed anatomical and functional information about the heart. It can accurately measure cardiac output by assessing blood flow through the great vessels. While highly accurate, cardiac MRI is less readily available and more expensive than echocardiography.

The choice of method for measuring cardiac output depends on the clinical context, the patient's condition, and the available resources. In critical care settings, the PAC is often the preferred method due to its accuracy and continuous monitoring capabilities. In less acute situations, echocardiography or cardiac MRI may be sufficient for assessing cardiac function and estimating cardiac output.

$$CO = \frac{VO_2}{C_aO_2 - C_vO_2}$$

$$CO = \text{cardiac output}$$

$$VO_2 = \text{oxygen consumption}\left(\text{ml/min}\right)$$

$$C_aO_2 = \text{arterial oxygen concentration}$$

$$C_vO_2 = \text{venous oxygen concentration}$$

Regulation and Dysfunction of Cardiac Output

To ensure adequate blood flow, cardiac output is variable and adjusts in response to fluctuating metabolic demands. Factors that influence changes in either stroke volume or heart rate will lead to proportional changes in cardiac output.

Stroke Volume

Stroke volume is influenced by factors such as ventricular contractility, preload, and afterload.

- *Preload*: The end-diastolic volume (EDV), or the amount of blood in the ventricle before contraction, directly influences stroke volume. Increased preload, as seen with greater EDV, leads to increased stroke volume and subsequently higher cardiac output.
- *Afterload*: The resistance the heart must overcome to eject blood, known as afterload, can significantly impact stroke volume. Conditions like chronic hypertension increase SVR, raising afterload and reducing stroke volume.
- *Contractility*: The force of ventricular contraction directly affects stroke volume. Increased contractility enhances the heart's ability to pump blood, leading to increased stroke volume.

Heart Failure

When disease states exceed the heart's capacity to compensate, there may be a reduction in its ability to maintain cardiac output, broadly defined as heart failure. The pathophysiology of heart failure depends on whether the failure is due to an inability to fill the ventricles with blood or to eject the blood once it is in the ventricles.

- *Systolic Heart Failure (HFrEF)*
  Systolic failure, or inadequate contractility, may arise from conditions such as coronary artery disease, previous myocardial infarctions, or long-standing arrhythmia. In systolic failure, there is typically a reduction in the ejection fraction, defined as the stroke volume divided by the EDV. Stroke volume, defined earlier, is the EDV minus the end-systolic volume (ESV). A failure of contractility will result in a larger ESV, owing to a reduced stroke volume compared to a non-pathological state.
- *Diastolic Heart Failure (HFpEF)*
  Alternatively, a reduction in preload will lead to decreased cardiac output due to a lower EDV and subsequent a lower stroke volume. Factors that may reduce diastolic filling include concentric hypertrophy and impaired relaxation, as seen with conditions like amyloidosis. In this case, the problem lies in ventricular filling rather than contractility hence the ejection fraction is preserved. The pathophysiology of heart failure with preserved ejection relates to inadequate cardiac output relative to the body's demands.

The symptomatology of both types of heart failure described above provides a framework to understand the role of cardiac output in end-organ perfusion.

Further Reading

Awad AS. Cardiac anesthesia: the basics of evaluation and management. Cham: Springer; 2021.

Bishop SP, Zhang J, Ye L. Cardiomyocyte proliferation from fetal- to adult- and from normal- to hypertrophy and failing hearts. Biology (Basel). 2022;11(6):880. https://doi.org/10.3390/biology11060880.

Boyette LC, Burns B. Physiology, pulmonary circulation. In: StatPearls [Internet]. Treasure Island: StatPearls Publishing; 2024. Available from: https://www.ncbi.nlm.nih.gov/books/NBK470401/.

Bradić J, Andjić M, Novaković J, Jeremić N, Jakovljević V. Cardioplegia in open heart surgery: age matters. J Clin Med. 2023;12(4):1698. https://doi.org/10.3390/jcm12041698.

Chaudhry R, Miao JH, Rehman A. Physiology, cardiovascular. In: StatPearls [Internet]. Treasure Island: StatPearls Publishing; 2024. Available from: https://www.ncbi.nlm.nih.gov/books/NBK459133/.

Cardiovascular Education (ecgwaves.com). ECG localization of myocardial infarction/ischemia and coronary artery occlusion (culprit). Available from: https://ecgwaves.com/ecg-localization-myocardial-infarction-ischemia-coronary-artery-occlusion-culprit/

Eisner DA, Caldwell JL, Kistamás K, Trafford AW. Calcium and excitation-contraction coupling in the heart. Circ Res. 2017;121(2):181–95. https://doi.org/10.1161/CIRCRESAHA.117.310230.

Hainsworth R. The importance of vascular capacitance in cardiovascular control. Physiology. 1990;5(6):250–7. https://doi.org/10.1152/physiologyonline.1990.5.6.250.

Keepers B, Liu J, Qian L. What's in a cardiomyocyte – and how do we make one through reprogramming? Biochim Biophys Acta Mol Cell Res. 2020;1867(3):118464. https://doi.org/10.1016/j.bbamcr.2019.03.011.

Mitchell JR, Wang JJ. Expanding application of the Wiggers diagram to teach cardiovascular physiology. Adv Physiol Educ. 2014;38(2):170–5. https://doi.org/10.1152/advan.00123.2013.

Mohan R, Boukens BJ, Christoffels VM. Lineages of the cardiac conduction system. J Cardiovasc Dev Dis. 2017;4(2):5. https://doi.org/10.3390/jcdd4020005.

Mulroney S. Netter's essential physiology. 2nd ed. Philadelphia: Elsevier; 2016.

Rossignol P, Hernandez AF, Solomon SD, Zannad F. Heart failure drug treatment. Lancet. 2019;393(10175):1034–44.

Sattar Y, Chhabra L. Electrocardiogram. In: StatPearls [Internet]. Treasure Island: StatPearls Publishing; 2024. Available from: https://www.ncbi.nlm.nih.gov/books/NBK459285/.

Seo DY, Kwak HB, Kim AH, Park SH, Heo JW, Kim HK, et al. Cardiac adaptation to exercise training in health and disease. Pflügers Arch. 2020;472(2):155–68. https://doi.org/10.1007/s00424-019-02365-8.

Vincent JL. Understanding cardiac output. Crit Care. 2008;12(4):174. https://doi.org/10.1186/cc6975.

Vives M, Hernandez A. Cardiac anesthesia and postoperative care in the 21st century. Cham: Springer; 2022.

Yancy CW, Jessup M, Bozkurt B, et al. 2017 ACC/AHA/HFSA focused update of the 2013 ACCF/AHA guideline for the Management of Heart Failure: a report of the American College of Cardiology/American Heart Association Task Force on Clinical Practice Guidelines and the Heart Failure Society of America. Circulation. 2017;136(6):e137–61. https://doi.org/10.1161/CIR.0000000000000509.

Blood Physiology and Oxygen Transport

3

Karina Braslavskaya, Vincent Reformato, and Enrique Pantin

Introduction

Blood, a specialized type of connective tissue, acts as a crucial transport medium within the cardiovascular system. It distributes essential substances like nutrients, gases, drugs, hormones, electrolytes, and metabolic waste products. This complex fluid matrix is composed of plasma, a protein-rich solution, and suspended cellular components, including erythrocytes (red blood cells, RBCs), white blood cells (WBCs), and platelets. These cellular and plasma constituents work together synergistically to perform four vital functions: transporting oxygen and other essential substances, facilitating hemostasis and blood clot formation, maintaining homeostasis, and defending against pathogens through immune responses. An average 70 kg adult has approximately 5 L of blood. Fifty-five percent of that volume is composed of plasma, while the rest is composed of cellular elements.

Blood Components and Their Functions

Blood consists of four main components, each with distinct functions. Plasma, the liquid portion, circulates nutrients, hormones, and waste and contains proteins essential for clotting and immune responses. WBCs are key to immune defense, platelets play a crucial role in clotting and healing, and RBCs transport oxygen to tissues and remove carbon dioxide from the body (see Fig. 3.1).

1. **Plasma the Soluble Components of Blood**

Plasma, the non-cellular component of blood, is a straw-colored, viscous solution composed of water (91%) and solids (9%), including electrolytes, plasma proteins, carbohydrates, and lipids.

Diversity and Roles of Plasma Proteins

The major proteins found in plasma are albumin, fibrinogen, globulins, and coagulation factors. Each protein has a specific function—some take part in the coagulation cascade to form a clot, while others help transport molecules.

- Albumin: This versatile transporter delivers a variety of molecules, including hormones, enzymes, fatty acids, and pharmaceuticals, throughout the circulatory system, ensuring their systemic availability.
- Fibrinogen: A primary agent in coagulation, fibrinogen initiates a series of biochemical events (coagulation proteins) following endothelial damage, culminating in clot formation, which is vital for hemostasis and tissue regeneration.
- Globulins: These proteins, especially immunoglobulins, play a critical role in the immune response by neutralizing pathogens and toxins. Other globulin subclasses are involved in lipid transport and hormonal modulation.

K. Braslavskaya · V. Reformato · E. Pantin (✉)
Department of Anesthesiology & Perioperative Medicine, Rutgers-Robert Wood Johnson Medical School, New Brunswick, NJ, USA
e-mail: vr247@rwjms.rutgers.edu

A. S. Awad, J. DiNardo (eds.), *Clinical Perfusion for Cardiac Surgery*, https://doi.org/10.1007/978-3-031-91163-7_3

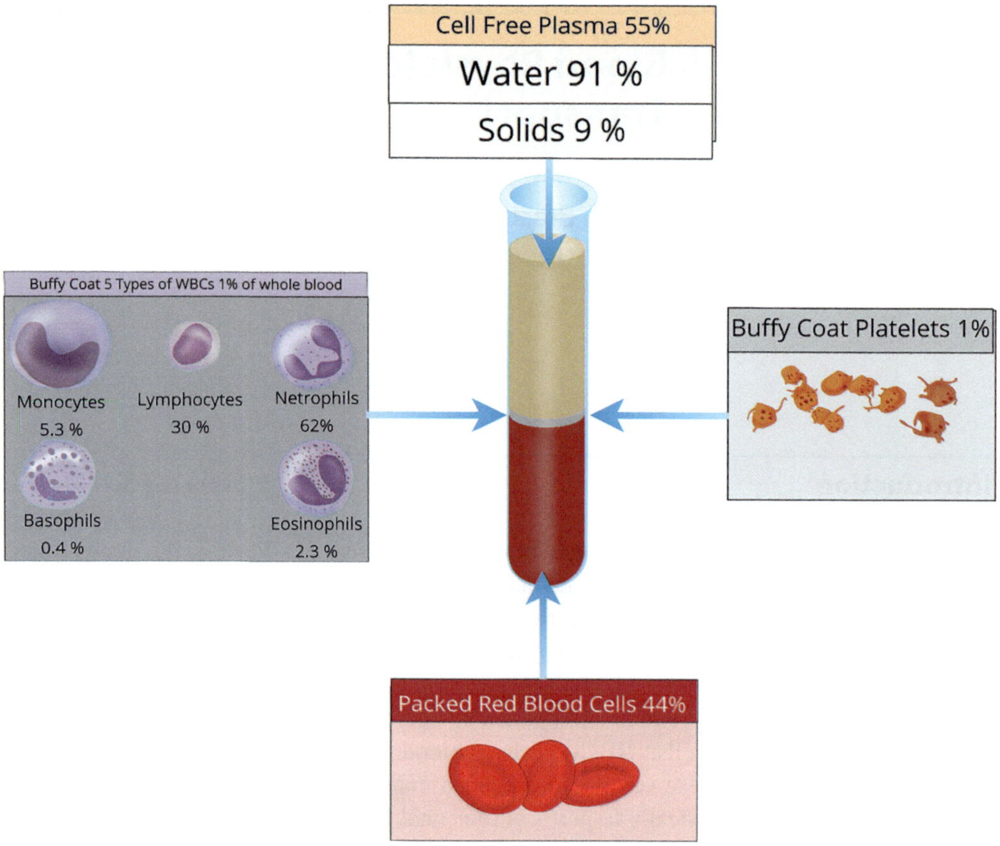

Fig. 3.1 Illustration of blood composition. This diagram depicts a test tube displaying the various components of blood, visually separating cell-free plasma 55%, Buffy coat of WBCs and Platelets 1%, and RBCs 44% to highlight their distinct proportions and roles within the circulatory system

Oncotic Pressure and Fluid Movement

The proteins within plasma also aid in maintaining the oncotic pressure within the vasculature. Oncotic pressure, also known as colloid osmotic pressure, is the pressure exerted by proteins in the blood on the capillary walls. It is an important force that regulates the movement of fluids between the blood vessels and surrounding tissues. Oncotic pressure is critical for maintaining the proper distribution of fluids in the body. When the oncotic pressure in the blood vessels is lower than the hydrostatic pressure (the force exerted by the blood on the capillary walls), fluid can leak out of the blood vessels and into the surrounding tissues, leading to edema. Conversely, when the oncotic pressure is higher than the hydrostatic pressure, fluids are drawn back into the blood vessels, helping to maintain the proper balance of fluids in the body.

Electrolytic Regulation and Function

The main electrolytes within plasma are sodium, chloride, calcium, potassium, and magnesium. These are osmotically active solutes, and they are essential for maintaining fluid balance and blood pressure. An increase or decrease in their concentration will impact the total blood volume. Electrolytes also play a key role in cell membrane physiology and pH regulation as they constantly move between blood, tissues, and interstitial space to maintain homeostasis.

Buffering Capacity and Blood pH

Plasma proteins and certain electrolytes also contribute significantly to the blood's buffering capacity, helping maintain pH within normal limits.

Blood Cellular components Types and Function

Leukocytes

Leukocytes or WBCs, play a crucial role in the body's defense system. All WBCs are produced in the bone marrow and can vary in diameter from 7 to 30 μm, depending on the type. They can be found anywhere in the body, blood, and lymphatic system but not inside healthy brains or some parts of the eye. Transported by the blood to areas of infection or injury, they work alongside antibodies and blood proteins to combat foreign agents and pathogens. In an adult human, the blood typically contains approximately 7,000 WBCs per microliter. Leukocytes are categorized into five types: neutrophils, eosinophils, basophils, lymphocytes, and monocytes.

- Neutrophils (7–15 μm), making up more than half of WBCs, are key to the immune system. They come as mature segmented or younger band forms, both loaded with enzymes to attack and neutralize pathogens. Crucial for internal defense, they constantly patrol the body, responding to invaders.
- Monocytes and Macrophages (15–30 μm): Monocytes are sparse in blood as they mostly reside in peripheral tissues. Here, they develop into larger macrophages, which are crucial for phagocytosis and antigen presentation to lymphocytes.
- Lymphocytes (7–15 μm) are granule-less cells divided into classes such as T and B lymphocytes. T cells, forming 70–80% of blood lymphocytes and maturing in the thymus, are vital for cell-mediated immunity. B cells, making up 10–15% and maturing in the bone marrow, produce antibodies for humoral immunity when activated by antigens and T cells. Natural killer cells are another type of lymphocyte.

Platelets

Platelets, nucleus-free fragments produced in the bone marrow from megakaryocytes, range from 150,000 to 450,000 per microliter of blood. Their production is regulated by thrombopoietin (TPO) and IL-3, with feedback mechanisms adjusting megakaryocyte activity to maintain platelet levels. Platelets, essential for hemostasis and approximately 2–3 μm in diameter, contain glycoprotein receptors, microtubules, and organelles like mitochondria and granules storing clotting factors and other substances. Their lifespan is about 10 days. During cardiopulmonary bypass (CPB), contact with the circuit's surfaces activates platelets and initiates the coagulation cascade. This activation, along with dilutional thrombocytopenia, leads to CPB-induced coagulopathy.

Erythrocytes

Erythrocytes, or red blood cells (RBCs) (6–8 μm), comprise the most abundant component of the total cell volume. In an adult human, the blood typically contains approximately five million RBCs per microliter of blood. The shape and size of the erythrocyte are vital to its function. Normal erythrocytes

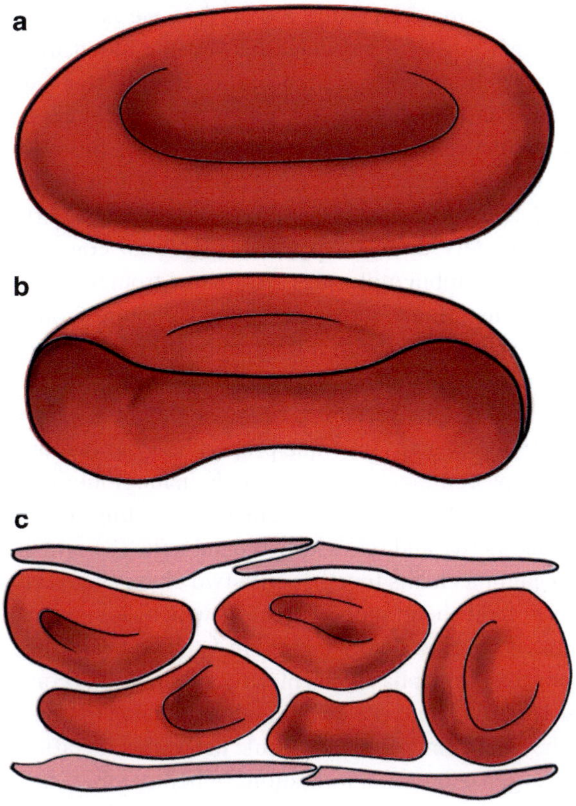

Fig. 3.2 Illustration of erythrocyte structure and organization. Image (**a**) displays a single erythrocyte, highlighting its distinctive biconcave disk shape. Image (**b**) provides a cross-sectional view of an erythrocyte, demonstrating its unique structure. Image (**c**) depicts multiple erythrocytes flowing within a small blood vessel, showcasing how their shape aids in efficient circulation

are biconcave disks (see Fig. 3.2). This unique shape optimizes the surface-to-volume ratio, enhancing the diffusion rate of gases and solutes, and allows the cells to navigate through small capillaries efficiently.

Erythrocytes are produced in the bone marrow and reach full maturity within 1–2 days after being released into circulation. The normal life span of erythrocyte is approximately 120 days. These cells lack a nucleus but possess enzymes that are essential for maintaining their function and biconcave shape. The majority of aged erythrocytes are sequestered and destroyed in the spleen. Additionally, some erythrocytes rupture within the circulatory system when their cell membranes become too fragile to maintain integrity.

Erythrocytes have three functions:

(a) Transporting oxygen from the lungs to various tissues.

Hemoglobin, the main component of the erythrocyte, binds oxygen to form oxyhemoglobin molecules, facilitating oxygen transport. Hemoglobin synthesis begins in the bone marrow, while the erythrocyte is maturing and finishes after being released into the bloodstream. Normal hemoglobin content is 14.0 g/dL for adult females and 15.0 g/dL for adult males. Hematocrit, meanwhile, refers to the fraction of the total blood volume that is composed of erythrocytes. It can be estimated using the formula Hct = Hgb × 3, as hematocrit is approximately three times the hemoglobin concentration. Hemoglobin molecules are created from heme protein chains. Heme molecules, which require iron for synthesis, combine with a polypeptide chain to form a hemoglobin subunit or chain. There are alpha, beta, gamma, and delta variations of the hemoglobin subunit, each of which gives it unique properties. Four hemoglobin chains combine to form a single hemoglobin molecule. Normal Hb is a tetramer, consisting of two α-subunits (α1 and α2) and two β-subunits (β1 and β2). Two gamma chains together with two alpha chains constitute fetal hemoglobin (HbF), which is normally replaced by adult hemoglobin (HbA) in the year following birth. Two alpha chains plus two delta chains constitute HbA-2. The types of hemoglobin chains that make up the final hemoglobin molecule determine the affinity for oxygen. Abnormal formations of hemoglobin lead to different physiologic characteristics and result in pathological disease states such as sickle cell anemia.

(b) Carrying carbon dioxide from tissues back to lungs

Erythrocytes are rich in the enzyme carbonic anhydrase (CA), which plays an important role in cellular respiration and in the transport of carbon dioxide produced during cellular respiration. During cellular respiration, carbon dioxide is produced as a waste product. CA catalyzes a reversible reaction between carbon dioxide and water to create bicarbonate and hydrogen ions. Bicarbonate ions are then transported in the plasma to the lungs. Once bicarbonate ions reach the pulmonary capillaries, the reverse reaction occurs. CA converts bicarbonate and hydrogen ion back to carbon dioxide and water, allowing it to be exhaled from the lungs as illustrated in Fig. 3.4.

(c) Serving as a vital component of the body's buffering system.

The bicarbonate ions generated by the action of CA contribute to maintaining the blood's pH balance. Furthermore, the hydrogen ions produced in the reaction are buffered by hemoglobin, which aids in maintaining the optimal pH for enzyme activity and oxygen transport.

Blood Types

Surgical procedures, particularly cardiovascular surgeries that directly manipulate the circulatory system, often result in significant blood loss. This frequently necessitates blood transfusions. However, blood is highly individualized, meaning not all donor blood is suitable for every patient, due to the risk of transfusion reactions. This compatibility is largely determined by specific antigens present on the surfaces of red blood cells, which define an individual's blood type.

A–B–O Blood Types

In a large percentage of people, two antigens—type A and type B—are present on the surfaces of RBCs. These antigens, known as agglutinogens, are mucopolysaccharides that are present on the surface of erythrocytes but are not contained within them. They can lead to RBC agglutination, which may trigger adverse reactions, and even death during blood transfusions. People may have type A, B, AB, or O blood, based on the presence or absence (type O) of these agglutinogens (Fig. 3.3). Additionally, blood plasma contains agglutinins that can react with different blood types, necessitating careful blood type matching.

Rh Blood Types

Besides the ABO system, there is the Rh system, with the primary agglutinogen being D (Rh positive). About 85% of people are Rh positive. Anti-D agglutinin in plasma is not naturally present but is formed upon exposure to the D agglutinogen.

To prevent transfusion reactions, blood must be typed and crossmatched, ensuring compatibility between donor and recipient blood. Mismatched transfusions can lead to dangerous agglutination and hemolysis, potentially fatal. In emergencies, where time is critical, O-negative blood, often referred to as the universal donor type, can be used for transfusion.

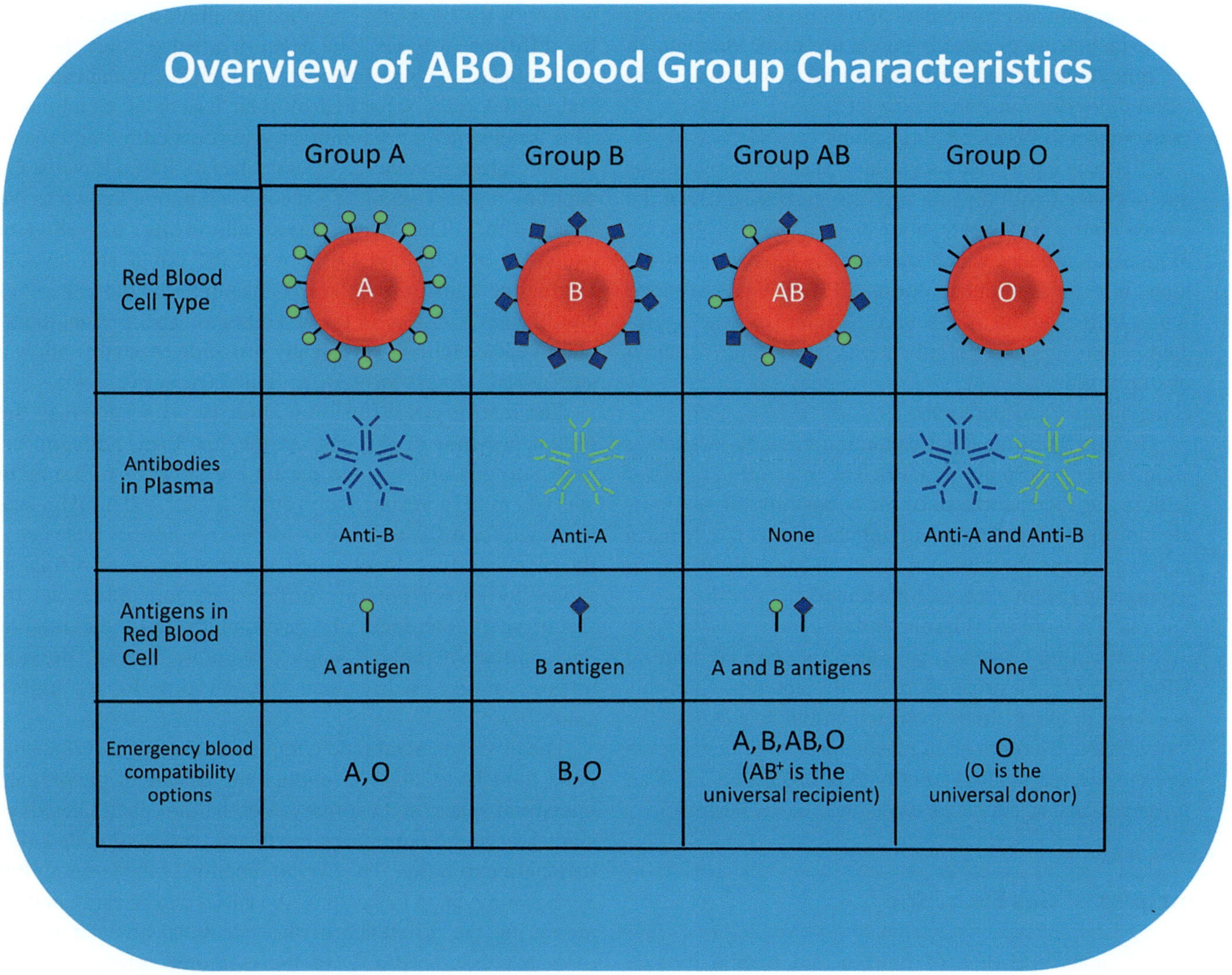

Fig. 3.3 Illustration of Table of ABO blood groups. Illustration of red blood cells, antigens, and antibodies, and a guide to emergency-compatible blood types

Blood Physiological Changes and Considerations During Cardiopulmonary Perfusion

CPB introduces significant alterations to blood physiology, necessitating an in-depth understanding and strategic approach to manage these alterations. While detailed discussions are provided in various sections of the book, this section will highlight the major physiological changes impacting blood during CPB.

1. Hemodilution

   One of the primary considerations in CPB is the management of blood volume. The use of a priming fluid in the bypass circuit can lead to hemodilution, diluting blood components, including medications dissolved in it. This dilution can impact the efficacy of blood components and must be carefully managed to maintain homeostasis. For in-depth details, see Chap. 19.

2. Hemolysis

   During CPB, erythrocytes face considerable stress, leading to hemolysis, the bursting of these cells. This hemolysis can result from mechanical forces within the bypass circuit, changes in osmolality and temperature, exposure to shear forces, and contact with hemolytic enzymes such as plasmin. Additionally, the use of intracardiac or intrapericardial suction subjects erythrocytes to further trauma. Historically, roller pumps, especially those not properly occlusive, and bubble oxygenators (no longer in use) with direct blood–gas interfaces, have been known to exacerbate hemolysis. The majority of hemolysis during CPB is attributed to suction systems. Although completely preventing this hemolysis is challenging, it can be minimized through meticulous suction techniques by the surgeon and controlled suction by the perfusionist, alongside the use of extracorporeal filtration. Maintaining erythrocyte integrity is essential for effective oxygen and carbon dioxide transport during CPB.

3. Leukocyte and Platelet Aggregations

   CPB can induce leukocyte and platelet aggregations due to contact with the non-physiological surfaces of the bypass circuit. This aggregation can lead to the formation of microaggregates, which are typically filtered out by the lungs but can accumulate during CPB. The use of blood filters in the circuit is essential to remove these aggregates and prevent complications like microvascular obstructions.

4. Coagulation Considerations

   The activation of the coagulation cascade is another significant concern during CPB. The interaction of blood with the artificial surfaces of the bypass circuit can initiate clot formation. The use of anticoagulants like heparin is standard, but their efficacy must be carefully balanced against the risk of excessive bleeding.

5. Oncotic Pressure and Plasma Proteins

   Maintaining oncotic pressure is crucial during CPB. The plasma proteins, primarily albumin, exert this pressure, drawing fluids from interstitial spaces into the vasculature. Disruptions in plasma protein concentration or excessive crystalloid solution administration can lead to issues such as edema or inadequate tissue perfusion.

Principles of Gas Exchange

The continuous exchange of oxygen and carbon dioxide between the lungs, blood, and tissues is a fundamental physiological process, crucial for maintaining cellular metabolism and overall homeostasis. Oxygen is necessary for cellular respiration, while carbon dioxide is a metabolic byproduct that needs to be removed from the body. The efficiency of this gas exchange process is essential for the functioning of organs.

Diffusion of Gases Through the Respiratory Membrane

Pulmonary arteries branch extensively, forming a dense, mesh-like network of capillaries that surround the alveoli, known as the alveolar–capillary network. This complex structure is made up of thin epithelial cells of the alveoli, endothelial cells of the capillaries, and their supporting matrix. The alveolar-respiratory membrane, closely associated with the capillary endothelium, plays a crucial role in the diffusion of gases. The network's barrier, only 1–2 μm thick, consists of type I alveolar epithelial cells and capillary endothelial cells, separated by their basement membranes. This arrangement, predominantly surrounded by air, creates an optimal environment for gas exchange. RBCs traverse the capillary network in under a second, a duration known as the transit time. This brief period allows for the efficient exchange of CO_2 and O_2 between the blood and alveoli. During the transit time, the gas tension in the blood reaches equilibrium with that in the alveolar gas. The internal diameter of each capillary is typically just wide enough to allow a single RBC to pass through, as illustrated in Fig. 3.4.

The rate of gas diffusion is directly proportional to the partial pressure of the gas. At the sea level, ambient air, with nitrogen and oxygen partial pressures of 600 mmHg and 160 mmHg, respectively, out of a total 760 mmHg, sets the stage for diffusion. Lipid-soluble respiratory gases easily permeate the alveolar cell membranes, with diffusion driven by partial pressure differences, and influenced by factors such as temperature, gas solubility, and thickness of the capillary-alveolar complex. Notably, carbon dioxide diffuses more readily than oxygen due to its higher solubility.

The alveolar membrane complex, including a surfactant-lined fluid layer, alveolar epithelium, basement membrane, interstitial space, and capillary endothelium, facilitates oxygen's journey to pulmonary blood and carbon dioxide's diffusion for expiration. The overall function of the lungs ability to allow oxygen to be taken by the RBCs can be estimated by measuring the difference of the calculated alveolar partial oxygen pressure (PAO2) to the measured arterial oxygen partial pressure (PaO2), this is called the "Alveolo-arterial oxygen gradient" = A-a gradient = PAO2 − PaO2.

$$\text{A-a gradient} = PAO_2 - PaO_2$$

where PAO2 = (P atmospheric-PH2O in the alveoli) FiO2-PaCO2/Respiratory quotient (if not measured, then estimated to be 0.8).

$$\begin{aligned} PAO2 &= (760\ \text{mmHg} - 47\ \text{mmHg})\ 0.21 - 40/0.8 \\ &= 100\ \text{mmHg} \end{aligned}$$

A-a gradient = PAO2 − PaO2 = 100 mmHg − 95 mmHg (normal value for a healthy patient breathing room air) = 5 mmHg

The normal A-a gradient stands below 10 mmHg on room air, and less than 100 if breathing 100% oxygen. This difference is a bit larger as we age.

Breathing, which brings air composed mainly of oxygen and nitrogen into the lungs, results in a mixture with existing

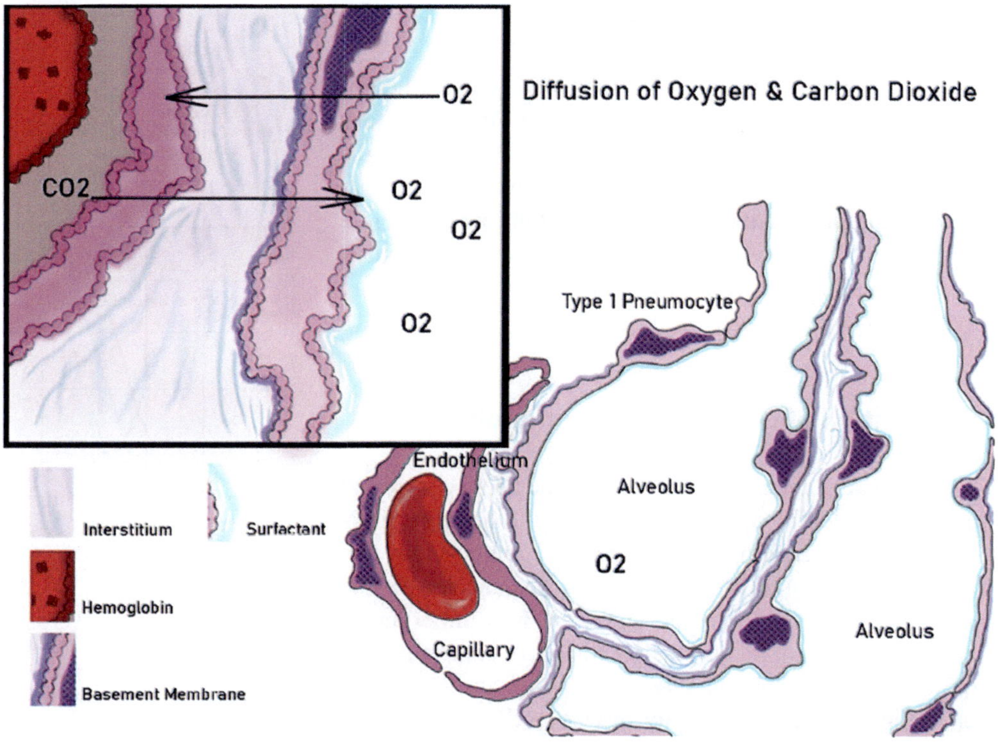

Fig. 3.4 Illustration of alveolar-respiratory membrane and capillary endothelium. This diagram depicts the intricate relationship between the alveolar-respiratory membrane and the capillary endothelium, highlighting the thin, permeable layers that facilitate efficient gas exchange between the alveoli and blood in the capillaries

gases. This composition is subject to variation depending on environmental factors like altitude, location, temperature, and humidity.

Diffusion of Gases Through Tissues

Gases exchange, nutrient delivery, and metabolic waste removal occur at the level of microcirculation, which comprises small blood vessels including arterioles, capillaries, and venules. Arterioles, diminutive branches of arteries, have the capacity to regulate blood flow to different parts of the body by contracting or dilating. Capillaries, the smallest blood vessels, form complex arrangements of vascular beds within tissues, facilitating the exchange of gases, nutrients, and waste products.

Substances transfer between plasma and tissues mainly via diffusion, either directly through the cell membranes or specialized intercellular pores in capillary walls. Gas movement is driven by differences in partial pressures, enabling molecules to move from higher to lower pressure areas as illustrated in Fig. 3.5. This process is known as diffusion. Cellular respiration, that is aerobic respiration for energy production, in all the major organs and tissues relies on the diffusion of gases into the blood passing through the lungs and delivered to the cells and ultimately to the mitochondria for ATP production.

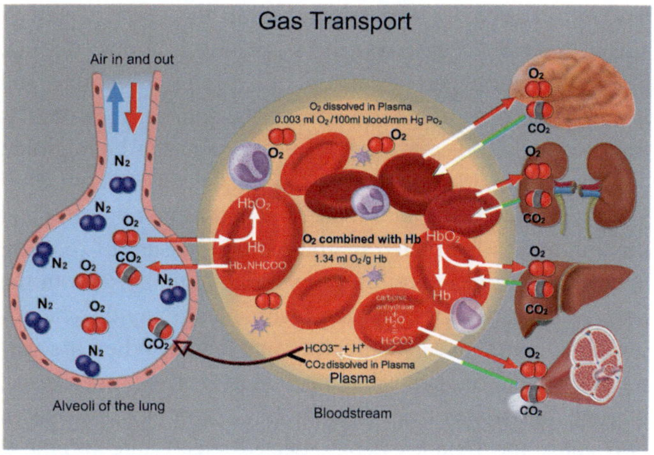

Fig. 3.5 This detailed illustration depicts the pathway of oxygen from the alveoli in the lungs through the circulatory system to different organs in the body, and its subsequent return carrying carbon dioxide. Oxygen in the blood is either dissolved in plasma or carried by hemoglobin as oxyhemoglobin (98–98.5%). It showcases the pivotal role of RBC, equipped with iron-rich hemoglobin, in transporting oxygen to essential organs such as the brain, liver, kidneys, and muscles and all tissues in general. Simultaneously, hemoglobin plays a crucial role in transporting carbon dioxide, a metabolic byproduct, back to the lungs for exhalation. Carbon dioxide travels in three forms: dissolved as a gas in plasma, bound to hemoglobin as carbaminohemoglobin, and dissolved in plasma as bicarbonate. This complex process, driven by the continuous flow of blood, exemplifies the sophisticated mechanisms of gas exchange and transport, characterized by hemoglobin-facilitated oxygen binding and diffusion across capillary membranes

Transport of Oxygen in the Blood

Oxygen is primarily transported in the blood bound to hemoglobin, a protein in RBC. Hemoglobin can bind up to four oxygen molecules, forming oxyhemoglobin. This binding is influenced by factors such as pH, carbon dioxide concentration, temperature, and the presence of 2,3-diphosphoglycerate (2,3-DPG). The oxygen–hemoglobin dissociation curve illustrates this relationship and is crucial in understanding oxygen delivery to tissues.

Combination of Oxygen with Hemoglobin

Oxygen loosely and reversibly binds to the heme compound within hemoglobin. Oxygen that is bound to hemoglobin is carried in its original molecular structure, composed of two oxygen atoms. This allows the oxygen to be quickly taken up and bound to hemoglobin and unloaded. It is important to note that hemoglobin also helps transport approximately 20% of carbon dioxide via direct binding. As discussed earlier in the chapter, the majority of carbon dioxide is transported in the form of bicarbonate ions.

Most of the oxygen that is transported from the lungs to tissues is bound to hemoglobin within the erythrocytes. A small portion of the oxygen is dissolved in the plasma. Normally, arterial partial pressure of oxygen is 95 mmHg, and it corresponds to about 1.5–3% of the total oxygen that is transported dissolved in blood. Thus, having a low hemoglobin content can significantly impact oxygen delivery to tissues.

Oxygen molecules are loosely bound to hemoglobin and this binding is facilitated by the partial pressure of oxygen. When the partial pressure of oxygen is high, as seen in the pulmonary capillaries, oxygen favors being bound to hemoglobin creating an oxyhemoglobin molecule. When the partial pressure of oxygen is low, such as in the tissue capillaries, oxygen dissociates from hemoglobin. Hemoglobin exists in two states: the T (taut—deoxygenated-tense) state and the R (oxygenated-relaxed) state. The two states differ in their affinity to bind oxygen. In an unbound state, hemoglobin exists in the T-state, and binding of oxygen occurs with low affinity. T-state hemoglobin requires a higher partial pressure of oxygen to facilitate the binding of an oxygen molecule. The binding of single oxygen induces a conformational change that destabilizes the T-state and facilitates the transition of the other subunits to the high-affinity R state. During this process, initial O_2 binding induces an alteration in hemoglobin from the taut to relaxed form, dissociating H+ protons and progressively increasing hemoglobin's affinity for oxygen at each of the remaining binding sites through positive cooperativity. This is the basis of the oxygen–hemoglobin dissociation curve (see Fig. 3.6).

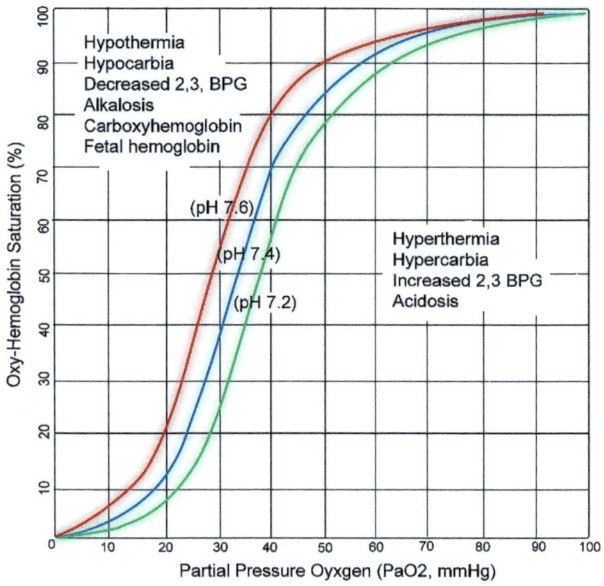

Fig. 3.6 Illustration of oxygen–hemoglobin dissociation curve; shift to the right caused by acidosis (decrease in pH) will result in lower oxyhemoglobin saturation leading to hemoglobin releasing more oxygen to the tissues

The Oxygen–Hemoglobin Dissociation Curve

The oxygen–hemoglobin dissociation curve demonstrates the increase in the percentage of oxygen bound to hemoglobin as the partial pressure of oxygen increases. Several factors can shift the curve either to the right or left. In acidic environments, hemoglobin undergoes an R to T conformational change. This shift from the higher oxygen affinity relaxed form to the lower oxygen affinity taut form releases oxygen in favor of the attachment of H+ protons. This favors dissociation of oxygen from hemoglobin at the tissue level. The rightward shift of the oxygen–hemoglobin dissociation curve in the presence of increases in the partial pressure of carbon dioxide, and/or decreased blood pH is known as the Bohr effect. In addition to pH, increased carbon dioxide concentration, increased temperature, and 2,3-DPG shift the curve to the right.

Alterations in Oxygen–Hemoglobin Dissociation During CPB

During CPB, the oxygen–hemoglobin dissociation curve can undergo significant changes due to various conditions. Factors such as hypothermia, increased pH, or reduced hemoglobin concentration can lead to increased oxygen–hemoglobin affinity. This change often results in diminished oxygen delivery across typical arterial and venous partial pressures of carbon dioxide (pCO_2). The presence of 2,3-DPG plays a pivotal role in these alterations. As organic phosphate, 2,3-DPG levels tend to drop in stored blood, crucially affecting the oxygen–hemoglobin dissociation curve. A deficiency in 2,3-DPG shifts the curve leftward, thereby decreasing oxygen release at standard arterial-venous pCO_2 levels. This shift is important to consider in the context of CPB, where maintaining optimal oxygen delivery is crucial.

Total Oxygen Content of Arterial Blood

The total amount of oxygen that is transported in the blood to tissues depends on several factors: concentration of oxygen in the air that is delivered to the lungs, partial pressure of oxygen in the lungs and tissues, efficiency of gas exchange in the lungs, and the ability of the cardiovascular system to deliver that oxygen. The total oxygen content of arterial blood (CaO_2) is determined by the oxygen saturation of hemoglobin, hemoglobin concentration, and the quantity that is dissolved in the plasma. The oxygen-carrying capacity formula delineates the contribution of each of these variables to CaO_2.

Oxygen saturation of hemoglobin refers to the percentage of hemoglobin molecules in erythrocytes that are bound to oxygen. The maximum amount of oxygen that can be carried by hemoglobin in the blood is about 1.39 mL of oxygen per gram of hemoglobin. However, even under normal conditions, a small portion of hemoglobin molecules are unable to bind oxygen because they exist in the reduced state of methemoglobin or are bound to carbon monoxide. Therefore, the empirical oxygen binding capacity of hemoglobin is stated to be 1.34 mL. In arterial blood, oxygen saturation is typically 97–99%. The amount of dissolved oxygen in the plasma is typically very small compared to the amount that is carried by the hemoglobin molecules. In a patient with hemoglobin of 15 g/dL, every 100 mL of blood would be able to carry approximately 20 mL of oxygen.

The formula below reflects the total oxygen carrying capacity in the blood.

$$CaO_2 = 1.34[Hgb](SaO_2 / 100) + 0.003PaO_2$$

1.34: Oxygen combining capacity (mL O_2/g Hgb)
Hgb: Hemoglobin concentration (g Hgb/100 mL of blood)
0.003: Solubility coefficient of oxygen (mL O_2/100 mL blood/mm Hg)

Similarities and Differences Between the Respiratory Membrane and the Membrane Oxygenator

The diffusion of gases in both the respiratory membrane and through a membrane oxygenator involves the movement of gases like oxygen (O_2) and carbon dioxide (CO_2) across a barrier. However, there are significant differences in the mechanisms and contexts in which these processes occur.

Similarities

In both the respiratory membrane and oxygenators, the fundamental principle underpinning gas exchange is diffusion, which is the movement of molecules from an area of higher concentration to one of lower concentration. This process is facilitated by the selective gas permeability characteristic of both systems, allowing only specific gases like oxygen O_2, CO_2, and inhaled anesthetics to pass through while restricting other substances. The driving force behind this diffusion in both scenarios is the difference in partial pressures of these gases across the membrane, dictating the direction and rate of gas movement. This similarity in the basic mechanics of gas exchange underscores the efficiency of both natural and artificial gas exchange processes as illustrated in Fig. 3.7.

Differences

The respiratory membrane in the lungs and the oxygenator used in CPB have distinct differences in their nature, gas transfer mechanisms, physiological regulation, and operational environments. The respiratory membrane is a biological structure made up of alveolar and capillary walls, extremely thin (about 0.5–1.0 μm) to facilitate efficient gas exchange. In contrast, an oxygenator in CPB employs an artificial membrane, specifically designed and engineered to optimize gas exchange in clinical settings.

Regarding the mechanism of gas transfer, the lungs rely on simple passive diffusion, dependent on partial pressure gradients. Conversely, an oxygenator's gas transfer, while also passive, is often enhanced mechanically, especially under high-flow conditions like those in CPB.

Physiologically, the rate of gas exchange in the lungs is regulated by altering breathing rate, respiration depth, and blood vessel perfusion. In the case of an oxygenator, gas

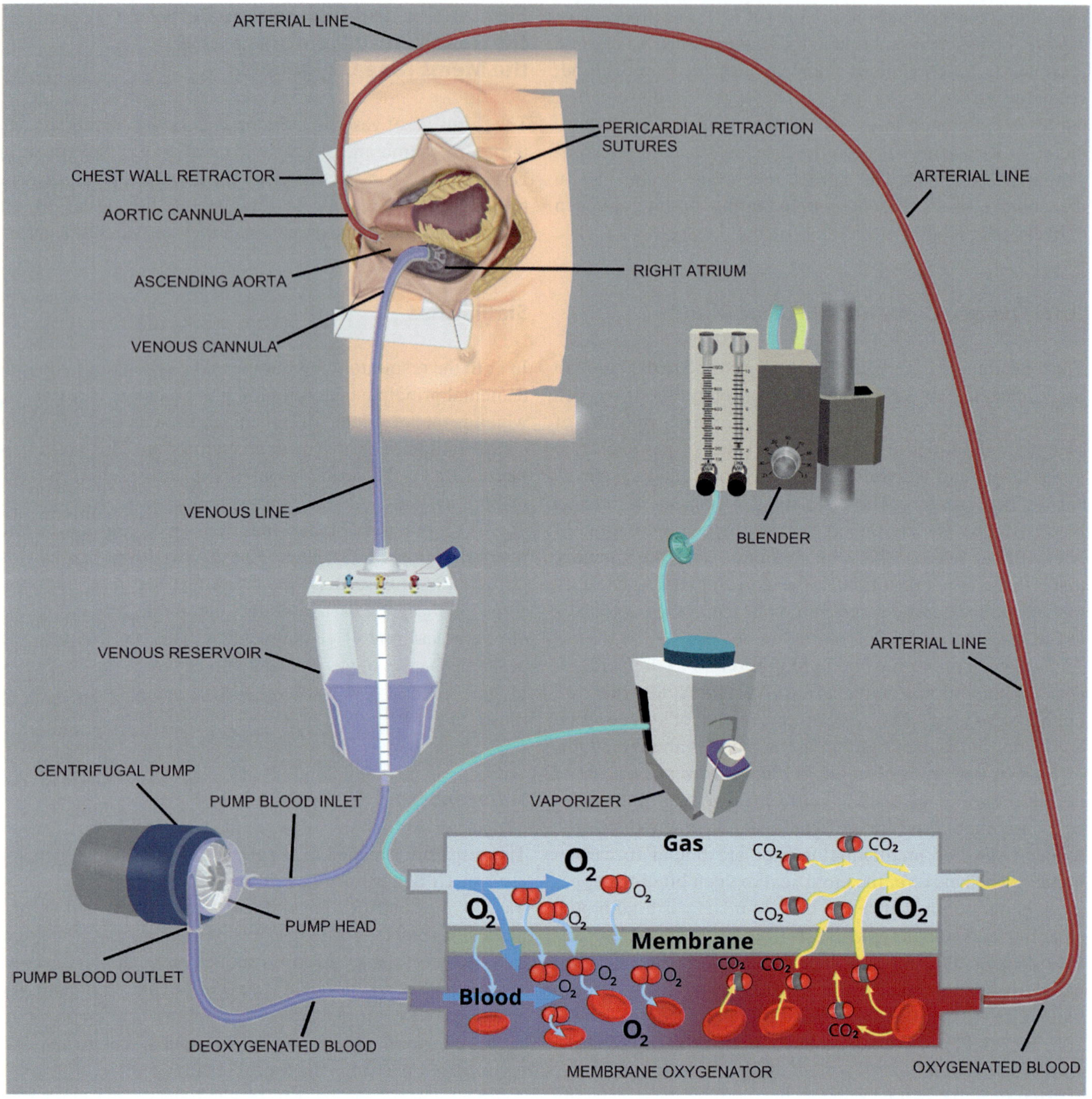

Fig. 3.7 This detailed illustration shows the CPB circuit, focusing on the oxygenator and its internal structure. The oxygenator, a key component of the circuit, is divided into two chambers by a semipermeable oxygenation membrane. Venous blood from the patient is directed into one chamber (the blood side shown here on the bottom of the oxygenator illustration), while a carefully controlled gas mixture, or fresh gas flow, passes through the other chamber (the gas side shown here on the top of the oxygenator illustration). This setup facilitates efficient gas exchange across the membrane: oxygen from the fresh gas flow diffuses into the patient's blood, oxygenating it, while carbon dioxide from the blood is removed and carried away by the sweep gas to be expelled to the room air or scavenging line. The gas mixture's composition in the fresh gas flow is adjusted by a blender, typically mixing air with oxygen. Additionally, the sweep gas is passed through the vaporizer of inhalation anesthetics before entering the oxygenator. The reoxygenated blood is then returned to the patient through the CPB's arterial line, completing the vital gas exchange process essential to CPB

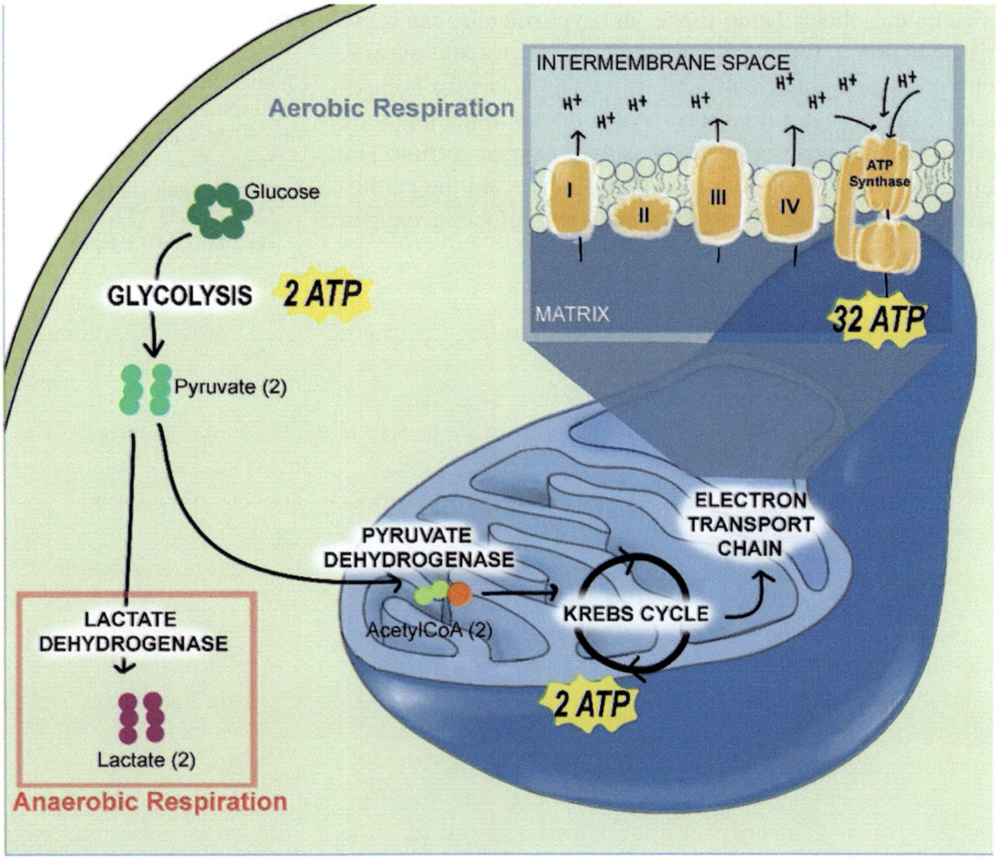

Fig. 3.8 Illustration of cellular respiration. This diagram shows the key stages of cellular respiration: glycolysis, the Krebs cycle, and the electron transport chain, emphasizing oxygen's role in energy (ATP) production. It also highlights anaerobic respiration, where the absence of oxygen leads to lactate production and less ATP

exchange is mechanically controlled by manually adjusting flow rates and pressures according to clinical requirements.

Lastly, the respiratory membrane operates within the body's natural physiological environment, influenced by factors such as body temperature, pH, and metabolic activities. On the other hand, an oxygenator functions in a controlled clinical environment, where external adjustments are made to ensure optimal gas exchange.

Understanding these differences is crucial for medical professionals, particularly in managing patients undergoing artificial oxygenation procedures like CPB.

Cellular Respiration

Cellular respiration, which is essential for the delivery of oxygen and removal of carbon dioxide at the tissue cellular level, plays a fundamental role in all life processes. Oxygen plays a key role in all life functions on a cellular level. Cellular respiration is the process that allows cells to convert glucose into energy, and there are three main cycles involved. The first cycle, glycolysis, breaks down glucose into two smaller pyruvate molecules. This is followed by the citric acid (Krebs) cycle, which converts pyruvate to carbon dioxide, water, NADH, and FADH, and energy in the form of Adenosine Triphosphate (ATP). Finally, the electron transport chain uses NADH and FADH2 from the citric acid cycle to create further ATP as part of oxidative phosphorylation. Oxygen is a crucial component for all three cycles as illustrated in Fig. 3.8.

In the absence of oxygen, however, cells will resort to anaerobic respiration. Anaerobic respiration begins with glycolysis, but pyruvate cannot be utilized in the citric acid cycle in the absence of oxygen, and consequently, lactate and small amount of ATP are produced. Overall, it is less efficient because it produces less energy for each molecule of glucose.

Tissues use oxygen to make energy to support all the various organ functions, and the metabolic waste is produced in the form of carbon dioxide.

Perfusion Limitation in Lung and Tissue Oxygen and Carbon Dioxide Exchange

The cardiovascular system is crucial for nutrient and gas delivery and waste removal, essential for aerobic respiration and homeostasis. Cardiac output, the volume of blood the heart pumps per minute, directly affects oxygen delivery to tissues. Reduced cardiac output, seen in conditions like cardiac failure, shock, hemorrhage, and hypovolemia, can cause tissue hypoxia. Blood, comprising erythrocytes and plasma, circulates gases, nutrients, and waste, and is key for homeostasis. Erythrocytes transport oxygen bound to hemoglobin, while plasma carries a smaller dissolved oxygen portion. The effective function of both blood physiology and the cardiovascular system is essential to maintain sufficient oxygen supply to sustain life.

Further Reading

Cloutier MM. Chapter 8 oxygen and carbon dioxide transport. In: Respiratory physiology. 2nd ed. Philadelphia: Elsevier; 2019.

Tibi P, McClure RS, Huang J, Baker RA, Kissoon K, Moffatt-Bruce S, et al. STS/SCA/AmSECT/SABM update to the clinical practice guidelines on patient blood management. Ann Thorac Surg. 2021;112(3):981–1004. https://doi.org/10.1016/j.athoracsur.2021.03.033. Epub 2021 Jun 30. PMID: 34217505.

Basic Cardiovascular Pharmacological Management During Cardiopulmonary Bypass

4

Eileen Kodack, Julie Wise, and Enrique Pantin

Introduction

Cardiopulmonary bypass (CPB), a type of extracorporeal circulation, is used during open heart surgeries to provide surgeons with a bloodless and motionless field for both non-beating heart and beating heart procedures. CPB involves arterial and venous cannulation, typically, in the ascending aorta and right atrium, respectively, with the placement varying by surgical approaches. Once on CPB, patients may experience an inflammatory response and/or hypotension due to decreased systemic vascular resistance (SVR), and hemodilution which, in extreme cases, can lead to coagulopathic states. While on CPB, it is vital to maintain adequate cerebral perfusion pressures, particularly in patients who have a previous diagnosis of cerebral vascular disease, carotid artery disease, and/or preexisting hypertension.

Principles of Clinical Pharmacology

Management of medications during CPB relies heavily on pharmacology, requiring a solid understanding of how drugs achieve effective concentrations at their sites of action. Consequently, this requires familiarity with two interwoven disciplines: *pharmacokinetics*, the study of drug movement within the body, and *pharmacodynamics*, the study of drug effects at specific concentrations. These interdependent disciplines shed light on how drugs are absorbed, distributed, metabolized, and excreted, and how these processes influence dose–response relationships. To illustrate pharmacokinetics principles and to simplify the complexities of drug movement, a two-compartment model is commonly employed. This model envisions the body as having two compartments: a central compartment, often represented by the blood volume, and a peripheral compartment, encompassing all other body tissues. Drugs enter the central compartment via administration and are progressively cleared through elimination processes like filtration and degradation. However, their pharmacologic actions predominantly occur in the peripheral compartment via diffusion processes. While this model simplifies the actual behavior of most drugs, it highlights key principles: drugs are administered and eliminated from the central compartment, but their pharmacologic actions usually occur in the peripheral compartment.

Following an intravenous injection, a drug's central compartment concentration initially declines rapidly due to distribution into the peripheral compartment, governed by the drug's apparent volume of distribution. As distribution plateaus, elimination becomes the primary determinant of central compartment concentration.

The duration of the elimination phase varies considerably, influenced by factors like body storages, diffusion rates, and elimination pathways. Notably, pharmacologic effects can persist even after a drug disappears from plasma due to slow diffusion away from the site of action or the presence of active metabolites.

Both distribution and elimination typically follow first-order kinetics, implying that the rate of concentration change is proportional to the current concentration. A deeper understanding of this model and the intricacy of pharmacokinetics is encouraged through further resources listed at the end of this chapter.

The Impacts of Cardiopulmonary Bypass on Pharmacology of Drugs

The effects of CPB on drugs are extensive and complex, influencing various aspects of their behavior within the body. This impact is attributed to a range of factors, including hemodilution, hypothermia, non-pulsatile blood flow, which tends to have influences on renal filtration functions,

E. Kodack · J. Wise · E. Pantin (✉)
Department of Anesthesiology & Perioperative Medicine, Rutgers-Robert Wood Johnson Medical School, New Brunswick, NJ, USA
e-mail: ek799@rwjms.rutgers.edu; wiseja@rwjms.rutgers.edu

A. S. Awad, J. DiNardo (eds.), *Clinical Perfusion for Cardiac Surgery*, https://doi.org/10.1007/978-3-031-91163-7_4

Table 4.1 The factors influencing drug behavior during CPB

Factor	Description
Hemodilution	CPB dilutes blood volume, which affects the concentration of unbound drugs (those available for action), potentially lowering their efficacy.
Hypothermia	Hypothermia during CPB can slow down drug metabolism and clearance, leading to prolonged drug action and increased potential for side effects.
Non-pulsatile blood flow	Compared to pulsatile flow, non-pulsatile flow during CPB can impact renal drug clearance, particularly for drugs excreted through glomerular filtration.
Bypassing the lungs	Drugs primarily eliminated by the lungs, such as volatile anesthetics, see their elimination halted during CPB, necessitating dosage adjustments While the design of the oxygenator can affect anesthetic uptake, the impact on polypropylene membrane oxygenators, commonly used during CPB, depends on a complex interplay of factors that lead to variable delivery of volatile anesthetics.
Changes in protein binding	CPB can affect the binding of some drugs to plasma proteins, altering the free fraction of the drug in circulation and consequently impacting their efficacy and side effect profile.

bypassing the lungs during circulation so that elimination of drugs by the lungs is halted and changes in protein binding. These elements collectively affect the *pharmacokinetics* (distribution, metabolism, elimination) and *pharmacodynamics* (action and effect) of drugs during CPB. Dosage adjustments, close effect monitoring, and switching to alternative drugs with less CPB interaction may be necessary in some cases. Notable changes in drug efficacy and behaviors during CPB are listed in Table 4.1.

1. Distribution: The increased blood volume from priming fluids and hemodilution during CPB can increase the distribution volumes for certain drugs, necessitating higher doses to attain the desired concentrations. So, it is a common practice to supplement muscle relaxation and midazolam at the initiation of CPB. Additionally, CPB can alter protein binding of certain drugs, which can affect their transportation. Reduced protein levels during CPB can change the amount of free drug available for action.
2. Metabolism: CPB can affect enzymes responsible for drug metabolism, especially hepatic enzymes during hypothermic perfusion. This alteration can impact drug clearance rates, potentially prolonging their action. Conversely, during the rewarming phase when hepatic enzymes become more active again, it is common practice to supplement with additional muscle relaxants and midazolam.
3. Elimination: Renal function may be temporarily impaired during CPB, affecting the elimination of drugs primarily excreted by the kidneys. Changes in blood flow and filtration rates in other organs, like the lungs, can also modify the elimination process for some drugs.
4. Pharmacodynamics: CPB can have both direct and indirect effects on drug activities. Directly, CPB can interact with certain drugs, altering their activity at the action site. For instance, hypothermia during CPB can reduce sensitivity to certain anesthetic agents or increase others, such as increasing volatile agent solubility and thus its tissue effect. Indirectly, the physiological changes induced by CPB, such as inflammation and hemodynamic alterations, can affect drug efficacy, necessitating adjustments in dosing or drug selection.

Choosing the Optimal Route for Drug Administration During CPB

Delivering medications effectively during CPB is crucial. While multiple routes exist, each with its own advantages and disadvantages, consideration is needed to select the most efficient and safe approach.

1. Arterial Outflow of the Oxygenator:

   This route offers the fastest and most complete delivery of drugs directly into the systemic circulation. However, concerns about inadvertent air bubbles or foreign body embolism made it the least favorable.
2. Central Venous Catheters:

   The convenience and familiarity of central venous catheters make them an appealing option for anesthesia providers. However, studies have demonstrated the potential for unpredictable drug delivery through this route. During CPB, drugs administered may get trapped in low-flow areas near the venous drainage cannulae. This can cause delayed drug entry into the systemic circulation and portions of the drug potentially sequestered in these low-flow areas. Furthermore, the timing of the drug's entry into the systemic circulation can become erratic and unpredictable, particularly influenced by the surgical manipulation of the heart.
3. The CPB Machine Sampling Manifold:

   To address the drawbacks associated with the two previous options, the manifold route is commonly employed (Fig. 4.1). This route utilizes a three-way stopcock manifold, serving as a port for both drawing blood samples and administering medications into the circulation. The arterial side of the manifold is connected to the arterial line of the CPB circuit via a one-way valve (Fig. 4.2), and the venous side of the manifold is directly connected to the venous line near the top of the hard-shell venous reservoir.

Calculating Drug Doses (Always Check Your Math Twice!)

To convert drug concentrations to milligrams (mg) or micrograms (μg) per milliliter (mL), please follow these steps:

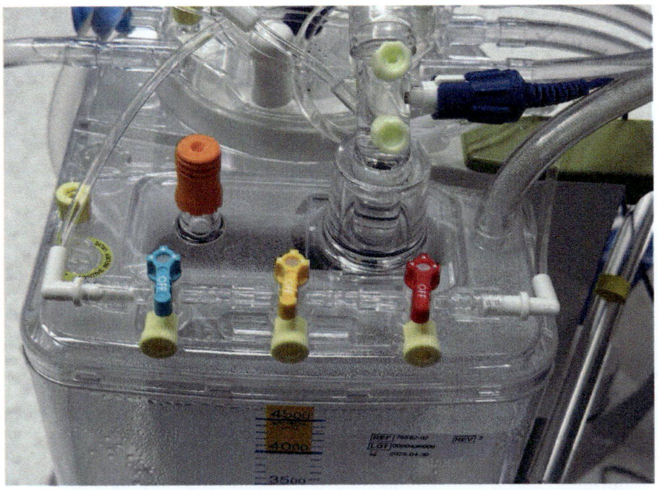

Fig. 4.1 Manifold with three ports for clinical use. This image showcases a manifold featuring three distinct ports—red, yellow, and blue—designed for efficient blood sampling and drug administration. The blue stopcock indicates the manifold's venous side, which is directly connected to the venous line near the top of the hard-shell venous reservoir. The red stopcock highlights the arterial side emerging from the oxygenator

1. *From grams per deciliter (g/dL)*:
   - A drug with "x"% concentration has x grams per deciliter (g/dL).
   - To convert to mg/mL, multiply "x" by 10 (since 1 g = 1000 mg and 1 deciliter = 100 mL).

2. *From ratio formats*:
   - For concentrations given as a ratio (e.g., 1:1000), convert to mg/mL by dividing 1000 mg by the ratio's denominator. For μg/mL, use 1,000,000 μg instead.

Examples:
- Lidocaine 2% means 2 g per deciliter (g/dL). To convert to mg/mL: 2 g by 10 = 20 mg/mL.
- Epinephrine 1:10,000. This ratio means 1 g of Epinephrine is dissolved in 10,000 mL of solution. To convert to mg/mL: divide 1000 mg/denominator or solution dissolved in, so 1000 mg/10,000 mL of solution = 0.1 mg/mL. To convert to μg/mL: multiple 1000/denominator so 1,000,000/10,000 = 100 μg/mL.

Calculating Infusion Rates (Did We Say, Always Check Your Math Twice?)

To convert calculate infusion rate, please follow these steps:

1. *Calculate Drug Concentration (μg/mL)*:
   - Multiply the amount of drug in the syringe or the infusion bag (in milligrams, mg) by 1000, then divide by the volume of the diluent (in milliliters, mL).
2. *Determine Desired Dose (μg/min)*:
   - Multiply the patient's weight in kilograms (kg) by the prescribed dose in micrograms per kilogram per minute (μg/kg/min).

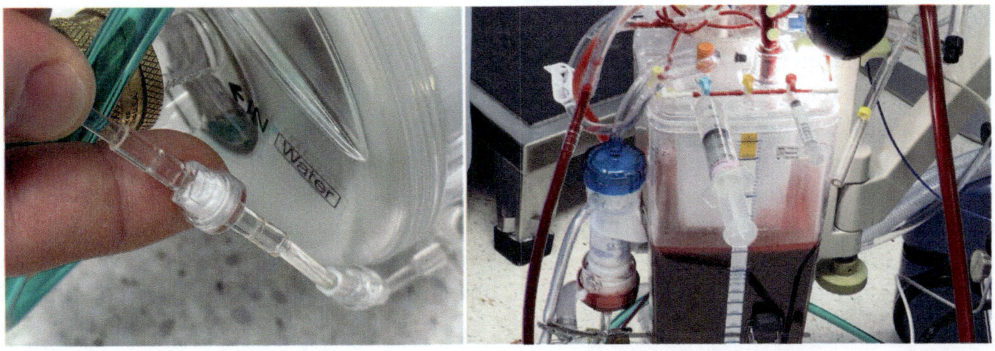

Fig. 4.2 Left Image: Arterial side of the manifold. This image displays the arterial side emerging from the oxygenator, featuring a one-way valve to prevent air bubbles from entering the oxygenator. Right Image: Manifold ports in use. In this image, the manifold's red port is connected to a syringe for blood sampling, the yellow port is designated for drug injections or drawing venous gas, and the blue port is attached to a vasopressor syringe for injections directed towards the venous line

3. *Find Infusion Rate (mL/min)*:
   - Divide the desired dose (in µg/min) by the drug concentration (in µg/mL).
4. *Convert Infusion Rate to mL/hour (mL/h)*:
   - Multiply the infusion rate (in mL/min) by 60.

Examples:

An 80 kg patient requires epinephrine infusion at 0.05 µg/kg/min. The infusion bag with a concentration of 4 mg in 250 mL 0.9% NS.

1. *Calculate Drug Concentration (µg/mL)*:
   - Concentration = (Drug in pump (mg) × 1000)/Diluent volume (mL).
   - For 4 mg in 250 mL: 4 mg × 1000/250 mL = 16 µg/mL

2. *Determine Desired Dose (µg/min)*:
   - Desired Dose = Patient weight (kg) × Dose (µg/kg/min).
   - For an 80 kg patient at 0.05 µg/kg/min: 80 kg × 0.05 µg/kg/min = 4 µg/min

3. *Find Infusion Rate (mL/min)*:
   - Infusion Rate = Desired dose (µg/min)/Concentration (µg/mL).
   - 4 µg/min/16 µg/mL = 0.25 mL/min

4. *Convert Infusion Rate to mL/hour (mL/h)*:
   - Infusion Rate (h) = Infusion rate (mL/min) × 60.
   - 0.25 mL/min × 60 = 15 mL/h

Vasopressors

Vasopressors are medications that constrict the patient's smooth muscle vasculature, thereby increasing SVR. The primary goal of this action is to increase the patient's mean arterial pressure. This is crucial to ensure adequate perfusion of the patient's vital organs. While on CPB, the perfusionist will administer vasopressors when necessary. Commonly used medications include phenylephrine, norepinephrine, and vasopressin with a goal of achieving a mean arterial pressure between 50 and 70 mmHg, as well as maintaining adequate flow rates related to body surface area once on CPB.

Phenylephrine HCl (Neosynephrine)

Phenylephrine is a pure alpha-1 adrenergic receptor agonist and non-catecholamine that primarily causes vasoconstriction. It increases both cerebral and coronary perfusion pressure and has a short duration of action (5–10 min). Since this medication increases blood pressure, it activates the carotid baroreflex, which then leads to reflex bradycardia. Furthermore, it can both increase or decrease cardiac output (CO) depending on specific clinical scenarios; increased afterload and reflex bradycardia can cause decreased cardiac output, whereas venoconstriction can increase preload and cardiac output. This vasoconstrictor is particularly useful in patients with coronary artery disease (CAD), aortic stenosis, and patients with hypertrophic obstructive cardiomyopathy.

Phenylephrine is used as both an intravenous (IV) infusion and bolus. The typical intravenous (IV) bolus dose is 50–200 mcg (1 µg/kg), and the typical infusion rate is 10–150 mcg/min and is titrated to effect. Different institutions may have premade syringes and infusions of phenylephrine. It is important to check the concentration before administering it to the patient as the concentrations may differ.

Mechanism of action:	A potent direct-acting agonist of alpha-1 adrenergic receptors, acting primarily as a vasoconstrictor without directly affecting cardiac function.
Dose:	Bolus: IV push 50–200 µg given every 1–2 min. Infusion dose: ranges from 10 to 150 µg/min.
Onset of action:	Effect achieved within seconds.
Dilution:	Mix 10 mg with 100 mL of NS or sterile water diluent to get a final concentration of 100 µg/mL for boluses or 16 or 50 mg in 250 mL NS to get a final concentration of 64 or 200 mcg/mL for continuous infusion.
Half-life:	Elimination 2–3 h through the liver and kidneys. However, the clinical impact of bolus administration is of short duration 5–10 min.
Hemodynamic effects:	Raises BP via elevating systemic vascular resistance but decreases HR and contractility.
Clinical usage:	Treatment of hypotension.

Ephedrine Sulfate

Ephedrine is a sympathomimetic medication that works both directly and indirectly. Ephedrine has a mild direct effect on activating alpha-1, beta-1, and beta-2 adrenergic receptors. It primarily works by indirectly inhibiting norepinephrine reuptake and displacing norepinephrine from storage vesicles. The norepinephrine that is released acts on postsynaptic alpha and beta receptors. Because norepinephrine binds both alpha and beta receptors, patients typically have an increase in both blood pressure and heart rate when ephedrine is administered without the reflex bradycardia seen with phenylephrine. Since ephedrine also activates beta-2 receptors causing smooth muscle vasodilation, the increase in blood pressure due to the activation of alpha-1 receptors is limited.

Although ephedrine's actions resemble epinephrine, ephedrine mainly works by indirect action and depends on the availability of norepinephrine in synaptic vesicles for full effect. With subsequent use of ephedrine, tachyphylaxis can occur due to the decrease in norepinephrine stores in the synaptic vesicles. This is not seen with epinephrine as this medication does not rely on catecholamine stores for effect. It is important to note that cocaine can inhibit the reuptake of norepinephrine and increase the cardiovascular effects of this medication; therefore, it should be avoided in patients who have recently used cocaine.

Ephedrine can increase heart rate, contractility, cardiac output, blood pressure, and SVR. Because ephedrine increases heart rate and afterload, it can lead to or exacerbate preexisting myocardial ischemia. Some of the other disadvantages of ephedrine include pulmonary vasoconstriction and possibly cardiac arrhythmias. Although this medication has some drawbacks, it is useful in patients with decreased SVR or low CO. It is typically given in 5–10 mg boluses through the patient's IV and lasts for 5–10 min. This medication can also be given intramuscularly (IM). If given IM, 25–50 mg is given, and it will last up to 1 h.

Mechanism of action:	Sympathomimetic with indirect dual alpha1 and beta1 agonist by releasing catecholamines.
Dose:	Bolus: IV push 5–10 mg given every 5–10 min.
Onset of action:	Effect was achieved within 30 s. Last 3–10 min.
Dilution:	Mix 50 mg in 1 mL with 9 mL of NS or sterile water diluent to get a final concentration of 5 mg/mL.
Half-life:	Elimination 3–6 h through the kidneys.
Hemodynamic effects:	Raises BP via elevating systemic vascular resistance, HR, and contractility.
Clinical usage:	Treatment of hypotension associated with bradycardia.

Norepinephrine (Levophed)

Norepinephrine is a potent vasopressor/inotrope that is commonly used during CPB, if hypotension is a problem. Norepinephrine is a direct alpha-1 and alpha-2 adrenergic receptor agonist with beta-1 adrenergic activity. It increases contractility, blood pressure, SVR, and pulmonary vascular resistance. Heart rate change can be variable. Given that CPB may cause vasoplegia and hypotension, norepinephrine can be given as boluses and/or as an infusion to increase the patient's SVR while on CPB or off CPB.

Bolus dose depends on the individual patient's response. Some patients are very sensitive to norepinephrine, so a small trial dose should be given to observe the effects on blood pressure and then titrated if needed. The typical bolus dose ranges from 4 to 32 mcg. For comparison's sake, roughly 8 mcg of norepinephrine is equivalent to 100 mcg of phenylephrine. The typical infusion dose ranges from 1 to 20 mcg/min. Norepinephrine can increase pulmonary vascular resistance (PVR), which can be detrimental in patients with pulmonary hypertension and/or decreased right ventricular (RV) function. A norepinephrine infusion should be connected to a central line as it can cause skin necrosis if it infiltrates into the subcutaneous tissue.

Mechanism of action:	Sympathomimetic with direct alpha1 and beta1 agonist.
Dose:	Bolus: IV push 4–32 μg. Infusion dose: ranges from 1 to 20 μg/min.
Onset of action:	Effect was achieved within 30 s. Last 1–2 min.
Dilution:	Mix 4, 8, or 16 mg with 250 mL of 5% dextrose to get a final concentration of 16, 32, or 64 μg/mL.
Half-life:	Elimination 2 min due to rapid metabolism by MAO and COMT in the synaptic cleft.
Hemodynamic effects:	Raises BP via elevating SVR, HR, and contractility. Causes vasoconstriction of the pulmonary arteries.
Clinical usage:	Low SVR-induced hypotension, as in septic shock.

Vasopressin (Pitressin)

Vasopressin is an anti-diuretic hormone that causes vasoconstriction primarily via V1a receptors. Peripheral V1a receptors that increase blood pressure are primarily located in the vascular smooth muscle. There are also V1a receptors in the skin, skeletal muscle, intestines, and adipose tissues Additionally, V1b receptors are found in the anterior pituitary and brain, mediating ACTH release, while V2 receptors in the kidneys are responsible for the antidiuretic effects. Vasopressin is effective in patients with severe acidosis, while other vasopressors are less effective because acidosis reduces calcium influx into the cells and decreases norepinephrine and epinephrine's affinity to bind with receptors. Of note, there are minimal or no functionally significant V1a receptors in the pulmonary vascular system so that PVR will not increase, and right heart function will not be affected. This medication is particularly useful in patients that are unresponsive to catecholamine vasoactive drugs. When vasopressin is combined with other vasoactive medications, it reduces the dose necessary to achieve adequate mean arterial pressure and can improve organ perfusion. High doses of vasopressin can lead to mesenteric ischemia and peripheral vascular insufficiency due to the constriction of blood vessels.

Vasopressin is administered as an infusion or as a bolus. The infusion dose typically ranges from 0.01 to 0.04 units/min, and the bolus dose ranges from 0.5 to 2 units (often used as a loading dose in refractory shock). Some patients can be very sensitive to vasopressin; it is imperative to give a smaller dose when first administering to prevent extreme hypertension. Additionally, this medication has a relatively longer half-life (10–20 minutes), which makes it more difficult to titrate compared to other cardiovascular medications with shorter half-lives (e.g., norepinephrine's 2–3 minutes). Furthermore, it should be known that vasopressin does not increase heart rate, which makes it an ideal choice in patients with ischemic cardiac disease.

Mechanism of action:	A hypothalamic hormone released from the pituitary into the bloodstream. Antidiuretic by activating V-2 receptors and vasoconstrictor through V-1 receptors in smooth muscle. Pulmonary, coronary, and cerebral circulations are largely spared.
Dose:	Bolus: 0.5–2 units. Infusion dose: 0.01–0.04 units/min (vasodilatory shock).
Onset of action:	Maximum effect achieved within 15 min.
Dilution:	Dilute 50 units in 250 mL of 0.9% normal saline for a 0.2 units/mL concentration or mix 100 units with 100 mL of 0.9% normal saline for a 1 unit/mL concentration.
Half-life:	Elimination through the liver and kidneys within 10–20 min.
Hemodynamic effects:	Elevates SVR.
Clinical usage:	Treats vasodilatory shock not responding to other drugs, vasoplegia syndrome post-CPB, diabetes insipidus, and upper gastrointestinal bleeding.

Methylene Blue (Methylthionine Chloride, Urolene Blue)

Methylene blue competes with guanylyl cyclase to decrease the amount of cGMP that is formed. Also, it inhibits nitric oxide synthase and reduces the production of NO, which causes vasodilation. A 2 mg/kg IV infusion over 20 min may be started, and it should not be given to patients with G6PD deficiency as hemolytic anemia can occur. Notably, methylene blue will interfere with the pulse oximetry and cause a falsely low SpO2 readings.

It should be noted that methylene blue should not be administered to patients taking serotonergic psychiatric medications as high levels of serotonin can build up in the brain and cause serotonin syndrome.

Mechanism of action:	It blocks nitric oxide synthase and guanylate cyclase, thereby reducing the relaxation of vascular smooth muscle.
Dose:	Infusion dose: IV 1–2 mg/kg over 5–20 min (Vasoplegic syndrome).
Onset of action:	Effect was achieved immediately.
Dilution:	10 mg/mL in 10 mL.
Half-life:	Elimination 5–6 h.
Hemodynamic effects:	Raises BP via elevation of SVR.
Clinical usage:	Treats vasodilatory shock not responding to other drugs, vasoplegic syndrome post-CPB.

Hydroxocobalamin (vitamin B12) Cyanokit)

Hydroxocobalamin is a newer treatment option for vasoplegia post-CPB or other vasoplegic states. Hydroxocobalamin inhibits guanylate cyclase, is a scavenger for nitric oxide, and inhibits NO synthase. Subsequently, it leads to less vasodilation. Cyanokit, which is used to treat cyanide poisoning, can be administered as a 5 g bolus over 15 min for 1–2 doses. The second dose can be given after 30 min if there is no response to the first dose. It is important to note that cyanokit can cause chromaturia that may last several weeks. If the patient is on hemodialysis, hydroxocobalamin can interfere with the hemodialysis machine and cause a false blood leak alarm, in addition, the plasma will turn red/red wine color, urine red, and the skin as well. This effect can last a couple of weeks.

Although there is no definitive treatment of vasoplegic syndrome, a balanced approach is to reduce the negative effects of each drug administered. After the catecholamine vasopressors have been started, and MAP goal is not reached, then the non-catecholamine agents such as vasopressin and methylene blue can be started. If that proves insufficient, then hydroxocobalamin may be considered.

Mechanism of action:	It inhibits guanylate cyclase, is a scavenger for nitric oxide, and inhibits NO synthase.
Dose:	5 g bolus over 15 min for 1–2 doses (Vasoplegic syndrome).
Onset of action:	Effect was achieved immediately.
Dilution:	5 g in 200 cc normal saline.
Half-life:	Elimination 26–31 h.
Hemodynamic effects:	Raises BP via elevation of SVR.
Clinical usage:	Treats vasodilatory shock not responding to other drugs, vasoplegic syndrome post-CPB.

Vasoplegic Syndrome

Vasoplegic syndrome, occurring post CPB, consists of low mean arterial pressure (MAP < 65 mmHg), normal to elevated cardiac index (CI > 2.2 L/min/m^2), normal right-sided pressures, and low SVR that is refractory to vasopressor support. Risk factors include preoperative ACE-inhibitors and beta-blockers, low preoperative ejection fraction, the need for vasopressors during CPB, and long duration of aortic cross-clamping. Some patients develop catecholamine-resistant vasoplegia—characterized by low SVR, normal or high cardiac output, and inability to maintain MAP >60 mmHg on high-dose vasopressors, such as norepinephrine.

The mechanism behind vasoplegic syndrome is thought to occur secondary to inflammatory cytokines, triggered by CPB. This activation can lead to increased inducible nitric oxide synthase activity, resulting in excessive vasodilation. The longer the patient is on CPB, the higher the concentration of nitric oxide synthase and the higher the level of nitric oxide. Nitric oxide can also inhibit ATP-sensitive potassium channels that inhibit calcium entry and vasoconstriction and contribute to low blood pressure.

Vasoplegia should first be treated with vasopressors such as phenylephrine, epinephrine, norepinephrine, and/or vasopressin. If these treatments are unsuccessful, then the administration of methylene blue or hydroxocobalamin may be considered.

Inotropic Drugs

Inotropic medications enable the patient's heart to contract more forcefully and efficiently. By increasing the amount of force that the heart can contract with, it enables the heart to increase its stroke volume and decrease its left ventricular end-diastolic pressure. Positive inotropic medications increase a patient's ejection fraction. Ejection fraction is calculated by taking the patient's stroke volume and dividing it by the end-diastolic volume.

Epinephrine HCl (Adrenaline)

Epinephrine, a powerful direct-acting inotropic medication, and a sympathomimetic catecholamine, mimics endogenous epinephrine and works on the same receptors. It is a direct-acting agonist at alpha-1 and 2, and beta-1 and 2 receptors. Epinephrine has different effects at varying doses. At low doses, epinephrine has a greater affinity for beta receptors, whereas at high doses it has more effect on alpha receptors than beta receptors. Due to its beta-agonist activity, heart rate and contractility will increase. The combination of these effects leads to an increase in CO. In addition, epinephrine's binding to alpha receptors causes vasoconstriction.

Although epinephrine has many positive effects, there are negative side effects, as well. At high doses, epinephrine can cause tachycardia, tachyarrhythmias, and skin necrosis if it extravasates into the extravascular tissue. Therefore, it is important to infuse it through a central line. Additionally, it increases plasma glucose by not only inhibiting insulin secretion from the pancreas but also stimulating glycogenolysis in the liver and muscles. Some epinephrine infusions are prepared in a solution of 5% dextrose and could further increase serum glucose levels. It is imperative to closely monitor patient's blood glucose levels while administering epinephrine, as hyperglycemia can cause impaired wound healing, infection, and osmotic diuresis.

During CPB, after the cross-clamp is removed, epinephrine and/or norepinephrine can be started in preparation to separate from bypass. If poor contractions of the right and/or left ventricles are seen on transesophageal echocardiography, or over the surgical drapes for the right ventricle, epinephrine should be preferably chosen. As the perfusionist fills the heart, the anesthesiologist can titrate these medications to a MAP depending on the heart's function prior to separating from bypass.

Epinephrine can be administered as an infusion or a bolus dose. Low-dose epinephrine (<3 mcg/min) can be started initially to stimulate cardiac function then titrated up or down depending on the effect it has on the patient's hemodynamics. While this medication is infusing, one should carefully monitor the patient's SVR, as it can impair cardiac function if SVR becomes too high.

Mechanism of action:	Sympathomimetic with direct dual alpha1&2 and nonselective beta agonist. Lower doses enhance heart rate (beta effects); higher doses cause vasoconstriction (alpha effects).
Dose:	Bolus: IV push 4–10 μg. Infusion dose: ranges from 3 to 20 μg/min.
Onset of action:	Effect achieved within seconds. Last 2–5 min.
Dilution:	Mix 4 mg with 250 mL of 5% dextrose to get a final concentration of 16 μg/mL.
Half-life:	Elimination 2 min due to rapid metabolism by MAO and COMT.
Hemodynamic effects:	Raises HR, and contractility in low dose. Raises SVR in high dose.
Clinical usage:	Bradyarrhythmia, heart transplant patients, low cardiac output, hypotension, bronchospasm, anaphylaxis.

Dobutamine (Dobutrex)

Dobutamine is a synthetic catecholamine that directly activates beta-1, beta-2, and alpha-1 receptors. Dobutamine is an inotrope and vasodilator (Inodilator). It increases cardiac contractility via its action on beta-1 receptors and decreases SVR via beta-2 agonism. Dobutamine is a useful inotropic drug because it increases stroke volume, cardiac output, contractility, heart rate, and blood pressure while reducing afterload by decreasing systemic and pulmonary vascular resistance, as well as left ventricular end-diastolic pressure. It is important to note that dobutamine can cause more tachycardia than epinephrine at equivalent doses.

Furthermore, dobutamine can cause hypotension if the decrease in SVR is not counteracted by an increase in cardiac output. Dobutamine is typically given as an infusion at doses of 2–20 mcg/kg/min.

Mechanism of action:	Sympathomimetic with direct beta1, beta2 and alpha1 agonist activities. However, it is predominantly a beta1 agonist.
Dose:	Bolus: IV push 4–32 μg. Infusion dose: ranges from 1 to 20 μg/kg/min.
Onset of action:	Effect achieved within 5–12 min. Last 10 min.
Dilution:	Mix 500 mg with 250 mL of 5% dextrose to get a final concentration of 2 mg/mL.
Half-life:	Elimination in 2 min through the liver by COMT.
Hemodynamic effects:	Raises CO via elevating HR, and contractility. Causes vasodilation of the pulmonary arteries.
Clinical usage:	Low cardiac output.

Milrinone (Primacor)

Milrinone is a phosphodiesterase 3 inhibitor (PDE-3) that increases cardiac inotropy, lusitropy (rate of myocardial relaxation), and peripheral vasodilation. It is considered an inodilator because it increases inotropy and causes vasodilation. PDE-3 inhibitors increase the amount of cyclic adenosine monophosphate in the myocardium, which then increases the amount of ionized calcium from the sarcoplasmic reticulum in the myocardium. This increase in calcium increases the heart's contractility and causes vasodilation.

Milrinone increases cardiac output and decreases SVR, PVR, preload, and afterload. It has very little effect on the heart rate. In comparison to dobutamine, milrinone is associated with less tachycardia, has a greater decrease in PVR which in turn increases RV ejection fraction, causes fewer arrhythmias, and results in less myocardial oxygen consumption. There is no tachyphylaxis associated with milrinone, and it can be used synergistically with beta-adrenergic receptor agonists. Given that milrinone lowers PVR and increases inotropy, it is a good choice for patients with right heart failure. However, milrinone should be used with caution in patients who are already hypotensive because it causes vasodilation and can further worsen the patient's blood pressures. Recent studies predominantly indicate that milrinone functions primarily as a modest inotrope. Its beneficial effects on stroke volume, which in turn enhances cardiac output, are largely attributed to vasodilation-induced reductions in arterial elastance (Ea), the "stiffness" of blood vessels. This occurs with minimal alteration in end-systolic elastance (Ees), a measure of the heart's intrinsic ventricular muscle stiffness at the end of systole, reflecting its contractile state independent of loading conditions. Therefore, the effectiveness of milrinone in augmenting stroke volume is greater when Ees is lower. This underscores the notion that stroke volume and cardiac output improvements are not directly synonymous with increased contractility.

A typical bolus dose of milrinone is 25–50 mcg/kg, given over 10 min once the cross-clamp is removed before separating from CPB. A maintenance infusion is then started at 0.25–0.75 mcg/kg/min depending on the patient's hemodynamics. Lower doses of the infusion should be started in patients with renal failure because milrinone is primarily excreted in the urine. If the creatinine clearance (CrCl) is <10 cc/min then the rate should be 0.2–0.23 mcg/kg/min. If the CrCl is between 10 and 30 cc/min, then the infusion should be set to 0.2–0.33 mcg/kg/min. The onset of action is usually within 5–15 min, and the half-life is about 2.3 h in patients with heart failure.

Mechanism of action:	Inodilator that blocks PDE III activity and prevents cAMP degradation.
Dose:	Bolus: IV push: 25–75 μg/kg. Infusion dose: ranges from 0.25 to 0.75 μg/kg/min.
Onset of action:	Effect achieved within 5–15 min. Last 2–5 h.
Dilution:	Prepared with 20 mg in 100 mL to get a final concentration of 200 μg/mL.
Half-life:	Elimination mainly through the kidney.
Hemodynamic effects:	Raises CO via increasing contractility. Causes vasodilation and lower systemic and pulmonary vascular resistance.
Clinical usage:	Low cardiac output heart failure. Right ventricular failure with pulmonary hypertension.

Vasodilator Drugs

Sometimes while on CPB, medications are necessary to lower a given patient's blood pressure, i.e., vasodilators.

Hydralazine (Apresoline)

Hydralazine is a direct vasodilator that mainly produces arterial vasodilation rather than venous dilation by reducing intracellular calcium in vascular smooth muscle in the coronary, cerebral, renal, and splanchnic vascular beds. Consequently, this vasodilation decreases blood pressure, SVR, and PVR. It also causes reflex tachycardia, increased CO due to decreases in afterload, and increased HR.

Hydralazine has a slow and variable onset of action. When given intravascularly, it can take 5–15 min to take effect, with peak effect at 20 min. Therefore, one should be patient when administering this medication. The IV dose of hydralazine is 2.5–5 mg every 15 min with a maximum dose of

20–40 mg. Hydralazine can be used for hypertension in patients without CAD and tachycardia.

Mechanism of action:	Promotes arterial vasodilation via smooth muscle relaxation.
Dose:	Bolus: IV push 5–20 mg.
Onset of action:	Effect achieved within 10–20 min. Last up to 10 h.
Half-life:	Elimination in 2–6 h from metabolism by liver and renal excretion.
Hemodynamic effects:	Lowers BP from afterload reduction.
Clinical usage:	Hypertension.

Nicardipine (Cardene)

Nicardipine, a dihydropyridine calcium channel blocker, acts primarily on the peripheral vasculature without causing myocardial depression. Nicardipine selectively inhibits L-type calcium channels in vascular smooth muscle cells, preventing calcium influx and contraction, ultimately resulting in vasodilation and reduced blood pressure. Nicardipine preserves cardiac output and stroke volume but can cause increases in heart rate due to reflex tachycardia. During CABG, nicardipine can be useful to dilate arterial conduits, reducing the incidence of vasospasm. It can also be useful in any open-heart surgery in patients with sustained hypertension.

Nicardipine is usually administered as an infusion. The typical starting dose is 2.5 mg/h and can be increased by 2.5 mg/h every 5 min with a maximum dose of 15 mg/h. It can also be administered as a bolus dose, 0.25–1.0 mg, as needed to acutely decrease blood pressure, as with most vasoactive medications, when administering a bolus always, start with a low dose to evaluate patient responsiveness. If nicardipine is administered through a peripheral IV, the site of infusion should be changed every 12 h to prevent phlebitis.

Mechanism of action:	It is a dihydropyridine calcium channel blocker.
Dose:	Bolus: IV push 0.25–1.0 mg. Infusion dose: ranges from 2.5 to 15 mg/h.
Onset of action:	Effect achieved within 1–3 min. Last 10–30 min after a bolus but 8 h after infusion discontinuation.
Dilution:	Preprepared bag with 40 mg in 200 mL NS with a final concentration of 0.2 mg/mL.
Half-life:	Elimination in 1–3 min from metabolism by liver and renal excretion.
Hemodynamic effects:	Lowers BP without notably diminishing myocardial contractility and has minimal impact on sinoatrial or atrioventricular nodal conduction.
Clinical usage:	Hypertension.

Clevidipine (Cleviprex)

Clevidipine, a short-acting dihydropyridine calcium channel blocker, works primarily on arterioles to rapidly decrease SVR, MAP, and increase stroke volume. Since the onset of action is rapid, it can be used to lower blood pressure prior to placing the aortic cannula or before its removal. The half-life of clevidipine is 1–3 min as it is metabolized by esterases in the blood. Its elimination is not influenced by renal or hepatic dysfunction. It is important to note that clevidipine is a milky white solution, so it should not be confused with propofol.

A cleviprex infusion should be started at 1–2 mg/h and is then titrated every 90 s. As the patient's mean arterial pressure reaches the set goal, the dose should be increased by less than half, and the time between each dose should lengthen to 5–10 min. Most patients are at a therapeutic dose at 4–6 mg/h. Since the half-life is approximately 1 min, the patient's BP should recover in 5–15 min if hypotension ensues.

Mechanism of action:	It is a dihydropyridine calcium channel blocker.
Dose:	Infusion dose: start at 1–2 mg/h and double every 1.5–5 min until target BP reached for maximum 32 mg/h.
Onset of action:	Effect achieved within 1–2 min. Last 10–15 min.
Dilution:	Preprepared bottle with 25 mg in 50 mL lipid emulsion to get a final concentration of 0.5 mg/mL.
Half-life:	Elimination in 2 min from rapid metabolism by ester hydrolysis in blood.
Hemodynamic effects:	Rapid drop of BP via decreasing systemic vascular resistance.
Clinical usage:	Hypertension.

Nitroglycerin (Tridil)

Nitroglycerin is a direct vasodilator of both arteries and veins but primarily causes venodilation. It produces nitric oxide, which in turn, activates guanylate cyclase to increase the amount of cyclic GMP. The increased cyclic GMP is responsible for vasodilation. When nitroglycerin is administered, the patient's heart rate and contractility may increase. Cardiac output, blood pressure, preload, SVR, and PVR all decrease. SVR and blood pressure decrease at high dosages. This drug can vasodilate both normal and post-stenotic coronary arteries, enhancing perfusion to the heart.

Nitroglycerin is a great option for patients with heart failure from myocardial ischemia—it decreases myocardial oxygen demand, left ventricular end-diastolic pressure, wall stress, preload, and may reduce PVR. At higher doses (>10 mcg/kg/min), it causes arterial vasodilation and can lead to decreased coronary artery perfusion and methemoglobinemia. Additionally, nitroglycerin can negatively inhibit hypoxic pulmonary vasoconstriction and increase intracranial pressure.

Nitroglycerin can be administered as an infusion or as a bolus. An infusion is usually started at 0.1 mcg/kg/min and titrated up to 7 mcg/kg/min. However, continuous infusions can lead to tachyphylaxis and reduce the effectiveness of the drug. For immediate and short-term blood pressure reduction in cases of hypertension, a bolus of 50–100 mcg can be given. During CPB, nitroglycerin infusion can induce venodilation, which reduces the blood volume available for the pump's reservoir.

Mechanism of action:	Vasodilator and venodilator via smooth muscle relaxation through conversion to nitric oxide and cGMP activation. Primarily venodilator.
Dose:	Bolus: IV push 50–100 μg. Infusion dose: ranges from 0.1 mcg/kg/min up to 7 mcg/kg/min.
Onset of action:	Effect achieved within 1 min. Last 1–10 min.
Dilution:	Preprepared bottle 50 mg with 250 mL of 5% dextrose to get a final concentration of 200 μg/mL.
Half-life:	Elimination 1–3 min from metabolism by liver and renal excretion.
Hemodynamic effects:	Coronary vasodilator, decrease BP via decreasing systemic vascular resistance, reflex increase in HR. Causes vasodilation of the pulmonary arteries.
Clinical usage:	Myocardial ischemia, hypertension.

Nitroprusside (Nipride, Nitropress)

Sodium nitroprusside is an ultra-short acting potent vasodilator of both the arterial and venous smooth muscle vasculature. It decreases SVR and preload and subsequently blood pressure. Clinical use of nitroprusside is limited by its toxic metabolite—cyanide. Typical infusion rates are from 0.5 mcg/kg/min with a maximum infusion rate of 10 mcg/kg/min. The maximum infusion rate should not last for more than 10 min, as this can lead to high levels of cyanide. It is important to note that hemolysis during CPB may cause overproduction of cyanide secondary to free hemoglobin release. If cyanide toxicity is suspected, it should be treated with hydroxocobalamin or sodium thiosulfate. It is a very potent dilator, and profound hypotension can ensue if not used carefully.

Mechanism of action:	Vasodilator and venodilator via smooth muscle relaxation through conversion to nitric oxide and cGMP activation.
Dose:	Bolus: IV push 4–32 μg. Infusion dose: ranges from 0.5 to 10 μg/kg/min.
Onset of action:	Effect achieved within 1 min. Last 1–10 min.
Dilution:	Preprepared with 50 mg in 250 mL 5% dextrose to get a final concentration of 200 μg/mL.
Half-life:	3–6 min.
Hemodynamic effects:	Decrease in BP via decreasing systemic vascular resistance, reflex increase in HR. Causes vasodilation of the pulmonary arteries.
Clinical usage:	Hypertension.

Nitric Oxide, inhaled (NO, iNO, INOmax)

Inhaled nitric oxide is an agent that selectively causes pulmonary vasodilation. After NO is inhaled, it diffuses across the alveolar-capillary membrane to activate guanylate cyclase. Then, guanylate cyclase converts GTP to cGMP, which causes vasodilation. Additionally, it can positively affect ventilation and perfusion matching as it vasodilates the well-ventilated regions of the lung.

Inhaled NO mixed with oxygen starts to cause pulmonary vasodilation in as little as 1–2 min. Therapeutic concentrations range from 0.05 to 80 parts per million, but the lowest effective concentration should be used. It can be started before separating from CPB in patients with pulmonary hypertension and is particularly useful in patients receiving a heart transplant. Pulmonary hypertension in heart transplant patients is a major cause of right heart failure, as the newly transplanted right ventricle is not accustomed to working against high pulmonary pressure. By starting NO during CPB, pulmonary vascular resistance will decrease, and right heart cardiac output will improve. In addition, inhaled NO can be used in newborns with diagnosed pulmonary hypertension.

Although inhaled NO has many positive effects, there are some potential side effects when using this medication. Inhaled NO can cause methemoglobinemia, the formation of nitrogen dioxide, rebound pulmonary hypertension, and inhibition of platelet aggregation. Methemoglobinemia is formed when inhaled NO combines with hemoglobin to form nitrosyl hemoglobin. This is then metabolized to methemoglobin. Studies have shown that at <80 PPM, this is a rare occurrence. However, methemoglobinemia is more apparent in neonates on inhaled NO than in adults because neonates have lower levels of the enzyme methemoglobin reductase. Nitrogen dioxide forms during spontaneous oxidation in the lungs. NO2 can then react with water in the lungs to form nitric acid. Similar to methemoglobinemia, NO_2 is insignificant if the inhaled NO is less than 80 ppm. Withdrawing inhaled NO abruptly can lead to rebound pulmonary hypertension. The inhaled NO suppresses endogenous endothelial NO synthetase formation. Therefore, inhaled NO should be weaned off slowly. Furthermore, inhaled NO can lead to decreased platelet aggregation by changes in intraplatelet cGMP levels.

Anesthetic Drugs

Anesthesia and Ventilation Shift to Perfusionists During CPB

When the cardiothoracic surgeon is ready to place the patient on CPB, the anesthesia team will turn off both the ventilator and the inhaled anesthetic, thus enabling the perfusionists to have full control over ventilation, perfusion, and anesthesia (with supervision). Oxygen, or oxygen–air mixture, and an inhaled anesthetic gas, usually sevoflurane or isoflurane, are delivered to the patient via the gas inflow of the membrane oxygenator; This acts as an artificial lung allowing the diffusion of oxygen or oxygen/air mixture and anesthetic vapor into the blood, while also taking the carbon dioxide from the blood into the gas exiting the membrane oxygenator. Usually, the anesthetic gases are inhaled by the patient; however, while on CPB, the volatile agent is taken up by the blood that passes through the membrane oxygenator instead of the lungs. The blood will then travel to the patient's brain to keep the patient anesthetized. To reduce occupational exposure, a scavenging unit is attached to the oxygenator gas exhaust port. It is important to note that nitrous oxide is not used during CPB to prevent an increase in the size of possible air emboli in the circuit. Volatile anesthetics have been shown to have cardioprotective effects when used before and during CPB by minimizing ischemia–reperfusion injury.

Total Intravenous Anesthesia

If the patient cannot have an inhaled anesthetic gas, due to a CPB circuit that has no vaporizer mounted on it, or due to a history of or risk factors for malignant hyperthermia, then a total intravenous anesthetic, usually with a propofol infusion, must be implemented. It should be noted that the free fraction of propofol in the plasma is influenced by hemodilution from the bypass circuit, the degree of absorption from the bypass circuit, the effect of hypothermia on the hepatic clearance of propofol, and plasma protein binding capacity. Propofol can be administered directly into the CPB circuit through the line connected to the venous reservoir or given through a central line or less ideally via a peripheral IV.

Maintenance of Anesthesia During CPB

Maintaining amnesia during CPB is of utmost importance, as cardiac surgery has a higher incidence of intraoperative awareness compared to other procedures. Subsequently, a bispectral index monitoring system (BIS monitor) is a useful tool available that can be used to assess the patient's depth of anesthesia. The BIS monitor collects electroencephalographic (EEG) data from the patient while asleep. An algorithm then interprets the data and displays a number on the monitor. The numbers range from 0 to 100, where 0 is flat EEG and 100 is awake. To prevent awareness under anesthesia, a goal BIS would be between 40 and 60. Anesthesia providers use the given information from the BIS to guide anesthetic dosages. Additionally, midazolam and dexmedetomidine are medications that can be used during CPB to decrease a given patient's chance of awareness.

It is important to note that during CPB, neuromuscular paralysis should be continuously monitored with a peripheral nerve stimulator to avoid the risk of a patient moving while on CPB. In addition, as CPB is initiated, the volume of distribution of the neuromuscular blocking agents increases as described earlier.

In summary, perfusionists and anesthesiologists should fully understand the impact of CPB on medication pharmacodynamics and pharmacokinetics to take care of these patients safely while on CPB.

Further Reading

Barash PG, Cullen BF, Stoelting RK, Cahalan MK, Stock MC. Clinical anesthesia. 7th ed. Philadelphia: Lippincott Williams & Wilkins; 2013.

Barry AE, Chaney MA, London MJ. Anesthetic management during cardiopulmonary bypass: a systematic review. Anesth Analg. 2015;120(4):749–69. https://doi.org/10.1213/ANE.0000000000000612. PMID: 25790208.

Hensley FA, Martin DE. Hensley's practical approach to cardiothoracic anesthesia. 6th ed. Philadelphia: Wolters Kluwer; 2019.

Kaplan JA. Essentials of cardiac anesthesia. 2nd ed. Philadelphia: Elsevier; 2018.

Part II

Cardiopulmonary Bypass Evolution and History

An Overview of Cardiopulmonary Bypass's Historic Development

5

Aric Johnson and Eugene A. Hessel II

Introduction

> If I have seen further, it is by standing on the shoulders of giants.
> —Isaac Newton

The development of cardiopulmonary bypass (CPB) is among one of the most important clinical advances in modern medicine. Less than a century ago operating on the heart routinely was thought impossible, and both congenital and acquired cardiac diseases were considered untreatable. This changed throughout the second half of the twentieth century with the development of CPB.

The birth of CPB is attributed to its first successful clinical use by John H. Gibbon Jr. in 1953. However, CPB as it exists today owes its development and success to the collective efforts of many brilliant minds. Similar to Newton's famous quote, many of these individuals built upon the knowledge and innovations of those who came before them. Throughout this chapter, we will discuss the early attempts and successes of CPB, as well as historical developments that have helped make CPB the remarkably safe and effective procedure that it has become today.

Early Attempts and Final Success (See also Table 5.1)

The thought that extra-corporeal circulation could support organ function was first suggested by a French physician, Julien Jean Le Gallois, whose work was centered on identifying parts of the body essential for life. In an 1812 publication, Le Gallois noted "But if the place of the heart could be supplied by injection—and if, for the regular continuance of this injection, there could be furnished a quantity of arterial blood, whether natural, or artificially formed, supposing such a formation possible—then life might be indefinitely maintained."

A major advancement in achieving what Le Gallois had conceptualized was accomplished by the German physiologists, Max von Frey and Max Gruber at the Leipzig Physiological Institute, when they constructed the first closed artificial circulation system. Prior to their invention, the perfusion circuit had to be interrupted in order to oxygenate the blood. Their machine demonstrated the possibility of removing venous blood, oxygenating it, and pumping it back into arterial circulation in one continuous circuit and was a precursor to the CPB machine later developed by Dr. John Gibbon.

Table 5.1 Steps in the early development of cardiopulmonary bypass

1812	Concept of extra-corporeal organ support introduced (Le Gallois)
1885	First conceptual drawing of heart-lung machine published (Frey and Gruber)
1900–1915	Discovery of blood types, anticoagulation, storage of blood, and blood transfusion (Landsteiner followed by many others)
1916	Discovery of heparin (McClean and Howell)
1934	Roller pump first used clinically (DeBakey)
1935	Successful use of heart-lung machine in cats; able to support for up to 117 min (Gibbon)
1937	Able to produce heparin (Best)
1937–1939	Protamine demonstrated to neutralize heparin (Chargraff and Olson)
1939	Long-term survival of cats using heart-lung machine during pulmonary artery occlusion (Gibbon)
1940	First clinical use of heparin (Murray)
1946	Benefits of hypothermia for cardiac surgery suggested (Bigelow)
1950	Silicone antifoam used to facilitate use of bubble oxygenator (Clark)
1951	IBM partners with Gibbon to develop the Gibbon Model II heart-lung machine
1953	First successful open-heart surgery using total cardiopulmonary bypass (Gibbon)
1955	First successful series of patients undergo open-heart surgery with total CPB (Kirklin et al. at Mayo Clinic and Lillehei et al. at University of Minnesota)

A. Johnson · E. A. Hessel II (✉)
Department of Anesthesiology & Perioperative Medicine, University of Kentucky, Lexington, KY, USA
e-mail: aric.johnson@uky.edu; ehessel@uky.edu

A. S. Awad, J. DiNardo (eds.), *Clinical Perfusion for Cardiac Surgery*, https://doi.org/10.1007/978-3-031-91163-7_5

John Gibbon Jr. was born in Philadelphia, Pennsylvania and earned his medical degree at Thomas Jefferson Medical College in 1927. In 1930, he undertook a 1-year surgical research fellowship at the Massachusetts General Hospital under the Chief of Surgery, Dr. Edward D. Churchill. During that year, Dr. Gibbon was assigned the task of monitoring a patient who had suffered a massive pulmonary embolism postoperatively. While observing her, he hypothesized that if only he could remove her venous blood, bypass her heart and lungs, oxygenate the blood, and then return it to her arterial system, she might be saved. Unfortunately, such technology did not exist, and the patient did not survive. However, this experience had a profound and lasting impact on Gibbon and forged an academic passion that he would pursue for the rest of his life.

In 1934–1935, he obtained a second fellowship under Churchill, and along with his wife Mary, set out to develop a viable heart-lung machine. He returned to Philadelphia in 1935 and continued working with his wife and Dr. John Y. Templeton. By 1939, they had successfully placed feline subjects on CPB; however, his research was interrupted by 4 years of military service during World War II. He returned to Philadelphia afterwards but struggled to develop a machine capable of pumping and oxygenating the larger volume of blood required to support a human. A fortuitous connection would help Gibbon solve this problem. A medical student working under him, E.J. Clark, had a family connection to the Chairman and CEO of International Business Machines (IBM), Thomas Watson. A meeting between Gibbon and Watson was arranged, and Watson was immediately intrigued by the idea. He assigned his chief engineer Gustav Malmros on the project, who helped incorporate Gibbon's designs into a larger machine. The initial apparatus was completed in 1949, weighed over 2000 pounds, and was too large to fit in the elevator at Jefferson Medical College. Cranes were ultimately used to hoist the machine to the appropriate floor.

Several years and prototypes later, the partnership between Gibbon and IBM resulted in a machine capable of supporting a human, employing a multiple vertical screen filming oxygenator, and after demonstrating a 90% survival in canines, Gibbon first attempted to use his CPB clinically on a 15-month-old child in February 1952. Unfortunately, the child had a patent ductus arteriosus instead of the anticipated atrial septal defect and died during surgery. However, his next patient, an 18-year-old had her atrial septal defect successfully repaired on May 6, 1953 after 26 min of full bypass. Thus, after 23 years, Dr. Gibbon had finally achieved the goal that he had first conceived as a resident physician.

Between 1952 and 1954, there was only one other successful open-heart surgery with the use of a heart-lung machine out of 16 attempts. This led to a feeling of hopelessness, and some hypothesized that humans were too sick to tolerate CPB. Gibbon himself offered to lead a movement to ban other attempts at open-heart surgery in the United States.

Fortunately, not everyone shared this pessimism. In 1954, Dr. C. Walton Lillehei and his team at the University of Minnesota began a remarkable series of cardiac surgeries with total CPB using another adult as the heart-lung machine. This was referred to as controlled cross-circulation, in which the adult's femoral artery and vein were connected to the child's arterial and venous systems, respectively. In most cases, the surgery was performed on a child with a parent sharing the same blood type, supplying the oxygenated blood. Over the next 16 months, they utilized this cross-circulation technique on 45 children with serious congenital heart defects (including ventricular septal defects, Tetralogy of Fallot, and atrioventricular canal defects), achieving a 62% survival rate. This demonstrated the potential for CPB to enable complex cardiac surgery, should a satisfactory heart-lung machine ever be developed.

By the spring of 1955, a team led by Dr. John Kirklin at the Mayo Clinic, just 90 miles south of the University of Minnesota, had created a modified version of the Gibbon Machine. The design for the IBM-Gibbon machine was patented, but IBM and Gibbon extracted no profit from it. Gibbon felt that his responsibility as a surgeon and researcher was to improve the care of patients rather than to make money, and as such, the design was made available to Kirklin at no charge. With this modified machine, Kirklin's team completed the first successful series of cardiac surgeries with the aid of a mechanical pump and oxygenator. This was followed later that year by a successful series by Lillehei, using a relatively simple heart-lung machine of their own design utilizing a bubble oxygenator, and by the fall of 1955, these two institutions were regularly performing open-heart surgery with mechanical CPB machines. The puzzle of open-heart surgery appeared to have finally been solved. Interestingly, the first successful use of CPB for a pulmonary embolectomy was accomplished in the spring of 1961, almost 30 years exactly after Gibbon's fateful experience.

Major Advances

The development of an effective CPB machine marked a major milestone in medical history. This achievement was accompanied by many other scientific advancements over a span of decades that helped make CPB the safe and effective procedure we know today. In this section, we will review some of the more notable developments (See also Tables 5.2 and 5.3).

Table 5.2 Early changes in the practice of CPB (1955–1960)

1. Addition of moderate hypothermia to CPB (Sealy 1957)
2. Use of median sternotomy instead of lateral thoracotomy (Julian and Lillehei 1957)
3. Rotating disc oxygenators introduced (Kay and Cross 1957)
4. Conversion from use of subclavian artery to femoral artery for arterial inflow (Lillehei 1959)
5. Use of roller pumps instead of finger pumps
6. Induced cardiac arrest with potassium (Melrose 1959; amongst others)
7. Introduction of hemodilution and asanguineous priming techniques (Panico and Neptune 1959; Zuhdi 1961; Cooley 1962)
8. Use of passive venous drainage (i.e., gravity) instead of active
9. Central venous cannulation instead of peripheral

History of Myocardial Protection and Cardioplegia

Early myocardial protection was limited but has evolved significantly, from early normothermic techniques to intermittent cross-clamping, fibrillatory arrest, topical hypothermia, and the development of specialized cardioplegia solutions with oxygenation (For a comprehensive exploration, refer to Chap. 28).

Table 5.3 Later developments in cardiopulmonary bypass: 1960–Present

Early-1960s	Disposable plastic bag bubble oxygenator (Gott)
1966	First journal devoted to CPB published (*Journal of Extra-corporeal Technology*)
1967	Intra-aortic balloon pump first used (Kantrowitz)
1968	AmSECT incorporated
Late-1960s	Hard shell disposable bubble oxygenator with integrated heat exchanger introduced (DeWall)
Late-1960s	Use of ascending aorta for arterial cannulation (McAlpine et al.; Parker)
1969	First baccalaureate program in perfusion offered at Ohio State University
1971	Establishment of the Texas Heart Institute School of Perfusion
Early-1970s	First commercially available disposable membrane oxygenators
1972	First certification examination for perfusionists
1973	Cold potassium cardioplegia (Gay and Ebert; many others)
1974	ABCP established by AmSECT
1975	Heparin and protamine monitoring with ACT introduced (Bull)
Mid-1970s	Commercially available microporous polypropylene disposable membrane oxygenator
1977	Perfusionists recognized by the American Medical Association as a profession
1978	Society of Cardiovascular Anesthesiologists (SCA) founded
1979	Introduction of bubble detector (Sarns) and arterial filter purge line (Baxter)
1981	Commercially available hollow fiber membrane oxygenators
1982	Implementation of arterial microfilters and minimizing use of cardiotomy suction, or processing it with cell savers
1982–1983	Retrograde delivery of cardioplegia (Menashe 1982; Grundy 1983)
1980's	Centrifugal pumps begin to replace roller pumps
1980's	Pulsatile flow advocated, and became available with roller and centrifugal pumps
Mid-1980s	Commercially available hollow fiber membrane oxygenators with extra-capillary flow
1985–1990	In-line monitoring of blood gases
1986	The journal *Perfusion* first published {EAH: Please move up to proper position in terms of date}
1987	Aprotinin shown to reduce perioperative bleeding (Royston; many others)
1990	Heparin-coated circuits introduced
1990	Retrograde cerebral perfusion used for cerebral protection during circulatory arrest (Ueda)
Early-1990s	Cerebral oximeter developed
Early-1990s	Antegrade cerebral perfusion advocated for cerebral protection during circulatory arrest
1991	European Board of Cardiovascular Perfusion established
1991	Use of modified ultrafiltration in infant surgery (Elliot and Naik)
1992	Epivascular scanning to assess atherosclerosis at arterial cannulation site (Kachoukos)
1995	Subclavian artery cannulation advocated for in patients with problematic ascending aorta (Sabik et al.)
1996	Port Access System introduced
1998	Retrograde autologous priming introduced as a blood conservation technique (Rosengart et al.)
2000	Augmented venous return introduced
2000	Minimized pump oxygenators first used
2007	Cerebral oximetry shown to improve outcome during coronary artery bypass grafting (Murkin)
2007	AmSECT established the International Consortium for Evidence-Based Perfusion
2011	AmSECT established a simulation task force
2011	AmSECT Mechanical Circulation Support Committee issues a position paper on the role of perfusionists

Oxygenators

The ability to effectively oxygenate blood is one of the most fundamental necessities for a heart-lung machine and the most challenging to solve. The earliest mechanical oxygenators were considered direct-contact oxygenators, in which blood is directly exposed to air. The most common direct-contact oxygenators included film and bubble oxygenators, both of which were used in early CPB machines.

The film oxygenator was first described by Frey and Gruber in 1885 (Fig. 5.1). *As mentioned earlier, vertical screen filming oxygenators were employed by Gibbon and Kirklin for their early cases.* Kay and Cross further advanced the film oxygenator through creation of their rotating disc oxygenator. This apparatus rotated multiple thin silicone-coated stainless-steel discs at approximately 120 RPM, in a horizontal cylindrical chamber through which blood flowed along the bottom (Fig. 5.2). As the discs rotated, they picked up a thin film of blood, allowing gas exchange to occur with the oxygen flowing through the top of the chamber. It became the favored oxygenator during the 1960s. However, like other filming oxygenators, the rotating disc oxygenators were cumbersome to clean and sterilize and required a large priming volume. They were largely replaced by disposable bubble oxygenators in the 1970s.

The first bubble oxygenator was built by Waldemar von Schroder of Strasbourg, France, in 1882. His machine introduced air into a venous reservoir. The increase in pressure from adding air into the venous reservoir then drove the blood into an arterial reservoir, which would then be pumped to the subject. This primitive bubble oxygenator was advanced in 1952 by Clarke, Gollan, and Gupta, and then improved upon again by Dr. Richard DeWall. DeWall's advancement included a novel helical coil defoaming chamber to help reduce the amount of bubbles that inevitably formed with bubble oxygenation (Fig. 5.3). DeWall's oxygenator was first used clinically by Lillehei and his team at the University of Minnesota in 1955. It was a simple yet efficient design that was rapidly improved upon with disposable

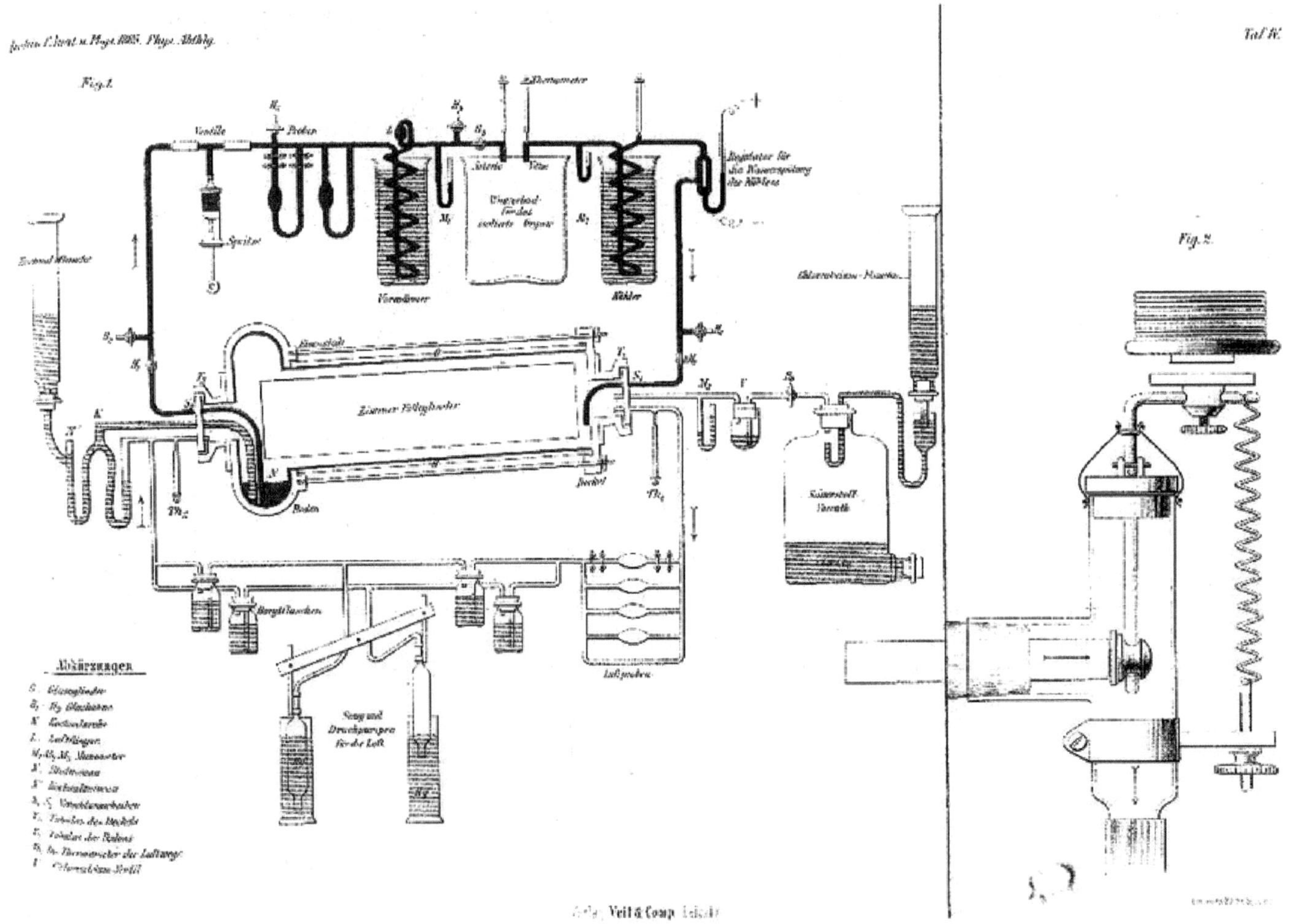

Fig. 5.1 The diagram published in 1885 by Frey and Gruber depicting their respiration apparatus. Note, the closed circuit contains a film oxygenator (Eisener Fullzylinder) and is driven by 10 mL syringes. (*Photo Credit*: Boettcher et al. 2003)

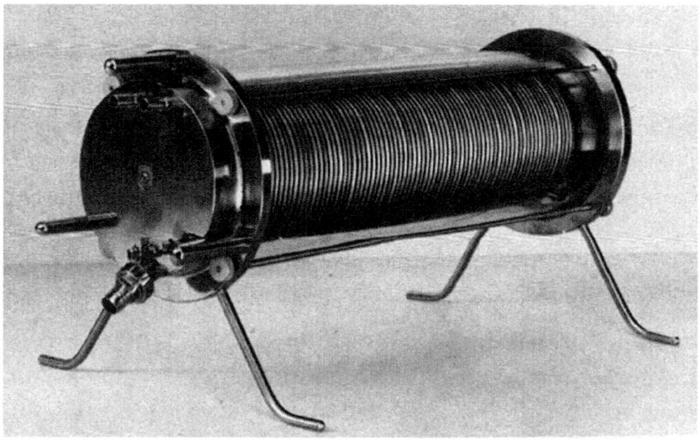

Fig. 5.2 Kay and Cross's rotating disc oxygenator. (*Photo Credit*: Hedland, KD. Remembering the disc oxygenator)

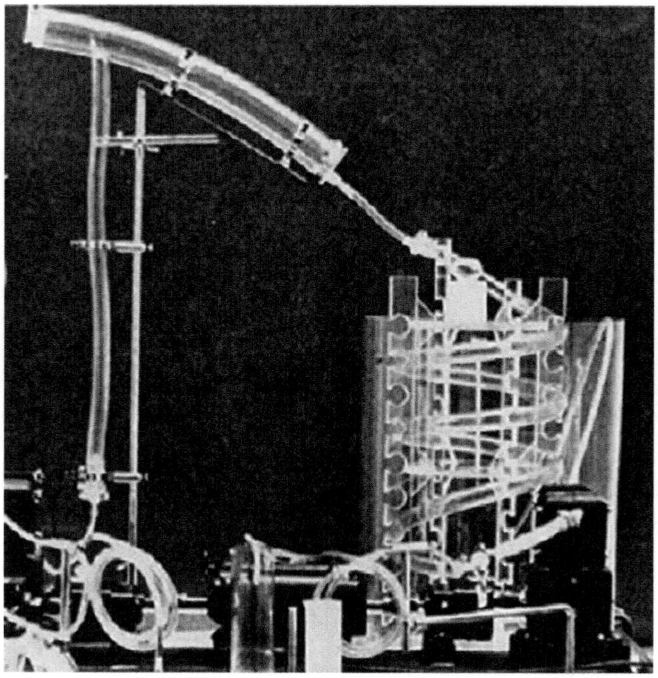

Fig. 5.3 Dewall bubble oxygenator. (*Photo Credit*: Hessel. Best Practice & Research Clinical Anaesthesiology 2015)

components and integrated heat exchangers. Bubble oxygenators were widely used through the 1970s.

A major drawback of direct-contact oxygenators is that they required exposure to 100% oxygen, thus limiting control over arterial oxygen partial pressure. Additionally, blood components suffer trauma through direct contact with air and the oxygenator surface. This trauma resulted in hemolysis of red blood cells as well as coagulopathies due to the destruction of platelets and clotting factors. As a result, the use of direct-contact oxygenators was limited to approximately 4 h.

The idea that a protective membrane could be placed between the blood and air to help prevent trauma to blood components was first proposed by Kolff and Berk in 1944, who noted that blood in their hemodialysis machine became oxygenated when exposed to aerated dialysate (Fig. 5.4). However, the development of this new membrane oxygenator (MO) was limited by finding a suitable material that offered both sufficient mechanical strength and gas exchange. Initially, Teflon was explored. It was not until the mid-1970s that an efficient MO became commercially available, initially made out of silicon rubber (e.g., Kolobow, Lande, and Travenol modulung), and then polypropylene (e.g., Travenol Adult TMO). In the 1980s, hollow fiber MOs were developed, which decreased the average distance over which gas exchange had to occur and virtually replaced all other oxygenators by 1994. In the early 2000s, a new nonporous diffusion membrane constructed from poly-(4-methyl-1-pentene) (PMP) was introduced, which is less likely to leak plasma after prolonged bypass (e.g., >6 h) and thus more suitable for long-term perfusion, such as patients requiring extra-corporeal membrane oxygenation. A limitation during anesthesia is that they do not allow the passage of volatile anesthetics. In recent years, some manufacturers have integrated screen microfilters into their MOs, perhaps eliminating the need for a separate arterial line microfilter.

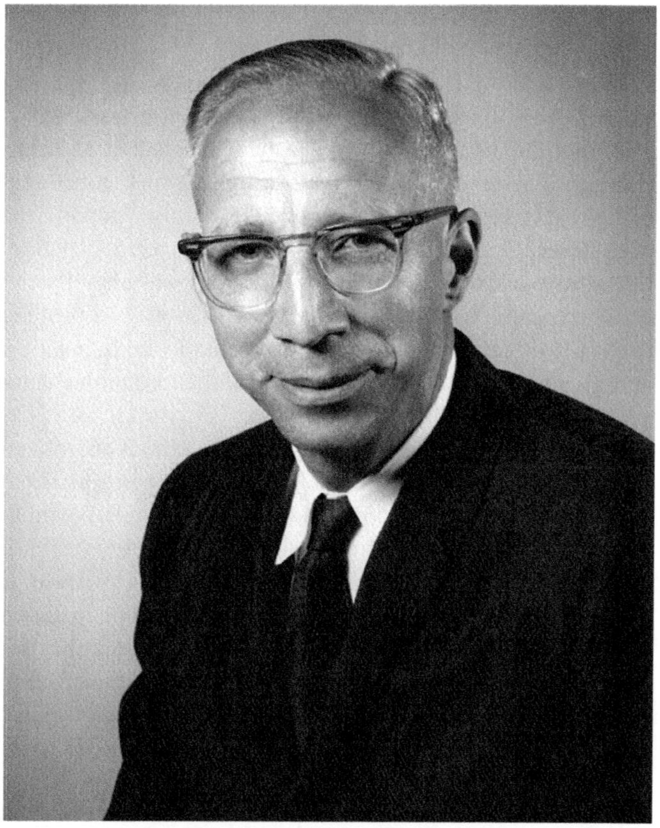

Fig. 5.4 Willem Johan Kolff (1911–2009), a pioneer of hemodialysis and artificial organs

Anticoagulation and Bleeding

Preventing blood from clotting and then reversing this effect were additional prerequisites for CPB. Heparin was discovered in 1916 by Jay McLean, a medical student at Johns Hopkins University, while he was searching for a procoagulant. The name "heparin" was derived from "hepar," the Greek word for liver, which was the source of its isolation. The ability of protamine to reverse heparin was also discovered serendipitously. While searching for a way to prolong heparin's effects, knowing that protamine extends insulin's duration, researchers surprisingly found that protamine actually reversed heparin's effects instead.

Heparin was administered by protocol without any objective monitoring for CPB cases until 1975 when Dr. Brian Bull of Loma Linda University advocated for objective monitoring through the use of activated clotting time (ACT) to guide heparinization and protamine reversal. The team at Loma Linda suggested a safe zone of 300–600 s but appeared to have arbitrarily set a target of 480 s—a threshold that has been widely accepted ever since, without much evidence to support it. By the end of the 1970s, objective monitoring for heparinization was employed by most institutions. Heparin-coated circuits were introduced in 1990, partly with the potential of reducing heparin requirements, but their use has remained controversial.

In 1987, Royston and other groups introduced the use of aprotinin to reduce perioperative bleeding, and soon, the use of aprotinin and synthetic anti-fibrinolytics during CPB became standard. Aprotinin was withdrawn from the market in 2007, following an analysis of a large randomized controlled trial (Blood Conservation Using Antifibrinolytic Therapy—BART), which demonstrated an increased risk of death with aprotinin, a risk not seen with other antifibrinolytic drugs. Since then, lysine analogues, such as tranexamic acid and epsilon amino caproic acid, have been routinely used as antifibrinolytics instead of aprotinin in many practices. However, the risks of aprotinin have been questioned, and its limited use is now approved in Canada, England, and Europe.

Arterial Pumps

Sigmamotor "finger" pumps were used in the earliest heart-lung machines, but they were soon replaced with roller pumps during the mid-1950s. Interestingly, the roller pump was first used clinically by DeBakey in 1934, specifically for a blood transfusion. In the 1980s, centrifugal pumps began to gain popularity due to their purported safety and ability to reduce blood trauma. Throughout the development of CPB, there has been an ongoing debate about the advantages of providing pulsatile flow, with numerous studies providing conflicting data.

Arterial Cannulation

Initially, most open-heart surgeries were performed through a transverse sternotomy bilateral anterior thoracotomy or a lateral thoracotomy approach, utilizing the subclavian artery for arterial cannulation. By the late 1950s, median sternotomy and femoral artery cannulation had replaced the aforementioned approach. However, femoral cannulation carried with it a significant incidence of retrograde dissection, and in the latter part of the 1960s, direct cannulation of the ascending aorta became standard. Femoral, axillary/subclavian, and innominate arteries remain alternative sites for cannulation today.

Venous Drainage

Initially, venous drainage was an active process and achieved through the use of a venous pump with the goal of matching venous and arterial flow; however, gravity drainage soon became standard. This remained true until the 1990s when augmented venous return was reintroduced to facilitate the long, narrow femoral venous cannulas used for minimally invasive cardiac surgery. This technique has become commonly employed for most cardiac surgical operations. Venous return can be augmented through the use of either pumps or vacuum applied to a hard shell venous reservoir. This allows for reduced priming volumes by utilizing smaller venous lines and for the heart-lung machine to be raised from the floor.

Temperature and pH Management

Before the successful development of CPB machines, Bigelow suggested that inducing hypothermia could reduce systemic oxygen requirement. During its early days, bypass was conducted at normothermia, as early machines lacked the ability to reliably cool and warm the patients. The first successful human operation during brief inflow occlusion, utilizing only moderate hypothermia without CPB, was performed by John Lewis at the University of Minnesota. Hypothermia was induced by wrapping an anesthetized 5-year-old patient in refrigerated blankets until her rectal temperature reached 28 °C. Following the repair of her atrial septal defect, she was then placed in a 45 °C water bath until her temperature increased to 36 °C. In 1959, Sealey introduced a heat exchanger to his DeWall oxygenator and began to utilize moderate hypothermia (28–32 °C) routinely, which quickly became standard of practice. Moderate hypothermia remained common until normothermic or "tepid" bypass became popular in the 1990s as a means to reduce the risk of cerebral hyperthermia during rewarming.

Deep hypothermic circulatory arrest (DHCA) was first introduced by Drew in 1959, although it was not widely adopted at this time due to concerns of neurological injury. It was reintroduced during the 1960s separately by Dillard and Barratt-Boyes to facilitate infant heart surgery and again by Griepp in 1975 for conducting aortic arch surgery. By the 1980s, it was widely accepted.

Until the 1980s during hypothermic CPB, temperature corrected (to patients actual temperature) pH and $PaCO_2$ were maintained at 7.40 and 40 mmHg, respectively (referred to as the "pH-stat strategy"). However, in 1982, Ream and colleagues advocated against this, suggesting that the natural respiratory alkalosis seen with hypothermia (due to increased solubility of CO_2 at lower temperatures) is preferred for normal physiology, and that patients should be alkalotic with a lower $PaCO_2$ when hypothermic. The "alpha-stat strategy," which keeps temperature uncorrected targeting a pH 7.40 and $PaCO_2$ 40 mmHg as measured at 37 °C, quickly became standard practice.

Hemodilution

Initially, heart-lung machines were primed with whole blood. In the late 1950s and early 1960s, hemodilution and asanguineous priming were introduced to reduce the negative effects associated with blood transfusion and to conserve this precious resource. As a result, hemodilution became a standard practice, sometimes to an extreme degree. The adoption of tepid bypass posed challenges to this practice, and several observational studies showed increased morbidity and mortality associated with low hematocrit during CPB. Techniques were subsequently implemented to reduce the severity of anemia due to hemodilution during CPB.

Hemofiltration was first described in 1979 by Darup as a way to remove excess crystalloid, raise hematocrit and plasma protein concentration, and to remove inflammatory mediators. Modified ultrafiltration (MUF) was introduced in 1991 by Naik, and in 1996, Journis advocated for zero-balance ultrafiltration (ZBUF). Other techniques to reduce priming volume and hence hemodilution included retrograde autologous priming, which allows for the patient's own blood to fill the extra-corporeal circuit displacing the priming solution, and miniaturized circuits. For comprehensive details on the different ultrafiltration techniques, please refer to Chap. 19.

Safety and Training

Perfusionists

Bypass machines were initially operated by surgeons and laboratory technicians. Gradually, these positions were filled by technicians with various backgrounds who received on-the-job training. The term "perfusionist" was first used by Bennett Mitchell in the early 1960s. As operations utilizing CPB became more common, the demand for perfusionists greatly increased, and in 1968, the American Society of Extra-corporeal Technology (AmSECT) was established. The first baccalaureate program in perfusion was created at Ohio State University in 1969, and in 1971, the famed Texas Heart Institute School of Perfusion opened. In 1974, the American Board of Cardiovascular Perfusion (ABCP) was formed and in 1977, perfusionists were recognized as a medical profession by the American Medical Association. In 1981, the ABCP proposed a plan to only allow examination and certification for graduates of accredited programs (as opposed to those who had received on-the-job training). In 1982, the Australasian Society of Cardiovascular Perfusionists (ASCVP) was formed, and in 1991, the European Board of Cardiovascular Perfusion was established. The field of clinical perfusion has continued to grow across the globe since, and many other countries have gone on to develop their own education and certification programs. Today, in the United States alone there are about 18 accredited perfusion training programs with over 4600 certified perfusionists.

Accident Surveys

Risk and risk containment have been concerns since the very beginning of clinical CPB. Interest in safety guidelines grew with the publication of the first national survey of perfusion accidents by Stoney et al., in 1980, and the 1981 report from the Utah Biomedical Test Laboratory on the safety and performance of CPB systems. Multiple subsequent surveys have been reported from the United Kingdom, the United States, France, and Australia/New Zealand. The information garnered from these surveys has led to additional educational efforts and the adoption of safe practice guidelines and safety equipment on bypass machines (such as low-level detectors, the Sarns air bubble detector and the Baxter Temptol arterial filter purge in 1979, and in-line monitoring of blood gases in the late 1980s). Periodically, AmSECT and the American Academy of Cardiovascular Perfusion (AACP) have issued statements, position papers, guidelines and checklists to further perfusion safety and performance especially addressing the adoption of newer technologies.

Evidence-Based Practice

The concept of basing medical practice on a critical review of the best evidence available in the medical literature was developed by David Sackett and his colleagues at McMaster

University in 1981. This group included GH Guyatt who is credited with coining the term "evidence-based medicine" (EBM). Unfortunately, as in many other fields of medicine, there remains a great need for high-level evidence to guide the practice of CPB, especially in high-risk patients. In the late 1980s, Mangano and colleagues initiated large multicenter studies involving thousands of patients, which have generated important observational data related to the conduct of cardiac surgery and CPB, as has the Northern New England Cardiovascular Disease Study Group. To promote EBM practice in CPB, AmSECT established the International Consortium for Evidence-Based Perfusion in 2007, and in 2017 published standards and guidelines for conduct of CPB, which were updated in 2023. In 2019, the combined European perfusionists, cardiac surgeons, and cardiac anesthesiologists published their own guidelines for conduct of CPB. The Australian and New Zealand College of Perfusionists host the annual "Perfusion Down Under." Other organizations host similar meetings and publish guidelines with the goal of encouraging best practice within the field.

Simulation

As in many other fields of medicine, the use of simulation for education and training has recently expanded into the practice of CPB. The idea of computer simulation for basic education in perfusion was first described by Riley and O'Kane at the Mayo Clinic in 1977. The use of simulation for bypass was greatly enhanced by the development of the "Orpheus" simulator by Morris and Pybus in 2007, and in the years since, many other low and high-fidelity simulators have been introduced. Many groups have demonstrated simulation's value in perfusion education, maintenance of core skills, practice of emergency situation responses, and the development of resource management. AmSECT subsequently established a Simulation Taskforce in 2011.

Further Reading

Boettcher W, Merkle F, Weitkemper HH. History of extra-corporeal circulation: the conceptional and developmental period. J Extra Corpor Technol. 2003;35(3):172–83.

Hessel EA. A brief history of cardiopulmonary bypass. Semin Cardiothorac Vasc Anesth. 2014;18(2):87–100. https://doi.org/10.1177/1089253214530045.

Hessel EA 2nd. History of cardiopulmonary bypass (CPB). Best Pract Res Clin Anaesthesiol. 2015;29(2):99–111. https://doi.org/10.1016/j.bpa.2015.04.006.

Holman WL, Timpa JG, Kirklin JK. Origins and evolution of extracorporeal circulation. J Am Coll Cardiol. 2022;79(16):1606–22. https://doi.org/10.1016/j.jacc.2022.02.034.

Jensen R. History of perfusion. J Extra Corpor Technol. 2003;35(4):270–3.

Lawrence AE, Palanzo DA. A brief history of the American Academy of Cardiovascular Perfusion. [Internet]. [cited 2024 Aug 4]. Available from: http://www.theaacp.com/AACP_History.pdf.

Lim MW. The history of extracorporeal oxygenators. Anaesthesia. 2006;61(10):984–95. https://doi.org/10.1111/j.1365-2044.2006.04796.x.

Romaine-Davis A. John Gibbon and his heart-lung machine. Philadelphia: University of Pennsylvania Press; 2016.

Stoney WS. Evolution of cardiopulmonary bypass. Circulation. 2009;119(21):2844–53. https://doi.org/10.1161/CIRCULATIONAHA.108.783164.

Part III

Adult Cardiopulmonary Bypass

6 Physiologic Changes and Inflammatory Response to Cardiopulmonary Bypass

Yvonne Fetterman, Grant Gagnon, and Benu Makkad

The Inflammatory Response

Introduction

CPB exposes the patient to multiple non-physiologic conditions that can trigger both humoral and cellular inflammatory responses. Factors such as blood exposure to non-biologic materials, mechanical blood component damage, endothelial dysfunction, hypothermia, heparinization, and ischemia–reperfusion contribute to this response. Surgical trauma, blood loss, and transfusions also play a role. However, clinical trials comparing off pump and on pump CABG show minimal differences in inflammation, suggesting CPB's limited impact. Yet, longer CPB duration correlates with increased morbidity and mortality.

The inflammatory response to CPB is divided into early and late phases. The early phase begins immediately upon blood contact with the CBP circuit, triggering the activation of coagulation and inflammation cascades as well as endothelial cells, immune cells, and platelets. The late phase, occurring during prolonged CPB exposure and weaning, involves heparin-protamine reversal effects, ischemia–reperfusion injury, endotoxemia, and coagulation derangements, leading to organ injury mediated by leukocytes, oxidative stress, cytokine release, and further complement activation.

Y. Fetterman (✉)
Department of Anesthesiology, Conemaugh Memorial Medical Center, Johnstown, PA, USA

G. Gagnon
NRP Specialist, Keystone Pefusion, Philadelphia, PA, USA

B. Makkad
Department of Anesthesiology, University of Cincinnati College of Medicine, Cincinnati, OH, USA

Humoral Inflammatory Response

Activation of the Contact System

The contact system, also known as the plasma kallikrein–kinin system, includes three serine proteinases—factor XII (Hageman factor), factor XI, and plasma prekallikrein (PPK)—and a cofactor, high-molecular weight kininogen (HK). Upon contact with negatively charged surfaces, such as those in the CPB circuit, factor XII is transformed into its active form, factor XIIa. This activation initiates the intrinsic coagulation cascade and activates factor XI. Factor XIIa also converts plasma prekallikrein (PPK) to plasma kallikrein (PK), which in turn activates additional factor XII, creating a positive feedback amplification loop. PPK and factor XI each form a heterodimer with HK. Like factor XII, HK binds to negatively charged surfaces, bringing PPK and factor XI in proximity to surface-bound factor XIIa, allowing for rapid activation of these molecules. Factor XIIa, Factor XIa, and PK all cleave HK releasing bradykinin (BK)—a potent vasoactive mediator that causes vasodilation, increases vascular permeability, contracts nonvascular smooth muscle, and stimulates fibrinolysis by promoting tissue plasminogen activator (tPA) release. Kallikrein also activates neutrophils and promotes fibrinolysis. Factor XIIa has a dual role, stimulating both fibrinolysis and coagulation, which highlights the delicate balance that exists between the pro-thrombotic and anti-thrombotic homeostatic mechanisms. The activation of the blood contact system inside a CPB circuit is illustrated below (Fig. 6.1).

Activation of the Coagulation Cascade

The coagulation system, essential for clot formation, comprises a cascade of plasma protein activations within two pathways: the intrinsic and extrinsic pathways. These pathways merge at clotting factor X to form the common pathway. During CPB, the intrinsic pathway is predominantly

A. S. Awad, J. DiNardo (eds.), *Clinical Perfusion for Cardiac Surgery*, https://doi.org/10.1007/978-3-031-91163-7_6

activated, as discussed earlier through the contact system. Factor XII is activated after contact with the non-endothelial surfaces of the CPB circuit. Factor XIIa then activates factor XI, which begins the intrinsic coagulation cascade. The extrinsic pathway, typically initiated via blood contact with tissue factor at the site of injury, is also activated during cardiac surgery, partly due to activated endothelial cell expression of tissue factor during CPB. Thrombin, a crucial component in the common pathway, not only amplifies the coagulation cascade and leads to fibrin formation but also plays a significant role in inflammatory signaling. It stimulates endothelial production of von Willebrand factor, causes the release of chemotactic and inflammatory cytokines, promotes neutrophil adhesion to endothelium, and activates platelets and mast cells. The interplay of key pathways—the contact system, the intrinsic pathway, the extrinsic pathway, the common coagulation pathway, and the fibrinolytic pathway—is illustrated in Fig. 6.2.

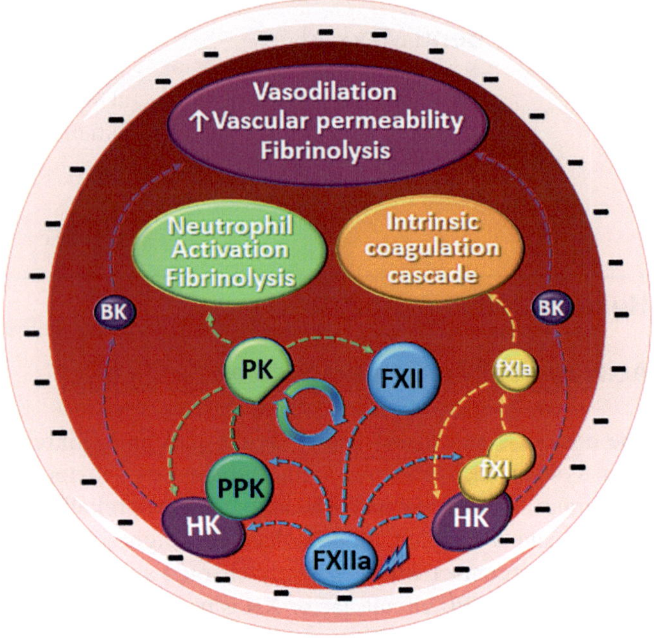

Fig. 6.1 The diagram illustrates the activation of the blood contact system inside a CPB circuit's negatively charged surface. It highlights factor XII (light blue circle) being activated (light blue oval) upon contact, which triggers the intrinsic coagulation cascade by activating factor XI (yellow), plasma prekallikrein (PPK) (dark green), and HK (purple). The release of bradykinin (dark purple) leads to increased vasodilation and vascular permeability, demonstrating the complex interactions that occur during CPB. Additionally, PK (light green), shown in the illustration, plays a critical role in neutrophil activation and the promotion of fibrinolysis

Heparin, widely used in cardiac surgery, exerts both anti-inflammatory and antithrombotic effects. It significantly enhances antithrombin III (ATIII) activity, boosting its ability to inhibit thrombin generation and clot formation by 500 to 1000-fold. ATIII predominantly inactivates factor Xa and thrombin in the coagulation cascade's final common pathway. Despite heparin use, thrombin formation persists in patients undergoing CPB. This ongoing thrombin activity can lead to thromboembolic complications or depletion of coagulation factors, leading to a consumptive coagulopathy.

Activation of the Fibrinolytic System

Activation of the contact and coagulation systems initiates fibrinolysis, a crucial process that prevents a state of unopposed thrombosis. Tissue plasminogen activator (tPA) converts plasminogen to plasmin, which in turn breaks down fibrin clots. Several factors, including BK, factor Xa, and

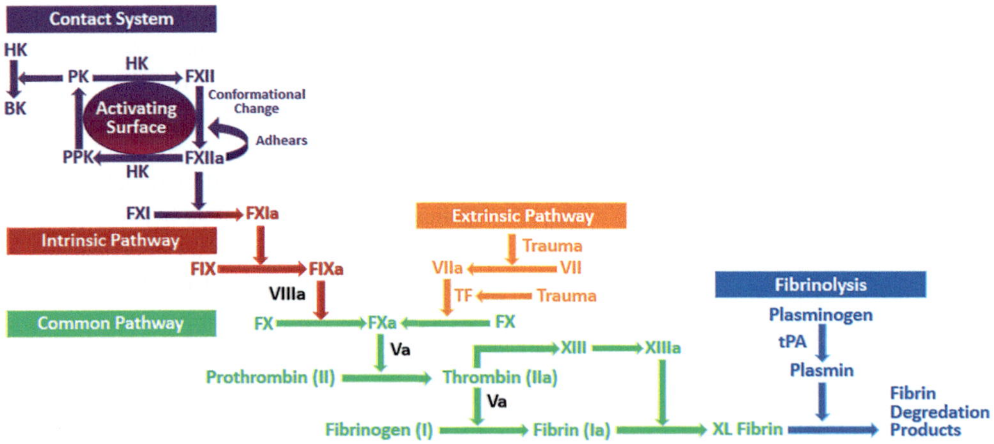

Fig. 6.2 The diagram illustrates the Humoral Inflammatory Responses during CPB, highlighting the interplay of key pathways. The contact system, depicted in purple, initiates the intrinsic coagulation pathway (shown in red), where activated factor XIIa begins the intrinsic coagulation cascade by activating factor XI. Concurrently, the extrinsic coagulation cascade (illustrated in yellow) is also activated. Both pathways converge at clotting factor X, leading into the common pathway (represented in green), culminating in clot formation with cross-linked fibrin (XL Fibrin). Additionally, the fibrinolysis pathway, shown in blue, functions to regulate and dissolve clots. This illustration captures the intricate balance between coagulation and fibrinolysis during CPB

thrombin, promote the release of tPA from the endothelium, and factor XIIa can directly convert plasminogen to plasmin. Kallikrein, another key molecule, releases BK from HK and enhances factor XII conversion, ultimately leading to factor Xa and thrombin generation. The degree of fibrinolysis has been positively correlated with increased perioperative bleeding. Fibrinolytic activity inherently dissolves clots, but further bleeding risk is conferred by its ability to hinder platelet aggregation by altering key glycoprotein Ib and IIb/IIIa receptors.

Activation of Complement

The complement system, integral to the innate immune system, enhances or "complements" antibody-mediated immunity with its network of plasma proteins, many of which are zymogens. These proteins trigger a proteolytic cascade, leading to pathogen opsonization and an inflammatory response. Complement activation is inherent in cardiac surgery, particularly during CPB, as well as following ischemic–reperfusion and heparin–protamine neutralization, and can occur via three pathways: classical, lectin a.k.a. mannan-binding lectin (MBL), and alternative. All pathways produce a C3 convertase and lead to the assembly of the membrane attack complex (MAC complex, C5b–C9), which causes osmotic cell lysis. The three pathways of complement activation are illustrated in (Fig. 6.3).

During CPB, blood contact with the non-endothelial surfaces primarily activates the alternative pathway, the primary means of complement activation attributed to CPB. Normally, small amounts of complement protein C3 undergo spontaneous hydrolysis and combine with another plasma protein, factor B. After factor B of this complex is cleaved by another plasma protein, factor D, the complex acts as a fluid-phase C3 convertase, which cleaves other C3 molecules to C3a and C3b. C3a circulates in the serum, but C3b must become surface-bound or it is quickly inactivated. C3b deposition normally occurs on the vascular endothelium; however, host cells contain complement regulatory proteins that destabilize C3b and prevent continuation of the alternative pathway. During CBP, the artificial surface of the bypass circuit does not possess complement regulatory proteins, and the alternative complement pathway may proceed uninhibited. C3b deposited on the CPB circuit is joined by factor B, which is then cleaved by factor D, producing the surface-bound C3 amplification convertase. This convertase greatly increases C3a and C3b production. Eventually C3b may combine with a C3 amplification convertase to produce a C5 convertase which leads to production of C5a, C5b, and the terminal complement products. The sequence of events detailing the activation of the alternative pathway of the complement system is shown in detail in (Fig. 6.4).

The classical pathway is activated by factor XIIa and heparin–protamine complexes, while endotoxin release from ischemic–reperfusion of the gut has been reported to activate

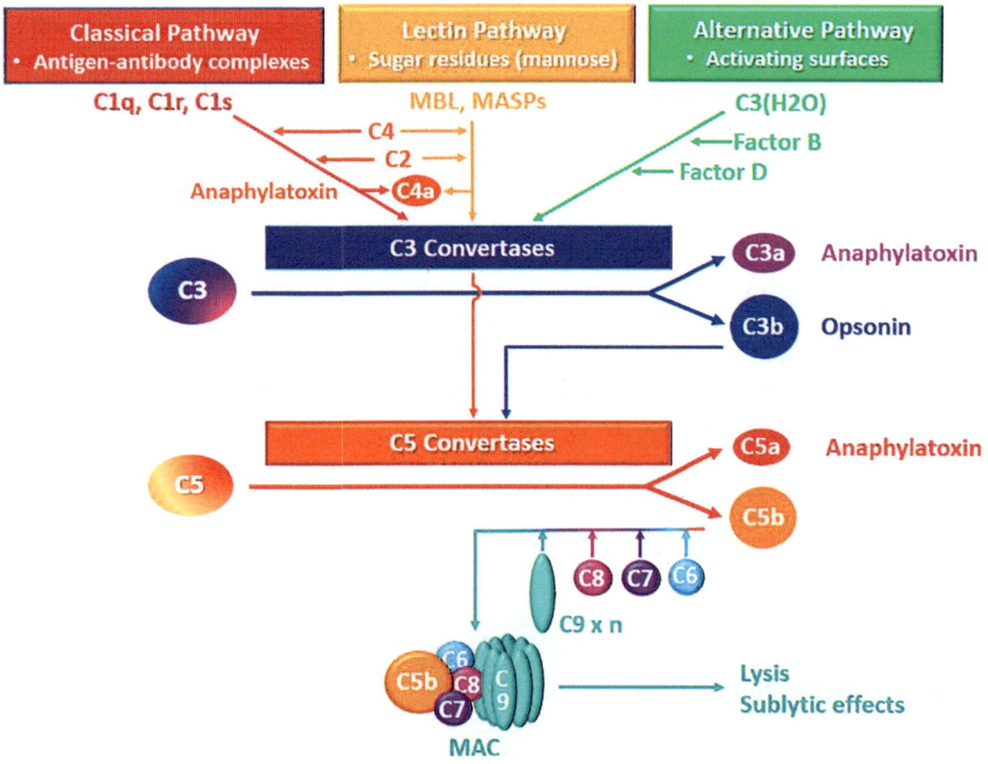

Fig. 6.3 The diagram illustrates the activation and interaction of the complement system. It depicts the three pathways of complement activation: the classical pathway (red box), the MBL pathway (yellow box), and the alternative pathway (green box). Each pathway leads to the formation of C3 convertase (blue box), which activates C5 convertase (orange box), culminating in the formation of the MAC. The MAC is responsible for the lysis effect on target cells. This detailed representation provides insights into the complex mechanisms of the complement system

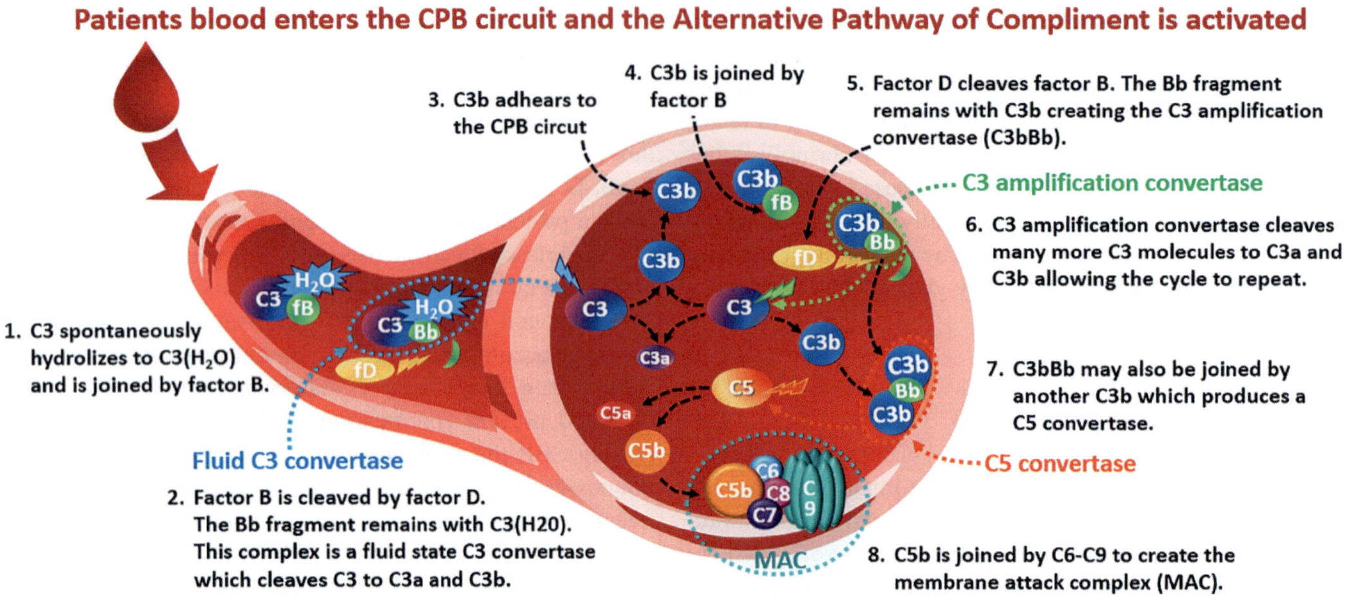

Fig. 6.4 The diagram illustrates the activation of the alternative pathway of the complement system, detailing the sequence of events in eight steps. These steps range from the initial blood exposure to non-endothelial surfaces to the formation of the MAC. This detailed representation provides insights into the complex mechanisms of the complement system

both the classical and alternative pathways. In the first 5 postoperative days, a second increase in classical complement activation is observed, which may be mediated by C-reactive protein production in response to heparin–protamine complexes. Activation of the MBL pathway has been reported in pediatric patients undergoing repair of congenital defects with CPB.

Complement fragments like C3a, C4a, and C5a (anaphylatoxins) modify vascular permeability and smooth muscle tone, inducing bronchoconstriction, hypotension, and fluid accumulation. C3a and C5a stimulate endothelial expression of adhesion molecules and mast cell release of histamine and TNF-alpha. C5a also directly influences neutrophils and monocytes, promoting endothelial adhesion, chemotaxis, degranulation, and superoxide generation.

Excessive complement activation is associated with hemodynamic instability, abnormal bleeding, postoperative organ dysfunction, including cardiac, renal, and hepatic dysfunction, as well as elevated morbidity and mortality. Please check Video 1 and Video 2 for the basics of the complement system:

Video 1 link: https://youtu.be/E4dZ5w3D9ZM?si=nurAab3oQoM0HBDC
Video 2 link: https://youtu.be/Uc4nq4Lazo4?si=1x8531Mr2HATXYLt

Ischemia–Reperfusion (I/R)

Reperfusion following ischemia, such as after aortic cross-clamp release, triggers an acute inflammatory response marked by a surge of inflammatory mediators. This I/R injury is mediated predominantly through endothelial–neutrophil interaction. Ischemia causes endothelial injury, resulting in neutrophil activation and sequestration upon reperfusion. Ischemic cells, already depleted of high-energy phosphates and antioxidant defenses, are further overwhelmed by reactive oxygen species (ROS) production during reperfusion. These ROS can damage cell membranes, denature proteins, disrupt local structures, or enter the circulation, intensifying the inflammatory response.

Global myocardial ischemic–reperfusion injury, particularly prevalent when coming off CPB, involves complement activation, as well as cytokine, chemokine, and adhesion molecule expression. These factors recruit neutrophils, monocytes, and other inflammatory cells, exacerbating damage to the ischemic myocardium. The longer the cardiac ischemia duration, the higher the levels of the pro-inflammatory cytokines IL-6 and IL-8. Notably, the heart itself is a significant producer of IL-6 and TNF-alpha, with cardiac myocytes capable of producing as much TNF-alpha as macrophages in response to endotoxin. Elevated TNF-alpha levels are associated with left ventricular dysfunction.

Endotoxemia

Endotoxin, a lipopolysaccharide (LPS) component of gram-negative bacterial cell walls, greatly contributes to the inflammatory response during CPB. Splanchnic vasoconstriction and hemodilution during CPB lead to bowel mucosal ischemia, which in turn may facilitate the translocation of endotoxin. Gut ischemia weakens tight junctions, potentially promoting endotoxin leak, though alternative sources are also suspected. An alternative explanation involves nonpulsatile flow during CPB, causing splanchnic vasoconstriction through the release of angiotensin II, with vasopressin levels increasing 20-fold.

Circulating endotoxin binds to serum-LPS binding protein, and this complex binds to macrophages, inducing cytokine production. Endotoxemia during CPB activates complement, stimulates the release of pro-inflammatory cytokines and nitric oxide, and increases postoperative oxygen consumption. Systemic endotoxin levels correlate with cardiovascular dysfunction after bypass. Individual responses to endotoxin vary, influenced by preexisting levels of immunoglobulin M antiendotoxin core antibody (IgM endocab), which neutralizes endotoxin. Low preoperative IgM endocab levels correlate with poor outcomes.

Cellular Inflammatory and Immune Response

Leukocytes

Leukocytes or white blood cells are a vital component of the immune system and include various cell types: neutrophils, lymphocytes, monocytes, eosinophils, and basophils. Initially, their levels decrease due to hemodilution from CPB circuit priming, but as CPB progresses, the number and activity of these cells increase, particularly neutrophils, monocytes, and lymphocytes, which are activated by exposure to CPB.

Neutrophils

Neutrophils, the primary cellular mediators of the inflammatory response, play a significant role in the inflammatory sequelae after CPB. The process begins within the CPB circuit, where blood contact with non-endothelial surfaces causes complement activation, predominantly through the alternative pathway, leading to a surge in levels of complement product C5a, which then activates neutrophils. Because the CPB circuit lacks the complement regulatory proteins of the vascular endothelium, complement-mediated neutrophil activation proceeds unopposed. The activated neutrophils are then reintroduced into the patient's bloodstream, where they interact with the patient's vascular endothelium and adhere to the endothelial walls via the interaction of a family of adhesion molecules known as *selectins*.

Neutrophil adherence to the endothelium, a key step in the progression of inflammation, occurs via a multistep process. Exposure to various physiologic stressors (bacteria, trauma, etc.) during the inflammatory process promotes expression of selectins. The initial C5a surge prompts rapid endothelial surface P-selectin expression from preloaded vacuoles, while later, cytokine release, particularly IL 1β and TNF α, promotes endothelial E-selectin production, which maintains primary neutrophil adhesion to the endothelium.

Neutrophil–endothelium interaction begins with low-affinity bonds involving P- and E-selectin on endothelial cells and L-selectin receptors on neutrophils, facilitating the rolling of neutrophils along the endothelial wall. L-selectin on neutrophils also contributes to interaction with other activated neutrophils to cause secondary neutrophil-to-neutrophil rolling.

Neutrophil adherence to the endothelium is strengthened by *integrins*, another family of cell surface adhesion molecules, each containing two subunits. Neutrophils express a subfamily of integrins consisting of the CD11 and CD18 subunits. While CD11a/CD18 expression remains relatively constant, CD11b/CD18 expression is influenced by cytokines such as IL-8 and C5a and increases substantially during CPB.

CD11b/CD18 integrins bind to the intercellular adhesion molecule (ICAM)-1, ICAM-2, and platelet endothelial cell adhesion molecule 1 (PECAM-1) expressed on the endothelial surface, priming neutrophils for degranulation. This tight adhesion may cause neutrophils to clump, resulting in microvascular occlusion and end-organ ischemia.

Neutrophils tightly bound to the endothelium then undergo conformational change and transmigrate into the interstitial space. They degranulate, releasing ROS and cytotoxic proteases, such as elastase and myeloperoxidase, which can damage the vascular endothelium and surrounding tissues. This process is modulated by chemokines, particularly platelet-activating factor and IL-8.

Degranulation releases both preformed and newly synthesized molecules, playing a significant role in ischemia–reperfusion injury. The stages of neutrophil activation during CPB are shown in Fig. 6.5.

Normally, during infection, neutrophils are drawn to sites of injury due to localized activation of complement and the coagulation cascade; however, in cardiac surgery and CPB, systemic distribution of circulating inflammatory mediators leads to ubiquitous activation of the endothelium and increased expression of adhesion molecules in all major organs. Leukocyte infiltration of tissue leads to widespread tissue damage and clinical or subclinical organ impairment.

Complement-activated neutrophils are implicated in pulmonary vasoconstriction following protamine administration and transfusion-related acute lung injury.

The endothelial cells return to their resting state and lose their adhesive properties when cytokines and C5a concentrations return to normal. This limits the inflammatory response in most patients undergoing cardiac surgery.

Endothelial Activation

Under normal conditions, the vascular endothelium regulates passage of molecules to and from the extravascular space and provides a conduit for blood flow to the capillary bed. The endothelium plays an important role in enabling leuko-

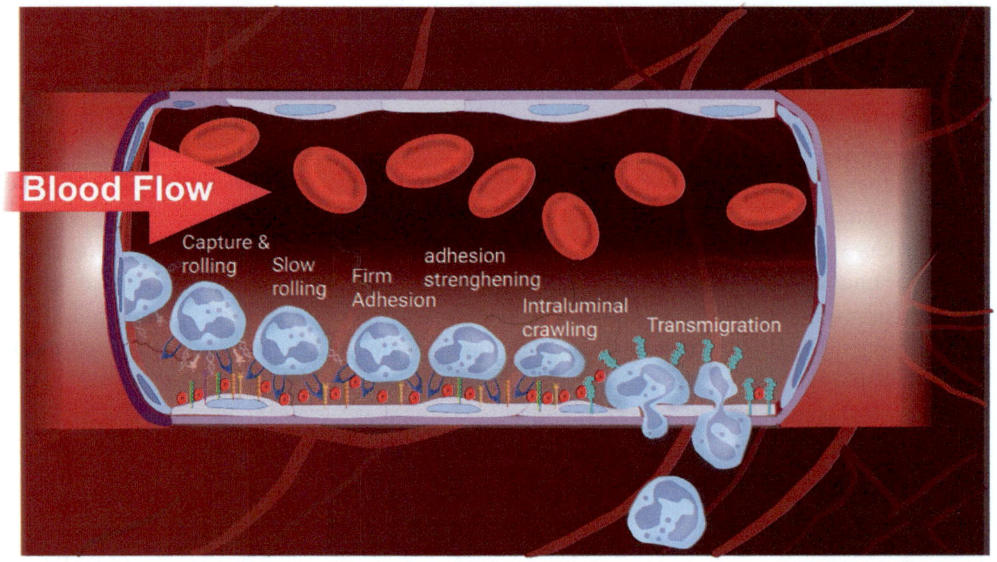

Fig. 6.5 The stages of neutrophil activation during CPB: This illustration depicts the sequential phases of neutrophil activation during CPB. Initially, neutrophils interact with the endothelium, rolling along the surface due to interactions with selectins. They then tightly bind to the endothelium through integrins, leading to conformational changes. Finally, neutrophils transmigrate either transcellularly or paracellularly into the interstitial space, playing a crucial role in the CPB-induced inflammatory response

cyte adhesion and migration into areas of inflammation, maintaining the fluidity of blood, regulating coagulation and thrombosis, and mediating vascular tone and permeability. During cardiac surgery, pro-inflammatory cytokines, thrombin, C5a, surgical trauma, I/R injury, and bacteria result in endothelial cell activation and increased endothelial expression of adhesion molecules. Neutrophil adhesion, activation, and degranulation can then ensue, leading to endothelial injury, diffuse capillary leak, tissue edema, and thrombosis. Additionally, leukocytes adherent to the vascular endothelium can clump, causing a leukocyte plug impairing or obstructing microcirculatory flow, leading to tissue ischemia.

Endothelial injury causes the release of tissue factor, which activates the extrinsic pathway of coagulation and can result in disseminated intravascular coagulation. In inflammatory states, the anticoagulant function of protein C is antagonized by TNF-α, leading to an enhanced procoagulant state.

The endothelium regulates local vascular tone by the production *and inactivation of vasoactive chemicals* such as nitric oxide (NO), prostacyclin, endothelin, and thromboxane A2. Reduced NO release due to pulmonary endothelial dysfunction is responsible for increased pulmonary vascular resistance following CPB.

Unlike local injury, the widespread endothelial injury following CPB can cause extensive activation of platelets as well as the coagulation and fibrinolytic systems, leading to diffuse fibrin deposition. Fibrin deposition in the microcirculation can occlude flow, leading to organ ischemia. In severe cases, disseminated intravascular coagulation, multiorgan failure (MOF), and death may ensue.

Thrombin, C5a, and the cytokines IL-1β and TNF-α are the primary endothelial cell activators during CPB. Please check Video 3 for the basics of the inflammatory response:

Video link 3: https://youtu.be/yIMz9pkT9xQ?si=h0C-MfSI80SKidTy

Platelets

Multiple factors contribute to both qualitative and quantitative deficits in platelets during CPB, which can contribute to hypocoagulability. Platelet numbers decrease by 30 to 50% on bypass as a result of hemodilution from crystalloid in the CPB circuit, platelet adhesion to the CPB circuit, mechanical destruction, organ sequestration, and consumptive coagulopathy.

Blood contact with the CPB circuit leads to activation of the fibrinolytic and coagulation systems, which generate plasmin and thrombin. Plasmin activates platelets and induces loss of platelet glycoprotein IIb (GpIIb) receptors, which are then deposited on the CPB circuit. Thrombin also activates platelets, which leads to platelet aggregation and release of thromboxane A2, plasminogen, and fibrinogen. Exposure of blood to the GpIIb receptors and fibrinogen deposited on the CPB circuit prompts platelets to activate and adhere to the bypass circuit, thus removing them from circulation. Additional factors that cause platelet activation include surgical wound creation, heparin administration, hypothermia, activated complement (C5b-9), leukotrienes, platelet-activating factor, and collagenases.

Altered expression of other surface molecules on platelets during CPB may explain some of the *qualitative deficits* observed. Glycoprotein Ib (Gp1b) and platelet endothelial cell adhesion molecule-1 (PECAM-1) are down-regulated, but expression of P-selectin is upregulated during CPB. Gp1b mediates platelet adhesion to endothelial cells via von Willebrand factor after tissue injury. PECAM-1 inhibits platelet reactivity and thrombosis. P-selectin is a transmembrane protein that mediates platelet adhesion with leukocytes and is considered a marker of platelet activation due to shear stress. Surface expression of P-selectin by platelets increases within 5 min of initiating CPB, and heparin administration further increases platelet P-selectin expression.

P-Selectin binds to P-selectin glycoprotein-1 (PSGL-1) on leukocytes, forming leukocyte conjugates. P-selectin interaction with monocytes leads to monocyte expression of tissue factor, which can trigger the extrinsic coagulation cascade. Surface-absorbed platelets, as platelet–leukocyte conjugates or platelet fibrin complexes, can sheer off to form microemboli.

Activated platelets express CD40 ligand (CD40L), which is structurally similar to TNF-alpha and induces the endothelium to secrete chemotactic molecules that attract neutrophils and monocytes and upregulate expression of additional adhesion molecules.

Hypothermia also plays a role in platelet dysfunction.

Both surgical improvements and technical innovations, such as improved membrane oxygenators and more biocompatible circuits, are aimed at reducing the inflammatory response and damage to blood components during CPB. These improvements may attenuate the deleterious effects of CPB on platelets. A recent small study by M. Törnudd et al. showed that both platelet number and function may be preserved following moderate CPB times. Platelet activation following protamine administration, in contrast, did show transient platelet dysfunction lasting up to 3 h postoperatively.

Monocytes

Activation of the monocytes with CPB occurs at a slower rate than neutrophil activation and is likely due to interaction with complement components C3b and C5b-9, soluble TF, and endotoxin, as well as contact with the CPB circuit. They have IgG and C3b receptors and possess migratory, chemotactic, pinocytic, and phagocytic capabilities. At the time of migration into the tissues, they differentiate into tissue macrophages.

Monocytes work alone or in conjunction with platelets to form platelet–monocyte conjugates and aid hemostasis. They can also increase the production and surface expression of tissue factor, which can activate factor VII and initiate the extrinsic coagulation pathway.

They play both a pro- and anti-inflammatory role depending on the signaling they receive, and monocytes are believed to play a role in the resolution of inflammation. When stimulated, they produce multiple cytokines, including IL-1, IL-2, IL-3, IL-6, and IL-8. Levels of these mediators peak some hours after CPB, suggesting monocyte impact on the inflammatory response may be largely in the early postoperative period. The overall balance of pro- and anti-inflammatory responses to CPB and cardiac surgery may influence the postoperative clinical course.

Consequences to Immunity

Lymphocyte count decreases with the commencement of CPB and remains low for 3–7 days after surgery. All types of lymphocytes, including B-lymphocytes, natural killer cells, T-helper cells, and T-suppressor lymphocytes, are affected. Decreased numbers and impaired function lead to a weaker cellular immune response and increase susceptibility to infection in the post-bypass period.

The large number of neutrophils activated during CPB demonstrate increased aggregability, release elastase, and generate free radicals in an oxidative burst up to 24 h post-CPB but show impaired oxidative function at 48 h after surgery. This biphasic pattern neutrophil function and activity suggests possible early tissue cytotoxicity followed later by neutrophil dysfunction.

Additionally, the phagosomes of reticuloendothelial Kupffer cells are greatly increased following CPB, which may lead to impairment of further phagocytic activity due to relative "overuse."

Mast Cells and Paneth Cells

Mast cells are tissue-fixed cells and are present in the perivascular spaces of the heart, lungs, skin, and intestine. They contain histamine and other inflammatory mediators in cytoplasmic granules. Activation of IgE receptors on their plasma membrane causes release of granular contents. Thrombin is a strong activator of mast cells through protease-activated receptors (PARs) and can have both pro- and anti-inflammatory effects. Mast cells and Paneth cells have been shown to mediate gut ischemic-reperfusion injury in a rodent model of CPB and hypothermic arrest.

Erythrocytes

Erythrocytes are subjected to both mechanical damage from CPB pumps and to sheer stress, which causes distortion of their biconcave shape. As a result, erythrocytes become more susceptible to destruction by complement, and they lose their deformability, making them less able to perfuse the microcirculation. Compromised blood flow, ischemic activation of endothelial cells, and hemoglobinemia impair tissue function.

Heparin–Protamine

With administration of protamine, heparin–protamine complexes activate complement, induce histamine release, cause the production of nitric oxide and thromboxane, and can lead to anti-platelet antibody formation. Anaphylactoid reactions can also occur, as can thromboxane-induced severe pulmonary hypertension in a minority of patients.

Clinical Significance

- The inflammatory response provoked during cardiac surgery and CPB can contribute to postoperative complications, including myocardial dysfunction, respiratory failure, renal and neurologic dysfunction, bleeding disorders, altered liver function, and MOF.
- Complement protein C5a, released after contact with the bypass circuit, is a potent stimulator of P-selectin expression by the vascular endothelium and may be responsible for sequestration of neutrophils in the pulmonary circulation seen after initiation of CPB.
- With release of the aortic cross-clamp, reperfusion of the ischemic heart releases inflammatory mediators which are distributed to other organs including the brain, kidney, and lungs. This can lead to a whole-body inflammatory response. Longer duration of ischemia increases levels of mediators such as TNF-alpha and interleukins. Higher levels of TNF-alpha correlate with left ventricular dysfunction. In one study, analysis of patients who developed systemic inflammatory response syndrome (SIRS) after cardiac surgery showed that patients with lower survival had substantially higher levels of IL-8 and interleukin-18 (IL-18).
- Patients with higher leukocyte counts following CPB are significantly more likely to develop atrial fibrillation, and postoperative atrial fibrillation is associated with high CD11b expression, indicating increased monocyte-macrophage activation. Additionally, levels of complement C4d–C-reactive protein complexes also correlate with postoperative arrhythmia after CABG.
- Activation of the classical complement pathway in response to heparin–protamine complexes is also associated with postoperative pulmonary shunt. Additionally, severe anaphylactoid reactions or thromboxane-induced severe pulmonary hypertension may result from the heparin–protamine interaction.
- Kidney injury is a frequent complication of cardiac surgery (5–30%) and correlates with the degree of inflammation. New-onset kidney failure is a poor prognostic sign following cardiac surgery.
- In contrast, immunosuppression associated with CPB can play a role in postoperative infectious complications.
- Depleted coagulation factors and dysfunctional platelets can lead to coagulopathy. Disseminated Intravascular Coagulation (DIC) can occur following CPB due to overactivation of thrombin, consumption of coagulation factors and platelets, and endothelial dysfunction. Antithrombin III (ATIII) levels can be as low as 40–50% and are commonly seen during CPB. This ATIII deficiency can also result from preoperative use of heparin, hemodilution, or CPB-related consumption.
- Sequestered leukocytes can lead to immune deficiency and infection postoperatively.

Hypothermia

Hypothermia Definitions

Hypothermia is defined as a core body temperature below 35 degrees Celsius (°C). Temperature ranges identifying four stages of hypothermia in cardiac surgery have been suggested, however, the values distinguishing mild, moderate, deep, and profound hypothermia differ from those of standard classifications (Table 6.1).

Protective Mechanisms of Hypothermia

Hypothermia decreases oxygen consumption in the heart and other vital organs. Historically, CPB has been performed under hypothermic conditions to protect vital organs such as the heart and central nervous system from ischemia. Biologic reaction rates change with temperature, which leads to an increase or decrease in the rate of total body oxygen consumption (VO_2) and carbon dioxide production (VCO_2). Hypothermia decreases reaction rates, VO_2, and VCO_2, while hyperthermia increases them. The Q10, or temperature coefficient, is the ratio describing the increase or decrease in metabolic reaction rates due to a temperature change of 10 °C. This ratio has been identified for VO_2. For every 10 degrees of temperature change, VO_2 changes by a factor of 2.6 in adults and a factor of 3.65 in infants. Thus, for VO_2, the Q10 is 2.6 for adults and 3.65 for infants. The protective mechanisms of hypothermia, however, are not limited to its effect on decreasing oxygen consumption. Hypothermia preserves high-energy phosphate stores necessary for cell integrity, accelerates recovery of protein synthesis, and has inhibitory effects on inflammation, free radical formation, and cell apoptosis, thus enhancing cell survival pathways. It has a unique role in protecting the central nervous system, particularly the brain, which is exquisitely sensitive to ischemia. Every patient undergoing CPB is likely to experience some degree of embolic phenomenon and cerebral hypoperfusion. Cerebral injury results in the release and uptake of

Table 6.1 Hypothermia: 1994 standard classification vs. suggested cardiac surgery stages

Hypothermia (°C)	1994 standard classification	Cardiac surgery definitions
Mild	32—35	28.1–34
Moderate	28–31.9	20.1–28
Deep	20.1–27.9	14.1–20
Profound	≤20	≤14

catecholamines and excitatory neurotransmitters such as glutamate that induce toxic levels of calcium to enter cells and potentiate ischemic damage. The cerebral metabolic rate ($CMRO_2$) is decreased 6–7% per degree of hypothermia; however, evidence suggests that the most important benefit of hypothermia on the ischemic brain is its ability to attenuate excitatory neurotransmitter release and hence an "excitotoxic cascade." Additionally, hypothermia inhibits blood–brain barrier dysfunction and decreases permeability in brain arterioles. Mild hypothermia has also been shown to inhibit the activation of peripheral leukocytes and brain microglia following brain insults. This inhibition is possibly due to the suppression of the pro-inflammatory transcription factor, Nuclear Factor kappa-light-chain-enhancer of activated B cells (NF-kB). Additionally, hypothermia helps decrease leukocyte adhesion in damaged areas.

Sixty percent of the total $CMRO_2$ is used for cerebral cell function (functional $CMRO_2$), and 40% is used solely to maintain cell integrity (structural $CMRO_2$). Temperature affects both functional and structural $CMRO_2$, while anesthetic drugs only affect functional $CMRO_2$.

Due to decreased oxygen demand, hypothermic CPB allows lower pump flows than normothermic CPB. This results in less blood trauma, better surgical field visualization, and a reduced embolic burden to the brain, which is the primary source of CNS injury in adult cardiac surgery. Unlike normothermic CPB, hypothermic CPB cools the systemic circulation. This cooling offers better myocardial protection by ensuring that blood returning from the pulmonary and bronchial circulations, as well as from non-coronary collaterals, does not re-warm the heart. In contrast, during normothermic CPB, systemic blood returning to the heart can compromise the protection offered by localized myocardial hypothermia, which is obtained with cold cardioplegia solution.

While hypothermia is neuroprotective, hyperthermia (greater than 37 °C) during CPB exacerbates cerebral ischemic injury. Elevated temperature increases metabolic activity and oxygen demand, which may overwhelm the brain's autoregulatory mechanisms in ischemic areas. Hyperthermia worsens intracellular acidosis, increases the release of excitotoxic neurotransmitters, enhances oxygen free-radicle production, and increases blood–brain barrier permeability. It also modulates protein kinase activity and destabilizes the cytoskeleton. Additionally, it's important to note that the solubility of gas in blood decreases as temperature increases. Rapid rewarming can lead to a gas suddenly escaping the dissolved state, forming bubbles that can embolize. Therefore, to prevent the formation of gaseous emboli, it is crucial to maintain the temperature difference between the arterial outlet and venous inflow at the oxygenator during CPB rewarming within a limit of 10 °C.

Hence, rewarming should occur slowly before weaning from CPB and avoid hyperthermia. Arterial outlet blood temperature should be less than 37 °C to avoid cerebral hyperthermia and minimize the risk of gas embolism. (Class 1, Level C).

Controversy and Deleterious Effects of Hypothermia

Despite its protective effects, the necessity of hypothermia during CPB was challenged in the early 1990s. Physiologic research demonstrated that cooling the heart below 27 °C, the temperature at which the heart arrests without cardioplegia, provided little additional protection. The largest determinant of myocardial oxygen consumption is electromechanical work, which can be terminated with chemical cardioplegic arrest. A chemically arrested heart at normothermia requires about 90% less oxygen than a normothermic beating heart. Additionally, chemically arresting the heart in conjunction with hypothermia reduces myocardial oxygen consumption by only an additional 5%. Furthermore, if continuous warm blood cardioplegia (which has greater oxygen-carrying capacity than crystalloid) is used to arrest the heart, the actual myocardial ischemic time is far less than the actual cross-clamp time. Hypothermia also impairs cerebral autoregulation, causes a left shift of the oxyhemoglobin dissociation curve, prolongs CPB times, and impairs coagulation. Moderate and deep hypothermia have been shown to cause platelet dysfunction and inhibit activated coagulation factors, while mild hypothermia is associated with the highest rate of fibrinolysis. The administration of antifibrinolytic drugs can be used to mitigate these effects. Table 6.2 outlines the key advantages and disadvantages of utilizing hypothermia during cardiac surgery.

Table 6.2 Hypothermia: advantages vs. disadvantages

Hypothermic CPB	
Advantages	Disadvantages
Decreases cerebral metabolic rate, decreases excitatory signaling, and limits ischemic insult	Impairs cerebral autoregulation
Inhibits apoptosis, preserves high-energy phosphate stores	Impairs platelets and coagulation, increases fibrinolysis
Decreased oxygen consumption	Left shift of oxy-hemoglobin dissociation curve
Attenuates inflammation	Impaired immunity
Enables lower pump flows: Less cerebral embolic load, less blood trauma	Prolonged CPB times

CPB and Hypothermia

Given that all organs must be considered during cardiac surgery, the optimal temperature for CPB remains controversial. CPB is still frequently conducted with nasopharyngeal temperatures of 25–32 °C; however, some centers may conduct CPB under mild hypothermic or normothermic conditions for certain operations to avoid the deleterious effects of hypothermia. Operations that require low flow or circulatory arrest, however, are performed with deep hypothermia (15–22 °C). A recent retrospective study evaluating 275 patients who underwent valve surgery compared normothermic CPB (34–36 °C) with mild, moderate, and deep hypothermic CPB. The results demonstrated that mild hypothermia (30–34 °C) was associated with the most favorable postoperative profile, as assessed by postoperative pulmonary artery pressures, left ventricular diameter, and the degree of decrease in postoperative renal function.

The timing of hypothermia appears to influence its protective effects on the heart. Benefit has repeatedly been demonstrated when hypothermia is initiated prior to an ischemic insult. However, hypothermia also confers marked benefit after myocardial ischemia if a target left atrial temperature 2–2.5 °C lower than normal is reached prior to coronary artery reperfusion. In an animal model, hypothermia initiated 10 min before reperfusion and maintained 2 h afterward significantly improved flow, decreased the "no flow" phenomenon (a phenomenon where flow in the microvasculature is still impaired despite coronary revascularization), and limited infarct size.

Deep Hypothermic Circulatory Arrest (DHCA)

Deep hypothermia in cardiac surgery is defined as temperatures below 20 °C. DHCA provides a bloodless field and helps prevent or mitigate ischemic injury of the central nervous system and crucial organs. It is used in various procedures, including ascending aortic surgeries such as type-A aortic dissection, complex aortic arch surgery, repair of complex congenital cardiac lesions, pulmonary embolism surgery, and in cardiac or thoracoabdominal aneurysm surgery. DHCA is particularly beneficial when pathology prohibits cross clamping of the aorta, such as with massive calcifications or a porcelain aorta.

While the heart abruptly decreases its oxygen consumption after mechanical cardiac arrest, which occurs even without cardioplegia solution at 27 °C, other organs decrease their oxygen consumption more gradually. Most organs have a Q10 near 2.0, and without deep hypothermia, are more susceptible to ischemia if perfusion is not maintained. Consequently, circulatory arrest is not initiated until temperatures are <20 °C.

The brain reaches its maximal reduction in metabolic rate and oxygen consumption when the electroencephalogram (EEG) becomes isoelectric. Traditionally, a temperature below 18 °C was believed necessary to achieve an isoelectric EEG. However, research has shown significant individual variability with an isoelectric EEG occurring anywhere between 10 °C and 27 °C. If EEG monitoring is feasible, it may facilitate surgery at a higher temperature, provided the EEG remains isoelectric.

At temperatures of 15 °C, 30 min of circulatory arrest is considered safe whereas at 10 °C, 40 min is the threshold duration after which the incidence and severity of neurologic complications significantly increase. Newer techniques, such as selective antegrade cerebral perfusion (SACP) and retrograde cerebral perfusion (RCP), allow maintenance of cerebral perfusion during circulatory arrest to the rest of the body and can enable surgery to proceed at increased core body temperatures. SACP surgery can be performed at body temperatures as high as 25–26 °C, which can significantly shorten rewarming and CPB times. Additionally, RCP has been shown to safely prolong circulatory arrest during deep hypothermia for up to 60 min.

Thermal Homeostasis Must Be Overcome in CPB

Humans are warm-blooded and therefore activate mechanisms to maintain tight control of temperature near 37 °C. Cold sensed by thermoreceptors triggers the hypothalamus to activate the sympathetic nervous system (SNS), which induces shivering and elevates heart rate and blood pressure, leading to overall increased oxygen consumption. Adequate anesthesia is required to blunt the sympathetic response and avoid increased heart rate and blood pressure, and a paralytic agent is needed to prevent shivering.

Hypothermia: Effect on pH and PCO2

Change in pH with Temperature

Water is the fundamental solvent for biological processes. It acts as both a weak acid and weak base, and thus a small percentage of it dissociates into hydrogen (H+) and hydroxide (OH−) ions in a temperature-dependent fashion. As temperature falls, there is a subsequent decrease in the kinetic energy of water molecules, which leads to less dissociation and reduced production of H+ ions. Therefore, hypothermia induces alkalosis, resulting in a left shift of the oxyhemoglobin dissociation curve and increased pK_a.

Arterial blood pH is more alkaline compared to water and parallels the pH changes of water as temperature varies.

Change in Partial Pressure of Carbon Dioxide (pCO2) with Temperature

Gases are more soluble in liquids, including biologic fluid, as temperature falls. Anyone who opens an agitated can of warm soda quickly realizes a substantial proportion of gas molecules vigorously escapes the solution. With cooling, there is decreased kinetic energy of dissolved gas molecules which leads to less gas molecules escaping the liquid. Thus, for a given total quantity of CO_2, as temperature falls, the amount of dissolved CO_2 *increases* and the pCO_2 *decreases*. Note that the previously described increase in pH (i.e. decreased hydrogen ion concentration [H+]) with a temperature decrease is NOT due to the decrease in pCO_2. In normothermic conditions, a decrease in PCO2 would imply a decrease in dissolved CO2 and thus an increase in pH. In hypothermia, a decrease in PCO2 is not due to a decrease in dissolved CO2; dissolved CO2 actually increases in hypothermia. Thus in hypothermia, the decrease in [H+] is due to a temperature induced increase in pK_a resulting in less [H+] dissociation and an alkaline drift.

> ***Further Explanation:***
> Dissolved CO2 reacts with H2O to produce carbonic acid (H2CO3):
>
> CO2 + H2O ←→ H2CO3 ←→ HCO3 + H+
>
> **Hypothermia induces a left shift**
>
> The decrease in H+ and pCO2 with hypothermia is NOT due to a decrease in the amount of dissolved CO2. In fact, the amount of dissolved CO2 is actually increased! The pCO2 is lower in hypothermia because the dissolved gas molecules have less kinetic energy. Under normothermic conditions, increased dissolved CO2 would typically lead to a more acidic environment. However, this does not occur in hypothermia because there is a left shift in reaction kinetics, resulting in less dissociation of carbonic acid into H+ despite an increase in dissolved CO2. (Note total CO2 has not changed .) Thus, temperature is the driving force behind the change in both pCO2 and pH.

Temperature Management: Alpha-Stat vs. PH-Stat Management

- *Alpha-stat management* is a pH management strategy during CPB where blood is allowed to follow its natural alkaline shift (parallel to water) as temperature drops. Hypothermia induces a left shift in reaction kinetics, and because no CO_2 is added to the system in alpha-stat management, blood becomes more alkaline. While the total CO_2 content in the system is kept constant, the partial pressure of CO_2 decreases due to increased gas solubility at lower temperatures. The net dissociation of proteins remains constant primarily because the pKa of histidine's imidazole group parallels the alkaline shift in blood pH during hypothermia (Fig. 6.6).
- *pH-stat management* is a pH management strategy during CPB where CO_2 is added to the circuit to counteract the increase in gas solubility and the left shift in reaction kinetics at colder temperatures, so that a $PaCO_2$ of 40 mmHg and a pH of 7.4 is maintained regardless of temperature.

Alpha-STAT Management

As mentioned, hypothermia causes a natural alkaline shift in the pH of neutral water (pN_{H2O}) and body fluids.

Blood and body fluids, which are slightly alkaline compared to water, parallel this alkaline drift as temperature drops (see Fig. 6.6). Buffering systems, particularly the imidazole group on histidine, a building block for proteins (see Fig. 6.7), maintain the relative alkaline state of body fluids as temperature varies.

At 37 °C, the pKa of imidazole is 6.8, which is close to normal intracellular pH, making imidazole an ideal buffer. Thus, at a temperature of 37 °C and normal intracellular pH, about half of the imidazole will remain unprotonated, and half will be protonated. *The ratio of unprotonated imidazole group to total imidazole group is a ratio known as alpha (α).* As temperature changes, the pKa of imidazole parallels the change in the pH of water and body fluids (see Fig. 6.6), so that *the* ratio of the unprotonated imidazole group to total imidazole group remains constant, a condition known as *alpha-stat*.

Alpha-stat management is a pH management strategy during CPB where blood is allowed to follow its natural alkaline shift (parallel to water) as temperature drops. The total CO_2 in the system is kept constant (no CO_2 is added), and the net dissociation of proteins also remains constant as temperature changes. Cellular transmembrane pH gradients, protein functioning, and enzyme activity, including the enzymes involved in cellular respiration, are closer to normal during alpha-stat management. This is because the arterial pH is allowed to drift in parallel with neutral water, and the pKa of proteins follows this same alkaline shift.

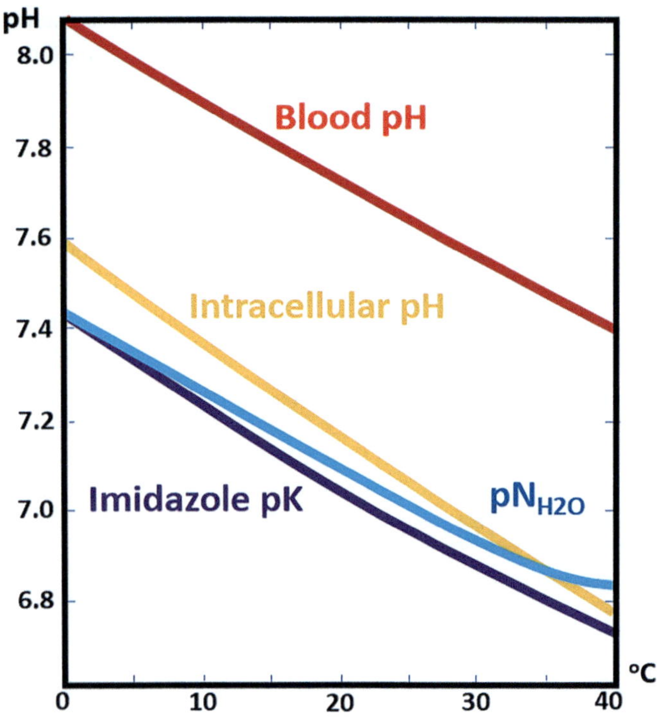

Fig. 6.6 Comparison of the pH of neutral water (pN_{H2O}), intracellular pH, Blood pH, and the pKaH of imidazole as temperature varies

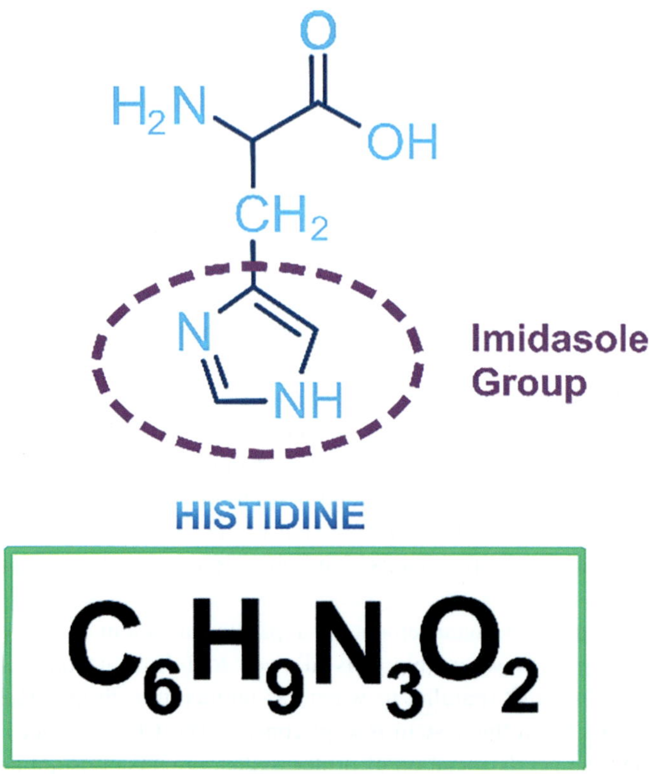

Fig. 6.7 Imidazole group on histidine

Although there is a left shift in the oxyhemoglobin dissociation curve with increased pH during alpha-stat management, this left shift is thought to be offset by the increased plasma content of dissolved oxygen during hypothermia. Additionally, while there is a reduction in cerebral blood flow resulting from decreased $PaCO_2$, the blood flow is still considered adequate. This adequacy is attributed to the flow exceeding the reduced metabolic demands from hypothermia. Furthermore, since autoregulation is preserved during alpha-stat, the coupling between cerebral blood flow and metabolic demand is maintained.

pH-Stat Management

Total body CO_2 is increased in pH-stat management, which leads to cerebral vasodilation and consequent loss of cerebral autoregulation (i.e., uncoupling of cerebral blood flow and cerebral metabolic rate). pH-stat management is argued to facilitate faster, more homogenous brain cooling and improved oxygen delivery by counteracting the left shift in the oxyhemoglobin dissociation curve that occurs in alpha-stat management.

Normally, blood gas samples are warmed to 37 °C and results are reported as *temperature uncorrected* (i.e., one not corrected to the patient's temperature). To report *temperature-corrected* results (those at the patient's hypothermic temperature), the blood gas analyzer uses an algorithm. This algorithm determines what the results would be at the current patient temperature, considering known changes in gas solubility in a closed sample during hypothermia. For the perfusionist, pH-stat management involves maintaining a pH of 7.4 and pCO_2 of 40 mmHg at the patient's current hypothermic temperature. This is typically achieved by using a temperature-corrected blood gas result and adding CO_2 to the CPB sweep gas to counteract the hypothermia-induced alkalosis. In contrast, the alpha-stat strategy requires that the patient's acid–base status be appropriately alkalotic for the degree of hypothermia. This is accomplished using a temperature uncorrected blood gas result. If an appropriate degree of alkalosis is present in a hypothermic patient, then a blood sample warmed to 37 °C in the blood gas analyzer should have a pH of 7.4 and pCO_2 of 40 mmHg.

What is Better, Alpha-Stat or pH-Stat? Refer to Table 6.3.

Adults

In 1995, three randomized controlled trials demonstrated better postoperative neurological and neuropsychological

Table 6.3 Alpha-Stat vs. pH-Stat

Alpha-STAT	pH-STAT
Cerebral autoregulation maintained	Causes cerebral vasodilation above metabolic demands
Decreased embolic load to brain	Loss of cerebral autoregulation
Maintains transcellular membrane pH gradients	Increased cerebral blood flow, volume, and embolic load
Reaction kinetics of respiratory enzymes function best when body fluid pH parallels the pH of water as temperature changes	Faster, more homogenous, and complete cerebral cooling
Alkaline pH may be beneficial before the ischemic insult of circulatory arrest in DHCA	Increased cerebral O_2 delivery due to correcting pH avoids a left shift in the Oxy-Hb dissociation curve that occurs with increased pH

outcomes with alpha-stat management compared to pH-stat management in cases involving mild to moderate hypothermia. Although conflicting data have been presented since, many believe that any potential benefits of excessive cerebral blood flow during hypothermic CPB are outweighed by an increased risk of cerebral micro- and macro-embolic load in adults. Consequently, most institutions adopt an alpha-stat strategy for adults to maintain cerebral autoregulation and limit cerebral embolic load.

Pediatrics

It is generally believed that pH-stat management provides better myocardial and cerebral protection in neonatal and infant cardiac surgery; however, improved neurocognitive development has not been consistently associated with either strategy. After deep hypothermic cardiac arrest in pediatric populations, pH-stat management has been shown to provide positive cerebral outcomes with more preserved cerebral autoregulation after the surgical procedure. The embolic risk is also thought to be low in neonatal and infant cardiac surgery. In cyanotic neonates and infants, pH-stat management shifts more blood flow toward the cerebral circulation and away from possible sources of aortopulmonary steal, such as a patent ductus arteriosus or major aortopulmonary collateral arteries. One potential advantage of pH-stat over alpha-stat management is the possibility of a shorter period of cooling to achieve the target brain temperature. Some studies have indicated decreased peak postoperative troponin levels, reduced ventilator dependence, and shorter ICU stays with pH-stat versus alpha-stat management; however, a randomized controlled trial of over 100 neonates and infants revealed that neither strategy was consistently associated with improved neurodevelopmental outcome.

Temperature Monitoring

During CPB, monitoring cerebral temperature is vital due to rapid core and peripheral temperature changes. Common monitoring sites include the tympanic membrane, esophagus, nasopharynx, pulmonary artery, and jugular bulb (JB). JB is the gold standard for monitoring cerebral perfusion, but it depends on correct probe positioning and is frequently not used. Intermediate sites like bladder and rectal temperatures may lag and be influenced by additional factors such as urine production and stool burden, often underestimating brain temperature during rewarming. Post-CPB, bladder temperature serves as a reliable noninvasive core temperature indicator. While mean esophageal, nasopharyngeal, and pulmonary artery temperatures have correlated with brain temperature, actual temperature at these sites may vary considerably. Thus, concurrent monitoring of esophageal, nasopharyngeal, and pulmonary artery temperatures is recommended. Arterial outlet temperature is a good surrogate for cerebral perfusion during CPB, though it may not precisely reflect distal perfusate temperature and may underestimate cerebral perfusate during rewarming by up to 0.67 °C. Pulmonary artery temperature, despite potential distortions from surgical factors, is useful for weaning from bypass. For detailed information, please refer to Chap. 13, "Various Monitoring Techniques Used During CPB."

Guidelines for Cooling and Rewarming

During CPB cooling and rewarming, as discussed in the "Protective Mechanisms of Hypothermia" section, changes in the solubility of gases in liquids have significant implications. To avoid gas emboli formation, it is recommended to maintain a temperature gradient of ≤ 10 °C between the arterial outlet and venous inflow, and to keep the arterial outlet temperature below 37 °C to prevent hyperthermia.

Some studies have shown better neurocognitive outcomes with slower rewarming, possibly due to avoidance of cerebral hyperthermia and more homogenous cerebral temperatures. JB oxygen saturation has also been observed to decrease less with slow rewarming strategies. Additionally, one small study indicated improved cardiac index, decreased lactate levels, better hemostasis, and shorter ICU stays with slow rewarming.

However, the benefits of slower rewarming must be weighed against the deleterious effects of prolonged CPB and surgical times. Therefore, Class IIa recommendations suggest that when the arterial outlet temperature is <30 °C during rewarming, it is reasonable to maintain a maximum temperature gradient between the arterial outlet and venous inflow on the oxygenator of less than 10 °C. When the arterial outlet temperature exceeds 30 °C in preparation for separation from bypass, the temperature gradient between the venous inflow and arterial outlet on the oxygenator should be 4 °C or less, with the temperature increase limited to 0.5 °C per minute or less.

Due to conflicting evidence, there is no specific temperature recommended for separation from CPB. Considerations include the need to avoid cerebral hyperthermia while also attempting to minimize coagulopathy.

Pharmacology in Hypothermia

The effects of hypothermia on various pharmacological drugs are discussed in Chap. 4.

CPB and Pharmacology

Chapter 4 provides a detailed discussion on the principles of clinical pharmacology and the impact of CPB on drug metabolism, elimination, concentration, and action, with a particular focus on the pharmacokinetics and pharmacodynamics of drugs during CPB, including specific individual drugs used.

Systems and Organs Dysfunction in CPB

Fluid Balance Disruption

CPB significantly disrupts fluid homeostasis, causing substantial shifts of fluid into the interstitial space. This phenomenon arises from multiple factors. Increased systemic venous pressure pushes fluid out of the vessels, while volume and osmotic changes due to hemodilution and protein dilution decrease the vasculature's ability to retain fluid. Additionally, adsorption of proteins to the CPB circuit and inflammation-induced increased capillary permeability further contribute to fluid leakage.

Hemodilution

Patient's blood volume mixes with the pump prime at the commencement of CPB. That will lead to hemodilution. This hemodilution is linked to a greater need for intraoperative transfusions and reduced coagulation factors. Low plasma protein concentration, below 45% of baseline, can lead to increased blood product use and longer ICU stays. For in-depth details, see Chap. 9 "Prime Solutions for the circuit and Hemodilution Reduction Strategies."

Renal Dysfunction

Renal function is compromised by factors such as hemodilution, microemboli, catecholamines, low perfusion pressure, diuretics, hypothermia, and hemolysis. Renal dysfunction due to CPB is detailed separately.

CPB Effect on Endocrine Function

Cardiac surgery often triggers stress-induced hyperglycemia (>140 mg/dl) due to inflammation, altered humoral responses, hormone surges, and altered insulin signaling. This is especially common in nondiabetic patients with weak hearts or long CPB use. Hyperglycemia after CPB surgery is more prevalent compared to non-CPB cases, and worse with hypothermia. Importantly, hyperglycemia increases postoperative risk of infection and end-organ dysfunction, and difficult glycemic control contributes to perioperative complications and deaths. Thyroid hormone levels also significantly drop after the initiation of CPB and return to normal within 24 h after surgery. For in-depth details, see Chap. 12 "Metabolic Derangements During Cardiopulmonary Bypass."

CPB and Pulmonary Effects

Bypassing the lungs during CPB inherently risks abnormal physiological changes, with prolonged pump time increasing the likelihood of postoperative pulmonary dysfunction. CPB can lead to Pump Lung, a form of acute respiratory failure characterized by pulmonary edema. This occurs from lung inflammation triggered by ischemic-reperfusion with blood carrying inflammatory mediators, particularly C3a, C4a, and C5a, as well as neutrophil sequestration and degranulation in the pulmonary vessels. Activated alveolar macrophages, which release TNF-alpha, Interleukin (IL)-6, IL-8, and superoxide dismutase, also contribute. The result is increased capillary permeability, leading to pulmonary edema which is further exacerbated by fluid shifts. CPB also diminishes the efficacy of natural surfactants, contributing to pulmonary dysfunction alongside general anesthesia and sternotomy effects. It leads to increased shunting, reduced compliance, decreased functional residual volume, and can precipitate Acute Respiratory Distress Syndrome (ARDS).

To minimize the occurrence of Pump Lung, perfusionists employ various strategies, primarily aimed at minimizing hemodilution and the inflammatory response. These strategies include using biocompatible coated equipment, reducing prime volumes, and potentially using leukocyte-depleting filters. Maintaining colloid osmotic pressure (COP) during bypass is crucial, often achieved by adding albumin to the pump prime. This addition not only maintains COP but also coats the circuit to prevent platelet adhesion and activation. Additionally, managing pulmonary artery pressure is vital to prevent distention of the heart and pulmonary vasculature. Effective measures include appropriate left ventricular venting and temporary reduction in pump flows. During bypass termination, careful management is essential to avoid overfilling the heart and pulmonary vasculature.

CPB and Cardiac Impact

Cardiac function alterations due to CPB are detailed separately.

CPB and Hemostatic Dysfunction

Bleeding and thrombotic complications during CPB are linked to the activation of platelets, plasma proteins, and the interplay of protamine and heparin. Normal bleeding times post-CPB, even with full heparin reversal, take 4–12 h to stabilize. Complications like DIC, Heparin-Induced Thrombocytopenia (HIT), and Thrombosis (HITT) are notable concerns.

CPB and Neurological Complications

The primary neurological risk during CPB is stroke, mainly caused by emboli released during aortic cannulation and clamping. Additionally, cognitive dysfunction, sometimes referred to as "pump head," can also occur.

Gastrointestinal Issues

While peptic ulceration is often more of a stress response than directly related to CPB, conditions like pancreatitis and mild jaundice are common post-CPB. This jaundice may stem from hepatic injury, excessive bilirubin production due to blood transfusions, or blood trauma. Typically, it is self-limiting and resolves within a week. Additionally, CPB can increase gut mucosa permeability, potentially leading to endotoxin translocation and exacerbating the inflammatory response.

Further Reading

Aljure OD, Fabbro M. Cardiopulmonary bypass and inflammation: the hidden enemy. J Cardiothorac Vasc Anesth. 2019;33:346–7.

Ballotta A, Saleh HZ, El Baghdady HW, et al. Comparison of early platelet activation in patients undergoing on-pump versus off-pump coronary artery bypass surgery. J Thorac Cardiovasc Surg. 2007;134:132–8.

Bartels K, Zakkar M. Imflammatory response to cardiopulmonary bypass. In: Gravlee GP, Davis RF, Hammon JW, Kussman B, editors. Cardiopulmonary bypass and mechanical support: principles & practice. 4th ed. Wolters Kluwer; 2016. p. 357–67.

Conlon JM. Bradykinin Peptides. Handb Biol Act Pept. 2013:321–5.

Davies LK, Reed H. Temperature management in cardiac surgery. In: Gravlee GP, Davis RF, Hammon JW, Kussman B, editors. Cardiopulmonary bypass and mechanical support: principles & practice. 4th ed. Philadelphia: Wolters Kluwer; 2016. p. 157–74.

Day JRS, Taylor KM. The systemic inflammatory response syndrome and cardiopulmonary bypass. Int J Surg. 2005;3:129–40.

Doenst T, Wijeysundera D, Karkouti K, Zechner C, Maganti M, Rao V, Borger MA. Hyperglycemia during cardiopulmonary bypass is an independent risk factor for mortality in patients undergoing cardiac surgery. J Thorac Cardiovasc Surg. 2005;130:1144.e1–8.

Engelman R, Baker RA, Likosky DS, Grigore A, Dickinson TA, Shore-Lesserson L, Hammon JW. The Society of Thoracic Surgeons, the Society of Cardiovascular Anesthesiologists, and the American Society of ExtraCorporeal Technology: clinical practice guidelines for cardiopulmonary bypass – temperature management during cardiopulmonary bypass. Ann Thorac Surg. 2015;100:748–57.

Englum BR, Andersen ND, Husain AM, Mathew JP, Hughes GC. Degree of hypothermia in aortic arch surgery – optimal temperature for cerebral and spinal protection: deep hypothermia remains the gold standard in the absence of randomized data. Ann Cardiothorac Surg. 2013;2:184–93.

Esper SA, Subramaniam K, Tanaka KA. Pathophysiology of cardiopulmonary bypass: current strategies for the prevention and treatment of anemia, coagulopathy, and organ dysfunction. Semin Cardiothorac Vasc Anesth. 2014;18:161–76.

Gravlee GP, Davis RF, Hammon JW, Kussman B. Cardiopulmonary bypass and mechanical support: principles and practice. 4th ed. TA – TT; 2016. https://worldcat.org/title/953604603

Gu YJ, van Oeveren W, Akkerman C, Boonstra PW, Huyzen RJ, Wildevuur CRH. Heparin-coated circuits reduce the inflammatory response to cardiopulmonary bypass. Ann Thorac Surg. 1993;55:917–22.

Hastings LA, Heitmiller ES, Nyhan D. Chapter 19 – Perioperative monitoring. In: Nichols DG, Ungerleider RM, Spevak PJ, Greeley WJ, Cameron DE, Lappe DG, Wetzel RC, editors. Critical heart disease in infants and children. 2nd ed. Philadelphia: Mosby; 2006a. p. 479–506.

Hastings LA, Heitmiller ES, Nyhan D. Chapter 19 – Perioperative monitoring. In: Nichols DG, Ungerleider RM, Spevak PJ, Greeley WJ, Cameron DE, Lappe DG, Wetzel RC, editors. Critical heart disease in infants and children. 2nd ed. Philadelphia: Mosby; 2006b. p. 479–506.

Hori D, Nomura Y, Ono M, Joshi B, Mandal K, Cameron D, Kocherginsky M, Hogue CW. Optimal blood pressure during cardiopulmonary bypass defined by cerebral autoregulation monitoring. J Thorac Cardiovasc Surg. 2017;154:1590–1598.e2.

Joshi B, Ono M, Brown C, Brady K, Easley RB, Yenokyan G, Gottesman RF, Hogue CW. Predicting the limits of cerebral autoregulation during cardiopulmonary bypass. Anesth Analg. 2012;114:503–10.

Jukema BN, de Maat S, Maas C. Processing of factor XII during inflammatory reactions. Front Med. 2016;3:1–7.

Kats S, Schönberger JPAM, Brands R, Seinen W, van Oeveren W. Endotoxin release in cardiac surgery with cardiopulmonary bypass: pathophysiology and possible therapeutic strategies. An update. Eur J Cardio-thoracic Surg. 2011;39:451–8.

Kefalogianni R, Kamani F, Gaspar M, Aw T, Donovan J, Laffan M, Pickering MC, Arachchillage DJ. Complement activation during cardiopulmonary bypass and association with clinical outcomes. eJHaem. 2022;3:86–96.

Kenne E, Nickel KF, Long AT, Fuchs TA, Stavrou EX, Stahl FR, Renné T. Factor XII: a novel target for safe prevention of thrombosis and inflammation. J Intern Med. 2015;278:571–85.

Klemperer JD, Klein I, Gomez M, Helm RE, Ojamaa K, Thomas SJ, Isom OW, Krieger K. Thyroid hormone treatment after coronary-artery bypass surgery. N Engl J Med. 1995;333:1522–7.

Levy JH, Tanaka KA. Inflammatory response to cardiopulmonary bypass. Ann Thorac Surg. 2003;75:S715. https://doi.org/10.1016/S0003-4975(02)04701-X.

Lichtenstein SV, Ashe KA, El Dalati H, Cusimano RJ, Panos A, Slutsky AS. Warm heart surgery. J Thorac Cardiovasc Surg. 1991;101:269–74.

Maillet F, Kazatchkine MD, Glotz D, Fischer E, Rowe M. Heparin prevents formation of the human C3 amplification convertase by inhibiting the binding site for B on C3b. Mol Immunol. 1983;20:1401–4.

McGuinness J, Bouchier-Hayes D, Redmond JM. Understanding the inflammatory response to cardiac surgery. Surgeon. 2008;6:162–71.

Michelson AD. Platelets. In: Elsevier science and technology books. 3rd ed. TA – TT; 2013. https://worldcat.org/title/828485716.

Moraes LA, Barrett NE, Jones CI, Holbrook LM, Spyridon M, Sage T, Newman DK, Gibbins JM. Platelet endothelial cell adhesion molecule-1 regulates collagen-stimulated platelet function by modulating the association of phosphatidylinositol 3-kinase with Grb-2-associated binding protein-1 and linker for activation of T cells. J Thromb Haemost. 2010;8:2530–41.

Muzic DS, Anesthesia C, Chaney MA. What's new with alpha-stat versus. Soc Cardiovasc Anesthesiol. 2006:2005–7.

Nussmeier NA. Management of temperature during and after cardiac surgery. Texas Heart Inst J. 2005;32:472–6.

Paparella D, Yau TM, Young E. Cardiopulmonary bypass induced inflammation: pathophysiology and treatment. An update. Eur J Cardio-thoracic Surg. 2002;21:232–44.

Rassias AJ. Intraoperative management of hyperglycemia in the cardiac surgical patient. Semin Thorac Cardiovasc Surg. 2006;18:330–8.

Roberts A, Duncan EC, Hargrave P, Kingery DR, Barnes J, Horstemeyer DL, Stahl RF. Complications of cardiopulmonary bypass from an Anesthesia perspective: a clinical review. HCA Healthc J Med. 2023;4:13–21.

Saad H, Aladawy M. Review article temperature management in cardiac surgery. Qatar Found J. 2013:45–62.

Stone GJ, Young WL, Smith CR, Solomon RA, Wald A, Ostapkovich N, Shrebnick DB. Do standard monitoring sites reflect true brain temperature when profound hypothermia is rapidly induced and reversed? Anesthesiology. 1995;82:344–51.

Taggart DP, Sundaram S, McCartney C, Bowman A, McIntyre H, Courtney JM, Wheatley DJ. Endotoxemia, complement, and white blood cell activation in cardiac surgery: a randomized trial of laxatives and pulsatile perfusion. Ann Thorac Surg. 1994;57:376–82.

Thiessen S, Vanhorebeek I, Van Den Berghe G. Glycemic control and outcome related to cardiopulmonary bypass. Best Pract Res Clin Anaesthesiol. 2015;29:177–87.

Tveita T, Sieck GC. Physiological impact of hypothermia: the good, the bad, and the ugly. Physiology. 2022;37:69–87.

Wahba A, Milojevic M, Boer C, et al. 2019 EACTS/EACTA/EBCP guidelines on cardiopulmonary bypass in adult cardiac surgery. Eur J Cardio-thoracic Surg. 2020;57:210. https://doi.org/10.1093/ejcts/ezz267.

Warltier DC, Laffey JG, Boylan JF, Cheng DCH. The systemic inflammatory response to cardiac surgery. Anesthesiology. 2002;97:215–52.

Warren OJ, Smith AJ, Alexiou C, Rogers PLB, Jawad N, Vincent C, Darzi AW, Athanasiou T. The inflammatory response to cardiopulmonary bypass: Part 1-Mechanisms of pathogenesis. J Cardiothorac Vasc Anesth. 2009;23:223–31.

Wu Y. Contact pathway of coagulation and inflammation. Thromb J. 2015;13:17. https://doi.org/10.1186/s12959-015-0048-y.

7 Fundamentals of Cardiopulmonary Bypass Machine Equipment

Kenneth John, Alex M. Chappell, Martin Kolodziejczak, and Andrew Maslow

Introduction

In 1935, Dr. John Gibbon designed a machine that could maintain a cat's life for 26 min. After modifications and innovations, the first person underwent successful open-heart surgery on May 6, 1953, during which the patient's cardiopulmonary functions were totally supported for 26 minutes. For more on the history of cardiopulmonary bypass (CPB) development, please refer to Chap. 5, "An Overview of Cardiopulmonary Bypass's Historic Development."

Since this time, there has been extensive research and innovation to improve the design, function, and application of the CPB machine. As discussed throughout this book, the CPB machine (Figs. 7.1 and 7.2), which bypasses the heart and lungs, impacts and activates multiple physiological systems. Although it is mainly used to facilitate cardiac surgical procedures, the CPB machine has been applied for surgeries on the lungs, liver, and brain. In addition, in the 1970s, case reports using CPB in nonsurgical patients over longer periods were the precursor to modern-day Extracorporeal Membrane Oxygenators (ECMO). Though CPB machine has evolved significantly over the last 70 years, the fundamental concepts remain the same.

In its most basic form, the CPB machine pulls blood from the patient prior to the pulmonary circulation, most often from the venous vasculature or the right side of the heart. It then drains the blood into a closed or open reservoir, filters it, ventilates and oxygenates it, warms or cools it, and returns it to the patient's arterial vasculature beyond the heart and lungs. In doing so, the CPB machine takes over the basic functions of the heart and lungs. Not only does the CPB machine sustain cardiopulmonary and vascular functions, but during cardiac surgery, it also through the infusion of cardioplegia provides the surgeon with a bloodless, motionless field to facilitate the surgical procedure.

It is imperative that those caring for cardiac surgical patients understand the functions and physiological impacts of the CPB machine. To achieve this, one must grasp the basic concepts and components of the CPB machine. The following chapter reviews the main or vital components of the CPB machine (Fig. 7.3).

K. John
Department of Anesthesiology and Critical Care Medicine, University of Florida College of Medicine, UF Health Shands Hospital, Gainesville, FL, USA
e-mail: kjohn2@anest.ufl.edu

A. M. Chappell
Cardiac Surgery Division, Department of Surgery, Children's Hospital of Philadelphia, Philadelphia, PA, USA
e-mail: achappell@keystoneperfusion.com

M. Kolodziejczak
Cardiac Surgery Division, Department of Surgery, Brown University, Providence, RI, USA

A. Maslow (✉)
Department of Anesthesiology & Perioperative Medicine, Brown University, Providence, RI, USA

A. S. Awad, J. DiNardo (eds.), *Clinical Perfusion for Cardiac Surgery*, https://doi.org/10.1007/978-3-031-91163-7_7

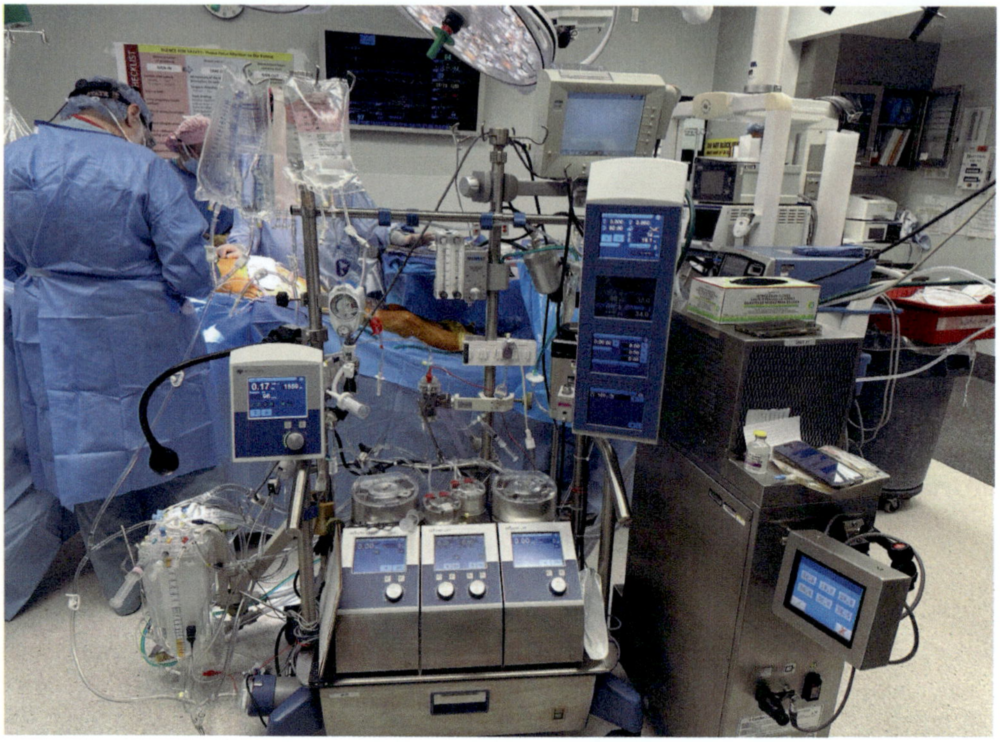

Fig. 7.1 This image displays a frontal view showcasing the readiness of fully set up cardiopulmonary bypass machines, primed and prepared for cardiac surgery procedure

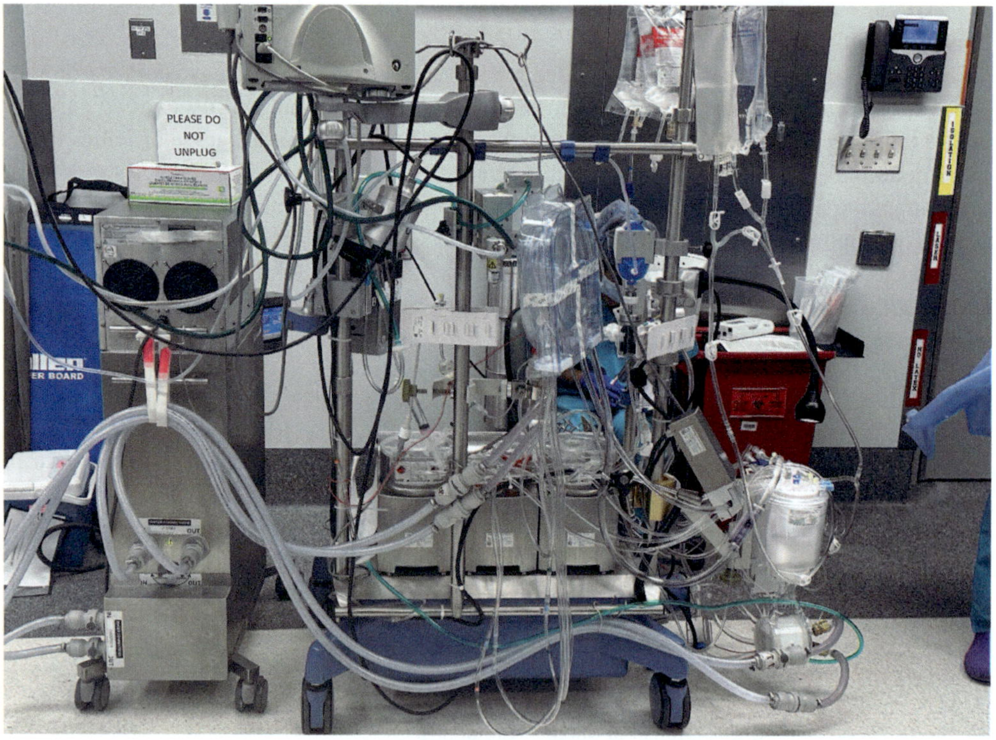

Fig. 7.2 An image displaying a back view of fully equipped cardiopulmonary bypass machines, meticulously set up, primed, and ready to facilitate cardiac surgery procedure

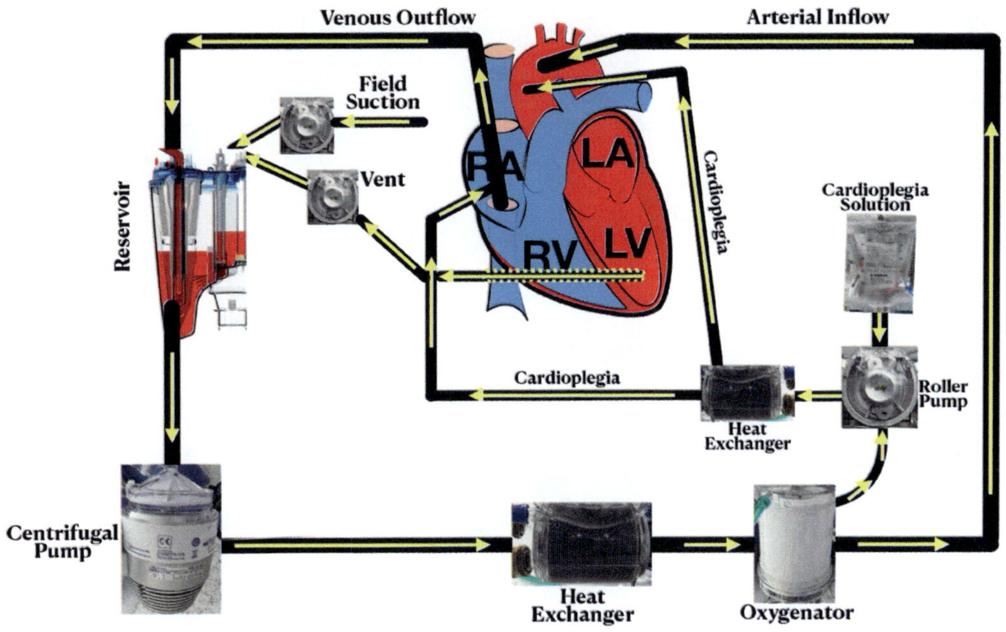

Fig. 7.3 This illustration shows a simplified CPB Machine and Circuit, depicting the key components and flow of blood during bypass surgery. The diagram highlights essential parts such as the oxygenator, arterial pump, venous reservoir, heat exchanger, and filters, all working together to maintain circulation and oxygenation, while the heart is stopped during surgery

The Cardiopulmonary Bypass Machine and Circuit

Deoxygenated blood (venous return) is removed from the body via one or two cannulae and passed into a reservoir of the CPB machine. Pumps then help drive the blood forward. Blood passes across a membrane/oxygenator/heat exchanger to exchange carbon dioxide for oxygen and to control temperature of the passing blood. Oxygenated blood is then returned to the patient via arterial cannulae, most often placed in the proximal aorta root a few centimeters distal to the aortic valve. Alternatively, the aortic cannula may be advanced to a more distal position or inserted in another portion of the aorta. Within this pathway, there may be air detectors, filters, and a temperature regulator.

While the machine itself is not disposable, the CPB circuit is replaced for each case. In between each case, the machine is cleaned and cared for according to guidelines. The Perfusionist and Bio-Medical staff ensure that equipment is used and maintained according to guidelines and in accordance with the manufacturer's specifications. This includes cleaning, disinfecting, and maintaining a properly functioning device between cases. The circuit, which includes internal surfaces that come into contact with the patient's blood, is therefore replaced between each case.

The bypass circuit is set up specifically for each case and can be tailored to the specific patient. The circuit is built with aseptic technique, preventing any opportunity for contamination. In adults, this task is easier as the bypass circuit generally remains the same regardless of the case or the patient. In pediatrics, however, the circuit lengths, tubing sizes, oxygenator sizes, and use of hemoconcentrators can vary from case to case, so the circuit is often built for the specific patient or case. Though it varies between institutions, research has shown dry, set up circuits maintain their sterility up to 60 days, while wet open circuits remain sterile for 5 days, and closed wet circuits remain sterile for up to 6 weeks.

Schematic of the CPB machine and circuit, as well as an actual CPB machine setup, can be referred to throughout the chapter as the components of the machine and circuit are discussed.

Pumps

The pump motor is the driving force of blood during CPB. It acts as the "heart" of the CPB machine, generating a gradient to move blood from its inlet to its outlet. The main systemic pump creates a pressure gradient to move blood from the reservoir toward the heat exchanger, the oxygenator, and finally to the arterial inflow cannula. There are two different types of pumps used in a CPB machine: a roller pump and a centrifugal pump.

Roller Pump

A roller pump, or a displacement pump, uses a peristaltic motion to generate flow by mechanically compressing the bypass circuit, thereby forcing blood/fluid forward (Fig. 7.4). Within the housing, two rotating arms are positioned 180 degrees from each other. These rotating arms compress, or occlude, the tubing filled with blood, forcing blood forward through the tubing i.e., positive displacement, creating flow. The more the tubing is compressed, the more blood that is

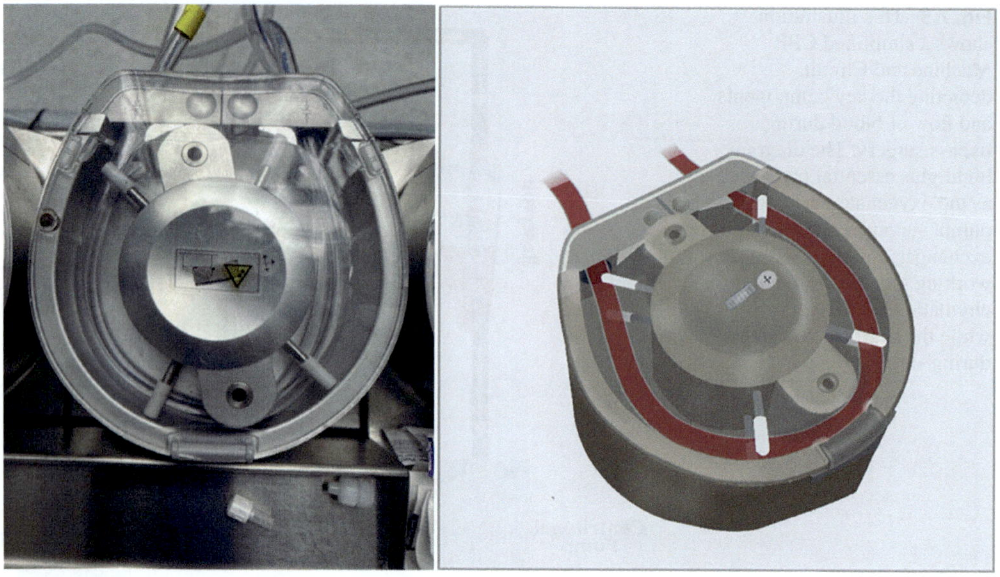

Fig. 7.4 Actual photo from the top of a roller pump ready for use (Left); on the right, detailed illustration of a roller pump

pulled or pushed through. However, excessive compression can cause trauma to the blood, leading to hemolysis, and spallation. Roller pumps can be used as the systemic pump as well as for generating flow in vents, suckers, cardioplegia and for a hemoconcentrator in the pediatric population. Depending on the patient population, patient size, and needs, the roller pump may be preferred.

Systemic roller pumps are widely used in the pediatric population. Their ability to deliver precise amounts of flows, while avoiding retrograde flows, allows the perfusionist to accurately deliver blood flows, such as 0.4 L/min. Additionally, the size of the tubing can be adjusted to tailor to the perfusionist's flow goals. The flow rate (Q) through a roller pump is determined by an equation that incorporates the pump's operational characteristics and the physical dimensions of the tubing. The equation is as follows:

$$Q = \pi \times (D/2)^2 \times (\text{RPM})$$

where

- Q is the flow rate, typically measured in liters per minute (L/min),
- π is the mathematical constant, approximately 3.14159,
- D is the internal diameter of the tubing, measured in meters,
- revolutions per minute (RPM) represents the revolutions per minute of the roller head.

This formula calculates the volume of blood moved per unit of time by considering the cross-sectional area of the tubing (derived from its diameter) and the speed at which the pump operates (RPM). The precision of roller pumps, coupled with the ability to select tubing of various diameters, provides perfusionists with a versatile tool for managing the circulatory needs of pediatric patients during cardiopulmonary bypass procedures.

While lower flows are easier to achieve with roller pumps, achieving larger flows can be more challenging. Roller pumps are less commonly used as systemic pumps in the adult population. As the internal diameter of the tubing increases, so does the prime volume of the boot (tubing in the raceway). Based on the configuration of the pumps, oxygenator, and reservoir, the length of the boot often results in a prime volume larger than that of a centrifugal configuration.

While most bypass cases run between 1 and 6 h on bypass, roller pumps are still used in longer scenarios, such as pediatric ECMO. ECMO runs could last from days to weeks, and during these prolonged runs, the durability of the tubing must be considered. Spallation is a side effect that occurs when tubing spends a prolonged amount of time in a roller pump. It is defined as the mechanical stress put on the tubing by repeated compression, leading to the deterioration of the tubing and the production of microparticles. Eventually, this deterioration can lead to a rupture of the tubing if it remains in the raceway too long. To combat spallation, different types of tubing can be used. Polyvinyl chloride (PVC) is the most common material of bypass tubing, and for short bypass runs, PVC is also used in the boot. For long ECMO runs, more durable tubing such as Super Tygon is the preferred tubing of use.

Centrifugal Pump

Centrifugal pumps are designed with a vaned impeller, typically made from biocompatible materials, encased in a durable shell. The impeller is magnetically coupled to an electric motor, enabling it to spin rapidly (Fig. 7.5). This action gen-

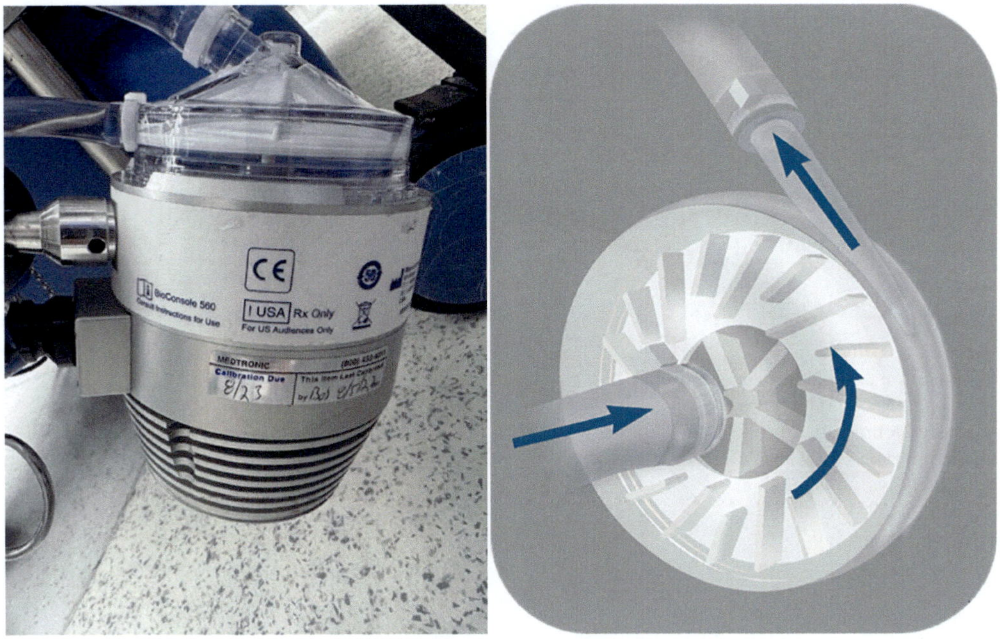

Fig. 7.5 Photo of centrifugal pump (Left) with attached pump head: On the right, an illustration of the pump head details the flow of operation, with arrows indicating the direction of the blood inlet from the venous reservoir (entering from the left in the center of the pump head) and the outlet towards the oxygenator (exiting to the top right)

erates centrifugal force, which converts to kinetic energy, thereby creating a pressure gradient that facilitates flow. Upon activation, the motor's speed, controlled by RPM, can be adjusted by the perfusionist to achieve the desired flow rate. The generated centrifugal propels blood from areas of higher pressure to lower or negative pressure regions.

Centrifugal pumps are recognized for their non-occlusive and non-compressive nature, which renders them less harmful to blood cells due to their pulseless flow.

Centrifugal pumps are entirely dependent on preload and afterload. The pump will only flow as much as it receives in preload. During CPB with an open reservoir, as long as there is blood in the reservoir, the pump should have adequate preload. Unlike the roller pump, the centrifugal pump is sensitive to afterload—the force that the pump must overcome. Contributors to afterload include patient's systemic arterial pressure or systemic vascular resistance and the resistance within the bypass circuit. This is determined by the length and width of the tubing, as well as the resistance created by the oxygenator and filters. At a set RPM, flow will decrease as afterload increases and vice versa.

There are a number of centrifugal pumps that vary depending on the anticipated duration extracorporeal support (ECMO; VADs). For longer use, pumps are designed to reduce heat, clot formation, and hemolysis. These pumps are often much more expensive than the centrifugal pumps build for short-term support or intraoperatively during CPB.

Both roller and centrifugal pumps can generate adequate flow, with no reported difference in hemolysis between the two. While both types of pumps can generate up to 7 L/min flow against an afterload pressure of 500 mmHg, the centrifugal pump is sensitive to afterload and will not pump against extreme resistance. By contrast, the roller pump will continue to pump regardless of resistance. Bypass machines may incorporate both such as centrifugal pumps may be used as the systemic pump to generate flow from the venous to the arterial side, while roller pumps may be used to deliver cardioplegia and for suction/aspiration.

The Cardioplegia Delivery System

Performing surgery on the cardiac system is more effectively facilitated by making the heart motionless. The cardioplegia delivery system serves a dual role: it not only induces a temporary cessation of cardiac activity but also offers protection and preservation to the myocardial cells. The delivery of cardioplegia involves a dedicated system, including a roller pump, cardioplegia line, pressure monitoring transducer, and heat exchanger (see Fig. 7.6). This system is integrated into CPB circuits. The system comprises several essential components.

Roller Pump A pump is essential for delivering cardioplegia to the heart, more specifically through coronary arteries, conduits, and/or the coronary sinus, which may have an internal diameter as small as 1–2 mm. To accommodate the delivery of cardioplegia through smaller tubing into these small vessels, tubing often required is 1/8 inch in diameter. Roller pumps enable finer adjustment of flow rates to accommodate the various ranges of cardioplegia: blood ratios (from 1:4 to 4:1). The structure and design of the roller pump have been discussed previously.

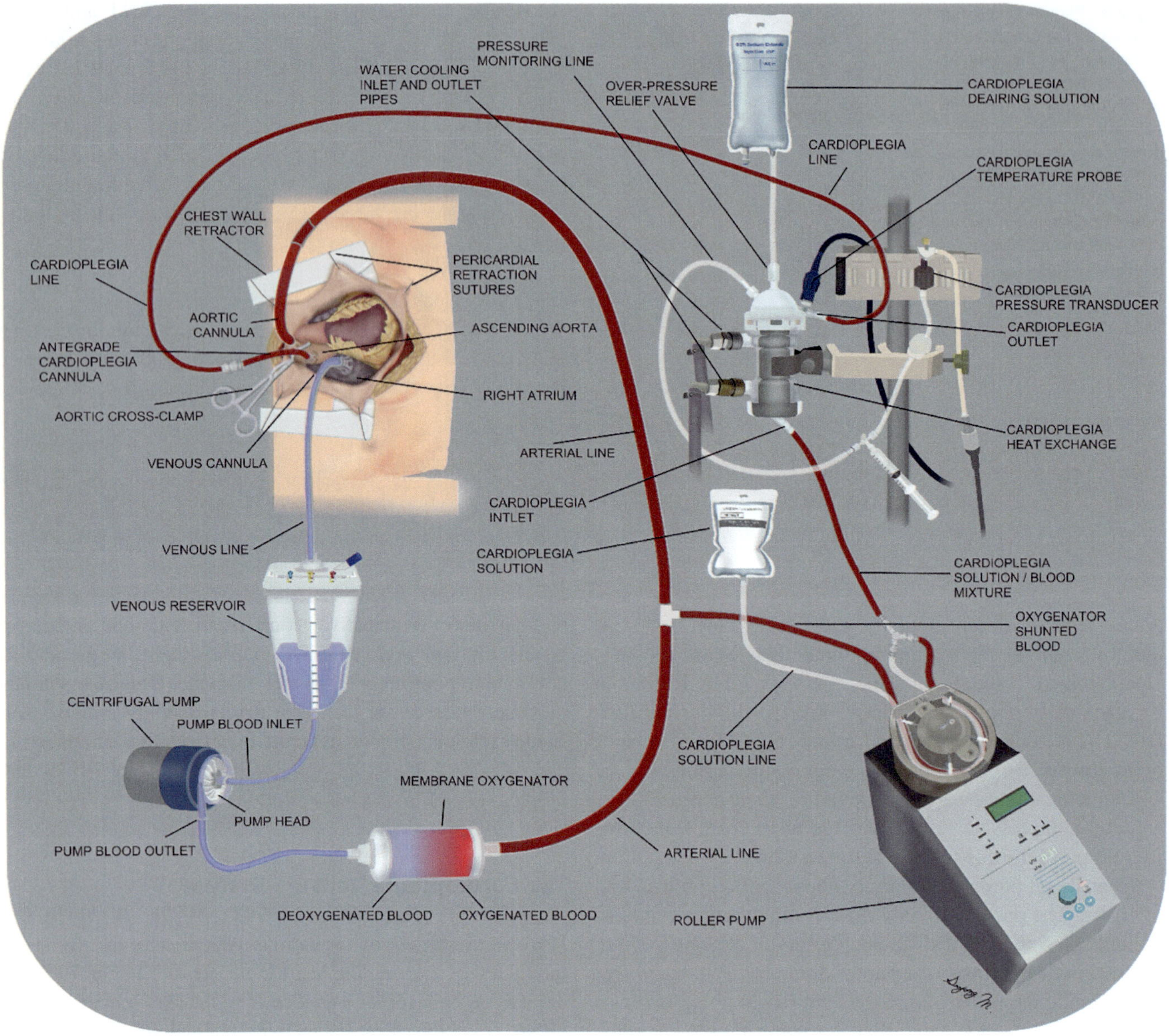

Fig. 7.6 This illustration displays the cardioplegia delivery system, highlighting key components integrated within CPB circuits. These include the roller pump, heat exchanger, the mixing of the cardioplegia solution with shunted blood from the oxygenator, the cardioplegia line, and the delivery cannula

Mixing Lines Here, the cardioplegia solution can be mixed with oxygenated blood shunted from the oxygenator.

Heat Exchanger Vital for adjusting the cardioplegia solution's temperature, the heat exchanger cools the solution to 4 °C after passing through the roller head, reducing the heart's metabolic demands during arrest or warming it to prepare for reactivation, thereby slowing O_2 consumption.

Cardioplegia Line From the heat exchanger, the temperature-adjusted cold cardioplegic solution is transported to the patient and delivered to the aortic root, coronary sinus, or directly to the coronary ostia, ensuring a smooth and uninterrupted flow.

Delivery Cannulae The final pieces of the system, the delivery cannulae, are meticulously selected and inserted to precisely administer the cardioplegia solution to the myocardium. Their sizes are crucial, influencing both pressure drop and maximum flow, with the selection typically tailored to the patient's requirements and surgeon's preference. There are three main routes for administering cardioplegia via these specialized cannulae.

- *Antegrade*: Antegrade cardioplegia delivers the cardioplegia solution directly into the aortic root, proximal to both the aortic cross-clamp and the aortic inflow cannula. A competent aortic valve alongside the aortic cross-clamp ensures that flow is blocked in both directions. This ensures all the cardioplegia solution exclusively is directed into the coronary arteries, maximizing myocardial protection. These cannulae are available in a variety of shapes and sizes, from simple slotted needles to more specialized designs like the dual-lumen aortic root cannula with a vent line or an extra arm for aortic root venting.
- *Direct Coronary Ostial*: Ostial cardioplegia is a technique that administers the solution directly into the coronary arteries, initiated after an incision is made and the aorta is opened. This method utilizes specialized coronary cannulae, each designed specifically for this precise task. The cannulae come in a wide range of designs and sizes, with each configuration tailored to different surgical needs. These handheld cannulae are prized for their maneuverability and are equipped with soft, malleable tips to ensure gentle and precise engagement with the coronary ostia. The most commonly used types of ostial perfusion cannulae include those with a balloon tip, ensuring a secure seal with the coronary ostium, and those with a basket tip and flange, providing effective delivery and secure placement within the coronary system.
- *Retrograde*: This method is commonly used in cases of an incompetent aortic valve or high-grade obstructive coronary artery disease that prevents effective myocardial protection. Retrograde cannulae, specialized devices for accessing the coronary sinus via the right atrium, are crucial for this approach. Once accurately positioned, sometimes with the guidance of echocardiography, a balloon near the cannula's tip is inflated to form a seal. This prevents the cardioplegic solution from leaking back into the right atrium. Such a setup allows the solution to flow retrogradely—against the normal direction of blood flow—through the heart's coronary venous system, effectively saturating the myocardium. There are two primary types of retrograde cannulae: one with a self-inflating balloon, simplifying the procedure for the surgical team, and another with a manually inflated balloon, providing more control and flexibility in certain scenarios.

Cardioplegia is given right after the aortic cross-clamp is applied, serving to both arrest the heart and cool it. This effect is achieved by delivering a high potassium solution (8–20 mEq/L), made up of a 4:1 mixture of crystalloid and blood, using the routes and cannulae discussed above.

The high potassium solution induces cardiac arrest by stopping the heart in diastole, i.e., when the myocardium is relaxed. Cardioplegia may be administered cold or at body temperature, with the cold approach commonly used to facilitate cardiac arrest while reducing myocardial metabolism and oxygen needs. The makeup of cardioplegia varies, but all formulations consist of the basic components:

1. High potassium (15–35 meq/L).
2. Electrolytes including Mg^{2+}, Ca^{2+}, Cl^-, Na^+.
3. Acid-base buffer to bind H^+ ions and reduce myocardial acidosis.
4. Dextrose and phosphate to provide nutrients to cardiomyocytes.
5. Mannitol to reduce myocardial cellular and tissue edema.

Please refer to Chap. 27 "Strategies of Myocardial protection During CPB" for more information.

Vent Pumps

Vents are used by surgeons to remove blood and/or air from specific parts of the heart, as well as to prevent chamber distention. Right ventricular distention can be managed by increasing venous return. However, left ventricle (LV) distention requires a vent. Left heart vents are most often inserted through the right upper pulmonary vein, so that the tip of the vent sits in the left atrium or LV (Fig. 7.7).

Alternatively, the antegrade cardioplegia delivery cannula, which rests in the aortic root, can be reversed and used as a vent (Fig. 7.8). Venting from the aortic root can be accom-

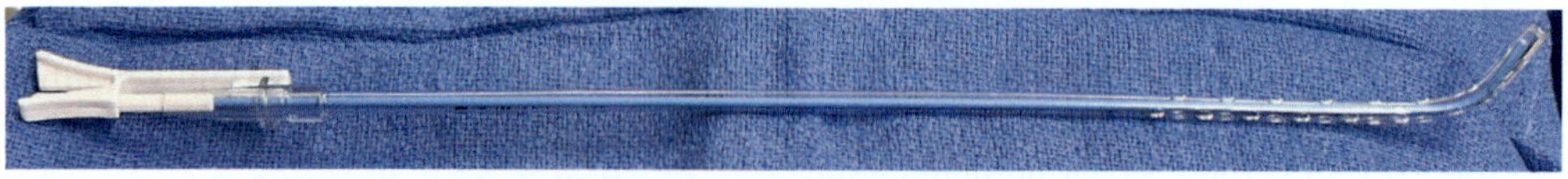

Fig. 7.7 This image displays an example of the left heart vent catheter, typically introduced via the right upper pulmonary vein

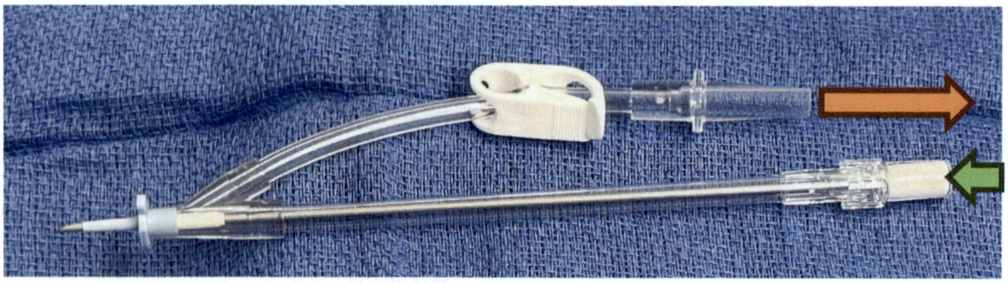

Fig. 7.8 Demonstrates a Y-shaped antegrade cardioplegia delivery cannula, designed for administering cardioplegia into the aortic root through its straight limb, while the system is secured with a white clamp. The green arrow indicates the direction of cardioplegia flow for myocardial preservation. Conversely, when the device functions as a vent, the cardioplegia line is clamped, the white clamp is opened, and suction is applied to the vent limb, as depicted by the orange arrow, illustrating the removal of blood and air from the aortic root

plished via a 14-gauge catheter placed proximal to the aortic cross-clamp and distal to a normally functioning aortic valve.

In some pediatric cases, an abnormal amount of collateral circulation may prevent the left side of the heart from being fully emptied, necessitating a vent in the left atrium. Valve surgery on the left side of the heart would require both an aortic root vent and a LV vent to both keep blood out of the surgeon's field of vision and to help de-air the heart while it is being closed. Coronary surgeries often require a root vent to help prevent blood from traveling down the coronary arteries into the anastomosis where the surgeon is sewing.

Vents are controlled by roller pumps, which pull the air and blood from the specified locations of the heart then push that blood back to the cardiotomy reservoir. Most CPB machines have one to two designated pumps for vents. The tubing inserted into vent pumps can range anywhere from 1/8 inch to 3/8 inch in diameter. The larger the tubing, the faster blood can be pulled from the heart. Of course, the size of the vent inserted into the heart itself is an additional limiting factor. The sizes of the vents themselves can range from 10 to 18 French. It is imperative that the tubing is inserted into the raceway so that the blood travels away from the heart. If inserted backwards, the pump could push air into the heart, leading to catastrophic air embolisms. To help prevent such events, one-way valves are included in vent tubing.

Sucker Pumps

Suckers are used during cardiac surgery to prevent excess blood loss away from the CPB machine. During surgery, the surgeon and assistants use suckers to direct any spilled blood in the surgical field away from the area of repair. Instead of wasting this blood, it is directed back to the cardiotomy reservoir, similar to the blood from the vents. Sucker pumps (Fig. 7.9) are also always roller pumps. Most CPB machines will have one to two designated pumps for suckers. Just like with vents, the tubing inserted into suckers also can range from 1/8 inch to 3/8 inch. This tubing often has a one-way valve for instances that it's used as an additional vent.

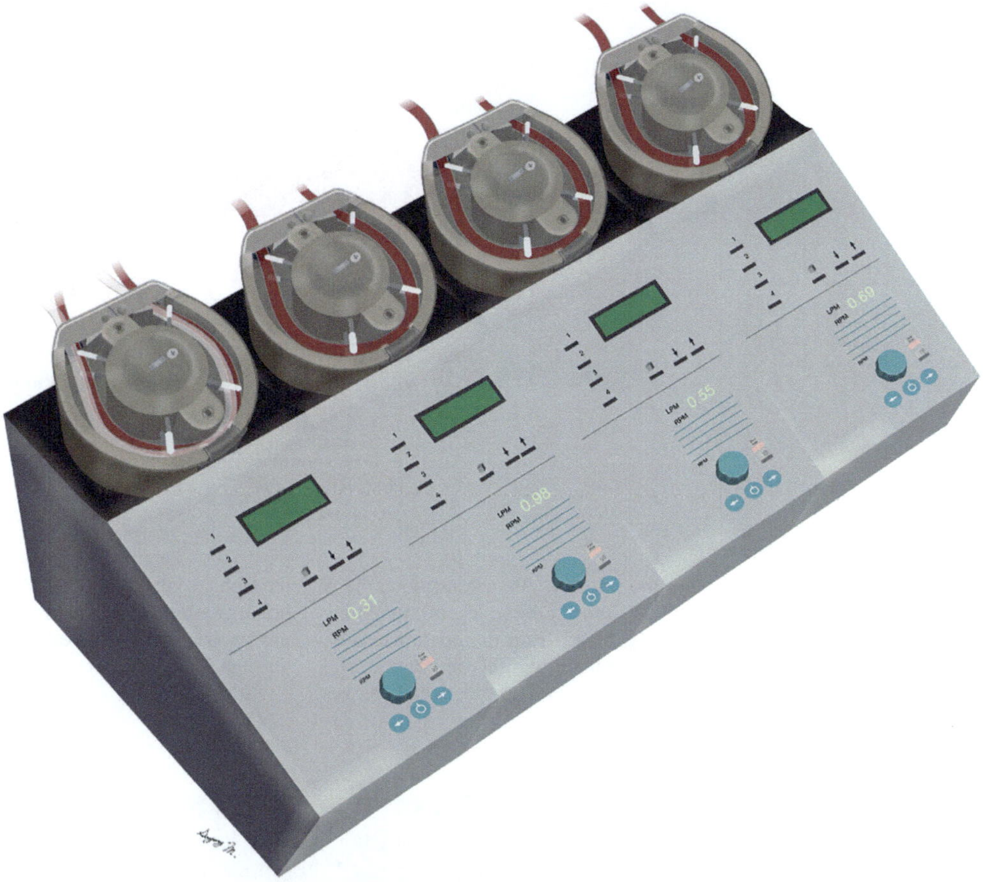

Fig. 7.9 Illustration of a CPB machine featuring four roller pumps: the leftmost roller pump is designated for cardioplegia delivery, ensuring precise administration of the cardioplegia solution, while the other three pumps are dedicated to vents and suckers

General Passage of Blood

The primary CPB circuit consists of several key components aligned in a specific order to facilitate blood circulation outside the body during cardiac surgery. Initially, blood is drawn from the right heart via a venous cannula, passing into a venous reservoir through wide-bore tubing. Simultaneously, blood collected from surgical suction, spilled in the surgical field, and from an active vent, is directed into the cardiotomy reservoir. This blood is then filtered before being combined with the venous blood in the venous reservoir. Subsequently, blood moves through a tube that passes through the main pump, which may be either a centrifugal or a roller pump. The main pump is essential for increasing both the flow and pressure of the blood as it advances to the arterial segment of the circuit. From there, the blood may pass through a heat exchanger and an oxygenator for gas exchange, essentially taking the place of the lungs. Finally, after oxygenation and temperature adjustment, the blood is routed through a smaller arterial tube and reintroduced into the patient's circulatory system via an arterial cannula positioned in the proximal aorta (Fig. 7.10).

Design and Tubing of the Bypass Circuit

The selection of tubing for the bypass circuit is crucial, as it must possess a wide enough diameter to support high blood flow rates without introducing undue resistance, which could lead to elevated pressures. The tubing and connectors used in the lines must be designed to withstand high internal pressures. The tubing comes in a sterile package delivered to the surgical area (Fig. 7.11). It is then uncoiled, and one end is passed across the field to the perfusionist, who assembles the circuit. This package includes a coil of tubing with large arterial and venous lines, along with four smaller diameter lines for the vent, cardioplegia, and suction devices. Each line is color-coded for easy identification: blue and red for the venous and arterial lines, respectively, and green, white, and orange for the vent and suction lines. The venous line typically consists of 1/2-inch internal diameter polyvinylchloride tubing (PVC), although certain circuits use 3/8-inch tubing, extending 4–6 feet in length. Continuous monitoring of mixed venous blood oxygen saturation is crucial. The in-line monitor for venous oxygen saturation, which provides accurate readings of venous SO2, Hct, and Hgb, should be

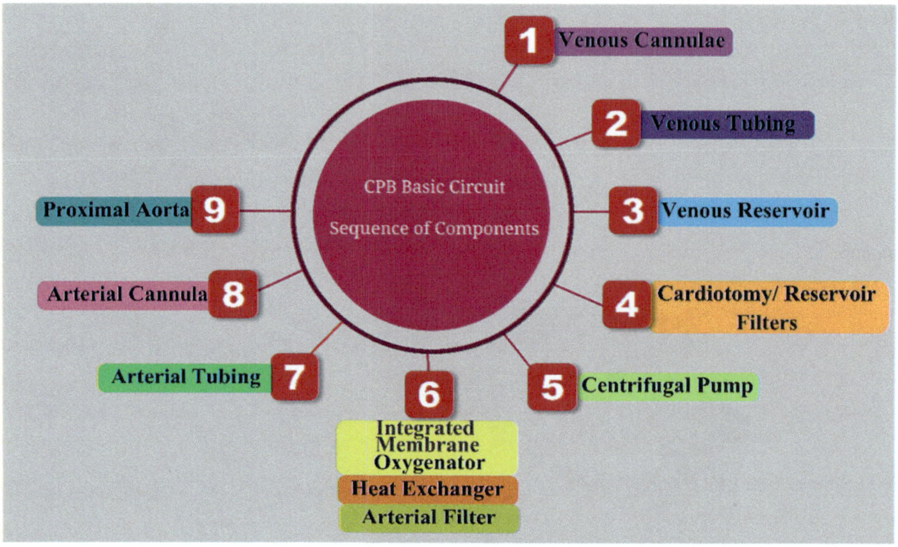

Fig. 7.10 This diagram displays the primary CPB circuit flow: (1) A venous cannula draws blood into (2) venous tubing, leading to (3) the venous reservoir. (4) Simultaneously, blood from the operative field, suction, and vent is directed into the cardiotomy reservoir, filtered, and merged with the venous reservoir blood. (5) The blood then passes through a centrifugal pump. (6) It proceeds through an integrated membrane oxygenator and heat exchanger, with an arterial filter facilitating gas exchange. (7) Processed blood is then routed via arterial tubing through (8) an arterial cannula into (9) the proximal aorta

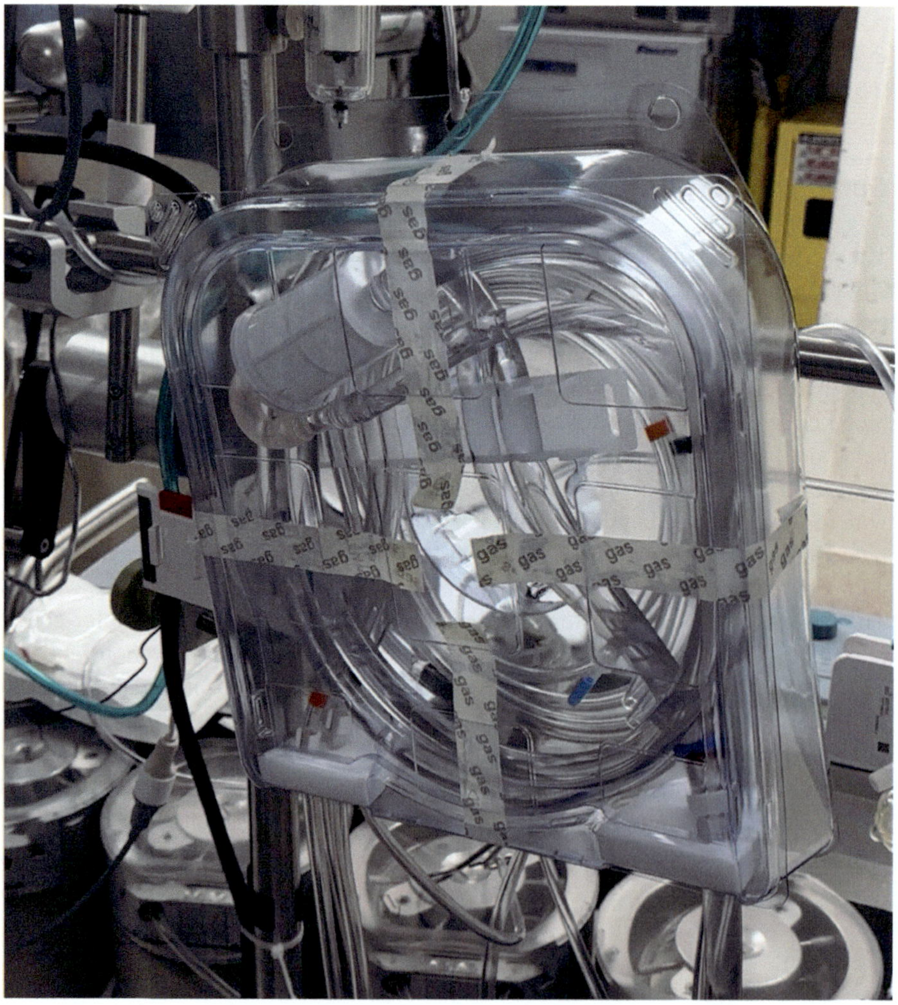

Fig. 7.11 This image displays sterile pre-packed kit ready for cardiac surgery: venous, arterial, suction, and vent lines being delivered to the surgical team, with key connections passed to the perfusionist for circuit assembly

ideally positioned about a foot before the venous reservoir. The arterial line, made of 3/8-inch internal diameter PVC tubing, extends from the oxygenator's outlet, passes through a flow probe that constantly measures the blood flow rate, and extends 8–10 feet to the arterial cannula.

Venous Cannulation

Venous return during CPB is crucial for maintaining optimal blood flow, governed by a pressure gradient that circulates blood within the CPB machine. Effective venous drainage, facilitated by selecting appropriate cannula options and cannulation sites, is influenced by various factors including cannula size, shape, and placement. These decisions must take into account patient needs, the surgical plan, and the choice between central or remote cannulation sites. Moreover, cannula positioning and myocardial retraction can impact drainage, presenting specific challenges in different surgical techniques, such as minimally invasive surgery. Factors like blood volume, vessel size, and potential complications, including cerebral venous congestion, necessitate careful evaluation.

In terms of cannula selection, it is important to consider the patient's flow requirements, which may not solely be based on body surface area (BSA) but also on other circumstances that might necessitate adjustments to the expected flow requirements. The selection process is guided by manufacturer data and the need to account for individual patient parameters. Additionally, considering the management of negative pressure through either gravity drainage or augmented techniques, with vessel size limitations in mind.

Site selection and cannulation technique are key, with central cannulation often involving the right atrium through single, dual-stage (Fig. 7.12), or bi-caval cannulae, each with its challenges such as Eustachian valve occlusion risk. Remote cannulation, targeting areas like the groin or neck, facilitates minimally invasive surgery but introduces risks, including femoral artery injury.

Cannulae are made of a flexible, wire-reinforced plastic, allowing some bending without kinking, accommodating the various needs and challenges presented during CPB.

Deoxygenated blood is removed either using a single cavo-atrial multi-orifice cannula or by using a two cannula (bi-caval), one placed in the inferior and the other superior vena cava (Fig. 7.13). It is anticipated that the superior vena cava will drain one-third of the patient's venous blood, compared to the two-thirds returned from the inferior vena cava. The single-stage technique is used for most surgical procedures, while the bi-caval technique is reserved for surgeries requiring entrance to the right atrium (RA) or left atrium (LA). Single cavo-atrial cannulae are the most efficient, while bi-caval cannulations, which help facilitate surgery through an atrial incision, are less efficient at decompression (Table 7.1).

Less common, a single multi-orifice cannula may be placed in the femoral vein and advanced so that the tip lies in the superior vena cava. Cannula selection depends on the surgical procedure, the approach, and the size of the patient. For most adults, these require 30–38 French cannula (>0.4-inch outer diameter). To secure connections between the patient and cannula and between cannula, purse strings sutures and tapes are used, respectively. Complications of venous cannulation include

1. Arrhythmias.
2. Atrial or caval tears/trauma.
3. Bleeding.
4. Caval obstruction/narrowing.

The efficacy of the venous drainage is gauged by the reservoir volume and the amount of volume in the cardiac chambers, more specifically the right side of the heart. In addition, the ability to cool and warm the heart with cardioplegia is related to the ability to keep the cardiac chambers empty of blood. This is a multi-orifice cannula with a hole at its tip and several proximal holes to allow drainage of inferior vena caval flow and all flows proximal, i.e., from the RA and superior vena cava.

A single cannula is inserted via the right atrial appendage, and the tip is directed toward and into the inferior vena cava. While most of the time, placement of the venous cannulae is performed via palpation, intraoperative echocardiography may help when there is a question (Fig. 7.14).

Fig. 7.12 This image displays a single cavo-atrial cannula

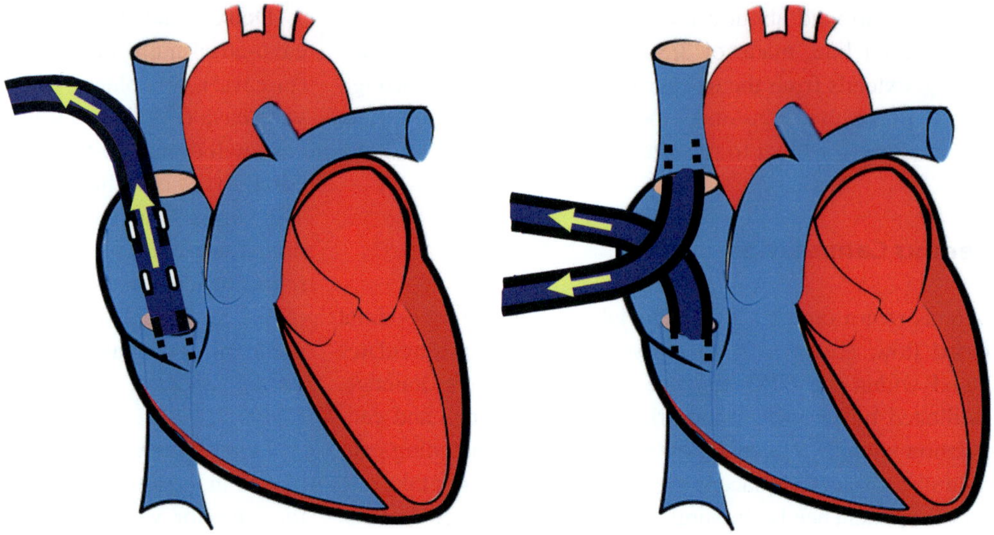

Fig. 7.13 This illustration displays a single cavo-atrial cannula (left) and bi-caval venous cannulation (right)

Table 7.1 Pros and cons of single vs. bi-caval cannulation

Feature	Bi-caval with tourniquet	Single: cavo-atrial
Atrial incisions	Good	Not preferred
Speed/ease of cannulation	More complex and time-consuming	Faster and simpler
Right heart exclusion	Allows for exclusion of the right heart from bypass	Not ideal
Right heart decompression	Provides optimal decompression of the right heart	Offers limited decompression
Caval drainage heart manipulation	Ensures optimal drainage, especially for complex cases and require more manipulation of the heart	Adequate drainage for most procedures with minimized manipulation
Drainage for all cardiac surgeries	Yes	No

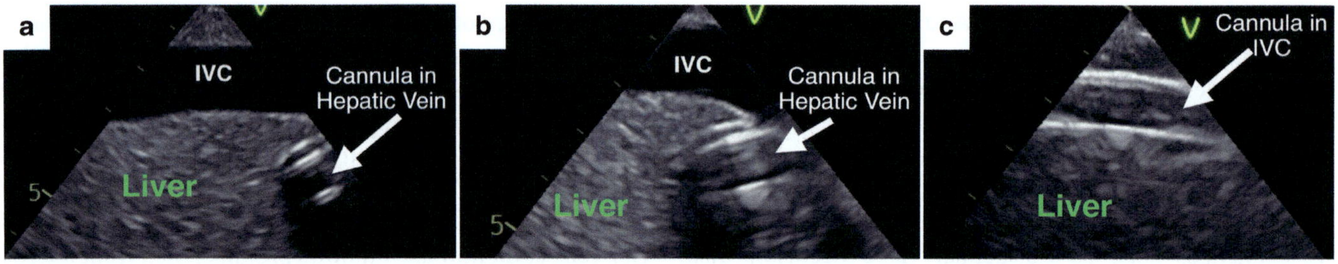

Fig. 7.14 This image displays TEE view, capturing the liver, inferior vena cava (IVC), hepatic vein, and the venous cannula. In panels A and B, the cannula is seen in the hepatic vein, while it is in the IVC in panel C

Venous Reservoir

The venous blood passes into the venous reservoir that lies immediately before the arterial pump. The reservoir acts as a capacitance chamber mirroring the venous system's role in the body and serves as a buffer to accommodate fluid shifts. Normally, 60–70% of a patient's total blood volume exists in the venous system, while less than 20% is resides in the arterial system. The remainder of the blood volume exists in capillaries, smaller vessels, and solid organs. The venous reservoir of the CPB system is designed to accommodate 60–70% of the patient's blood volume, typically 4 liters or less. This capacitance system has the capability to manage shifts in blood volumes as necessary. Additionally, the reservoir acts as a collection point for all vents and suckers placed in the surgical field. Without it, any change in drainage would directly affect the arterial output delivered to the patient. The volume within the venous reservoir serves as a buffer against these minor fluctuations, ensuring a consistent uninterrupted flow of arterial blood.

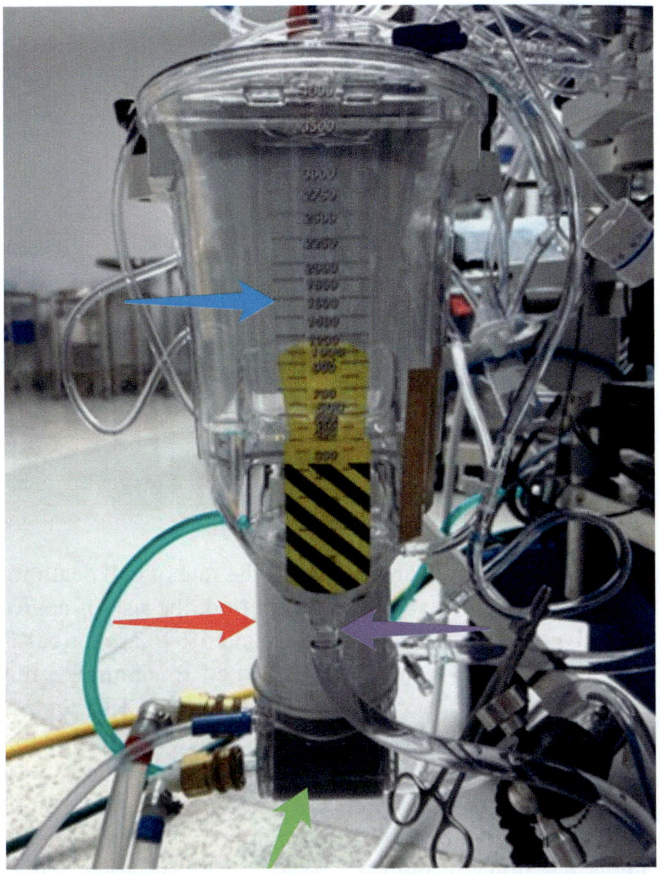

Fig. 7.15 This image displays a hard-shell graduated venous reservoir (blue arrow). The purple arrow points to the reservoir output, while the red arrow points to the membrane oxygenator. The green arrow points to the heat exchanger

Venous flow to the CPB circuit can be passive, moving down a pressure gradient created by gravity, augmented by a centrifugal pump, or it can utilize suction to create negative pressure. However, negative pressure from suction may lead to hemolysis, emboli, platelet damage, thrombin generation, and fibrinolysis.

Types of Reservoirs

There are two types of venous reservoirs on the market: a bag-like closed system (soft-shell) or a hard-shell open reservoir (Fig. 7.15). The closed venous reservoir, made from a polyvinyl chloride bag, has the advantage of preventing air from being drained into the pump, or worse, the patient. However, this soft-shell bag reservoir cannot manage air from the venous line, vents or suckers and requires a separate cardiotomy reservoir. It is also limited in the amount and types of reservoir filtration it can provide. In contrast, the more commonly used hard-shell open venous reservoir system, made of polycarbonate, can handle any air entrained in the suckers, vents, or venous line. It can utilize venous-assisted vacuum and incorporates a more complex filtration system. The biggest disadvantage of the hard-shell open system is the blood–air interface, which can lead to significant blood activation. This interface also allows the reservoir to be emptied, necessitating close monitoring by the perfusionist. Additionally, safety measures like level sensors and bubble detectors must be included to prevent the reservoir from draining and a massive air emboli event from occurring.

Included inside the open reservoir are two types of filters: depth and screen filters. These work together to filter out micro-emboli larger than 20 microns, preventing potential harm to the patient. At the top of the open reservoir, the venous line, vents, and suckers are all aseptically attached by the perfusionist during the assembly of the pump. There is one outlet at the bottom of the reservoir, designed to reduce the risk of air emboli. This outlet is, once again, attached to tubing by the perfusionist and leads to the arterial pump.

There are two types of reservoirs found in the CPB circuits: (1) cardiotomy reservoirs and (2) venous reservoirs. The larger of the two, the venous reservoir, allows for the collection of the intravascular blood returning via the venous cannula(s). The cardiotomy reservoir collects blood spilled in the surgical field and returned through suckers and from drainage vents placed in the cardiac chambers, helping to keep chambers empty and reduce wall stress, which could lead to myocardial ischemia. The majority of CPB circuits utilize an integrated cardiotomy reservoir/venous reservoir. In this integrated reservoir, cardiotomy blood is collected, filtered, and defoamed before mixing with the filtered venous blood. This setup also allows vacuum to be applied to augment venous drainage beyond what can be achieved through gravity alone, a process known as vacuum-assisted venous drainage. Circuits that use this integrated hard-shell reservoir are commonly known as "open systems."

A less commonly used system utilizes separate venous and cardiotomy reservoirs and is referred to as a soft venous reservoir system. Augmentation of blood return in this setup cannot utilize vacuum-assist; instead, it utilizes a centrifugal pump to move blood toward the soft-venous reservoir, a process known as kinetic-assisted venous drainage. Circuits that use a soft-venous reservoir are called "closed systems."

Drugs, fluids, and blood can be added to the reservoir. Several avenues allow for suction or aspirate blood and gas from open chambers (e.g., ventricle, aorta, atrium), the pericardium, and the surgical field, all of which are directed to the venous reservoir.

Quick Prime Line

Attached to the top of the venous reservoir, the quick prime line functions as its name suggests. It enables the perfusionist to rapidly add large volumes to the reservoir, both before and during CPB. Initially, the line is used to prime the circuit, eliminating any air. During bypass, it facilitates the addition of tailored volumes, such as crystalloids (e.g., plasmalyte and normal saline) or blood products, quickly and efficiently.

Recirculation Line

Although not a standard feature in all CPB circuits, the recirculation line is commonly included in most. This line attaches to a port post-oxygenator and returns to a port on top of the venous reservoir. Serving as a crucial safety mechanism, the recirculation line can mitigate the risk of air emboli reaching the arterial pump. In such events, a distal clamp may be applied to the arterial line, briefly coming off bypass, while simultaneously opening the clamp on the recirculation line. This setup allows any undesired air to be diverted back to the open reservoir, away from the patient. Furthermore, the recirculation line can supply blood to the cardioplegia circuit or the hemoconcentrator, provided that all access points are situated proximal to the clamp on the closed recirculation line.

Heat Exchanger

The heat exchanger is essential for adjusting temperatures to meet the requirements of the surgical procedure and is critical to the overall conduct of CPB. A CPB machine typically includes two heat exchangers: one to adjust the systemic flow temperature that is in line with the oxygenator and a separate one to regulate the temperature of the cardioplegia solution. Both operate on the same principle. They adjust the temperature of the systemic flow (i.e., the patient) and the cardioplegia to not only meet the procedural needs but also to ultimately return the patient to normal homeostatic state.

Systemic adjustments to the patient's temperature are made to significantly lower the body's metabolic rate (Fig. 7.16), thereby dramatically reducing the oxygen demand. This allows the patient to tolerate significantly longer periods of CPB, which may involve reductions in systemic flow or complete cessation of circulation (known as Deep Hypothermic Cardiac Arrest, DHCA). During DHCA, the patient's body temperature can be cooled to as

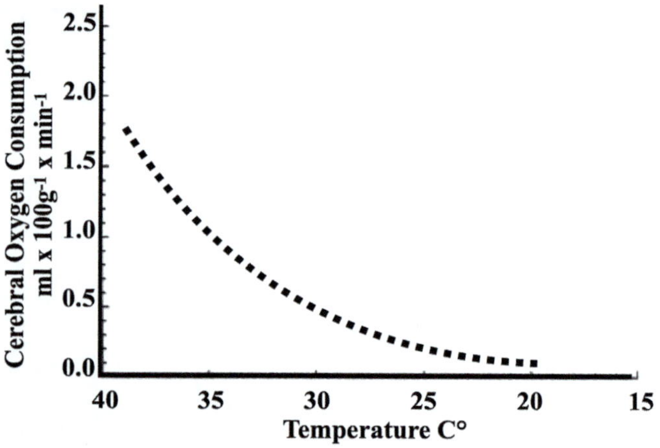

Fig. 7.16 This graph displays changes of cerebral oxygen consumption with temperature

low as 18 °C, significantly slowing the rate of cell death for up to 45 min. However, after this period, the risk of neurocognitive injury increases from around 5% to around 10%. Various measures can be implemented to minimize this risk, highlighting the complex interplay of CPB components during DHCA preparation. Once the desired low temperature is reached, the system recirculates for approximately 20 min to ensure uniform and homogenous cooling. To improve uniformity, the perfusionist might adjust gas flows to induce a degree of hypercarbia, which causes cerebral vascular dilation and facilitates homogenous cooling of the brain. Other strategies include maintaining cerebral flow using perfusion catheters, either through antegrade perfusion via the carotid artery or retrograde perfusion through the jugular vein.

While cooling the patient plays a crucial role in patient management, the rewarming phase is equally or more critical in preventing adverse outcomes. The duration of rewarming can vary, taking anywhere from 1 to 2 h depending on the patient's lowest temperature during CPB. The rate of rewarming is critical in preventing injuries, with a particular focus on preventing cerebral/neurologic damage. During this phase, the perfusionist will carefully adjust the perfusate temperature to maintain it within 10 °C difference of the patient's monitored temperature (for example, esophageal, nasopharyngeal, bladder, or rectal). During this phase, α-stat blood gas management is practiced. Once the patient's temperature reaches approximately 30 °C, the perfusate gradient is reduced to 4–5 °C. Rewarming rates can vary, typically ranging from less than 0.1 °C/min to 0.4 °C/min, depending on the degree of hypothermia experienced during CPB. The rewarming rate tends to be slower following more severe hypothermia. The target systemic "core" temperature varies by institution but is generally aimed at approximately

36.5 °C. Some data suggest that maintaining a lower "core" temperature between 35.5 and 36.0 °C might be associated with better neurologic outcomes. While not the focus here, decisions as to which patient temperature best reflects core and brain temperature is debated, along with whether it is best to focus on core or brain temperature. For more information on hypothermia management, please refer to Chap. 6, "Physiologic Changes and Inflammatory Response to Cardiopulmonary Bypass."

The type of surgery, the duration of the procedure, and the patient's comorbidities are key factors in deciding the extent to which the patient should be cooled. Institutional guidelines or individual surgeon preferences also play a significant role in determining temperature management strategies. Variations in maintaining systemic and cardioplegia temperatures range from "Warm Patient-Warm Cardioplegia" to "Cool Patient-Cool Cardioplegia," reflecting different approaches to thermal regulation during surgery.

Investigators have reported the use of warm cardioplegia at temperatures of 35–37 °C, placing greater emphasis on inducing hyperkalemia to maintain cardiac asystole. In contrast, cold cardioplegia temperatures typically range between 4 and 15 °C, with most falling below 10 °C. Proponents of the former approach argue that it better maintains and/or facilitates the return of cardiac functions but requires continuous (or nearly continuous) delivery of cardioplegia. Advocates for the latter approach highlight the significant reduction in myocardial oxygen requirements and the ability to tolerate of longer periods of aortic cross-clamping. Lowering the heart's temperature to 4–8 degrees also helps in maintaining an asystolic state, particularly when combined with hyperkalemic cardioplegia. Ultimately, the goal is to return cardiac perfusion to normal homeostatic state, ensuring the proper function of cardiac enzymes, ionic channels, and contractile elements.

After leaving the reservoir, blood and fluids pass through a heat exchanger before reaching the oxygenator. The heat exchanger has the capability to either cool or warm the blood. Hypothermia, induced by cooling, allows the body to tolerate reduced flows by reducing tissue metabolic rate and oxygen consumption. When hypothermia is no longer desired, the heat exchanger is utilized to rewarm the patient's blood and body. The rate of rewarming is maintained below 0.2 °C/min and typically targets a temperature of 36.5 °C to prevent cerebral ischemia. Temperatures are kept below 40 °C to prevent denaturation of proteins.

The heat exchanger modifies blood temperature by convection. A stainless-steel interface separates the coolant (water or propylene glycol; Figs. 7.17 and 7.18) on one side from the blood on the other. This design allows the perfusionist to precisely control the blood temperature, thereby regulating the patient's overall temperature.

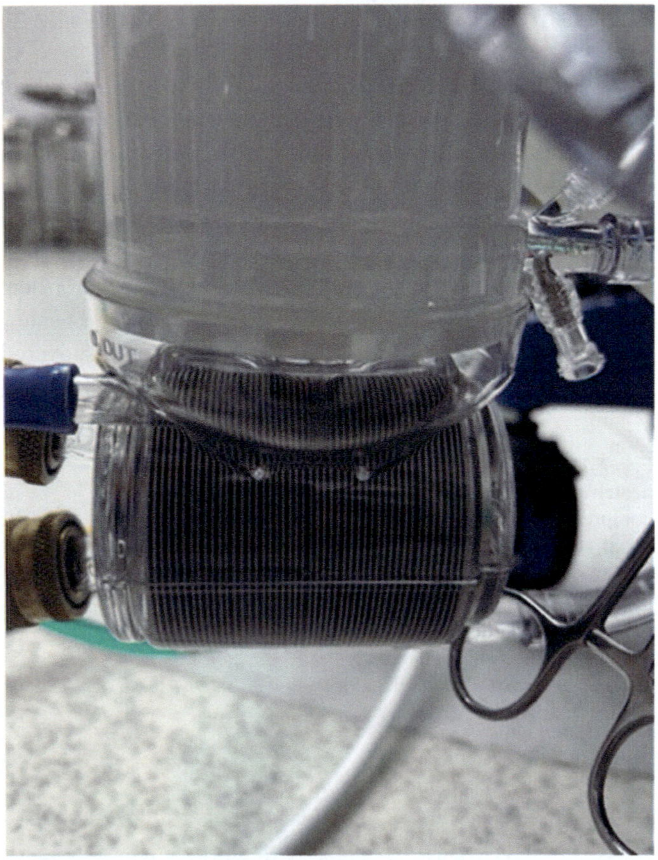

Fig. 7.17 This image showcases the heat exchanger, which is strategically positioned beneath the oxygenator in the CPB circuit. The heat exchanger uses coils to either warm or cool the blood through the process of convection. By adjusting the temperature of a fluid that circulates within these coils, the heat exchanger effectively regulates the blood temperature as it passes through, ensuring that it meets the specific requirements of the patient's physiological state during surgery

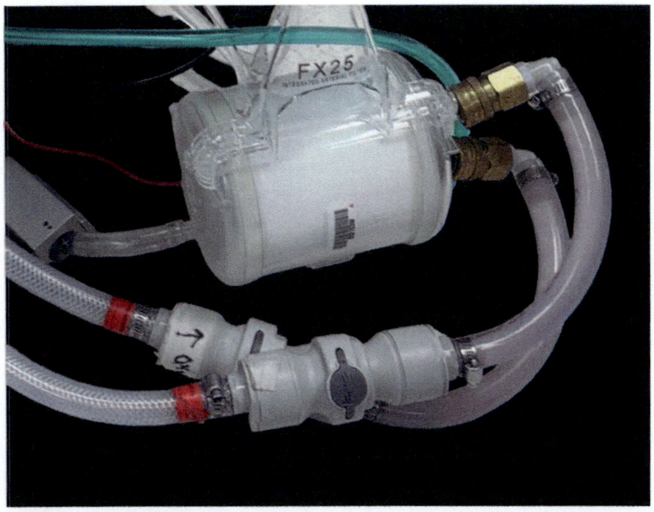

Fig. 7.18 This image showcases a next-generation oxygenator that offers seamless blood gas exchange and integrated heat management. It simplifies setup and provides clinicians with greater control during CPB procedures

The Heater-Cooler

The heater-cooler (see Fig. 7.19) is distinct from heat exchangers. The heater-cooler lies outside the CPB circuit (i.e., no in-line with blood flow). It is a water-based system that adjusts temperature-controlled water through tubing connected to the oxygenator/heat exchanger of the bypass circuit. The heater-cooler pumps the temperature-controlled water through tubing connected to the oxygenator/heat exchanger of the bypass circuit. In 2016, the current heater-cooler technology came under fire when it was discovered that they had a potential to infect patients with nontuberculous mycobacteria. In these instances, mycobacteria-coated intrinsic surfaces within the heater-cooler were aerosolized by the internal fans. The aerosolized bacteria had potential to travel to the patient leading to could-be infections. Cleaning regimens in IFUs and protocols have since been changed, and new heater-coolers have been designed. Not only are there new water-based heater-coolers on the market, but companies have designed heater-coolers using propylene glycol to help attenuate the possible cross-contamination risks. In addition, the heater-cooler may be placed on the non-patient side of the CPB machine to further reduce any airborne contamination.

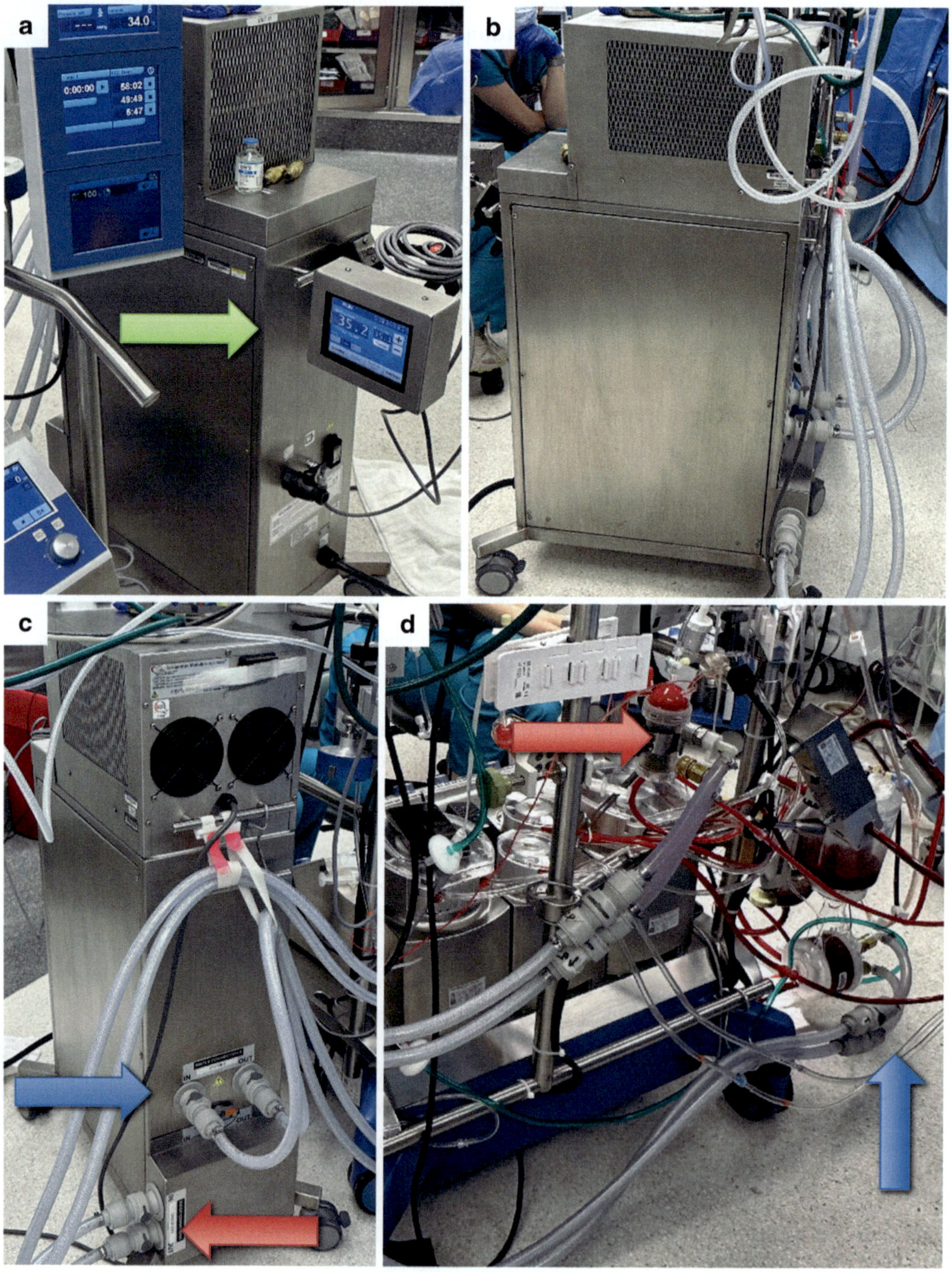

Fig. 7.19 Exploring the heater-cooler system: A comprehensive view. Image **a**: Front view of the heater-cooler system, highlighting the temperature control screen indicated by a green arrow. Image **b**: Side perspective showing the cardioplegia and oxygenator heat exchanger inflows and outflows, illustrating the system's complexity and integration. Image **c**: Rear view of the heater-cooler system, with a blue arrow marking the heat exchanger inflows and outflows, and a red arrow showcasing the cardioplegia inflows and outflows, emphasizing the system's vital connections. Image **d**: Detailed focus on the integration of the system, where a blue arrow points to the heat exchanger inflows and outflows positioned beneath or within the oxygenator, and a red arrow directs attention to the cardioplegia heat exchanger inflows and outflows, highlighting the precision in setup and operation

Oxygenator

The oxygenator (Fig. 7.20), serving as the "lung" of the CPB machine, permits the exchange of oxygen (O_2) and carbon dioxide (CO_2). Gas exchange is driven by pressure gradients, with the blood O_2 and CO_2 levels indicated by the partial pressures of venous oxygen and carbon dioxide (PvO2 and PvCO2), return to the reservoir from the venous cannula, reflecting the patient's metabolic rate. Gas exchange occurs as gases move down a gradient across the oxygenator's membranes. Two types of oxygenators are used for adult patients: microporous polypropylene (PPL) and non-porous polymethylpentene (PMP). Both utilize hollow fiber membrane technology for oxygenation, which is biocompatible, minimizing hemolysis, platelet activation, and protein denaturation. The fibers, with an internal diameter of 100–200 μm, are designed to enhance gas exchange by allowing blood to flow around them, while gas moves within or through them, facilitating CO_2 removal and O_2 addition (Fig. 7.21). The key distinction between these two types of oxygenators lies in their specific membrane materials that separate the blood and gas compartments. This difference in material significantly impacts their capacity for durability and efficiency. PMP oxygenators, known for their long-lasting gas exchange capabilities, have non-porous fibers that prevent plasma leaks, making them ideal for extended use in procedures like ECMO. However, their inability to facilitate the exchange of volatile anesthetics limits their compatibility with procedures using CPB machines. In contrast, PPL oxygenators, while more com-

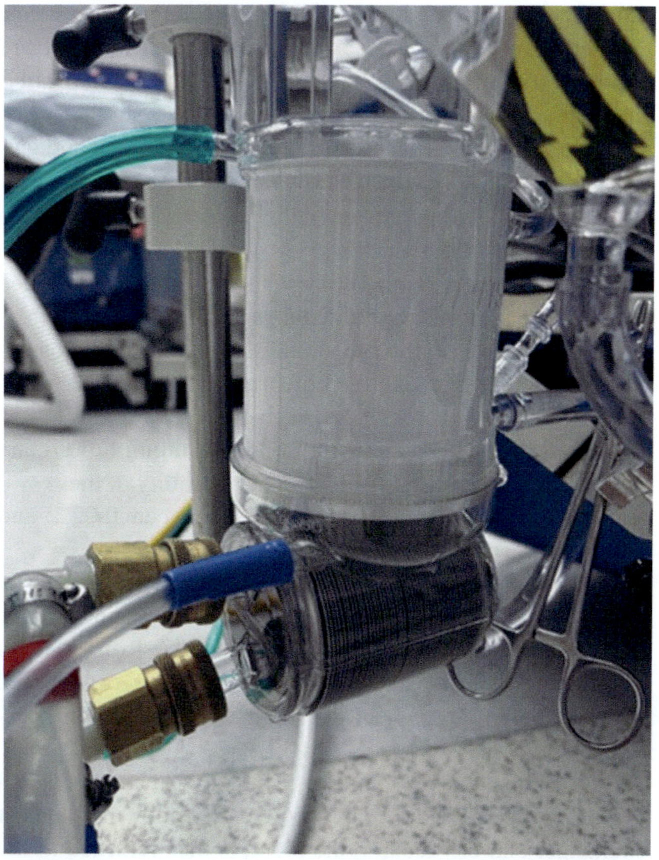

Fig. 7.20 This image displays the oxygenator with its multiple sheets of microporous polypropylene fibers allowing blood to interface with gas

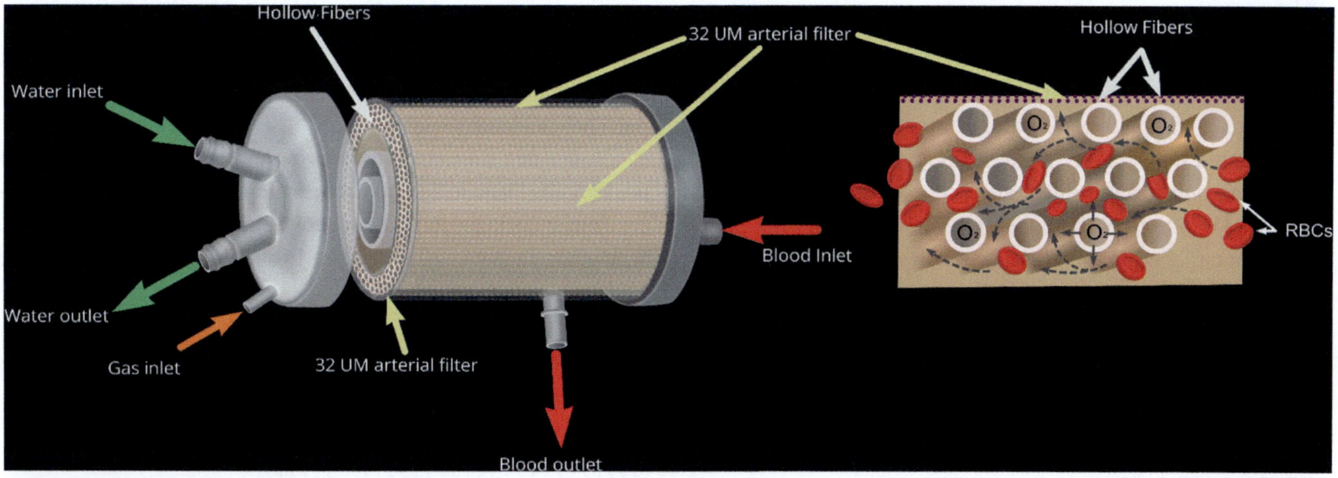

Fig. 7.21 Illustration depicting the structure of a membrane oxygenator integrated with a heat exchanger and arterial filter on the left. The right side of the illustration reveals the oxygenator's core feature: hollow fibers with diameters ranging from 100 to 200 micrometers. These fibers facilitate a unique interaction between blood and gas; blood circulates around the fibers, while oxygen and carbon dioxide transfer occur within or through these fibers, enabling a critical gas exchange process

monly used, may see a reduction in performance over time due to plasma leakage from extended use. Both PPL and PMP oxygenators are engineered from polypropylene and polymethylpentene, creating a thin, capillary-like structure that increases the interaction surface area between blood and gas, thus enhancing gas exchange efficiency.

After the initiation of bypass, the patient's blood coats the membrane material, reducing stress on the blood and improving gas exchange. A high-O_2 low-CO_2 gas mixture is applied to the oxygenator side opposite the incoming blood, optimizing O_2 infusion into the blood and CO_2 removal. Adjusting the gas flow by adjusting the flow meter increases the gradient and therefore increases gas exchange.

The oxygenator can transfer up to 470 ml/min of O_2 and remove up to 350 ml/min of CO_2. The reliability of these systems is high, with malfunction rates between 0.02% and 0.26%.

Recent innovations include the integration of the arterial line filters within oxygenators. Similar to the original design of arterial line filters, these screen filters range from 30 to 40 microns in size and exist as a last line of defense. Integrated arterial filters help prevent micro air emboli, clot, and particulate emboli.

The oxygenator is monitored using oxygen analyzers and assessing arterial and venous blood tests. Following the heat exchanger and oxygenator, the blood is then returned to the patient via cannulae placed in the aorta (Please see Fig. 3.7).

Arterial Cannula

Blood is returned to the systemic circulation from the oxygenator through arterial line tubing and then via the aortic cannulation. Possible locations for cannula placement include ascending aorta, femoral artery, or the axillary artery. The cannula may feature a curved or straight tip (Fig. 7.22), depending on the anatomical and procedural requirements of the vessel to which blood is being returned. A curved tip cannula, when placed in the ascending aorta, directs flow toward the aortic arch, while a straight tip cannula is typically advanced further into the arterial vessel, for example, femoral artery.

Complications to be aware of during arterial cannulation include

1. Bleeding from difficult insertion.
2. Ascending aortic wall injury—hematoma or dissection (0.01–0.09%).
3. Malposition reducing flow to a major vessel.
4. Femoral artery injury.
   (a) Retrograde dissection (0.2–1.3%).
   (b) Late stenosis.
   (c) Thrombosis.
   (d) Infection.
5. Air embolism.
6. Plaque embolization.

For further details, please refer to Chap. 25, "Mechanical Complications of Cardiopulmonary Bypass."

The selection of the arterial cannula size is influenced by the patient's size, estimated metabolic rates, and the desired flow rates. A larger cannulae allows for higher flow while minimizing the risk of blood cell trauma. The criteria for size selection include the patient's age, weight, and/or BSA, allowing for an optimized match between cannula size and patient needs. Larger cannulae enable more substantial blood flow at higher rates, with a 3/8″ line commonly used in adults and sizes as small as 1/8″ utilized in pediatric patients. However, the maximum size of the cannula is ultimately determined by the size of the patient's blood vessels. Achieving a balance between cannula size and vessel size, and the required flow rates to meet metabolic demands is crucial, taking into account both the risk of trauma to blood components and the specifics of the patient's anatomy.

Flow rates thought tubing or cannulae are determined by the Hagen–Poiseuille equation, which provides a mathematical framework to understand how changes in size, pressure, and other factors influence the flow of fluid through a tube (Table 7.2).

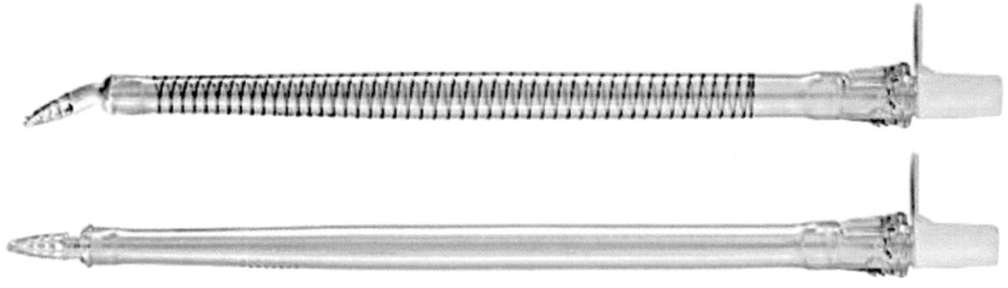

Fig. 7.22 This image displays Curved (top) and straight (bottom) aortic cannula utilized in the cardiopulmonary bypass system to return blood to the patient

Table 7.2 Different examples of arterial cannulae are chosen based on patient BSA

Different examples of arterial cannulae for aortic cannulation			
BSA (m^2)	Size (mm)	Size (French)	Max flow (L/min)
<1.3	5.0–5.3	15–16	2.5–3.2
1.3–<2.0	5.7–6	17–18	4.0–4.5
2.0–2.4	7.0	20–22	6.0
>2.5	8.0	24	8.0

The larger the cannulae, the greater amount of flow that can pass without causing harmful trauma to the cellular components

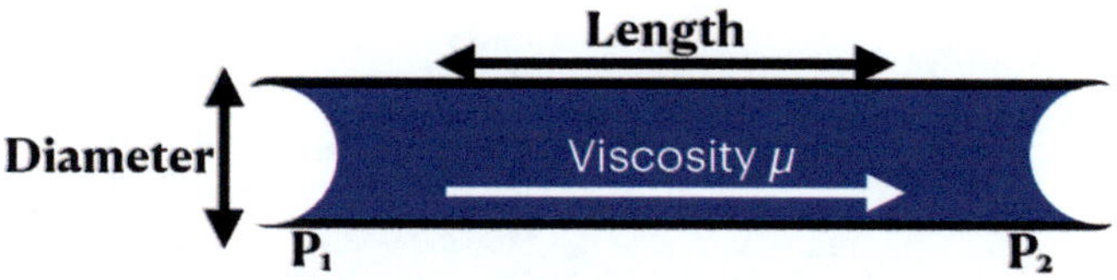

$$Q = \text{Flow Rate}$$

$$Q = \frac{\Delta P \times \pi \times r^4}{8 \times L \times \mu}$$

$$\Delta P = P_1 - P_2$$

Arterial Line Filters

While arterial line filters are less common in modern CPB circuit configurations, they are still present in some setups. Just like the integrated versions, arterial line filters serve as a crucial last line of defense. These filters are designed to capture any particulates, clots, or air bubbles that may bypass the cardiotomy filters and oxygenator. The filter pore size typically ranges from 30 to 40 microns.

Before the initiation of CPB and during the priming process, the arterial line is connected to the venous line, creating a continuous loop. This setup allows the perfusionist to prime the circuit effectively, incorporating blood (if necessary), and adding prime drugs, all while recirculating the prime solution. Within this arterial-venous loop lies a pre-bypass filter, which has a pore size of 0.2–5 microns, targeting particulate matter remaining from the manufacturing process. Due to its small pore size, this filter is removed before the addition of prime drugs and blood products.

The Gas Supply System and the Oxygen/Air Blender in CPB Machines

The gas supply system is an essential component of the CPB machine. The O_2/air blender takes a supply of air, O_2, and sometimes CO_2, blends these gases together to achieve a specific mixture, delivering it at a controlled flow rate. The blender (Fig. 7.23) has two to three different settings. One is the FiO_2, which ranges from 21 to 100%, and the other is the flow rate. Additionally, CO_2 can be introduced to manage blood pH levels, especially during procedures that involve hypothermia or require deep hypothermic circulatory arrest.

Modern CPB machines feature blending units and flow meters that are digitally controlled, allowing for precise regulation of the sweep gas flow. Continuous monitoring of inspired O_2 is crucial to ensure that patients are not exposed to a hypoxic gas mixture. Alongside the blending system, an inhaled anesthetic vaporizer works in conjunction to administer anesthesia directly into the gas flow.

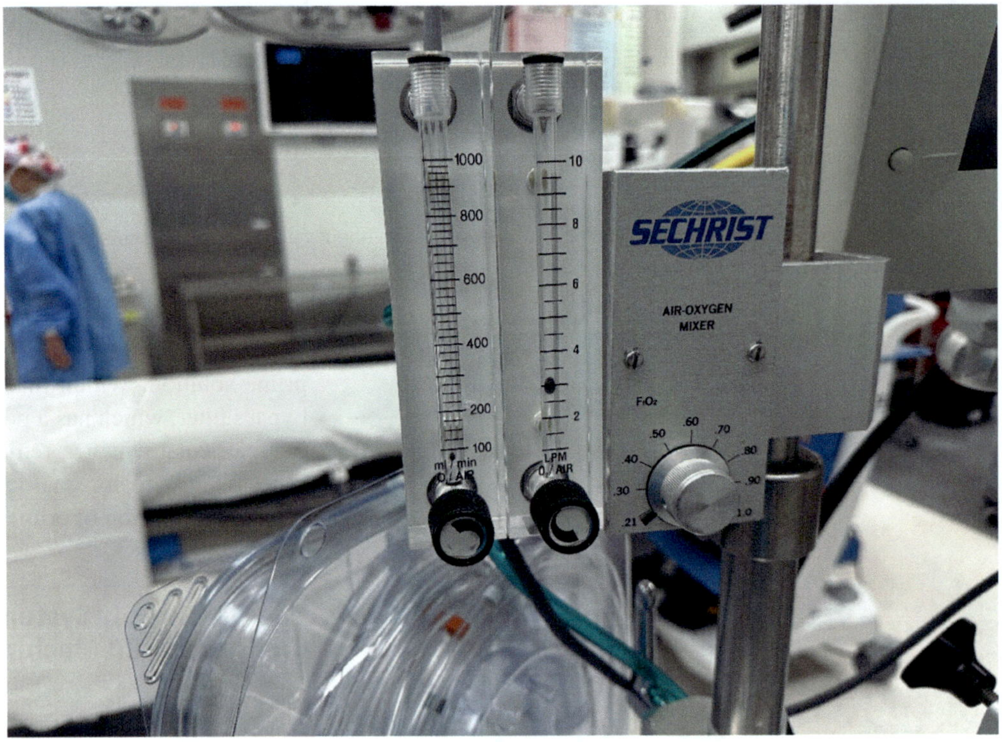

Fig. 7.23 This image displays an O_2/air blender on a CPB machine, which mixes air, O_2, and, optionally, CO_2 to achieve desired FiO_2 levels ranging from 21% to 100% and specific flow rates, paired with an inhaled anesthetic vaporizer

Inhaled Anesthetic Vaporizer

The vaporizer (Fig. 7.24) delivers inhaled anesthesia to patients during periods when it cannot be adequately or accurately provided by the mechanical ventilator. During CPB, a dedicated vaporizer, attached to the CPB machine and in-line with the oxygen flow to the oxygenator, ensures the continuous provision of inhaled anesthetic to the patient. This system can administer any of the commonly used inhalation agents, such as isoflurane, sevoflurane, and desflurane. In addition to providing anesthesia, these inhalation agents have vasodilatory effects and can be used to manage blood pressure during the CPB period.

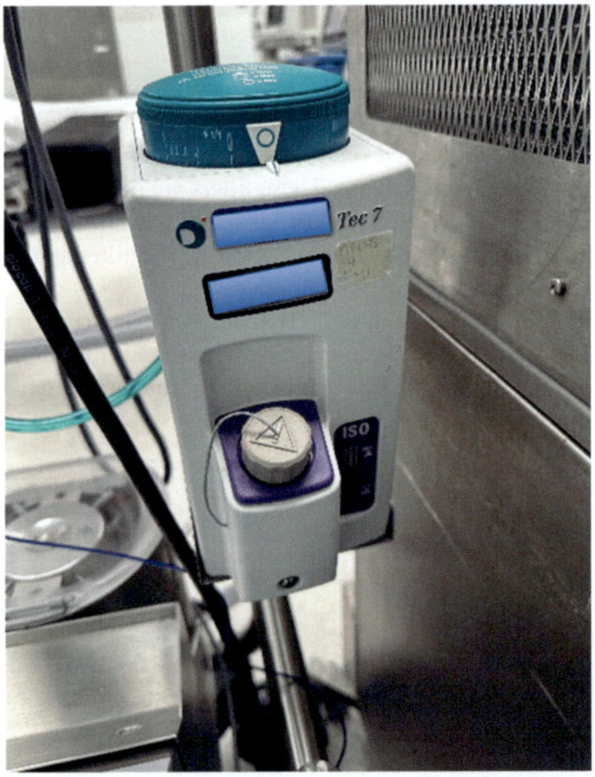

Fig. 7.24 This image showcases an integrated vaporizer within the CPB circuit, specifically designed to administer isoflurane. The vaporizer seamlessly integrates with the CPB machine to ensure the precise delivery of this inhaled anesthetic, essential for maintaining anesthesia during surgeries

Flow Measurement in CPB Machines

CPB machines measure blood flow using either ultrasonic (Fig. 7.25) or electromagnetic principle, with ultrasonic flow probes being more common. The concept of transit time involves measuring how long it takes for ultrasonic signals to travel through the blood in a CPB machine. A transit-time probe consists of two piezoelectric crystals, one located upstream and the other is located downstream on the tubing. A pulse is emitted from both crystals. The pulse traveling in the same direction of the blood will arrive at its destination within the flow probe slightly faster than the pulse traveling the opposite direction of the blood. The difference in the

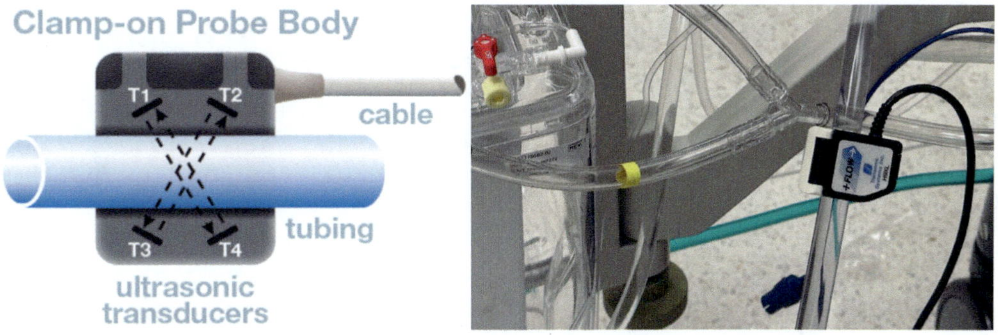

Fig. 7.25 Left illustration: Clamp-on ultrasonic flow probe featuring ultrasound transducers on either side of a tube, showcasing the setup for transit-time flow measurement. Image courtesy of Spectrum Medical. Right photo: Clamp-on ultrasonic flow probe securely positioned around arterial line tubing, designed for precise blood flow measurement in a fully setup CPB circuit ready for a CPB run

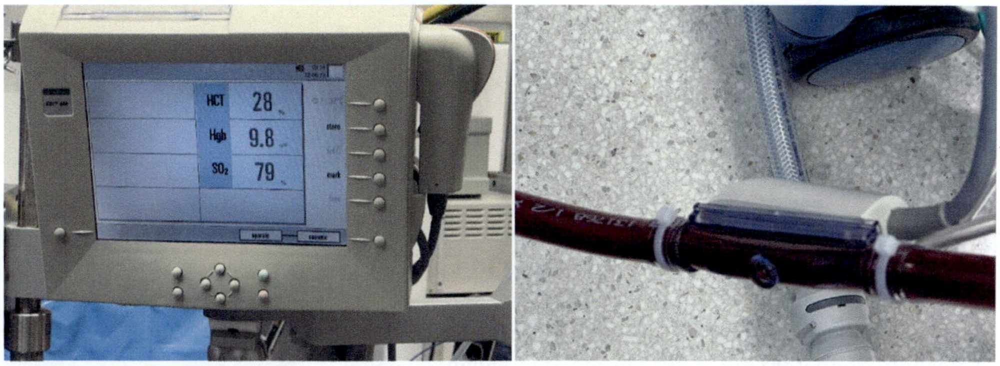

Fig. 7.26 Left photo: The Terumo CDI 500 blood parameter monitoring system, showcasing real-time numeric values on its display: HCT 28, Hgb 9.8, and SVO_2 79. Right photo: Features the CDI (Hemoglobin/Saturation) H/S cuvette securely attached to the probe head, integral for precise blood parameter measurements

pulse travel times or "phase delay" allows a determination of blood flow rate.

Continuous In-Line/Online Metabolic Monitoring

The distinction between in-line and on-line monitoring lies in the method and location of analysis or measurement. In-line monitoring employs sensors or cuvettes directly placed in the blood's flow path, allowing for direct contact and continuous measurement of parameters such as blood gases. This method ensures real-time data but necessitates regular calibration and maintenance to ensure accuracy. In-line blood gas monitoring requires cuvettes or sensors to be placed somewhere within the perfusion circuitry. Examples of in-line blood parameter monitoring devices include the Terumo CDI 500 (Fig. 7.26) and CDI 550. Conversely, online monitoring employs non-invasive techniques, attaching probes externally to tubing to infer parameters through indirect means, offering continuous data with less maintenance due to the absence of direct blood contact. While online methods minimize maintenance challenges, they may face limitations in measurement accuracy and parameter range compared to the direct approach of in-line monitoring. Online monitoring places probes on the outside of the tubing to monitor parameters continuously. An example of an online blood parameter monitoring device is the Spectrum Medical's M System.

Continuous blood gas monitoring, or at a minimum, continuous venous oximetry, provides the perfusionist with a real-time insight into the patient's metabolism. Blood gas and metabolic monitoring can be performed intermittently at 10–15 min intervals or more frequently, depending on the patient's needs. After the initial CPB blood gas assessments, analyzers can be calibrated based on the blood gas results. For all machines, venous oximetry and in-line hematocrit are calibrated.

For continuous monitoring, the analyzer then tracks metrics such as PO_2, PCO_2, Base excess, pH, K, SVO_2, HCT, and Hb. With these data, many workstations can now calculate oxygen delivery (DO_2), oxygen consumption (VO_2), and carbon dioxide production (VCO_2), all of which provide the perfusionist an understanding of patient perfusion.

Temperature Probes

Multiple temperature probes are utilized on the CPB machine to monitor the various temperature adjustments that occur during cardiac surgery. These probes are strategically positioned at the cardioplegia outflow, the arterial outflow, and the venous inflow to the reservoir (Fig. 7.27).

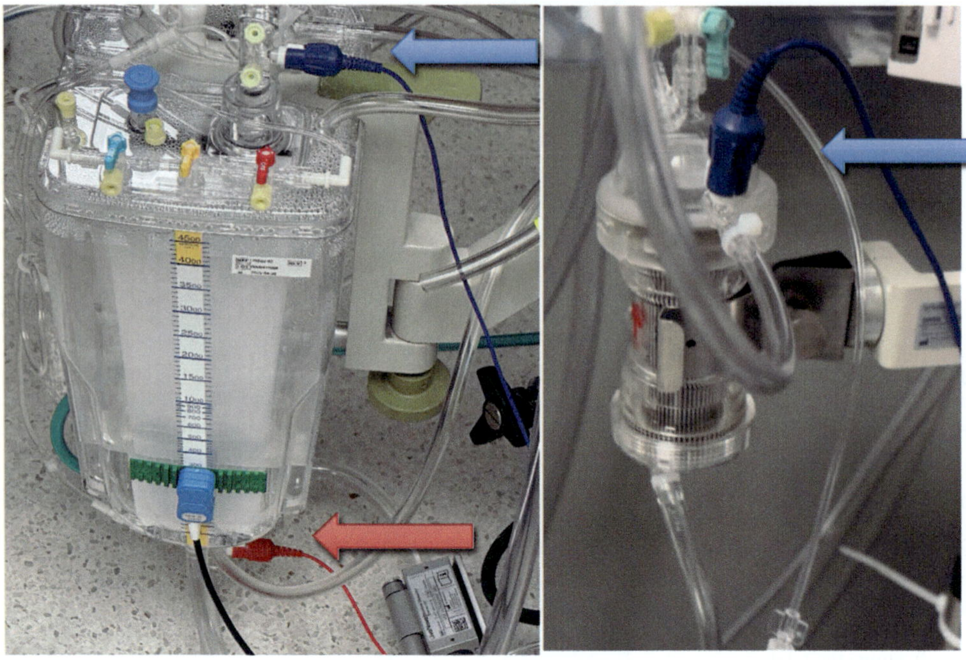

Fig. 7.27 Left photo: A blue temperature probe at the venous inflow to the reservoir and a red temperature probe at the arterial outflow, each indicated by corresponding colored arrows. Right photo: The blue temperature probe at the cardioplegia outflow, highlighted by a blue arrow, showcasing the critical monitoring points on the CPB machine for precise temperature management during cardiac surgery

Venous-Assisted Vacuum Regulator in CPB Systems

A vacuum regulator (Fig. 7.28), designed to enhance venous drainage, is a common feature on numerous CPB machines. Historically, gravity has been the principal force facilitating venous drainage. Bypass circuits were designed to position the venous reservoir as close to the ground as possible, optimizing this gravitational advantage. However, the adoption of augmented venous drainage techniques has emerged to address challenges associated with poor venous drainage, which can occur with long femoral cannulas or smaller venous cannulas in general. Additionally, augmented venous drainage supports the miniaturization of bypass circuits by allowing the venous reservoir to be positioned higher, thereby shortening both the arterial and venous lines. Various methods of augmented venous drainage have been employed, including kinetic centrifugal pumps, roller pumps, and vacuum regulators, with vacuum-assisted venous drainage now being the predominant method in the field.

Despite the apparent benefits of enhancing venous drainage, several safety concerns arise. The introduction of micro air bubbles into the venous line—whether through the purse string sutures of the venous cannula, any defects in the heart itself, or excessive negative pressure—presents a significant risk. Furthermore, applying negative pressure directly to the reservoir itself can pose its own set of challenges. Especially in systems utilizing a centrifugal pump head, any instance where the negative pressure in the reservoir surpasses the positive pressure generated by the pump head can lead to massive de-priming events. To mitigate such events, the vacuum regulator is set no more than −30 to −40 mmHg.

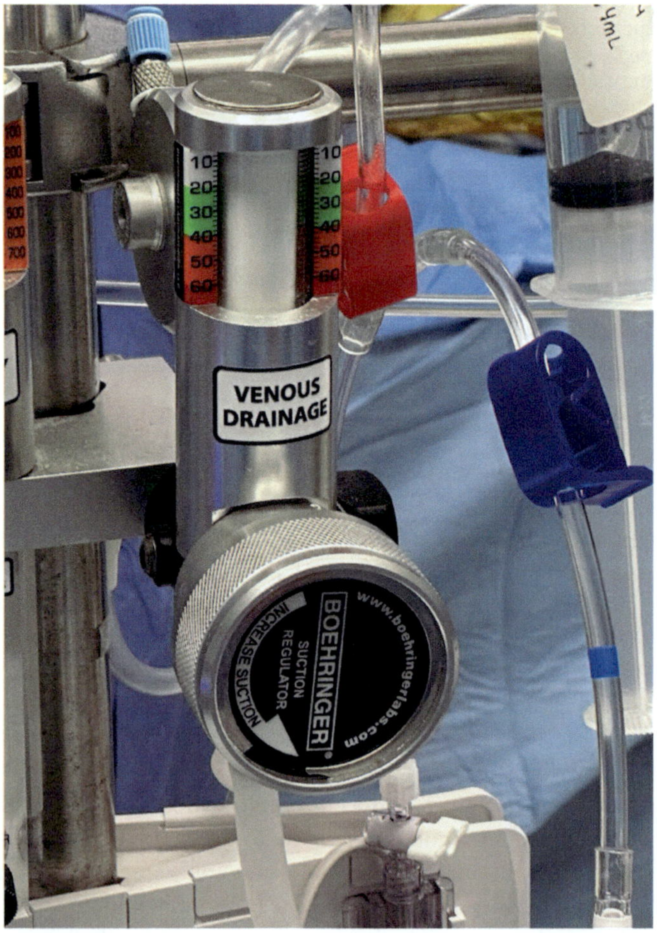

Fig. 7.28 This image showcases an example of a vacuum regulator, calibrated from 0 to –60 mmHg. The white zone spans from 0 to –20 mmHg, indicating minimal or no vacuum application. The green zone spans from –20 to –40 mmHg, indicating safe vacuum levels for enhanced venous drainage. The orange zone, from –40 to –60 mmHg, signals caution, and the red zone, above –60 mmHg, denotes critical vacuum levels requiring immediate attention

Pressure Transducers in CPB Circuits

Pressure transducers provide a real-time visualization of all the internal pressures within the CPB circuit, essential for identifying and mitigating potential issues. Constant monitoring of these pressures helps reduce the possibility of safety-related incidents, which can include

- Over pressurization anywhere within the circuit leading to tubing rupture.
- Excessive negative pressure causing cavitation, which can result in air being drawn out of solution.
- Excessive negative pressure within the venous reservoir.
- Excessively high positive pressure in the venous reservoir.
- Aortic dissection.
- Excessive hemolysis.
- Clot formation within the circuit.
- Circuit malfunctions.
- Coronary artery and sinus damage during cardioplegia delivery.

To ensure comprehensive monitoring, pressure transducers are connected to several critical areas, including the arterial line, the venous reservoir, and the cardioplegia delivery system (Fig. 7.29) as well as any other areas where roller

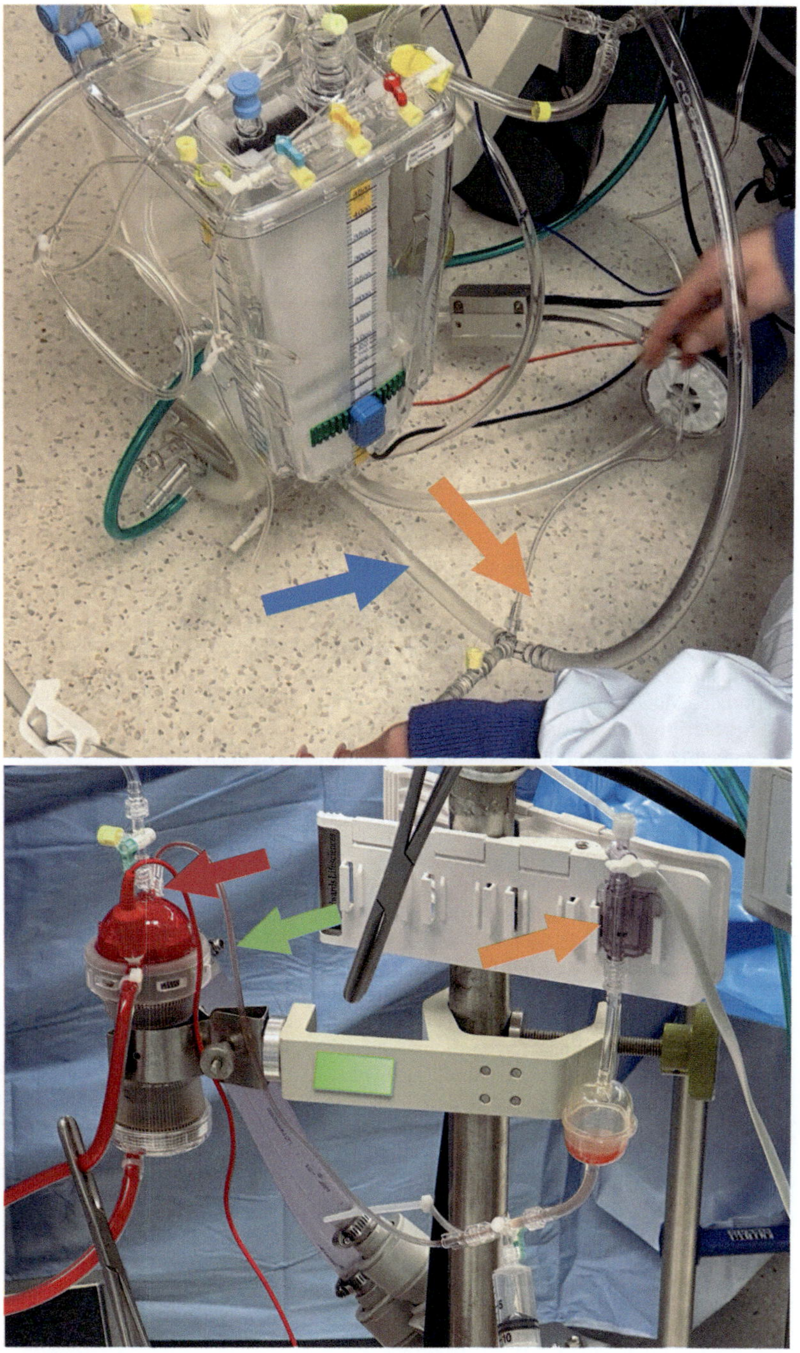

Fig. 7.29 Two images for the most common locations of pressure monitoring transducers in CPB circuits: Top Image: A photo of a pressure monitoring line (orange arrow) connected to the oxygenator outlet (blue arrow) for monitoring arterial line pressure in CPB circuits. Bottom Image: Depiction of a pressure monitoring line (red arrow) connected to the cardioplegia delivery system, with pressure monitoring line (green arrow) linked to the transducer (orange arrow) to monitor cardioplegia line pressure.

pumps regulate blood flow, such as the Modified Ultrafiltration (MUF) Circuitry. The system is designed to automatically adjust the pumps that are tied to these pressure transducers; for example, the cardioplegia pump slows or stops when a preset pressure is hit.

Further Reading

AmSECT. American society of ExtraCorporeal technology standards and guidelines for perfusion practice. StandardView. 2017;6(2):9.

Ashraf S, Butler J, Tian Y, Cowan D, Lintin S, Saunders NR, Watterson KG, Martin PG. Inflammatory mediators in adults undergoing cardiopulmonary bypass: comparison of centrifugal and roller pumps. Ann Thorac Surg. 1998;65(2):480–4. https://doi.org/10.1016/S0003-4975(97)01349-0.

Britanica. Kinetic Pumps, 1996. https://www.britannica.com/technology/waterwheel-engineering

Brolhorst J, Peterson B, Holt DW. Flow awareness as a new safety device for cardiopulmonary bypass. J Extra Corpor Technol. 2019;51(1):20–5.

Brown WR, Moody DM, Challa VR, Stump DA, Hammon JW. Longer duration of cardiopulmonary bypass is associated with greater numbers of cerebral microemboli. Stroke. 2000;31(3):707–13. https://doi.org/10.1161/01.str.31.3.707.

Charrière J, Pélissié J, Verd C, Léger P, Pouard P, de Riberolles C, Longrois D. Survey: retrospective survey of monitoring/safety devices and incidents of cardiopulmonary bypass for cardiac surgery in France. J Extra Corpor Technol. 2007a;39(3):142–57. discussion 158–9

Charrière J, Pélissié J, Verd C, Léger P, Pouard P, de Riberolles C, Menestret P, Hittinger M, Rougé P, Longrois D. Analysis of incidents, monitoring and safety devices of cardiopulmonary bypass for cardiac surgery for the year 2005 in France. Annales Françaises d'Anesthésie Et De Réanimation. 2007b;26(11):907. https://doi.org/10.1016/j.annfar.2007.09.025.

Chilton V, Klein A. Equipment and monitoring. In: Ghosh IS, Falter F, Cook D, editors. Cardiopulmonary bypass (Cambridge clinical guides). Cambridge: Cambridge University Press; 2009. p. 1–22. https://doi.org/10.1017/CBO9780511635564.002.

Conolly S, Arrowsmith JE, Klein AA. Deep hypothermic circulatory arrest. Cont Educ Anaesth Crit Care Pain. 2010;10(5):138–42. https://doi.org/10.1093/bjaceaccp/mkq024.

Deptula J, McGrath C, Preston T, Miller H, Yen B, Munari L, Setty SP. Sterility and performance of open and closed extracorporeal circuits after long-term dry-wet setups. Perfusion. 2021;36(2):130–7. https://doi.org/10.1177/0267659120937898.

Eckert E, Münch F, Göen T, Purbojo A, Müller J, Cesnjevar R. Comparative study on the migration of di-2-ethylhexyl phthalate (DEHP) and tri-2-ethylhexyl trimellitate (TOTM) into blood from PVC tubing material of a heart-lung machine. Chemosphere. 2016;145:10–6. https://doi.org/10.1016/j.chemosphere.2015.11.067.

Engelman R, Baker RA, Likosky DS, et al. The Society of Thoracic Surgeons, the Society of Cardiovascular Anesthesiologists, and the American Society of Extracorporeal Technology: clinical practice guidelines for cardiopulmonary bypass temperature management during cardiopulmonary bypass. Ann Thorac Surg. 2015;100(2):748–57.

Gravlee GP, Davis RF, Utley JR, Ovid Technologies I. Cardiopulmonary bypass: principles and practices. 3rd ed. Lippincott Williams & Wilkins; 2007.

Guimarães DP, Caneo LF, Matte G, Carletto LP, Policarpo VC, Castro AVCX, Miranda MHC, Costa PS, Jatene MB, Cestari I, Jatene FB. Impact of vacuum-assisted venous drainage on forward flow in simulated pediatric cardiopulmonary bypass circuits utilizing a centrifugal arterial pump head. Rev Bras Cir Cardiovasc. 2020;35(2):134–40. https://doi.org/10.21470/1678-9741-2019-0311.

Hessel E. A., 2nd (2014). A brief history of cardiopulmonary bypass. Semin Cardiothorac Vasc Anesth, 18(2), 87–100. doi:https://doi.org/10.1177/1089253214530045

Hessel E II, Shann K. Blood pumps, circuitry, and cannulation techniques in cardiopulmonary bypass. Thoracis Key. 2016; https://thoracickey.com/blood-pumps-circuitry-and-cannulation-techniques-in-cardiopulmonary-bypass/

Hori D, Everett AD, Lee JK, et al. Rewarming rate during cardiopulmonary bypass is associated with release of glial fibrillary acidic protein. Ann Thorac Surg. 2015;100(4):1353–8. https://doi.org/10.1016/j.athoracsur.2015.04.006.

Ismail A, Semien G, Miskolczi SY. Cardiopulmonary bypass. In: StatPearls. StatPearls Publishing; 2023.

Iwahashi H, Yuri K, Nose Y. Development of the oxygenator: past, present, and future. J Artif Organs. 2004;7:111–20.

Junior FUV, Antunes N, de Oliveira PP, Filho LMS, Vilarinho KAS, Costa ET. Does the roller pump adjustment in cardiopulmonary bypass settings influence hemolysis? Int J Artif Organs. 2017;40(3):118–22. https://doi.org/10.5301/ijao.5000570.

Kato S, Kusama Y, Abe K, Shibamoto T. Study for the quantification of the roller pump occlusion on the cardio-pulmonary bypass: definition factors of the roller pump occlusion on stable the roller pump operation. Jpn J Extra-Corporeal Technol. 2019;46(4):382–7. https://doi.org/10.7130/jject.46.382.

Kumari S (2013) A retrospective comparison of the clinical impact of use of roller pump or centrifugal pump for cardiopulmonary bypass in patients undergoing coronary artery bypass grafting.

Landoni G, Lomivorotov VV, Nigro Neto C, Monaco F, Pasyuga VV, Bradic N, Lembo R, Gazivoda G, Likhvantsev VV, Lei C, Lozovskiy A, Di Tomasso N, Bukamal NAR, Silva FS, Bautin AE, Ma J, Crivellari M, Farag AMGA, Uvaliev NS, MYRIAD Study Group. Volatile anesthetics versus total intravenous anesthesia for cardiac surgery. N Engl J Med. 2019;380(13):1214–25. https://doi.org/10.1056/NEJMoa1816476.

Lim MW. The history of extracorporeal oxygenators. Anaesthesia. 2006;61(10):984–95.

Machin D, Allsager C. Principles of cardiopulmonary bypass. Contin Educ Anaesth Crit Care Pain. 2006;6(5):176–81. https://doi.org/10.1093/bjaceaccp/mkl043.

Matte GS, del Nido PJ. History and use of del Nido cardioplegia solution at Boston Children's Hospital. J Extra Corpor Technol. 2012;44(3):98–103.

McMillan J, Bago M, McDonald M. Heat exchanger integrity in various concentrations of hydrogen peroxide: an experimental analysis and review of methods to examine integrity of membrane oxygenator heat exchangers. The Australian and New Zealand College of Perfusionists Gazette, 2019. https://epublishbyus.com/ebook/10048363/F143-166335-1-ANZCP_Gazette-DEC18-V5-EPU B.pf

Mick SL, Robich MP, Houghtaling PL, Gillinov AM, Soltesz EG, Johnston DR, Blackstone EH, Sabik JF. del nido versus buckberg cardioplegia in adult isolated valve surgery. J Thorac Cardiovasc Surg. 2015;149(2):626–636.e5. https://doi.org/10.1016/j.jtcvs.2014.10.085.

Miller AL, Theodore D, Widrich J. Inhalational anesthetic. [Updated 2023 May 1]. In: StatPearls [Internet]. Treasure Island: StatPearls Publishing; 2023. Available from: https://www.ncbi.nlm.nih.gov/books/NBK554540/.

Mongero L, Stammers A, Tesdahl E, Stasko A, Weinstein S. The effect of ultrafiltration on end-cardiopulmonary bypass hematocrit during cardiac surgery. Perfusion. 2018;33(5):367–74. https://doi.org/10.1177/0267659117747046.

Murphy GS, Hessel EA 2nd, Groom RC. Optimal perfusion during cardiopulmonary bypass: an evidence-based approach. Anesth Analg. 2009a;108(5):1394–417. https://doi.org/10.1213/ane.0b013e3181875e2e.

Murphy GS, Hessel EA, Groom RC. Optimal perfusion during cardiopulmonary bypass: an evidence-based approach. Anesth Analg. 2009b;108(5):1394–417. https://doi.org/10.1213/ane.0b013e3181875e2e.

Nagase K, Kohori F, Sakai K. Oxygen transfer performance of a membrane oxygenator composed of crossed and parallel hollow fibers. Biochem Eng J. 2005;24(2):105–13. ISSN:1369-703X. https://doi.org/10.1016/j.bej.2005.02.003.

Pan Y, Li Y, Li Y, Li J, Chen H. Fatigue of red blood cells under periodic squeezes in ECMO. Proc Natl Acad Sci USA. 2022;119(49):e2210819119. https://doi.org/10.1073/pnas.2210819119.

Riley JB. Arterial line filters ranked for gaseous microemboli separation performance: an in vitro study. J Extra Corpor Technol. 2008;40(1):21–6.

Sarkar M, Prabhu V. Basics of cardiopulmonary bypass. Indian J Anaesth. 2017;61(9):760–7. https://doi.org/10.4103/ija.IJA_379_17.

Schaadt J. Fiber manufacturing, membrane classification, and winding technologies associated with membrane oxygenators. J Extra Corpor Technol. 1998;30(1):30–4. https://doi.org/10.1051/ject/199830130.

Segers PA, Heida JF, de Vries I, Maas C, Boogaart AJ, Eilander S. Clinical evaluation of nine hollow-fibre membrane oxygenators. Perfusion. 2001;16(2):95–106. https://doi.org/10.1177/026765910101600203.

Snyder EJ, Mcelwee DL, Harb HM, Cullen JA, Tackel IS, Baumgart S, Iskandarani B, Elkind A, Shaker M. Investigation of fatigue failure of S-65-HL super tygon roller pump tubing. J Extra Corpor Technol. 1996;28(2):79–87. https://doi.org/10.1051/ject/199628279.

Soliman R, Fouad E, Belghith M, Abdelmageed T. Conventional hemofiltration during cardiopulmonary bypass increases the serum lactate level in adult cardiac surgery. Ann Card Anaesth. 2016;19(1):45–51. https://doi.org/10.4103/0971-9784.173019.

Spectrum Medical. Quantum perfusion systems, 2023a. https://www.spectrummedical.com//brochures/perfusion-technologies/quantum-perfusionsystems_web_5-23-18.pdf. Accessed Aug 2023.

Spectrum Medical. Flow and bubble detection, 2023b. https://www.spectrummedical.com/en/quantum-perfusion-for-the-icu-cath-lab-and-transport/quantum-perfusion-icu-transport/quantum-ventilation-system/flow-bubble-detection

Tagaya M, Matsuda M, Ryugo M, Takasaki T, Kurita S, Handa H, Hara K. Is using an open-reservoir cardiopulmonary bypass circuit after 6 days on standby safe? Interact Cardiovasc Thorac Surg. 2016;22(2):155–60. https://doi.org/10.1093/icvts/ivv302.

TERUMO Cardiovascular. CAPIOX Cardiotomy Reservoirs, 2023a. https://www.terumocv.com/products/ProductDetail.aspx?groupId=1&familyID=6&country=1. Accessed Aug 2023.

TERUMO Cardiovascular. CDI® Blood Parameter Monitoring System 550, 2023b. https://www.terumocv.com/cdi550/. Accessed Aug 2023.

Tschaut RJ, editor. First edition. Pabst Science Publishers; 2020. Print: ISBN:978-3-95853-545-9, eBook:ISBN 978-3-95853-546-6

Wang S, Rosenthal T, Kunselman AR, Ündar A. Evaluation of different diameter arterial tubing and arterial cannulae in simulated neonatal/pediatric cardiopulmonary bypass circuits. Artif Organs. 2015;39(1):43–52. https://doi.org/10.1111/aor.12446.

Zangrillo A, Garozzo FA, Biondi-Zoccai G, Pappalardo F, Monaco F, Crivellari M, Bignami E, Nuzzi M, Landoni G. Miniaturized cardiopulmonary bypass improves short-term outcome in cardiac surgery: A meta-analysis of randomized controlled studies. J Thorac Cardiovasc Surg. 2010;139(5):1162–9. https://doi.org/10.1016/j.jtcvs.2009.07.048.

Ziganshin BA, Elefteriades JA. Deep hypothermic circulatory arrest. Ann Cardiothorac Surg. 2013;2(3):303–15. https://doi.org/10.3978/j.issn.2225-319X.2013.01.05.

Zorrilla-Vaca A, Núñez-Patiño RA, Torres V, Salazar-Gomez Y. The impact of volatile anesthetic choice on postoperative outcomes of cardiac surgery: a meta-analysis. BioMed Res Int. 2017, 2017:Article ID 7073401, 12 pages. https://doi.org/10.1155/2017/7073401.

Cardiopulmonary Bypass Hardware Assembly and Setting Up the Circuit

8

Alex Chappell and Celia Gagnon

Introduction

The cardiopulmonary bypass machine (CPB), first used in 1953 by John Heysham Gibbon Jr., was designed with the purpose of giving the surgeon a bloodless, motionless field during heart surgery. Over the years, through improvement, ingenuity, and innovation, the CPB machine has also been adapted for surgeries on the lungs, liver, and brain. Although the CPB machine has evolved significantly over the last 70 years, its fundamental concepts remain unchanged.

The CPB pulls blood from the patient (typically from the venous vasculature or the right side of the heart), drains it into a closed or open reservoir, filters it, oxygenates it, adjusts its temperature (warming or cooling), and then returns it to the patient's arterial vasculature beyond the heart and lungs. This shunting of blood away from the patient to the CPB machine and back allows for hemodynamic stability while the heart or lungs are operated on. To fully understand the concepts and complexities of CPB, it is essential to first grasp the components of the machine and how sterile, single-use disposables are assembled to perform CPB.

Hardware and Disposables in CPB

In the context of CPB, we distinguish between two key categories:

Supplementary Information The online version contains supplementary material available at https://doi.org/10.1007/978-3-031-91163-7_8.

A. Chappell (✉)
Perfusion Services, Cardiac Surgery Division, Department of Surgery, Children's Hospital of Philadelphia, Philadelphia, PA, USA

Pediatrics, Keystone Perfusion Services, Philadelphia, USA
e-mail: achappell@keystoneperfusion.com

C. Gagnon
Perfusion Services, Cardiac Surgery Division, Department of Surgery, Children's Hospital of Philadelphia, Philadelphia, PA, USA
e-mail: achappell@keystoneperfusion.com

Hardware

The hardware of the CPB machine refers to the equipment that remains intact and reusable from case to case and is not discarded after use on a patient. Each hardware component plays a specific role in CPB, which we will discuss individually. This equipment is typically maintained by a Biomedical Engineering department, responsible for performing preventive maintenance according to the equipment's Instructions for Use (IFU). It is essential to review all IFUs to ensure the equipment is used, cleaned, and maintained correctly over time. The hardware of a pump generally is not removed or changed on a case-by-case basis. However, while the hardware remains consistent between cases, variations may exist between institutions depending on the overall goals of bypass, the types of surgeries performed, and the patient populations being treated.

One-Time-Use Disposables

"One-time-use disposables" refer to the components of the CPB circuit that are used for a single patient and discarded after each surgical case. The bypass circuit is customized for each procedure and can be tailored to the specific needs of the patient. The circuit is assembled using aseptic techniques to prevent contamination. In many cases, the CPB machine can be set up in advance. For adults, this process is generally simpler, as the bypass circuit remains fairly consistent across different cases. In pediatric cases, however, variations in circuit length, tubing size, oxygenator size, and the use of hemoconcentrators often require the circuit to be customized for each patient. While practices may vary between institutions, some studies suggest that dry, closed pre-set circuits can maintain sterility for up to 60 days, while wet, open circuits can do so for up to 5 days. According to the Extracorporeal Life Support Organization (ELSO) guidelines, pre-assembled and primed Extracorporeal Membrane Oxygenation (ECMO) systems (as an example of wet closed

A. S. Awad, J. DiNardo (eds.), *Clinical Perfusion for Cardiac Surgery*, https://doi.org/10.1007/978-3-031-91163-7_8

circuits) can be safely stored for up to 30 days but only if specific conditions are strictly adhered to.

Illustrative Diagrams and Photos

Figure 7.3 is a referenced diagram that illustrates the equipment, disposables, and blood flow path during CPB. It effectively highlights the fundamental concepts of a CPB circuit. Following the diagram are two series of photos demonstrating the setup of a CPB system. While the overall concepts and functions of the machine and circuitry remain consistent, the finer details can vary significantly. There is no single, universally accepted method for constructing a bypass circuit; this chapter provides an example of how both adult and pediatric cardiopulmonary circuits can be assembled.

Preparation for Assembly

Sterilization and Safety Checks

Before assembling the CPB circuit, it is critical to ensure that all components are sterile and intact. Disposables used for constructing a CPB circuit typically come in sterilized packs. Always check the expiration date and inspect the packaging's integrity for any holes, tears, or the presence of foreign objects or fluids. Ensure all tools and components are sterilized according to institutional protocols to prevent any potential contamination and harm to the patient.

Workspace Preparation

A clean and organized workspace is essential for assembling the CPB circuit. Regardless of whether the assembly takes place in a designated setup room or directly in the operating room, the area must be thoroughly cleaned and disinfected beforehand. Gather all necessary components of the circuit, prioritizing those with sooner expiration dates. This may include the circuit components themselves, fluids required for priming, safety devices, blades, alcohol swabs for cutting tubing to specific lengths, clamps, and other necessary items. Arrange all components and disposables in the sequence in which they will be opened and assembled (Fig. 8.1).

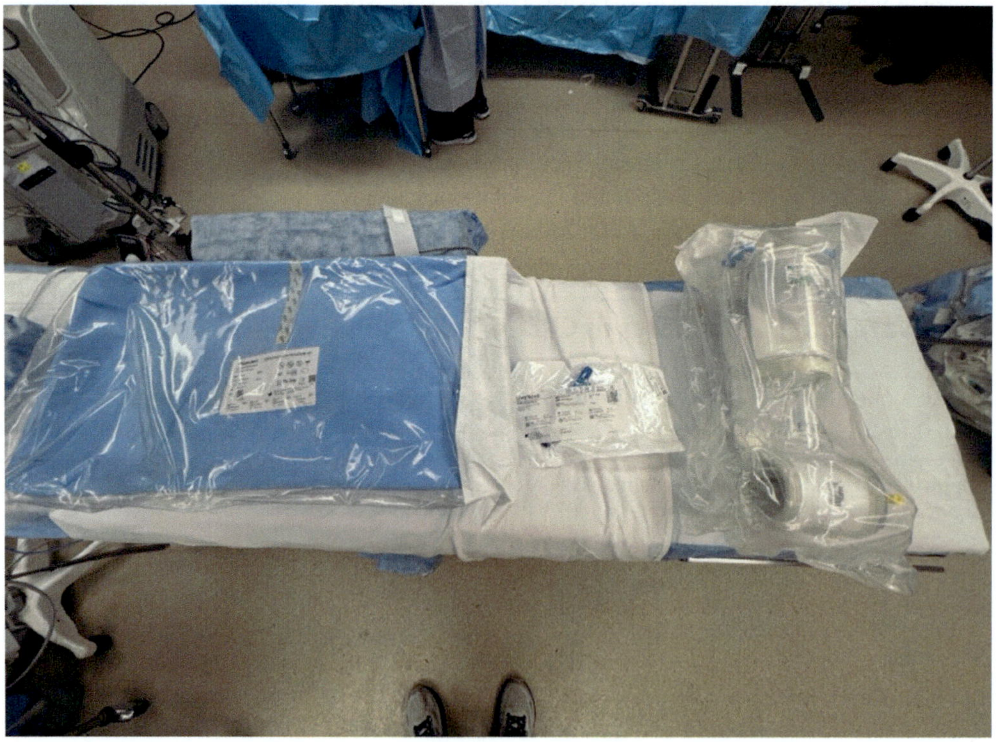

Fig. 8.1 A clean, disinfected workspace is essential for CPB circuit assembly. Gather components by expiration date and arrange them in assembly order for efficiency and safety

Setup of the CPB Machine

Once all single-use disposables have been gathered, it is time to assess the CPB machine. Meticulously inspect all the equipment, including roller pumps, safety devices, clamps, and monitors. Determine if anything is missing or broken, if so resolve the issue appropriately before putting the CPB machine into service. Items to look for include.

- Centrifugal motor or arterial roller pump.
- Cardioplegia pump(s).
- Vent pumps.
- Sucker pumps.
- Reservoir/oxygenator holder.
- Arterial line filter holder (if applicable).
- Hemoconcentrator holder.
- Manifold holder (if applicable).
- Oxygen/air blender.
- Inhaled anesthetic vaporizer.
- Heater–Cooler.
- Flow probes.
- Continuous in-line/online monitoring.
- Venous-assisted vacuum regulator.
- Temperature probes.
- Pump monitors.
- Level sensor.
- Pressure transducers.
- Bubble detector.
- Electronic clamps (if applicable).
- Tubing clamps.

Evaluate the cleanliness of the pump. Although every pump should be wiped down post-bypass, it is imperative that the CPB machine be free of any blood or other sources of contamination. Once the CPB machine has been thoroughly examined, single-use disposables can be placed on the pump.

Assembly of the CPB Circuit

Assembling a CPB circuit requires special care, diligence, and attention to detail. Mistakes made during the setup can affect the quality of care provided to the patient and may lead to safety concerns. For new perfusionists and perfusion students, it is imperative to practice building the circuit as much as possible. Being able to assemble your institution's CPB circuit quickly and efficiently is crucial in emergency situations. Below, you will find two examples of bypass circuit setups. The blue-outlined photos on the left depict an example of an adult circuit, while the red-outlined pictures on the right illustrate an example of a pediatric pump.

Step-by-Step Guide to Assembling the Circuit (Figs. 8.1, 8.2, 8.3, 8.4, 8.5, 8.6, 8.7, 8.8, 8.9, 8.10, 8.11, 8.12, 8.13, 8.14, 8.15, 8.16, 8.17, 8.18, 8.19, 8.20, 8.21, and 8.22)

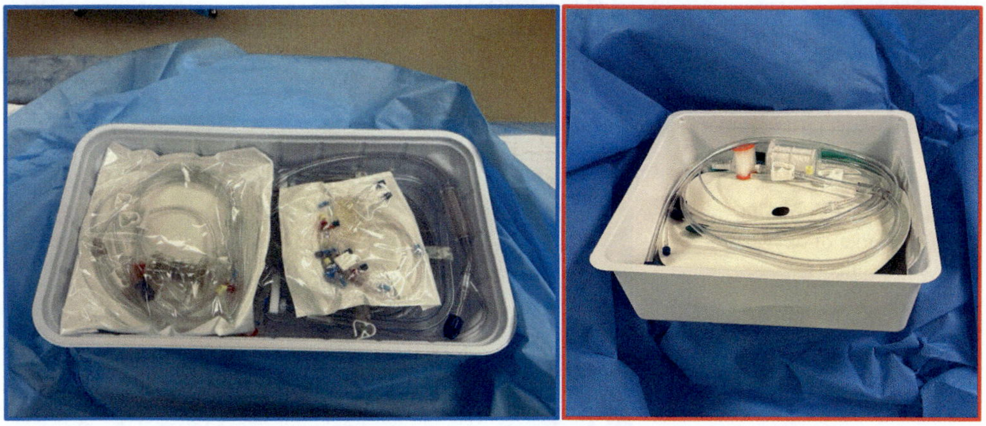

Fig. 8.2 Open pump pack

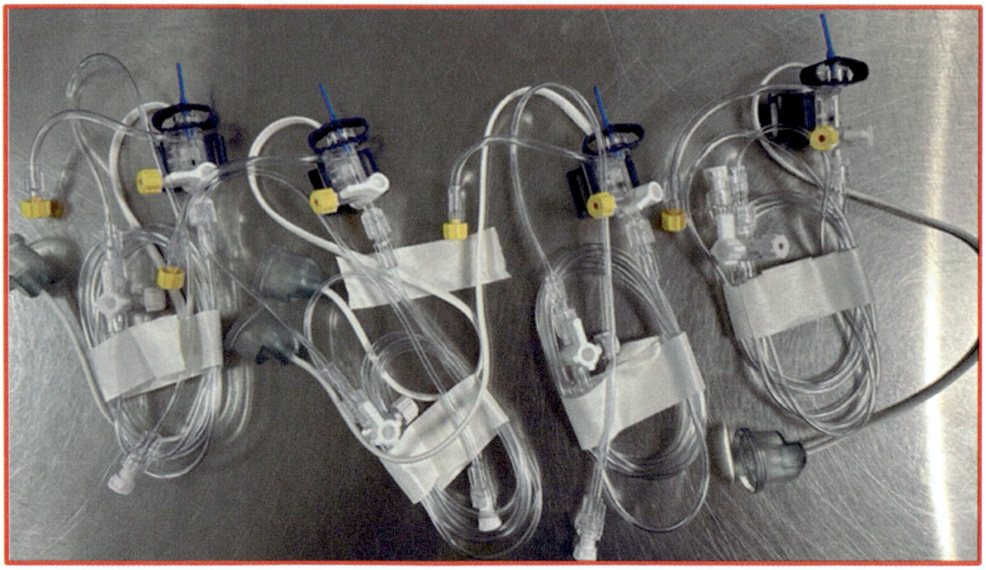

Fig. 8.3 Assemble pressure transducers (if applicable)

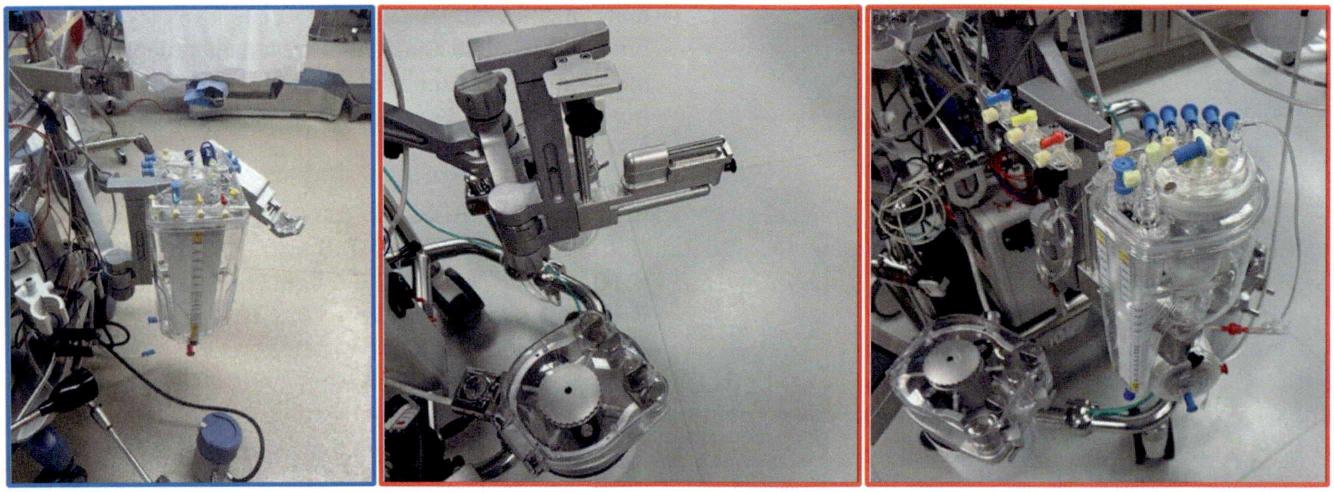

Fig. 8.4 Attach reservoir to the reservoir/oxygenator holder

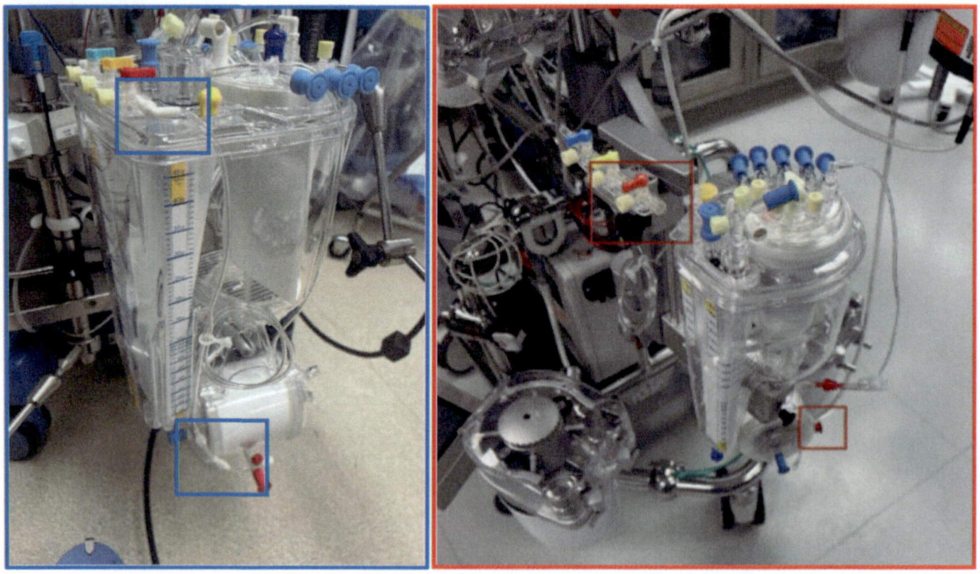

Fig. 8.5 Attach manifold tubing to outlet of oxygenator and venous inlet

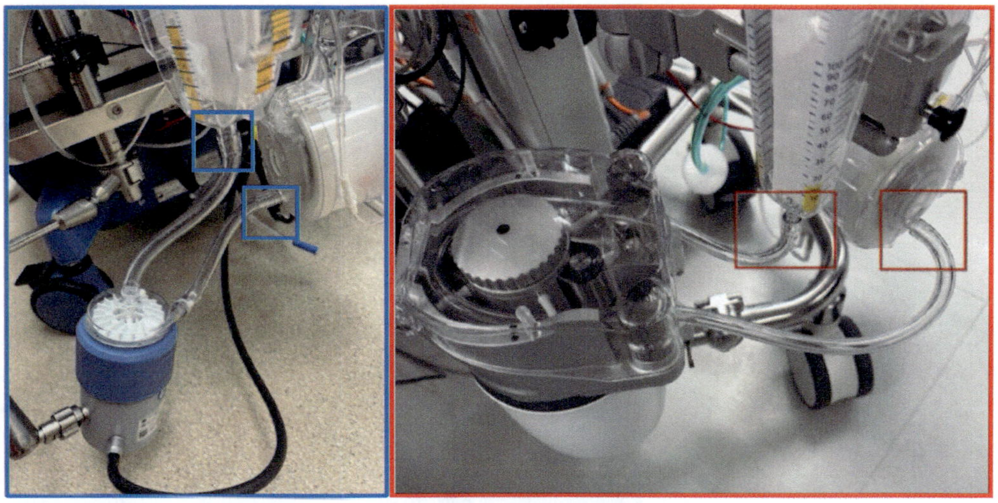

Fig. 8.6 Attach centrifugal head or arterial raceway tubing to the outlet of reservoir and inlet of oxygenator

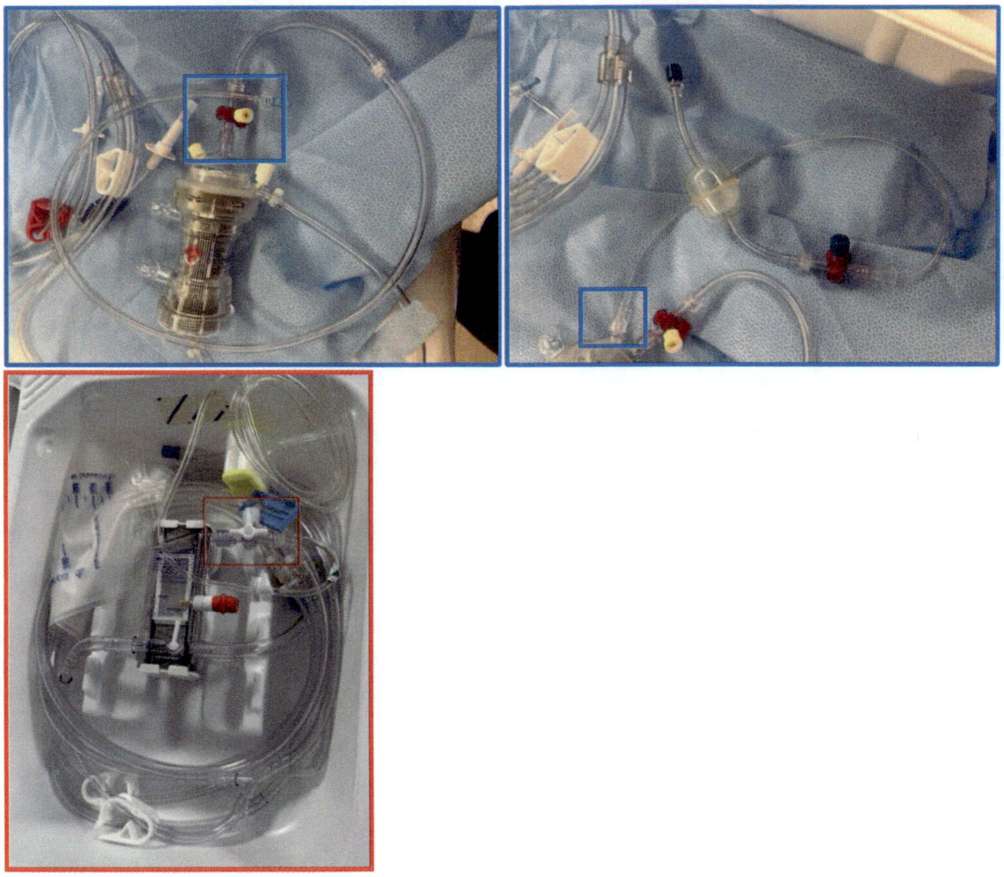

Fig. 8.7 Attach recirculation line and pressure line to cardioplegia heat exchanger

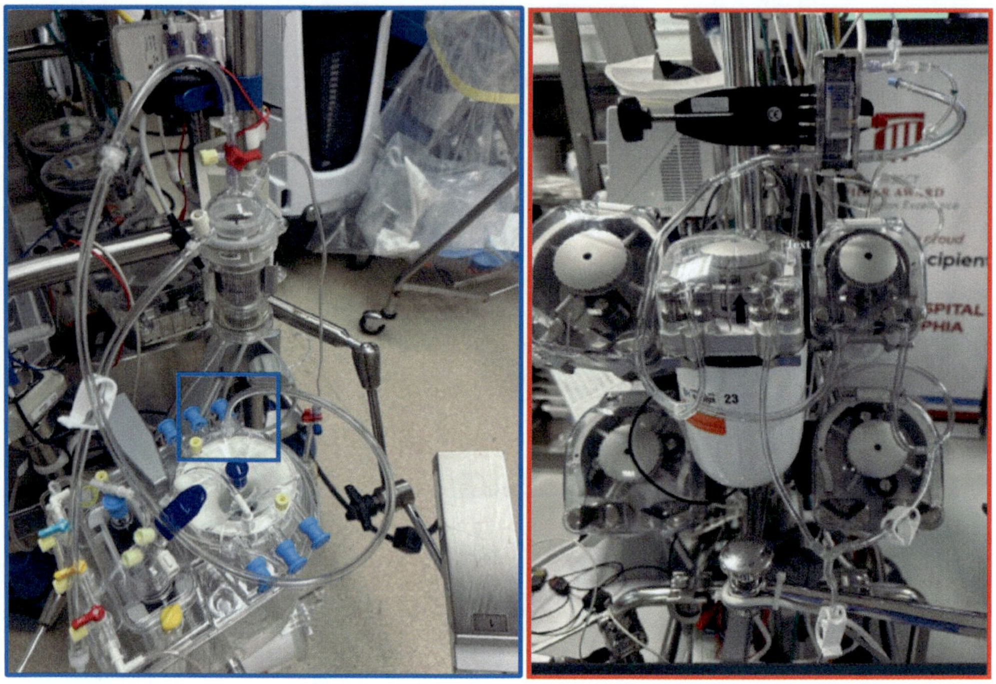

Fig. 8.8 Place cardioplegia heat exchanger in its holder and attach recirc line to reservoir

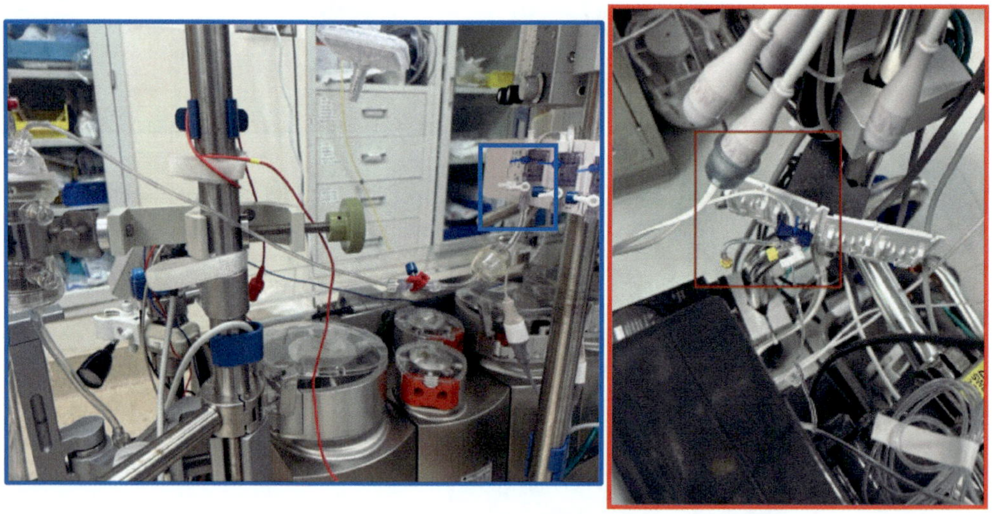

Fig. 8.9 Attach pressure line and pressure dome to the cardioplegia heat exchanger

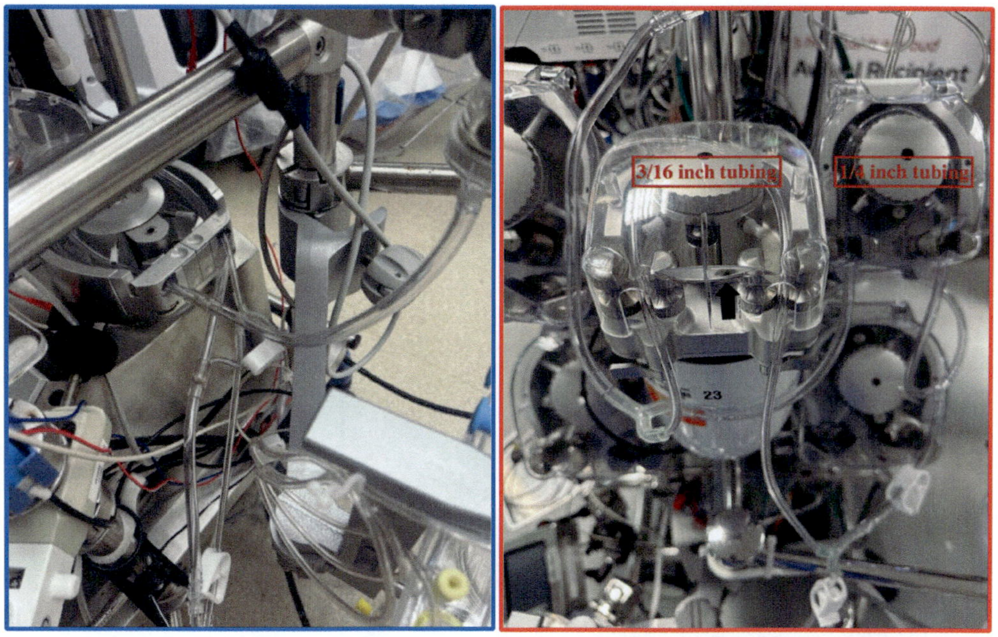

Fig. 8.10 Place cardioplegia tubing into its designated raceway(s)

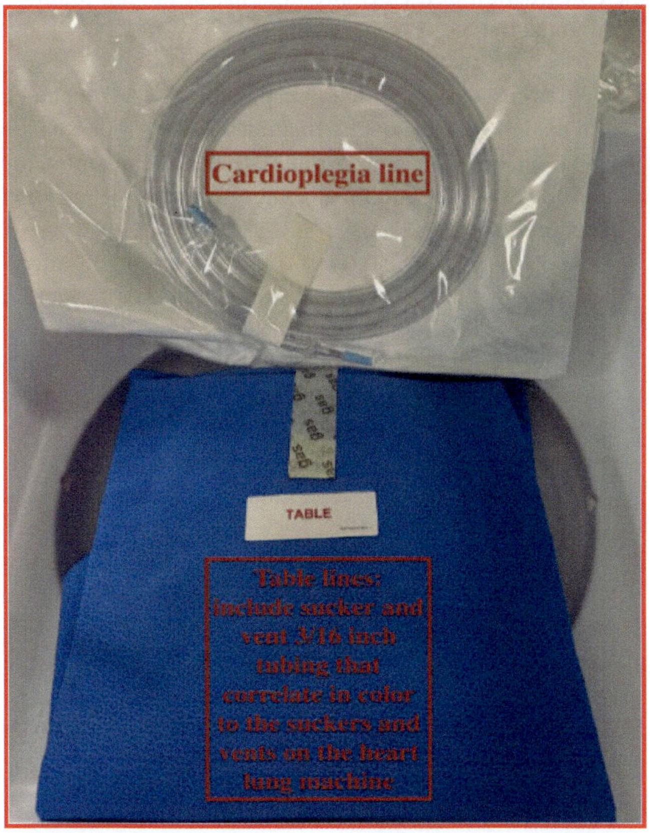

Fig. 8.11 Pediatric example only—Give the circulating nurse sterile suckers, vents, and cardioplegia line (these lines get passed back to perfusion and are connected just prior to initiation of bypass)

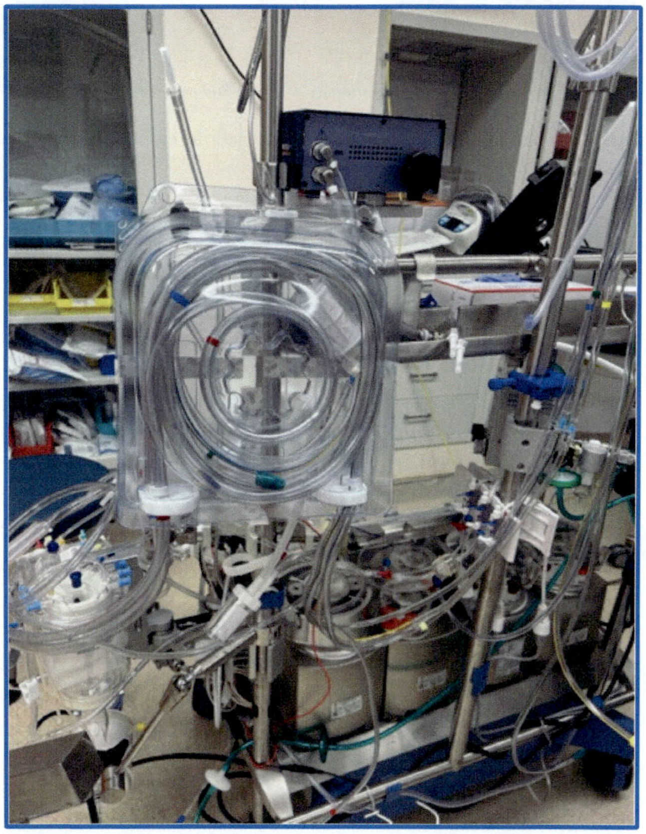

Fig. 8.12 Adult Example Only- Hang sterile table lines on pump in convenient location (if applicable)

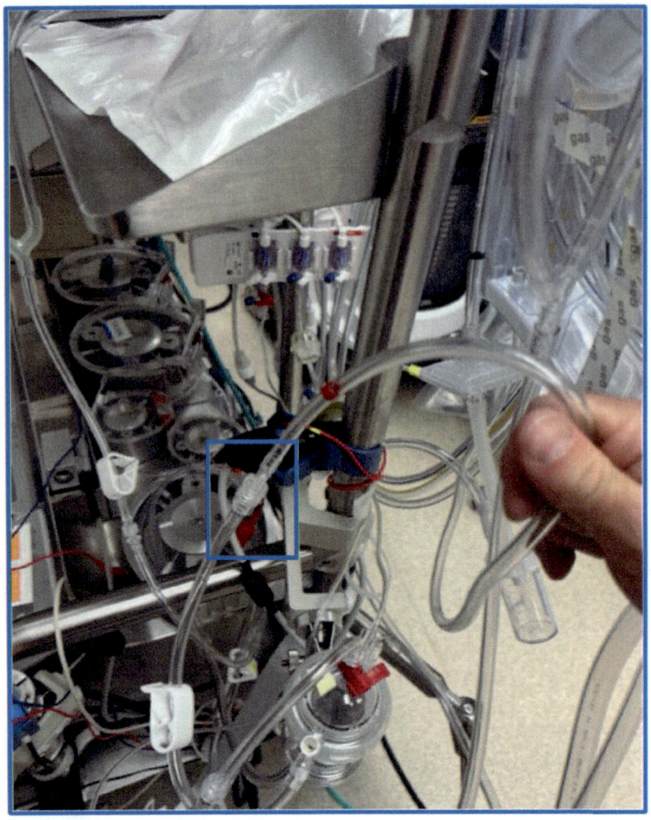

Fig. 8.13 Adult example only—Connect sterile cardioplegia line to the outlet of cardioplegia heat exchanger

Tips for Efficient and Safe Assembly

- Always ensure that your hands are clean. The use of gloves can help prevent contamination of the circuit.
- Ensure every connection is performed aseptically. Once caps are removed from the ends of tubing, connectors, or Luer locks, do not set them down or allow them to touch anything other than their designated connections. In a controlled manner, attach the tubing or Luer lock to the correct location.
- Push tubing connections fully onto the connectors, ensuring they pass the second barb (the small ridges or raised edges on the connectors), to guarantee a secure fit.
- Hand-tighten all Luer lock connections as tightly as possible.
- If cuts need to be made to adjust the length of tubing, ensure a sterile blade is used and the desired area is cleaned with alcohol. While it may sometimes be necessary, try to avoid cutting into the circuit whenever possible. Every time the circuit is altered, the risk of contamination increases.
- Systematically build your pump the same way each time, creating a routine. Following a routine when constructing a circuit will help prevent mistakes and increase efficiency during times of emergencies.
- Double-check each connection after completing the build.
- Trace the blood's path through the circuit to confirm the build's completeness.
- Check the occlusion settings of all roller pumps on the CPB machine.

Common Pitfalls and How to Avoid Them

While there are numerous mistakes that can be made during the construction of a CPB circuit, a list of the top pitfalls is highlighted below.

1. Contamination of the circuit can be highly detrimental to the patient. Since contamination is often not visually apparent, it is easy to overlook. To prevent contamination, carefully inspect and ensure the integrity of every connection made.
2. Loose connections can result in air entrainment, circuit leaks, inaccurate pressure measurements, or leakage of venous-assisted vacuum.
3. Making incorrect connections will alter the proper path of blood, most likely rendering the bypass circuit useless. Always trace the path of blood to ensure the circuit is constructed correctly. Critical connections, such as the green oxygen tubing, are essential for the proper functioning of CPB.
4. Placing the tubing for suckers, vents, cardioplegia pumps, or the arterial head pump in the incorrect direction can have serious consequences. Arrows placed on the roller pump, along with diligent double-checks, can help prevent this error.
5. Incorrect pump occlusions can hinder the blood's ability to flow correctly or cause hemolysis.

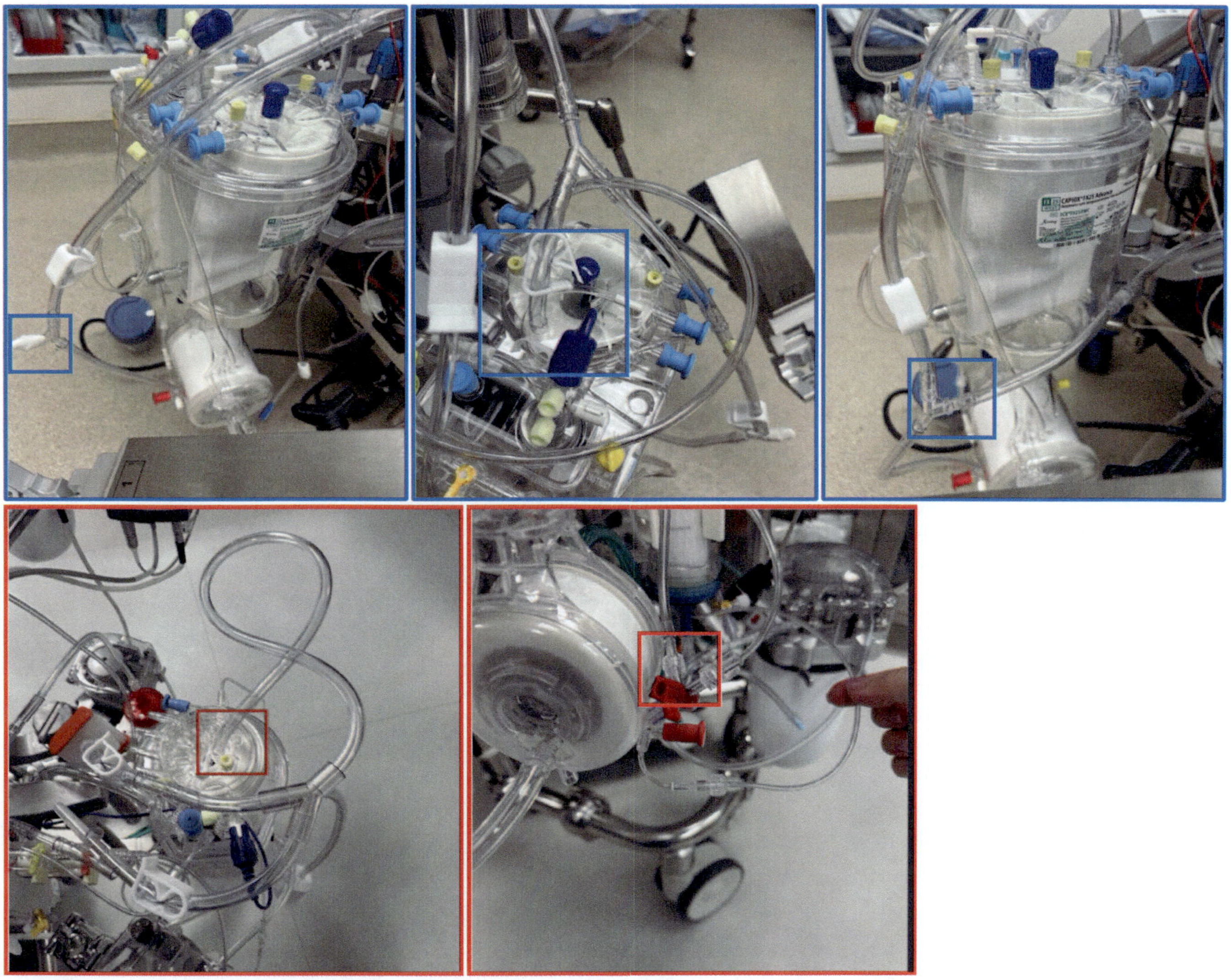

Fig. 8.14 Attach quick prime line, the cardioplegia line, and, if present (adult example) the recirculation line

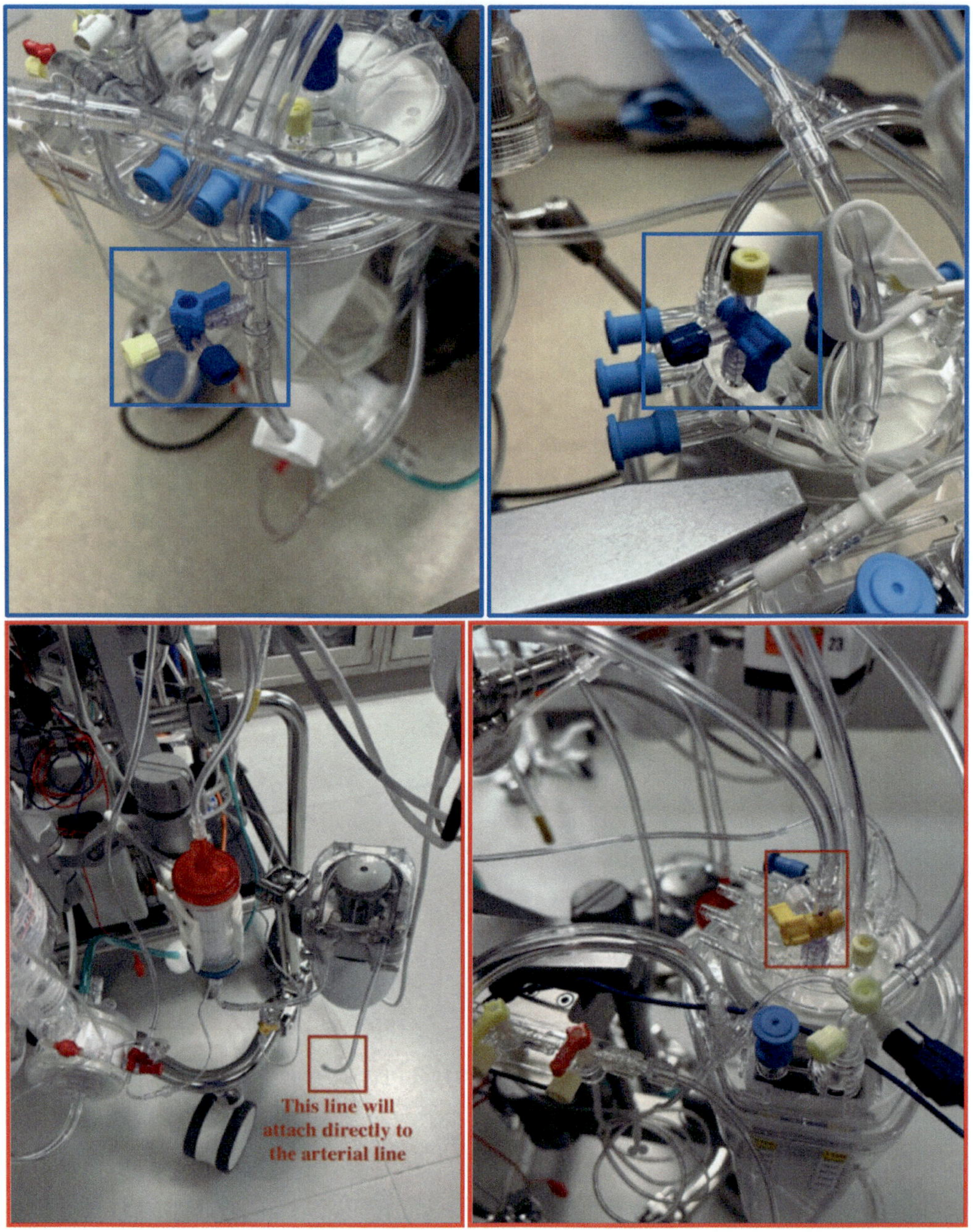

Fig. 8.15 Attach three-way stopcocks to allow for hemoconcentrator addition during the bypass run OR attach the inlet and outlet of the hemoconcentrator

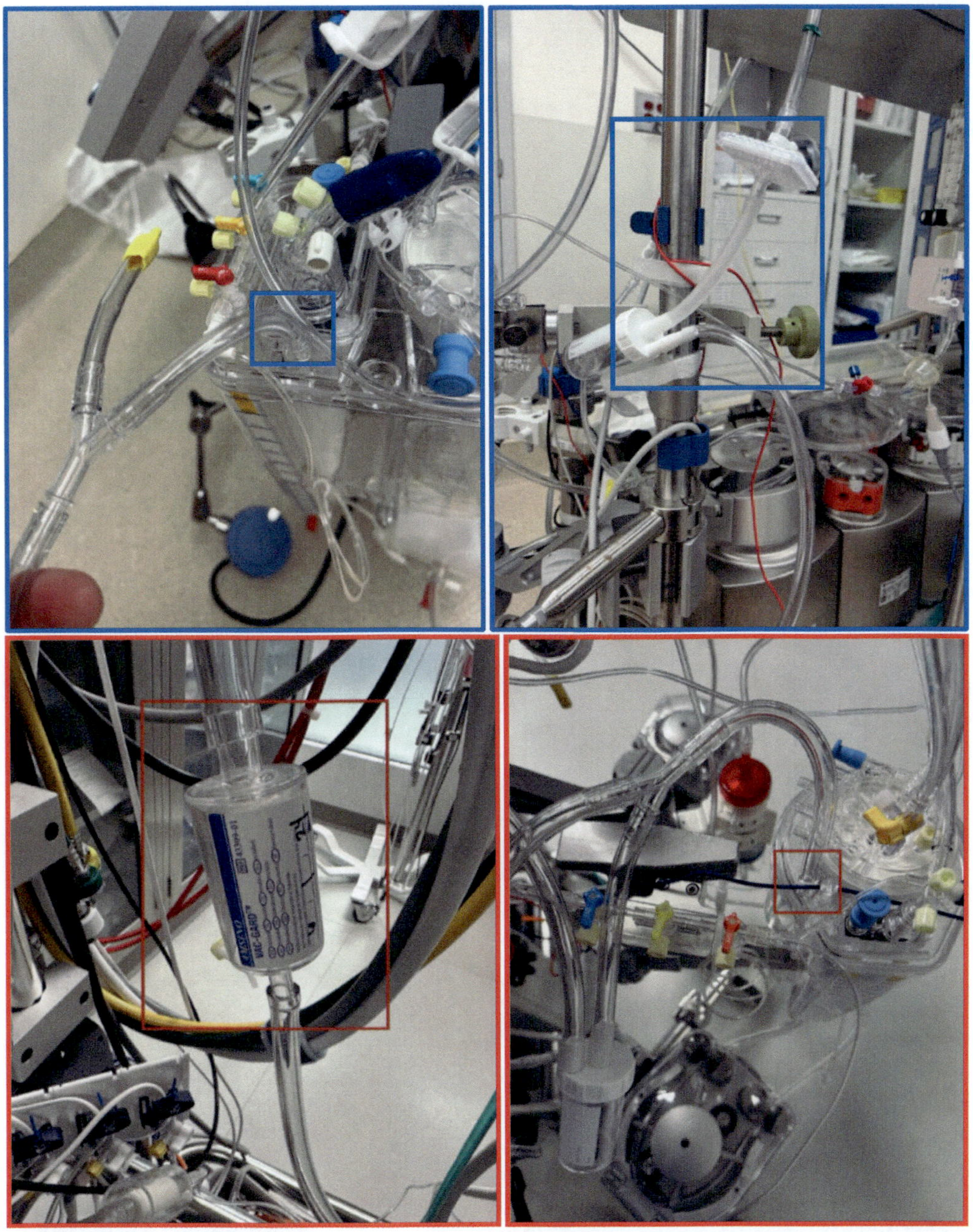

Fig. 8.16 Attach venous-assisted vacuum line to the reservoir and vacuum regulator

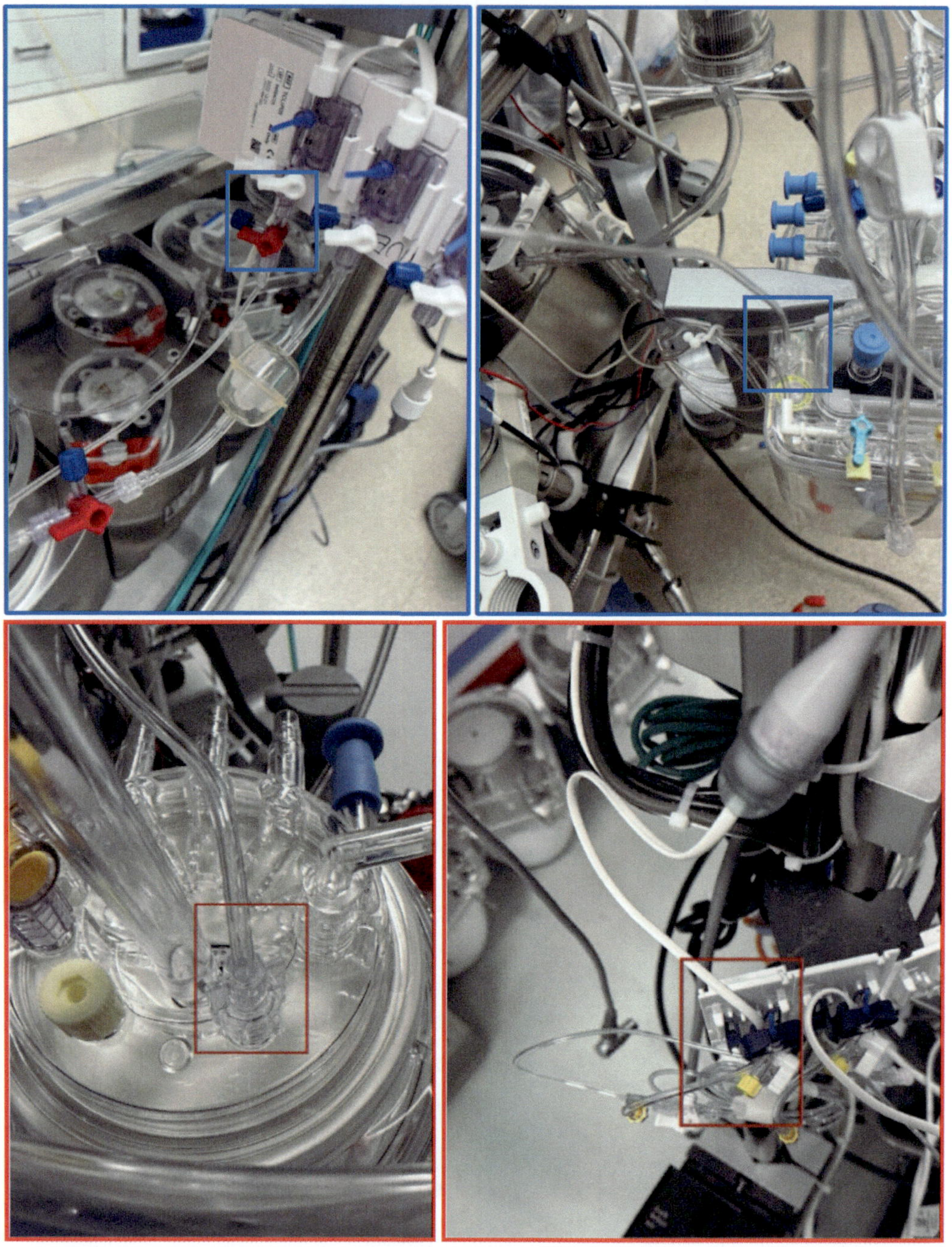

Fig. 8.17 Attach reservoir pressure tubing to the venous reservoir and pressure transducer

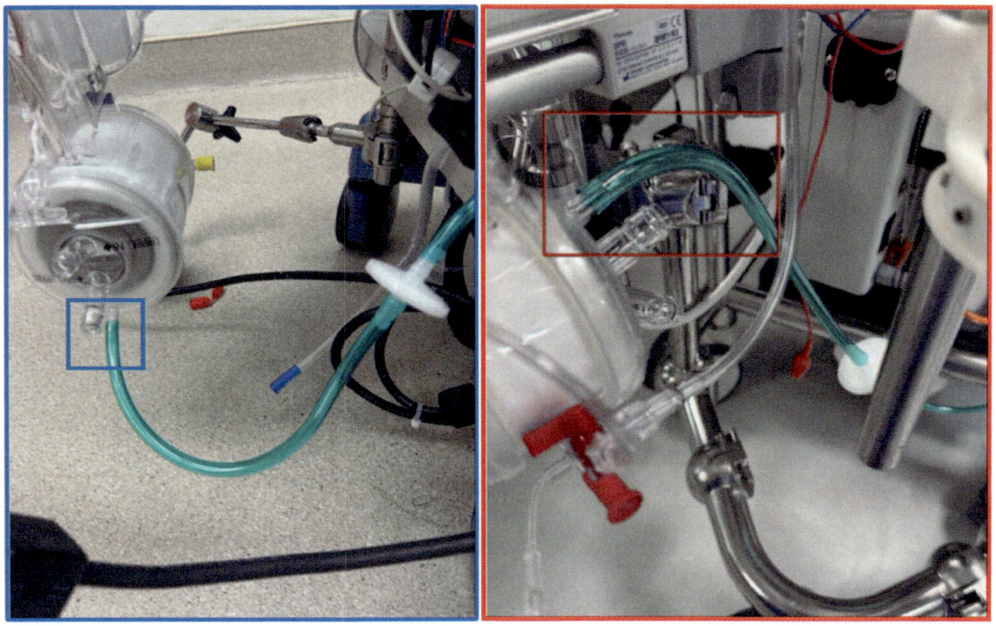

Fig. 8.18 Attach green oxygen tubing to the oxygenator

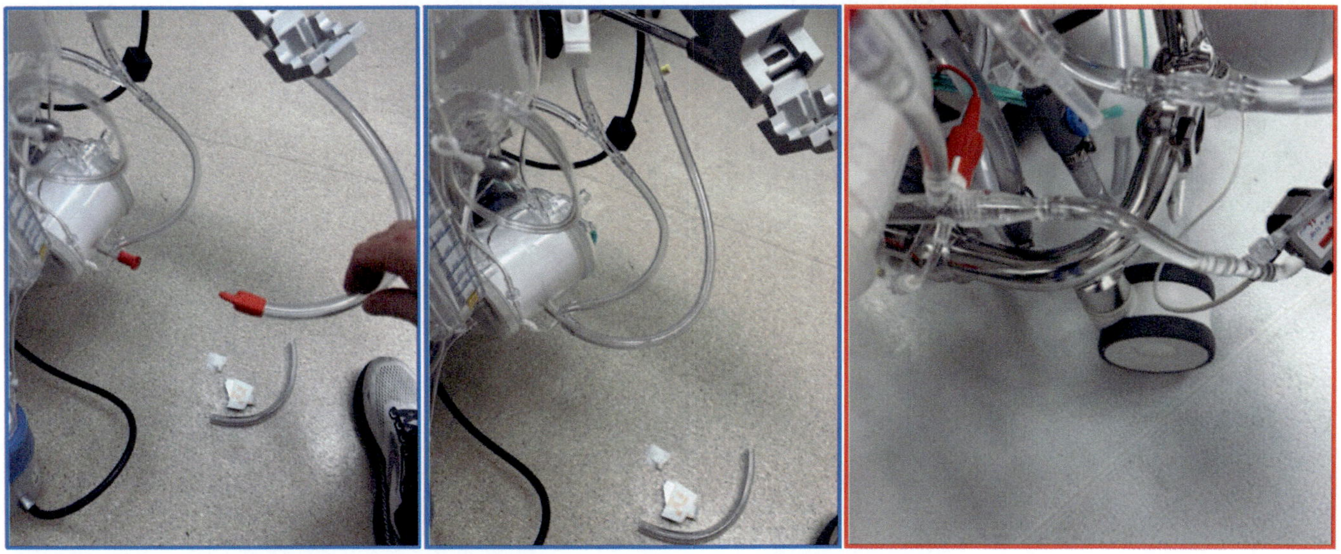

Fig. 8.19 Connect arterial line to the outlet of oxygenator

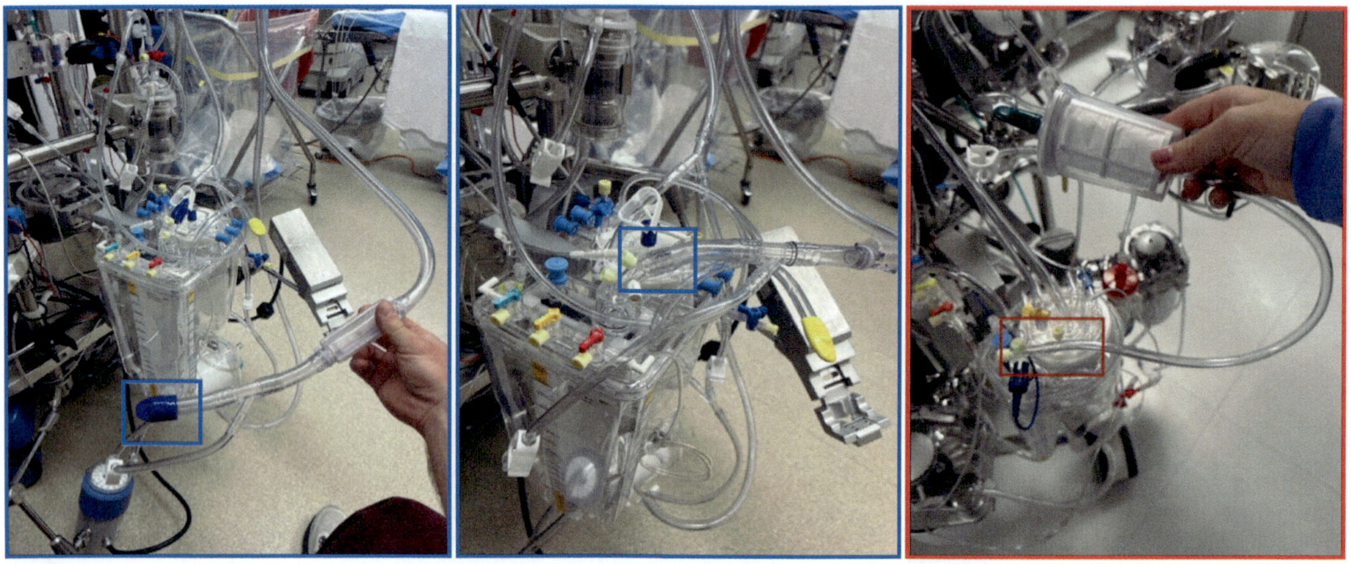

Fig. 8.20 Connect venous line to the inlet of the venous reservoir

Fig. 8.21 Connect the arterial pressure line to the arterial line and its pressure transducer

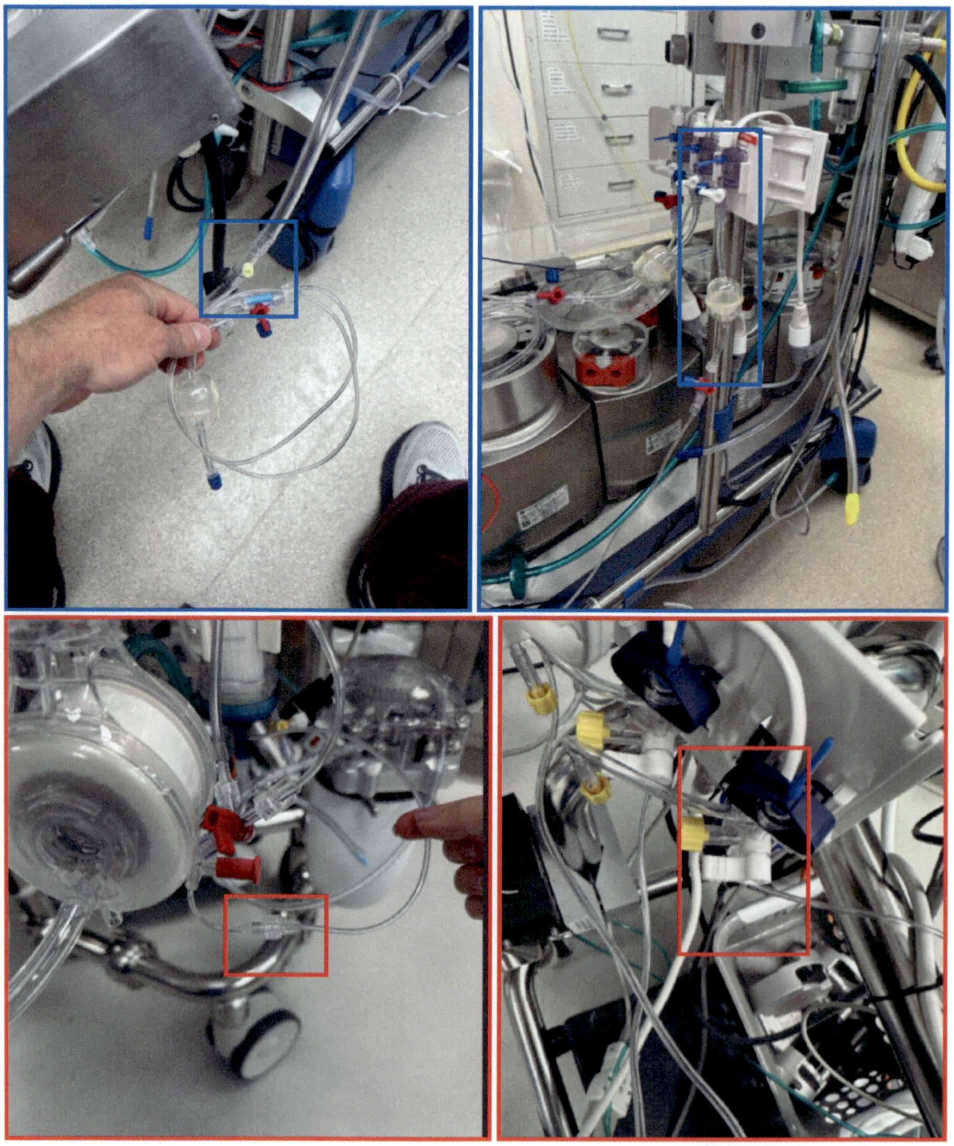

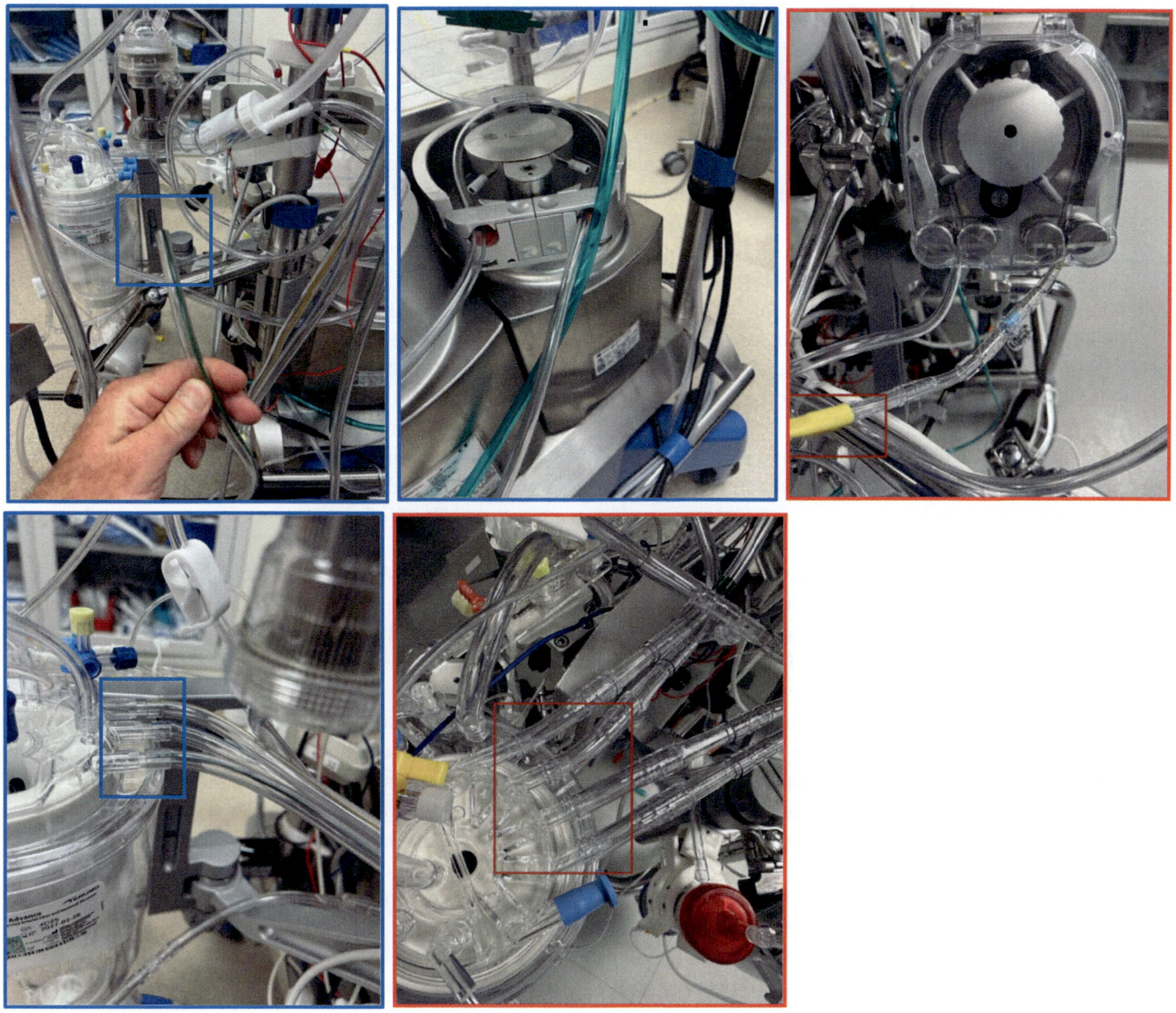

Fig. 8.22 Place suckers and vents in their respective raceways and connect to the venous reservoir

Priming the CPB Circuit

Priming the CPB circuit is a critical step to ensure the system is free of air and ready for use. While the specific solutions and additives used for priming a circuit are discussed in Chap. 9, only a few remarks on special situations will be outlined below.

Selection of Priming Fluid

- *Isotonic/pH Balanced Crystalloid Solution*: Typically used for priming, such as Plasmalyte A or Normosol R.
- *Additives*: While each institution may use different variations of additives in their CPB prime, we will focus on some of the most commonly used ones, whether added directly to the pump or administered by anesthesia providers. A total of 25% albumin helps maintain oncotic pressure; heparin prevents clot formation; sodium bicarbonate, a buffer, counteracts metabolic acidosis and helps restore physiological pH balance; mannitol acts as both an oxygen-free radical scavenger and an osmotic diuretic; furosemide (Lasix) is a loop diuretic; cefazolin (Ancef) is a first-generation cephalosporin antibiotic; tranexamic acid (TXA) and aminocaproic acid (Amicar) are antifibrinolytic agents; and methylprednisolone (Solu-Medrol) reduces inflammatory response.

Process of Priming and Air Removal (De-Airing)

1. *Preparation and Assemble Circuit Components*
   - Assemble the CPB circuit with the appropriate tubing, oxygenator, and filters. Verify that all components are sterile, properly connected, and securely fastened, ensuring that all tubing connections are tight (using zip ties as needed).
   - Perform a carbon dioxide (CO_2) flush (optional, based on institutional preference) to fill the tubing and components. This displaces nitrogen, as CO_2 is more soluble, and helps reduce the risk of bacterial growth.
   - Ensure that the oxygenator's integrated heat exchanger has been water-tested for leaks before adding any fluid to the circuit.
   - Use a prebypass filter (0.2–10 μm) to remove any particulates from the prime, ensuring the filter is removed prior to blood priming.
2. *Fill the Reservoir*

   Start by clamping the reservoir outlet line, then fill the main reservoir with the selected priming fluid (e.g., crystalloids or blood, if required), ensuring the minimum required prime volume is achieved. It is crucial to monitor the level to prevent underfilling or overfilling, as either can affect the priming process and circuit performance.
3. *Removing the Clamp from the Reservoir Outlet*

   Once the reservoir is filled, remove the clamp from the reservoir outlet line to allow the fluid to flow into the circuit.
4. *Initial Gravity Pump Head Priming*

   Allow the priming fluid to flow by gravity from the reservoir into the centrifugal pump head, which helps displace any trapped air within the pump. Centrifugal pumps are commonly utilized in adult practice. If priming with a roller arterial pump, commonly used in pediatric practice, this step can be skipped.
5. *Oxygenator/AV Loop Priming*
   - Isolate the oxygenator and AV Loop: Prime the oxygenator and AV loop first. As the priming fluid begins to fill the oxygenator, gently tap the oxygenator housing a few times. This tapping action helps to dislodge any air bubbles that may be trapped within the fine mesh of the oxygenator's membrane.
   - Pressurize the Oxygenator: Achieve oxygenator pressurization by gradually increasing the revolutions per minute (RPM) of the pump head while partially clamping the venous line to raise pressure within the oxygenator. Ensure the purge line is open to allow any trapped air to be expelled during this process. Complete fluid filling and air removal from the oxygenator are crucial, as any remaining air pockets can significantly impair gas exchange efficiency during the procedure.
6. *Circuit Priming*
   1. *Sequential Priming*
      - Once the oxygenator has been successfully primed and is free of air, proceed to prime each additional section of the pump sequentially. Remove the clamp on the arterial line and gradually increase the RPM of the pump to pressurize the entire circuit. This step helps move fluid through the system, expelling any remaining air in the following order:
        - From the outlet of the oxygenator to the arterial line, through the pre-bypass filter, and finally to the venous line.
        - Recirculation Line: Next, prime the recirculation line, which allows blood to bypass the patient's heart and lungs during CPB.
        - Pressure Monitoring Lines: Prime the lines connected to pressure transducers.
        - Cardioplegia System: Finally, prime the cardioplegia system.
        - Filters: During the sequential priming process, ensure that any additional filters (such as arterial line filters or pre-bypass filters) are also primed to prevent air or debris from entering the circuit.
   2. *Tap Connectors and Tubing*: Tap on all tubing and connectors to dislodge and release trapped air bubbles. Monitor closely for any remaining air.
   3. *Visual Inspection*: Conduct a thorough visual inspection of the entire circuit for any remaining air bubbles. Ensure that all sections are free of air and completely secure before proceeding.

Adjustments Based on Patient-Specific Needs

1. *Blood Priming*
   - *Low Hematocrit Patients*: Consider adding donor blood to the priming solution for patients with low hematocrit to maintain adequate oxygen-carrying capacity.
   - *Autologous Blood Priming*: For patients with sufficient blood volume, use the patient's own blood for priming to minimize exposure to donor blood and maintain consistency in hematologic parameters.
2. *Electrolyte and pH Adjustments*
   - *Patient-Specific Adjustments*: The electrolyte composition and pH of the priming fluid should be tailored to the individual patient's needs. This is particularly important in pediatric cases, where physiological differences and smaller blood volumes demand greater precision. Patients with preexisting electrolyte imbalances or acid-base disorders may also require modifications to the priming solution.

Adjustments typically involve altering levels of sodium, potassium, and bicarbonate to maintain proper electrolyte balance and pH.

3. *Temperature Control*
   - *Thermal Adjustment*: Warm or cool the priming fluid to match the patient's body temperature, ensuring thermal compatibility and reducing the risk of temperature-induced complications during the procedure.

By following this detailed priming procedure, you can ensure that the CPB circuit is thoroughly de-aired and prepared for safe operation, tailored to the individual needs of each patient.

Safety and Quality Control

CPB is a critical component of cardiac surgery, enabling surgeons to perform procedures that would not be possible without the perfusionist, heart-lung machine (HLM), and associated circuitry. However, with its importance comes the risk of catastrophic safety events, which can potentially cause harm or death to the patient (please refer to Chaps. 26 and 27). To help mitigate these risks, various safety devices and checks are employed for the HLM, as detailed in Chaps. 13 and 31. In addition to these safety devices and checks, every aspect of the CPB circuit is designed with safety in mind—from the design of the oxygenator and its de-airing properties to the customizability of the alarms. In this section, we will focus on only a few key safety measures, touching on their importance in conducting CPB effectively and safely.

Leak Testing the Circuit (Performed Before Priming)

The integrity of the heat exchanger within the oxygenator must be verified through a leak test. A defective heat exchanger could allow water to cross over and contaminate the patient's blood.

1. *Connecting the Heat Exchanger*
   - *Setup*: Attach the heat exchanger to the oxygenator and cardioplegia delivery system.
   - *Priming the Lines*
     (a) Open and prime the lines after connecting them.
     (b) Activate the lines at normal support for a few minutes before circuit priming.
     (c) Note: Detecting a heat exchanger leak is more challenging if the circuit is primed before connecting the heat exchanger lines.
2. *Leak Detection*
   - *Initial Inspection*: During the priming process, carefully inspect the circuit for any leaks from the heat exchanger into the oxygenator.
3. *Signs of Leakage*
   - *Hemolysis and Elevated Potassium*: If a leak goes undetected while the system is supporting the patient, signs may include hemolysis and elevated serum potassium levels.
   - *Reservoir Volume and Hematocrit*: A slow increase in reservoir volume accompanied by a decrease in hematocrit can also indicate a potential leak in the system.

Checking the Occlusion of All Roller Pumps

1. *For Fluid Filled Tubing*
   - *Preparation*
     (a) Close all shunts.
     (b) Clamp the outflow tubing leaving the roller pump.
   - *Pressurization*
     (a) Briefly turn on the roller pump to pressurize the line.
   - *Pressure Monitoring*
     (a) Monitor the pressure within the tubing.
   - *Occlusion Assessment*
     (a) Properly occluded roller pumps should allow pressure to diffuse 1–2 mmHg every second.
2. *For Non-fluid Filled Tubing (vents/suckers)*
   - *Setup*
     (a) Clamp the inlet of the tubing leading into the roller pump.
   - *Pump Activation*
     (a) Turn on the roller pump.
   - *Monitoring and Observation*
     (a) Watch for the tubing collapsing on itself within the roller pump.
   - *Occlusion Test*
     (a) Stop the roller pump.
     (b) The collapsed tubing should slowly expand over 5–10 seconds.

Connecting all Safety Devices/Safety Checks

- *Activate and Attach the Level Sensor*
- The level sensor is attached to the front of the venous reservoir and positioned at the minimum desired blood volume (Fig. 31.7). This device prevents scenarios where the reservoir empties completely, which could result in air being pumped to the patient, potentially causing catastrophic interruptions in flow, stroke, or ischemia. The level sensor is linked to a servo-regulation system, which automatically adjusts the pump's speed or operation based

on pressure readings. If the reservoir level drops too low, the servo-regulation system can either slow down the pump to reduce blood flow or activate an electronic clamp to completely cut off arterial flow. This allows venous drainage to catch up, refilling the reservoir and preventing significant air entrainment.

- *Attach, Prime, and Zero Pressure Transducers*
- Pressure transducers provide real-time monitoring of internal pressures within the CPB circuit, helping to reduce the possibility of safety events. These devices detect issues such as
  - Over-pressurization, which can cause tubing rupture.
  - Excessive negative pressure, which can lead to cavitation and air entrainment.
  - Excessive positive or negative pressure within the venous reservoir.
  - Aortic dissection.
  - Excessive hemolysis.
  - Clot formation within the circuit.
  - Circuit malfunctions.
  - Coronary artery and sinus damage during cardioplegia delivery.

Pressure transducers are connected to various parts of the pump, including the arterial line, venous reservoir, and cardioplegia circuit. They help regulate pumps associated with these areas, such as slowing or stopping the cardioplegia pump when a pre-set pressure is reached. Once the transducers are thoroughly primed, turn the stopcock on the transducer off to the patient and open it to air. Using the monitor, select the option to zero the transducer.

Within the pressure menu, the perfusionist can see the pressure thresholds at which the pump will alarm and servo-regulate. The chosen pressure depends on the type of pump, the type of case, and the size of the patient.

- *Placement of Bubble Detectors*
- Bubble detectors are placed in areas where blood is being delivered to the patient, typically after the venous reservoir and before the arterial pump head. If automatically triggered, it will stop the arterial pump to prevent air from being delivered to the patient. Recently, bubble detectors have also been designed for the cardioplegia line to prevent air from being introduced into the coronary arteries during cardioplegia delivery (Fig. 31.6).
- *Place Tubing in Electronic Clamps (if applicable)*
- Electronic clamps provide an additional layer of safety for both arterial and venous lines. When connected to pressure sensors, bubble detectors, and level sensors, an arterial line clamp can automatically close in response to a safety event, preventing potential harm to the patient (Fig. 31.9).
- *Ensuring Proper Function of the O_2/Air Blender*
- An essential component of the CPB machine, the O_2/Air blender mixes air, O_2, and sometimes CO_2 in a specific ratio and delivers it at a prescribed flow rate. For the blender to function properly, it requires a constant supply of these medical gases. Typically, medical air hoses are connected to the wall, tapping into the hospital's centralized medical air, O_2, and CO_2 supplies. Each hose uses color-coded hoses with unique connections to prevent errors.
  1. The blender has two to three different settings
     - Fraction of Inspired Oxygen (FiO2): This setting controls the percentage of oxygen blended into the airflow, ranging from 21% to 100%.
     - Flow Rate: This setting determines the speed at which the medical air flows through the oxygenator.
  2. Types of Blenders

     There are various types of blenders available. For many years, the Sechrist analog blender was the most commonly used, but electronic blenders made by specific HLM manufacturers are becoming increasingly more prevalent.
  3. Testing Procedures
     - To test the Sechrist blender: Turn on the vaporizer, physically remove the oxygen tubing from the oxygenator, and check for airflow from the O_2 tubing.
     - To test electronic blenders: Observe the electronic display for error messages and listen for alarms. These electronic systems provide an additional layer of protection with built-in gas analyzers and alarms, alerting the perfusionist to any faults in the air supply or the blender itself.

Connect All Monitoring Systems

Effective data capture in a CPB circuit is crucial for ensuring patient safety, enhancing operational efficiency, and supporting ongoing improvements in cardiac surgery practices. Advanced monitoring technologies and automated data management systems play a vital role in this process. By continuously capturing and analyzing real-time data, such as flow rates, pressures, oxygenation levels, and temperature, healthcare providers can make informed decisions and promptly address any issues that arise. In addition to the safety devices described above, attach the following devices/probes:

- *Place a flow probe on the arterial line*
- Especially important in a non-occlusive centrifugal pump, the flow probe allows the perfusionist to see the exact amount of flow going to the patient.
- *Attach temperature probes*

- Multiple temperature probes are used on the CPB machine due to the many temperature manipulations that can occur with cardiac surgery. Temperature probes are located at the cardioplegia outflow, arterial outflow, and venous inflow to the reservoir.
- *Attach any in-line/online monitoring*
- Considered by many as a standard of care, continuous blood gas monitoring gives the perfusionist a real-time view of the patient's blood gases. After the first blood gas measurement is obtained on bypass, the analyzer can be calibrated based on the results. The analyzer then tracks parameters such as PO_2, PCO_2, Base excess, pH, K, SVO_2, HCT, and Hbg. With these readings, many workstations can now calculate DO_2, VO_2, and VCO_2, providing the perfusionist with a detailed view of the patient's perfusion status. In-line blood gas monitoring requires cuvettes to be placed within the perfusion circuit, while online monitoring places probes on the outside of the tubing to monitor parameters continuously.

Additionally, comprehensive event logging and integration with electronic health records (EHR) facilitate postoperative analysis and research, contributing to improved patient outcomes and the development of best practices. Ensuring data accuracy, maintaining equipment, protecting patient privacy, and achieving system interoperability are essential considerations for successful data capture in CPB circuits.

Further Reading

AmSECT. American Society of ExtraCorporeal technology standards and guidelines for perfusion practice. StandardView. 2017;6(2):9.

Ashraf S, Butler J, Tian Y, Cowan D, Lintin S, Saunders NR, Watterson KG, Martin PG. Inflammatory mediators in adults undergoing cardiopulmonary bypass: comparison of centrifugal and roller pumps. Ann Thorac Surg. 1998;65(2):480–4. https://doi.org/10.1016/S0003-4975(97)01349-0.

Britanica. Kinetic Pumps. 1996. https://www.britannica.com/technology/waterwheel-engineering

Brolhorst J, Peterson B, Holt DW. Flow awareness as a new safety device for cardiopulmonary bypass. J Extra Corpor Technol. 2019;51(1):20–5.

Charrière J, Pélissié J, Verd C, Léger P, Pouard P, de Riberolles C, et al. Survey: retrospective survey of monitoring/safety devices and incidents of cardiopulmonary bypass for cardiac surgery in France. J Extra Corpor Technol. 2007a;39(3):142–57. discussion 158–9

Charrière J, Pélissié J, Verd C, Léger P, Pouard P, de Riberolles C, Menestret P, Hittinger M, Rougé P, Longrois D. Analysis of incidents, monitoring and safety devices of cardiopulmonary bypass for cardiac surgery for the year 2005 in France. Annales Françaises d'Anesthésie Et De Réanimation. 2007b;26(11):907. https://doi.org/10.1016/j.annfar.2007.09.025.

Chilton V, Klein A. Equipment and monitoring. In: Ghosh S, Falter F, Cook D, editors. *Cardiopulmonary bypass* (Cambridge clinical guides). Cambridge: Cambridge University Press; 2009. p. 1–22. https://doi.org/10.1017/CBO9780511635564.002.

Deptula J, McGrath C, Preston T, Miller H, Yen B, Munari L, Setty SP. Sterility and performance of open and closed extracorporeal circuits after long-term dry-wet setups. Perfusion. 2021;36(2):130–7. https://doi.org/10.1177/0267659120937898.

Engelman R, Baker RA, Likosky DS, et al. The Society of Thoracic Surgeons, the Society of Cardiovascular Anesthesiologists, and the American Society of Extracorporeal Technology: clinical practice guidelines for cardiopulmonary bypass temperature management during cardiopulmonary bypass. Ann Thorac Surg. 2015;100(2):748–57.

Gravlee GP, Davis RF, Utley JR, Ovid Technologies I. Cardiopulmonary bypass: principles and practices. 3rd ed. Lippincott Williams & Wilkins; 2007.

Guimarães DP, Caneo LF, Matte G, Carletto LP, Policarpo VC, Castro AVCX, Miranda MHC, Costa PS, Jatene MB, Cestari I, Jatene FB. Impact of vacuum-assisted venous drainage on forward flow in simulated pediatric cardiopulmonary bypass circuits utilizing a centrifugal arterial pump head. Rev Bras Cir Cardiovasc. 2020;35(2):134–40. https://doi.org/10.21470/1678-9741-2019-0311.

Hessel EA 2nd. A brief history of cardiopulmonary bypass. Semin Cardiothorac Vasc Anesth. 2014;18(2):87–100. https://doi.org/10.1177/1089253214530045.

Hessel E II, Shann K. Blood pumps, circuitry, and cannulation techniques in cardiopulmonary bypass. Thoracis Key; 2016. https://thoracickey.com/blood-pumps-circuitry-and-cannulation-techniques-in-cardiopulmonary-bypass/

Ismail A, Semien G, Miskolczi SY. Cardiopulmonary bypass. In: StatPearls. StatPearls Publishing; 2023.

Kato S, Kusama Y, Abe K, Shibamoto T. Study for the quantification of the roller pump occlusion on the cardio-pulmonary bypass: definition factors of the roller pump occlusion on stable the roller pump operation. Jap J Extra-Corporeal Technol. 2019;46(4):382–7. https://doi.org/10.7130/jject.46.382.

Kumari S. A retrospective comparison of the clinical impact of use of roller pump or centrifugal pump for cardiopulmonary bypass in patients undergoing coronary artery bypass grafting. 2013

Lee WH Jr, Rubin JW, Huggins MP. Clinical evaluation of priming solutions for pump oxygenator perfusion. Ann Thorac Surg. 1975;19(5):529–36. https://doi.org/10.1016/s0003-4975(10)64428-1.

Machin D, Allsager C. Principles of cardiopulmonary bypass. Continuing Educ Anaesth Crit Care Pain. 2006;6(5):176–81. https://doi.org/10.1093/bjaceaccp/mkl043.

Matte GS, del Nido PJ. History and use of del Nido cardioplegia solution at Boston Children's Hospital. J Extra Corpor Technol. 2012;44(3):98–103.

McMillan J, Bago M, McDonald M. Heat exchanger integrity in various concentrations of hydrogen peroxide: an experimental analysis and review of methods to examine integrity of membrane oxygenator heat exchangers. The Australian and New Zealand College of Perfusionists Gazette. Jan 2019. https://epublishbyus.com/ebook/10048363/F143-166335-1-ANZCP_Gazette-DEC18-V5-EPUB.pf

Mick SL, Robich MP, Houghtaling PL, Gillinov AM, Soltesz EG, Johnston DR, Blackstone EH, Sabik JF. del nido versus buckberg cardioplegia in adult isolated valve surgery. J Thorac Cardiovasc Surg. 2015;149(2):626–636.e5. https://doi.org/10.1016/j.jtcvs.2014.10.085.

Miller AL, Theodore D, Widrich J. Inhalational Anesthetic. [Updated 2023 May 1]. In: StatPearls [Internet]. Treasure Island (FL): StatPearls Publishing; 2023 Jan-. Available from: https://www.ncbi.nlm.nih.gov/books/NBK554540/

Murphy GS, Hessel EA, Groom RC. Optimal perfusion during cardiopulmonary bypass: an evidence-based approach. Anesth Analg. 2009;108(5):1394–417. https://doi.org/10.1213/ane.0b013e3181875e2e.

Nagase K, Kohori F, Sakai K. Oxygen transfer performance of a membrane oxygenator composed of crossed and parallel hollow fibers. Biochem Eng J. 2005;24(2):105–13. ISSN 1369-703X. https://doi.org/10.1016/j.bej.2005.02.003.

Pan Y, Li Y, Li Y, Li J, Chen H. Fatigue of red blood cells under periodic squeezes in ECMO. Proc Natl Acad Sci USA. 2022;119(49):e2210819119. https://doi.org/10.1073/pnas.2210819119.

Riley JB. Arterial line filters ranked for gaseous microemboli separation performance: an in vitro study. J Extra Corpor Technol. 2008;40(1):21–6.

Sarkar M, Prabhu V. Basics of cardiopulmonary bypass. Indian J Anaesth. 2017;61(9):760–7. https://doi.org/10.4103/ija.IJA_379_17.

Spectrum Medical. Quantum perfusion systems. 2023a., https://www.spectrummedical.com//brochures/perfusion-technologies/quantum-perfusionsystems_web_5-23-18.pdf. Accessed August 2023.

Spectrum Medical. Flow and bubble detection. 2023b. https://www.spectrummedical.com/en/quantum-perfusion-for-the-icu-cath-lab-and-transport/quantum-perfusion-icu-transport/quantum-ventilation-system/flow-bubble-detection

Tagaya M, Matsuda M, Ryugo M, Takasaki T, Kurita S, Handa H, Hara K. Is using an open-reservoir cardiopulmonary bypass circuit after 6 days on standby safe? Interact Cardiovasc Thorac Surg. 2016;22(2):155–60. https://doi.org/10.1093/icvts/ivv302.

TERUMO Cardiovascular. CAPIOX Cardiotomy Reservoirs. 2023a. https://www.terumocv.com/products/ProductDetail.aspx?groupId=1&familyID=6&country=1. Accessed August 2023.

TERUMO Cardiovascular. CDI® Blood Parameter Monitoring System 550. 2023b. https://www.terumocv.com/cdi550/. Accessed August 2023.

Tschaut RJ, editor. First Edition, Pabst Science Publishers. 2020. Print: ISBN 978-3-95853-545-9 eBook: ISBN 978-3-95853-546-6.

Wang S, Rosenthal T, Kunselman AR, Ündar A. Evaluation of different diameter arterial tubing and arterial cannulae in simulated neonatal/pediatric cardiopulmonary bypass circuits. Artif Organs. 2015;39(1):43–52. https://doi.org/10.1111/aor.12446.

Zangrillo A, Garozzo FA, Biondi-Zoccai G, Pappalardo F, Monaco F, Crivellari M, Bignami E, Nuzzi M, Landoni G. Miniaturized cardiopulmonary bypass improves short-term outcome in cardiac surgery: a meta-analysis of randomized controlled studies. J Thorac Cardiovasc Surg. 2010;139(5):1162–9. https://doi.org/10.1016/j.jtcvs.2009.07.048.

Prime Solutions for the Circuit and Hemodilution Reduction Strategies

9

Jason Cohen

Introduction

The cardiopulmonary bypass (CPB) system, a cornerstone in cardiac surgery, necessitates meticulous preparation to ensure its optimal functioning and patient safety. One critical preparatory step involves priming the CPB circuit with a fluid solution. This priming of CPB circuit with a fluid solution serves to rapidly achieving adequate flow rates on initiation of CPB, thus preventing the risk of air embolism. Priming fluid fills both venous and arterial limbs of the circuit and maintains an adequate reserve volume in the venous reservoir to ensure that air is not entrained into the arterial side of the circuit during initiation of CPB. The optimum composition of the CPB priming solution is still a matter for debate. Currently used priming solutions provide a fluid that when mixed with blood is capable of maintaining oxygen delivery, carbon dioxide, and physiological homeostasis.

Historical Perspective of CPB Priming

Historically, fresh heparinized homologous whole blood was the primary fluid used to prime CPB circuits (Fig. 9.1), with the goal of preserving a high hematocrit (Hct) and closely matching the patient's own rheological characteristics, both considered crucial for optimal oxygen delivery during surgery. However, because CPB circuits in the early days were large and had voluminous circuits, along with the risk of excessive hemodilution and its potential to jeopardize organ perfusion, crystalloids and colloids were not considered viable priming fluids.

Priming CPB circuits with whole blood presented several drawbacks, including the risk of transfusion-related complications such as infectious disease transmission and allergic reactions. Additionally, whole blood priming was associated with an increased risk of capillary leak syndrome, potentially exacerbated by an elevated histamine load in the prime. This syndrome has been implicated in both transient postoperative arrhythmias and pulmonary dysfunction, posing significant concerns.

Moreover, the need for substantial amounts of blood for priming CPB circuits often dictated the scheduling of cardiac surgeries based on the availability of donor blood. Typically, 7–10 units of heparinized blood were needed for each CPB circuit, with heparin being used to prevent clot formation and avoid the risks of citrate toxicity associated with stored blood products. Additionally, the use of stored blood raised concerns about its altered rheological properties and diminished capacity for oxygen delivery to the tissues.

Non-blood priming, a concept that revolutionized CPB practices, was first introduced in 1959. This innovative approach combined hemodilution with controlled hypothermia to reduce the body's oxygen consumption and demand, thereby demonstrating that non-blood primes could be used safely and effectively. Today, this practice has been widely adopted, with non-blood primes and moderate hemodilution constituting the standard protocol in the majority of medical centers.

While priming practices have evolved over time, the use of blood priming has remained relevant and vital in specific scenarios. Its significance is most notable in pediatric cardiac surgeries. Given their smaller blood volumes, children are especially vulnerable to hemodilution effects. Blood priming acts as a safeguard against this susceptibility, preserving an elevated Hct level and guaranteeing consistent oxygen delivery during the bypass. Furthermore, adult patients who have decreased Hct levels before surgery, possibly due to conditions such as anemia, can benefit greatly from blood priming.

Supplementary Information The online version contains supplementary material available at https://doi.org/10.1007/978-3-031-91163-7_9.

J. Cohen (✉)
Department of Clinical Perfusion, Cooper University Hospital Care, Camden, NJ, USA

A. S. Awad, J. DiNardo (eds.), *Clinical Perfusion for Cardiac Surgery*, https://doi.org/10.1007/978-3-031-91163-7_9

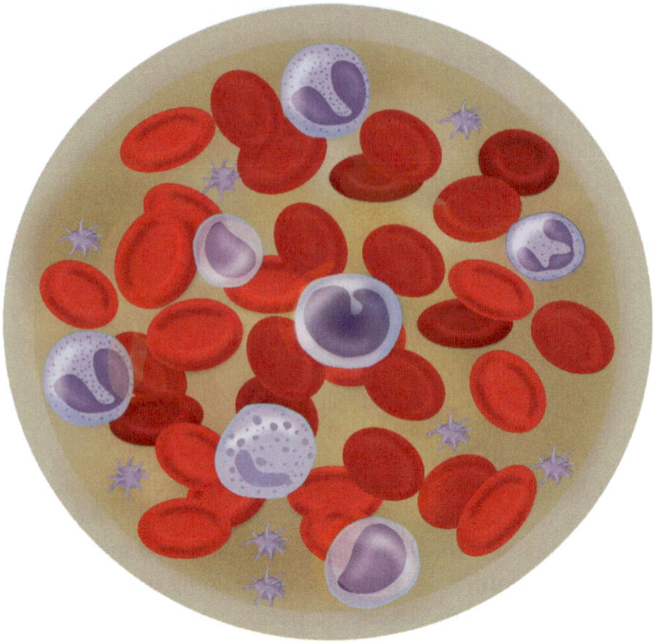

Fig. 9.1 Fresh heparinized homologous whole blood was the primary choice for priming CPB circuits in the early days of cardiac surgeries

Hemodilution

Recent advances in CPB circuit priming techniques have been heavily influenced by research on the benefits of hemodilution. Hemodilution is the deliberate reduction of the Hct, the percentage of red blood cells in blood, by increasing the plasma volume. This dilutes the blood and has become an integral part of the multidisciplinary strategy to optimize CPB. Collaboration among surgeons, anesthesiologists, and perfusionists to balance the patient's flow, perfusion, and oxygen delivery needs is essential.

Hemodilution during CPB offers several physiological benefits:

- Reduced blood viscosity: Decreased viscosity enhances blood flow, which can help to offset the effects of hypothermia. Hypothermia often leads to vasoconstriction, increased plasma viscosity, and reduced red blood cell plasticity.
- Enhanced regional blood flow: Dilution helps distribute blood more evenly across different body regions.
- Optimized oxygen delivery: Despite the dilution of red blood cells, improved flow can enhance oxygen delivery to tissues.
- Reduced reliance on blood products: It minimizes the need for transfusions, lowering the risk of transfusion-related complications.
- Better flow at lower pressures: Especially during hypothermic states, hemodilution can maintain adequate flow without requiring high perfusion pressures.

For patients with low preoperative Hct, a hybrid approach using both blood and non-blood components can be considered to maintain the balance between Hct levels and fluid volume.

Hemodilution Calculations

Hemodilution calculations are an essential step before implementing any CPB priming plan.

They are performed for all patients prior to surgery to estimate the post-dilution Hct, which is influenced by the dilutional effects of the priming solution. This preemptive calculation is crucial for identifying patients whose post-dilution Hct might approach borderline levels, which could jeopardize adequate oxygen-carrying capacity. To calculate Hct, we first need to estimate blood volume.

Estimating Blood Volume (EBV)

Accurate estimation of a patient's EBV is essential for effective use of hemodilution during cardiopulmonary bypass (CPB). EBV varies based on age, sex, weight, and height. Here is a general method for estimating EBV:

- Adults
  - Men: EBV is approximately 70 milliliters per kilogram (mL/kg) of body weight.
  - Women: EBV is about 65 mL/kg of body weight.

For a more precise calculation, the following formulas can be used.

- Men: $\text{EBV} = 0.3669 \times (\text{Height in meters})^3 + 0.03219 \times \text{Weight in kg} + 0.6041$.
- Women: $\text{EBV} = 0.3561 \times (\text{Height in meters})^3 + 0.03308 \times \text{Weight in kg} + 0.183$.

These formulas, derived from Nadler's method, take into account the patient's body build.

- Children:
  - Newborns: Approximately 85 mL/kg of body weight.
  - Children: Ranges from 70 to 75 mL/kg of body weight.

Application in Hemodilution

Once the EBV is calculated, it is used in the hemodilution formula to determine the appropriate amount of priming volume required to achieve the target Hct on CPB. It is important to note that the EBV should be calculated as closely as possible to the patient's actual volume status, considering factors that may cause deviation from normal values.

Using EBV in Hemodilution Calculations

With the EBV estimated, it can be plugged into the hemodilution formula:

$$HCT_{CPB} = \frac{(\text{Pre operative HCT} \times \text{EBV})}{(\text{EBV} + \text{Priming Volume})}$$

This calculation helps to predict the post-dilution HCT, guiding the perfusion team on how much priming solution should be used to avoid excessive hemodilution while maintaining adequate oxygen-carrying capacity.

Patient Variability and HCT Targets

Cardiac surgical patients vary widely in their ability to tolerate hemodilution. Determining the ideal HCT level during CPB is a complex issue with no one-size-fits-all approach. The recommended HCT range of 21–25% during CPB is based on the balance between maintaining adequate oxygen delivery and minimizing the risks associated with hemodilution. The tolerance to HCT levels during CPB is influenced by a multitude of factors, including patient age, baseline HCT levels, and the type of surgical procedure being performed. Additionally, these guidelines are based on the recognition that different organ systems have varying abilities to tolerate anemia during CPB. Consequently, this necessitates a tailored approach to priming strategies, which takes into account the unique needs of each patient.

Practical Considerations

In practice, clinicians may adjust these estimations based on the patient's clinical condition and preoperative HCT levels. It is also important to consider the patient's fluid status preoperatively, as dehydration or fluid overload can significantly alter the EBV. Close monitoring of the patient's hemodynamics and HCT levels during CPB is necessary to make real-time adjustments as needed.

Current Perspective on CPB Priming

As advancements in cardiac surgery continue, CPB priming methods have become more sophisticated. Varying amounts of crystalloids, colloids, and additives are used in combination for best results in each patient based on a number of physiological parameters including starting and desired HCT on CPB, body surface area, type of procedure, and the target cooling temperature.

One notable evolution in this field is the incorporation of techniques such as retrograde autologous priming (RAP), venous autologous prime, vacuum-assisted venous drainage (VAVD), and hybrid models of priming. These methods align with the ongoing trend to reduce the risks of traditional priming solutions while enhancing patient outcomes.

1. Hybrid models of priming are becoming increasingly popular, as they offer the potential to balance the benefits of blood with the risk management and volume control offered by other solutions. For example, some hybrid priming strategies involve using a combination of blood, crystalloids, and colloids to achieve the desired HCT level and electrolyte balance. And hybrid models of blood and non-blood components in patients with low preoperative HCT level.
2. VAVD is a technique in CPB surgery that enhances venous return to the CPB machine by using vacuum assistance for priming the CPB circuit, aiding de-airing, and boosting venous return efficiency. Unlike traditional methods dependent on gravity, VAVD uses regulated negative pressure for optimized venous drainage. This offers benefits like reduced risk of air embolism, greater positional flexibility for the CPB machine, and improved venous return across various surgical contexts. However, it is crucial to monitor the vacuum levels to prevent complications like hemolysis. In essence, VAVD is an advanced CPB priming method that, when used judiciously, maximizes the benefits while minimizing risks.
3. RAP and venous antegrade priming (VAP) are modern techniques developed to address the hemodilution typically associated with CPB initiation. The fundamental principle of these methods is to utilize the patient's own blood instead of relying solely on external priming solutions when launching CPB. One of the standout benefits of these techniques is their potential to drastically reduce the volume of exogenous priming solutions.

   The technique unfolds in several systematic steps

   - Setup: As with traditional CPB procedures, the circuit is first primed with the selected solution. This ensures that the CPB's equipment is ready and that there are no air bubbles that might pose a risk to the patient.

- Cannulation: Once primed, the patient is then cannulated to allow for blood to be diverted through the CPB machine.
- Unclamping the arterial line: After removing the arterial line clamp, blood is allowed to drain passively into the circuit.
- Displacement through Retrograde Flow: With everything in place, the patient's own blood is directed retrograde into the arterial limb of the CPB circuit. This means the blood flows in a direction opposite to what would be its natural course. As this happens, the priming solution in the circuit gets displaced.
- Collection of Displaced Fluid: The displaced priming solution doesn't reenter the patient's system. Instead, it is redirected and collected in a separate reservoir.
- VAP: After releasing the venous line clamp, blood drains antegradely through the venous cannula into the venous reservoir.
- During RAP and VAP in CPB, maintaining arterial pressure is crucial. To counteract potential hypotension, anesthesia providers often use the Trendelenburg position to enhance venous return and arterial pressure. Additionally, vasoconstrictors can further stabilize arterial pressure.

4. Tolerating Lower HCT Levels in Selected Cases

In certain circumstances, such as when avoiding blood transfusions is desired, patients may be able to tolerate lower HCT levels if it is clinically acceptable. The feasibility of this approach depends on maintaining cerebral oximetry readings at or above baseline, which ensures sufficient oxygen delivery to the brain. Additionally, patients are closely monitored for any signs of increased blood lactate levels, which could indicate inadequate oxygenation and tissue perfusion.

5. Miniaturized Extracorporeal Circulation (MECC) Systems.

MECC represents a significant advancement in the field of cardiac surgery, specifically addressing the challenges associated with priming volumes in traditional CPB circuits. By substantially reducing the foreign surface area and the amount of priming fluid required, MECC systems aim to lessen the inflammatory response and the dilution of blood components typically seen with larger volume circuits. This approach minimizes the systemic inflammatory response and the associated coagulation disturbances, potentially reducing the need for blood transfusions and improving overall patient outcomes.

6. Use of hemoconcentrator to remove plasma water from the blood. Please refer to Chap. 19 ultrafiltration and leukofiltration for more information.

Steps for Priming the Circuit

Priming the CPB circuit is a meticulous process that prepares the circuit for its role in temporarily taking over the heart and lung functions during cardiac surgery. Proper priming ensures adequate flow rates, eliminates air, and provides an environment suitable for the patient's blood. Here are the typical steps involved in priming the CPB circuit (please refer to the video for steps for priming the circuit):

1. *Circuit Inspection*
   - Before introducing any priming solution, visually inspect the entire circuit, including the oxygenator, arterial filter, reservoirs, tubing, and connectors, to ensure that there are no defects or leaks.
   - Ensure that all the clamps are in place and that the circuit components, like the oxygenator and arterial filter, are correctly positioned and secured.
2. *Selection of Priming Solution*
   - Depending on the surgical team's decision and the patient's clinical status, choose the priming solution. This could be crystalloids, colloids, blood, or a combination thereof.
3. *Introducing the Priming Solution*
   - Gradually infuse the selected priming solution into the venous reservoir.
   - Release the clamp on the reservoir outlet line and let gravity fill the centrifugal pump head, oxygenator, and arterial filter.
   - Continuously monitor the solution flow, ensuring there are no air bubbles and that all components get filled without any obstruction.
4. *De-airing the Circuit*
   - While filling, carefully tilt, tap, and manipulate the circuit to remove any trapped air bubbles.
   - Particular attention should be paid to the oxygenator, arterial filter, and connectors, where air is most likely to get trapped.
   - For further de-airing, some circuits have a vent on the arterial filter that can be opened to allow trapped air to escape.
   - Unclamp the arterial line and gradually raise the arterial flow to five Lpm. Periodically clamp and unclamp the arterial line near the oxygenator outlet to expel air through the purge ports.
   - Decrease the flow to 200 ml/min and then re-clamp the arterial outlet.
   - Once more, gently tap the arterial oxygenator from bottom to top to aid in releasing air through the purge ports. After dislodging any air, unclamp the oxygenator's arterial outlet, raise the flow to five lpm, and ensure all air is removed from the entire CPB system (Fig. 9.2).

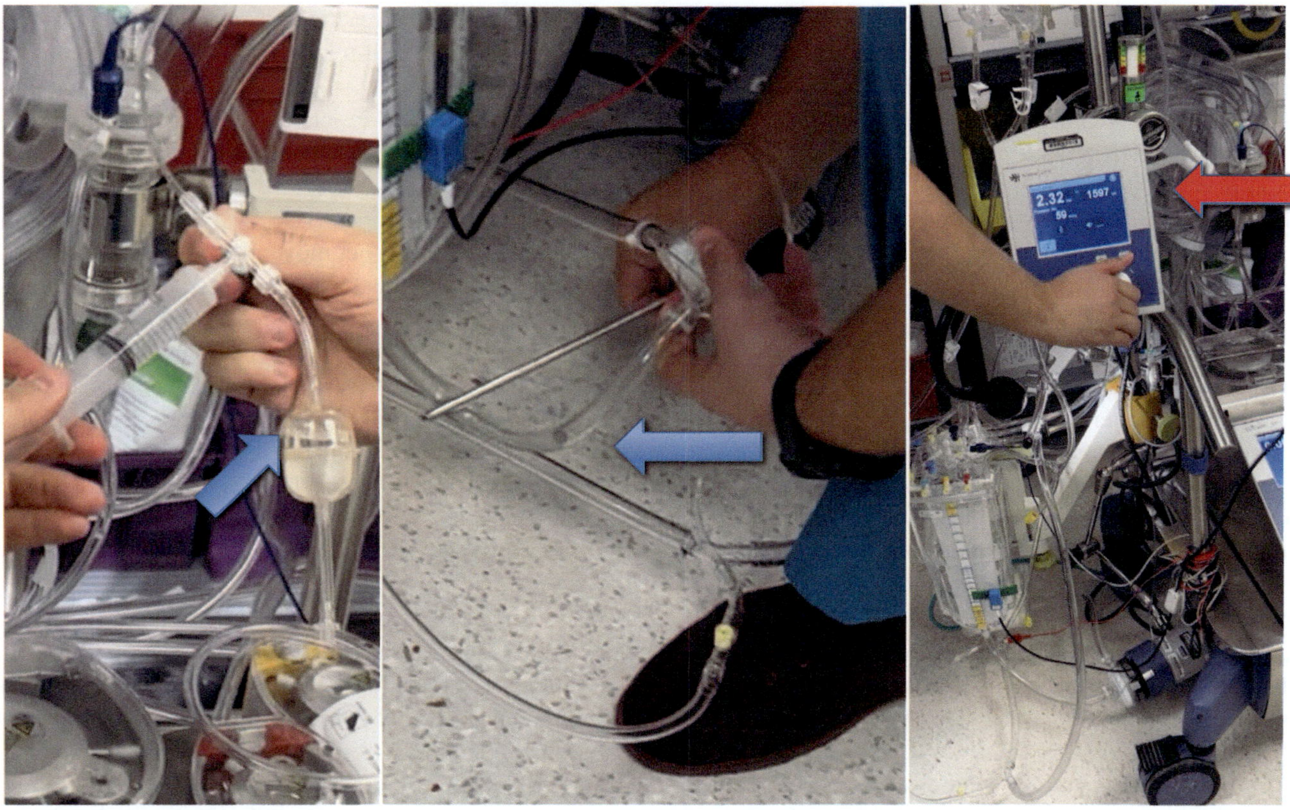

Fig. 9.2 A meticulous clinical perfusionist expertly primes the CPB circuit, exercising utmost precision and careful attention to eliminate all air bubbles, essential for a safe and successful procedure

5. *Temperature Regulation*
   - Adjust the temperature of the heat exchanger to the desired level and ensure the priming solution reaches the target temperature.
6. *Additives and Medications*
   - Introduce any necessary additives to the priming solution, such as electrolytes, bicarbonate, mannitol, or anticoagulants (e.g., heparin), as per the hospital protocol.
7. *Final Checks*
   - Ensure that the level of the priming solution in the venous reservoir is appropriate and that there is adequate reserve.
   - Check all pressure monitors and flow sensors to ensure they're functioning properly.
   - Conduct a final visual inspection to confirm there is no air in the circuit and that all connections are secure.
8. *Connect to the Patient*:
   - Once the circuit is fully primed, and all checks are satisfactory, the CPB circuit can be connected to the patient, typically via cannulation of the appropriate vessels but only after achieving full anticoagulation and reaching the target activated clotting time (ACT).

Throughout the priming process, sterility must be maintained to prevent any contamination. Furthermore, the exact steps and procedures might vary slightly based on the specific CPB machine model, the surgeon's preferences, or institutional protocols.

Classification of the Priming Solutions

A solution is a homogeneous mixture of two or more substances in which one substance, known as the solute, is dissolved in another, called the solvent. In simpler terms, solutions are liquids that contain dissolved substances.

Types of Priming Solutions

In the context of priming, solutions are broadly classified based on solute size into crystalloid and colloidal solutions.

1. Crystalloid solutions consist of small molecules dissolved in water, many of which can move across cell membranes. The permeability of solutes across cell mem-

branes depends on their size, charge, and the specific properties of the cell membrane.

2. Colloidal solutions are characterized by the suspension of large molecular weight particles like proteins or hydroxyethyl starches (HES) in a crystalloid solution. Common examples are albumin and HES. Due to their larger molecular size, these particles remain in the circulatory system longer, making them effective for increasing blood volume and pressure.

Crystalloid Solutions

Crystalloids are water-based solutions that contain electrolytes and other solutes.

Crystalloid solutions can be used alone or in combination with other fluids, such as blood and colloids, to create a priming solution for CPB. The choice of crystalloid solution and the composition of the priming solution will depend on a number of factors, including the patient's age, medical history, and the type of CPB procedure being performed.

Here are some of the benefits of using crystalloid solutions in CPB priming:

- Cost-effective: Crystalloid solutions are relatively inexpensive compared to other priming fluids, such as blood and colloids.
- Readily available: Crystalloid solutions are widely available in most hospitals.
- Easy to store and transport: Crystalloid solutions can be stored and transported at room temperature.
- Low risk of adverse reactions: Crystalloid solutions are generally safe and well-tolerated.

Crystalloid solutions are classified into three categories based on solute concentration relative to plasma:

- Isotonic: These solutions have the same osmolality as plasma, leading to no net movement of water across cell membranes due to equal osmotic pressure inside and outside the cells.
- Hypotonic: With lower osmolality than plasma, hypotonic solutions cause water to move into cells, potentially leading to cell swelling and rupture, a process known as hemolysis in red blood cells.
- Hypertonic: These solutions have higher osmolality than plasma, causing water to move out of cells, which can lead to cell shrinkage and dehydration.

Where tonicity is closely related to osmolality, specifically refers to the effective osmolality of a solution (Fig. 9.3).

Additionally, crystalloid solutions can be classified as buffered/balanced or unbuffered/unbalanced, depending on whether their electrolyte composition mirrors that of human plasma. The specific compositions of the various crystalloid solutions, along with their classification as balanced or unbalanced, are detailed in Table 9.1.

Unbalanced/Unbuffered Crystalloid Priming in CPB

Unbalanced or unbuffered crystalloid solutions, typically lacking bicarbonate or bicarbonate precursors, do not closely

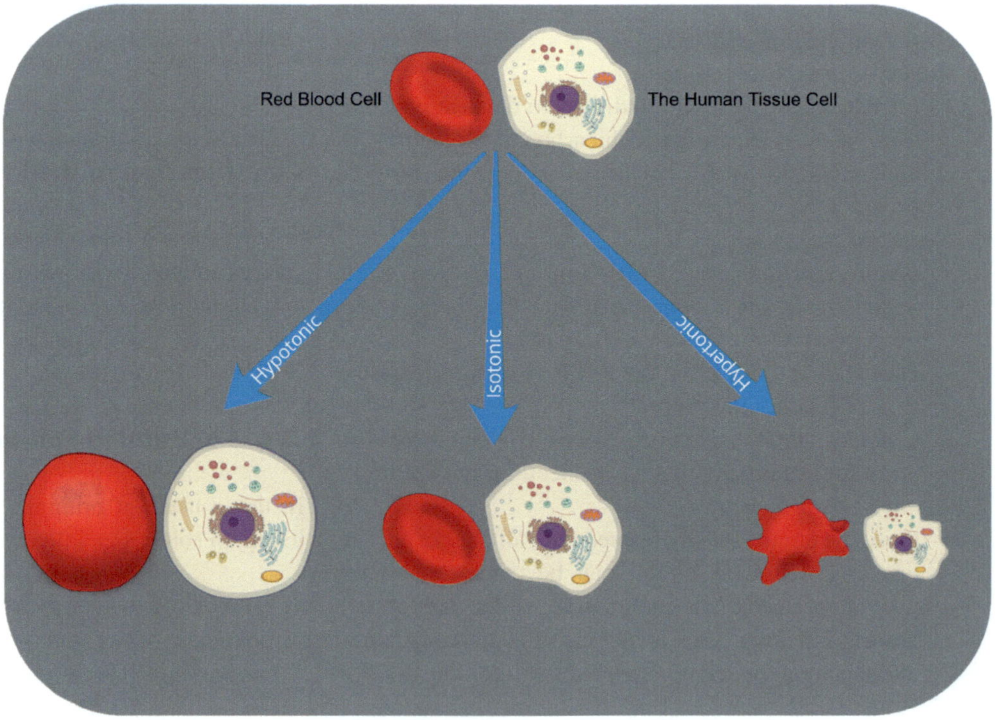

Fig. 9.3 Illustration demonstrating the impact of fluid tonicity on human tissue cells and red blood cells. It shows cells swelling in a hypotonic solution, shrinking in a hypertonic solution, and remaining unchanged in an isotonic solution. This comparison effectively highlights the effects of isotonic, hypotonic, and hypertonic solutions on cells

Table 9.1 Comparison of crystalloid solutions used for CPB priming with plasma composition

Solution	Osmolality (mOsm/L)	PH	Na + (mEq/L)	Cl- (mEq/L)	K+ (mEq/L)	Ca2+ (mEq/L)	Mg2+ (mEq/L)	HCO3-	Acetate (mEq/L)	Lactate (mEq/L)	Gluconate (mEq/L)	Balanced/ Unbalanced
Plasma	290	7.4	142	105	4.5	3	2	24	0	1	0	Balanced
D5W	253	5	0	0	0	0	0	0	0	0	0	Unbalanced Hypotonic
Normal saline 0.9% NaCl	308	5.7	154	154	0	0	0	0	0	0	0	Unbalanced Isotonic
Lactated ringer's	275	6.2	130	110	4	3	0	0	0	28	0	Balanced Hypotonic
Hartmann's solution	279	6.5	131	111	5	2	0	0	0	29	0	Balanced
Plasmalyte A	294	7.4	140	98	5	0	3	0	27	0	23	Balanced Isotonic
Normosol-R	295	7.4	140	98	5	0	3	0	27	0	23	Balanced Isotonic
Isolyte S	295	7.4	141	98	5	0	3	0	27	0	23	Balanced Isotonic

Note that D5W starts as isotonic but becomes hypotonic as the body metabolizes the dextrose. Ringer's lactate exhibits a marginally lower osmolarity compared to plasma, yet this variation is typically insufficient to classify it as hypotonic in a clinical setting. Similarly, NaCl displays a slightly higher osmolarity than plasma, but this difference is generally not substantial enough to consider it as hypertonic in clinical use match the body's natural plasma electrolyte composition and can cause metabolic acidosis when used in large volumes due to their typically higher chloride content and lower pH compared to blood plasma.

1. *Normal Saline (NaCl) or 0.9% Sodium Chloride*

   NaCl, also known as physiological saline, is a sterile and isotonic solution, consisting of sodium chloride dissolved in water. With an osmolality close to 308 mOsm/L, it closely aligns with the osmolality of blood plasma, making it a widely used and affordable option in medical settings. Its isotonic nature is crucial for maintaining fluid balance and minimizing the risk of hemolysis. However, despite these benefits, normal saline has its drawbacks. It does not contain bicarbonate precursors, which are vital for blood pH regulation. Moreover, it lacks other critical electrolytes such as potassium, calcium, and magnesium, which can lead to electrolyte imbalances during CPB.

2. *Dextrose Priming in CPB*

   Dextrose, or glucose, is a carbohydrate that is essential for energy production in the body. D5W, or 5% dextrose in water, is initially isotonic when administered, but becomes hypotonic as the dextrose is metabolized. It was one of the first crystalloid solutions adopted for priming the CPB machine after the transition away from using blood for priming. This solution lacks electrolytes or bicarbonate, and therefore, it is not classified as a balanced crystalloid. When metabolized in vivo, the byproducts can contribute to an acidifying effect on the body's pH balance.

   Dextrose priming offers certain advantages such as

- Reduced mechanical damage to erythrocytes: Dextrose can help to reduce the mechanical damage to red blood cells that can occur during CPB.
- Enhanced diuresis: Dextrose can help to increase urine output during and after CPB.
- Reduced fluid needs: A crystalloid prime with dextrose can help to reduce the need for fluids before and after CPB.

However, there are also some downsides to dextrose priming:

- Metabolic acidosis: The metabolism of dextrose can dilute plasma bicarbonate, potentially leading to systemic metabolic acidosis.
- Hyperglycemia: The CPB process itself can elevate serum glucose and insulin levels, and introducing dextrose to the prime might exacerbate hyperglycemia. This poses particular risks for diabetic patients.
- Neurological complications: Glucose-rich priming solutions have been linked to an increased risk of neurological complications related to CPB.

Balanced/Buffered Crystalloid Priming in CPB

Balanced crystalloid solutions are specifically designed to closely resemble the body's natural plasma electrolyte balance and pH. They contain a blend of electrolytes, including sodium, potassium, calcium, and chloride, along with bicarbonate precursors such as lactate, acetate, or gluconate. Examples of balanced crystalloids include Plasmalyte A (Baxter Healthcare), Normosol-R (Hospira), Isolyte-S (B. Braun Medical), Lactated Ringer's solution, and Hartmann's solution (Baxter Healthcare). In contrast, unbalanced crystalloids, like Normal Saline and D5W, may have an electrolyte composition that differs from plasma. Once D5W is administered and metabolized, it essentially becomes hypotonic. These properties of balanced crystalloids render them an ideal choice for priming CPB circuits and Extra Corporeal Membrane Oxygenation (ECMO) devices.

Balanced crystalloid priming offers several advantages over other priming fluids, such as blood and normal saline. These advantages include

- Prevention of Metabolic Acidosis: Balanced crystalloid solutions contain bicarbonate precursors, which help buffer the blood and prevent metabolic acidosis. Metabolic acidosis can occur during CPB due to the accumulation of lactic acid and other acidic byproducts, which result from reduced tissue perfusion and anaerobic metabolic processes.
- Maintenance of Electrolyte Balance: Balanced crystalloid fluids contain a mix of electrolytes, including sodium, potassium, chloride, calcium, and magnesium, similar to those found in plasma. This helps maintain electrolyte balance and prevent imbalances that can lead to complications.
- Lower Risk of Hyperglycemia: Compared to D5W, crystalloid fluids are less likely to cause hyperglycemia or elevated blood sugar levels.
- Cost-Effectiveness: Balanced crystalloid fluids are generally more affordable than other priming fluids, such as blood or colloids, making them a more cost-effective option.

Plasmalyte is often the preferred balanced crystalloid fluid for priming because it contains acetate and gluconate, which contribute to bicarbonate production. Bicarbonate is an important buffer for maintaining acid-base balance and preventing metabolic acidosis during CPB and ECMO. It also contains magnesium, which is an essential intracellular cation that plays an important role in cellular energy transfer processes and is often depleted during CPB and ECMO, so providing it as the prime solution can help to prevent complications such as arrhythmias and myocardial dysfunction.

Diabetic patients are cautioned against large volumes of lactate-containing fluids, as lactate may be converted into glucose in vivo through the gluconeogenic pathway.

This table shows that all of the crystalloid solutions listed contain sodium and chloride. However, they vary in their concentrations of other electrolytes, such as potassium, calcium, and lactate (Table 9.1; Fig. 9.4).

Colloid Solutions

Blood Plasma

Plasma, the liquid component of blood, is essential for numerous physiological functions, including transporting oxygen and nutrients to tissues, removing waste, regulating blood pressure, and aiding in blood clotting. Its water, protein, electrolyte, and nutrient content are vital for these roles. The efficacy of using plasma in CPB priming, however, remains a topic with mixed evidence.

The impact of CPB priming volume on blood volume in newborns and infants is significant due to their small size,

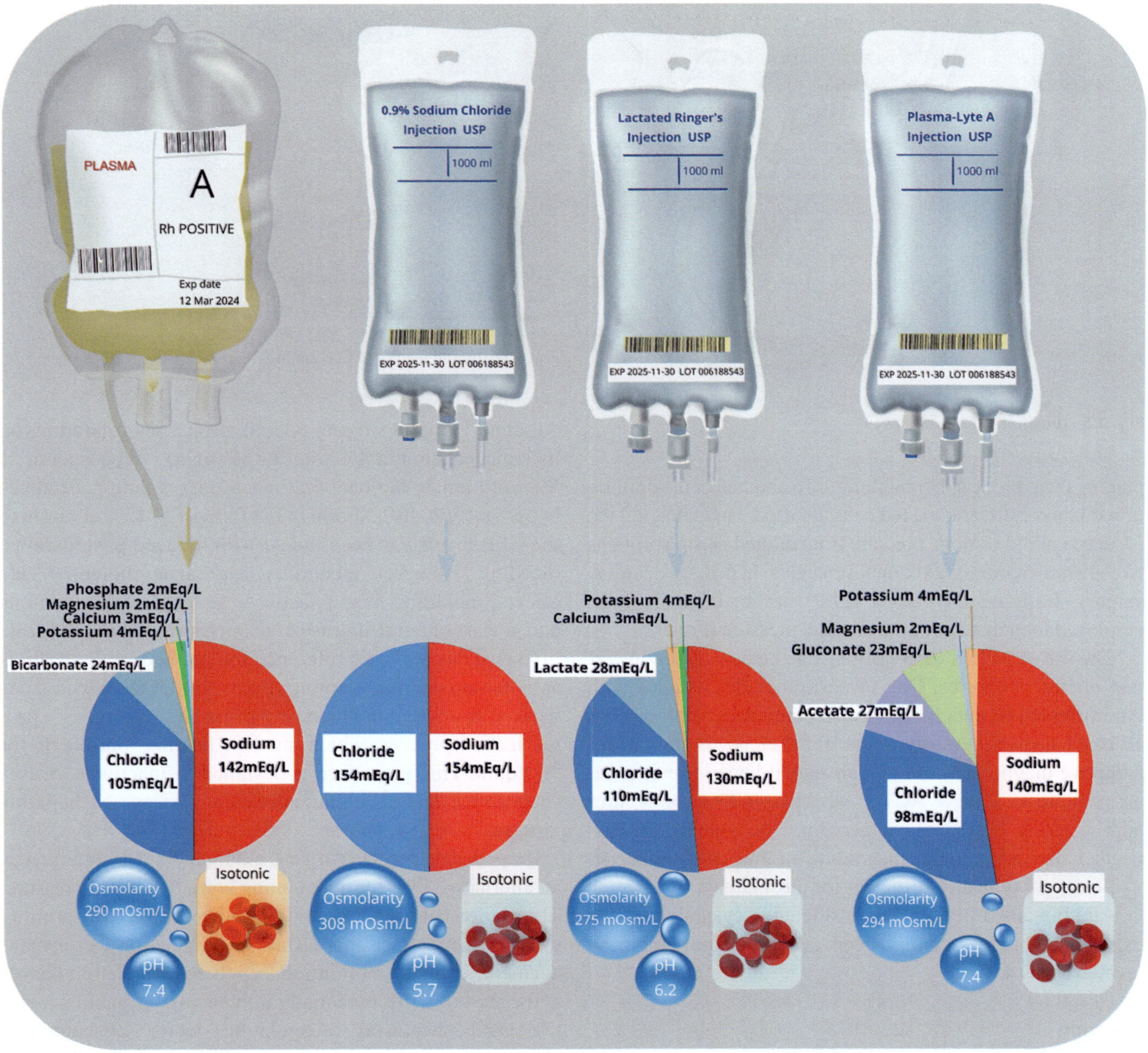

Fig. 9.4 Illustration comparing electrolyte content in human plasma and various intravenous crystalloid solutions used for CPB priming

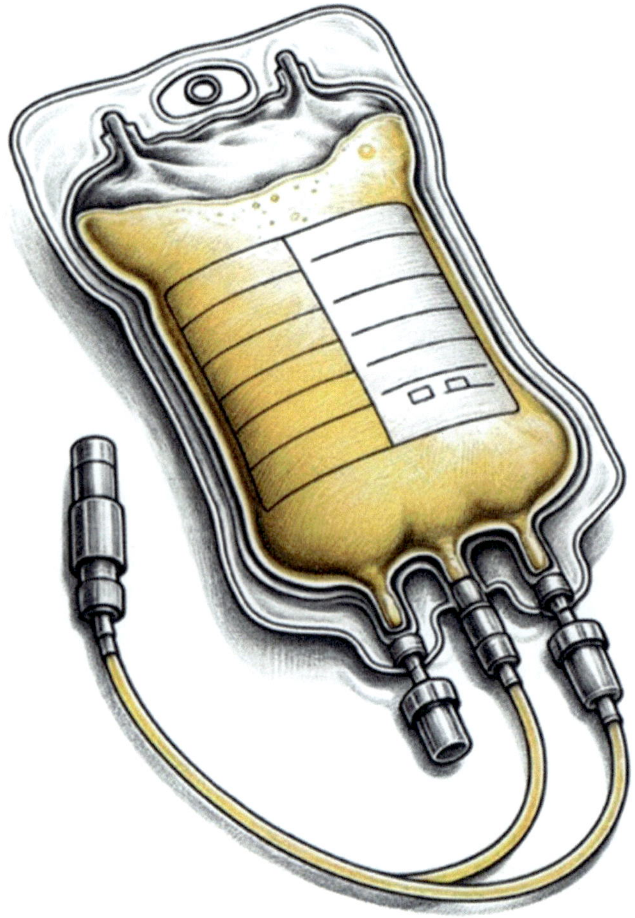

Fig. 9.5 Illustration for human FFP

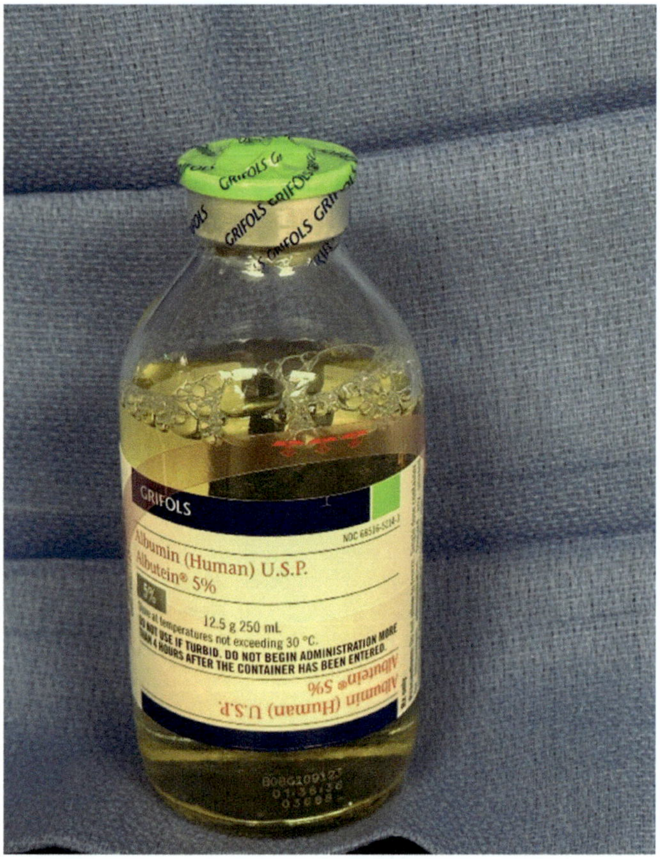

Fig. 9.6 Image for 250 CC Human Albumin 5%

making them prone to hemodilution. To counteract the dilution of red blood cells, packed red cells are used, but managing the reduced colloid osmotic pressure from diluted plasma proteins like albumin requires additional strategies. In pediatric cardiac surgery, fresh frozen plasma (FFP) has traditionally been employed to maintain colloid osmotic pressure (Fig. 9.5).

The use of FFP in CPB priming can be considered in certain clinical scenarios. One scenario includes patients with Antithrombin III deficiency when recombinant Antithrombin III is not available. Antithrombin III deficiency is often a presumptive diagnosis based on substantial heparin resistance, e.g., failure to achieve ACT greater than 400 seconds after administering 800 U/kg of heparin. The volume of FFP needed depends on the magnitude of the deficiency, but 2–3 units are typically sufficient for most adults.

Additionally, FFP may be considered in cyanotic patients experiencing polycythemia, specifically when the hematocrit level exceeds 45%.

Albumin

Albumin (Fig. 9.6), constituting 75–80% of plasma oncotic pressure, is essential for maintaining plasma volume. Albumin exhibits varying oncotic properties depending on its concentration: a 4% solution is slightly hypo-oncotic, a 5% solution is iso-oncotic, and a 25% solution becomes hyper-oncotic. Its addition in the form of 5–25% albumin to the CPB prime has been linked with reduced postoperative bleeding. However, albumin usage carries potential side effects, including anaphylactic or anaphylactoid reactions and a risk of viral disease transmission. Additionally, its high cost has led to a preference for synthetic colloid fluids as alternatives for priming fluids in CPB. Albumin is derived from human blood or plasma and undergoes a pasteurization process, which involves heating it at 60 °C for 10 hours. This procedure is designed to inactivate viruses such as the human immunodeficiency virus and hepatitis viruses.

In pediatric cardiac surgery, albumin 5% has emerged as an alternative FFP for maintaining colloid osmotic pressure. The choice between FFP and 5% albumin for CPB priming reflects two distinct approaches to coagulation factor management. Utilizing FFP introduces these coagulation factors at the start of CPB, potentially influencing thrombin generation and increasing coagulation factor consumption. Conversely, priming with albumin allows for controlled dilution of coagulation factors, potentially minimizing thrombin generation and reducing coagulation factor consumption. In adult CPB circuit priming, the key advantage of using albumin, in addition to maintaining colloid osmotic pressure, lies in its ability to form a natural coating layer on the oxygenator and CPB circuit. This action prevents the patient's fibrinogen from forming its own coating layers. When fibrinogen adheres, it can lead to platelet adhesion via the glycoprotein IIb/IIIa receptor, resulting in the consumption of both fibrinogen and platelets. Priming with albumin, therefore, and its subsequent adsorption onto the circuit surface, can effectively reduce the consumption of these critical blood components.

Dextran

Dextran solution, naturally occurring polysaccharide, is available in different molecular weights and oncotic properties: 70 kDa (6% iso-oncotic) and 40 kDa (10% hyper-oncotic). It is a polysaccharide produced from sucrose by a Gram-positive, facultatively anaerobic bacterium. The plasma volume increase, achieved by mobilizing water from extracellular to intravascular space, is approximately 100% for 6% dextran 70 and 175% for 10% dextran 40, with the plasma expansion effect lasting between 3 and 5 hours. Dextran 40 offers potential benefits as a colloid solution for CPB priming, including colloid osmotic pressure maintenance, reduced blood viscosity, and leukocyte adhesion reduction. However, its use requires careful consideration of potential risks such as anaphylactoid reactions, coagulation impairment, and volume overload. The decision to use dextran should be made on an individualized basis, taking into account patient factors, the specific clinical situation, and the availability of alternative colloid options. Typical dosage of dextran 40 solution ranges from 1 to 2 g/kg (10–20 mL/kg), with a maximum limit of 2 g/kg (20 mL/kg). The volume of the solution used depends and varies with the capacity of the pump oxygenator.

Gelatins

Gelatin, a protein derived from collagen, can be used as a colloid solution in CPB priming. It is effective in maintaining colloid osmotic pressure, aiding in expanding blood volume during CPB. Additionally, gelatin's capacity to coat the CPB circuit and oxygenator may play a role in reducing platelet adhesion and thrombus formation; however, it has a relatively high incidence of anaphylactoid reactions compared with other colloids. For this reason, gelatins are not commonly used.

Hydroxyethyl Starch

Hydroxyethyl starch (HES), a synthetic colloid derived from hydroxyethylated glucose polymers, was once employed as a plasma volume expander. However, its association with increased mortality and acute kidney injury in critically ill patients led to its withdrawal from clinical use in the United States by the Food and Drug Administration.

Additional Components in the Circuit Prime

Besides crystalloids and colloids, several additives can be included in the priming solution to enhance outcomes and minimize side effects during CPB. These additives and their effects are listed below.

Heparin is used in CPB priming to enhance anticoagulation and offer an additional safety factor in case of inadequate systemic heparinization. Typically, a dose of between 5000 and 10,000 units is added to the pump before the initiation of CPB, ensuring effective anticoagulation during the procedure.

Magnesium sulfate, typically added to the CPB priming solution at 2 grams and another 2 grams post aortic cross-clamp removal, offers numerous benefits in cardiac surgery. It helps by decreasing postoperative arrhythmia rate by maintaining cardiac electrical stability, reducing myocardial stunning, and has vasodilatory effects that improve myocardial perfusion. Additionally, its neuroprotective properties can lower the risk of neurological complications.

Mannitol is commonly used in CPB, though its effectiveness is not robustly evidenced. As an osmotic diuretic, it prevents cerebral edema by drawing fluids into the intravascular space. It helps maintain colloid osmotic pressure, crucial for fluid balance during CPB. Additionally, mannitol acts as an oxygen free radical scavenger, protecting against cellular damage from reactive oxygen species generated during CPB. It also offers renal protection by promoting renal perfusion and safeguarding kidney tubules, which is especially beneficial for patients with pre-existing renal issues facing increased risks during CPB. Typically, a dose of 12.5 grams is administered right after the removal of the aortic cross-clamp. In cases involving circulatory arrest, the usual dose is increased to 25 grams.

Corticosteroids, such as methylprednisolone, are used in CPB in some centers to mitigate the systemic inflammatory response triggered by the CPB circuit. Their role is to suppress pro-inflammatory cytokines, reduce leukocyte migration, and stabilize cell membranes, which may reduce the severity of Systemic Inflammatory Response Syndrome (SIRS) and improve clinical outcomes. They are also used with the intention of lowering the incidence of postoperative atrial fibrillation and acute kidney injury, although these benefits are theoretical and not yet conclusively confirmed. A notable drawback of adding steroids to the CPB prime is that they can cause hyperglycemia. The usual dose is 250 micrograms in the prime for CPB, which is increased to 1 gram in cases involving circulatory arrest.

Bicarbonate Sodium bicarbonate serves as a buffer if unbalanced solutions and colloids are used in CPB priming.

It helps maintain pH balance, especially important in cases of circulatory arrest, where a 50 mEq ampoule is typically added to the prime. However, caution is needed as excessive volumes can lead to hypernatremia.

Calcium is typically added to the prime in CPB when citrated blood is used, particularly in pediatric procedures, to counteract hypocalcemia caused by citrate ions binding to calcium in the blood. Citrate prevents clotting but also chelates calcium. The dosage varies based on patient factors and citrated blood volume, but 100–200 mg of calcium per liter of citrated blood is a general guideline.

Lasix In cases of circulatory arrest, Lasix is often added to the prime, typically in a dosage of 20–40 mg.

The selection of priming fluids for CPB varies from institution to institution, and the choice is influenced by various factors, including patient characteristics, cost considerations, ease of use, and the desired clinical outcomes. The preference for crystalloid solutions, either alone or in combination with colloids, stems from their lower cost and ease of administration. However, the use of colloids has gained traction due to their ability to maintain colloid osmotic pressure and expand blood volume, which can be beneficial for patients with low blood volume or those at risk of fluid overload. Many cardiac centers use routinely a combined strategy of crystalloid and albumin in the priming.

Further Reading

Miles LF, Coulson TG, Galhardo C, Falter F. Pump priming practices and anticoagulation in cardiac surgery: results from the global cardiopulmonary bypass survey. Anesth Analg. 2017;125(6):1871–7. https://doi.org/10.1213/ANE.0000000000002052. PMID: 28614119

Niemi TT, Miyashita R, Yamakage M. Colloid solutions: a clinical update. J Anesth. 2010;24(6):913–25. https://doi.org/10.1007/s00540-010-1034-y. Epub 2010 Oct 17. PMID: 20953964

Semler MW, Kellum JA. Balanced crystalloid solutions. Am J Respir Crit Care Med. 2019;199(8):952–60. https://doi.org/10.1164/rccm.201809-1677CI. PMID: 30407838; PMCID: PMC6467313

Zarychanski R, Abou-Setta AM, Turgeon AF, Houston BL, McIntyre L, Marshall JC, Fergusson DA. Association of hydroxyethyl starch administration with mortality and acute kidney injury in critically ill patients requiring volume resuscitation: a systematic review and meta-analysis. JAMA. 2013;309(7):678–88. https://doi.org/10.1001/jama.2013.430. Erratum in: JAMA 2013 Mar 27;309(12):1229

Goal-Directed Perfusion Throughout Various Stages of Cardiopulmonary Bypass

10

Karl D. Hillenbrand and Eugene A. Hessel

Introduction

The main goal of cardiopulmonary bypass (CPB) during cardiac surgery is to provide adequate blood flow, perfusion, and oxygen to all tissues and organs (Fig. 10.1). This requires adequate oxygen delivery (systemic blood flow times arterial oxygen content) and mean arterial pressure (see discussion in Chap. 14, on "Monitoring adequacy of perfusion during CPB"). Other goals include (1) avoiding venous hypertension and distension of the right and left heart, (2) minimizing micro-embolism and avoiding macro-embolization, (3) minimizing activation of inflammation and stress response, (4) minimizing activation of coagulation, (5) minimizing myocardial ischemia, (6) minimizing return of unprocessed cardiotomy drainage, and (7) optimizing surgical exposure.

In the following sections, we suggest items that require your attention during various stages of CPB to assure goal-directed perfusion (GDP). Many of these topics are discussed in detail in other chapters, but they are consolidated here for a more focused approach (*see* Table 10.1).

Prior to starting CPB, adequate systemic anticoagulation, most commonly with heparin, should be administered, and its effect confirmed using the activated clotting time (ACT) or some other appropriate measure. Groups vary as to what ACT is adequate for CPB, but most require an ACT >400 and many aim for >480 seconds.

One should observe arterial, venous, and any other cannulation given the risk of air embolism, bleeding, or arrhythmias; the presence of which will require prompt intervention.

If a pulmonary artery catheter (PAC) is in place, it should be withdrawn into the main pulmonary artery. This precaution is necessary because hypothermia can stiffen the catheter, increasing the risk of pulmonary artery perforation.

K. D. Hillenbrand · E. A. Hessel (✉)
Department of Anesthesiology & Perioperative Medicine, University of Kentucky, Lexington, KY, USA
e-mail: ehessel@uky.edu

If using retrograde autologous priming (RAP), there may be a need for vasopressors and/or Trendelenburg position while the patient is partially exsanguinated.

Depending on the volume of CPB prime, and if RAP was used, drug effect site concentrations may fall considerably at the initiation of CPB. This may necessitate redosing certain medications, particularly hydrophilic ones such as nondepolarizing muscle relaxants.

A plan must also be developed for continuing to ensure adequate anesthesia. This involves either initiating or continuing total intravenous anesthesia (TIVA) or transitioning responsibility for volatile anesthetic uptake from the lungs/anesthesiologist to the oxygenator/perfusionist. Many practitioners will use a processed EEG monitor such as the BIS or SedLine to ensure adequate yet not excessive anesthesia. This is particularly important as signs of light anesthesia, such as sweating and tachycardia, are masked on CPB.

The role of temperature in providing optimal GDP, particularly outside the context of deep hypothermia used during circulatory arrest, remains a controversial topic. While some groups utilize moderate hypothermia (28–32° C), others use normothermia or "tepid" (34–36° C) temperature management. Hypothermia may offer neuroprotection, reduce the systemic blood flow required, and increase tolerance to anemia, it is also associated with prolonged durations of CPB and the risk of hyperthermia during rewarming. During the cooling and warming phases, brain temperature is most accurately estimated from the nasopharynx, while the temperature of the rest of the body can be gauged using bladder or rectal measurements. The Society of Thoracic Surgeons, The Society of Cardiovascular Anesthesiologists, and The American Society of ExtraCorporeal Technology (AmSECT) have published guidelines on temperature management during CPB, which are recommended for reference. For more information on temperature management and hypothermia, please refer to Chap. 6. Also see Engelman et al. (2015) for further details.

Early after the onset of CPB, and before cross-clamping the aorta and administering cardioplegia, one should monitor

A. S. Awad, J. DiNardo (eds.), *Clinical Perfusion for Cardiac Surgery*, https://doi.org/10.1007/978-3-031-91163-7_10

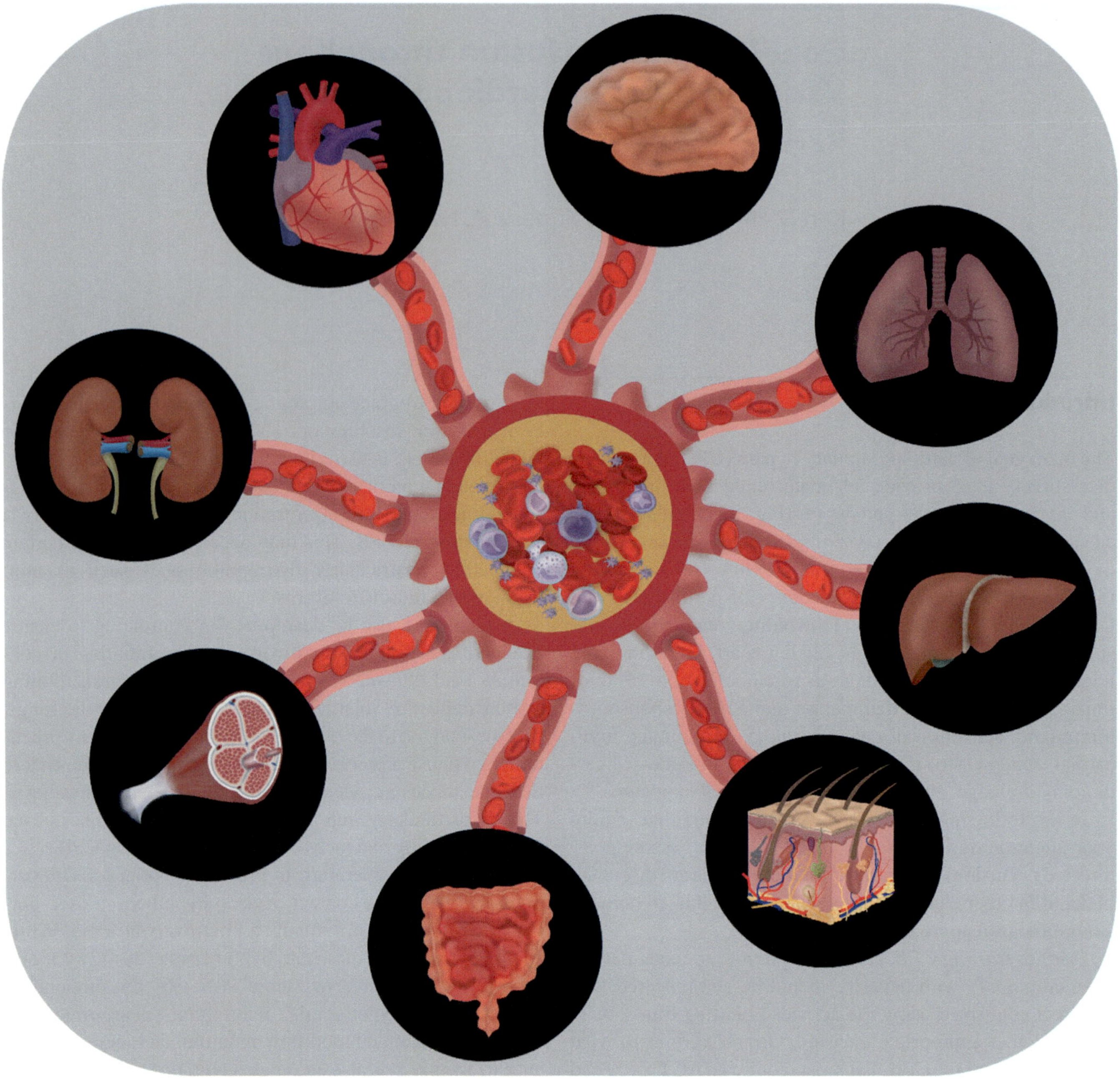

Fig. 10.1 Illustration of perfusion utilizing a CPB machine during cardiac surgery, highlighting the central role of CPB in delivering adequate blood flow, perfusion, and oxygen to vital organs, including the heart, brain, lungs, liver, kidneys, gastrointestinal tract, skin, and muscles

for about 2 minutes to assure (1) that perfusionist is able to maintain the desired flow with adequate venous return, and no loss of volume, (2) there is adequate arterial oxygenation (oxygenator function), (3) acceptable mean arterial pressure (MAP) (≥50 mm Hg or higher, depending on local criteria) with no evidence of arterial dissection, (4) acceptable mixed venous oxygen saturation (>75%), (5) there is adequate decompression of right and left heart along with low systemic venous pressures, (6) appropriate arterial line pressure from heart-lung machine (per the perfusionist), and (7) acceptable hematocrit level (≥21% or higher, depending on local criteria), if this parameter is immediately available. These issues should be resolved and dealt with before proceeding. If not immediately resolved, one can resume ventilation and weaning off CPB can be considered.

Throughout peri-bypass period, the anesthesiologist must ensure adequate anesthesia, including hypnosis, analgesia, muscle relaxation, and administration of prophylactic antibiotic for surgical site infection. Suppression of the stress response to CPB is achieved by maintaining desired systemic

Table 10.1 Goals during various stages of CPB

Stage	Goals	Key points
Prior to CPB	Achieve adequate anticoagulation	Administer heparin or alternative anticoagulant Check ACT
	Withdraw PAC into main PA	Avoid perforation of the PA.
	Observe cannulation	For risk of air embolism, bleeding, or arrhythmias
	Observe during RAP	Use vasopressors and/or Trendelenburg position to mitigate
	Plan anesthesia and pre-bypass drugs	To ensure adequate anesthesia (TIVA or volatile anesthetic)
Early CPB	Observe for 2 minutes after going on CPB and before cross-clamping and cardioplegia.	Adequate flow Adequate arterial oxygenation Acceptable MAP Acceptable mixed venous saturation Adequate decompression of right and left heart Appropriate arterial line pressure in CPB machine Acceptable hematocrit level
Throughout CPB	Maintain adequate anesthesia and redose the antibiotic after 4 hrs	Ensure patient comfort and prevent awareness
	Monitor the frequency of cardioplegia, vital signs parameters.	Deliver adequate cardioplegia for myocardial protection Track MAP, pump flow, oxygen delivery, temperature, mixed venous oxygen, acid-base status, and blood chemistries
	Be aware of CO_2 flooding	Manage sweep flow through the oxygenator
Aortic cross-clamp application	Temporarily reduce pump flow	Reduce the risk of iatrogenic aortic injury
	Adequate venting	Minimize ventricular distention
	Monitor cardioplegia	Promptly achieve cardiac arrest
Cross-clamp removal	Trendelenburg position	Prevention of air embolism in case the heart starts ejecting.
	Be prepared for pacing	To achieve an adequate heart rate in cases of slow rate or absence of spontaneous electrical activity
	Monitor for LV distention	Identify potential complications early
Prior to CPB weaning	Ensure adequate de-airing	TEE for the presence of air Gentle compression of the ventricles Use vent lines to actively remove air
	Assess ventricular function and filling	TEE is used for real-time assessment of ventricular function CVP and PCWP data Direct visual assessment of the RV
	Prepare medications and fluids	Anticipate potential needs during weaning
	Re-expand lungs and resume ventilation	Transition back to mechanical ventilation

flow, oxygen delivery, arterial pressure, and adequate hypnosis and analgesia. The use of corticosteroids is recommended by some but not strongly supported by clinical studies.

It is important to monitor the frequency of cardioplegia administration, both for its critical role in myocardial protection and as possible cause of transient hypotension while on CPB due to the potassium load. Detection of ECG activity may indicate the need of additional administration, but it should be correlated with visible heart activity. This is because numerous mechanical parts in the CPB circuit, especially the roller pumps, can create ECG artifacts; grounding of the CPB machine may be necessary.

Often, the surgical field is flooded with carbon dioxide to reduce the severity of air embolism, given carbon dioxide's higher blood solubility compared to nitrogen. However, the carbon dioxide may also be sucked into the heart-lung machine, resulting in hypercarbia if not compensated for by increasing the sweep flow through the oxygenator.

One must be continually cognizant of arterial pressure, systemic flow from the heart-lung machine, mixed venous oxygen saturation fluid balance and its management, management of anticoagulation, hematocrit, glucose, and acid-base status. If abnormalities are detected, assist the perfusionist in evaluating and managing these issues.

When the surgeon applies the aortic cross-clamp, the surgeon will typically ask the perfusionist to temporarily reduce arterial flows. This practice allows for precise and careful application of the cross-clamp, potentially reducing the chance of an iatrogenic aortic injury or damage to the nearby pulmonary artery.

When the aortic cross-clamp is removed, the surgeon often requests the Trendelenburg position. One must observe for left ventricular (LV) distension, and the surgeon may request pacing of the heart through temporary epicardial pacing wires.

In anticipation of coming off CPB, one must prepare for pacing if requested. Additionally, it is important to have prepared protamine, along with any indicated blood and procoagulation products, intravascular volume agents, vasoactive and inotropic drugs. The anesthesiologist may

Table 10.2 Perturbations and complications during CPB: prevention, detection, and management

Problem	Potential causes	Detection	Management
Hypotension (MAP < 50–80 mmHg)	Inadequate arterial flow, shunting, aortic dissection, anemia, vasodilators, excessive anesthesia, allergies, sepsis, vasoplegia. See Table 10.2	Verify pressure accuracy (central location), blood gas, and ECG.	Vasopressors, corticosteroids, methylene blue, hydroxocobalamin, angiotensin II, and vitamin C.
Hypertension (MAP > 80 mmHg)	Rewarming from deep hypothermia, inadequate anesthesia	Rule out inadequate anesthesia-BIS monitor	Systemic vasodilators
Inadequate venous return	Venous cannula malposition/kinking, hypovolemia, air lock, inadequate patient elevation	Monitor pressure, observe drainage	Reposition cannula, administer fluids, remove air lock, adjust patient position
Low arterial oxygenation (<95%)	Oxygenator malfunction, excessive oxygen demand	Monitor blood color, arterial oxygen saturation, and cerebral oximetry	Check oxygenator flow/function, consider inline sensors.
Low mixed venous oxygen saturation (<75%)	Inadequate oxygen delivery (anemia, low arterial oxygenation, low flow), excessive demand (sepsis, malignant hyperthermia)	Monitor oxygen saturation, blood gas	Evaluate and optimize oxygen delivery (anemia management, flow adjustment, etc.).
Low oxygen delivery (DO_2 < 275 ml/min/M2)	Reduced flow, anemia, and poor oxygenation	Monitor DO_2, blood gas, and hemoglobin	Increase flow, manage anemia, consider packed RBCs (with caution)
Low cerebral oximetry (NIRS)	Inadequate supply vs. demand. See Table 10.3	Monitor NIRS, follow Denault algorithm steps. Table	Increase CO_2, increase flow, increase BP, and transfuse blood
Low hematocrit	Blood loss and hemodilution	Monitor hemoglobin and hematocrit.	Diuresis/hemoconcentration, packed RBCs (carefully).
Metabolic acidosis/lactic acidosis	Inadequate oxygen delivery and organ ischemia	Monitor blood gas and lactate	Optimize oxygen delivery, consider specific interventions based on source
Hyperkalemia	Cardioplegia and cell breakdown	Monitor potassium levels	Diuresis/ultrafiltration, insulin/dextrose, beta-agonists, and calcium chloride (temporary).
Hyperglycemia	Stress response and cardioplegia solution.	Monitor blood glucose	Intravenous insulin, consider reducing dextrose in cardioplegia
Oliguria	Hypotension, non-pulsatile flow and high CVP	Monitor urine output and fluid balance.	Manage hemodynamics and optimize fluid replacement.
Hematuria	Transfusion reaction and urinary tract bleeding	Monitor urine color and hemoglobin.	Investigate cause and adjust anticoagulation/ consult urology

assist with de-airing, for example, by using Trendelenburg position, and perform its assessment with TEE. Finally, one must resume ventilation following recruitment maneuvers, before coming off bypass. TEE will help assess volume status and cardiac function.

For information regarding the *role of anesthesiologist during emergence* from CPB and in the early post-CPB period, please refer to Chap. 11.

Further *details on monitoring during CPB* can be found in Chap. 13.

An important goal of providing optimal GDP is *detecting and correcting perturbations in vital hemodynamics* or blood chemistry (*see* Table 10.2).

Hypotension

Hypotension is a major concern during CPB. The lower limit of acceptable MAP during CPB remains controversial and likely varies from patient to patient based on their associated morbidities. Recent European guidelines recommend maintaining MAP between 50 and 80 mm Hg. (See Kunst et al. 2019) If hypotension is observed, one must first assure that pressure measurement is accurate. As discussed in Chap. 14, radial artery pressure is often falsely low when coming off bypass due to rewarming and vasodilation. Consider verifying the pressure at a more central location, such as the brachial or femoral artery, or using a needle or catheter in the ascending aorta. If low, the differential includes inadequate arterial flow, shunting in the bypass circuit, aortic dissection, anemia, inadvertent administration of vasodilators, excessive anesthesia, allergic reactions (anaphylaxis), sepsis, and "idiopathic" vasoplegia. The latter occurs in 10–20% of cases and may require administration of vasopressors such as phenylephrine, norepinephrine, vasopressin, and occasionally epinephrine. If vasoplegia persists despite these measures, the administration of corticosteroids, methylene blue (with caution for serotonin syndrome), hydroxocobalamin, or angiotensin II should be considered. Vitamin C is also advocated by some (*see* Table 10.3).

Table 10.3 Potential causes of low pressure during and immediately after CPB

Potential causes of low pressure during and after CPB		
Category	Cause	Description
Blood flow issues	Inadequate arterial flow	Circuit or pump malfunction
	Shunting in the bypass circuit	The circuit diverts blood away from the patient
	Aortic dissection	Tears in the aortic wall
	Iatrogenic vasodilation	Administration of vasodilator medications.
Blood properties	Anemia	Low red blood cell count leading to low viscosity and low pressure
	Excessive anticoagulation	Increased bleeding tendency can lead to blood volume loss and lowered pressure.
Anesthesia and reactions	Excessive anesthesia	Depth of anesthesia can impact pressure
	Allergic reactions (anaphylaxis)	Severe allergic response leading to vasodilation and lowered pressure.
Infectious and inflammatory	Sepsis	Systemic inflammatory response or infection can affect heart function and vascular tone.
	"Idiopathic" vasoplegia	Vasodilation and low pressure despite seemingly normal conditions

Hypertension

Hypertension (MAP >80 mm Hg) is less commonly encountered during CPB, but it can put stress on suture lines, the heart, increase washout of cardioplegia, and cause decreased forward flow in CPB machines that utilize a centrifugal pump. Hypertension is occasionally seen during rewarming from deep hypothermia, one should rule out inadequate anesthesia as a cause and then consider administration of a systemic vasodilator.

Inadequate Venous Return

The perfusionist may experience inadequate venous return. The differential diagnosis includes malposition or kinking of the venous cannula and hypovolemia. If gravity drainage is used, an "air lock" or inadequate elevation of the patient above the venous reservoir can also contribute to this issue. In cases of augmented venous return, inappropriate vacuum level or kinetic flow may be considered.

Low Arterial Oxygenation

Low arterial oxygenation (<95%) can suggest a malfunctioning oxygenator or excessive oxygen demand. Appropriate color change in the blood between the venous and arterial cannula should be continuously monitored due to pulse oximetry's inability to function under pulseless CPB. Some CPB circuits are equipped with inline arterial oxygenation sensors, allowing for continuous monitoring of arterial oxygen saturation. While cerebral oximetry mainly reflects cerebral venous saturation, a low reading may suggest a fall in arterial oxygenation.

Low Mixed Venous Oxygen Saturation

Low mixed venous oxygen saturation (< 75%) suggests inadequate oxygen delivery to meet oxygen demand. Differential diagnosis includes inadequate oxygen delivery due to anemia, low arterial oxygenation, low arterial flow, or excessive oxygen demand. If arterial oxygenation is reduced, an evaluation of oxygen flow through the oxygenator, as well as the function of the oxygenator, is required. Excessive oxygen demand could be due to factors such as sepsis, malignant hyperthermia, inadequate anesthesia and muscle relaxation, or an excessively large patient for the oxygenator and cannula sizes.

Low Oxygen Delivery (DO_2)

DO_2 (less than approximately 275 ml/min/M^2). Maintaining an adequate oxygen delivery is now recommended as an important goal of perfusion because when low it is associated with adverse outcomes, especially acute kidney injury (AKI) (See Magruder et al. 2022; Peng et al. 2022). Causes of low DO_2 include reduced systemic blood flow, inadequate blood oxygenation, and severe anemia. Prevention of anemia during CPB is key, and raising flow is often the best remedy. Although giving packed RBCs will improve calculated DO_2, its effectiveness in enhancing tissue oxygenation or oxygen consumption is questionable. AmSECT Standard 9.2 states that "Indexed Oxygen delivery and consumption calculations shall be utilized to evaluate and optimize gas exchange."

Table 10.4 Management steps for low cerebral oximetry during CPB

Step number	Action	Notes/details
Step number: 1	Rule out mechanical issues	Check for malposition or obstruction of arterial and venous cannulae; assess head and neck position.
Step number: 2	Ensure adequate MAP	Adjust the pump flow to maintain Consider adding vasopressors
Step number: 3	Verify systemic oxygenation	Check oxygen levels and adjust oxygenator function as necessary
Step number: 4	Ensure adequate hemoglobin	Monitor hemoglobin levels; manage accordingly
Step number: 5	Ensure adequate pump flow	Adjust pump settings to maintain optimal flow
Step number: 6	Decrease cerebral O2 consumption	Avoid hyperthermia, deepen anesthesia, and consider hypothermia induction
Step number: 7	Consider pulsatile flow	Evaluate the need for pulsatile blood flow to improve cerebral perfusion

Low Cerebral Oximetry (NIRS)

A drop in NIRS 20% or more from baseline, either bilaterally or unilaterally, suggests an inadequate supply versus demand. A commonly used algorithm was proposed by Denault et al. in 2007. This includes the following steps. Step (1), rule out mechanical malposition or obstruction of the arterial and venous cannula or head or neck position; (2), ensure adequate MAP; (3), verify systemic oxygenation; (4), ensure adequate hemoglobin concentration; (5), ensure adequate pump flow; (6), decrease cerebral oxygen consumption by avoiding hyperthermia, increasing depth of anesthesia, and possibly inducing hypothermia; and (7), consider adding pulsatile blood flow (*see* Table 10.4).

Low Hematocrit

The definition of critically low hemoglobin/hematocrit during bypass remains controversial. The key focus should be on the prevention of anemia during bypass. However, if levels fall below local thresholds, options include diuresis or hemoconcentration or administration of packed red blood cells. It is important to note that the latter option is associated with the standard risks of blood transfusion. Furthermore, the administration of packed red blood cells has been linked to a dose-dependent increase in morbidity and mortality, so the decision to transfuse must be made carefully.

Metabolic Acidosis/Lactic Acidosis

Metabolic acidosis/lactic acidosis may be ominous. It could be a sign of inadequate oxygen delivery or organ ischemia, especially in the gut or liver. The anesthesiologist and perfusionist should work together to ensure adequate oxygen is being delivered to the body's tissues. However, especially in the setting of aortic dissection extending into the abdominal branches, sometimes there may be limitations to what can be done to improve the situation while on CPB.

Hyperkalemia

Hyperkalemia is commonly encountered due to the administration of cardioplegia. It is usually transitory and begins improving before coming off CPB. Diuresis or zero balance ultrafiltration (ZBUF) can be used to lower the potassium levels. Similarly, standard therapies such as the combination of insulin and dextrose, which trigger potassium uptake into the cells or beta-agonists that stimulate potassium uptake into skeletal muscle, are also effective. If the potassium remains high while attempting to wean off CPB or establish a rhythm after cross-clamp removal, calcium can be administered as a temporizing measure. Persistent hyperkalemia rarely requires dialysis.

Hyperglycemia

Hyperglycemia is frequently encountered even in nondiabetic patients. Guidelines recommend maintaining glucose levels <180 given its association with various morbidities, but achieving this can be challenging. Contributing factors include steroid administration, the stress response to surgery and CPB, and the large glucose load delivered to the patient in some cardioplegia solutions. Consequently, many patients require intravenous insulin administration during bypass to try to help regulate glucose levels.

Oliguria

Oliguria is variably encountered while on CPB. Its presence is associated with post-operative AKI; however, merely transforming the kidney injury from oliguric to polyuric does not improve outcomes. Its origin may be related to the hypotension and non-pulsatile flow encountered on CPB as well as increased CVP from inadequate drainage, which can cause "back pressure" on the kidney. Therefore, ensuring optimal hemodynamics may help reduce post-operative

AKI. Conversely, some patients may experience brisk diuresis while on CPB due to mannitol and glucose, which may be found in the pump prime and cardioplegia solution. This situation will necessitate diligent fluid replacement, as urine volumes can be quite substantial.

Hematuria

Hematuria or hemoglobinuria is not uncommon and may be a sign of a transfusion reaction or bleeding in the urinary tract associated with anticoagulation and urinary bladder catheterization. Hemoglobinuria most commonly occurs during prolonged duration bypass with extensive use of cardiotomy suction, which can lead to red blood cell rupture and trauma.

Finally, *the anesthesiologist plays a crucial role in the early detection and assistance with the management of serious complications of CPB.* These include (1) arterial dissection, (2) massive gas embolization, (3) oxygenator failure, (4) pump failure, and (5) electrical failure. These complications are discussed in detail in Chapters 24 and 25.

Managements during emergence from CPB are discussed in Chap. 11.

More details regarding *monitoring during CPB* are discussed in Chaps. 13 and 14.

Further Reading

American Society of ExtraCorporeal Technology. Standards and Guidelines for Perfusion Practice. 2023. Available from: https://www.amsect.org/Portals/0/AmSECT_Perfusion_S%26G_2023%20Ratified%20021023_Digital%20edition.pdf

Cheung AT. Management of CPB. UpToDate Aug 2023.

Denault A, et al. A proposed algorithm for the intraoperative use of cerebral near-infrared spectroscopy. Semin Cardiothorac Vasc Anesth. 2007;11(4):274–81.

Engelman R, et al. Clinical practice guidelines for cardiopulmonary bypass—temperature management during cardiopulmonary bypass. J Cardiothorac Vasc Anesth. 2015;29(4):1104.

Gibbs NM, et al. Management of CPB. In: Gravlee GP, et al., editors. Hensley's practical approach to cardiothoracic anesthesia. 6. 2019 Wolters Kluwer/Lippincott Williams & Wilkins Health, Philadelphia

Grocott H, et al. CPB Management and organ protection. In: Kaplan JA, et al., editors. Kaplan's cardiac anesthesia. 7. 2016. Elsevier

Kunst G, et al. 2019 EACTS/EACTA/EBCP guidelines on cardiopulmonary bypass in adult cardiac surgery. BJA. 2019;123:713–57.

Magruder JT, Weiss SJ, DeAngelis KG, et al. Correlating oxygen delivery on cardiopulmonary bypass with Society of Thoracic Surgeons outcomes following cardiac surgery. J Thorac Cardiovasc Surg. 2022;164(3):997–1007.

Murphy GS, Hessel EA 2nd, Groom RC. Optimal perfusion during cardiopulmonary bypass: an evidence-based approach. Anesth Analg. 2009;108(5):1394–417.

Peng K, et al. Society of cardiovascular anesthesiologists clinical practice update for management of acute kidney injury associated with cardiac surgery. Anesth Analg. 2022;135(4):744–56.

Termination of Cardiopulmonary Bypass

11

Donghwan Lee, Nathan Minie, and Michael G. Fitzsimons

Introduction

The process of weaning a patient from cardiopulmonary bypass (CPB) is a critical stage in the management of individuals undergoing procedures requiring extracorporeal support. The process of weaning entails the gradual transition from mechanical pump-assisted circuitry and pulmonary support provided by CPB to that of the native heart and lungs. Accomplishing this process necessitates a multistep approach and extensive communication among an interdisciplinary team, including surgeons, anesthesiologists, perfusionists, and operating room nurses. This section aims to explore the weaning process from CPB and discuss the perioperative management involved to ensure successful patient outcomes.

Physiological Changes Associated with Cardiopulmonary Bypass

CPB is associated with multiple physiologic changes impacting nearly every organ system (Table 11.1). For comprehensive details, please refer to Chap. 6, "Physiologic Changes and Inflammatory Response to Cardiopulmonary Bypass." These changes can impact weaning from extracorporeal support. Many of these changes are induced to protect the body during extracorporeal circulation such as hypothermia, anticoagulation, and hemodilution, while others are the results of contact of blood with the circuitry that make up the bypass system. Chap. 6 "Physiologic Changes and Inflammatory Response to Cardiopulmonary Bypass" provides a detailed discussion on physiologic changes during CPB.

Table 11.1 Negative effects of CPB

Negative effects of CPB
Hypothermia
Inflammation
Hemodilution
Profound anticoagulation
Ischemia/reperfusion injury
Vasodilation
Myocardial dysfunction
Electrolyte imbalance: hypocalcemia and hyperkalemia

Preparation

Preparation for separation from cardiopulmonary bypass (CPB) begins as early as the review of the history and physical examination of the patient. Various patient and surgical factors may make the weaning process more complex, necessitating extra preparation (Table 11.2). Therefore, it is critical to take these factors into account when preparing a plan for separation from CPB. Factors complicating the weaning process can be divided into patient-specific or surgical factors.

Checklists serve as a guide to ensure all necessary steps of a process are considered or completed, whether during preparation or actual performance. The subsequent section will present a detailed discussion of an organ-specific checklist, elucidating the essential measures and factors to be considered to accomplish a successful CPB termination.

D. Lee · M. G. Fitzsimons (✉)
Department of Anesthesia, Critical Care, and Pain Medicine, Massachusetts General Hospital, Boston, MA, USA
e-mail: DLEE75@MGH.HARVARD.EDU; MFITZSIMONS@mgh.harvard.edu

N. Minie
Perfusion Services, Cardiac Surgery Division, Department of Surgery, Massachusetts General Hospital, Boston, MA, USA
e-mail: NMINIE@mgh.harvard.edu

A. S. Awad, J. DiNardo (eds.), *Clinical Perfusion for Cardiac Surgery*, https://doi.org/10.1007/978-3-031-91163-7_11

Table 11.2 Factors predicting difficulty with weaning

Patient factors	Surgical factors
Advanced age	Increased CPB duration and aortic cross clamping
Renal disease	Emergency procedures
Anemia (low hemoglobin)	Complexity of the surgical procedure, e.g., multiple valve interventions
Elevated partial thromboplastin time (PTT)	Inadequate myocardial protection
Previous myocardial infarction (MI)	Incomplete surgical repair, residual valvular regurgitation or stenosis, or uncorrected shunts can impede successful weaning
Reduced left ventricular ejection fraction (LVEF)	Excessive bleeding during surgery
Procedures associated with repeat sternotomy	Intraoperative surgical complications like injury to cardiac structures
Left ventricular diastolic dysfunction	
Right ventricular dysfunction	

General Considerations

Temperature

Hypothermia may prove detrimental to patient outcome during the weaning process by worsening coagulopathy and myocardial function, potentiating the effects of muscle relaxants, and prolonging time to extubation in the intensive care unit. Adequate warming during the final stages of bypass is the most efficient means to reduce problems. Gradual rewarming to a naso- or oropharyngeal temperature of 37 °C and a bladder temperature of 35.5 °C is recommended. It is also crucial to prevent the cerebral temperature from exceeding 37 °C, as this might lead to an increased cerebral metabolic rate and potential neurological injury. The temperature measured in the head may read higher than that measured in the bladder or rectum due to the proximity of the aortic cannula to the great vessels of the arch as well as the higher relative blood flow to the brain. Bladder or rectal temperatures alone may underestimate the cerebral temperature. Measures such as forced-air warming, fluid warming, and increasing the temperature of the room may help to reduce temperature loss after termination of bypass but are less effective than adequate warming via bypass.

Neurological Consideration

Anesthesia

A plan should be formulated beforehand to ensure continuous maintenance of anesthesia into the post-bypass period. Perfusionists should communicate with the anesthesia team before any anesthetics administered through the bypass circuit are stopped. The doses of anesthetics and muscle relaxants often decrease during bypass due to the effects of induced hypothermia. However, as the patient is warmed during the final stages of bypass, an anesthetic requirement may increase. Ensuring a steady and uninterrupted supply of anesthetic is of paramount importance, and, if necessary, supplementing with medications such as benzodiazepines, narcotics, and muscle relaxants is warranted. Volatile anesthetics delivered from the anesthesia machine or total intravenous anesthesia (TIVA) is used to maintain anesthesia during the weaning process. Although most patients are sedated and remain intubated immediately after CPB, an increasing number of patients are managed via a "Fast Track" or Enhanced Recovery After Surgery (ERAS) pathway, which includes a plan for early extubation.

Cardiovascular Preparation

Monitors

The anesthesiologist will assure that all monitors necessary during weaning are working properly. Pressure transducers should be "leveled" and "zeroed" to assure the most accurate measures. The volume on the pulse oximeter should be audible to the entire team. A functioning EKG allows detection of ischemia or arrhythmias. If the accuracy of the monitored pressure is questioned, a more precise monitor should be established such as a femoral artery catheter.

Adjuvant Drugs

The anesthesiologist must ensure that intravenous and inhaled medications necessary for the weaning process are available and prepared for delivery. Antiarrhythmic medications, inotropic agents, insulin, and vasoactive infusions are commonly needed. Inhaled agents such as epoprostenol and inhaled nitric oxide (iNO) may be necessary for patients with right heart failure or pulmonary hypertension. These drugs should be readily accessible to avoid distraction during the weaning process.

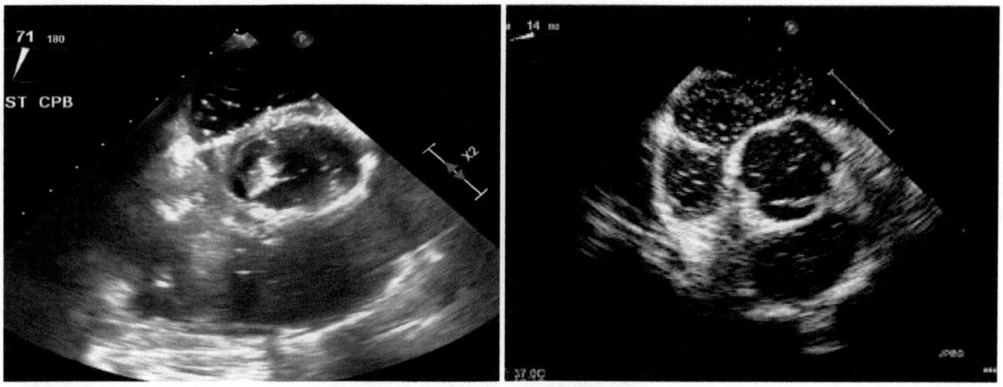

Fig. 11.1 This image displays TEE view, capturing the presence of air within the heart chambers during partial CPB. TEE aids in the critical de-airing process by allowing assessment of the amount and location of residual air in the heart. This step is crucial for the safe removal of air bubbles, thus preventing the risk of air embolism in cerebral vessels and coronary arteries

Air Removal (De-Airing)

Air may accumulate in the chambers of the heart or aortic root during cardiac procedures, especially those requiring entry into the left atrium, ventricle, or aorta. Initiation of lung ventilation may force air that has accumulated in the pulmonary veins to enter the heart. Failure to adequately de-air the heart may allow air embolization to the great vessels, resulting in neurologic ischemia, or to the coronary arteries, leading to myocardial ischemia, arrhythmias, and ventricular dysfunction. The right coronary artery is most vulnerable when a patient is supine for surgery due to the superior position of the vessel.

Partial CPB allows the heart to mobilize any remaining intracardiac air, which may then be removed through the antegrade cardioplegia cannula by reversal of flow (venting of the aortic root). The surgeon may manually agitate the heart to force out any residual air. Patients are typically positioned in Trendelenburg position during de-airing to reduce entry into the central nervous system (CNS). Transesophageal echocardiography (TEE) is performed during the de-airing process to assess the amount and location of air remaining in the heart (see Fig. 11.1).

Rhythm

A stable heart rhythm facilitates weaning by maximizing cardiac output. Surgeons commonly attach temporary epicardial pacemaker wires to the right atrial appendage and the right ventricle. Normal sinus rhythm is preferred, but if the rate is not adequate, atrial pacing is initiated generally at a rate of approximately 80–90 beats per minute. A-V pacing or V pacing are less ideal. Patients with chronic atrial fibrillation may only achieve a ventricular paced rhythm. Arrhythmias such as ventricular fibrillation, ventricular tachycardia, or atrial fibrillation with a rapid ventricular response require treatment with defibrillation, cardioversion, or antiarrhythmic medications.

Rate

A heart rate between 80 and 90 beats/min is preferred to optimize the balance between cardiac output and coronary diastolic perfusion time. Epicardial pacing may be required to reach optimal heart rate.

Vascular Resistance

Systemic vascular resistance (SVR) plays a crucial role in myocardial workload and oxygen balance. An elevated SVR can increase afterload, leading to an increased workload and oxygen consumption of the heart. A low SVR can result in inadequate tissue perfusion and hypotension, necessitating treatment with vasopressors. Vasoplegia is common after cardiopulmonary bypass. Factors associated with vasoplegia include heart transplantation, prolonged cardiopulmonary bypass, preoperative ACE inhibitors, preoperative use of heparin, and patients on mechanical circulatory assist. Vasoplegia refractory to conventional treatment with phenylephrine, norepinephrine, or vasopressin may require escalation to methylene blue.

Aortic Cross-Clamp Removal (Reperfusion)

Myocardial reperfusion occurs when the aortic cross clamp is removed, allowing blood flow to the coronary arteries and myocardium and washout byproducts of anaerobic metabolism, including potassium associated with cardioplegia. This process restores high-energy ATP levels and allows the cooled heart to warm up to systemic temperature. The rapid temperature change and potassium washout can increase the risk of reperfusion-associated ventricular fibrillation (VF). Patients who require defibrillation for VF may need higher doses of inotropic agents due to reduced myocardial performance. The administration of lidocaine before cross-clamp removal may decrease the occurrence of VF and reduce the need for defibrillation. Reperfusion should result in return of a spontaneous heartbeat (see Fig. 11.2). If a heart rhythm does not return, pacing may be initiated.

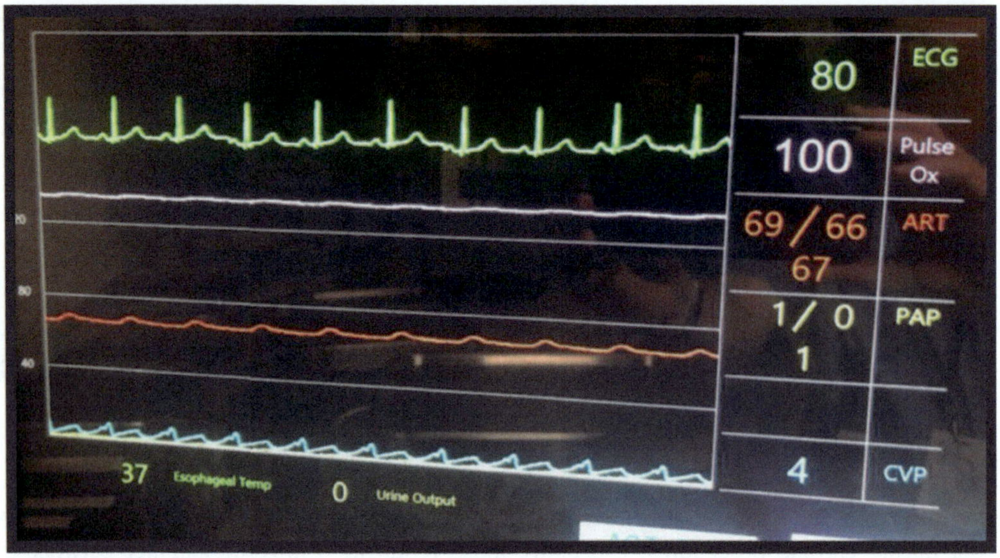

Fig. 11.2 This image displays the monitor screen immediately following the removal of the aortic cross clamp. The monitor indicates the heart beginning to beat on its own, as in this case, or with the aid of a pacemaker when needed. Continual venous drainage maintains a low central venous pressure (CVP) and PA pressure, as indicated here by PA 1 (in yellow) and CVP 4 (in blue)

Pulmonary Considerations

Oxygenation/Ventilation

Ventilation must be resumed prior to beginning the weaning process. The lungs should be manually reinflated to recruit atelectatic segments prior to resumption of mechanical ventilation. Resumption of ventilation may reveal bronchospasm, atelectasis, mucus plugging, blood in the airway, or a kinked endotracheal tube. Patients with preexisting lung disease may require additional treatments such as positive end-expiratory pressure (PEEP), bronchodilators, or pressure control ventilation to ensure adequate oxygenation and ventilation. Pulmonary problems should be addressed prior to weaning to avoid unnecessary distraction. The presence of blood or secretions may require bronchoscopy.

Hematologic Considerations

Hemoglobin

Hemoglobin (Hb) levels should be closely monitored and maintained at 7–8 g/dL or higher. In cases where Hb falls below 7 g/dL, transfusion should be considered, as severe anemia can compromise the delivery of oxygen to myocardial tissues.

Coagulation

One of the notable adverse effects of the CPB circuit is the development of coagulopathy beyond that induced by heparin administration, including platelet depletion and dysfunction. This can lead to increased bleeding after bypass. Blood products should be immediately available for those patients likely to require transfusion including females, those with pre-existing coagulopathy, renal insufficiency, longer procedures, procedures associated with repeat sternotomy, and patients receiving anticoagulants prior to surgery. Coagulation status and platelet function studies, including activated clotting time (ACT), heparin assays, or thromboelastography (TEG), are generally assessed after protamine administration, but platelets count and prothrombin (PT) can be assessed prior to protamine.

Metabolic Considerations

Electrolytes

Electrolytes abnormalities should be identified and corrected prior to separation from CPB.

- Acid-base abnormalities: Metabolic acidosis is commonly seen during the prolonged CPB cases. The cause should be continually sought and corrected. Severe base deficits (> −8 mmol/L) should be corrected with sodium bicarbonate to minimize depression of myocardial function or reduction in the effectiveness of inotropic drugs.
- Potassium (normal 4–5.5 mmol/L): Hypokalemia may potentiate arrhythmias. Hyperkalemia can affect heart rhythm and contractility. Potassium level below 4 mmol/L or above 6.0 mmol/L must be treated. Pharmacologic management of hyperkalemia includes insulin and dextrose or the administration of furosemide. Perfusion may perform zero-balance ultrafiltration.

- Ionized calcium (normal 1.09–1.3 mmol/L): Ionized calcium levels may decrease due to the hemodilution or transfusion of citrate-containing blood products. Hypocalcemia can contribute to cardiac arrhythmias, impaired contractility, impaired clotting function, and vasodilation. Supplemental calcium may be administered after aortic cross-clamp removal to maintain the ionized calcium level above 1.1 mmol/L.
- Lactate (normal 0.5–2.5 mmol/L): Lactate values and trends are indicative of the adequacy of end-organ perfusion and should be monitored closely.

Chapter 12 "Metabolic Management during CPB" provides a detailed discussion on the electrolyte's abnormalities during CPB.

The Weaning Process

Weaning a patient from CPB is a team effort. Clear, closed-loop communication is required between the cardiac surgeon, anesthesiologist, and perfusionist from the phase of interoperative preparation through the actual act of weaning into the post-weaning period. The use of a checklist reduces the incidence of missed steps critical to a process.

The pre-weaning checklist consists of components that are most effectively managed while on bypass (warming) or require transition from the bypass system to the anesthesia team (ventilation, medications, and anesthetics). Team members should verbally review and confirm completion of the tasks on the pre-weaning checklist (Table 11.3).

Weaning from CPB begins with the surgeon or perfusionist partially reducing venous drainage that allows blood to return to the right atrium and resultant filling chambers of the heart (see Fig. 11.3).

As the heart fills with blood and contraction occurs, pulsatility is noted on the CVP and pulmonary artery pressure (PAP) waveforms (see Fig. 11.4). Filling and ejection of blood from the left ventricle are indicated by pulsatility in the arterial waveform (radial, femoral, or brachial). The perfusionist or surgeon will incrementally reduce venous return to the reservoir while continuing to return blood through the aortic cannula to maintain blood pressure adequate to perfuse the heart and peripheral tissues. Arterial blood flow from the bypass system is reduced as ejection from the heart is sufficient to maintain a sufficient perfusion pressure.

Once the left ventricle (LV) is adequately filled and is ejecting a sufficient stroke volume, venous return is ceased, arterial flow from the bypass circuit via the aortic cannula is stopped, and the patient is considered "off bypass" (see Fig. 11.5). The perfusionist must verbally communicate this to the team. A minimum amount of blood is circulated through the bypass system (see Fig. 11.6). A clamp is applied to the arterial line when flow is ceased (see Fig. 11.7).

Throughout the weaning process, the anesthesiologist and surgeon are continually assessing ventricular function and hemodynamic status. The function of the right ventricle is directly visualized and assessed with TEE. The LV is primarily assessed with TEE for overall function, wall motion abnormalities, and the presence of any residual air within the chambers. The EKG is assessed for the presence of ischemic changes and arrhythmias. The CVP, PAP, and TEE are monitored to guide the adequacy of blood volume within the heart. Hemodynamic goals are targeted during the weaning process (Table 11.4). Once satisfactory hemodynamic status is achieved, the surgeon inspects the surgical site for residual bleeding. The anesthesiologist and surgeon review TEE imaging and hemodynamic data to assure that surgical intervention is complete before proceeding to protamine administration and vascular decannulation.

Table 11.3 Pre-weaning checklist

Component	Issues
Patient temperature	Warming adequate for termination of CPB
Laboratory values	Hemoglobin, lactate, potassium, calcium, and arterial blood gas values reviewed
Vacuum-assisted venous drainage (VAVD)	VAVD off
Circuit shunts	Circuit shunts off
Ventilation (gas exchange)	Initiated by anesthesia team
Administration of vasopressor and inotropic agents	Transitioned to management by anesthesia team
Anesthesia	Anesthetic administration transitioned to anesthesia team

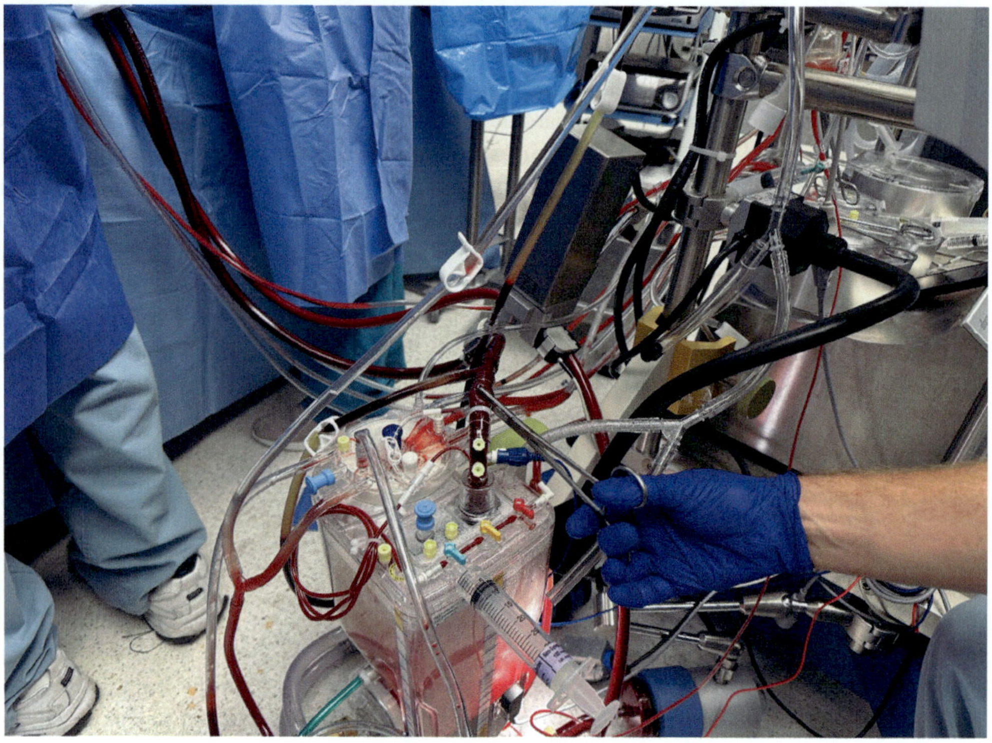

Fig. 11.3 In this image, a skilled perfusionist is carefully applying a partial clamp to the venous return line during the weaning process. This crucial step enables controlled filling of the heart, allowing it to eject blood efficiently. The perfusionist's precision in manipulating the venous return is vital for a smooth transition and weaning from CPB support

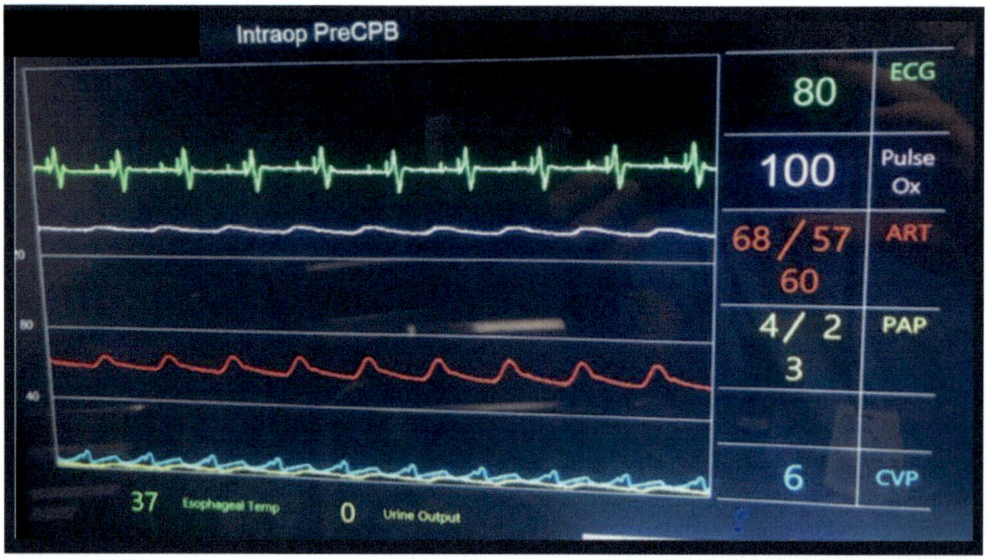

Fig. 11.4 The image captures the moment while still on bypass, demonstrating partial filling of the heart and generation of pulsatility: Placement of a partial clamp on the venous line by the perfusionist reduces the amount of blood returning to the hard-shell reservoir. Blood fills the heart, which can now eject blood into the aorta and contributes to the pressure resulting in pulsatility on the arterial line tracing and the pulse oximeter. The heart rhythm is atrioventricular pacing

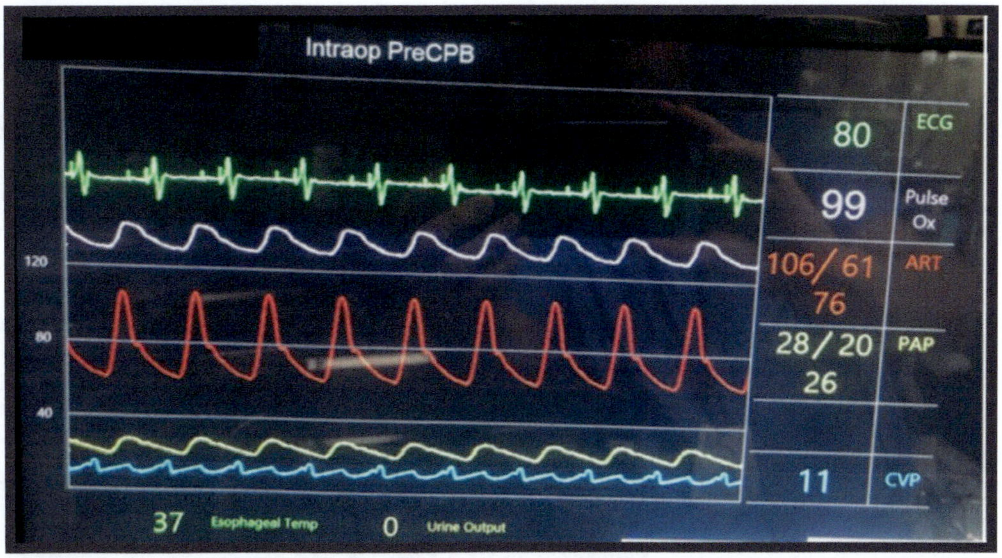

Fig. 11.5 This image shows the monitor screen immediately following the discontinuation of cardiopulmonary bypass. With the bypass deactivated, blood is no longer diverted to the hard-shell venous reservoir and is instead returned to the heart. This change is evident in the noted pulsatility of the CVP, PA, and arterial tracings on the monitor. The heart's rhythm is maintained through atrioventricular pacing (AV pacing), ensuring stable cardiac function post-bypass

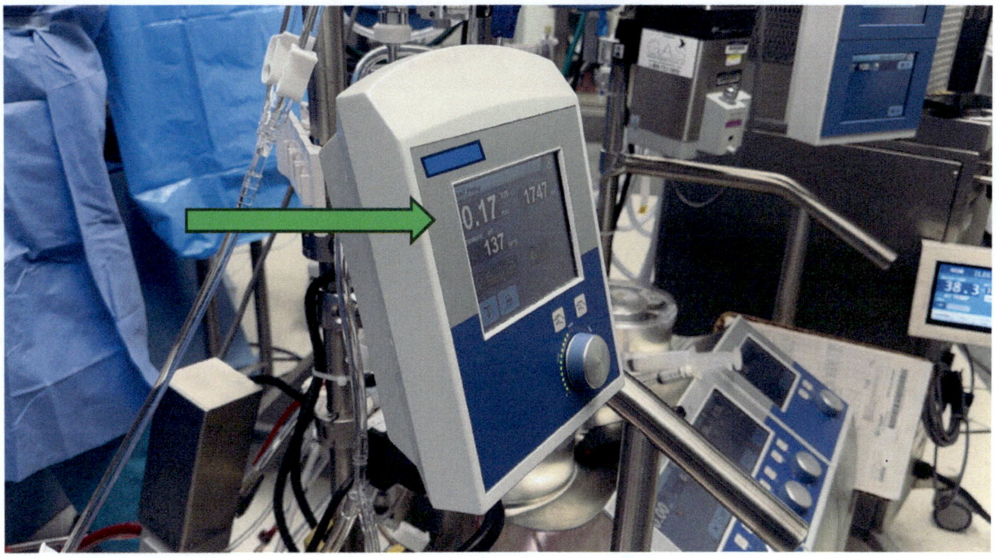

Fig. 11.6 This photo captures the crucial moment when the patient is successfully weaned off CPB. While the patient no longer receives blood flow from the bypass circuit, a minimal flow is maintained through the circuit to ensure stability. In this specific instance, the flow rate is maintained at a minimal rate of 0.17 liters per minute, as displayed in the image

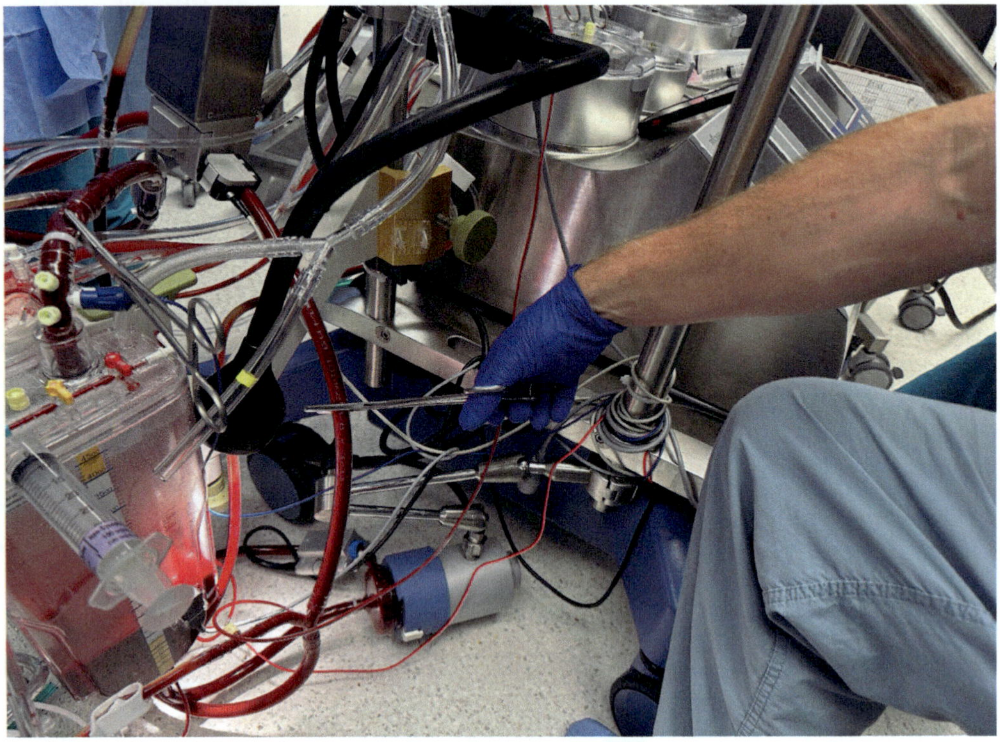

Fig. 11.7 Captured in this image is a critical juncture in cardiac surgery: the moment a patient is fully weaned off CPB and after pumping the blood in the venous reservoir. The skilled perfusionist is seen carefully clamping off the arterial inflow line

Table 11.4 Hemodynamic targets during weaning

Hemodynamic parameter	Target
Heart rate (HR)	80–90 beats/min, pacing of either RA, RV, or both maybe necessary
Mean arterial pressure (MAP)	60–90 mmHg
Cardiac index (CI)	2.0–2.4 L/min/m^2
Mixed venous oxygen saturation (SvO2)	65–75%
Preload	Adequate end-diastolic volume in LV and RV observed on TEE

Left Ventricular Vent and Cardioplegia Cannula Removal

There are several cannulas that are removed as part of the weaning process. Removal of unnecessary cannula prior to actual weaning allows focus to be placed on the critical mechanics of the process. The left ventricular vent is removed after it has served its purpose to facilitate the removal of additional fluid and entrained air in the left heart chambers. The retrograde cannula is removed during the rewarming process after it is determined that no additional cardioplegia is necessary. The antegrade cardioplegia cannula may be removed before, during, or after weaning from cardiopulmonary bypass depending upon the need to evacuate air that has entered the aortic root from the heart.

Venous Decannulation and Administration of Residual Blood from the Reservoir

After the perfusionist communicates to the team that the patient is "off bypass," the surgeon can remove the venous cannula and suture the cannulation site. Blood in the venous tubing is returned to the venous reservoir. Blood remaining within the venous reservoir can then be returned to the patient via by administering small aliquots of 100–200 mL via the aortic cannula as directed by the anesthesiologist and surgeon. The blood pressure is monitored during administration.

Protamine Administration

The reversal of the anticoagulation effect induced by heparin is achieved through the administration of protamine. Protamine is a small protein that neutralizes the anticoagulant effects of heparin by forming a stable protamine–heparin complex.

Protamine administration holds crucial importance during the weaning and decannulation process and should be considered a "point of no return." In practical terms, a "point of no return" signifies that substantial modifications to the procedural plan may be necessary, including the potential need for a repeat administration of heparin prior to the re-

Table 11.5 Protamine adverse reactions

Phenotypes of protamine adverse reactions		
Type of reaction	Mechanism	Clinical manifestation
Type I rapid administration	Histamine release from mast cells	Systemic hypotension
Type IIA anaphylactic reaction.	IgE and IgG4 antibodies on mast cells or basophils recognize an antigen (protamine), and this induces a cascade of reactions with the release of inflammatory mediators	Systemic hypotension, bronchospasm, and skin and mucous membrane reactions
Type IIB immediate anaphylactoid reactions.	IgE- and non-IgE-mediated mechanisms	Hypotension, bronchospasm, and both RA and LA pressures are generally low
Type IIC delayed anaphylactoid reactions noncardiogenic pulmonary edema	Delayed and association with protamine unclear	Massive pulmonary capillary leak, pulmonary edema, and decreased pulmonary compliance
Type III catastrophic pulmonary hypertension	Possible thromboxane A2	Bronchospasm, pulmonary hypertension, RV failure, and systemic hypotension

initiation of CPB. Clear and definitive two-way, closed-loop verbal communication of protamine administration to the entire team is critical. Practicing closed-loop communication as part of a system ensures that all team members are well-informed and prepared for the subsequent steps in the procedure. Two-way communication also allows team members a final opportunity to voice concerns.

Before administering protamine, the surgical team must ensure that the patient's myocardial function is adequate, bleeding is well controlled, and there is no anticipated need to emergently reinitiate CPB. The appropriate dose of protamine may vary among centers, but typically 1.0–1.3 mg of protamine is given for each 100 units of heparin administered or a dose calculated through an automated system. Excessive protamine administration may paradoxically worsen coagulopathy.

Protamine administration is associated with several potential adverse reactions, most of which are mild, but others can be catastrophic (Table 11.5). A common practice is to administer an initial "test dose" of 10–20 mg of protamine and monitor for adverse physiologic effects. Protamine can cause vasodilation and negative inotropic effects, so it is suggested that the remainder of the dose be administered slowly. Catastrophic reactions to protamine include anaphylactic and anaphylactoid reactions as well as catastrophic pulmonary vasoconstriction and non-cardiogenic pulmonary edema. These reactions may require repeat administration of heparin and a return to CPB. Thus, it is crucial for all team members to communicate and act accordingly during this period.

Arterial Decannulation

Removal of the aortic cannula is timed to occur nearly concurrently with protamine administration. A cautious approach is taken to prevent the formation of clot at the tip of the aortic cannula with the potential for systemic embolization.

It is crucial to maintain the systolic blood pressure (SBP) within a range of 90–100 mmHg at the time of aortic decannulation and tying of sutures at the site of cannulation. This is done to minimize the risk of aortic dissection and bleeding. The anesthesiologists may administer small boluses of short-acting medications such as nitroglycerin, change anesthetic concentrations, or adjust temporary pacemaker settings to control blood pressure during aortic cannula removal.

In Fig. 11.8, witness the dynamic collaboration of surgeon, anesthesia provider, and perfusionist as they navigate the weaning of CPB.

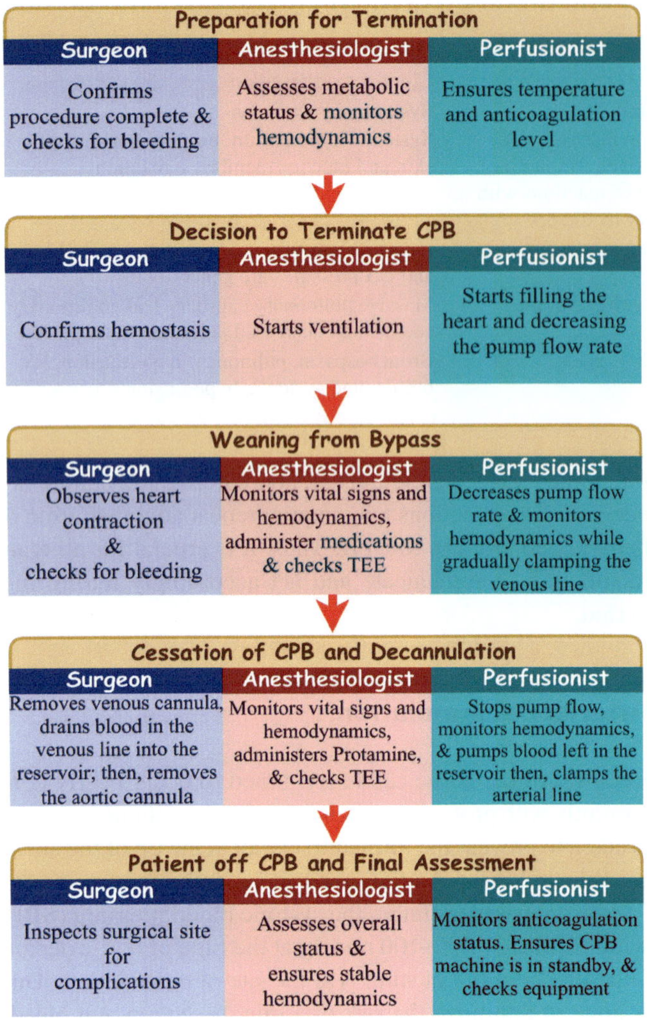

Fig. 11.8 This schematic diagram illustrates the coordinated roles of the surgical team during the weaning process from CPB. It highlights the critical interplay between the surgeon, anesthesia provider, and perfusionist

Failure to Wean and Return to Cardiopulmonary Bypass

Failure to wean from cardiopulmonary bypass may occur for multiple reasons. Prior to protamine administration and aortic decannulation, a return to CPB requires reestablishing venous return to the reservoir and initiation of arterial flow through the aortic cannula. If protamine has been already administered, a significantly higher repeat dose of heparin (about 500 units/kg) may be needed to return to bypass. After heparinization, aortic and venous cannulation must occur. Emergent return to bypass requires that all team members rapidly perform critical tasks. Checklists should not be ignored, and additional help should be summoned.

Table 11.6 Team reassessment after failure to wean from bypass

Team member	Check
Surgeon	Assess coronary grafts for adequate flow by visual inspection or flow probe Assess the integrity of surgical anastomosis Check cannulation and aortotomy sites for bleeding Check pacing wires Additional de-airing maneuvers Place additional monitors if needed (i.e., femoral arterial line or left atrial line)
Anesthesiologist	Address acid-base, electrolyte, and hemoglobin status Adjust vasopressors and inotropic agents or add additional agents Consider initiation of pharmacologic means to reduce pulmonary vascular resistance (if necessary) Zero and level the monitors and address any potential discrepancies from expected pressures Optimize pacing Assure blood products are available Address any airway issues (bronchospasm, blood in airway, pulmonary edema, etc.)
Perfusion team	Confirm adequacy of rewarming Assess the availability of fluid in venous reservoir for next attempt at weaning Review acid-base and hemoglobin status Confirm that shunts and vacuum-assisted venous drainage are off

A return to bypass allows the entire team to reassess the situation and make further interventions to increase the chance of a successful wean (Table 11.6). Indicators that weaning may be unsuccessful may be evident to the entire team or recognized by teams separately.

There are multiple factors that may prevent successful weaning. Surgical factors include bypass graft or valve repair/replacement compromise, excessive bleeding from sites of anastomosis or surgical access, ventricular dysfunction, vasoplegia and inability to maintain an adequate blood pressure, pulmonary hypertension with right ventricular compromise, and pulmonary complications preventing adequate oxygenation and ventilation. Appropriate management may avoid the need for postoperative mechanical support (Table 11.7).

Most situations requiring a return to CPB can be managed successfully and are followed by subsequent successful weaning. Despite appropriate measures, a small percentage of patients cannot be weaned from CPB despite pharmacological support and require temporary mechanical support. Please refer to Chaps. 32, 33, and 34 for comprehensive review of *IABP*, *Extracorporeal membrane oxygenation (ECMO)*, Temporary ventricular assist devices (VADs), and Impella.

Table 11.7 Potential problems identified during or after weaning from bypass

Complications	Potential causes(s) or risk factors	Treatment(s)
Surgical or technical failure with compromise of bypass grafts	Graft kink Graft thrombosis Inadequate revascularization	Inspection/graft revision Add additional graft(s) Increased perfusion pressure
Left ventricular dysfunction	Inadequate protection Graft inadequacy Metabolic disarray Coronary compromise or ligation	Graft inspection/revision/addition Addition of inotropic agents Increase perfusion pressure Biventricular pacing Electrolyte correction Temporary mechanical support (intra-aortic balloon pump (IABP), Impella, ECMO)
Right ventricular dysfunction	Inadequate protection Graft inadequacy Increased pulmonary resistance Metabolic disarray Coronary compromise Air embolization	Graft inspection/revision Addition of inotropic agents Institution or inhaled vasodilators Electrolyte correction Temporary mechanical support (ProtekDuo™, Avalon, Impella® RP or Flex)
Valve problems	Residual/new stenosis Paravalvular leak Excessive valvular regurgitation	Review TEE Direct measurement of pressure gradients Surgical repair or replacement
LV outflow tract obstruction with systolic anterior motion (SAM)	Hypovolemia Tachycardia Hypercontractility Mitral valve repair	Slow heart rate (reduce pacing rate) Maintain filling Administer beta-blockage
Vasoplegia	Pre-op ACE-I Pre-op heparin Emergency surgery Prior MI Sepsis/infection	Addition of vasoconstrictor (vasopressin and phenylephrine) Consider alternative management (methylene blue)
High airway pressures	Anaphylaxis Protamine Latex Hypothermia Inadequate anesthesia ETT malposition, blood in ETT, or kinked ETT	Check ETT for kink Suction Beta-agonists Steroids Deepen anesthesia

Further Reading

Kahan A. Weaning from cardiopulmonary bypass and management of difficulties. In: Awad MD, MBA, A.S., editors. Cardiac anesthesia. Cham: Springer; 2021. https://doi.org/10.1007/978-3-030-51755-7_17.

Cui WW, Ramsay JG. Pharmacologic approaches to weaning from cardiopulmonary bypass and extracorporeal membrane oxygenation. Best Pract Res Clin Anaesthesiol. 2015;29(2):257–70. https://doi.org/10.1016/j.bpa.2015.03.007. Epub 2015 Apr 1. PMID: 26060034

Licker M, Diaper J, Cartier V, et al. Clinical review: management of weaning from cardiopulmonary bypass after cardiac surgery. Ann Card Anaesth. 2012;15(3):206–23. https://doi.org/10.4103/0971-9784.97977. PMID: 22772515

Barry E, Chaney A, London J. Anesthetic management during cardiopulmonary bypass: a systematic review. Anesth Analg. 2015;120(4):749–69. https://doi.org/10.1213/ANE.0000000000000612.

Monaco F, Di Prima AL, Kim JH, et al. Management of challenging cardiopulmonary bypass separation. J Cardiothorac Vasc Anesth. 2020;34(6):1622–35. https://doi.org/10.1053/j.jvca.2020.02.038. Epub 2020 Feb 29. PMID: 32276758

Lombard W, Grichnik P. Update on management strategies for separation from cardiopulmonary bypass. Curr Opin Anaesthesiol. 2011;24(1):49–57. https://doi.org/10.1097/ACO.0b013e328342064a.

Korelidis G, McFadyen R, Fang CC, Qsous G, Zamvar V. Difficulty weaning from cardiopulmonary bypass following an aortic valve replacement. Cureus. 2023;15(7):e42692. https://doi.org/10.7759/cureus.42692. PMID: 37649947; PMCID: PMC10465131

Fitzsimons MG, Mark JB, Nussmeier NA. Weaning from cardiopulmonary bypass, UpToDate.com

Denault AY, Tardif JC, Mazer CD, Lambert J, BART Investigators. Difficult and complex separation from cardiopulmonary bypass in high-risk cardiac surgical patients: a multicenter study. J Cardiothorac Vasc Anesth. 2012;26(4):608–16. https://doi.org/10.1053/j.jvca.2012.03.031. Epub 2012 May 11. PMID: 22578975

Winterhalter M, et al. Cardiopulmonary bypass in cardiac surgery: a prospective randomized trial. J Cardiothorac Vasc Anesth. 2008;22:406–13.

McKinlay KH, Schinderle DB, Swaminathan M, Podgoreanu MV, Milano CA, Meisser RH, El-Moalem H, et al. Predictors of inotrope use during separation from cardiopulmonary bypass. J Cardiothorac Vasc Anesth. 2004;18:404–8.

Mekontso-Dessap A, Houel R, Soustelle C, Kirsk M, Thebert D, Loisance DY. Risk factors for post-cardiopulmonary bypass Vasoplegia in patients with preserved left ventricular function. Ann Thorac Surg. 2001;71:1428–32.

Park KW. Protamine and protamine reactions. Int Anesthesiol Clin. 2004;42(3):135–45.

Baraka A, Kawkabani N, Dabbous A, Nawfal. Lidocaine for prevention of reperfusion ventricular fibrillation after release of aortic cross-clamping. J Cardiothorac Vasc Anesth. 2000;14:531–3.

Doll N, Kiaii B, Borger M, Bucerius J, Kramer K, Schmidt DV, Walther T, Mohr FW. Five-year results of 219 consecutive patients treated with extracorporeal membrane oxygenation for refractory postoperative cardiogenic shock. Ann Thorac Surg. 2004;77:151–7.

Metabolic Derangements During Cardiopulmonary Bypass

12

Vikas Mishra, Tzonghuei H. Chen, and Andrew Maslow

Introduction

Intraoperative metabolic changes in the cardiac surgical patient occur due to the impact of extracorporeal circulation. The cellular and tissue trauma, blood interaction with foreign materials, a non-pulsatile state, hemodilution, with or without systemic hypothermia, activate inflammatory, coagulation, and complement systems, as discussed in detail in Chap. 6 "Physiologic Changes and Inflammatory Response to Cardiopulmonary Bypass." These systemic disturbances result in altered oxygen delivery and consumption, acid–base imbalance, impaired glucose metabolism, electrolyte disturbances, and alterations in drug pharmacokinetics.

Delivery of oxygen is related to hemoglobin concentration, oxygen saturation (SaO_2) and arterial oxygen levels (PaO_2), perfusion pressure, and cardiac output. During cardiopulmonary bypass (CPB), the latter is equivalent to "pump" flow. Upon initiation of CPB, the patient's blood is mixed with the CPB prime solution, resulting in a reduced hemoglobin concentration. Although oxygen content may decline, viscosity also declines, leading to improved tissue perfusion. Balance between oxygen delivery and demand is reflected by mixed venous oximetry, acid–base balance, and serum lactate levels.

To match reductions in oxygen content and delivery, metabolic demand is reduced by administering general anesthesia and muscle relaxation and, when applicable, systemic hypothermia. For detailed information about hypothermia during CPB, please see Chap. 6.

Temperature Management

Application of therapeutic hypothermia is guided by institutional protocols and preferences and can be altered based on individual patient or case needs. Estimated reductions in oxygen consumption (VO_2) are 7% per decrease in every 1 °C body temperature. Hypothermia increases electrolyte loss by inducing diuresis, which results from volume shifts from the peripheral to central circulation. This leads to increased central blood volume and pressure through hormonal and hemodynamic pathways and is further compounded by impaired renal tubular function. Hypokalemia, hypocalcemia, hypomagnesemia, and hypophosphatemia are discussed later in this chapter. During rewarming, caution is necessary to monitor, prevent, and/or manage potential rebound increases in these electrolytes.

While hypothermia plays an important role in maintaining oxygen balance, the process of rewarming has significant consequences and should be accomplished slowly (0.2–0.5 °C/min) to minimize neurologic risks associated with rapid rewarming. Otherwise, patients may suffer from stroke, neuronal apoptosis, and neuronal cell death.

End-organ oxygen and nutrient delivery are dependent on CPB flow and perfusion pressure. Under normothermic conditions, CPB flow typically equals a cardiac index greater than 2.4 L/min/m^2 or a flow rate of 50–70 ml/kg/min. Flows can be reduced if VO_2 is reduced, as in the case of hypothermia. The impact of hypothermia extends beyond oxygen demands to include end-organ function and drug metabolism.

$$DO_2 = CI \times CaO_2 \times 10$$

where DO2 is the oxygen delivery (in mL O_2/min), CI is the cardiac index (in L/min/m^2), CaO_2 is the arterial oxygen content (in mL O_2/dL), and the factor 10 is used to convert dL to L for consistency in units.

DO_2 is approximately determined by pump flow CI, CaO_2, and perfusion pressure.

V. Mishra
Department of Anesthesiology & Perioperative Medicine, Inova Fairfax Medical Center, Falls Church, VA, USA

T. H. Chen · A. Maslow (✉)
Department of Anesthesiology & Perioperative Medicine, Brown University, Providence, RI, USA

A. S. Awad, J. DiNardo (eds.), *Clinical Perfusion for Cardiac Surgery*, https://doi.org/10.1007/978-3-031-91163-7_12

Perfusion pressure, the difference between arterial and venous pressure, is essential for effective DO_2. It drives blood flow, ensuring oxygen and nutrients reach tissues. Even with adequate cardiac output and oxygen content, low perfusion pressure can hinder oxygen delivery due to insufficient blood flow. Thus, while perfusion pressure isn't explicitly mentioned in the DO_2 calculation, it plays a vital role in the overall process of DO_2.

$$CaO_2 = \left(Hgb \times 1.34 \times SaO_2 / 100\right) + \left(0.0031 \times PaO_2\right)$$

$$\begin{aligned} CaO_2 &= Hgb\left(gm/dl\right) \times 1.34\, O_2 / gm/dl \times SaO_2 \times 1/100 \\ &+ PaO_2 \times 0.003 \text{ at normothermia} \end{aligned}$$

$$\begin{aligned} CaO_2 &= Hgb\left(gm/dl\right) \times 1.34\, O_2 / gm/dl \times SaO_2 \times 1/100 \\ &+ PaO_2 \times 0.003 \text{ at hypothermia} \end{aligned}$$

where:

CaO_2 is the arterial oxygen content (mL O_2/dL), Hgb is the hemoglobin concentration (g/dL), 1.34 is the amount of oxygen (in mL) carried by one gram of hemoglobin, SaO_2 is the arterial oxygen saturation (%), PaO_2 is the partial pressure of oxygen in arterial blood (mmHg), 0.003 is the solubility coefficient of oxygen in blood (mL O_2/dL blood/mmHg), accounting for the oxygen dissolved in plasma.

Hemodilution

Hemodilution leads to reduced hemoglobin levels and, as a result, decreased oxygen content. These changes are compensated by either sustained or increased blood flow, a reduction in VO_2, and improvements in end-organ microcirculation due to reduced viscosity. Although blood transfusion can increase oxygen content, the optimal hemoglobin, or even the "nadir hematocrit" at which adverse outcomes increase, is a subject of ongoing discussion and debate. Maintaining a hemoglobin ≥ 6 gm/dl is reasonable even while considering the potential adverse effects of blood transfusion. Depending on the patient and procedure, the "minimum hemoglobin" level may be different. For in-depth details on hemodilution, see Chap. 9, "Prime Solutions for the Circuit and Hemodilution Reduction Strategies." While these changes are expected to occur, the best management approach is guided by tissue reaction, metabolic performance, or acid–base balance. When tissue oxygen demands are not met, glucose is broken down into pyruvate, which, via the anaerobic pathway, yields fewer high-energy phosphates and produces lactic acid. In the absence of oxygen, metabolic acidosis develops, affecting all other metabolic systems.

Acid–Base Management During CPB

Acid–base management during CPB can be employed purposefully and reactionary. The former refers to the manipulation of arterial carbon dioxide (CO_2) to alter cerebral vascular tone and flow especially during deep hypothermia. Oxygen and carbon dioxide become more soluble in blood with reduced temperature:

$$PaO_2 \text{ decreases by } 7.2\% \text{ for each } 1\,°C.$$
$$PaCO_2 \text{ decreases by } 4.5\% \text{ for each } 1\,°C.$$
$$pH \text{ increases by } 0.015 \text{ for each } 1\,°C.$$

Blood gas analysis is typically performed at 37 °C. For hypothermic patients, results are adjusted to account for changes in oxygen and CO_2 solubility at lower temperatures. This "corrected" analysis, known as pH-stat management, alters $PaCO_2$ and pH levels to reflect respiratory alkalosis and guides CO_2 administration to normalize these values. In contrast, α-stat management does not adjust for hypothermia, maintaining a balance in hemoglobin functionality across temperatures. While pH-stat management enhances cerebral oxygen delivery during hypothermia, its routine use is limited due to potential neurocognitive risks, particularly during high-risk procedures like aortic manipulations. It's generally employed in specific clinical scenarios. For in-depth details on arterial blood gas analysis and management during hypothermia, including pH-stat and α-stat strategies, refer to Chaps. 6 and 31.

Aside from pH-stat management, respiratory acidosis or alkalosis is common, typically mild, and treated by adjusting the sweep speed of the oxygenator gas flow. Exceptions are CO_2-producing or CO_2-introducing conditions. Examples of the former are conditions that increase metabolic rate, such as light anesthesia, seizures, and malignant hyperthermia. CO_2 introduction occurs during endovascular vein harvest, where CO_2 is entrained to improve visualization during dissection and may persist into the CPB period.

Metabolic alkalosis is uncommon. In contrast, mild metabolic acidosis often occurs at the onset of CPB due to hemodilution. Thereafter, with increasing CPB duration, serum lactate levels typically rise but uncommonly higher than 2–3 mmol/L. A dilutional acidosis occurs because of the crystalloid used in the CPB prime solution. Normal saline, lactated ringers, and plasmalyte have pH values of 5.7, 6.2, and 7.4, respectively (Fig. 9.4). This type of acidosis is readily corrected by adding sodium bicarbonate or another buffer solution.

Lactic acidosis can be described as Type A (anaerobic) or Type B (aerobic). Both are due to reduced oxygen delivery. The latter may be associated with glucose metabolism and catecholamines. Hypothermia, which increases Oxy-Hgb affinity, increases lactate levels. When coupled with a reduced clearance by the liver and kidneys, lactate levels rise. It is uncommon for lactate levels to rise higher than 3 mM or for the pH < 7.3. Lactate levels >5 mM are reflective of end-organ ischemia and are associated with increased adverse outcomes. Management includes increasing CPB flows to improve end-organ perfusion, administering bicarbonate to bind H^+, and increasing gas flows or sweep speeds to create a respiratory alkalosis to balance the pH. Whether vasopressors are a cause of lactic acidosis or should be administered to improve end-organ perfusion pressures is decided per individual case.

Endocrine Abnormalities

Thyroid Hormones

CPB triggers a significant drop in triiodothyronine (T3) levels (40–50%), returning to normal within 24 hours post-surgery, which has notable implications for cardiac function and metabolism. The temporary "euthyroid sick syndrome" induced by CPB, as described by Holland et al. (1991), is characterized by depressed levels of T3 and free T3 and increased reverse T3 but normal thyroid-stimulating hormone, thyroxine, and free thyroxine levels. This syndrome impacts cardiac function and metabolism.

Multiple studies have provided valuable insights into the effects of T3 on cardiac performance and its impact on vulnerable populations. Klemperer et al. (1995) discovered that perioperative T3 administration in coronary artery bypass surgery patients improved cardiac output and reduced systemic vascular resistance, although it did not affect the overall outcome of the surgery. Expanding on this, Reichert and Verzino (2001) emphasized the alterations in thyroid hormone levels induced by CPB and suggested potential benefits of T3 supplementation for improved cardiac outcomes. In a similar vein, Sinci et al. (1994) experimentally demonstrated the ability of T3 to enhance the recovery of ventricular contractile force, heart work, and heart rate following global ischemia, indicating its potential benefits for postoperative myocardial function. Additionally, focusing on vulnerable groups, Mitchell et al. (1992) observed a more significant decrease in both T3 and thyroxine (T4) levels in infants weighing less than 5 kg undergoing CPB. This finding underscores the heightened susceptibility of this demographic to thyroid hormone fluctuations during such procedures. While these studies suggest potential benefits of T3 supplementation for cardiac performance, its overall impact on surgical outcomes and the need for standard postoperative therapy remain unclear. Further research is needed to determine the optimal approach for managing T3 during and after CPB.

Hyperglycemia

Hyperglycemia (≥180 mg/dl or ≥10 mM) is not uncommon during CPB due to increased catecholamines, glucagon levels, stress hormones (e.g., cortisol), and the inclusion of glucose (e.g., dextrose) in the cardioplegia. Catecholamine levels are elevated by hypothermia and non-pulsatile flow. The use of heparin throughout CPB leads to an increase in free fatty acid buildup, which in turn increases insulin resistance and reduces glucose uptake. The occurrence of hyperglycemia is anticipated, especially for those with a known history of diabetes and/or those with insulin resistance.

Hyperglycemia is associated with adverse outcomes for cardiac surgical patients. A glucose ≥15 mM or 270 mg/dl in healthy subjects was found to increase blood pressure, heart rate, catecholamine levels, platelet aggregation, and blood viscosity. These are thought to be related to reduced nitric oxide levels and affect end-organ flow, perhaps most significantly to the myocardium. Hyperglycemia and/or insulin resistance are associated with increased free fatty acids, oxygen free radicals, and impaired myocardial utilization of glucose. In diabetic patients, glucose levels greater than 180 mg/dl have been associated with adverse outcomes, while in non-diabetics, adverse outcomes are linked to even higher glucose levels, exceeding 250 mg/dl. Whether the complication is related to any specific glucose level, impaired glucose utilization, or both isn't clear. Older data described the benefits of glucose-insulin-potassium (GIK) solutions on cardiac function. The co-administration of GIK cocktail (200 g/L glucose, 66.7 U/L insulin, and 80 mM KCl) has been associated with improved outcome. This benefit occurs even with higher recorded glucose levels, underscoring the value of directly delivering glucose substrate to the heart tissue alongside insulin.

Although recommendations suggest a glucose less than 180 mg/dl on postoperative day one, the optimal level of glucose during CPB to reduce adverse outcomes remains unclear. Data reports that microvascular harm and vascular constriction occur with significantly elevated glucose levels (≥270 mg/dl). Most would agree on maintaining glucose levels below 220 mg/dl during the intraoperative period, but there is uncertainty about whether to initiate insulin prophylactically or in response to elevated glucose levels. However, Chaney et al. demonstrated that insulin resistance occurs at the onset of CPB. Despite high doses of insulin, high glucose levels persisted, which was then followed by hypoglycemia after separation from CPB. Hypokalemia (<3.5 mM or meq/L) can result from insulin therapy and is associated with arrhythmias. For patients in whom hyperglycemia is anticipated, successful, and safe management of perioperative glucose levels is facilitated by starting insulin prior to CPB while closely monitoring glucose and potassium levels.

Electrolyte Abnormalities

Electrolyte abnormalities are common during and immediately after CPB and are assessed every 15 minutes during CPB using intraoperative point-of-care tests. Magnesium (Mg^{2+}), calcium (Ca^{2+}), potassium (K^+), and sodium (Na^+) are critical to generate neuromuscular activity. Transmembrane electrical potentials play a crucial role in determining and maintaining internal/external ion concentrations and regulating ion movement in and out of cells. At rest, a negative membrane potential is necessary to maintain a high ratio of intracellular to extracellular potassium levels across open K-channels. A higher K_{in}/K_{out} ratio renders the resting membrane potential more negative, ranging between −40 and − 80 mV. Either spontaneously (in pacemaker cells, such as SA and AV nodes) or in response to a stimulus (in myocardial cells), the transmembrane potential becomes less negative and reaches the threshold potential, and an action potential is generated, causing muscle contraction or the propagation of the electrical pulse. For myocardial cells, in response to a stimulus, a threshold (approximately −40 mV) is reached and sodium channels open, generating an action potential that reaches the sarcoplasmic reticulum, stimulating T-tubules to open Ca^{2+}channels, thereby making calcium available to the myocardial contractile elements. Calcium binds with troponin, enabling actin and myosin to bind together, resulting in shortening, or contraction, of the muscle fiber.

The resting membrane potential for the pacemaker cells can be described as "unstable" because it spontaneously depolarizes at a "pre-specified" pacemaker rate, primarily due to a slow influx of sodium. When the threshold is reached, calcium channels open, initiating an action potential.

Subsequently, in both myocardial and pacemaker cells, repolarization occurs through the involvement of sodium, potassium, and calcium channels. This process returns the transmembrane potential back to the resting potential and restores the transmembrane potential along with electrolyte/ion concentrations. Any alterations in ion concentrations can have an impact on action potential generation and muscle contractility.

Potassium (Table 12.1)

Regulation of normal serum K^+ levels (3.5–5.0 mM or mEq/L) is critical for a host of vital functions, including maintaining cellular-membrane potential, propagating action potentials, regulating vascular tone and blood pressure, maintaining acid–base homeostasis, and supporting insulin metabolism. Potassium is almost entirely intracellular (98%), with the serum levels maintained within a narrow range of 3.5–5.0 mM through transmembrane movement coupled with renal and gastrointestinal handling. Potassium homeostasis involves a complex array of processes that balance membrane potential, ionic gradients, osmolality, and acid–base balance. This includes sodium/potassium (Na/K) ATPase pumps as well as several proteins and hormones. While insulin, epinephrine, aldosterone, and glucocorticoids promote potassium uptake into cells, renal tubules are responsible for roughly 90% of its excretion. Aside from Na/K exchange, potassium is also important in the body's management of acid–base balance. Under acidic conditions,

Table 12.1 Causes and management of hypo- and hyperkalemia

	Hypokalemia (<3.5 mEq/L)		Hyperkalemia > 5.0 mEq/L	
Causes	Losses/excretion	Diuretics or diuresis Hypothermia (cold) Hyperaldosteronism Low Mg2+	Decreased excretion	Renal failure Aldosterone ACE inhibitors
	No change in absolute mEq	Hemodilution	Increased intake	Oral/intravenous Cardioplegia
	Cellular shift	Insulin $Beta_2$ agonists Alkalosis	Cellular shift	Low insulin Trauma Beta blockers Acidosis
Management	Mg2+ Hold diuretics Administer potassium		Sodium bicarbonate Lasix Hypertonic solution Glucose Insulin Calcium chloride	

H+ can move intracellularly for exchange with K+. During CPB, all these functions are either utilized or affected.

During CPB, multiple variables contribute to changes in serum potassium levels, which have a significant impact on transmembrane electrical potential and ion currents in both cardiac and non-cardiac functions. Hypokalemia less than 3.5 mM lowers the transmembrane electrical potential, resulting in a larger action potential, increased myocardial irritability, hyperexcitability, and ectopy. Hypokalemia is often accompanied by hypomagnesemia, making myocardial arrhythmias more likely. By contrast, hyperkalemia, which raises the resting membrane potential, reduces activation and causes cardiac and non-cardiac muscle weakness. A less negative transmembrane potential results in a smaller action potential. When the serum (extracellular) potassium concentration is even higher, there is no action potential, and the muscle does not contract. This forms the basis for hyperkalemic cardioplegic arrest. Cardioplegia solutions vary and range from 9 to 36 mM. Solutions may be warm or varying degrees of cold. Hypothetically, this reduces myocardial injury during CPB by maintaining a relaxed state with lower metabolic demands. Changes in serum K^+ are frequent during cardiac surgery with CPB. While hyperkalemic cardioplegia solutions are administered to induce cardiac arrest and may result in elevated levels of potassium during CPB, hypokalemia often occurs soon after separation.

CPB related temperature changes alter serum K^+. Hypothermia lowers potassium by shifting K^+ intracellular and by inducing a diuresis. Care must be taken to avoid overcorrecting hypokalemia. Upon rewarming, serum K^+ may increase from intracellular stores.

Although hyperkalemic cardioplegia helps protect the myocardium, it's worth noting that hyperkalemia can also cause microvascular dysfunction and is associated with postoperative myocardial dysfunction. Hyperkalemia can cause heart block, increased QRS duration, causes dysrhythmias, and poses a risk of malignant ventricular arrhythmias.

Hyperkalemia/Electrocardiogram

Peaked T waves (5.5–6.5 mM)
P wave widening/flattening (6.5–7.0 mM)
PR prolongation
Bradyarrhythmias; Sinus, AV Block, Junctional/Ventricular escape rhythms (7.0–9.0 mM)
Conduction delays
QRS widening

Severe Hyperkalemia (>9.0 mM)

Ventricular fibrillation
Pulseless electrical activity
Wide complex
Asystole (Fig. 12.1).

Corrections of hyperkalemia are urgent if not emergent given the risk of cardiac arrest. Corrections can be categorized as follows:

1. *Moving Potassium into Cells*: Those that move potassium into the cells such as insulin and glucose. B2-adrenergic agonists like albuterol can also be used for this purpose.
2. *Counter Immediate Effects*: Those that counter the immediate effects such as sodium bicarbonate, calcium chloride, and hemodilution.
3. *Removing Potassium from the Body*: Those that help to remove potassium from the body such as loop diuretics such as furosemide. The first two groups can be accomplished quickly, while the Lasix induced diuresis requires 30–60 minutes.
4. *Emergent Dialysis*: Emergent dialysis is a definitive option but requires preparation and time.

Disturbances in potassium homeostasis can increase the occurrence of arrhythmias, especially atrial tachyarrhythmias and, less frequently, ventricular arrhythmias. These are a major source of morbidity and mortality following cardiac surgery. Hypokalemia often results from diuresis, insulin administration, and increased aldosteronism. Because a serum potassium less than 3.5 mM (mEq/L) increases the risk of atrial and ventricular arrhythmias, supplementation to maintain levels above 4.0 or even 4.5 mM is part of routine care. In contrast to managing hyperkalemia, hypokalemia cannot be corrected quickly for the risk of developing acute hyperkalemia. Potassium administration is typically limited to no more than 60 mEq/hour.

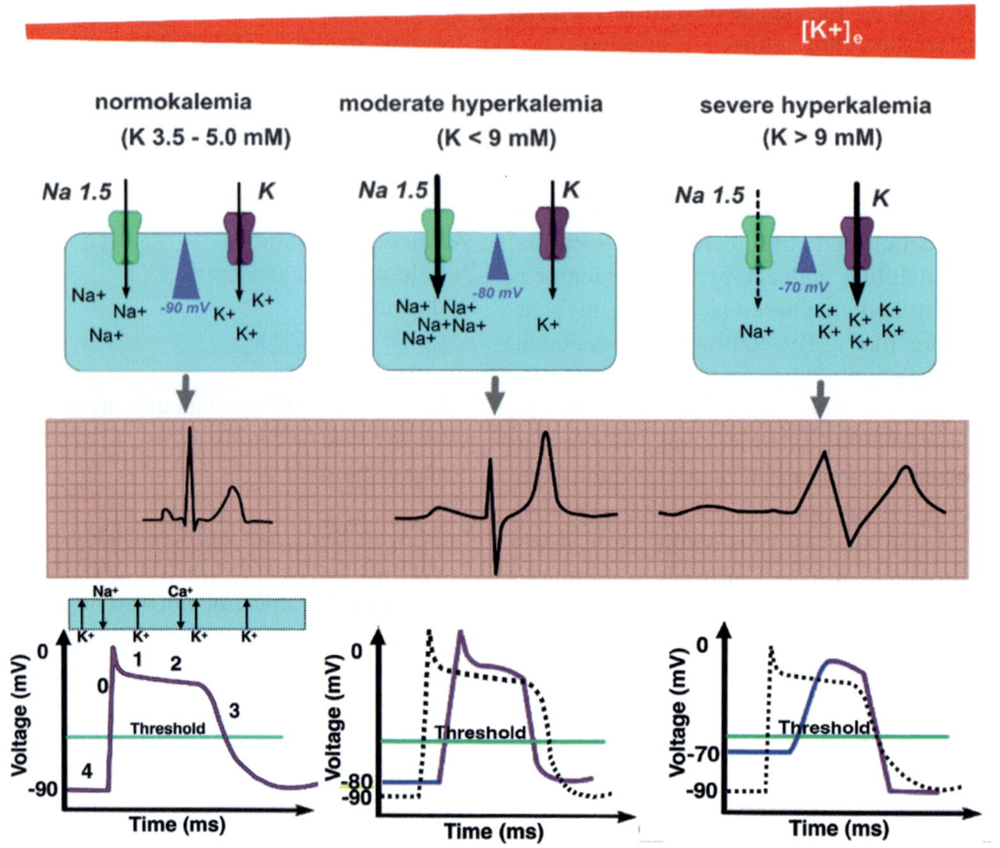

Fig. 12.1 This illustration demonstrates the impact of hyperkalemia on cardiac electrical activity and its potential to induce arrhythmias, structured in three sections: The top section displays the Na and K channels. The middle section depicts changes in the ECC, illustrating the electrical activity alterations due to hyperkalemia. The bottom details changes in the action potential, highlighting the impact on cardiac electrical activity. As extracellular potassium increases, it diminishes the potassium gradient across the cell membrane and lowers the resting membrane potential, represented by the green line. This causes the membrane voltage to become less negative, approaching −80 mV and nearing the threshold potential. Consequently, this facilitates the initiation of an action potential and heightening myocyte excitability, as evidenced by T wave peaking on the ECG. A further rise of potassium impairs sodium voltage-gated channels (Nav1.5) (closed green gate), crucial for the rapid influx of sodium ions during the action potential's depolarization phase. This surge in potassium also activates inwardly rectifying potassium channels (wider purple gate), thus slowing down impulse conduction, diminishing the electrical signal, and potentially rendering cells unresponsive to electrical triggers (refractory). ECG changes in hyperkalemia begin with peaked T waves due to synchronized repolarization across the ventricular wall, followed by broadening and flattening of the P wave and eventual disappearance as the QRS complex widens from slowed conduction. Severe hyperkalemia (>9.0 mmol/L) risks heart block, asystole, and ventricular arrhythmias

Sodium

Normal serum sodium (Na+, 135 to 145 mM or mEq/L) is important for fluid balance, osmolality, blood pressure control, and neuromuscular function. Serum sodium levels are the main contributor to serum osmolality (normal range: 275 to 295 mOsm/kg), which directs water across cell membranes that are not permeable to sodium. A low serum osmolality will direct water into the cell causing cell swelling and edema, while a high serum osmolality will draw water out of the cell causing cellular dehydration (Fig. 9.3).

Sodium excretion is controlled by the renin-angiotensin-aldosterone system (RAAS) and atrial natriuretic peptide (ANP). The RAAS, which is activated by factors like low blood volume, low blood pressure, and indirectly by low sodium in the distal tubules of the kidney, ultimately stimulates sodium reabsorption in the distal tubules and collecting ducts through a cascade of renin, angiotensin II, and aldosterone release. ANP peptide is secreted in response to increased atrial blood volume and atrial stretch. It inhibits RAAS and directly reduces sodium reabsorption in the collecting ducts. An imbalance in Na + excretion and reabsorption can lead to dysnatremia, which occurs in up to 24% of cardiac surgical patients. While chronic (lasting more than 48 hours) sodium abnormalities may be well tolerated, acute changes (occurring in less than 48 hours) can have devastating consequences, including but not limited to neurologic dysfunction.

Perioperative hyponatremia (Na + <135 mM), affecting 1 in 7 heart surgery patients, can trigger complications such as confusion, seizures, and even death. It often stems from fluid overload or diuretic use, raising risks of stroke, kidney failure, and atrial fibrillation.

Hyponatremia during CPB arises from impaired sodium reabsorption in the renal tubules as a consequence of hypothermia and cold diuresis. Other contributing factors include administration of hyponatremic dextrose-based priming solutions and cardioplegia, blood transfusions, and activation of the RAAS and release of ADH during non-pulsatile blood flow. The occurrence of hyperglycemia further worsens hyponatremia by drawing water out of cells into the bloodstream.

Management depends on the severity and acuity of hyponatremia. Rapid changes in sodium levels within 48 hours are associated with greater risks of complications and adverse outcomes such as neurocognitive and motor dysfunction. The shift of free water into the cells causing swelling and dysfunction of astrocytes leads to dysfunction. Rapid correction can cause devastating neurologic consequences, including osmotic demyelination syndrome. Upon initiation of CPB, the patient's blood mixes with the CPB priming solution. Careful selection of CPB prime and cardioplegia solutions can help avoid worsening or rapid correction of hyponatremia. Correction of severe hyponatremia (< 120 meq/L) starts with correction of half the deficit followed by a slower correction of Na + toward normal. If possible, hyponatremia should be corrected prior to surgery with free water restriction and administration of normal (0.9%) or hypertonic (3%) saline or administration of loop diuretics that result in urine excretion with sodium concentrations of approximately 65–75 mM or 0.45% saline fluid.

Hypernatremia (Na more than 145 mM) leads to a hyperosmolar state and cellular dehydration. Depending on acuity and severity, patients may present with neurologic dysfunction such as irritability, confusion, muscle weakness, seizures, and coma. Severe cases (Na^+ > 160 mM) may be associated with cerebral vascular rupture and intracranial or subarachnoid hemorrhage, all due to acute brain volume contraction. In cardiac surgical patients, hypernatremia occurs due to hypotonic fluid loss, which may be due to loop diuretics, especially in combination with water restriction, or from the administration of solutions high in sodium, such as sodium bicarbonate ($NaHCO_3^-$), 0.9%, or 3% saline. A hypernatremic CPB prime with added hypertonic (3%) saline, $NaHCO_3^-$, and mannitol initially increases serum osmolality and worsens cellular dehydration. Subsequently, an osmotic diuresis can lead to natriuresis and significantly decrease Na^+ concentration. Careful selection and preparation of the CPB prime can prevent exacerbations and/or rapid changes in sodium concentrations.

Hypernatremia is managed with free water or hypotonic fluid administration. These can be coupled with the use of loop diuretics, which typically stimulate excretion of urine with a sodium concentration equivalent to 0.45% saline. Correction should be limited to a maximum of 10 mM over the first 24 hours.

Calcium

Calcium ($Ca^{2+)}$, an essential divalent cation, acts as both a primary activator and a cofactor in various bodily functions, including muscle contraction, nerve impulse conduction, regulation of cardiac electrophysiology, blood clotting, and fluid balance. Ninety-nine percent of the body's calcium is stored in bone and teeth, providing structure and contributing to mineralization. Serum calcium levels are primarily regulated by dietary intake, and parathyroid hormone (PTH), which increases levels. Thyroid hormones, specifically calcitonin, play a smaller role in decreasing levels. Calcium is dynamically exchanged with bone stores. In the serum, calcium exists in three forms: protein-bound (mainly to albumin and globulin, accounting for 45%), chelated (bound to substances like phosphate and citrate, making up 15%), and ionized (the biologically active form, constituting about 51%). When assessing Ca^{2+}levels, ionized Ca^{2+} (iCa^{2+}) is a more indicative measure than total $Ca2^+$ levels. If, however, total Ca^{2+}levels are measured, then they should be accompanied by albumin levels to help determine the amount of free Ca^{2+}. For each decrease in albumin of 1 gm/dl, the serum total Ca2+ decreases by approximately 0.8 mg/dL (or about 0.2 mM).

Total serum calcium levels decrease during CPB due to factors such as hemodilution from crystalloid prime, calcium binding with citrate, hypothermia, and surgical trauma to cells. Heparin is associated with reduced iCa^{2+} helping to explain the reduction in blood pressure with its administration. While it is known that serum and ionized calcium levels decline with CPB, it is not evident what is the optimal timing when to administer (i.e., during or after CPB) Ca^{2+} and at what dose. During CPB, prolonged ischemia leads to elevated intracellular Ca^{2+} levels triggering the activation of phospholipases, nucleases, and proteases that begin degrading organelles, cytoskeletal protein, and cellular DNA. Mitochondria may be particularly sensitive to higher intracellular Ca^{2+} resulting in significant dysfunction. However, adequate $Ca^{2+}$is necessary for pacemaker properties, generation of action potentials, and binding of Troponin-C to permit Actin and Myosin cross-bridges to form and the muscle to contract. Muscle relaxation is an active process that requires the removal of calcium from the myofilaments in the presence of oxygen and ATP. A normally functioning sarcoplasmic reticulum is essential for the regulation of Ca^{2+} movement to and from the myofilaments (Table 12.2).

Hypocalcemia, defined as a total calcium level less than 8.5 mg/dL (see Table 12.3), shortens the QT interval and may predispose the patient to bronchospasm and arrhythmias. It can also lead to severe cardiovascular depression that is refractory to inotropes. Ca^{2+}administration, such as with calcium chloride (CaCl), can reduce the need for inotropic medications immediately after CPB. While Ca^{2+} itself is not an inotrope, it is the final common pathway in the mechanism of action for all inotropes. However, Ca^{2+} may also induce vasoconstriction of the coronary and internal mammary arteries. Despite the fact that calcium overload is harmful to myocardial cells, administration of Ca^{2+} at a dose of 5–15 mg/kg (CaCl) appears safe and is associated with transient improvement in hemodynamic parameters.

While Ca^{2+} administration is beneficial for the treatment of moderate reductions in contractility or for vasoplegia, other vasoactive medications can be equally effective in achieving the same goals by utilizing or increasing the sensitivity to the already present Ca^{2+}. Avoiding high iCa^{2+} levels minimizes or prevents dysfunction associated with Ca^{2+}. High intracellular Ca^{2+} impairs myocardial repolarization–relaxation coupling (i.e., diastolic dysfunction) and can cause myocardial contraction band necrosis/injury. While "stone heart" syndrome is described, evidence supporting its association with calcium administration is limited, and its occurrence is uncommon if not rare. However, there is no benefit in administering excess calcium. Furthermore, upon coronary reperfusion, there is an increase in oxygen free radicals, which increases intracellular Ca^{2+}. This combination of oxygen free radicals and excess Ca^{2+} impairs sarcolemmal Ca^{2+}-ATPase pump, resulting in the release of Ca^{2+}. However, reduced sequestration causes Ca^{2+} overload and impaired excitation-contraction–relaxation coupling.

Perhaps less appreciated are the effects on primary and secondary coagulation. After release from delta granules, Ca^{2+} (coagulation factor IV) acts to activate platelet functions. Calcium acts as a cofactor for multiple coagulation proteins, being a necessary component for normal coagulation including but not limited to the prothrombinase complex conversion of prothrombin to thrombin which subsequently cleaves fibrinogen to form fibrin, the necessary coagulation factor for clot stabilization and strengthening. Patients with hypocalcemia tend to experience greater blood loss and a

Table 12.2 Serum calcium levels: a comparison

Feature	Ionized calcium ($iCa2^+$)	Total calcium (total $Ca2^+$)
Normal range (mM)	1.1–1.4	2.2–2.6
Normal range (mg/dL)	4.4–5.6	8.8–10.4
Hypocalcemia	<8.5 mg/dL (<2 mM)	–
Severe hypocalcemia (potentially fatal)	<6.0 mg/dL (<1.6 mM)	–
Hypercalcemia	>10.5 mg/dL (>2.6 mM)	–
Severe hypercalcemia (critically high and potentially fatal)	>15.1 mg/dL (>3.7 mM)	–

Table 12.3 Causes and management of hypo- and hypercalcemia

Serum $Ca2^+$ level (see Table 12.2) (Mg/dL)	Causes	Clinical features	Treatment
Hyper-$iCa2^+$ (>10.5)	Hypoparathyroidism. Vitamin D Acidosis (iCa^{2+}) Cancer.	Polyuria. Anxiety/depression. Bone pain/weakness. Nausea/vomiting. Muscle weakness. Arrhythmia/↓QT, stone heart. Renal failure. Lethargy/confusion, coma.	Hydration. Calcitonin. Biphosphonate. Diuretics. Steroid.
Normal $iCa2^+$ (>4.4–5.6)	Regulated by Parathyroid hormone. Vitamin D. Calcitonin.	Asymptomatic.	N/A (maintain balance).
Hypo-iCa2+ (<8.5)	Vitamin D deficiency. Mg^{2+} deficiency. Acute pancreatitis. Kidney failure. Alcoholism. Intestinal malabsorption	Muscle spasm/cramps. Neuromuscular irritability, tetany. Paresthesia, numbness, seizures, laryngospasm. Cognitive impairment. ↑QT, syndrome MI/HF.	CaCl2, ca gluconate. PTH (if appropriate).

higher incidence of severe bleeding after cardiac surgery than normocalcemic patients.

Acute clinical changes in Ca^{2+} are best reflected by iCa^{2+} levels. Data support cautiously maintaining iCa^{2+} while highlighting its beneficial effects on coagulation and acknowledging the transient hemodynamic effects. High levels of iCa^{2+} adversely affect heart function and the response to other inotropes. In a survey of 100 medical centers from 32 countries, 88% reported administering calcium salts intraoperatively, with 71% citing hemodynamic support as the reason. Ca2+ was the first-line medication for hemodynamic support in 23% of respondents. Moreover, 78% indicated that the amount of Ca^{2+} administered is guided by iCa^{2+} levels, with dosing ranging from less than 5 mg/kg to more than 15 mg/kg, with the majority between 5 and 15 mg/kg.

Magnesium

$Mg2^{+}$, a ubiquitous divalent cation, plays vital roles throughout the body, including in the central and peripheral nervous systems, heart, and skeletal muscles. $Mg2^{+}$ acts as an antagonist to Ca^{2+} and possesses anti-inflammatory properties. It is estimated to be a cofactor for more than 600 enzyme reactions, an activator in another 200, and is necessary for DNA/RNA structure, stability, function, and activity.

Serum Mg^{2+} represents only about 1% of the total body Mg^{2+}; therefore, blood levels of Mg2+ may not reflect a depleted state. Although filtered by the kidneys, over 95% is reabsorbed, typically in the thick ascending limb of Henle, with reabsorption potentially hindered by diuretic-induced diuresis.

Given $Mg2^{+}$'s widespread physiological functions, organ dysfunction is commonly associated with $Mg2^{+}$ deficiency, or hypomagnesemia, which is found in a large range of acute and chronic end-organ dysfunction. While hypomagnesemia is noted in chronic ailments, it is unclear if $Mg2^{+}$ administration alters outcomes. In the perioperative period, hypomagnesemia occurs commonly because of fluid losses replaced with non-Mg^{2+} containing fluids. It is particularly common during cardiac surgery and CPB, such that routine supplementation is commonplace before and after CPB, and as a part of cardioplegia (Table 12.4).

Proposed benefits of Mg^{2+} administration include improved neurocognitive, cardiovascular, and pulmonary function. By blocking other cations, notably Ca^{2+}, $Mg2^{+}$ acts as an N-methyl-D-Aspartate (NMDA) antagonist. A Mg^{2+} deficiency is associated with neuronal excitability and irritability, cognitive dysfunction, and seizures. $Mg2^{+}$administration is effective in reducing neuronal excitation and seizures in patients with a history of epilepsy, patients with pre-eclampsia, and patients without a preexisting risk. $Mg2^{+}$ also increases gamma aminobutyric acid (GABA) stimulation contributing to sedation, and reduces the release of Substance P, thus reducing pain, inflammatory mediators, and inflammation. Although it seems evident how these benefits apply to the cardiac surgical patient, conclusive data is still lacking.

During CPB, the lungs are deflated, resulting in atelectasis, inflammation, and injury. $Mg2^{+}$ administration may be beneficial by antagonizing the effects of Ca^{2+}-related bronchiole constriction, regulating/inhibiting the release of histamine and acetylcholine, and through anti-inflammatory effects. $Mg2^{+}$ administration is associated with bronchodilation and vasodilation.

$Mg2^{+}$ influences cardiac metabolism, Ca^{2+} homeostasis, vascular tone/resistance, and cardiac output, largely due to its antagonism of Ca^{2+}. Considering that the CPB period represents an ischemic period followed by a reperfusion with possible injury, important benefits of Mg^{2+} include anti-inflammatory effects, coronary vasodilating effects (and/or anti-spasm), and anti-arrhythmic effects, particularly by affecting Ca^{2+} and K^{+} influx/efflux during phase 2 and phase 3 of the cardiac electric cycle. Mg^{2+} also possesses anti-platelet aggregation properties, which might be beneficial after coronary procedures. While cardiac dysfunctions, arrhythmias, and adverse outcome are associated with hypomagnesemia, data vary as to the outcomes benefits of supplemental $Mg2^{+}$. For the patient requiring CPB, it is assumed that Mg^{2+} levels are low, and reliance on serum levels underestimates the incidence of hypomagnesemia. Compared to a deficient state, hypermagnesemia is uncommon as a disease entity and more commonly the result of ingestion or administration (Table 12.5).

A survey from 24 hospitals revealed that 20% of anesthesiologists routinely administer $Mg2^{+}$ in the cardiac surgical

Table 12.4 Serum levels of normal, hypo-, and hypermagnesemia

$Mg2^{+}$ serum level	mg/dL	mM	mEq/L
Severe Hypermagnesemia	>12	>5	>10
Moderate Hypermagnesemia	5–12	2–5	4–10
Therapeutic target	3.6–4.9	1.5–2	3–4
Normal	1.7–3	0.7–1.2	1.4–2.4
Moderate hypomagnesemia	1.2–1.7	0.5–0.7	1.0–1.4
Severe hypomagnesemia	<1.2	<0.5	<1.0

Table 12.5 Causes and management of hypo- and hypercalcemia

Serum Mg^{+} level (mg/dL) (see Table 12.4)	Causes	Clinical features	Treatment
Severe hyper-Mg^{2+} (>12)	Ingestion: Moderate Mg overdose. Chronic laxative use.	Muscle weakness. Paralysis. Respiratory distress. Heart block, bradycardia, hypotension. Delirium, coma, death.	Ca^{2+} salts. Dialysis (severe cases).
Moderate hyper-Mg^{2+} (5–12)	Ingestion: Overdose of Mg supplements. Laxatives.	Hyporeflexia Lethargy Confusion Flush Nausea, vomiting Bradycardia Prolongation of ECG intervals	Supportive care. Monitor electrolytes. Consider chelating agents for severe cases.
Normal (1.7–3)	N/A	Asymptomatic	N/A (maintain balance)
Moderate hypo-Mg^{2+} (1.2–1.7)	Diuretics: Loop and thiazide diuretics. Proton pump inhibitors. Some cancer medications. General diseases.	Neuromuscular irritability Muscle spasms Tremor Hypocalcemia Hypokalemia	Mg^{2+} supplements. Address underlying cause.
Severe hypo-Mg^{2+} (<1.2)	Poor intake. Malnutrition. Alcoholism. Chronic diarrhea. Severe vomiting.	Tetany Nystagmus Seizures Psychosis Arrhythmias	IV/oral Mg^{2+} Address underlying cause. Treat electrolyte imbalances (K^{+} if needed).

patient. Among these, 76% administer 2–4 gm (8–16 mmol) during CPB for arrhythmia prophylaxis, myocardial protection, and suspected hypomagnesemia. Additionally, 36% administer $Mg2^{+}$ after CPB, while 24% do so both during and after CPB. Finally, 32% administer Mg^{2+} prior to CPB. The primary stated reasons for Mg2+ include arrhythmia prophylaxis, myocardial protection, and neuroprotection. However, only 36% of the respondents assess $Mg2^{+}$ levels.

Drug Metabolism

The initiation and progress of CPB impact serum drug levels and metabolism due to the combined effects of hemodilution, non-pulsatile flow, hypothermia, altered renal and hepatic perfusion and function, acid–base abnormalities, protein binding, impaired enzymatic metabolism of medications, isolation of the lungs from circulation, and uptake of drugs by the CPB circuit.

The detailed discussion on the impact of CPB on drug pharmacokinetics and pharmacodynamics is extensively covered in Chap. 4, “Basic cardiovascular pharmacology used in CPB.” Briefly, the initiation of CPB involves mixing 1500–2000 ml of crystalloid solution with the patient’s blood, leading to immediate changes in serum drug levels, volume distribution, and protein binding. This hemodilution decreases drug concentrations by up to 50% and affects plasma drug-binding proteins. Heparin administration also alters drug-protein binding dynamics. The effects of CPB on drug concentrations are multifaceted, including impacts from hemodilution, hypothermia, acidosis, changes in organ perfusion, and interaction with CPB circuit components. These factors variously influence the metabolism and efficacy of different drugs, including opioids, anesthetics, and neuromuscular blocking agents, altering their pharmacokinetic profiles and necessitating careful management during and after CPB.

Further Reading

Baraka AS, Baroody MA, Haroun ST, Sibai AA, Nawfal MF, Dabbous AS, Taha SK, el-Khatib RA. Effect of alpha-stat versus pH-stat strategy on oxyhemoglobin dissociation and whole-body oxygen consumption during hypothermic cardiopulmonary bypass. Anesth Analg. 1992;74(1):32–7. https://doi.org/10.1213/00000539-199201000-00006. PMID: 1734795

Barry AE, Chaney MA, London MJ. Anesthetic management during cardiopulmonary bypass: a systematic review. Anesth Analg. 2015;120:749–69.

Bolli R. Mechanism of myocardial “stunning”. Circulation. 1990;82(3):723–38. https://doi.org/10.1161/01.cir.82.3.723. PMID: 2203553

Braunwald E. Heart failure. JACC Heart Fail. 2013;1(1):1–20. https://doi.org/10.1016/j.jchf.2012.10.002. Epub 2013 Feb 4. PMID: 24621794

Butterworth JF 4th, Zaloga GP, Prielipp RC, Tucker WY Jr, Royster RL. Calcium inhibits the cardiac stimulating properties of dobutamine but not of amrinone. Chest. 1992;101(1):174–80. https://doi.org/10.1378/chest.101.1.174. PMID: 1729065

Canaday S, Rompala J, Rowles J, Fisher J, Holt D. Chronic severe hyponatremia and cardiopulmonary bypass: avoiding osmotic demyelination syndrome. JECT. 2015;47:228–30.

Chaney MA, Nikolov MP, Blakeman BP, Bakhos M. Attempting to maintain normoglycemia during cardiopulmonary bypass with insulin may initiate postoperative hypoglycemia. Anesth Analg. 1999;89:1091–5.

de Baaij JH, Hoenderop JG, Bindels RJ. Magnesium in man: implications for health and disease. Physiol Rev. 2015;95(1):1–46. https://doi.org/10.1152/physrev.00012.2014. PMID: 25540137

Demers P, Elkouri S, Martineau R, Couturier A, Cartier R. Outcome with high blood lactate levels during cardiopulmonary bypass in adult cardiac operation. Ann Thorac Surg. 2000;70(6):2082–6. https://doi.org/10.1016/s0003-4975(00)02160-3. PMID: 11156124

Doenst T, Wijcysundera D, Karkouti K, Zechner C, Maganti M, Rao V, Borger MA. Hyperglycemia during cardiopulmonary bypass is an independent risk factor for mortality in patients undergoing cardiac surgery. J Thorac Cardiovasc Surg. 2005;130(4):1144. https://doi.org/10.1016/j.jtcvs.2005.05.049. PMID: 16214532

Fitzsimons MG, Agnihotri AK. Hyponatremia and cardiopulmonary bypass. J Cardiothorac Vasc Anesth. 2007;21(2):273–5.

Gedney JA, Ghosh S. Pharmacokinetics of analgesics, sedatives, and anaesthetic agents during cardiopulmonary bypass. Br J Anaesth. 1995a;75:344–51.

Gedney JA, Ghosh S. Pharmacokinetics of analgesics, sedatives and anaesthetic agents during cardiopulmonary bypass. Br J Anaesth. 1995b;75(3):344–51. https://doi.org/10.1093/bja/75.3.344. PMID: 7547056

Giugliano D, Marfella R, Coppola L, Verrazzo G, Acampora R, Giunta R, Nappo F, Lucarelli C, D'Onofrio F. Vascular effects of acute hyperglycemia in humans are reversed by L-arginine. Evidence for reduced availability of nitric oxide during hyperglycemia. Circulation. 1997;95(7):1783–90. https://doi.org/10.1161/01.cir.95.7.1783. PMID: 9107164

Hall RI. Cardiopulmonary bypass and the systemic inflammatory response: effects on drug action. J Cardiothorac Vasc Anesth. 2002;16(1):83–98.

Hogue CW Jr, Palin CA, Arrowsmith JE. Cardiopulmonary bypass management and neurologic outcomes: an evidence-based appraisal of current practices. Anesth Analg. 2006;103(1):21–37. https://doi.org/10.1213/01.ANE.0000220035.82989.79. PMID: 16790619

Holland FW 2nd, Brown PS Jr, Weintraub BD, Clark RE. Cardiopulmonary bypass and thyroid function: a euthyroid sick syndrome. Ann Thorac Surg. 1991;52(1):46–50. https://doi.org/10.1016/0003-4975(91)91416-s. PMID: 2069461.

Janelle GM, Urdaneta F, Martin TD, Lobato EB. Effects of calcium chloride on grafted internal mammary artery flow after cardiopulmonary bypass. J Cardiothorac Vasc Anesth. 2000;14(1):4–8. https://doi.org/10.1016/s1053-0770(00)90046-6. PMID: 10698383

Kant S, Sellke FW, Feng J. Potassium and cardiac surgery. In: Physiology. IntechOpen; 2022. https://doi.org/10.5772/intechopen.99735.

Kant S, Banerjee D, Sabe SA, Sellke F, Feng J. Microvascular dysfunction following cardiopulmonary bypass plays a central role in postoperative organ dysfunction. Front Med (Lausanne). 2023;10:1110532. https://doi.org/10.3389/fmed.2023.1110532. PMID: 36865056; PMCID: PMC9971232

Kersten JR, Toller WG, Tessmer JP, Pagel PS, Warltier DC. Hyperglycemia reduces coronary collateral blood flow through a nitric oxide mediated mechanism. Am J Physiol Heart Circ Physiol. 2001;281:H2097–104.

Khan FW, Fatima B, Lahr BD, Greason KL, Schaff HV, Dearani JA, Daly RC, Stulak JM, Crestanello JA. Hyponatremia: an overlooked risk factor associated with adverse outcomes after cardiac surgery. Ann Thorac Surg. 2021;112:91–8.

Kho C, Lee A, Hajjar RJ. Altered sarcoplasmic reticulum calcium cycling – targets for heart failure therapy. Nat Rev Cardiol. 2012;9(12):717–33. https://doi.org/10.1038/nrcardio.2012.145. Epub 2012 Oct 23. PMID: 23090087; PMCID: PMC3651893

Klemperer JD, Klein I, Gomez M, Helm RE, Ojamaa K, Thomas SJ, Isom OW, Krieger K. Thyroid hormone treatment after coronary-artery bypass surgery. N Engl J Med. 1995;333(23):1522–7. https://doi.org/10.1056/NEJM199512073332302. PMID: 7477166.

Kruger C, Sidebotham D, Brown AJ, Singh H, Merry AF. Timely bolus insulin for glucose control during cardiopulmonary bypass. J Extra Corpor Technol. 2012;44(1):34–8.

Lazar JL. Glycemia control during coronary artery bypass graft surgery. Int Schol Res Network: ISRN Cardiology. 2012;2012 https://doi.org/10.5402/2012/292490.

Leong XF, Cheng M, Jong B, Hwang NC, Roscoe A. Sodium abnormalities in cardiac surgery with cardiopulmonary bypass in adults: a narrative review. J Cardiothorac Vasc Anesth. 2021;35(11):3374–84. https://doi.org/10.1053/j.jvca.2020.07.047. Epub 2020 Jul 17. PMID: 32888797

Levine M, Nikkanen H, Pallin DJ. The effects of intravenous calcium in patients with digoxin toxicity. J Emerg Med. 2011;40(1):41–6. https://doi.org/10.1016/j.jemermed.2008.09.027. Epub 2009 Feb 6. PMID: 19201134

Li M, Dai Y, Hu S, et al. The association between preoperative blood calcium and postoperative blood loss in patients undergoing heart valve replacement surgery. Perfusion. 2022; https://doi.org/10.1177/02676591221140239.

Lomivorotov VV, Guvakov D, Belletti A, Boboshko V, Shmyrev V, Kunst G, Stoppe C, Akselrod B, Kamenshchikov N, Efremov S, Chernyavskiy A, Landoni G. Current practice of calcium use during cardiopulmonary bypass weaning: results of an international survey. J Cardiothorac Vasc Anesth. 2020;34(8):2111–5. https://doi.org/10.1053/j.jvca.2020.02.010. Epub 2020 Feb 12. PMID: 32173209

Maslow AM, Schwartz CS, Bert A, Hurlburt P, Gough J, Stearns G, Singh AK. Endovascular vein harvest: systemic carbon dioxide absorption. J Cardiothorac Vasc Anesth. 2006;20(3):347–52. https://doi.org/10.1053/j.jvca.2006.02.001. PMID: 16750734

Mets B. The pharmacokinetics of anesthetic drugs and adjuvants during cardiopulmonary bypass. Acta Anaesthesiol Scand. 2000;44:261–73. https://doi.org/10.1034/j.1399-6576.2000.440308.x.

Mitchell IM, Pollock JC, Jamieson MP, Donaghey SF, Paton RD, Logan RW. The effects of cardiopulmonary bypass on thyroid function in infants weighing less than five kilograms. J Thorac Cardiovasc Surg. 1992;103(4):800–5. PMID: 1548924

Noguchi S, Saito J, Hashiba E, Kushikata T, Hirota K. Lactate level during cardiopulmonary bypass as a predictor of postoperative outcomes in adult patients undergoing cardiac surgery. JA Clin Rep. 2016;2(1):39. https://doi.org/10.1186/s40981-016-0064-3. Epub 2016 Nov 24. PMID: 29492434; PMCID: PMC5813764

Nola GT, Pope S, Harrison DC. Assessment of the synergistic relationship between serum calcium and digitalis. Am Heart J. 1970;79(4):499–507. https://doi.org/10.1016/0002-8703(70)90255-3. PMID: 5418023

Palmer BF, Clegg DJ. Physiology and pathophysiology of potassium homeostasis. Adv Physiol Educ. 2016;40:480–90.

Palta S, Saroa R, Palta A. Overview of the coagulation system. Indian J Anaesth. 2014;58(5):515–23. https://doi.org/10.4103/0019-5049.144643. PMID: 25535411; PMCID: PMC4260295

Polderman KH, Girbes ARJ. Severe electrolyte disorders following cardiac surgery: a prospective controlled observational study. Crit Care. 2004;8(6):R459–66. https://doi.org/10.1186/cc2973.

Polderman KH, Peerdeman SM, Girbes ARJ. Hypophosphatemia and hypomagnesemia induced by cooling in patients with severe head injury. J Neurosurg. 2001;94(5):697–705.

Reichert MG, Verzino KC. Triiodothyronine supplementation in patients undergoing cardiopulmonary bypass. Pharmacotherapy. 2001 Nov;21(11):1368-74. https://doi.org/10.1592/phco.21.17.1368.34425. PMID: 11714210..

Roscoe A, Ahmed AB. A survey of peri-operative use of magnesium sulphate in adult cardiac surgery in the UK. Anaesthesia. 2003;58(4):363–5. https://doi.org/10.1046/j.1365--2044.2003.03082_1.x. PMID: 12688270

Rosen DA, Rosen KR. Elimination of drugs and toxins during cardiopulmonary bypass. J Cardiothorac Vasc Anesth. 1997;11(3):337–40.

Schmittinger CA, Dünser MW, Torgersen C, Luckner G, Lorenz I, Schmid S, Joannidis M, Moser P, Hasibeder WR, Halabi M, Steger CM. Histologic pathologies of the myocardium in septic shock: a prospective observational study. Shock. 2013;39(4):329–35. https://doi.org/10.1097/SHK.0b013e318289376b. PMID: 23376953

Seghrouchni A, Atmani N, Moutakiallah Y, Belmekki A, El Bekkali Y, Houssa MA. Does severe hyperlactatemia during cardiopulmonary bypass predict a worse outcome? Ann Med Surg (Lond). 2021;73:103198. https://doi.org/10.1016/j.amsu.2021.103198. PMID: 35070281; PMCID: PMC8767239

Sinci V, Soncul H, Gunaydin S, Halit V, Gokgoz L, Tatlican O, Yener A, Bilgehan A, Ersoz A. The effects of thyroid hormones on the heart following global ischemia. A clinical and experimental study. Jpn Heart J. 1994;35(4):443–54. https://doi.org/10.1536/ihj.35.443. PMID: 7967049.

Soleimanpour H, Rahmani F, Golzari SE, Safari S. Main complications of mild induced hypothermia after cardiac arrest: a review article. J Cardiovasc Thorac Res. 2014;6(1):1–8. https://doi.org/10.5681/jcvtr.2014.001. Epub 2014 Mar 21. PMID: 24753824; PMCID: PMC3992725

Stokes DL, Wagenknecht T. Calcium transport across the sarcoplasmic reticulum: structure and function of Ca2 + -ATPase and the ryanodine receptor. Eur J Biochem. 2000;267(17):5274–9. https://doi.org/10.1046/j.1432-1327.2000.01569.x. PMID: 10951184

Teloh JK, Dohle DS, Sönmez S, et al. Transient dilutional acidosis but no lactic acidosis upon cardiopulmonary bypass in patients undergoing coronary artery bypass grafting. Arch Med Sci. 2017;13(3):585–90. https://doi.org/10.5114/aoms.2016.58144.

Udensi UK, Tchounwou PB. Potassium homeostasis, oxidative stress, and human disease. Int J Clin Exp Physiol. 2017;4(3):111–22. https://doi.org/10.4103/ijcep.ijcep_43_17. PMID: 29218312; PMCID: PMC5716641

Wahr JA, Parks R, Boisvert D, et al. Preoperative serum potassium levels and perioperative outcomes in cardiac surgery patients. JAMA. 1999;281(23):2203–10. https://doi.org/10.1001/jama.281.23.2203.

Warwick R, Palmer K, Johnson I, Poullis M. Preoperative hyponatremia and cardiopulmonary bypass: yet another factor for cerebral dysfunction? JECT. 2010;42:52–6.

Young R. Perioperative fluid and electrolyte management in cardiac surgery: a review. J Extra Corpor Technol. 2012;44(1):P20–6.

Zacchia M, Abategiovanni ML, Stratigis S, Capasso G. Potassium: from physiology to clinical implications. Kidney Dis (Basel). 2016;2(2):72–9. https://doi.org/10.1159/000446268.

Zaloga GP, Strickland RA, Butterworth JF 4th, Mark LJ, Mills SA, Lake CR. Calcium attenuates epinephrine's beta-adrenergic effects in postoperative heart surgery patients. Circulation. 1990;81(1):196–200. https://doi.org/10.1161/01.cir.81.1.196. PMID: 2153475

Zhao K, Zhang Y, Li J, Cui Q, Zhao R, Chen W, Liu J, Zhao B, Wan Y, Ma XL, Yu S, Yi D, Gao F. Modified glucose-insulin-potassium regimen provides cardioprotection with improved tissue perfusion in patients undergoing cardiopulmonary bypass surgery. J Am Heart Assoc. 2020;9(6):e012376. https://doi.org/10.1161/JAHA.119.012376. Epub 2020 Mar 10. PMID: 32151220; PMCID: PMC7335515

Part IV

Monitoring During Cardiopulmonary Bypass

Various Monitoring Techniques Used During Cardiopulmonary Bypass

13

Sanjay Dwarakanath and Eugene A. Hessel II

Introduction

Cardiopulmonary bypass (CPB) represents a cornerstone technique in cardiac surgery, enabling operations on a standstill heart. The inherent complexity of this procedure presents a multitude of physiological challenges, demanding meticulous monitoring by anesthesiologists and perfusionists. The objective is to uphold the patient's physiological homeostasis throughout the operation, a task that requires both a foundational understanding of basic monitoring principles and the adept application of advanced monitoring strategies. The role of anesthesiologists and perfusionists is critical, extending beyond merely administering anesthesia and conducting CPB; they must continuously evaluate the patient's physiological condition before, during, and after CPB. The American Society of Anesthesiologists' (ASA) Standard 1 for Basic Anesthetic Monitoring emphasizes the need for qualified anesthesia personnel to be present throughout all anesthesia administrations, a guideline that is relevant in the context of CPB. Similarly, AMSECT highlights the necessity for qualified perfusionists to operate the CPB machine. According to Standard 2.1, a perfusionist who is board-certified by the American Board of Cardiovascular Perfusion or demonstrates equivalent qualifications and competency shall conduct CPB. CPB, however, introduces additional unique monitoring requirements due to its complexity. This chapter explores advanced monitoring techniques crucial during CPB, highlighting both the broad responsibilities and specific tasks essential for maintaining patient stability throughout surgery. Several of these monitoring techniques are discussed in greater detail within other chapters of this book; however, for the sake of comprehensiveness, an overview will be provided herein.

Key monitoring responsibilities include:

S. Dwarakanath · E. A. Hessel II (✉)
Department of Anesthesiology & Perioperative Medicine, University of Kentucky, Lexington, KY, USA
e-mail: sanjay.d@uky.edu; ehessel@uky.edu

1. *Adequacy of Anesthesia:* Monitor for appropriate levels of hypnosis and depth of anesthesia, muscle relaxation, and the administration of prophylactic antibiotic for surgical site infection (SSI).
2. *Conduct of CPB and Complications Detection:* Ensuring the smooth operation of CPB equipment and vigilant detection of any arising complications.
3. *Adequacy of Heparinization:* Closely observing coagulation status to maintain appropriate anticoagulation.
4. *Surgical Field and Activity Observation:* Monitor the surgical team's course of the procedure and observe any significant events.
5. *Hemodynamic Status Monitoring:* A cornerstone of intraoperative monitoring, providing essential data on blood pressure, cardiac output, and tissue perfusion to ensure adequate organ perfusion.
6. *Adequacy of perfusion:* Ensuring that tissue perfusion is maintained at optimal levels throughout the procedure.
7. *Facilitating Communication:* Maintain continuous communication between the anesthesia provider, the surgeon, and the perfusionist to ensure cohesive team operation.
8. *Maintenance of Physiological Homeostasis:* Monitoring and regulating hematocrit, acid–base status, electrolytes, and glucose levels.
9. *Temperature Monitoring*: Managing body temperature to support metabolic needs during surgery, whether through normothermia or controlled hypothermia.
10. *Oxygenation Monitoring*: Monitoring oxygen saturation and assessing arterial blood gases to verify sufficient oxygen delivery and carbon dioxide removal.

Monitoring Depth of Anesthesia

The anesthesiologist is responsible for ensuring that the patient is adequately anesthetized during CPB. This includes administering or monitoring the administration of anesthetic

A. S. Awad, J. DiNardo (eds.), *Clinical Perfusion for Cardiac Surgery*, https://doi.org/10.1007/978-3-031-91163-7_13

agents (intravenous or volatile) and other hypnotic drugs, narcotics, and muscle relaxants. One must then assess the adequacy of the depth of anesthesia. Aids for this assessment include processed EEG (e.g., BIS), monitoring expired agent concentration from the membrane oxygenator (see further discussion subsequently), objective NMB monitoring, as well as interpreting hemodynamic signs. Anesthesiologists also commonly assume responsibility for ensuring adequate administration of antibiotics for SSI prevention and control of blood glucose.

Conduct of CPB

The cardiac surgical team should be aware of how CPB is being conducted. Parameters to be cognizant of include:

1. Flow rate
2. Sweep flow and inspired oxygen saturation
3. Adequacy of venous returned and any losses
4. Administration of fluids, blood, and colloids
5. Administration of any vasoactive agents
6. Use and amount of ultrafiltration
7. Use of augmented venous return
8. Adequacy of heparinization throughout the duration of CPB. (see also Chaps. 15 and 17)

Monitoring the Status of the Patient

Basic hemodynamic parameters to be monitored include mean arterial pressure (MAP), central venous pressure (CVP), and pulmonary artery pressure (PAP) if a pulmonary artery catheter is in place.

Due to the non-pulsatile nature of arterial pressure during CPB, it is most commonly monitored from a catheter in the radial artery. However, in about 35% of cases, the mean radial artery pressure is ≥10 mm Hg below central aortic or femoral pressure, and systolic radial artery pressure is ≥25 mm Hg below central aortic or femoral pressure. This has led some teams to use the brachial or femoral artery for monitoring arterial pressure.

Pressure in the superior vena cava (SVC), usually measured using CVP, is an important determinant of the jugular venous pressure and, thus, cerebral perfusion pressure. It is usually monitored via a catheter placed in the internal jugular or subclavian vein with the tip positioned in the SVC or from the CVP port of a pulmonary artery catheter. However, it is important that this monitoring site be located cephalad to the venous cannula draining the SVC. This is particularly important when using bicaval cannulation for venous drainage and when the left ventricle (LV) is elevated to work on the posterior surface of the heart.

Hematocrit/hemoglobin, glucose, potassium, calcium, acid/base status, and lactate should be monitored at least every 30 min. Some of these may be provided continuously by inline monitors on the extracorporeal circuit. Please refer to Chap. 7 for more information.

ECG is monitored throughout CPB to detect arrhythmias and evidence of ischemia during critical phases such as cannulation, the start of CPB, and after unclamping the aorta. Additionally, it is observed with the administration of cardioplegia to assure asystole and to detect the recurrence of activity between doses.

The adequacy of cerebral perfusion is of critical concern and requires continuous monitoring. Adequate cerebral perfusion is typically achieved by maintaining adequate cerebral perfusion pressure (calculated as MAP minus CVP), arterial oxygen content (dependent on hemoglobin and oxygen saturation), and systemic blood flow. However, objective assessment of brain function is crucial. Several approaches have been advocated, including raw and processed EEG (e.g., BIS), transcranial Doppler, and jugular venous saturation. Notably, the use of NIRS cerebral oximetry has become almost a standard of practice during CPB for both adults and children, particularly for procedures affecting the aortic arch vessels. Several different commercial devices are available, and the choice varies with each cardiac surgical team. Baseline values should be measured on room air. A 20% decrease in baseline values is considered significant. Hence, the trend is often more beneficial than a single value at a given time. Strategies to improve cerebral perfusion may include raising MAP, systemic blood flow, $PaCO_2$, FiO_2, and hematocrit. Additionally, adjusting the temperature, repositioning the patient's head, and increasing the depth of anesthesia may be considered. While these approaches frequently improve measured values, there is yet to be conclusive evidence that they directly translate to better clinical neurologic outcomes. Asymmetric declines in cerebral oxygenation (i.e., on one side compared to the other) are particularly concerning and warrant investigation for evidence of impaired perfusion to the cerebral arteries. NIRS is particularly helpful in guiding management during deep hypothermic circulatory arrest and antegrade cerebral perfusion.

Adequacy of Perfusion

Parameters advocated for, in addition to adequate flow and MAP, include oxygen delivery (DO2), oxygen consumption, carbon dioxide production, mixed venous oxygen saturation, base deficit and lactic acid levels, cerebral oximetry (NIRS), and urine output.

DO2, calculated from arterial oxygen content and systemic blood flow, is a parameter some CPB machines include in their monitoring modules. Ideally, this value should be maintained around or above 275 ml/min/m^2.

Monitoring mixed venous oxygen saturation in the venous return line is a standard parameter required of perfusionists, with the target should be ≥75%. The defining and monitoring of perfusion adequacy are more thoroughly discussed in Chaps. 10 and 14.

Monitoring Expired Gases from the Oxygenator of the Extracorporeal Circuit (ECC)

Such monitoring is comparable to the monitoring of end-tidal gases before and following CPB. It measures expired oxygen content, PCO_2, and agent concentration. Data from multiple studies show a reasonable correlation with arterial measurements of volatile anesthetic concentrations and $PaCO_2$. This monitoring can confirm that gas, especially oxygen, is flowing through the membrane oxygenator (MO), potentially helping to identify oxygenator failure. It also offers insights into arterial CO_2 levels, adequacy of sweep gas flow, and clues to arterial anesthetic vapor, ensuring the patient receives adequate anesthetic agents by the perfusionist. Its use is recommended by the 2019 European guidelines for CPB. It can be easily accomplished by attaching the expired gas monitor line, which runs from the patient's airway circuit to the anesthesia machine, to the expired outlet of the MO after initiating CPB (Fig. 13.1 and 13.2).

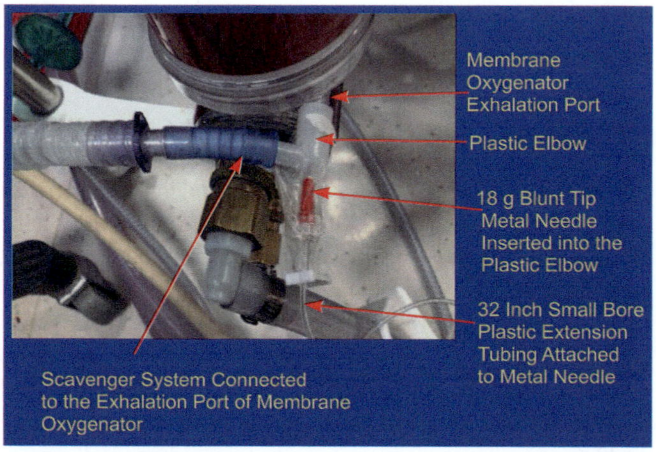

Fig. 13.1 System setup for accessing expired gas from the MO. The scavenger system is connected to the MO's exhalation port via a plastic elbow, with an 18-gauge blunt-tip metal needle inserted into the elbow and secured with a small Telfa dressing. A 32-inch small-bore plastic extension tubing links the metal needle to the display monitor, enabling real-time monitoring of anesthetic agent, CO_2, and oxygen concentrations during CPB

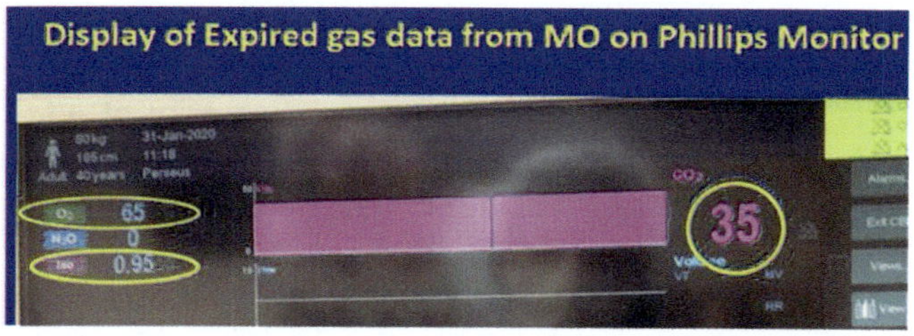

Fig. 13.2 Display of expired gas concentration data from the membrane oxygenator (MO) on the Philips monitor, showing real-time levels of anesthetic agent, CO_2, and oxygen concentrations during CPB

"The Two-Minute Drill"

It is critical to ensure that everything is functioning properly before committing the patient to be dependent on support by the ECC once the aorta is cross-clamped and the heart arrested.

Problems such as oxygenator failure, arterial dissection, and blood loss may take a couple of minutes to become apparent. If discovered before aortic cross-clamping and heart arrest, one can simply resume patient ventilation and come off CPB to solve the problem. Once the heart is arrested, resolving these issues becomes more problematic. Therefore, during this 2-min period of observation, one should ensure that:

1. Targeted flow is achievable.
2. Venous return is adequate, and volume is not being lost.
3. Oxygenation is adequate (out of oxygenator).
4. Arterial pressure is acceptable (to rule out dissection).
5. Both the right and left hearts are decompressed.
6. Systemic venous pressure is Low, especially in SVC.
7. Arterial line pressure is acceptable.
8. Venous saturation is acceptable.

Role of TEE in Monitoring Conduct of CPB

TEE is employed during most cardiac surgeries to assess the presence of abnormalities leading to the surgery and the adequacy of the surgical repair or procedure. What is often underappreciated is the role of TEE in guiding the conduct of CPB. TEE proves invaluable throughout the procedure, particularly in the following stages:

A. In anticipation of CPB, that is, early in the case.
   1. Detect anatomic abnormalities that could affect the conduct of CPB:
      (a) Assess the aorta for atherosclerosis (via TEE and epi-aortic scanning).

See the discussion below on the use of epi-aortic scanning.
   (b) It identifies the presence and severity of aortic regurgitation to plan for the route of cardioplegia delivery.
   (c) TEE can identify atrial septal defect (ASD) or patent foramen ovale (PFO) using two-dimensional and color flow imaging with agitated saline contrast and the Valsalva maneuver if needed.
   (d) A large coronary sinus (if >11 mm) may be a clue to the presence of a persistent left SVC.
   (e) TEE can identify a patent ductus arteriosus (PDA).
   (f) It can also identify a large Eustachian valve, a prominent Chiari network, or a right-sided cor triatriatum.
2. TEE can also detect intra-cardiac devices (e.g., electrodes) or masses (thrombi, vegetations, tumors) that could affect cannulation.

B. In preparation for using CPB, Ensure proper placement of the following:
   1. Arterial cannula.
   2. Venous cannulas (especially those placed via peripheral sites, e.g., from the femoral vein into the right atrium). First, confirm the guidewire's placement in the right atrium, and then ensure that the cannula's tip is positioned correctly within the atrium.
   3. Guide the surgeon to place the retrograde cardioplegia cannula in the coronary sinus.
   4. For left ventricular venting, guide the surgeon to pass the LV vent through the right superior pulmonary vein and into either the left atrium or left ventricle.
   5. Left atrial cannula (e.g., for left-sided heart bypass).
   6. Femoral artery inflow cannula (confirm that guidewire is intraluminal in descending aorta).
   7. Assist with placing the IABP (intra-aortic balloon pump) in the appropriate position.

C. During CPB
   1. Ensure adequate decompression of the LV (as this is more reliable than PAP or the surgeon's assessment).
   2. Differential diagnosis of low arterial pressure on CPB (e.g., rule out arterial dissection, particularly when using femoral artery inflow).
   3. Assess for possible malperfusion of cerebral vessels.
   4. Some practitioners use TEE to assess flow in the alimentary and renal arteries.

D. Toward the end of CPB
   1. Assess for the presence of residual air and ensure adequacy of de-airing.
   2. Assess ventricular and valvular function.
   3. Check for any pleural blood or fluid.

E. Early post-CPB
   1. Check for residual air.
   2. Evaluate the filling of the left and right sides of the heart.
   3. Assess the contractility of left and right ventricles.
   4. Evaluate the results of the surgical repair/procedure.
   5. Rule out aortic injury or evidence of dissection.

F. During sternal closure
   1. Check for evidence of tamponade.
   2. Check for wall motion abnormalities suggestive of CABG graft occlusions.

G. Before the end of the case
   1. Rule out evidence of an aortic dissection or tear
   2. Conduct a final assessment of filling, ventricular function, and valvular function.

The indications and use of epi-aortic scanning remain controversial. TEE is unable to assess atherosclerosis in the more distal portion of the ascending aorta, where cannulation, cross-clamping, and anastomosis are performed. In contrast, epi-aortic scanning has been shown to be much more sensitive than palpation in detecting atheroma in the ascending aorta. This information could guide the surgeon in the conduct of CPB and potentially reduce the risk of atheroembolism and adverse cerebral events. Thus, many authorities and guidelines recommend obtaining epi-aortic examinations in all patients or at least in those over 50 years old and in those who have evidence of significant atherosclerosis in the proximal ascending, transverse, or proximal descending aorta on TEE, if the surgeon agrees and will act on this information. However, this is not commonly practiced.

Detection of Complications

The anesthesiologist, as a member of the cardiac surgical team, plays a crucial role in assisting the surgeon and perfusionist with the detection, evaluation, and management of complications associated with CPB. Common problems include hypotension, hypertension, loss of volume, anemia, metabolic acidosis, and hyperglycemia. More severe problems include arterial dissection, systemic air embolism, oxygenator failure, and cannula misplacement or dislodgement. By observing the surgical field and the parameters just reviewed, one can assist with the early detection of these problems.

To facilitate monitoring, the use of checklists is recommended. Consider the following checklists, which cover timelines before, during, and after CPB from the anesthesia provider's perspective. See also Chap. 30 on safeguards and checklists for additional checklists recommended for perfusionists.

A. *Prior To Going On CPB*
   1. *Calculate:* Determine the expected hematocrit on CPB and assess the need for RBC priming (check with the surgeon).
   2. *Anticoagulation:* Administer heparin and ensure that the desired level of anticoagulation (ACT) is achieved.
   3. *Pulmonary Artery Catheter*: Withdraw the catheter (≥5 cm to <50 cm) to prevent wedging. Confirm the position with TEE.
   4. *Monitoring Lines:* Check pressure monitoring lines and transducers (are they properly zeroed?).
   5. *Urinary Catheter:* Empty the reservoir.
   6. *Patient Assessment:* Examine the patient's face and eyes.
   7. *Venous/Arterial Cannulas and ECC Lines:*
      (i) *Confirm:* Ensure that no air is present in these lines.
      (ii) *Verify:* Check for normal pulsatile pressure in the arterial inflow line, including pressure during test inflow.
      (iii) *Assess:* Confirm proper line positioning using TEE or epi-aortic scanning.
      (iv) *Monitor:* (If bicaval cannulation is used) check SVC pressure via the side-port of the IJ introducer and ensure that it is within normal range.
   8. *Anesthetic Agents*: Consider administering an additional bolus of anesthetic agents.
   9. *Collaboration with Perfusionist*: Discuss the following:
      (a) Anesthetic requirements.
      (b) Management goals for hematocrit, arterial pressure, flow, temperature, and pH/$PaCO_2$ (e.g., alpha-stat vs. pH-stat) in consultation with the surgeon.
      (c) Intravascular volume status.
   10. *Nitrous Oxide (If used):* Discontinue several minutes before the start of CPB.

B. *Early after going on CPB ("2 Minute Drill")*
   (See earlier section on the "Two-Minute drill" for details)
   1. Ventilator & Anesthesia
      When on full bypass or at targeted full flow
      (a) Turn off the vaporizer.
      (b) Place the ventilator on manual mode with 4 cm PEEP and fresh gas flow at 2 L/min air, without oxygen.
      (c) If the lungs obstruct the surgeon's access, disconnect the circuit from the anesthesia machine.
   2. *Medications & Fluids:*
      (a) Discontinue vasoactive and inotropic infusions and fluid administration.
      (b) Continue drug runner and antifibrinolytic.
   3. *Glucose & Insulin*: Manage per protocol.
   4. *Patient Assessment*:
      (a) Check face for symmetry and color change while going on CPB.
      (b) After full flow, assess eyes for venous or arterial congestion and pupil size.
      (c) Monitor cerebral oximetry (if used).
   5. *Arterial Pressure:* Maintain an acceptable arterial pressure (50–80 mm Hg). If it is low, use TEE to rule out aortic dissection.
   6. *Systemic Arterial Inflow:* Ensure that the line pressure on the heart-lung machine is acceptable (as per the perfusionist).
   7. *Achieving Full Flow:*
      (a) Ensure the ability to achieve and maintain full flow (as determined by the perfusionist) (>2.2 L/min/M^2).
      (b) Confirm adequate venous return.
      (c) Verify a stable venous reservoir volume (no excessive volume loss).
   8. *Oxygenation:* Ensure full oxygenation (check arterial line PO_2 or saturation and the color of blood in the arterial line; venous oxygen saturation can be used as a surrogate).
   9. *Ventricular Decompression:*
      (a) Visually confirm adequate emptying of the right ventricle.
      (b) Use TEE to assess the left ventricles.
   10. *CVP:* Maintain low CVP, especially in the SVC with bicaval cannulation.
      (a) Confirm the proper location of the pressure monitoring site.
      (b) Briefly occlude the SVC venous drainage line to verify that venous pressure rises rapidly.
   11. *PAP:* Maintain low PA pressure.
   12. *Mixed Venous Saturation:* Aim for >70–80% (consult with the perfusionist).
   13. *Excessive LV Distension*: If present, consider the following causes:
      (a) Inadequate systemic venous drainage.
      (b) Aortic regurgitation.
      (c) PDA.
      (d) Persistent left superior vena cava.
   14. *Cerebral Oximetry:* Monitor cerebral oximetry closely and intervene as discussed earlier.

15. *ECG:* Ensure there are no ischemic changes or new-onset arrhythmias on the ECG.
16. *Anesthesia:* Confirm adequate levels. Consider the following:
    (a) Monitor BIS closely.
    (b) Check the level of expired agent concentration from the oxygenator.
    (c) Collaborate with the perfusionist to determine the dose of the inhalation agent being administered.
    (d) For TIVA, confirm the dose being administered.
17. *Non-Invasive Monitoring:* Turn off the non-invasive BP and SpO2. Switch the monitor mode to 'perfusion' to silence alarms that are not required.

C. *Immediately following aortic cross-clamping and administration of cardioplegia*:
   1. Confirm prompt arrest of the heart.
   2. Assess for and rule out LV distension.
   3. Ensure carbon dioxide gas is insufflated by the surgeon into the open cardiac chambers during CPB.

D. *During warming*
   1. Maintain arterial inflow temperature ≤ 37 °C and nasopharyngeal temperature ≤ 37.5 °C.
   2. Anticipate the potential need for additional anesthetic agents and muscle relaxants.
   3. Be prepared to manage vasoplegia.

E. *Removal of aortic cross-clamp*
   1. The surgeon may request the Trendelenburg position.
   2. Closely monitor for cardiac distension.
   3. Assess cardiac rhythm.
   4. Consider the need for pacing.

F. *Prior to coming off CPB*
   1. *Systemic Vascular Resistance (SVR)*: Anticipate SVR and assess the potential need for vasoconstrictors based on MAP, pump flow, and calculated SVR during CPB.
   2. *Assess Ventricular Function:*
      (a) Right Ventricle: Evaluate visually.
      (b) LV: Assess with TEE.
   3. *Evaluate Surgical Repair:* Ensure adequacy of surgical repair, especially after valve surgery and congenital heart surgery; regional wall function after CABG).
   4. *Manage Intra-cardiac Air and Adequacy of De-airing:*
      (a) Ventilate lungs: A recruitment maneuver will dislodge trapped air.
      (b) Positioning: Employ the Trendelenburg position to prevent air from ejecting into the circulation, especially to the right coronary artery and carotid arteries.
   5. *Manage Ventilation:*
      (a) Resume ventilation of the lungs (80% oxygen, PEEP of 5) after a recruitment maneuver.
      (b) Consider suctioning and administering a bronchodilator.
      (c) Administer an inhalational agent for bronchodilation.
   6. *Removing LV Vents*: After intracardiac air is cleared from the LV, verify that the surgeon has removed the vents or discontinued suction.
   7. *Caval Tapes/Tourniquets:* Verify that the surgeon released them.
   8. *Lab Values:* Ensure appropriate hematocrit, potassium, calcium, magnesium, and acid–base status.
   9. *ECG Assessment*: Verify good pattern, rate, and rhythm.
   10. *Pacing Leads*:
       (a) Check pacing leads for their ability to pace, threshold, and the size of the R-wave and P-wave.
       (b) Pace as necessary, in the following order of preference: atrial, A-V sequential, and then ventricular pacing.
       (c) Discuss the optimal rate with the surgeon.
   11. *Coagulation Status:*
       (a) Consider checking the platelet count, fibrinogen levels, and conducting viscoelasticity testing.
   12. *Coagulation Reversal:* Calculate the protamine dose and have it ready to administer.
   13. *Inotropes/Vasoactive Drugs:* Prepare infusions or ensure they are running (discuss with the surgical team).
   14. *Coagulation Products:* Order coagulation products (e.g., FFP, platelets, cryoprecipitate, rFVIIa, DDAVP, PPC, etc.) if deemed indicated (discuss with the surgical team).
   15. *Volume Management:* Prepare intravascular volume expanders and check volume lines.
   16. *Temperature:* Confirm adequate rewarming (bladder or PA temperature > 35-37 °C as per local protocol).
   17. *Monitoring Lines:* Check the position and zeroing of pressure monitor lines and transducers.
   18. *Insulin:* Consider reducing the infusion.
   19. *Anesthetic Agents:* Unless there is very poor cardiac function and the patient is receiving high-dose narcotic anesthesia, the use of volatile anesthetic agents typically continues, despite some practitioners choosing to discontinue them.
   20. Non-invasive Monitoring: Activate the non-invasive BP and SpO_2 monitoring. Switch the monitor mode to cardiac.

G. *Early after coming off CPB*
   1. *Ventilation:* Immediately confirm patient ventilation.
      (a) Check end-tidal CO_2 (ET > 20 mm Hg ensures adequate ventilation and cardiac output).
   2. *Oxygenation:* Verify adequate arterial oxygen saturation.
   3. *Blood Pressure:*
      (a) Check MAP, systolic, and diastolic.
      (b) Verify accuracy when the radial artery pressure is low by comparing it with aortic root measurements or arterial line pressure from the CPB machine.
   4. *Cardiac Function:*
      (a) Assess filling pressures, cardiac output, and mixed venous oxygen saturation.
      (b) Visual inspection of the right ventricle function.
      (c) Examine the LV using TEE.
   5. *TEE Examination:* Conduct a comprehensive TEE examination.
   6. *Medications:* Confirm vasoactive and inotropic infusions as well as anesthetic administration.
   7. *Anticoagulation Reversal Management*:
      (a) Discontinue field suction to the CPB machine when starting protamine, opting to stop field suction at the beginning of protamine administration rather than waiting until a certain dose was infused (e.g., 1/3rd or 1 mg/kg) has been administered; this approach is a perfusion standard approved by the STS.
      (b) Obtain verbal confirmation from the perfusionist and surgeon.

Further Reading

Gibbs NM, et al. Management of CPB. In: Gravlee GP, et al., editors. Hensley's practical approach to cardiothoracic anesthesia. 6th ed. Wolters Kluwer; 2019. Chapter 7.

Grocott H, et al. CPB management and organ protection. In: Kaplan JA, et al., editors. Kaplan's cardiac anesthesia. 7th ed. Elsevier; 2017. Chapter 31.

Hessel EA, Groom RC. Guidelines for conduct of cardiopulmonary bypass. J Cardiothorac Vasc Anesth. 2021;35(1):1–17.

Jacquet-Lagrèze M, et al. Can we trust radial artery pressure monitoring for cardiac surgery? Can J Anaesth. 2022;69(11):1319–26.

JohnBull EA, et al. Perianesthetic monitoring. Chapter 5. In: Bartels K, et al., editors. Hensleys's practical approach to cardiothoracic anesthesia. 7th ed. Wolters Kluwer; 2024.

Kunst G, et al. 2019 EACTS/EACTA/EBCP guidelines on cardiopulmonary bypass in adult cardiac surgery. Br J Anaesth. 2019;123(5):713–57.

Milne B, et al. Neuromonitoring and neurocognitive outcomes in cardiac surgery: a narrative review. J Cardiothorac Vasc Anesth. 2022;35(8):2098–113.

Oh AR, et al. Risk factors for femoral-to-radial artery pressure gradient after weaning from cardiopulmonary bypass: a historical cohort study. Can J Anaesth. 2022 Nov;69(11):1330–9.

Svenmarker S, et al. Central venous oxygen saturation during cardiopulmonary bypass predicts 3-year survival. Interact Cardiovasc Thorac Surg. 2013;16(1):21–6.

Svenmarker S, et al. A retrospective analysis of the mixed venous oxygen saturation as the target for systemic blood flow control during cardiopulmonary bypass. Perfusion. 2018;33(6):453–62.

Monitoring Adequacy of Perfusion During Cardiopulmonary Bypass

14

Chao Ji, Shyamal Asher, Geoffrey Hayward, and Andrew Maslow

Introduction

Maintaining adequate perfusion to vital organs is crucial during cardiopulmonary bypass (CPB). Inadequate perfusion during CPB can lead to adverse outcomes, such as end-organ dysfunction, prolonged recovery time, and increased morbidity and mortality. Organs of special concern include the heart, brain, kidneys, liver, lungs, and gastrointestinal tract. Specific end-organ monitoring is not commonly performed. Given that the term "adequate perfusion" during CPB remains poorly defined, it is more accurate to think of the perfusion quality as a continuum, ranging from inadequate, to adequate, to optimal. Optimal perfusion during CPB is defined as providing the best long-term patient outcome with minimal disruptions to all organ systems. The focus of this chapter will be on the key variables affecting perfusion and the most common methods of monitoring adequacy of perfusion during CPB.

Physiologic Variables Affecting Perfusion

Maintaining adequate perfusion during CPB depends on an appropriate balance between tissue oxygen supply and demand. The key variables involved in this balance include blood flow (or CPB flow), oxygen content, and metabolic demand, with the latter being partly controlled by the depth of anesthesia and temperature.

C. Ji
Department of Anesthesiology & Perioperative Medicine, Rhode Island Hospital, Providence, RI, USA

S. Asher · G. Hayward · A. Maslow (✉)
Department of Anesthesiology & Perioperative Medicine, Brown University, Providence, RI, USA

CPB Flow

CPB flow rates vary based on individual perfusionist experience and institutional preferences. Several factors influence safe flow rates. Initially, a patient's body surface area and their blood oxygen content guide flow rate selection, aiming to achieve a flow rate that reflects a typical cardiac index of exceeding 2.2 L/min/m^2. However, during hypothermic CPB with depressed metabolic rates, successful outcomes have been achieved with flow rates as low as 1.2 L/min/m^2.

Modern CPB pumps offer both pulsatile and non-pulsatile flow options. Early mechanical pumps only delivered non-pulsatile flow, establishing it as the standard practice. Research has since compared the effects of pulsatile perfusion on various outcomes, including mortality, neurological dysfunction, myocardial infarction, renal injury, inflammatory mediator release, and mechanical and pharmacological circulatory support requirements. While non-pulsatile flow may be associated with decreased microcirculatory perfusion to the skin and splanchnic vasculature, pulsatile flow might be associated with lower systemic catecholamine levels. The data on which approach provides better end-organ flow remains inconclusive. Due to concerns about cell trauma with pulsatile flow, non-pulsatile CPB flow remains the standard of care in most cardiac centers.

Temperature

Inducing systemic hypothermia is a common strategy during CPB to balance the body's oxygen demand with oxygen delivery. By decreasing metabolic rate and oxygen demand, systemic hypothermia increases the body's tolerance to ischemia. This aligns with the Q10 temperature coefficient, which is defined as a decrease in metabolic rate as temperature drops by 10° C. However, it's important to note that systemic hypothermia can also increase blood viscosity, potentially impairing oxygen delivery to tissues. This is

A. S. Awad, J. DiNardo (eds.), *Clinical Perfusion for Cardiac Surgery*, https://doi.org/10.1007/978-3-031-91163-7_14

reflected by a leftward shift of the oxygen-hemoglobin dissociation curve.

Hematocrit/Hemoglobin

Hemodilution anemia commonly occurs with the onset of CPB. The degree of hemodilution anemia depends on the patient's starting hematocrit and the priming volume used in the CPB circuit. Hemodilution during CPB has both advantages and disadvantages. The advantages include a decreased risk of hypertensive episodes during higher bypass flow rates and an improved microcirculatory flow due to a reduction in blood viscosity. The disadvantages include decreases in oxygen content, systemic blood pressure, and oxygen delivery to tissues. Multiple studies have reported that a "restrictive" transfusion policy, most often defined by a transfusion trigger of less than 23%, is non-inferior to liberal transfusion practices. Although a nadir hematocrit—below which adverse outcomes increase—is ill-defined, propensity score analyses suggest that a hematocrit of less than 21% may be associated with increased neurological injury, renal injury, and mortality. Therefore, transfusion decisions should be tailored to each case type, case conditions, and patient requirements. For example, data support maintaining a higher hematocrit of 30% for cases involving profound hypothermic CPB. While avoiding severe hemodilution is supported, the benefits and risks of PRBC transfusion require careful consideration, as blood bank products have been associated with greater adverse outcomes, including infection. Hematocrit levels as low as 15–18% have been reported to be "safe." Fontana et al. hemodiluted non-cardiac surgical patients to a hemoglobin level of 3 gm/dl (hematocrit of approximately 9%) without increasing lactate levels, provided that normovolemia was maintained. Although the hematocrit is used as a transfusion threshold, it is best to make transfusion decisions in the context of other measures of perfusion.

Oxygen Delivery

Balancing oxygen demand and delivery, and therefore tissue perfusion, is key to CPB management. In the absence of end-organ monitoring and a determination of tissue metabolic rates, "optimal" oxygen delivery (DO_2) is difficult to measure. DO_2 is equal to the pump flow rate multiplied by the arterial oxygen content, "CaO_2." This is reflected in the equation:

$$DO_2 = CO \times CaO_2$$

which can be rewritten as

$$DO_2 = CO \times (1.34 \times Hgb \times SaO2) + (0.0031 \times PaO_2)$$

SaO_2 represents the arterial oxygen saturation
PaO_2 represents the partial pressure of arterial oxygen.

Normal indexed DO_2 in adults is 500 ml/min/m^2 (ranging between 300 and 600 ml/min/m^2), and it is higher for newborns and pediatric patients, which may exceed 600 ml/min/m^2. By comparison, normal oxygen consumption (VO_2) is 150 ml/min/m^2). The onset of CPB is associated with a decrease in DO_2 due to hemodilution, compensated for by an increase in tissue oxygen extraction, termed "flow-independent oxygen consumption." However, once tissue oxygen extraction reaches its maximum, critical DO_2, or the minimum DO_2 required to satisfy the metabolic oxygen demand, is achieved. Given individual variability and the impact of viscosity and rheology during hemodilution, determining a nadir DO_2 is challenging. However, some reports suggest that 200 ml/min/m^2 may be a threshold below which oxygen debt, tissue ischemia and injury, and metabolic acidosis occur. Both DO_2 and oxygen demand can be adjusted: DO_2 increases with oxygen content and flow, while oxygen demand decreases with increased anesthetic depth and lower temperature. Although regional variability (i.e., end-organ differences) exists, specific tissue perfusion monitoring is difficult. Instead, assessment of tissue perfusion is largely based on generalized parameters.

Monitoring Adequacy of Perfusion

The adequacy of perfusion and managing oxygen demand/delivery balance for each specific vital organ system during CPB is not feasible, considering the duration and limitations of the perioperative arena. Instead, monitoring and clinical decisions are based on surrogate monitors that reflect total body oxygen balance. Generally, monitors that reflect moment-to-moment changes receive greater emphasis and attention.

Mean Arterial Pressure and Central Venous Pressure

Monitoring and maintaining mean arterial pressure (MAP) is a major component of managing systemic perfusion during CPB. Although an optimal MAP goal to ensure "adequate" perfusion during CPB has yet to be established, a MAP target on CPB is 50–70 mmHg. Fifty mmHg is the lower limit of cerebral autoregulation. Proponents of higher MAP goals (greater than 70 mmHg) emphasize the benefits of enhanced tissue perfusion during CPB. Ultimately, the optimal MAP during CPB should be individualized for each patient after an assessment of their comorbid conditions. Higher pressures may be beneficial in elderly and/or hypertensive patients to theoretically reduce the risk of neurocognitive dysfunction, which has devastating consequences. Although a desired range of MAP is stated, these values vary per the individual patient and CPB management. For example, cerebral autoregulation, presumed to be autoregulated between a MAP of 50–150 mmHg, may be adequate for a MAP as low as 20–30 mmHg under hypothermic conditions and during hemodilution. Lower ranges of MAP reduce bleeding, blood trauma, and embolic load.

Although important, maintaining a systemic perfusion pressure is only part of what drives blood flow to end-organs. Perfusion is intimately related to pressure, flow, and resistance, as shown by the following equations:

$$\text{MAP} - \text{CVP} = \text{SVR} \times \text{CO}$$

$$\text{CO} = \left(\text{MAP} - \text{CVP}\right) / \text{SVR}$$

CO is cardiac output
CVP is central venous pressure
SVR is systemic vascular resistance

An elevated CVP or venous congestion may be more detrimental to perfusion than a low MAP. A recent study found that incremental elevations of the CVP, especially those greater than 12 mmHg, were associated with renal injury and were stronger predictors of poor perfusion than intraoperative hypotension (MAP <60 mmHg). Together, maintaining systemic perfusion relies on optimizing MAP, CVP, and flow rates.

Cerebral Monitoring Approaches and Cerebral Oximetry

Inadequate cerebral perfusion during cardiac surgery can result in devastating postoperative neurological complications. Prior to the advent of non-invasive cerebral oximetry, intraoperative monitoring of cerebral tissue oxygenation was limited by the invasive, time-intensive, unreliable, and costly nature of existing techniques. Examples of invasive cerebral perfusion monitoring include jugular venous oxygen saturation ($SjvO_2$) and continuous brain tissue oxygen ($PbtO_2$) monitoring. $SjvO_2$ measurements can be obtained by direct puncture of the jugular bulb or by placing catheters in a high position in the jugular vein for repeated sampling. $SjvO_2$ monitoring more accurately reflects whole-brain rather than regional, blood oxygen saturation. The duration of $SjvO_2$ monitoring increases the risks of hematoma and venous thrombosis.

Non-invasive cerebral oximetry uses near-infrared spectroscopy (NIRS) to monitor regional oxygen saturation in the frontal cortex (Fig. 14.1).

For a detailed overview of comprehensive cerebral monitoring approaches, see Fig. 14.2.

NIRS involves a monitor and adhesive probes strategically placed on the forehead, overlying the frontal cortex. These probes contain a light source and light detector. The emitted near-infrared light penetrates the skull to a depth of approximately 2–2.5 cm, reaching the underlying frontal cortex. Interactions with the tissue (reflection, refraction, etc.) alter the light, and these changes are analyzed by the cerebral oximeter monitor, which calculates cerebral oxygenation according to the Beer-Lambert laws, which relate to the absorption and penetration of light through substances at varying concentrations and depths. It's essential to establish baseline cerebral oximeter values prior to administering anesthesia. Values within 60–80% are generally considered normal, though 55–60% may be acceptable in certain cardiac patients. For an overview of the basic physics principles behind cerebral and tissue oximetry, refer to the schematic diagram in Fig. 14.3.

Proponents of NIRS monitoring highlight its value in providing a safe and non-invasive estimate of cerebral oxygen balance. Intraoperative decreases from baseline have been associated with worsening neurologic outcomes, and patients experiencing a 30% decrease from baseline exhibited significantly higher rates of neurocognitive dysfunction 1 month after coronary artery bypass grafting (CABG). Other studies have also found an associated higher risk of stroke. However, the mechanisms by which these adverse neurologic events

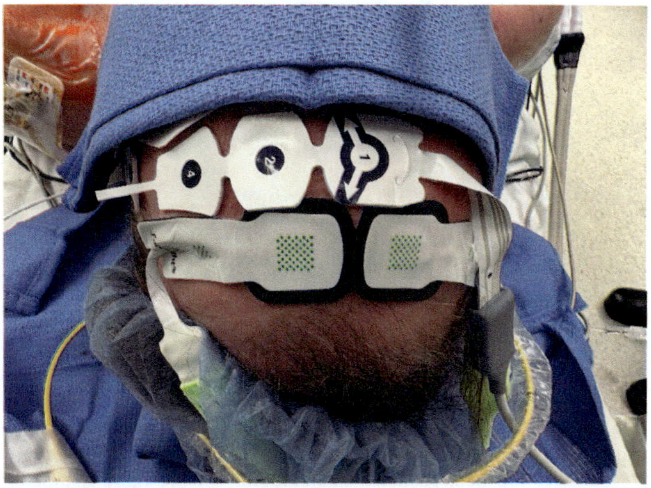

Fig. 14.1 In a clinical setting, this image captures a patient during a CPB procedure, featuring non-invasive NIRS monitoring stickers and a BIS monitor strip on the forehead, placed on the patient's forehead, tools essential for advanced monitoring of cerebral oxygenation and anesthesia depth

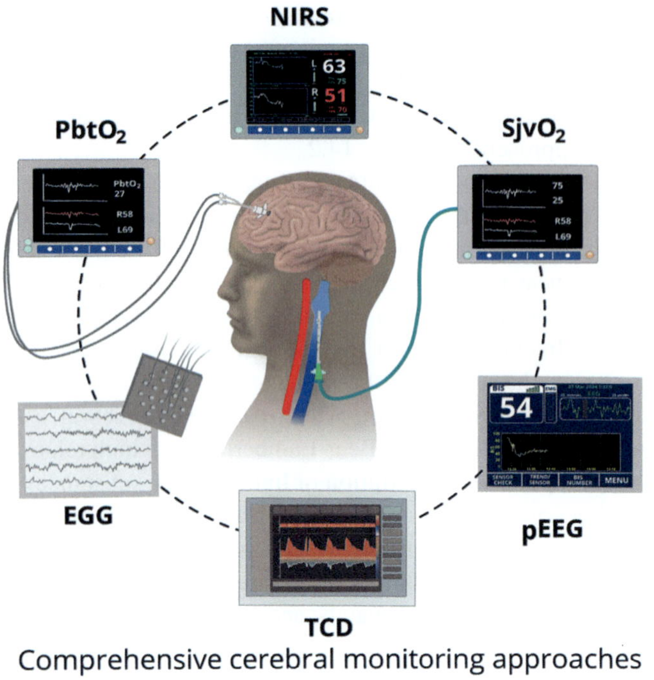

Fig. 14.2 Illustrative comparison of cerebral perfusion monitoring modalities. This figure presents an array of invasive techniques, such as internal jugular bulb venous oxygen monitoring ($SjvO_2$) and brain tissue oxygenation ($PbtO_2$), alongside non-invasive methods, including electroencephalography (EEG), processed EEG (pEEG), NIRS, and transcranial Doppler (TCD)

develop during cardiac surgery are complex and intertwined, with cerebral hypoxemia and microemboli both playing critical roles. During cardiac surgery, microemboli, consisting of air, atheromas, lipids, and platelet-fibrin thrombi, are showered into millions of small capillaries and arterioles, especially in the watershed areas of the brain. It is thought that adequate cerebral blood flow and its associated factors can lyse and wash out these microemboli. Proponents also argue that NIRS cerebral oximetry fills a niche, since there is no other easily performed, non-invasive cerebral monitoring technique. Currently, there has been no evidence of harm by NIRS-guided interventions, aside from the associated cost.

Arguments against its use highlight the variability in what is considered normal and abnormal values, as well as the lack of robust evidence for improved clinical outcomes with NIRS-guided interventions. There is a large variability in baseline values among different patients. Normal or near normal cerebral oximetry values can be found in patients who have died after prolonged cardiac arrest. This could be due to residual blood sequestered in the cerebral venous vasculature of a non-metabolizing brain or persistent extracranial circulation. Abnormal values may include absolute values of <50–55% or reductions of 15–20% from baseline values. Algorithms aimed at increasing cerebral oximetry values generally involve increasing systemic blood pressure, enhancing perfusion flow, cooling the patient, administering

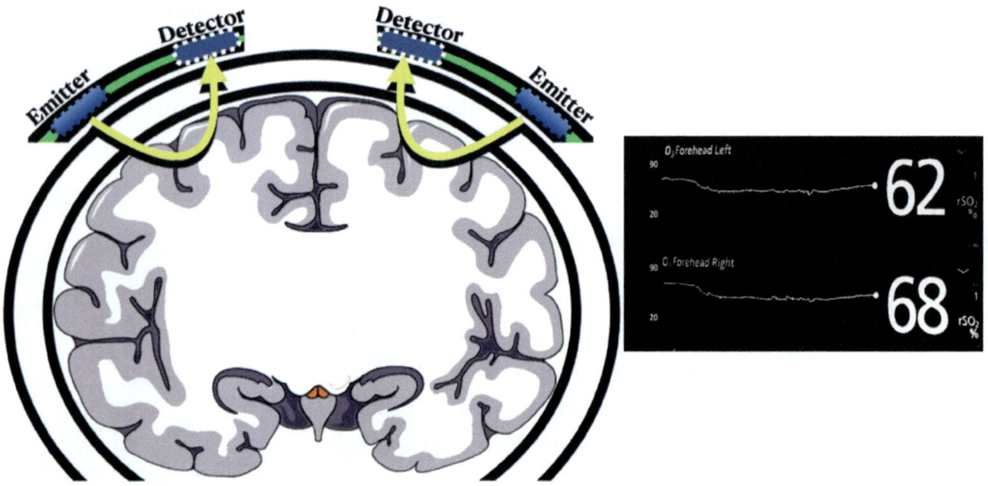

Fig. 14.3 Cerebral Oximetry in Action: This image illustrates the principles of cerebral oximetry. On the left, a human brain is shown with cerebral oximeter stickers attached to the forehead. These stickers contain light emitters and detectors. The emitted near-infrared light penetrates the skull and brain tissue, where it's absorbed differently by oxygenated and deoxygenated hemoglobin. On the right, a monitor screen displays the calculated cerebral oxygenation values for each hemisphere, derived using the Beer–Lambert law. This law relates the absorption of light to the properties of the material through which it travels, allowing for the estimation of oxygen saturation in the brain tissue. The image demonstrates how non-invasive cerebral oximetry provides real-time monitoring of brain oxygenation, crucial for patient safety during procedures that may affect cerebral perfusion.

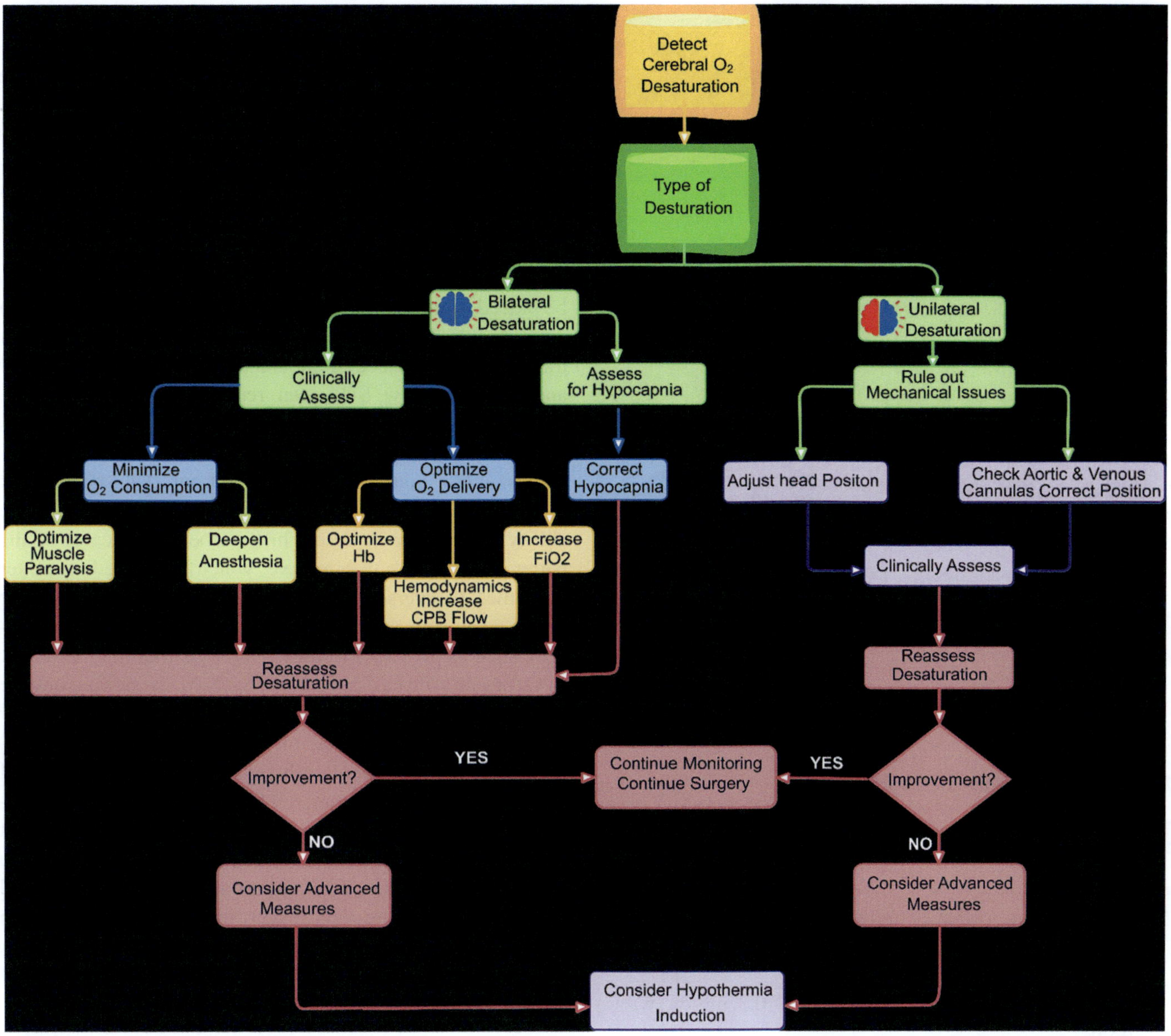

Fig. 14.4 This diagram illustrates algorithms for managing unilateral and bilateral cerebral desaturation, outlining strategies to optimize cerebral oximetry values during cardiopulmonary bypass

blood transfusions, and optimizing acid–base status (Fig. 14.4) (Table 10.3).

For more information about the algorithm proposed by A Denault, et al. for managing low cerebral oximetry during CPB, please refer to Chap. 10, "Goal-Directed Perfusion Throughout Various Stages of Cardiopulmonary Bypass." During CPB, up to 67% of patients will experience a 10–20% decline in cerebral oximetry values. Even though 60–90% of patients respond to management, it remains unclear if their outcomes improve. Positive predictive value and specificity of cerebral oximetry are below 30%, but sensitivity has been found to be as high as 75%. If used, cerebral oximeter values should be interpreted in the context of all other available clinical data.

Urine Output

Renal perfusion is autoregulated over a range of blood pressures by the neurohormonal system. Blood pressures outside of this range may increase the risk of renal hypoperfusion. Currently, there are no intraoperative clinical monitors that directly measure renal perfusion. The most used surrogate during CPB is urine output. Urine output reflects kidney function (Fig. 14.5).

Renal hypoperfusion during CPB can result in acute kidney injury (AKI). Please refer to Chap. 29, "Strategies of Kidney protection During CPB," for the Kidney Disease: Improving Global Outcomes (KDIGO) definition of

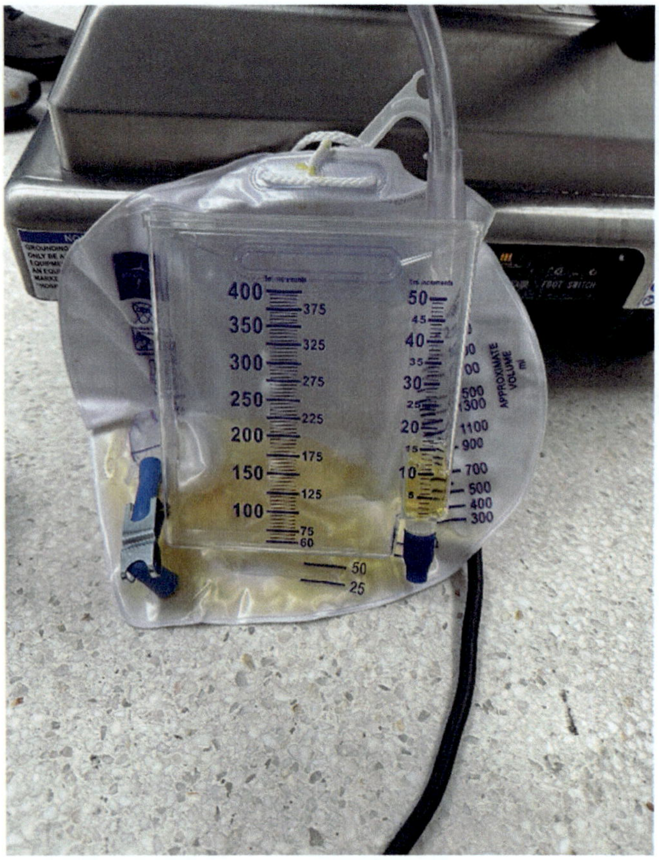

Fig. 14.5 In a clinical setting, this image captures urine collection bag during CPB procedure, serving as a key indicator of kidney function through monitoring urine output, the primary surrogate for reflecting kidney function

AKI. According to that definition, AKI is characterized by any of the following:

- An increase in serum creatinine of ≥0.3 mg/dL within 48 h
- An increase in serum creatinine by ≥1.5 times baseline
- A urine output of <0.5 mL/kg/hour for 6 h

Monitoring urine output during CPB may facilitate timely interventions, as decreases in urine output typically precede increases in serum creatinine levels. A urine output rate less than 1.5 mL/kg/hour has been associated with an increased risk of AKI. Paradoxically, excessive urine output (>4 mL/kg/hour) has also been linked to increased AKI risk. This diuresis is likely results from the effects of hypothermia, and/or inflammation-induced tubular damage sustained during CPB. However, it is important to note that urine output is a poor predictor of overall outcomes during cardiac surgeries, and its predictive value is even less reliable during CPB.

In-line Venous Oxygen Saturation

Venous oxygen saturation (SvO_2) is a measurement of the oxygen content in the blood returning from the whole body. When oxygen supply fails to meet oxygen demand, it is expected that the SvO_2 will be abnormal, reflecting an imbalance of systemic hemodynamics and oxygen delivery. CPB circuits typically are equipped with a continuous, in-line SvO_2 monitor (Fig. 7.26). This monitor samples venous blood draining from the surgeon's venous cannula and can be placed in the right atrium or superior and/or inferior vena cava. A normal SvO_2 is greater than 70–75%. Values lower than this range reflect an imbalance between oxygen supply and demand. Low SvO_2 can represent reduced delivery, increased oxygen extraction, or both. Clinical data suggests that SvO_2 values below 60% are associated with adverse outcomes, while goal-directed interventions that successfully increase SvO_2 are associated with improved outcomes. The ability to increase SvO_2 might be a better indicator of the patient's cardiovascular reserve, which itself predicts better outcomes. Conversely, SvO_2 values greater than 80% can be observed during situations with decreased oxygen extraction, such as general anesthesia and hypothermia. However, SvO_2 monitoring has limitations. SvO_2 can be normal despite microcirculatory impairment. Additionally, there is no clear consensus on the optimal monitoring frequency of SvO_2 (continuously or intermittently) or the relative importance of intraoperative values compared to those obtained postoperatively in the Intensive Care Unit (ICU). Finally, the target SvO_2 for goal-directed therapy remains under debate, with some advocating for ≧60% and others for ≧70%. Reported benefits of achieving target SvO_2 include fewer end-organ complications, reduced time on mechanical ventilation, shorter ICU and hospital length of stay, and lower mortality rates.

Carbon Dioxide Gap

Goal-directed therapies are geared toward optimizing oxygen delivery and balance within end-organs to prevent hypoperfusion, ischemia, oxygen debt, and tissue hypoxia/dysoxia. While hemodynamic data and goals are important, they don't fully capture tissue or microcirculatory dysfunction. Metabolic data, such as serum lactate levels or venous blood gas analyses, are considered better reflections of overall end-organ tissue dysfunction. Notably, though arterial blood gas analysis is often used to assess tissue metabolic function, it might be a better indicator of pulmonary gas exchange rather than end-organ function specifically. Venous blood, in the same patient, typically has higher CO_2 levels and a lower pH, while arterial blood gas analysis mainly reflects oxygenation and minute ventilation. The CO_2 gap (the difference between arterial and venous CO_2) has been studied as a potential prognostic indicator.

$$CO_2 \text{ gap} = \text{Venous } CO_2 - \text{Arterial } CO_2$$

During anaerobic metabolism, pyruvate is converted into lactate to generate high-energy phosphates in the absence of oxygen. Although this process is less efficient than aerobic metabolism, it allows tissues to function temporarily while in oxygen debt. If perfusion is adequate, tissues can recover. The Cori Cycle ultimately reconverts lactate to glucose in the liver. Anaerobic metabolism leads to an increased production hydrogen ions, which are largely buffered by the bicarbonate system, resulting in greater CO_2 production (VCO_2). The pulmonary system then removes this excess carbon dioxide, as reflected in the $PaCO_2$ value. If VCO_2 exceeds the body's buffering ability and clearance capacity, $PvCO_2$ increases.

$$VCO_2 = \text{cardiac output} \times \left(CvCO_2 - CaCO_2\right)$$

Where VCO_2 is the venous carbon dioxide production, $CvCO_2$ is the venous carbon dioxide content, and $CaCO_2$ is the arterial carbon dioxide content.

Substituting PCO_2 (partial pressure of carbon dioxide) for CCO_2 (carbon dioxide content).

$$VCO_2 = \text{cardiac output} \times \left(PvCO_2 - PaCO_2\right) / k$$

Where VCO_2 is the venous carbon dioxide production, $PvCO_2$ is the venous partial pressure of carbon dioxide, $PaCO_2$ is the arterial partial pressure of carbon dioxide, and k = coefficient

$$PCO_2 \text{ gap} = k \times VCO_2 / \text{Cardiac Output}$$

Under normal conditions, the CO_2 gap ranges from 4 to 6 mmHg. Under conditions of reduced cardiac output, CO_2 clearance decreases, leading to a widened PCO_2 gap. This rise in tissue CO_2 might be an early indicator of tissue oxygen debt. In critical care settings, the CO_2 gap indirectly reflects cardiac output, end-organ perfusion, microcirculatory dysfunction, and tissue acidosis. Some studies suggest that a CO_2 gap exceeding 8 to10 mmHg may be a better predictor of outcomes than either serum lactate or SvO_2.

Lactate

Although acid–base balance is carefully monitored during CPB, pH changes can result from a host of variables, including ventilation. Metabolic acidosis is not uncommon during CPB and might be more indicative of fluids administered and other iatrogenic interventions than poor tissue perfusion. Lactate, a byproduct of anaerobic metabolism, is routinely measured as a point-of-care test during CPB. It is widely regarded as a good marker of inadequate tissue perfusion. Normal lactate levels typically range from 0.5–2 mmol/L, with hyperlactatemia defined as >2 mmol/L, and lactic acidosis defined as >4 mmol/L. Lactic acidosis is associated with an increased risk of various complications, including postoperative low-output cardiac syndrome, renal insufficiency, gastrointestinal complications, blood transfusion requirements, extended ICU length of stay, and overall postoperative morbidity and mortality. A lactate level exceeding 5 mmol/L measured immediately after coming off CPB has been linked to an eight-fold greater mortality risk compared to normal lactate levels. Time on CPB is a key factor influencing intraoperative lactate production. 96 minutes on CPB has been identified as predictive of hyperlactatemia during CPB. Importantly, persistent hyperlactatemia is considered a greater risk factor for adverse outcomes than transient elevations. Currently, there is a lack of consensus on interpreting intraoperative lactate levels within the 2–4 mmol/L range or the timing of peak lactate elevations. Furthermore, the significance of the differential uptake and release of lactate by various organs and its relationship to the development of organ dysfunction during CPB remains unclear. To date, no universally accepted recommendations exist on the optimal timing and frequency of perioperative lactate checks.

Table 14.1 summarizes the various measures used to assess tissue perfusion during CPB. Although listed individually, changes in individual case management often incorporate two or more values. For example, a hematocrit of 18% alone does not necessarily require transfusion if other perfusion variables are within acceptable ranges.

Clinical Pearls

- Safe flow rates during CPB are determined by several factors: acid–base balance, blood oxygen content, BSA, depth of anesthesia, oxygen consumption, neuromuscular blockade, temperature goals, and organ tolerance to ischemia.
- Hematocrit levels below 21% have been associated with increased neurological injury, renal injury, and mortality.
- Critical DO_2 during CPB is the minimum amount of DO_2 oxygen delivery needed to satisfy the metabolic oxygen demand.
- Hypothermia decreases the body's oxygen demands and increases organs' tolerance to ischemia.

Table 14.1 Measures utilized to assess perfusion during CPB

Measure	Typical range	Considerations
Systemic perfusion		
Systemic flow rates	2.0 to 2.5 L/min/m^2	Adjust pump flow to maintain a target flow rate based on body surface area (BSA), aiming for a cardiac index of >2 L/min/m^2.
MAP	50-70 mmHg (80 mmHg for select cases)	Lower targets may be acceptable with adequate organ perfusion.
Hematocrit	> 18% (during CPB)	Optimal level during CPB is debated; consider patient and procedure-specific factors.
Cerebral perfusion		
Cerebral oximetry (NIRS)	60–80% or < 30% change from baseline	Monitor trends and decreases from baseline.
Renal perfusion		
Urine output	0.5–1.5 cc/kg/hr. (during CPB)	Oliguria can indicate renal hypoperfusion. However, polyuria more than 4 cc/kg/hr. is considered a potential sign of tubular dysfunction.
Metabolic markers		
In-line SvO_2	70–75%	Low SvO_2 suggests increased oxygen extraction or reduced oxygen delivery.
Lactate	0.5-2 mmol/L	Elevated lactate indicates anaerobic metabolism. Time on CPB and persistence are important factors.
CO_2 Gap ($PvCO_2$—$PaCO_2$)	< 8–10 mmHg	Widened gap may indicate reduced cardiac output and tissue perfusion.

- Non-invasive oximeters use NIRS to monitor regional oxygen saturation in the frontal cortex.
- In-line SvO_2 can be normal despite microcirculatory impairment.
- A normal CO_2 gap (around 8 mmHg) suggests blood flow is likely adequate but does not inform on the adequacy of tissue oxygenation.
- Time on CPB is a key determinant of intraoperative lactate production.
- A urine output rate of <1.5 mL/kg/hour and > 4 mL/kg/hour have been associated with an increased risk of AKI.

Further Reading

Alston RP, Cormack L, Collinson C. Metabolic acidosis developing during cardiopulmonary bypass is related to a decrease in strong ion difference. Perfusion. 2004 May;19(3):145–52. https://doi.org/10.1191/0267659104pf751oa.

Chen T, Pan T, Luo X, Wang D. High central venous-to-arterial CO_2 difference is associated with poor outcomes in patients after cardiac surgery: a propensity score analysis. Shock. 2019;52:583–9.

Cormack LG, Collinson CV, Alston RP. Metabolic acidosis and cardiopulmonary bypass: hypoperfusion or iatrogenic? Crit Care. 2002;6(Suppl 2):2. https://doi.org/10.1186/cc1806.

Duebener LF, Sakamoto T, Hatsuoka S, Stamm C, Zurakowski D, Vollmar B, Menger MD, Schäfers HJ, Jonas RA. Effects of hematocrit on cerebral microcirculation and tissue oxygenation during deep hypothermic bypass. Circulation. 2001 Sep 18;104(12 Suppl 1):I260–4. https://doi.org/10.1161/hc37t1.094912.

Fontana JL, Welborn L, Mongan PD, Sturm P, Martin G, Bünger R. Oxygen consumption and cardiovascular function in children during profound intraoperative normovolemic hemodilution. Anesth Analg. 1995 Feb;80(2):219–25. https://doi.org/10.1097/00000539-199502000-00003.

Goonasekera CDA, Carcillo JA, Deep A. Oxygen delivery and oxygen consumption in pediatric fluid refractory septic shock during the first 42 h of therapy and their relationship to 28-day outcome. Front Pediatr. 2018;6:314. https://doi.org/10.3389/fped.2018.00314.

Holm J, Håkanson RE, Vánky F, Svedjeholm R. Mixed venous oxygen saturation is a prognostic marker after surgery for aortic stenosis. Acta Anaesthesiol Scand. 2010;54:589–95.

Holm J, Håkanson E, Vánky F, Svedjeholm R. Mixed venous oxygen saturation predicts short- and long-term outcome after coronary artery bypass grafting surgery: a retrospective cohort analysis. Br J Anaesth. 2011;107:344–50.

Kaakinen TI, Ikäläinen T, Erkinaro TM, et al. Association of low mixed venous oxygen saturations during early ICU stay with increased 30-day and 1-year mortality after cardiac surgery: a single-center retrospective study. BMC Anesthesiol. 2022;22:322. https://doi.org/10.1186/s12871-022-01862-8.

Kunst G, Milojevic M, et al. 2019 EACTS/EACTA/EBCP guidelines on cardiopulmonary bypass in adult cardiac surgery. Br J Anaesth. 2019;123(6):713–57. https://doi.org/10.1016/j.bja.2019.09.012.

Loor G, Li L, Sabik JF 3rd, Rajeswaran J, Blackstone EH, Koch CG. Nadir hematocrit during cardiopulmonary bypass: end-organ dysfunction and mortality. J Thorac Cardiovasc Surg. 2012 Sep;144(3):654–662.e4. https://doi.org/10.1016/j.jtcvs.2012.03.058. Epub 2012 Apr 14.

Moore CC, Yu S, Aljure O. A comprehensive review of cerebral oximetry in cardiac surgery. J Card Surg. 2022;37:5418–33. https://doi.org/10.1111/jocs.17232.

Moussa MD, Durand A, Leroy G, Vincent L, Lamer A, et al. Central venous-to-arterial PCO2 difference, arteriovenous oxygen content and outcome after adult cardiac surgery with cardiopulmonary bypass. Eur J Anaesthesiol. 2019;36:279–89.

Murphy GS, Hessel EA 2nd, Groom RC. Optimal perfusion during cardiopulmonary bypass: an evidence-based approach. Anesth Analg. 2009;108(5):1394–417. https://doi.org/10.1213/ane.0b013e3181875e2e.

Pölönen P, Ruokonen E, Hippeläinen M, Pöyhönen M, Takala J. A prospective, randomized study of goal-oriented hemodynamic therapy in cardiac surgical patients. Anesth Analg. 2000;90:1052–9.

Sarkar M, Prabhu V. Basics of cardiopulmonary bypass. Indian J Anaesth. 2017 Sep;61(9):760–767. https://doi.org/10.4103/ija.IJA_379_17. PMID: 28970635; PMCID: PMC5613602.

Shastri L, Kjaergaard B, Rees SE, Thomsen LP. Changes in central venous to arterial carbon dioxide gap (PCO_2 gap) in response to acute changes in ventilation. Brit Med J. 2021;8:e000886. https://doi.org/10.1136/bmjresp-2021-000886.

Zamparelli R, De Paulis S, Martinelli L, Rossi M, Scapigliati A, Sciarra M, Meo F, Schiavello R. Pulsatile normothermic cardiopulmonary bypass and plasma catecholamine levels. Perfusion. 2000 Jun;15(3):217–23. https://doi.org/10.1177/026765910001500306.

Monitoring the Status of Anticoagulation

15

Stanley Desire, Michelle Gorgone, and Andrew Maslow

Introduction

Cardiopulmonary bypass (CPB), a cornerstone in cardiac surgery, allows surgeons to perform life-saving procedures by temporarily taking over the heart and lungs. However, this powerful tool presents a unique challenge: the meticulous monitoring and regulation of anticoagulation.

Cardiac surgery and CPB activate the inflammatory and coagulation systems. The interaction between blood cells and the foreign surfaces of the CPB system places the patient at significant thrombotic risk via activation of pro-thrombotic factors. Anticoagulation is used to prevent thrombotic events associated with the use of an extracorporeal CPB circuit. Although CPB has been in use since the 1950s, it is only recently that evidence-based guidelines for CPB anticoagulation have been delineated. These guidelines are not just a set of instructions; they represent a culmination of decades of clinical experience, research, and technological advancements. Despite this, there is variability in the use, dosing, monitoring, and reversal of anticoagulation as it relates to surgery with CPB. Building upon the detailed exploration and foundational knowledge presented in Chap. 17, this chapter briefly revisits the anticoagulation medications, their dosing, and the rationale behind these choices. To achieve effective anticoagulation management during CPB, a variety of devices were utilized, encompassing both established and emerging point-of-care technologies. Additionally, several other devices offering various modalities for monitoring, based on non-activated clotting time (ACT) measurement, were also employed. Following the successful completion of the CPB run, meticulous attention must be paid to safe and efficient strategies for anticoagulation reversal, facilitating a seamless return to normal hemostasis.

Anticogulant Options for CPB

Although unfractionated heparin (UFH) is used in almost all patients, the details of management vary as regards dosing, patient response, and reversal. For patients with heparin-induced thrombocytopenia/thrombosis (HITT), UFH can only be used in certain circumstances, and other modalities, such as the direct thrombin inhibitors like bivalirudin and argatroban or platelet inhibitors, have to be utilized. As illustrated below in (Fig. 15.1), the anticoagulants that inhibit thrombin formation work at different points in the hemostatic pathway. For a more in-depth review of anticoagulant options, please refer to Chap. 17.

Unfractionated Heparin (UFH)

UFH is the most commonly utilized anticoagulant because it is effective, easily reversible, well tolerated, and inexpensive. Derived from porcine intestine, UFH is a sulfated glycosaminoglycan with varying polymer lengths. Its half-life ranges from 60–90 min, and it's primarily cleared by the reticuloendothelial system, with minor renal elimination.

UFH works by binding to antithrombin III (ATIII), inhibiting factors IIa and Xa, and preventing thrombin-mediated actions. For CPB, UFH is dosed at 300–500 U/kg, with the exact amount guided by point-of-care tests.

Heparin resistance, often due to ATIII deficiency, can complicate anticoagulation as UFH anticoagulant effects require ATIII as a cofactor. ATIII deficiency can be due to a variety of factors, some of which are listed below (Table 15.1). In such cases, ATIII can be replenished, or alternative antico-

S. Desire
Department of Anesthesiology & Perioperative Medicine, Massachusetts General Hospital, Boston, MA, USA
e-mail: SDesire@lifespan.org

M. Gorgone · A. Maslow (✉)
Department of Anesthesiology & Perioperative Medicine, Brown University, Providence, RI, USA

A. S. Awad, J. DiNardo (eds.), *Clinical Perfusion for Cardiac Surgery*, https://doi.org/10.1007/978-3-031-91163-7_15

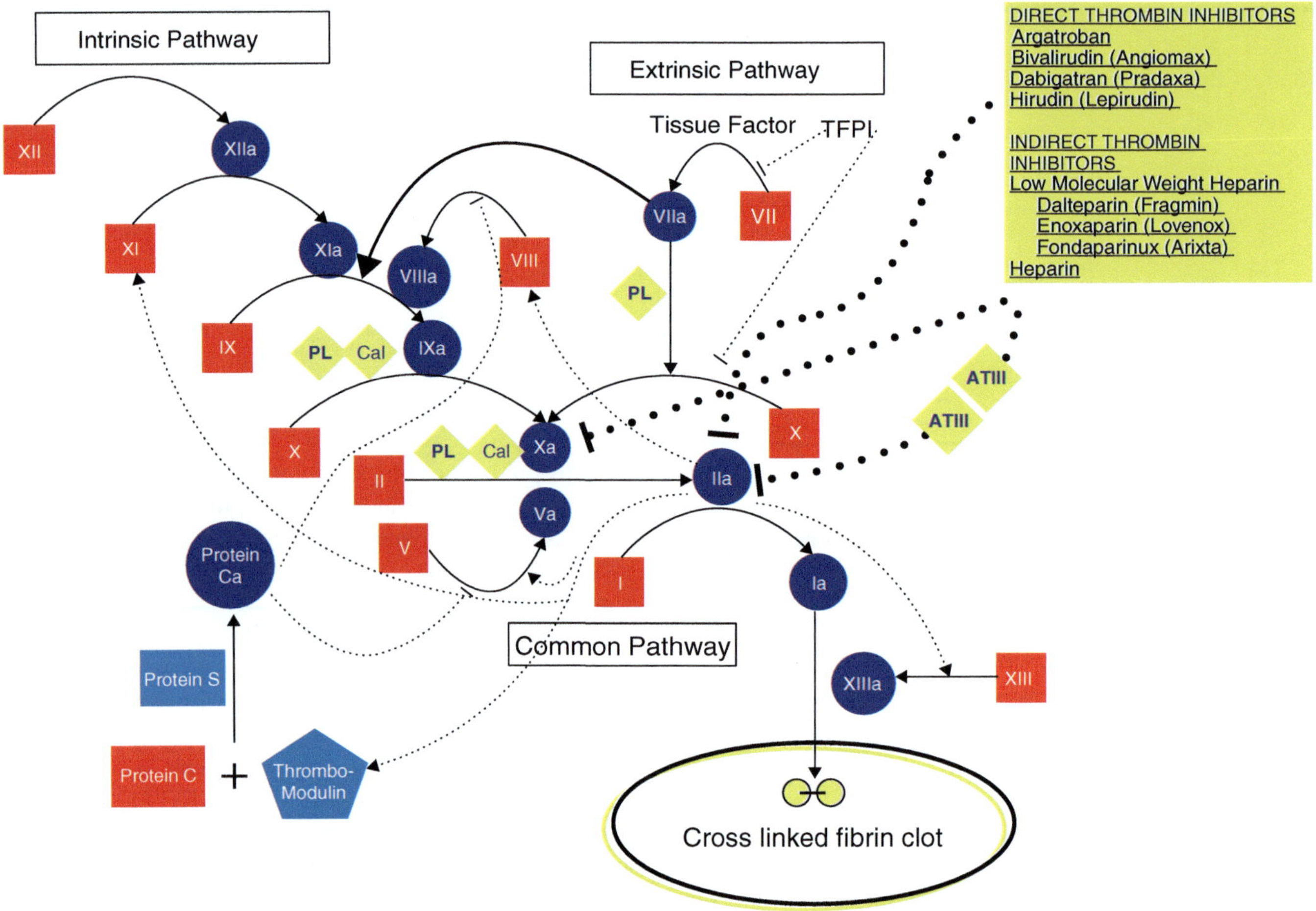

Fig. 15.1 A summary of the coagulation cascade. Factor activation is indicated by solid arrows. Inhibition is indicated by a line with a shorter line at a right angle. The extrinsic pathway (tissue factor) is activated upon endothelial cell damage and begins the cascade. Activated factor VII (VIIa) (all factors are denoted without activated notation in this figure for simplicity). VIIa catalyzes factor X to its activated form. Once factor II (thrombin) is converted from prothrombin to thrombin by Xa, it activates several coagulation factors (dotted arrows). The end goal result is conversion of inactive factor I (fibrinogen) to its active form, fibrin, so that it may from fibrin strands, crosslink via catalyzation by XIIIa, and stabilize the platelet plug that will ultimately form. Unfractionated heparin is typically administered to provide anticoagulation. Smaller heparin molecules (<18 disaccharides) can directly inhibit Xa, while an >18 disaccharides molecule's interaction with ATIII inhibits IIa. Direct thrombin inhibitors (argatroban and bivalirudin) inhibit Xa directly

Table 15.1 Causes of decreased ATIII activity

Drug induced	Increased consumption	Dilution	Decreased synthesis	Increased elimination	Other
Heparin	Disseminated intravascular coagulation	CPB	Liver dysfunction	Nephrotic syndrome	Genetic
	Sepsis				

agulants like factor Xa inhibitors, which are reversible with andexanet alfa, may be used.

Regardless of the reason, if heparin cannot be used, other anticoagulant agents should be explored.

Patients with heparin hypersensitivity or HITT require different anticoagulants. See Chap. 21 for more discussion of HITT. HITT, characterized by antibodies against heparin-platelet factor 4 complexes, leads to thrombosis and is diagnosed via immunologic and functional tests. In patients with a history of HITT with undetectable antibodies who require cardiac or vascular surgery, care must be taken to minimize exposure to heparin, using it only when necessary and for the shortest acceptable duration perioperatively. Patients who are HITT antibody positive should postpone surgery until the antibodies clear, which typically occurs after 60–90 days. If urgent or emergent cardiac or vascular surgery is needed in patients with a positive HITT antibody titer, alternative anticoagulation should be used intraoperatively.

Bivalirudin

Bivalirudin, a bivalent direct thrombin inhibitor (DTI), effectively binds to both circulating and clot-bound thrombin, unlike UFH. It is particularly useful in patients with ATIII deficiency, as it requires no cofactors. Metabolized through proteolytic cleavage and renal mechanisms, bivalirudin has a short half-life of about 25 min (see Fig. 15.1). The half-life increases significantly in patients with renal impairment. It can be used as an alternative for anticoagulation in cardiac surgery, especially in patients with HITT.

Bivalirudin rapidly induces anticoagulation, elevating aPTT, thrombin time, and ACT. However, despite ECT's better accuracy for bivalirudin levels, its lack as a point-of-care (POC) test reduces its use in cardiac surgery. ACT is used to monitor therapeutic coagulation in the OR. Bivalirudin is administered in patients with HITT undergoing cardiac surgery in lieu of UFH. Bivalirudin, primarily cleared by the kidneys, is administered using a protocol of an initial loading dose, maintenance infusion, and CPB prime. The target ACT is typically 2.5 times the baseline. To prevent thrombosis, blood pooling in the chest should be avoided and preferably directed to a cell saver.

Argatroban

Argatroban, a DTI reversibly inhibits thrombin and is monitored intraoperatively using ACT. With a half-life of about 50 min, it differs from bivalirudin in its primarily hepatic excretion, making it suitable for patients with end stage renal disease (ESRD) but requiring caution in liver disease. Limited data exist on its use in cardiac surgery with CPB, with a suggested dosing schedule in Table 15.3.

Other Alternatives

In terms of UFH alternatives in the setting of HITT and CPB, bivalirudin has the most body of evidence as a UFH alternative, but other less-studied anticoagulation options exist without consensus on their efficacy and safety in the setting of CPB. These include the removal of heparin-PF4 antibodies via plasmapheresis followed by re-administration of UFH and the use of anti-platelet agents such as the glycoprotein IIb/IIIa (GPIIb/IIIa) receptor antagonist tirofiban, the $P2Y_{12}$ inhibitor cangrelor, or intravenous epoprostenol (prostacyclin or prostaglandin I_2) with and without UFH (see Chaps. 17 and 21).

Devices for Anticoagulation Monitoring

Activated Clotting Time

The ACT, originally described in 1966 as the *Activated Coagulation Time in Whole Blood*, was performed using 1 mL of whole blood in a glass tube with diatomatous earth as a contact activator. In current practice, a small sample of whole blood is added to a cartridge or tube containing a contact activator, typically celite or kaolin, to assess the speed of clot formation initiated by the intrinsic coagulation pathway. Clot formation, as determined by the ACT represents the interaction of plasma coagulation factors, platelets, and erythrocytes. Consequently, the ACT is influenced by factors such as platelet count and platelet function, factor deficiencies, fibrinogen levels, anti-platelet and anticoagulant medications, hypothermia, and inhibitors of contact activation such as aprotinin.

Intraoperatively, ACT is the gold standard for monitoring anticoagulation for CPB. The ACT measurement is typically obtained using POC methods, with a normal ACT range of 80–130 s, though some variation is acceptable.

Determining the optimal ACT for CPB has been a subject of debate and extensive study since the 1960s. Early experiments demonstrated no clot formation in the CPB circuit when an ACT of 300 s was maintained. However, this threshold was later challenged following animal studies that detected fibrin formation on cannulae during CPB with an ACT sustained between 300 s and <350 s. Consequently, the threshold was increased to 400 s, a decision supported by safe completion of CPB in five pediatric patients with a goal of ACT ≥400 s. Currently, an ACT ≥480 s is widely adopted to ensure a safety margin above the established 400-s threshold.

There are many POC devices available to measure ACT (Fig. 15.2). The ACT result profile obtained is specific to each device, even if the same reagent is used across different devices. Thus, the target ACT ranges vary for each device. However, the concept behind all devices is the same. A sample of the patient's whole blood is activated to begin clot formation by a contact activator such as silica, kaolin, or celite. The time it takes the blood to reach a predetermined level of clot formation is the ACT. In the Hemochron Response device, 2 mL of patient whole blood is added to a glass tube containing a small iron bar at the bottom, along with the contact activator, either celite or kaolin. The device rotates the tube in alternating clockwise and counterclockwise directions through a magnetic detector. The ACT is the time it takes for stable clot formation to pull the iron bar up and away from the bottom of the tube, breaking the magnetic field. The newer Hemochron Signature Elite device uses a 0.15 mL micro-sample of the patient's blood placed on a cuvette. The device precisely mixes a combination of silica, phospholipid, and kaolin as activators with the blood sample and shuttles the mixed sample back and forth between optical sensors. It calculates the ACT based on the time it takes for the shuttling speed to decrease to a predetermined threshold, indicating increased viscosity caused by clot formation. Table 15.2 provides a list of some common POC ACT devices, along with their activators and distinguishing features.

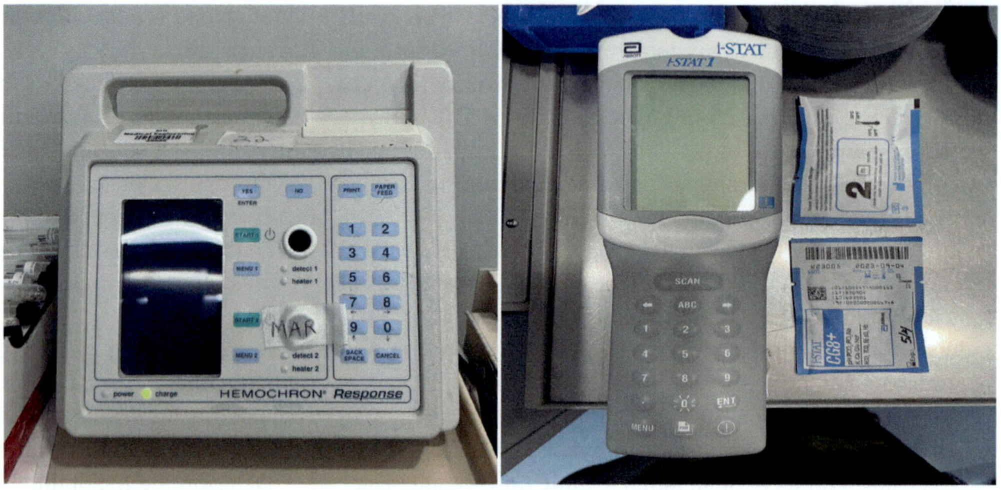

Fig. 15.2 Commonly used ACT POC devices at the author's institution. Left: Hemochron Response machine. Right: Abbott i-STAT machine with two cartridge packages shown

Table 15.2 Commonly used anticoagulation devices

Manufacturer	Device	Reagent	Comments
Werfen	Hemochron Signature line	Kaolin	Handheld, single-channel unit capable of performing several coagulation tests on whole blood
		Celite	Can compute ACT, aPTT, and PT
		Phospolipid	Has poor inter-instrument reliability
Medtronic	HMS Plus	Kaolin	A six-channel instrument that automatically dispenses a blood sample from a syringe into an assay cartridge
			Can measure HDR, heparin concentration, platelet function, ACT, and can calculate protamine dose based on a specific cartridge and patient via a whole blood sample
	ACT Plus	Kaolin	A two-channel instrument designed to calculate the ACT of whole blood
Abbott laboratories	i-STAT	Celite kaolin	A battery-operated, handheld sample analyzer that can perform various diagnostic tests on whole blood, including ACT
			Uses test-specific disposable cartridges
			Good inter-instrument reliability
			Higher cost
Helena laboratories	Cascade Abrazo	Celite	A handheld sample analyzer with an intuitive touchscreen interface
			Can be used to monitor ACT or warfarin therapy
			Not available in the US

Adapted from Bagai et al.

Table 15.3 Anticoagulant options: Dose, maintenance, goals, and reversal

Anticoagulant	Initial Dose	Maintenance	Desired ACT	Reversal
UF heparin	300–500 U/kg	Re-dose based on ACT and heparin concentration levels	>480, recheck every 30 min while on CBP	Protamine: 1 mg of protamine for every 100 U of UFH
Bivalirudin	1 mg/kg bolus +50 mg added to the CPB circuit	2.5 mg/kg/h infusion	2.5x baseline	None available: ½ life is 25 min
Argatroban	5 mg bolus	5 μg/kg/min infusion	>480	None available: ½ life is 50 min

Heparin Dose Response Relationship

The Medtronic HMS Plus (HMS Plus Hemostasis Management System®; Medtronic, Minneapolis, MN) is the only POC system currently available that can generate a patient heparin dose response (HDR) relationship. This test utilizes cartridges with increasing, predetermined UFH concentrations. Patient whole blood is added to each cartridge, and by plotting the patient's high range ACT (HR-ACT) against the known heparin concentration in each cartridge, an individualized UFH dose response curve is generated (Fig. 15.3). Generally, a minimum heparin concentration >2 U/ml, associated with an ACT >350 s, is desired prior to instituting CPB. When using the HDR-Hepcon system, the required doses of heparin and protamine to achieve therapeutic targets differ from those determined by using ACT alone.

Heparin Dose Response (HDR) Test

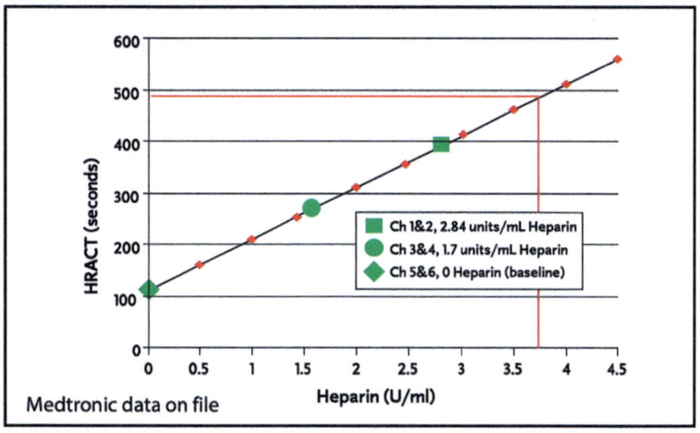

Fig. 15.3 An example of a patient HDR relation. This is used to determine the amount of UFH required to reach a target ACT in a particular patient

Other Modalities for Monitoring Anticoagulation

Given the wide variation of ACT results and differences between various technologies, alternative methods for assessing heparin activity have been considered. These methods do not directly measure the plasma concentration of UFH; instead, they are functional assays that provide indirect estimates. Such methods include anti-Xa assays and protamine sulfate titration assays. While there are assays that directly measure the plasma concentration of heparin, they are not clinically useful as they also measure heparin molecules lacking anticoagulant activity.

Anti-Xa Activity

The reference standard for monitoring of UFH's anticoagulation effects is the measurement of anti-Xa activity, as factor Xa is a key target of UFH. In the chromogenic procedure, a sample of the patient's blood is mixed with a known amount of factor Xa. The heparin in the plasma binds to ATIII and forms a complex with factor Xa. The residual factor Xa is detected by adding a substrate that is cleaved by factor Xa, releasing a colored compound that can be detected by a spectrophotometer. The amount of residual factor Xa is inversely proportional to the amount of heparin in the plasma. These assays typically incorporate an excess of ATIII, making them insensitive to ATIII deficiency in the patient's blood. While laboratory devices can effectively assay anti-Xa activity in plasma, their suitability for POC testing is limited, reducing their utility in the operating room.

Whole Blood Heparin Concentration

Relying solely on an ACT assay may result in an overestimation of heparin concentration, as factors such as hypothermia, anemia, and hypofibrinogenemia can cause falsely elevated ACT values during CPB. Therefore, using both ACT and heparin concentration assays together may help prevent the underdosing of UFH. In addition, whole blood heparin concentration assays show a closer correlation with plasma anti-Xa activity (considered the gold standard) compared to ACT assays alone. Finally, when heparin concentration assays are utilized, they have been associated with a significant reduction in thrombin formation, fibrinolysis, and neutrophil activation.

Currently, the Medtronic HMS Plus (HMS Plus Hemostasis Management System®; Medtronic, Minneapolis, MN) is the only POC system available that provides both an ACT and heparin concentration (activity) assay. The UFH concentration is determined using a heparin/protamine titration (HPT) assay. The HPT method measures clotting times, induced by kaolin and enhanced by the addition of a fixed dose of thromboplastin, in several channels containing varying concentrations of protamine. Assuming a protamine to UFH neutralization ratio of 1:1, the first channel to clot indicates the point where the protamine to UFH concentration ratio is closest to unity. From this data, the whole blood UFH concentration is determined.

Maintenance of Anticoagulation on Bypass

An ACT is typically drawn and measured 3–5 min after administering the initial bolus of UFH. An ACT is then measured every 15–20 min to ensure the target value (>400–450 s) is maintained. Some institutions redose heparin at fixed intervals in the absence of heparin concentration assays, even when ACT levels are adequate, although there is limited data to support this practice. The timing of such redosing would depend greatly on the patient's baseline ACT and heparin sensitivity.

There is less standardization regarding the non-heparin alternatives. As previously mentioned, two large studies have proposed protocols for using bivalirudin. For CPB, an initial 1 mg/kg bolus +50 mg added to the CPB circuit followed by a 2.5 mg/kg/h infusion with additional boluses as needed to maintain an ACT that is at least 2.5 times that of the baseline value. For argatroban, which is rarely used in CPB, the recommendations include a 5 mg bolus followed by 5 μg/kg/min during CPB, with a target ACT of ≥480 s.

Reversal of Anticoagulation

Perhaps the most favorable characteristic of UFH for CPB anticoagulation management is the ability to quickly fully reverse its anticoagulant effects with protamine sulfate.

There are several approaches to the neutralization of UFH with protamine.

- Reverse extrapolation. Some centers use 1.0 mg of protamine for each 100 USP units of UFH estimated to be present at the termination of CPB. This ratio is based on the in vitro protamine to UFH neutralization ratio, which ranges from 1:1 to 1.3:1. Upon CPB termination, an ACT is obtained, and reverse extrapolation of the patient's UFH dose–response curve is performed to correlate the ACT with the amount of UFH present. This method has been criticized because the ACT obtained at the termination of CPB is prolonged by factors other than UFH, such as CPB-induced platelet dysfunction and hemodilution. This could lead to an overestimation of the UFH present at the termination of CPB, resulting in a larger-than-necessary dose of protamine.
- Empiric dosing. Some centers simply administer a fixed dose. This method does not rely on any post-CPB assessment of residual UFH effect, such as ACT, to determine the protamine dose. Nonetheless, these methods have been shown to result in adequate UFH reversal. In the case of the fixed-dose regimen, UFH reversal is obtained at much lower protamine doses than predicted by the reverse extrapolation method. The protamine dose is determined either based on the patient's weight regardless of the UFH dose or by administering 1.0 mg of protamine for each 100 USP units (1.0 mg) of UFH given at the onset of CPB.
- Anti-factor Xa assay. The anti-factor Xa assay for UFH is utilized to calculate the protamine dose, considering the patient's blood volume and a neutralization ratio of 1:1, equating 1.0 mg of protamine for every 100 U of UFH. Despite the fact that not all UFH present in blood exerts an anticoagulant effect and needs to be neutralized, this method has been shown to provide adequate UFH reversal with low doses of protamine.
- In vitro protamine titration. The heparin/protamine titration test (HPT, Medtronic Hemotec®) facilitates in vitro protamine titration. The channel that clots first indicates where the protamine concentration most closely matches the heparin concentration in the patient's whole blood sample. Assuming a 1:1 protamine-to-UFH neutralization ratio, the results of this test are used in combination with an estimate of the patient's blood volume to determine the appropriate protamine dose to neutralize circulating UFH. The absolute clotting time is not important, only the determination of the channel with the appropriate protamine concentration. Therefore, the determination should be independent of non-UFH factors that prolong the ACT. This method results in adequate UFH reversal with lower doses of protamine than those predicted by the reverse extrapolation based solely on a post-CPB ACT.

Regardless of which dosing method is used, it is prudent to limit the total amount of protamine given to less than 2.6 mg of protamine per 100 U of UFH, as doses above this ratio have been shown to lead to inhibition of platelets, prolongation of ACT values, and an increased risk of bleeding. Protamine should also be given slowly to minimize hypotension caused by rapid administration. For a detailed description of the phenotypes of protamine reactions, refer to Table 11.5.

There have been documented attempts at utilizing other drugs for heparin neutralization, such as methylene blue, hexadimethrine, PF4, vancomycin, and heparinase 1, but none of these options have been proven equivalent to protamine in terms of the safety profile and efficacy. Andexanet alfa, a newer reversal agent developed for oral direct factor Xa inhibitors, has demonstrated near full reversal of UFH in in vitro studies. Although promising, further studies are needed to derive conclusive results about its efficacy.

When an alternative to UFH has been utilized for anticoagulation, there exist many challenges. For non-UFH options, finding reversal agents that offer the rapid, reliable reversal comparable to protamine for UFH remains a challenge. When DTIs are utilized, treating post-CPB coagulopathy often involves administering recombinant factor VIIa, prothrombin complex concentrates, and blood products to restore hemostasis. In addition, bivalirudin can be eliminated via ultrafiltration and dialysis when necessary (Fig. 15.3).

Further Reading

Asher S, Maslow A, Mishra V, Flaherty D, Hayward G, Whiteneck S, Cheves T, Sweeney J. A pilot study to assess the clinical onset of IV heparin in interventional cardiology and cardiac surgery. J Cardiothorac Vasc Anesth. 2022;36(12):4281–8. https://doi.org/10.1053/j.jvca.2022.07.030.

Bagai J, Beavers C. Anticoagulation monitoring during cardiac procedures: considerations for anticoagulation safety, 2020. https://scai.org/anticoagulation-monitoring-during-cardiac-procedures-considerations-anticoagulation-safety

Levy JH, Ghadimi K, Kizhakkedathu JN, Iba T. What's fishy about protamine? Clinical use, adverse reactions, and potential alternatives. J Thromb Haemost. 2023; https://doi.org/10.1016/j.jtha.2023.04.005.

Li H, Serrick C, Rao V, Yip PM. A comparative analysis of four activated clotting time measurement devices in cardiac surgery with cardiopulmonary bypass. Perfusion. 2021;36(6):610–9.

Malviya, et al. Alternatives to heparin anticoagulation for cardiopulmonary bypass and extracorporeal membrane oxygenation. Med Res Arch [S.l.]. 2021. ISSN:2375-1924. Available at: https://esmed.org/MRA/mra/article/view/2528. Date accessed Mar 24 2023;9(8) https://doi.org/10.18103/mra.v9i8.2528.

Ojito JW, Hannan RL, Burgos MM, Lim H, Huynh M, Velis E, Arocha M, Tirotta CF, Burke RP. Comparison of point-of-care activated clotting time systems utilized in a single pediatric institution. J Extra Corpor Technol. 2012;44(1):15–20.

Revelly E, Scala E, Rosner L, Rancati V, Gunga Z, Kirsch M, Ltaief Z, Rusca M, Bechtold X, Alberio L, Marcucci C. How to solve the conundrum of heparin-induced thrombocytopenia during cardiopulmonary bypass. J Clin Med. 2023;12:786. https://doi.org/10.3390/jcm12030786.

Shore-Lesserson L, Baker RA, Ferraris V, Greilich PE, Fitzgerald D, Roman P, Hammon J. STS/SCA/AmSECT clinical practice guidelines: anticoagulation during cardiopulmonary bypass. J Extra Corpor Technol. 2018;50(1):5–18.

Ural K, Owen C. Pro: the Hepcon HMS should be used instead of traditional activated clotting time (ACT) to dose heparin and protamine for cardiac surgery requiring cardiopulmonary bypass. J Cardiothorac Vasc Anesth. 2016;30(6):1727–9. https://doi.org/10.1053/j.jvca.2016.07.001.

Part V

Basics of Blood Management

Hematocrit and Transfusion Management During Cardiopulmonary Bypass

16

Dima Daaboul and James DiNardo

Introduction

The decision to transfuse erythrocytes and other blood products during the conduct of cardiopulmonary bypass (CPB) is a complicated one. In adults, there is robust data demonstrating that anemia, particularly low nadir hematocrit (Hct), during CPB is associated with increased morbidity and mortality. However, erythrocyte transfusion during CPB is also linked with high morbidity and mortality. Further complicating the decision-making is evidence that combined exposure to both anemia and erythrocyte transfusion increases the risk of adverse outcomes following cardiac surgery more than either exposure alone.

Consequences of Hemodilution

Hemodilution during hypothermic CPB has traditionally been considered advantageous because it offsets the increase in blood viscosity induced by hypothermia and promotes microvascular flow. In addition, systemic hypothermia reduces whole-body and cerebral oxygen consumption by 5–6% for each 1 °C decrease in body temperature, offsetting the reduced oxygen delivery associated with lower red cell mass and oxygen-carrying capacity. Moderate hemodilution (Hct 25%) does increase cerebral blood flow by decreasing cerebral vascular resistance, with the effect being most evident at normothermia. However, with extreme hemodilution (Hct <20%), the beneficial effects of increased cerebral blood flow are drastically outweighed by the reduction in blood oxygen-carrying capacity.

In circumstances where the volume of the CPB prime is large relative to the patient's blood volume, red cell mass, and plasma volume, an asanguineous prime may lead to an unacceptably low Hct and diminished levels of coagulation factors on CPB. In this case, erythrocytes and/or plasma may have to be added to the prime to achieve a target CPB Hct and to prevent dilution of coagulation factors. The acceptable target CPB Hct and the degree of coagulation factor dilution that is tolerated vary from institution to institution.

With currently available technology, the smallest typical CPB prime volume for neonatal use is approximately 215 mL. Estimated blood volume (EBV) based on weight is shown in Table 16.1. Given that the EBV of a 4.0 kg neonate is approximately 340 ml, 63% dilution of the patient's blood volume is expected upon initiation of CPB with this circuit.

The hematocrit on CPB can be accurately predicted in the following manner when the pump is primed with an asanguineous solution:

1. Calculate the patient red cell mass (RCM_P) using the formula:

$$\text{RCM}_{\text{P}} = \text{Patient hematocrit}(\text{Hct}) \times \text{EBV}$$

2. Determine the Hct on CPB using the formula:

$$\text{Hct on CPB} = \text{RCM}_{\text{P}} / (\text{EBV} + \text{prime volume})$$

For example, in a 4.0 kg neonate with a Hct of 40% using the circuit described above, the expected CPB Hct would be 24%.

The CPB red cell mass (RCM_{CPB}) necessary to obtain a target Hct on CPB can be determined as follows:

$$\text{RCM}_{\text{CPB}} = \left[(\text{desired Hct on CPB}) \times (\text{EBV}_{\text{P}} + \text{prime volume})\right] - \text{RCM}_{\text{P}}$$

D. Daaboul · J. DiNardo (✉)
Department of Anesthesiology, Critical Care and Pain Medicine, Cardiac Anesthesia, Boston Children's Hospital, Boston, MA, USA
e-mail: dima.daaboul@childrens.harvard.edu; James.DiNardo@childrens.harvard.edu

A. S. Awad, J. DiNardo (eds.), *Clinical Perfusion for Cardiac Surgery*, https://doi.org/10.1007/978-3-031-91163-7_16

Table. 16.1 Estimated patient blood volume based on body weight

Estimated patient blood volume	
Patient weight (kg)	Blood volume (ml/kg)
<10	85
10–20	80
20–30	75
30–40	70
>40	65

The volume of prime blood necessary to obtain a target Hct on CPB can be determined as follows:

$$\text{Volume necessary} = (\text{RCM}_{\text{CPB}}) / \text{Hct of prime blood}$$

The volume of blood prime necessary to obtain the desired RCM_{CPB} will depend on whether packed cells or whole blood are used in the prime. A unit of packed cells typically has an Hct of 70%, while a unit of whole blood typically has an Hct of 40%. The 4.0 kg neonate described here would have to have the CPB circuit primed with 75 mL of whole blood to reach a target CPB Hct of 30%.

Transfusion Thresholds—Adults

Erythrocyte transfusion thresholds to treat reduced hemoglobin (Hb) concentration during and after cardiac surgery have been evaluated in multiple institutional series and more importantly in several large, randomized trials. The important randomized trials are:

- Transfusion Requirements in Cardiac Surgery (TRICS) III
- Transfusion Indication Threshold Reduction (TITRe2)
- Transfusion Requirements After Cardiac Surgery (TRACS)
- Cleveland Clinic (USA) and SAL Hospital (India) trial

It is important to point out that only the TRICS III, TRACS, and the Cleveland Clinic trials evaluated transfusion during both CPB and in the postoperative period while the TITRe2 trial analyzed data only for postoperative erythrocyte transfusion. In the aggregate, and as demonstrated in several meta-analyses, these studies show no difference in adverse outcomes defined as acute myocardial infarction, cerebrovascular accidents, pulmonary morbidity, acute kidney injury (AKI), postoperative infection, and 30-day mortality between groups managed with a restrictive versus a liberal transfusion strategy. Across these studies, the restrictive transfusion strategy is defined as a target Hb ranging from 7.0 to 8.0 g/dL (Hct 21–24%) while the liberal strategy targets range from 8.5 g/dl in the non-ICU(intensive care unit) setting to 9.5 g/dL in the operating room or ICU (Hct 25.5–28.5%).

Hemoglobin concentration alone should not be used as a sole treatment endpoint to mitigate cardiac surgery related adverse effects. It is more physiologically sound to consider reduced Hb concentration as a component of low systemic oxygen delivery (DO_2) on CPB. DO_2 measured in mL O_2/min/m^2 is calculated as follows: Indexed Oxygen delivery = DO2i (mL/min/m²) = 10 × pump flow index (L/min/m²) × [(hemoglobin (g/dL) × SaO_2 (%) × 1.36) + (PaO_2 (mmHg) × 0.003)]

$$DO_2 = \left[\left(Hb\,g/\text{L} \times 1.34\text{mLO}_2\right)/\,g\,Hb \times SpO_2/100\right)\right] + \left[\left(PaO_2 \times 0.03\text{mLO}_2/\text{L}/\text{mmHg}\right) \times \text{Pump flow in L}/\text{min}/\text{m}^2\right]$$

In addition, the ability to measure the oxygen saturation of the venous line (SvO_2) and to calculate the oxygen extraction ratio (O_2ER), defined as VO_2/DO_2, affords an opportunity to further define the target Hb level at which to initiate erythrocyte transfusion. This is important, because both VO_2 and the DO_2 necessary to match metabolic demand decrease as body temperature decreases. It has been determined that the CPB DO_2 necessary to match metabolic demands decreases with body temperature on CPB by 23 mL/min/m^2/°C. The DO_2 necessary at 37 °C is 350 mL/min/m^2 and at 27 °C, it is 120 mL/min/m^2. Therefore, at 37 °C a Hb of 11.7 g/dL (Hct 34%) would require a CPB flow of 3 L/min/m^2, while at 27 °C a Hb of 11.7 g/dL (Hct 34%) would require a CPB flow of 1.1 L/min/m^2.

A recent study comparing mild and moderate hemodilution during CPB in adult cardiac patients favors mild hemodilution, with Hct maintained above 25%. Moderate hemodilution (Hct 21–25%) was associated with a higher incidence of postoperative neurological complications and neurocognitive dysfunction when compared to the more conservative mild hemodilution strategy. That said, the decision to transfuse erythrocytes during CPB in adults should not be based solely on absolute values, but should be individualized based on physiologic parameters and a determination of the relationship between VO_2 and DO_2. Erythrocytes should only be transfused when the Hb values fall below a threshold considered critical to maintain an adequate DO_2. As regards the prevention of AKI in adults, consensus statements recommend target DO_2 values above 280–300 mL/min/m^2. During CPB, PRBC transfusions are effective if the SvO_2 falls below 68% and/or the O_2ER exceeds 39%. Existing guidelines recommend transfusing packed red blood cells when Hct is < 18% (Hb < 6 g/dl). For Hct levels between 18-24% (Hb 6-8 g/dl), clinical indicators -including DO_2-

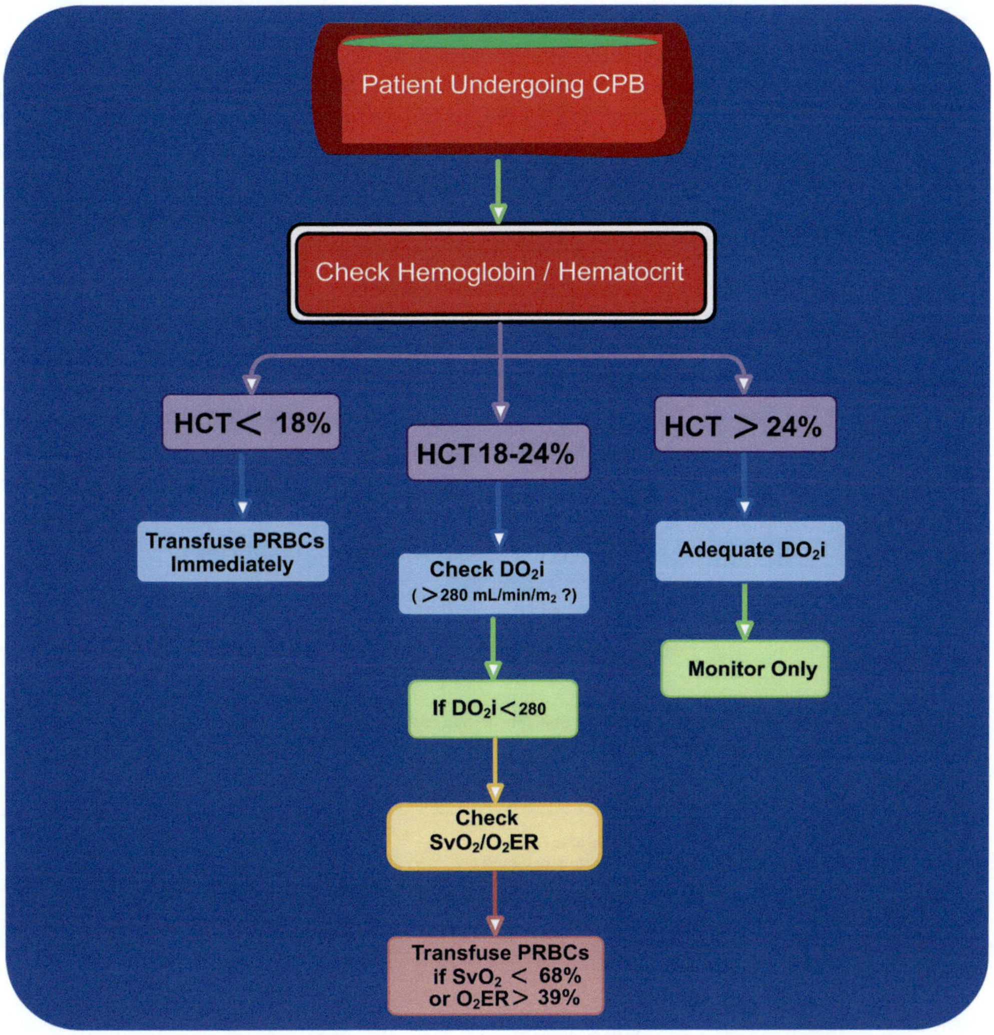

Fig. 16.1 Transfusion decision-making for adults flowchart during CPB: A step-by-step guide to assessing hematocrit levels, oxygen delivery, and clinical indicators for erythrocyte transfusion

should guide decision-making. Transfsuion is indicated if DO_2 is < 273 ml/min/m^2, SVO_2 is < 68%, and/or O_2ER > 39%. When Hct is > 24% (Hb > 8 g/dl), transfusion is generally not recommended if DO_2 is adequate, and continued monitoring is advised. see Fig. 16.1 for more illustration.

Fresh frozen plasma (FFP) should not be used prophylactically during CPB to reduce perioperative blood loss. It should only be considered to treat antithrombin deficiency and improve heparin responsiveness in the absence of antithrombin concentrate, recognizing that antithrombin III concentrate is the preferred treatment for antithrombin deficiency.

Transfusion Thresholds—Children

In 2003, a randomized trial involving 147 patients was conducted, wherein 74 infants were assigned to a lower-Hct strategy (target of 20%) at the onset of low-flow CPB and 73 to a higher-Hct strategy (target of 30%). The lower-Hct group exhibited higher intraoperative fluid balance and higher serum lactate levels 60 minutes after cessation of CPB. Additionally, they had lower nadirs of cardiac index in the first 24 hours and, at age 1 year, worse psychomotor development index (PDI) scores, although mental development index (MDI) scores were similar between groups. Because it was felt that determination of an optimal target Hct level could not be determined from these results, a second randomized trial of target Hct 25% versus 35% in a similar study population was conducted. In this trial, there were 124 patients, of whom 56 were assigned to a medium-Hct strategy (target of 25%) at the onset of low-flow CPB and 68 to a higher-Hct strategy (target of 35%). Both treatment groups had similar serum lactate levels 60 minutes after cessation of CPB, nadirs of cardiac index in the first 24 hours, PDI scores, and MDI scores, although the 25%Hct group had higher intraoperative fluid balance. The conclusion of this trial was that hemodilution to Hct levels of 35% compared with 25% had marginal clinical benefits and no increased risks.

Analysis of the data from both trials concluded that Hct level at the onset of low-flow CPB of approximately

24% or higher was associated with higher PDI scores and reduced lactate levels. Consequently, most centers generally target a Hct of approximately 25%. However, because the effects of hemodilution vary according to diagnosis, age at operation, bypass variables such as pH acid–base management strategy and flow rate, it is impossible to declare a universally "safe" hemodilution level.

In 2015, the Pediatric Critical Care *T*ransfusion and *A*nemia E*x*pertise *I*nitiative (TAXI) was created in collaboration with the Pediatric Critical Care Blood Research Network (BloodNet), the Pediatric Acute Lung Injury and Sepsis Investigators (PALISI), the AABB, and the Society for Critical Care Medicine (SCCM). It is a panel comprised of experts in pediatric critical care and transfusion medicine, organized to synthesize data regarding blood transfusion in critically ill pediatric patients or those at risk for critical illness. The panel collaborated to develop evidence-based recommendations. In areas where evidence-based recommendations could not be formulated, expert-based consensus statements were generated.

Within the TAXI recommendations, particular attention is given to patients with congenital heart disease (CHD), with specific consideration given to pathophysiologic subtypes and the presence or absence of cyanosis. However, there is no explicit guidance on the management of Hb values during CPB. Nonetheless, Fig. 16.2 illustrates how the erythrocyte transfusion thresholds for children with CHD differ from those of other critically ill children. As regards erythrocyte transfusion thresholds for children on CPB, DO_2 values greater than 350 mL/min/m^2 on CPB have been recommended to mitigate the risk of AKI. It is also considered reasonable to transfuse erythrocytes if SvO_2 is below 68% and/or the O2ER exceeds 39% once the CPB pump flow has been optimized.

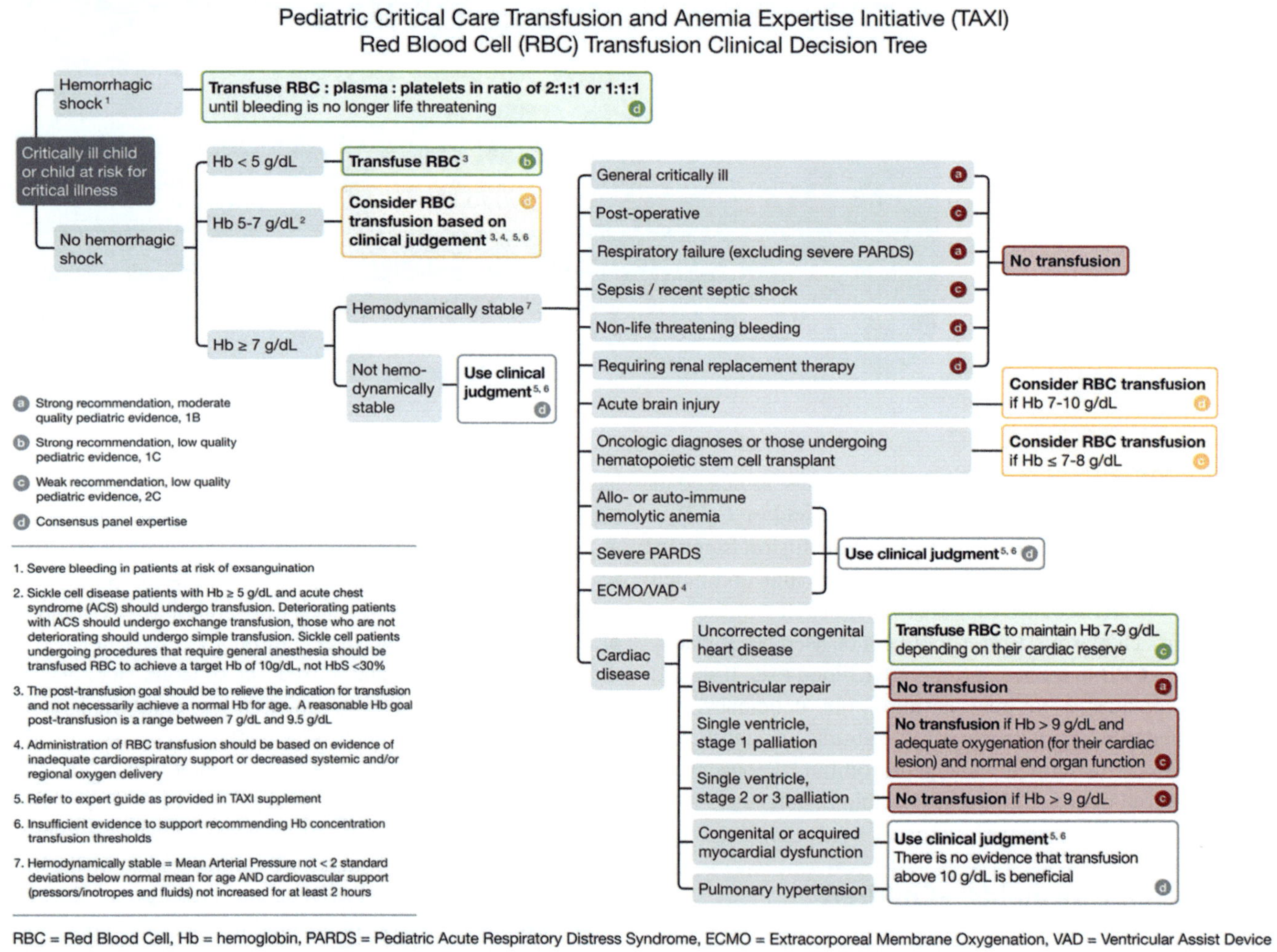

Fig. 16.2 TAXI RBC Transfusion Decision Tree for Critically Ill Children. This decision tree outlines the guidelines for erythrocyte transfusion in pediatric critical care settings, based on the recommendations by the Pediatric Critical Care TAXI. (Reproduced with permission from Valentine et al. (2018))

Strategies to Avoid Transfusion on CPB

A comprehensive review of blood conservation techniques during CPB is covered in Chap. 18. These techniques are the first step in limiting or avoiding transfusion of erythrocytes on CPB. Initial treatment during CPB to manage an Hb lower than the desired target can be reduction of hemodilution due to the CPB prime by performing hemoconcentration through removal of fluid by ultrafiltration when CPB circuit volume is adequate. It was demonstrated in one study that high-volume (>32 mL/kg) continuous ultrafiltration (CUF) during CPB increased the risk of AKI; however, this has not been substantiated in a large systemic review and meta-analysis. Nonetheless, large-volume CUF should be used cautiously, particularly in patients at risk for AKI. For more details on ultrafiltration, please refer to Chap. 19.

If further treatment is needed for a low Hb resulting in reduced DO_2, available salvaged blood and/or reinfusion of blood units harvested via normovolemic hemodilution should be undertaken prior to administration of allogeneic erythrocytes.

Further Reading

Cheruku SR, Raphael J, Neyra JA, Fox AA. Acute kidney injury after cardiac surgery: prediction, prevention, and management. Anesthesiology. 2023;139(6):880–98. https://doi.org/10.1097/ALN.0000000000004734.

Cholette JM, Willems A, Valentine SL, et al. Recommendations on RBC transfusion in infants and children with acquired and congenital heart disease from the pediatric critical care transfusion and anemia expertise initiative. Pediatr Crit Care Med. 2018;19(9S Suppl 1):S137–48. https://doi.org/10.1097/PCC.0000000000001603.

Chow JH, Mazzeffi MA, Tanaka KA. Teaching an old dog new TRICS: re-evaluating transfusion triggers in high-risk cardiac surgery. J Thorac Dis. 2018;10(2):674–7. https://doi.org/10.21037/jtd.2018.01.78.

Cook DJ, Oliver WC Jr, Orszulak TA, Daly RC, Bryce RD. Cardiopulmonary bypass temperature, hematocrit, and cerebral oxygen delivery in humans. Ann Thorac Surg. 1995;60(6):1671–7. https://doi.org/10.1016/0003-4975(95)00648-6.

Garg AX, Shehata N, McGuinness S, et al. Risk of acute kidney injury in patients randomized to a restrictive versus liberal approach to red blood cell transfusion in cardiac surgery: a substudy protocol of the transfusion requirements in cardiac surgery III noninferiority trial. Can J Kidney Health Dis. 2018;5:2054358117749532. Published 2018 Jan 3. https://doi.org/10.1177/2054358117749532.

Hajjar LA, Vincent JL, Galas FR, et al. Transfusion requirements after cardiac surgery: the TRACS randomized controlled trial. JAMA. 2010;304(14):1559–67. https://doi.org/10.1001/jama.2010.1446.

Jonas RA. Hematocrit trial. J Thorac Cardiovasc Surg. 2005;129(5):1200–2. https://doi.org/10.1016/j.jtcvs.2004.09.039.

Jonas RA, Wypij D, Roth SJ, et al. The influence of hemodilution on outcome after hypothermic cardiopulmonary bypass: results of a randomized trial in infants. J Thorac Cardiovasc Surg. 2003;126(6):1765–74. https://doi.org/10.1016/j.jtcvs.2003.04.003.

Mazer CD, Whitlock RP, Fergusson DA, et al. Restrictive or liberal red-cell transfusion for cardiac surgery. N Engl J Med. 2017;377(22):2133–44. https://doi.org/10.1056/NEJMoa1711818.

Mistry N, Shehata N, Carmona P, et al. Restrictive versus liberal transfusion in patients with diabetes undergoing cardiac surgery: an open-label, randomized, blinded outcome evaluation trial. Diabetes Obes Metab. 2022;24(3):421–31. https://doi.org/10.1111/dom.14591.

Padmanabhan H, Siau K, Curtis J, et al. Preoperative anemia and outcomes in cardiovascular surgery: systematic review and meta-analysis. Ann Thorac Surg. 2019;108(6):1840–8. https://doi.org/10.1016/j.athoracsur.2019.04.108.

Pagano D, Milojevic M, Meesters MI, et al. 2017 EACTS/EACTA Guidelines on patient blood management for adult cardiac surgery. Eur J Cardiothorac Surg. 2018;53(1):79–111. https://doi.org/10.1093/ejcts/ezx325.

Patel NN, Murphy GJ. Evidence-based red blood cell transfusion practices in cardiac surgery. Transfus Med Rev. 2017;31(4):230–5. https://doi.org/10.1016/j.tmrv.2017.06.001.

Reeves BC, Pike K, Rogers CA, et al. A multicentre randomised controlled trial of Transfusion Indication Threshold Reduction on transfusion rates, morbidity and health-care resource use following cardiac surgery (TITRe2). Health Technol Assess. 2016;20(60):1–260. https://doi.org/10.3310/hta20600.

Soliman R, Saad D, Abukhudair W, Abdeldayem S. The neurocognitive outcomes of hemodilution in adult patients undergoing coronary artery bypass grafting using cardiopulmonary bypass. Ann Card Anaesth. 2022;25(2):133–40. https://doi.org/10.4103/aca.aca_206_20.

Spiess BD. Transfusion of blood products affects outcome in cardiac surgery. Semin Cardiothorac Vasc Anesth. 2004;8(4):267–81. https://doi.org/10.1177/108925320400800402.

Tibi P, McClure RS, Huang J, et al. STS/SCA/AmSECT/SABM update to the clinical practice guidelines on patient blood management. Ann Thorac Surg. 2021;112(3):981–1004. https://doi.org/10.1016/j.athoracsur.2021.03.033.

Valentine SL, Bembea MM, Muszynski JA, et al. Consensus recommendations for RBC transfusion practice in critically ill children from the pediatric critical care transfusion and anemia expertise initiative. Pediatr Crit Care Med. 2018;19(9):884–98. https://doi.org/10.1097/PCC.0000000000001613.

Wahba A, Milojevic M, Boer C, et al. 2019 EACTS/EACTA/EBCP guidelines on cardiopulmonary bypass in adult cardiac surgery. Eur J Cardiothorac Surg. 2020;57(2):210–51. https://doi.org/10.1093/ejcts/ezz267.

Wahba Gudrun A, Filip K, Henrik De S, et al. 2024 EACTS/EACTAIC/EBCP Guidelines on cardiopulmonary bypass in adult cardiac surgery. Eur J Cardiothorac Surg. 2025;67(2). https://doi.org/10.1093/ejcts/ezae354.

Wilkinson KL, Brunskill SJ, Doree C, Trivella M, Gill R, Murphy MF. Red cell transfusion management for patients undergoing cardiac surgery for congenital heart disease. Cochrane Database Syst Rev. 2014;(2):CD009752. Published 2014 Feb 7. https://doi.org/10.1002/14651858.CD009752.pub2.

Willems A, Harrington K, Lacroix J, et al. Comparison of two red-cell transfusion strategies after pediatric cardiac surgery: a subgroup analysis. Crit Care Med. 2010;38(2):649–56. https://doi.org/10.1097/CCM.0b013e3181bc816c.

Wypij D, Jonas RA, Bellinger DC, et al. The effect of hematocrit during hypothermic cardiopulmonary bypass in infant heart surgery: results from the combined Boston hematocrit trials. J Thorac Cardiovasc Surg. 2008;135(2):355–60. https://doi.org/10.1016/j.jtcvs.2007.03.067.

Anticoagulation for Cardiopulmonary Bypass

17

Heather Lander and Michael Eaton

Hemostasis

The balanced interaction between vascular endothelium, the soluble coagulation proteins, and platelets is responsible for maintaining blood fluidity and hemostasis when vascular integrity is compromised. The coagulation cascade model, first described in the 1960s, outlines the interplay of the intrinsic and extrinsic pathways. An injury to the endovascular lining results in exposure of the extracellular matrix, which is comprised of tissue factor (TF), von Willebrand factor (vWF), collagen, and fibronectin.

The exposure of subendothelial components results in a multifactorial process. Firstly, platelets attach to the site of injury and become activated. This activation leads to a conformational change, exposing negatively charged phospholipids that serve as binding sites for plasma factors, which simultaneously release procoagulants such as fibrinogen, coagulation factors, and vWF. Glycoprotein IIb/IIIa receptors on the platelet surface are also exposed, leading to fibrinogen binding, platelet aggregation, and the formation of a platelet plug. Figure 17.1.

The plasma protein-mediated coagulation pathway is also initiated with platelet activation. Historically, the coagulation cascade was described as two separate pathways—the extrinsic and intrinsic—that converge on a common pathway, resulting in thrombin activation and the formation of an insoluble clot. However, the newer coagulation model more accurately represents the interrelatedness of the intrinsic and extrinsic pathways, regulatory proteins, and cellular elements.

The platelet plug provides an active matrix for the assembly of activated coagulation factors, resulting in the formation of an insoluble clot. The extrinsic pathway of the coagulation cascade is initiated by the exposure of subendothelial TF after vascular injury. The exposed TF binds to and activates factor VII, forming a complex. This complex then activates factors IX and X, which converge on the "final common pathway." The intrinsic pathway is initiated by the exposure of factor XII to a foreign surface, important in CPB as the circuit may serve as such a surface, resulting in the activation of XII. Activated XII then initiates a cascade by activating factor XI, which activates IX, leading to the amplification and convergence on the common pathway.

The common pathway represents convergence of intrinsic and extrinsic pathways with the activation of factor X. Activated factor X then activates factor II (prothrombin) in the presence of cofactor V, cleaving prothrombin to form thrombin. Thrombin then triggers the cleavage of fibrinogen into fibrin, and the fibrin monomers then cross-link and form a stable, insoluble clot. Thrombin also initiates other pro- and anticoagulant pathways, including the amplification of platelet activation and the activation of inhibitor protein C and fibrinolysis by plasmin. To gain a deeper understanding of the coagulation cascade, please refer to Figs. 6.2 and 15.1. These figures will provide visual aids that enhance the comprehension of the concepts presented in the respective chapters.

H. Lander (✉) · M. Eaton
Department of Anesthesiology & Perioperative Medicine, University of Rochester, Rochester, NY, USA
e-mail: heather_lander@urmc.rochester.edu; michael_eaton@urmc.rochester.edu

A. S. Awad , J. DiNardo (eds.), *Clinical Perfusion for Cardiac Surgery*, https://doi.org/10.1007/978-3-031-91163-7_17

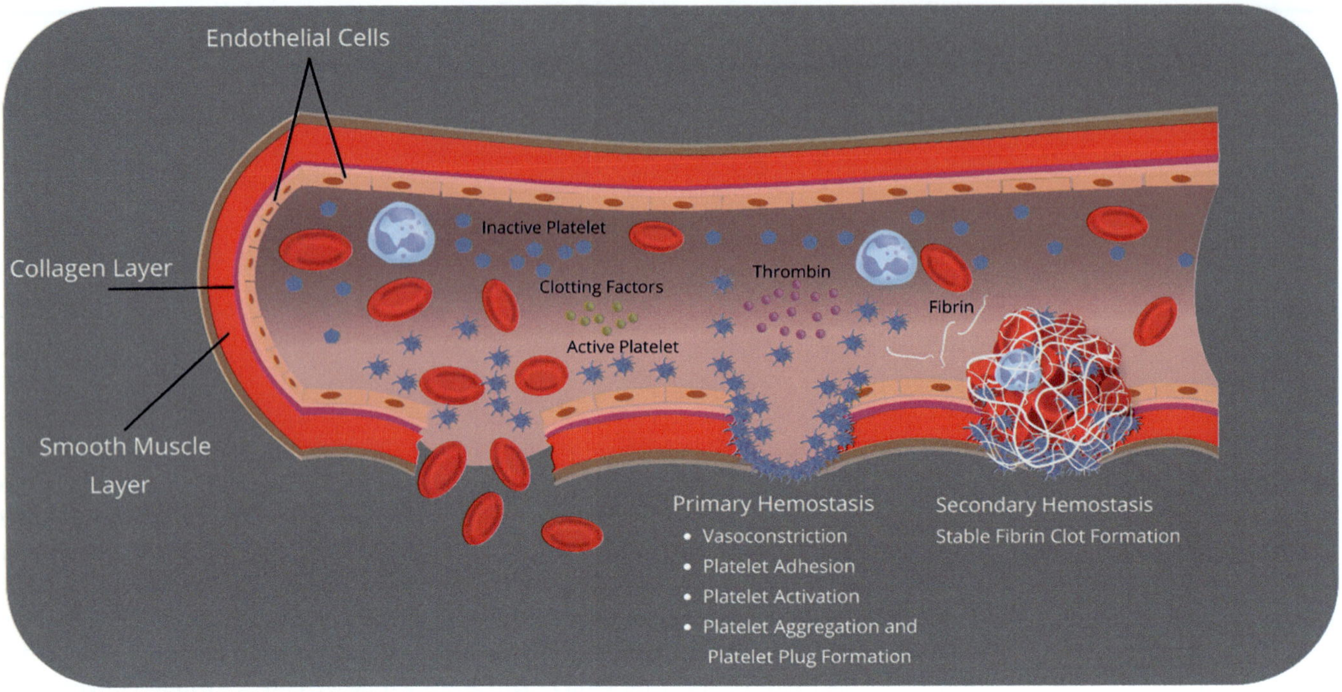

Fig. 17.1 The stages of primary and secondary hemostasis: the formation of a platelet plug followed by the development of a stable fibrin clot

Heparin

History

Heparin is the most ubiquitous and widely used anticoagulant for CPB (Fig. 17.2). It was first discovered in 1916 by Jay McLean, a medical student at the time, who found that this molecule prevented coagulation during an experiment. Subsequent studies by Chargaff and Olson identified protamine, a peptide capable of neutralizing heparin and reversing anticoagulation.

This discovery of an anticoagulant that could be quickly and reliably reversed facilitated the first successful cardiac surgery with cardiopulmonary bypass (CPB) at Jefferson Hospital in 1953. Since this historic surgery, investigators have been working to identify methods to monitor, refine, and avoid complications associated with heparin use and post-bypass bleeding.

Pharmacology

Heparin consists of acidic polysaccharides that are highly sulfated and therefore negatively charged. Heparin preparations utilized for CPB are an unfractionated mixture of molecules with a range of molecular weights, averaging around 15,000 Daltons and ranging from 3000 to 30,000 Daltons. Historically derived from animal source such as bovine lung or porcine intestinal mucosa, bovine-sourced heparin was removed from the US market in the 1990s following the outbreak of bovine spongiform encephalopathy.

Heparin's mechanism of action is primarily to potentiate and enhance the activity of antithrombin III (AT). Under normal conditions, AT is a glycoprotein that functions as a slow inhibitor of coagulation by inactivating thrombin, factor X, and factor IX. A specific pentasaccharide sequence is required for heparin to function as an anticoagulant, which is present on only approximately one-third of heparin molecules. This sequence enables heparin to bind to AT and initiate a conformational change in AT. This change converts AT to a rapid inhibitor, on the order of 1000-fold faster at inhibiting thrombin, factor X, and factor IX. While the pentasaccharide sequence alone (synthesized and marketed as fondaparinux) is capable of activating antithrombin and inhibiting factor Xa, only a molecule exceeding 5000 Daltons may simultaneously bind Xa and thrombin and strongly inhibit the latter. Heparin also binds cofactor II and slowly inactivates thrombin independent of AT, which is particularly relevant in patients with congenital AT deficiency because these patients often have a higher concentration of cofactor II.

Heparin is also known to bind platelets; however, this interaction is only partially understood. Studies have demonstrated that heparin can both activate and inhibit platelets. There appears to be a relationship between heparin molecular weight and its interaction with platelets. Low-molecular-weight heparin has minimal interaction with platelets, while high-molecular weight heparin preparations exhibit a greater degree of interaction and activation of platelets.

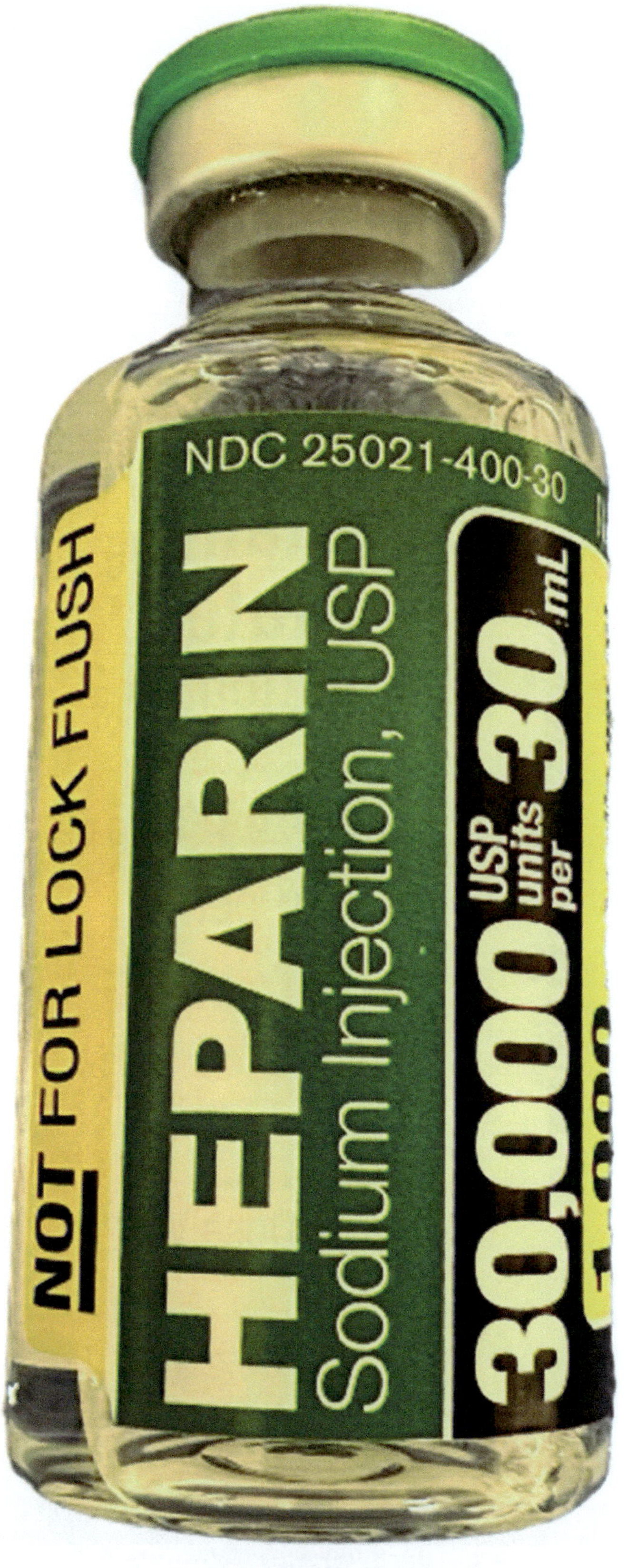

Fig. 17.2 Large vial of unfractionated heparin, containing 30,000 units, commonly used in CPB procedures

Heparin is poorly absorbed by the gastrointestinal tract, so it is administered subcutaneously for antithrombotic prophylaxis or intravenously for higher potency anticoagulation, including CPB. Its maximal anticoagulant effect occurs within 5 min of a central venous bolus. Heparin exhibits some degree of redistribution to endothelial cells, which may help explain heparin rebound following anticoagulation despite an appropriate dose of protamine for neutralization.

Heparin is primarily metabolized and cleared rapidly by endothelial cells and macrophages, which internalize and depolymerize it into smaller molecules, thereby inactivating its function. Additionally, heparin is metabolized slowly by the liver, with renal clearance of its desulfated fragments.

UFH is a heterogeneous mixture of molecules with different affinities for AT and therefore with different anticoagulant potentials. This, coupled with interindividual differences in AT activity and other factors, means that dosing must be individualized and effects measured. Additionally, heparin has a variable duration of action, as its clearance is related to molecular size. High-molecular-weight heparin molecules are cleared more rapidly than low-molecular-weight molecules, which presents challenges because the high-molecular-weight molecules are often the most active. These characteristics explain why there can be differences between the degree of anticoagulation and the quantifiable heparin level.

Dosing Considerations

Therapeutic anticoagulation for CPB with UFH is most commonly achieved by weight-based dosing. Alternatively, a dose–response titration can be performed to produce a patient-specific dosing strategy. Typically, the prime volume of the CPB pump includes heparin to prevent a drop in anticoagulant effect with initiation of CPB.

The Society of Thoracic Surgeons (STS), the Society of Cardiovascular Anesthesiologists (SCA), and the American Society of ExtraCorporeal Technology (AmSECT) published Clinical Practice Guidelines in 2018 on Anticoagulation during CPB. They recommend, as a Class IIa Recommendation (Level of Evidence C), that bolus administration of UFH based on weight is reasonable for heparin dosing and initiation.

However, they also acknowledge that individual responses to heparin are heterogeneous and require a therapeutic functional test prior to the initiation of CPB, regardless of bolus dose used.

Weight-based methods most commonly involve the bolus administration of heparin with an initial bolus of 300–400 U/kg. Given the variability in response to heparin among patients, coagulation testing should be performed prior to initiating CPB to determine the adequacy of anticoagulation. This is typically done using the activated clotting time (ACT), but other methods are available (see Chap. 15). Additional boluses of heparin are often required to maintain anticoagulation, according to the results of intermittent testing.

Bull and colleagues first identified the utility of heparin dose–response testing in the 1970s, publishing two landmark papers. These papers highlighted the inadequacy of the empirical heparin dosing prevalent at the time and demonstrated improvements in the adequacy of anticoagulation and reversal using heparin dose-response curves. They identified wide variability in heparin responsiveness and helped set the stage for the development of target anticoagulation levels for CPB. Subsequently, automated or semiautomated dose-response systems have been developed and marketed, including the Hemochron RxDx (International Technidyne, Edison, N.J.) and the Hepcon Heparin Management System (HMS) (Medtronic, Minneapolis, MN). The Hepcon HMS was adopted by many centers as a more sophisticated system to manage heparin and protamine dosing. Experience demonstrated that using the Hepcon resulted in higher heparin doses and lower protamine doses without significant effects on bleeding or transfusion.

Monitoring Methods for Anticoagulation

Monitoring adequacy of anticoagulation before, during, and after CPB is essential to avoid life-threatening complications. Please refer to Chap. 15 for in-depth discussion of this topic.

Reversal of Anticoagulation

(i) Protamine and Dosing.

Similar to the variability in heparin dosing, there is also variability in heparin reversal strategies with protamine. Protamine is a polycationic protein, alkaline in nature, obtained from the sperm of salmon and other fish. It primarily binds to and neutralizes heparin, forming a stable ion pair and ceasing heparin's anticoagulant activity (Fig. 17.3). The neutralized complex is then cleared by the reticuloendothelial system. In isolation, protamine has a weak anticoagulant effect. This consideration is crucial post-CPB as un-neutralized heparin can result in bleeding, but excessive administration of protamine in excess can also result in bleeding.

Dosing methodologies vary by institution, but there are three primary approaches: (1) Fixed protamine:heparin ratio dosing (2) ACT-based reversal methods (3) Titration method.

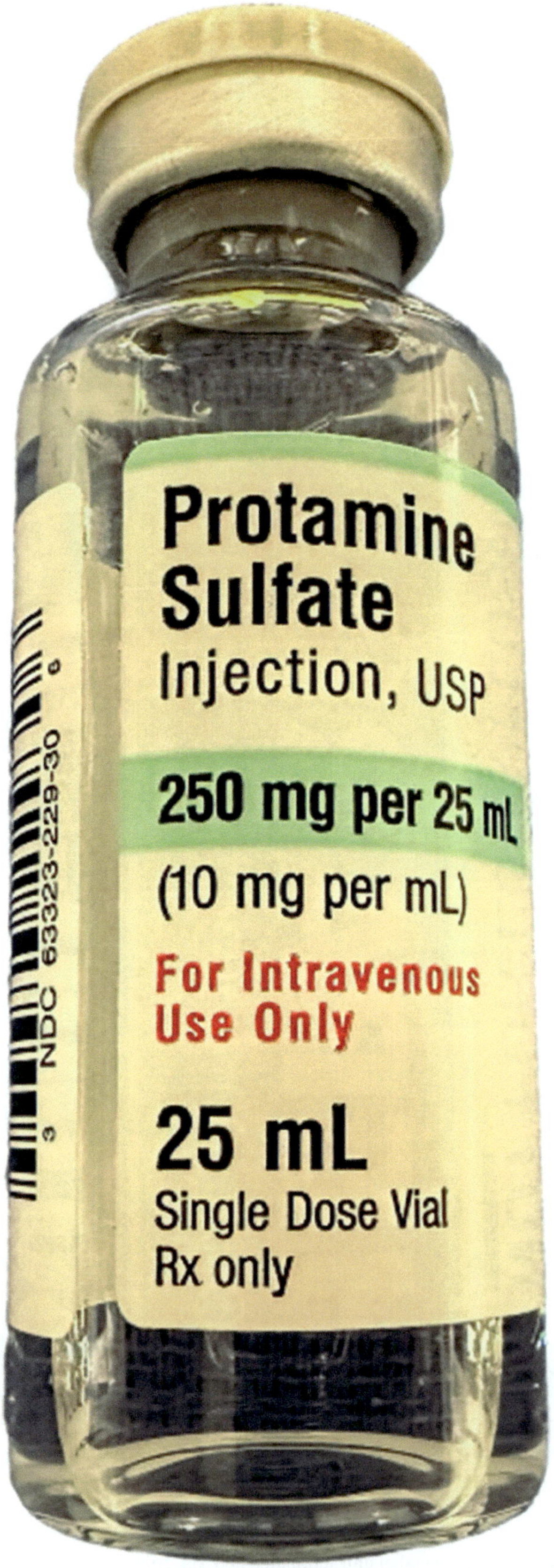

Fig. 17.3 Large vial of protamine sulfate, containing 250 mg, commonly used for heparine reversal in CPB procedures

(1) Fixed protamine:heparin ratio dosing is typically based upon a set ratio of initial heparin dose in a 1:1 ratio. For example, 1 mg of protamine is administered for every 100 U of heparin administered before initiation of CPB. This is arguably the simplest approach. However, it can result in an overdose of protamine administration as heparin is metabolized over time or in an underdose if additional heparin was administered while on CPB, which is not accounted for in this model.

According to the STS/SCA/AmSECT Clinical Practice Guidelines, a Class IIa recommendation (Level of Evidence C) suggests keeping the protamine/heparin ratio below 2.6 mg of protamine per 100 units of heparin. Exceeding this ratio may compromise platelet function, prolong ACT, and increase the risk of bleeding.

(2) ACT-based reversal methods, first described by Bull et al. in the 1970s, determine the protamine dose by considering the patient's weight, initial heparin dose, and ACT level at baseline, before CPB, and before administering protamine. However, since ACT values don't consistently align with heparin levels during CPB, this method might not yield a more accurate dose than the fixed ratio approach. Studies have found no significant differences in total blood loss or transfusion requirements with this method.

(3) The titration method employs an automated technique to determine protamine dosing. It calculates the patient's heparin level by mixing blood samples with increasing concentrations of protamine across multiple channels. The first channel to clot indicates the optimal protamine dose for neutralizing the patient's heparin. According to the 2018 STS/SCA/AmSECT Clinical Practice Guidelines, using this titration method to calculate the protamine dose for heparin reversal is advantageous. This approach is linked to decreased bleeding and reduced blood transfusion needs (Class IIa Recommendation, Level of Evidence B).

(ii) Heparin Rebound and Management:

In cases of prolonged CPB or when high doses of heparin are administered, heparin rebound may occur. This phenomenon is characterized by detectable blood levels of heparin after apparent neutralization by protamine, likely attributed to heparin's retention in body fat and plasma proteins. Notably, this rebound is prominent with heparin doses exceeding 400 IU/kg, necessitating higher doses of protamine for effective reversal. This persistence of heparin is observable immediately, as well as 2–4 h after protamine administration, as confirmed by anti-Xa and viscoelastic measurements. However, standard monitoring methods such as ACT and activated partial thromboplastin time (APTT) often fail to detect this residual heparin. Clinically, the implementation of a continuous protamine infusion post-CPB has been shown to significantly reduce chest tube blood loss, although it does not necessarily decrease the need for blood transfusions. The 2018 STS/SCA/AmSECT Clinical Practice Guidelines recommend managing heparin rebound with a Class IIb Recommendation. This involves administering a low-dose protamine infusion, specifically at 25 mg/h, for up to 6 h following the conclusion of CPB, as part of a comprehensive blood conservation strategy (Level of Evidence C).

(iii) Alternatives

While protamine is the only available drug used to reverse heparin, the alternatives that have been investigated include platelet factor 4 (PF4), methylene blue, hexadimethrine, vancomycin, and heparinase I.

1. PF4, a natural polypeptide, found in platelets alpha granules, effectively reverses heparin anticoagulation after CPB and may cause fewer allergic reactions.
2. Heparinase I is an enzyme from *Favobacterium heparinum*, also reverses heparin by breaking it into smaller fragments.

Despite these investigations, no alternative has yet matched protamine's safety in reversing heparin after CPB.

Heparin Resistance

Heparin resistance is defined by the need to administer a larger dose of heparin to attain an appropriate level of anticoagulation for CPB. While there is no clear cutoff, heparin resistance is indicated if a patient has received ≥500–600 U/kg of heparin and fails to achieve the target ACT. Depending on the degree, heparin resistance may or may not need to be treated prior to the initiation of CPB.

There are both clinical and patient factors that increase the risk of a patient experiencing heparin resistance. These include acquired and congenital AT deficiency, thrombocytosis, and sepsis.

AT deficiency can be either acquired or congenital and is defined by an AT level below 80%. Acquired AT deficiency, more common than congenital, often results from decreased hepatic synthesis (due to liver pathology), increased excretion (gastrointestinal or renal pathology), increased consumption (as in disseminated intravascular coagulation), dilution, or drug induction. Congenital AT deficiency, which is autosomal dominant, includes Type I, a quantitative defect leading to reduced AT concentration, and Type II, a qualitative defect that results in non-functional AT. Congenital AT deficiency is often clinically manifested by recurrent venous thromboembolism at a young age, often following an infection, surgery, or pregnancy.

Thrombocytosis can also result in heparin resistance. Platelets bind and degranulate upon contacting the nonendothelial surface of the bypass circuit, releasing platelet factor 4 (PF4), a cationic substance that potentiates platelet aggregation and neutralizes the anticoagulant effect of heparin-AIII complexes. This reaction can necessitate higher heparin dosing to overcome the pro-coagulant effect. Similarly, in sepsis, activated neutrophils release a multitude of heparin-binding proteins, reducing the amount of bioavailable heparin. Treating the underlying cause of sepsis, in combination with administering additional heparin, is essential.

Historically, AT deficiency was treated with administration of fresh frozen plasma (FFP); however, the risks of transfusion-related reactions and infection were not negligible. Two formulations of AT concentrate are available in the USA: recombinant antithrombin III, which is genetically engineered and derived from the milk of goats modified to produce human antithrombin, and AT concentrate, a preservative-free, lyophilized preparation sourced from human serum. They are the preferred treatment for AT deficiency-induced heparin resistance.

The management of heparin resistance often varies by institution but typically includes four potential interventions. The first is simply to administer additional heparin. If that fails to raise the ACT acceptably, a second step would be to administer AT concentrate. If the ACT remains subtherapeutic, administration of FFP may be considered. A final consideration would be whether to utilize an alternative anticoagulant or accept the subtherapeutic ACT and proceed with CPB without further intervention. A randomized controlled study by Koster et al., published in 2003, found that treating heparin resistance with AT, hirudin, or tirofiban decreased fibrin generation compared to no additional treatment.

Heparin-Induced Thrombocytopenia

(i) Heparin-induced thrombocytopenia (HIT) is a serious immune-mediated condition where heparin-PF4 complexes cause platelet aggregation and thrombocytopenia, often leading to widespread intravascular thrombosis and potential end-organ damage. Approximately 5–10% of hospitalized patients with HIT die due to related complications, making prompt diagnosis and treatment vital.

(a) *Pathophysiology of HIT*

HIT involves the formation of immunoglobulin G antibodies that bind ultra-large complexes of heparin and PF4. These large immune complexes bind to Fc receptors on platelets and monocytes, triggering cellular activation and release of pro-coagulant molecules, producing a pro-thrombotic state often resulting in both venous and arterial thrombosis.

(b) *Diagnosis of HIT*

The classic feature of HIT is a reduction in platelet count of more than 30% compared to baseline that occurs between 5 and 10 days after the start of heparin. HIT immunoglobulin G antibodies are short-lived and typically persist for 40–100 days before declining. Re-exposure to heparin after initial HIT takes 4–10 days for new antibody formation.

Diagnosis involves both clinical and laboratory assessments. Clinically, the 4Ts scoring system is commonly used (Table 17.1). A low score on this system highly negates HIT, while a high score necessitates further testing. The initial laboratory tests include HIT antibodies using an immunoglobulin G-specific immunoassay such as the enzyme-linked immunosorbent assay (ELISA). High optical density in ELISA strongly indicates HIT, but confirmatory

Table 17.1 4Ts scoring system for HIT probability assessment

4T's Categories	0 points	1 point	2 points
Thrombocytopenia (decrease in platelets)	Nadir $<10^9/l$ <30%	Nadir 10–$19^9/l$ 30–50%	Nadir $\geq 20^9/l$ >50%
Timing of platelet decrease	≤4 days without recent exposure	5–10 day decrease, but not clear After 10 days ≤1 day if previous heparin exposure in past 30–100 days	Clear onset 5–10 days ≤1 day if previous heparin exposure within 30 days
Thrombosis or other sequelae	None	Progressive thrombosis Non-necrotizing skin lesions Suspected thrombosis (not proven)	New, confirmed thrombosis Skin necrosis Acute systemic reaction after IV heparin bolus
Other causes of thrombocytopenia	Definite	Possible	None

Probability Score: Low Probability: 1–3 points, Intermediate Probability: 4–5 points, High Probability: 6–8 points tests such as the serotonin release assay or heparin-induced platelet aggregation assay are recommended, though not always available.

Once HIT has been diagnosed, treatment is focused on mitigating the severity of thrombosis. This involves stopping all heparin exposure and initiating an alternative, non-heparin anticoagulant. Often, platelet counts begin to recover in 48–72 h and return to baseline within 2 weeks. Clinical bleeding is rare, and caution should be taken with administering platelets, as this can precipitate thrombosis in patients with HIT. Additionally, a non-heparin anticoagulant should be started, and the primary choices are the direct thrombin inhibitors such as lepirudin, argatroban, and bivalirudin. The patient should be on a direct thrombin inhibitor until platelets have stabilized at or above 150,000/mm^3 at which time the patient can be initiated on warfarin.

Heparin Alternatives

(a) Heparin remains the primary method of anticoagulation for CPB. However, there are clinical situations, such as active HIT, heparin, or protamine allergy, where the use of heparin and/or protamine is contraindicated, and an alternative anticoagulant strategy is necessary. Danaparoid, ancrod, hirudin, and synthetic hirulogs have been explored as alternatives.

(i) Danaparoid, derived from heparin production, combines heparin sulfate, dermatan sulfate, and chondroitin sulfate. Its anti-Xa activity has a half-life of 25 h and minimal heparin cross-reactivity. It is used in CPB for HIT patients. Danaparoid's lack of a reversal medication and only partial correction of coagulation with FFP and platelets make it challenging for CPB use. It was discontinued in the US market in 2002.

(ii) Ancrod, a defibrinogenating agent from pit viper venom. It affects fibrinogen and fibrin formation, with an initial half-life of 3–5 h. Achieving full anticoagulation for CPB can take up to 12 h, requiring significant FFP and cryoprecipitate for reversal. Ancrod is no longer marketed in the USA.

(iii) Hirudin, a protein from leech saliva, is a direct thrombin inhibitor (DTI) used in CPB. It prevents clot formation and was available as recombinant hirudin (Refludan) until 2012. Its half-life is around 30–60 min, and ACT or APTT can monitor low concentrations used for treating HIT. However, the higher concentrations needed for CPB require alternate monitoring, such as the unavailable ecarin clotting time. While used in human CPB, its association with excessive postoperative bleeding limits its practical use.

(iv) Synthetic DTIs such bivalirudin and argatroban have been used as alternatives to heparin for anticoagulation for CPB in humans.

1. *Bivalirudin* is a synthetic peptide analogue of hirudin that binds both the catalytic site and the anion binding site of thrombin. It has a relatively short 25-min half-life and is primarily metabolized by enzymatic degradation in the plasma with enough renal excretion that impaired glomerular filtration significantly prolongs its duration of action. Bivalirudin is the most commonly used alternative to heparin for patients undergoing cardiac surgery and is recommended for this purpose in national guidelines. Reported experience with bivalirudin suggests that problems with thrombosis and bleeding are common. Initial Bivalirudin Administration: Administer a 1 mg/kg bolus dose followed by adding 50 mg to the CPB circuit. For maintenance, infuse at a rate of 2.5 mg/kg/hr.
2. *Argatroban* is a univalent non-peptide DTI that inhibits thrombin by binding to its catalytic site. Argatroban is eliminated primarily via hepatobiliary metabolism and thus may be preferred in patients with renal insufficiency. Its elimination half-life is approximately 45 min. Published use of argatroban in CPB is limited to a few case reports and a small case series. Complications, including both thrombosis and excessive bleeding, are described in most cases. Initial Argatroban Dosing: Begin with a 5 mg bolus dose, followed by a maintenance infusion at a rate of 5 µg/kg/min.

Both bivalirudin and argatroban result in a concentration-dependent inhibition of both free and clot-bound thrombin, contributing not only to prevention of clot formation but also decreasing the stability of existing thrombi and promoting fibrinolysis. Monitoring anticoagulation for both drugs during CPB is covered in detail in Chap. 15, "Monitoring the Status of Anticoagulation." Both agents lack a reversal agent, and elimination may be enhanced somewhat with dialysis of modified ultrafiltration. Although these medications have been found effective for anticoagulation for CPB for the most part, bleeding and thrombotic complications are common and limit their use beyond urgent necessity.

(v) *Platelet Inhibitor*

Since the pathophysiology of HIT involves diffuse platelet activation and aggregation, it is possible to prevent thrombosis when using heparin for CPB in a patient with HIT by first administering a potent platelet inhibitor. This strategy has been used successfully in a few case reports and small case series using several different platelet inhibitors, including cangrelor, tirofiban, iloprost, and epoprostenol. While the limited data show this to be a viable strategy for successful CPB, numbers are too small to evaluate safety.

(vi) Recently, therapeutic plasma exchange (TPE) or plasmapheresis has gained acceptance as a therapy for patients with HIT requiring CPB. TPE decreases HIT antibody titers by 50–84% and allows the use of conventional heparin anticoagulation with ACT monitoring. This simplifies CPB management compared to using bivalirudin. A case series from Duke involving 24 HIT patients managed with TPE reported successful CPB and surgeries without intraoperative incidents. However, two patients experienced postoperative thromboembolic events potentially linked to HIT. TPE requires complex equipment and expertise, takes several hours to decrease HIT antibody levels, and may not be well tolerated in hemodynamically tenuous patients. TPE is a promising therapy for HIT patients needing CPB, but appropriate use, potentially including additional TPE or anticoagulation with a DTI postoperatively, requires further study.

Coagulation Adjuvants

Cardiac surgery involving CPB activates coagulation, inflammation, and fibrinolysis (see Chap. 6). Fibrinolysis significantly contributes to postoperative blood loss and the subsequent need for transfusion. Inhibiting fibrinolysis is, therefore, a critical component of blood loss management. Chap. 18 details blood conservation strategies and coagulation adjuvants used in cardiac surgery involving CPB, emphasizing the importance of fibrinolysis inhibition in managing postoperative blood loss and reducing transfusion requirements. Key pharmacologic strategies include:

- *Antifibrinolytics:* These agents, essential for inhibiting fibrinolysis and subsequent fibrin degradation, have proven effective in reducing transfusion requirements.
  - *Aprotinin:* A serine protease inhibitor, aprotinin faced controversy over safety concerns and was temporarily removed from the market. It is no longer available in the USA.
  - *Tranexamic acid (TA) and epsilon aminocaproic acid (EACA):* These widely used synthetic lysine derivatives prevent excessive plasmin formation, thereby reducing bleeding and transfusion needs. TA, being more potent, is associated with a higher risk of seizures at elevated doses.

    For a comprehensive understanding, refer to Chap. 18 for an in-depth discussion on these strategies.

Summary

Anticoagulation for CPB remains primarily achieved with heparin as an anticoagulant and protamine to reverse its effect. Monitoring is most commonly accomplished with the ACT utilizing cartridge-based technology. Clinical practice guidelines published in 2018 remain a reliable evidence-based guide. It is imperative to consider individualized approaches for high-risk patients given the complex interaction of inflammation, coagulation, and fibrinolysis during CPB. Further research is necessary to develop and refine alternative anticoagulants and reversal agents for patients with contraindications to heparin and protamine.

Further Reading

Achneck HE, Sileshi B, Parikh A, Milano CA, Welsby IJ, Lawson JH. Pathophysiology of bleeding and clotting in the cardiac surgery patient: from vascular endothelium to circulatory assist device surface. Circulation. 2010;122(20):2068–77.

Ammar T, Fisher CF. The effects of heparinase 1 and protamine on platelet reactivity. Anesthesiology. 1997;86(6):1382–6.

Andersson LO, Barrowcliffe TW, Holmer E, Johnson EA, Söderström G. Molecular weight dependency of the heparin potentiated inhibition of thrombin and activated factor X. Effect of heparin neutralization in plasma. Thromb Res. 1979;15(3–4):531–41.

Barrowcliffe TW. History of heparin. Handb Exp Pharmacol. 2012;207:3–22.

Boer C, Meesters MI, Veerhoek D, Vonk ABA. Anticoagulant and side-effects of protamine in cardiac surgery: a narrative review. Br J Anaesth. 2018;120(5):914–27.

Boneu B, Caranobe C, Sie P. Pharmacokinetics of heparin and low molecular weight heparin. Baillieres Clin Haematol. 1990;3(3):531–44.

Broadwin M, Grant PE, Robich MP, et al. Comparison of intraoperative tranexamic acid and epsilon-aminocaproic acid in cardiopulmonary bypass patients. JTCVS Open. 2020;3:114–25.

Bull BS, Huse WM, Brauer FS, Korpman RA. Heparin therapy during extracorporeal circulation. II. The use of a dose-response curve to individualize heparin and protamine dosage. J Thorac Cardiovasc Surg. 1975a;69(5):685–9.

Bull BS, Korpman RA, Huse WM, Briggs BD. Heparin therapy during extracorporeal circulation. I. Problems inherent in existing heparin protocols. J Thorac Cardiovasc Surg. 1975b;69(5):674–84.

Cartwright B, Mundell N. Anticoagulation for cardiopulmonary bypass: part one. BJA Educ. 2023a;23(3):110–6.

Cartwright B, Mundell N. Anticoagulation for cardiopulmonary bypass, part 2: alternatives and pathological states. BJA Educ. 2023b;23(7):256–63.

Chan T, Hwang NC, Lim CH. A statistical analysis of factors predisposing patients to heparin resistance. Perfusion. 2006;21(2):99–103.

Chargaff EOK. Studies on the chemistry of blood coagulation. J Biol Chem. 1937;122:153–67.

Chen Y, Phoon PHY, Hwang NC. Heparin resistance during cardiopulmonary bypass in adult cardiac surgery. J Cardiothorac Vasc Anesth. 2022;36(11):4150–60.

Cohn LH. Fifty years of open-heart surgery. Circulation. 2003;107(17):2168–70.

Crawley JT, Zanardelli S, Chion CK, Lane DA. The central role of thrombin in hemostasis. J Thromb Haemost. 2007;5(Suppl 1):95–101.

DeAnda A Jr. Aprotinin and cardiac surgery. J Thorac Cardiovasc Surg. 2008;135(3):492–4.

Demma L, Levy JH. A case series of recombinant platelet factor 4 for heparin reversal after cardiopulmonary bypass. Anesth Analg. 2012;115(6):1273–8.

Dyke CM, Smedira NG, Koster A, et al. A comparison of bivalirudin to heparin with protamine reversal in patients undergoing cardiac surgery with cardiopulmonary bypass: the EVOLUTION-ON study. J Thorac Cardiovasc Surg. 2006;131(3):533–9.

Follis F, Filippone G, Montalbano G, et al. Argatroban as a substitute of heparin during cardiopulmonary bypass: a safe alternative? Interact Cardiovasc Thorac Surg. 2010;10(4):592–6.

Gundry SR, Drongowski RA, Coran AG, Kirsh MM, Klein MD. Failure of automated protamine titration to determine the protamine reversal dose of systemic heparin: comparison with other methods. Curr Surg. 1986;43(2):110–2.

Guo Y, Tang J, Du L, et al. Protamine dosage based on two titrations reduces blood loss after valve replacement surgery: a prospective, double-blinded, randomized study. Can J Cardiol. 2012;28(5):547–52.

Hage A, Louzada M, Kiaii B. Sepsis-induced heparin resistance during extracorporeal membrane oxygenation. CMAJ. 2019;191(10):E283–e285.

Hirsh J. Heparin. N Engl J Med. 1991;324(22):1565–74.

Hoffman MM, Monroe DM. Rethinking the coagulation cascade. Curr Hematol Rep. 2005;4(5):391–6.

Hogan M, Berger JS. Heparin-induced thrombocytopenia (HIT): review of incidence, diagnosis, and management. Vasc Med. 2020;25(2):160–73.

Koster A, Fischer T, Gruendel M, et al. Management of heparin resistance during cardiopulmonary bypass: the effect of five different anticoagulation strategies on hemostatic activation. J Cardiothorac Vasc Anesth. 2003;17(2):171–5.

Koster A, Faraoni D, Levy JH. Argatroban and Bivalirudin for perioperative anticoagulation in cardiac surgery. Anesthesiology. 2018;128(2):390–400.

Koster A, Nagler M, Erdoes G, Levy JH. Heparin-induced thrombocytopenia: perioperative diagnosis and management. Anesthesiology. 2022;136(2):336–44.

Lemmer JH Jr, Despotis GJ. Antithrombin III concentrate to treat heparin resistance in patients undergoing cardiac surgery. J Thorac Cardiovasc Surg. 2002;123(2):213–7.

Levi M, Cromheecke ME, de Jonge E, et al. Pharmacological strategies to decrease excessive blood loss in cardiac surgery: a meta-analysis of clinically relevant endpoints. Lancet. 1999;354(9194):1940–7.

Levy JH, Cormack JG, Morales A. Heparin neutralization by recombinant platelet factor 4 and protamine. Anesth Analg. 1995;81(1):35–7.

Linkins LA, Dans AL, Moores LK, et al. Treatment and prevention of heparin-induced thrombocytopenia: antithrombotic therapy and prevention of thrombosis, ninth ed.: American College of Chest Physicians Evidence-Based Clinical Practice Guidelines. Chest. 2012;141(2 Suppl):e495S–530S.

Northam KA, Parker WF, Chen SL, et al. Evaluation of 4Ts score inter-rater agreement in patients undergoing evaluation for heparin-induced thrombocytopenia. Blood Coagul Fibrinolysis. 2021;32(5):328–34.

Nuttall GA, Smith MM, Smith BB, Christensen JM, Santrach PJ, Schaff HV. A blinded randomized trial comparing standard activated clotting time Heparin management to high target active clotting time and individualized Hepcon HMS Heparin management in cardiopulmonary bypass cardiac surgical patients. Ann Thorac Cardiovasc Surg. 2022;28(3):204–13.

Olin DA, Urdaneta F, Lobato EB. Use of danaparoid during cardiopulmonary bypass in patients with heparin-induced thrombocytopenia. J Cardiothorac Vasc Anesth. 2000;14(6):707–9.

O-Yurvati AH, Laub GW, Southgate TJ, McGrath LB. Heparinless cardiopulmonary bypass with ancrod. Ann Thorac Surg. 1994;57(6):1656–8.

Rao LV, Rapaport SI. Activation of factor VII bound to tissue factor: a key early step in the tissue factor pathway of blood coagulation. Proc Natl Acad Sci USA. 1988;85(18):6687–91.

Revelly E, Scala E, Rosner L, et al. How to solve the conundrum of Heparin-induced thrombocytopenia during cardiopulmonary bypass. J Clin Med. 2023;12(3):786.

Riess FC, Poetzsch B, Madlener K, et al. Recombinant hirudin for cardiopulmonary bypass anticoagulation: a randomized, prospective, and heparin-controlled pilot study. Thorac Cardiovasc Surg. 2007;55(4):233–8.

Runge M, Møller CH, Steinbrüchel DA. Increased accuracy in heparin and protamine administration decreases bleeding: a pilot study. J Extra Corpor Technol. 2009;41(1):10–4.

Shigeta O, Kojima H, Hiramatsu Y, et al. Low-dose protamine based on heparin-protamine titration method reduces platelet dysfunction after cardiopulmonary bypass. J Thorac Cardiovasc Surg. 1999;118(2):354–60.

Shore-Lesserson L, Reich DL, DePerio M. Heparin and protamine titration do not improve haemostasis in cardiac surgical patients. Can J Anaesth. 1998;45(1):10–8.

Shore-Lesserson L, Baker RA, Ferraris VA, et al. The society of thoracic surgeons, the society of cardiovascular anesthesiologists, and the American society of ExtraCorporeal technology: clinical practice guidelines-anticoagulation during cardiopulmonary bypass. Anesth Analg. 2018;126(2):413–24.

Sniecinski RM, Chandler WL. Activation of the hemostatic system during cardiopulmonary bypass. Anesth Analg. 2011;113(6):1319–33.

Stafford-Smith M, Lefrak EA, Qazi AG, et al. Efficacy and safety of heparinase I versus protamine in patients undergoing coronary artery bypass grafting with and without cardiopulmonary bypass. Anesthesiology. 2005;103(2):229–40.

Staples MH, Dunton RF, Karlson KJ, Leonardi HK, Berger RL. Heparin resistance after preoperative heparin therapy or intraaortic balloon pumping. Ann Thorac Surg. 1994;57(5):1211–6.

T. S. Patient Blood Management: Coagulation. In: Miller's Anesthesia. 8th ed. Philadelphia: Elsevier:1868–1880.

von Segesser LK, Mueller X, Marty B, Horisberger J, Corno A. Alternatives to unfractionated heparin for anticoagulation in cardiopulmonary bypass. Perfusion. 2001;16(5):411–6.

Walenga JM, Bakhos M, Messmore HL, et al. Comparison of recombinant hirudin and heparin as an anticoagulant in a cardiopulmonary bypass model. Blood Coagul Fibrinolysis. 1991;2(1):105–11.

Wanat-Hawthorne A, Tanaka K, Angona R, Feng C, Eaton M. Survey of practice pattern in patients with Heparin-induced thrombocytopenia requiring cardiopulmonary bypass. Anesth Analg. 2021;133(5):1180–6.

Wang J, Ma HP, Zheng H. Blood loss after cardiopulmonary bypass, standard vs titrated protamine: a meta-analysis. Neth J Med. 2013;71(3):123–7.

Weiss HJ, Turitto VT, Baumgartner HR, Nemerson Y, Hoffmann T. Evidence for the presence of tissue factor activity on subendothelium. Blood. 1989;73(4):968–75.

Westaby S. Aprotinin: twenty-five years of claim and counterclaim. J Thorac Cardiovasc Surg. 2008;135(3):487–91.

Wilcox JN, Smith KM, Schwartz SM, Gordon D. Localization of tissue factor in the normal vessel wall and in the atherosclerotic plaque. Proc Natl Acad Sci USA. 1989;86(8):2839–43.

Wilds SLCL, Dearing JP. Activated clotting time and cardiopulmonary bypass, III. Effect of high plate- let count on heparin management. J Extra-Corp Technol. 1982;14:322–4.

Williams MS, Ng'alla LS. Heparin therapy leads to platelet activation and prolongation of PFA-100 closure time. J Cardiovasc Pharmacol Ther. 2005;10(4):273–80.

Williams RD, D'Ambra MN, Maione TE, Lynch KE, Keene DF. Recombinant platelet factor 4 reversal of heparin in human cardiopulmonary bypass blood. J Thorac Cardiovasc Surg. 1994;108(5):975–83.

Xiao Z, Théroux P. Platelet activation with unfractionated heparin at therapeutic concentrations and comparisons with a low-molecular-weight heparin and with a direct thrombin inhibitor. Circulation. 1998;97(3):251–6.

Zulys VJ, Teasdale SJ, Michel ER, et al. Ancrod (Arvin) as an alternative to heparin anticoagulation for cardiopulmonary bypass. Anesthesiology. 1989;71(6):870–7.

Blood Conservation Techniques

18

Dima Daaboul and James DiNardo

Introduction

Blood conservation for surgical patients is part of a broader practice of "patient blood management," (PBM), which encompasses multidisciplinary and interdisciplinary practices aimed at conserving a patient's blood and minimizing transfusion during and after cardiac surgery. Ideally, PBM starts in the preoperative period, weeks before the surgical procedure in elective. This approach includes patient participation and patient-centered decision-making to optimize outcomes. It involves identifying high-risk patients and surgeries, managing and treating pre-existing anemia, and optimizing coagulation. The majority of blood conservation strategies are implemented through intraoperative management, with efforts to conserve the patient's own blood volume through pharmacologic and non-pharmacologic measures. These efforts must also extend into the postoperative period, focusing on minimizing iatrogenic blood loss and continuing anemia management when needed.

Complications of Blood Transfusion

1-Infectious Risks

Advancements in donor screening and laboratory testing since the 1980s have dramatically reduced the risk of transfusion transmitted infections. However, microbial contamination during collection, processing and storage remains a concern, albeit infrequent. Transfusion-associated sepsis (TAS) is particularly associated with platelets transfusion which are stored at room temperature and more prone to bacterial proliferation. TAS accounts for about 10% of allogeneic blood transfusion (ABT)-related deaths in the USA.

2-Acute Hemolytic Transfusion Reactions

Acute hemolytic transfusion reactions can be immune or non-immune in origin. Immune reactions are typically caused by transfusion of ABO- or antigen-incompatible red blood cells due to patient identification errors, leading to hemolysis and symptoms such as fever, chills, hypotension, and potentially severe complications like renal failure or shock. Diagnosis relies on clinical presentation and serological testing, and management is supportive. Non-immune reactions result from physical or chemical damage to red blood cells due to incompatible solutions or improper storage

3-Allergic Transfusion Reactions

Allergic transfusion reactions typically occur within four hours of blood component administration and are most frequently associated with platelet transfusions. Most reactions are mild, presenting with symptoms such as rash, pruritus, urticaria, and localized angioedema. However, in rare cases, these reactions can be severe and life-threatening, manifesting as anaphylaxis, characterized by systemic symptoms including bronchospasm, respiratory distress and hypotension.

Supplementary Information The online version contains supplementary material available at https://doi.org/10.1007/978-3-031-91163-7_18.

D. Daaboul · J. DiNardo (✉)
Department of Anesthesiology, Critical Care and Pain Medicine, Cardiac Anesthesia, Boston Children's Hospital, Boston, MA, USA
e-mail: dima.daaboul@childrens.harvard.edu; James.DiNardo@childrens.harvard.edu

A. S. Awad, J. DiNardo (eds.), *Clinical Perfusion for Cardiac Surgery*, https://doi.org/10.1007/978-3-031-91163-7_18

4-Transfusion-Related Acute Lung Injury (TRALI):

TRALI is an acute, non-cardiogenic pulmonary edema that typically develops within 6 hours of transfusion. It is characterized by sudden respiratory distress, hypoxemia, and bilateral pulmonary infiltrates on imaging, in the absence of left atrial hypertension, differentiating it from cardiogenic pulmonary edema. It is most frequently associated with plasmacontaining blood products, such as fresh frozen plasma (FFP). Supportive therapy, including supplemental oxygen and mechanical ventilation is often but not always effective

5-Transfusion-Associated Cardiac Overload (TACO)

TACO results from fluid overload due to excessive or rapid transfusion, leading to pulmonary edema and respiratory compromise It is often mistaken for TRALI due to similar presentations. However, echocardiography and clinical evaluation aid in distinguishing between the two. TACO is typically associated with elevated BNP levels, positive fluid balance, and responsiveness to diuretics.

6-Transfusion-Related Immunomodulation (TRIM)

TRIM refers to the immune-suppressive effects of allogeneic transfusions, particularly the inhibition of cell-mediated immunity, which may increase the risk of postoperative infections and tumor recurrence. Donor white blood cells are thought to contribute to this effect, leading to the wide spread adoption of leukoreduction, especially in surgical and immunocompromised populations.

Factors that Increase the Risk of Bleeding or Transfusion during Cardiac Surgery

- Age over 75 years.
- Female gender.
- Small size body.
- Preoperative anemia.
- Preoperative thrombocytopenia.
- Preoperative coagulopathy.
- Preoperative elevated liver enzymes due to congestive heart failure.
- Use of anticoagulant medications.
- Use of antiplatelet medications.
- Re-do surgery.
- Renal insufficiency.
- Combined coronary artery bypass graft (CABG) and valve surgery.
- Emergency surgical procedures.
- Prolonged cardiopulmonary (CPB) time.
- Preoperative cardiogenic shock or the use of assist devices.

Preoperative Management

Identifying and Treating Preoperative Anemia

Anemia is frequently encountered in cardiac surgical patients, particularly among those at the extremes of age and those with multiple comorbidities and chronic diseases. The prevalence of anemia in this population is estimated to be 30–40%, with severe anemia occurring in about 10% of cases.

The World Health Organization (WHO) defines anemia as a hemoglobin (Hb) level less than 12 g/dl in adult non-pregnant females, less than 11 g/dl in adult pregnant females, and less than 13 g/dl in adult males. For children, it is defined as Hb less than 11 g/dl for those under 6 years of age, Hb < 11.5 g/dl for ages 6–11 years, and Hb <12 g/dl for ages 12–14 years. Severe anemia is defined as Hb < 8 g/dl, or < 7 g/dl in younger children and pregnant women.

Several studies have shown an association between anemia and increased morbidity, such as stroke and renal dysfunction, as well as increased length of hospital stay and mortality following cardiac surgery. The risks associated with anemia are independent of those associated with transfusion. Since anemic patients are more likely to receive blood transfusions during cardiac surgery, their risk of increased morbidity and mortality is compounded, but it remains difficult to isolate the risk attributable to each exposure. Notably, the severity of anemia is directly correlated with mortality risk, with each 1 g/dl decrease in hemoglobin concentration linked to an increased mortality risk. This has prompted suggestions to standardize the definition of anemia to <13 g/dl for both women and men, as women are at higher risk for anemia-related adverse outcomes.

Table 18.1 Expected laboratory findings in different forms of iron deficiency and anemia

Condition	Hemoglobin	Ferritin	Serum Iron/TSAT	TIBC	CHr	Hepcidin[a]
Iron deficiency without anemia	Normal	Decreased	Decreased	Increased	Decreased	Decreased
IDA	Decreased	Decreased	Decreased	Increased	Decreased	Decreased
AI/iron sequestration	Decreased	Increased	Normal or decreased	Decreased	Normal or decreased	Increased
Mixed anemia (AI/IDA)	Decreased	Normal	Decreased	Variable	Decreased	Normal

Abbreviations: AI, anemia of inflammation; CHr, reticulocyte hemoglobin content; IDA, iron deficiency anemia; TIBC, total iron-binding capacity; TSAT, transferrin saturation
[a]Hepcidin testing not widely available

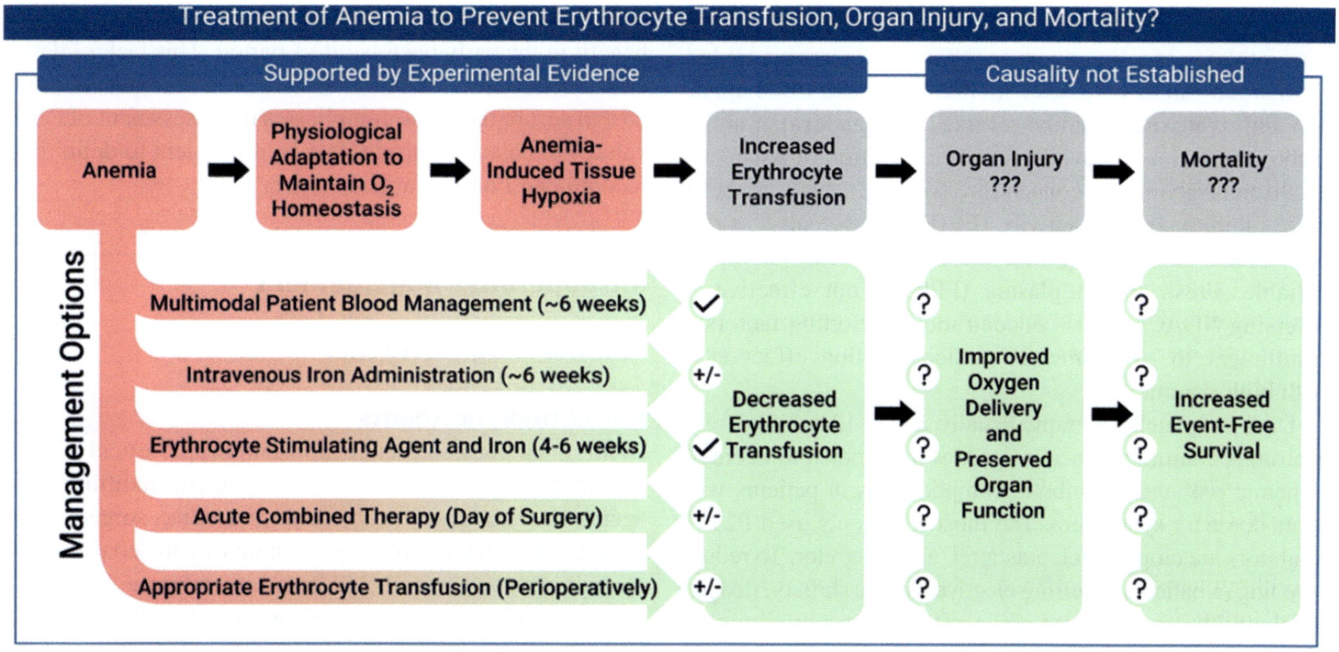

Fig. 18.1 Established management options to treat perioperative anemia as well as the estimated time required for treatment are shown with the transition of red to green arrows. Options that have been shown to reduce erythrocyte transfusion are shown with a check mark, while those where the effect of the treatment on transfusion requirements is equivocal are shown with a +/− designation. As indicated by the question mark designation, none of these treatments to reduce erythrocyte transfusion has been demonstrated to reduce organ injury or mortality. In addition, enthusiasm for the use of erythropoietin-stimulating agents (ESA) must be tempered by the equivocal evidence of an increased incidence of thrombotic cardiovascular events associated with ESA administration to treat anemia. Hare, G. M. T. & Mazer, C. D. Anemia: Perioperative Risk and Treatment Opportunity. *Anesthesiology 135*, 520–530 (2021). (Reproduced with permission)

Efforts to identify and treat preoperative anemia should be made whenever possible. Iron deficiency anemia is the most common type, affecting about half of the cardiac surgical patients. Table 18.1 summarizes the laboratory test results used to define the type of anemia present.

Warner MA, Shore-Lesserson L, Shander A, et al. Perioperative Anemia: Prevention, Diagnosis, and Management Throughout the Spectrum of Perioperative Care. (Reproduced with permission).

As summarized in Fig. 18.1, anemia induces physiologic adaptations to limit tissue hypoxia and often triggers the need for erythrocyte transfusion. While certain management options are clearly effective in reducing the need for erythrocyte transfusion, as indicated by a check mark (✓), the impact of others remains equivocal, denoted by a plus/minus symbol (+/−). Furthermore, it is not entirely clear, as indicated by a question mark (?), as to whether a reduction in erythrocyte transfusion mitigates end-organ injury or mortality.

Management of Anticoagulant Medications

Nonvitamin-K antagonist oral anticoagulants (NOACs) are the preferred alternatives over the vitamin K antagonist, warfarin, for stroke prevention in nonvalvular atrial fibrillation and in the treatment of venous thromboembolism. The most encountered agents are dabigatran, a direct thrombin inhibitor, and the factor Xa inhibitors: apixaban, betrixaban, edoxaban, and rivaroxaban. In patients requiring emergent cardiac surgery with recent ingestion of a NOAC or laboratory evidence of a NOAC effect, administration of the reversal antidote specific to that NOAC is recommended. Dabigatran can be reversed with idarucizumab, while apixaban and rivaroxaban can be reversed with andexanet alpha. If these agents are unavailable, administration of a 4-factor prothrombin complex concentrate (4FPCC), such as factor eight inhibitor bypass activity (FEIBA) or Kcentra, is recommended, recognizing that the response can be highly variable. Fresh frozen plasma (FFP) is not effective in reversing NOACs, as its concentration of clotting factors is insufficient to overcome the anticoagulation effect even with high volume.

Dual-antiplatelet therapy, usually a P2Y12 inhibitor and aspirin, is commonly encountered, as it is known to decrease ischemic risk and thrombotic complications in patients with acute coronary syndromes. The most commonly used P2Y12 inhibitors are clopidogrel, prasugrel, and ticagrelor. To reduce bleeding in patients requiring elective cardiac surgery, ticagrelor should be discontinued preoperatively for a minimum of 3 days, clopidogrel for 5 days, and prasugrel for 7 days.

Preoperative Autologous Donation (PAD)

PAD involves repeated blood donation to obtain four units of blood, each approximately 450 ml, starting about 35 days prior to surgery. The last donation should take place at least 48–72 hours before the operation to allow for blood volume equilibration. Donated units are collected in citrated phosphate dextrose blood bags and conventionally stored under appropriate conditions in the blood bank. Iron and erythropoietin therapy may be used to increase the concentration of hemoglobin between donations; however, this adds to the cost of PAD and may not always be effective. Although PAD is stored as whole blood, the activity of platelets and levels of coagulation factors decline during storage. PAD minimizes risks such as viral transmission, immune-mediated hemolysis, and febrile or allergic reactions. Importantly, there is no immunomodulatory effect associated with re-transfusion, and avoiding TRIM may contribute to a reduced incidence of perioperative infections.

Contraindications to PAD include unstable angina, severe ischemic heart disease, severe aortic stenosis, anemia, cyanotic heart disease, and uncontrolled hypertension. Furthermore, the logistics of PAD, requiring repeated phlebotomy prior to surgery, limit its use to elective surgeries. Despite these efforts, up to 50% of pre-donated blood often remains unused. This wastage, combined with the administrative costs of the PAD program, results in a higher cost per unit of blood compared to allogeneic blood.

While patients participating in PAD may exhibit higher postoperative hemoglobin levels, there is no clear clinical benefit in the early postoperative period. This lack of definitive benefit, along with the considerable effort and additional cost to secure the units, complicates the assessment of PAD's value. On balance, current data is insufficient to definitively recommend PAD in cardiac surgery.

Intraoperative Management

Pharmacological Agents

Antifibrinolytic Agents

Lysine analogues, such as epsilon aminocaproic acid (EACA) and tranexamic acid (TXA), are synthetic antifibrinolytic agents that are extensively used in cardiac surgery. They work by attenuating fibrinolysis, inhibiting the conversion of plasminogen to plasmin, and, to a lesser degree, by directly inhibiting plasmin activity. Consequently, they enhance hemostasis by inhibiting clot lysis and stabilizing clot formation.

Several studies have compared TXA and EACA with each other and against a placebo. These studies have generally shown the superiority of these agents over placebo in reducing blood loss during cardiac surgery, as well as in reducing the need for blood transfusions and reexploration due to bleeding. However, there is no convincing evidence favoring one agent over the other in either cardiac or noncardiac surgery. While the administration of TXA has been associated with seizures, this association remains questionable. The studies in question were not sufficiently powered to definitively detect this side effect. Nevertheless, the use of antifibrinolytic agents plays a major role in blood conservation strategies across all patient ages.

Desmopressin (DDAVP)

Desmopressin, 1-deamino-8-D-arginine vasopressin (DDAVP), is a synthetic vasopressin analogue that stimulates the release of von Willebrand factor from endothelial cells. As such, it is used to prevent and treat hemorrhage in

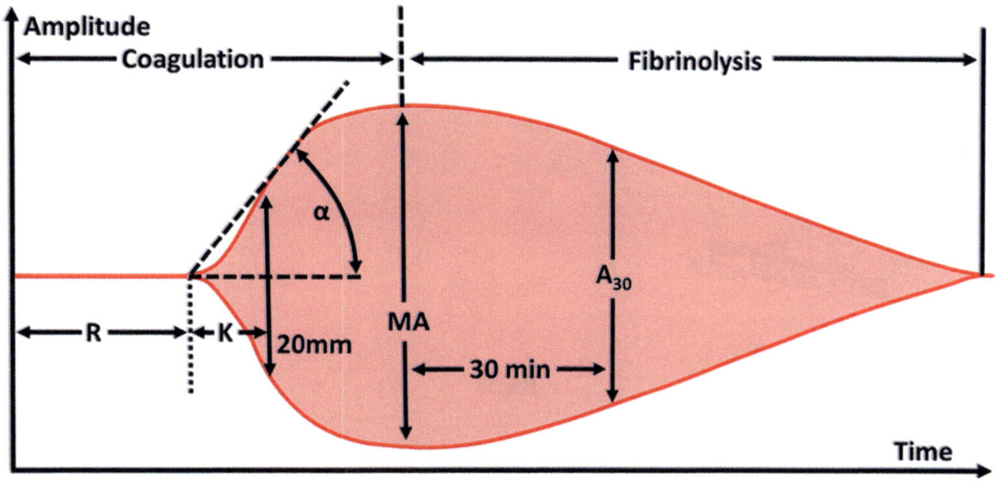

Fig. 18.2 TEG parameters as it appears on TEG courtesy of Mikael Häggström, M.D.

patients with mild hemophilia A and type 1 von Willebrand disease. Additionally, DDAVP may be effective in treating platelet dysfunction associated with conditions such as uremia or prolonged CPB, particularly when these defects are confirmed by platelet function testing.

Topical Hemostatic Agents

In addition to intravenous agents, topical hemostatic agents, such as gelatin sponges or topical thrombin are frequently employed in cardiac surgery. These agents play a significant role in the multimodal approach to blood conservation, aiding in controlling bleeding directly at the surgical site.

Point-of-Care (POC) Testing

Post-CPB coagulopathic bleeding, often multifactorial, may arise from factors beyond inadequate systemic heparin reversal, such as hemodilution, hypothermia, and activation of coagulation pathways. Traditional "shotgun therapy" involves transfusing FFP, cryoprecipitate, and platelets. However, viscoelastic POC tests such as Thromboelastogram (TEG) and Rotational Thromboelastometry (ROTEM) provide dynamic whole blood clotting analysis, guiding targeted transfusion post-bypass and visualizing clot formation and lysis.

While there are many devices available, such as Quantra, Sonoclot, ClotPro, and ReoRox G2 assay, the two main types of viscoelastic POC tests are:

1. TEG: Thromboelastogram (TEG®), developed by Dr. Hellmut Hartert in 1948, is a diagnostic tool that uses a pin and cuvette to measure clot strength and dynamics and analyze blood clotting. In TEG, a small blood sample in a cuvette is warmed to body temperature and oscillated to simulate venous blood movement. A pin, suspended in the sample by a torsion wire, moves in response to clot formation, generating a signal that is translated into a diagram showing clot formation and lysis. The degree of pin motion correlates with clot strength. The graph generated by this movement depicts various stages of clot formation, providing a detailed visual representation of the clotting process. For a more comprehensive understanding, please refer to Fig. 18.2, which illustrates these stages.
2. The advanced TEG® 6 s uses an automated, multichannel system with four assays to measure clot viscoelasticity through resonance. It involves a citrated blood sample mixed with reagents in four channels. The blood's vertical motion in response to vibrations is measured using LED illumination and a sensor, providing a readout of clot dynamics based on resonant frequencies. Higher resonant frequencies in the output indicate stronger clot formation.
3. Rotational Thromboelastometry (ROTEM): Rotational thromboelastometry (ROTEM®) is a diagnostic tool for analyzing blood coagulation, similar to thromboelastogram (TEG) but with a key difference: in ROTEM, the pin rotates within a stationary cuvette containing an activated whole blood sample. ROTEM is available in three versions: ROTEM-gamma, ROTEM-delta, and the automated ROTEM-sigma. The sigma model uses prefilled cartridges with four parallel channels. ROTEM employs various assays such as NATEM, INTEM, EXTEM, FIBTEM, APTEM, and HEPTEM, each involving different activators or inhibitors, with INTEM, EXTEM, FIBTEM, and APTEM being the most commonly used. These assays provide detailed information on blood coagulation based on the specific assay and reagents used (Fig. 18.3).

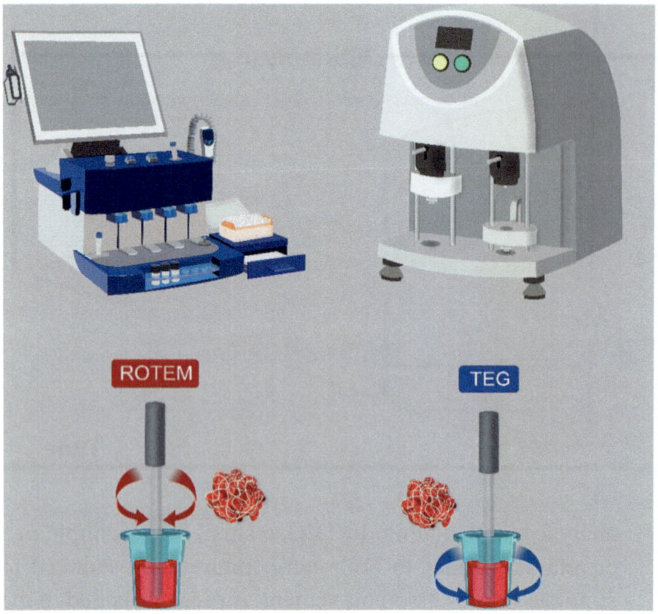

Fig. 18.3 Featuring the two most prevalent point-of-care devices: On the left, ROTEM (thromboelastometry) illustrates a pin descending into a cup with a whole blood sample at 37 °C, where the pin oscillates, red arrows, while the cup remains stationary. On the right, TEG (thromboelastography) shows a pin descending into a cup with a whole blood sample at 37 °C, in this setup, the cup oscillates, blue arrows, while the pin is stationary, demonstrating the unique principles of how each device operates

Interpretation of Viscoelastic Graphs Guides Targeted Transfusion Therapy Based on Specific Abnormalities

1. Treatment Recommendations Based on TEG Graph Analysis
   - Administer FFP when R time is prolonged.
   - Give cryoprecipitate or fibrinogen concentrate if the alpha angle is below 65 degrees, indicating fibrinogen deficiency.
   - Provide Platelets ± Cryoprecipitate for a Maximum Amplitude (MA) under 55 mm, which suggests platelet dysfunction and/or fibrinogen deficiency.
   - Use antifibrinolytic agents, such as aminocaproic acid or tranexamic acid, when the fibrinolysis (LY-30) exceeds 5%.
2. Treatment Recommendations Based on ROTEM Graph Analysis
   - Administer FFP when clotting time (CT) is extended, specifically if INTEM CT exceeds 240 seconds or EXTEM CT surpasses 100 seconds.
   - Provide cryoprecipitate or fibrinogen concentrate if the FIBTEM clot firmness amplitude at 10 minutes (A10) drops below 11 mm, indicating a fibrinogen deficiency.
   - In cases where FIBTEM A10 is above 10 mm but EXTEM A10 is below 40 mm, suggesting platelet dysfunction, administer Platelets.
   - Use an antifibrinolytic, such as aminocaproic acid or tranexamic acid, when the EXTEM maximum lysis (ML) exceeds 15%, indicating increased fibrinolysis.

Goal-directed transfusion algorithms incorporating these tests aim to reduce bleeding and transfusion in cardiac surgery. Use of viscoelastic devices such as TEG and ROTEM is becoming increasingly common. TEG/ROTEM-guided algorithms for treating microvascular bleeding are increasingly used, as shown in Fig. 18.4, while non-TEG/ROTEM algorithms are presented in Fig. 18.5. Institutions may adapt these algorithms, particularly concerning the trigger levels for transfusion of packed red cells (PRBC), platelet count, fibrinogen concentration, FFP, as well as the use and dosage of recombinant activated factor VII (rFVIIA), PCC, and desmopressin in cases of refractory bleeding.

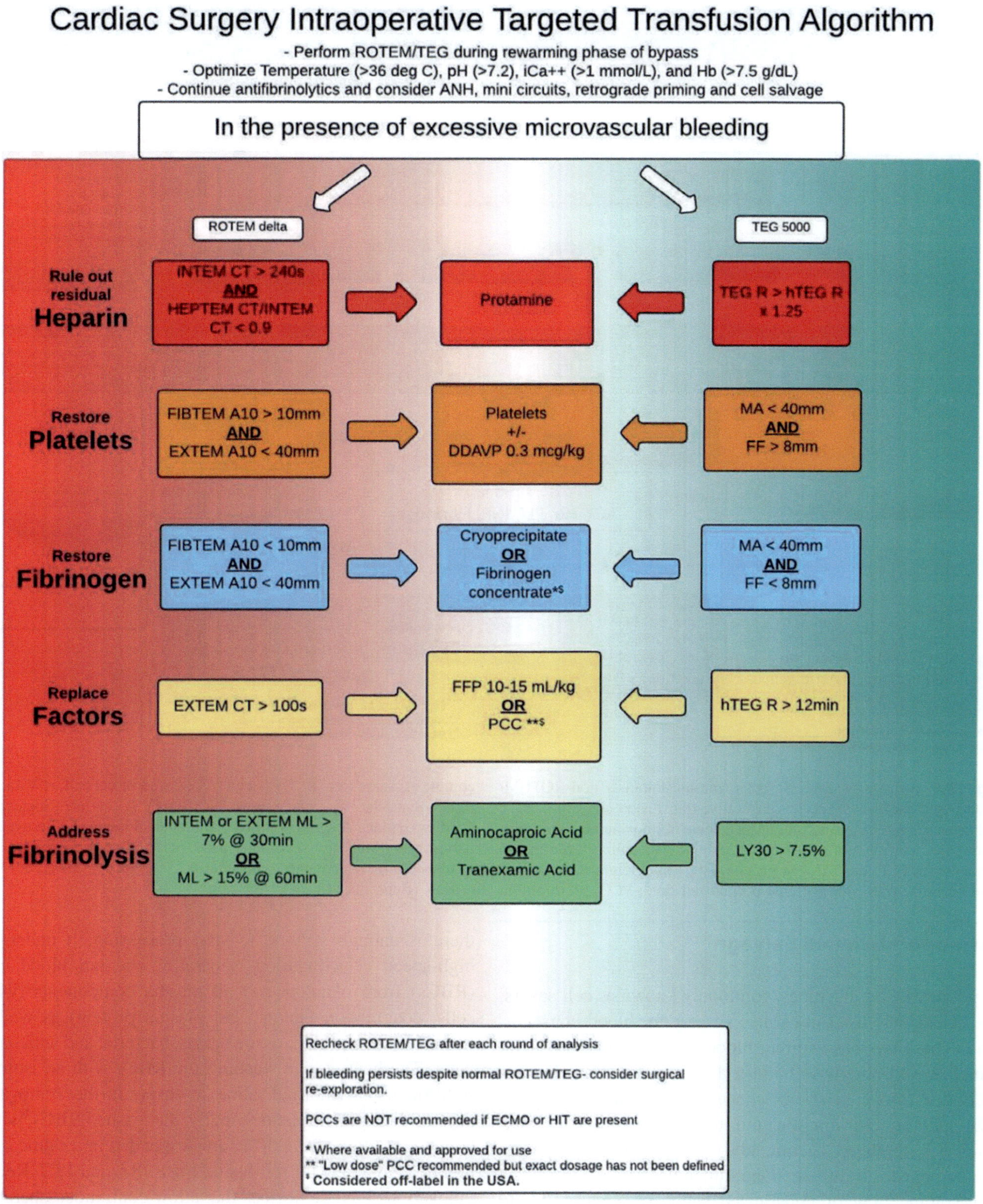

Fig. 18.4 Society of cardiovascular anesthesiologists ROTEM/TEG-based cardiac surgery intraoperative transfusion algorithm. ANH indicates acute normovolemic hemodilution; A10, amplitude at 10 minutes; CT, clotting time; DDAVP, 1-deamino-8-d-arginine vasopressin; ECMO, extra corporeal membrane oxygenation; EXTEM, extrinsic pathway thromboelastometry; FIBTEM, fibrinogen-based thromboelastometry; FF, functional fibrinogen; FFP, fresh-frozen plasma; Hb, hemoglobin; HEPTEM, heparinase thromboelastometry; HIT, heparin-induced thrombocytopenia; hTEG, heparinase thromboelastography; iCA++, ionized calcium; INTEM, intrinsic pathway thromboelastometry; LY30, clot lysis at 30 min; MA, maximum amplitude; ML, maximum lysis; PCC, prothrombin complex concentrate; R, reaction time; ROTEM, rotational thromboelastometry; TEG, hromboelastography Raphael, J. et al. Society of Cardiovascular Anesthesiologists Clinical Practice Improvement Advisory for Management of Perioperative Bleeding and Hemostasis in Cardiac Surgery Patients. *Anesthesia Analgesia* 129, 1209–1221 (2019). (Reproduced with permission)

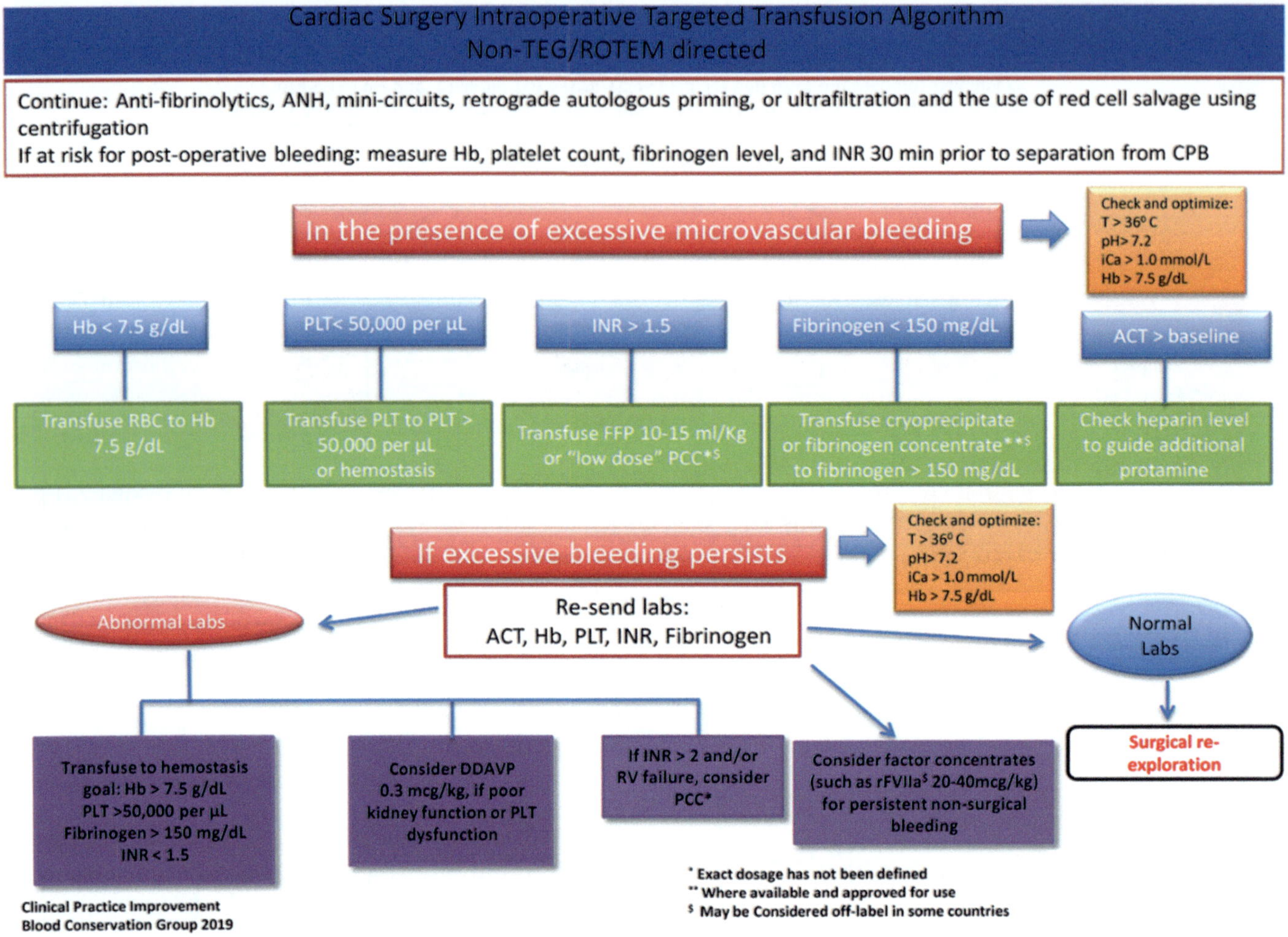

Fig. 18.5 Society of cardiovascular anesthesiologists non-ROTEM/TEG-based cardiac surgery intraoperative transfusion algorithm. ACT indicates activated clotting time; ANH, acute normovolemic hemodilution; CPB, cardiopulmonary bypass; DDAVP, 1-deamino-8-d-arginine vasopressin; FFP, fresh-frozen plasma; Hb, hemoglobin; iCA++, ionized calcium; INR, international normalized ratio; PCC, prothrombin complex concentrate; PLT, platelets; RBC, red blood cell; rFVIIa; RV, right ventricle; T, temperature. Raphael, J. et al. Society of Cardiovascular Anesthesiologists Clinical Practice Improvement Advisory for Management of Perioperative Bleeding and Hemostasis in Cardiac Surgery Patients. *Anesthesia Analgesia* 129, 1209–1221 (2019). (Reproduced with permission)

Intraoperative Cell Salvage

Autotransfusion machines, commonly known as cell savers, are extensively used in cardiac surgery for blood conservation. These devices aspirate blood from the surgical field, which would otherwise be lost, and then process it by collecting it into a reservoir, concentrating and washing the RBCs, before returning them to the patient. The system features a specialized suction line equipped with a double-lumen collection catheter. One lumen delivers a continuous low-volume flow of heparinized saline or a citrate-based anticoagulant to prevent clot formation during blood suctioning that takes place simultaneously through the second lumen via negative suction pressure. To avoid damage to the erythrocytes, the suction pressure is usually kept below −100 to −150 mmHg. Once the blood is collected in a reservoir and there is enough volume to start processing, it undergoes high-speed centrifugation, separating the red blood cells (RBCs) from platelets and all plasma components (white cells, coagulation factors, and plasma protein) as well as from free hemoglobin, tissue debris, bacteria, and anticoagulants. The next step is washing the RBCs with an isotonic solution, usually normal saline, to ensure further removal of any residual contaminants. Finally, the washed RBCs, with a hematocrit often above 50%, are suspended in a saline solution in a bag ready for reinfusion Figs. 18.6 and 18.7. Recent innovations include devices that allow continuous operation and smaller centrifugation bowls (55–70 ml), which permit use in pediatric patients. Please refer to Video 18.1 for guidance on the setup and assembly of the cell saver.

Cell salvage can be utilized during the entirety of the procedure, from skin incision to the administration of heparin

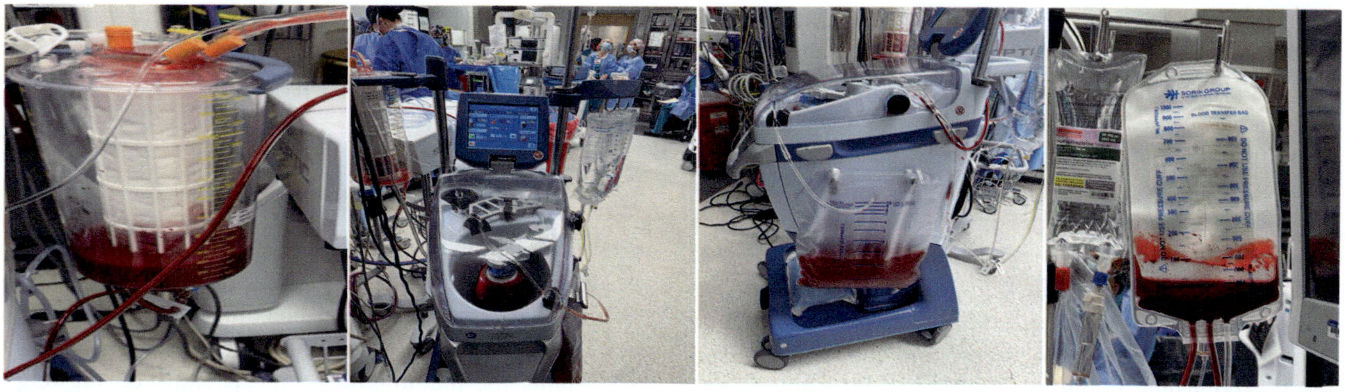

Fig. 18.6 Stages of cell salvaging system function: (1) Left—collection of blood into the reservoir with filtration; (2) Second from left—concentration of blood through high-speed centrifugation; (3) Third from left—washing process of RBCs, with waste being directed to a separate bag; (4) Far right—salvaged blood with hematocrit above 50% in a collection bag, ready for reinfusion

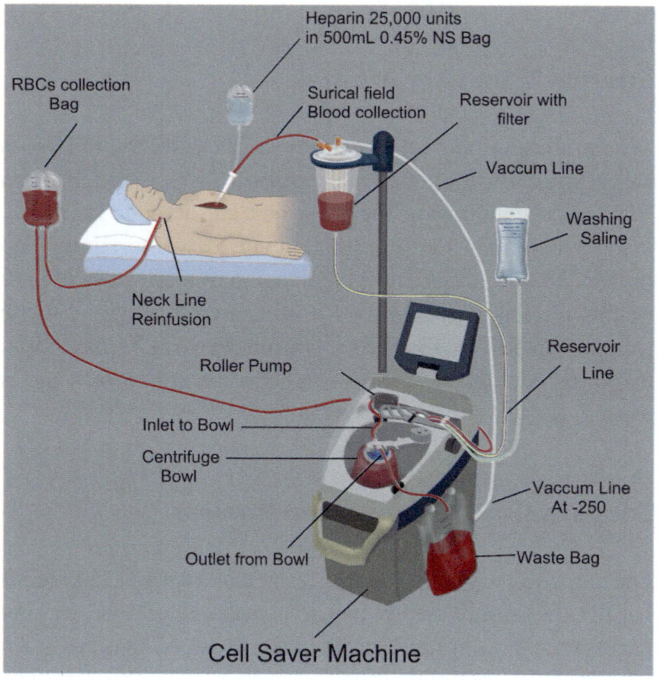

Fig. 18.7 Cell saver machine configuration: Illustrating the process from blood collection in the surgical field, through the washing phase, to the final collection in the reinfusion bag, ensuring safe and efficient autologous blood recovery

and then from the administration of protamine until skin closure. During anticoagulation for CPB (from administration of heparin until the administration of protamine), it is recommended that the surgeons utilize cardiotomy suction to return shed blood directly to the CPB circuit to preserve platelets and plasma proteins, including coagulation factors. Following removal of the arterial cannula, residual blood in the CPB circuit can be salvaged for re-transfusion. Caution should be exercised with gross bacterial contamination and certain topical hemostatic agents, such as Avitene, Surgicel, and Gelfoam, as they are relatively contraindicated for use with cell saver systems.

It is recommended that the salvaged, washed blood be re-infused back to the patient within 8 hours of collection. Prompt reinfusion ensures improved RBC quality and a better oxygen-carrying capacity. This blood is believed to have a higher concentration of 2,3-DPG (2,3-diphosphoglycerate) than banked RBCs, leading to a rightward shift of the oxygen dissociation curves and a decrease in hemoglobin-oxygen affinity and greater oxygen unloading at the tissue level, as illustrated in Fig. 3.6.

When transfusing cell-salvaged blood, one must be aware of the potential for reinfusion hypotension, a complication whose incidence and underlying cause remain not fully understood. Bradykinin release or hypocalcemia are considered potential contributing factors. In addition, it should be emphasized that cell salvaged blood contains mainly RBCs and lacks platelets or clotting factors. Consequently, it should be treated like allogeneic RBC transfusion in terms of the need for supplemental blood products and clotting factors if required, especially in the case of massive transfusion.

While meta-analysis and several observational studies suggest a reduced need for homologous blood transfusion associated with intraoperative blood salvage in adults, no effects on mortality and morbidity have been clearly demonstrated. The evidence supporting the use of cell salvage to reduce ABT is compelling, and it is recommended that cell salvage be used routinely in pediatric patients having cardiac surgery with CPB support. The 2021 update to the Clinical Practice Guidelines on Patient Blood Management, issued by the Society of Thoracic Surgeons (STS), the Society of Cardiovascular Anesthesiologists (SCA), the American Society of ExtraCorporeal Technology (AmSECT), and the Society for the Advancement of Blood Management (SABM), advocates for red cell salvage, classifying it as a Class I recommendation with a Level of Evidence A.

Acute Normovolemic Hemodilution (ANH)

ANH is consistently utilized in only a minority (17%) of adult cardiac centers. ANH involves the withdrawal of whole blood from the patient intraoperatively, just before the start of surgery, with the intent to re-infuse the harvested autologous blood following termination of CPB. The blood is typically collected by gravity drainage through a large-bore intravenous line into citrate-phosphate-dextrose bags and then stored either at room temperature with an agitated device to prevent clotting or in a blood cooler. Isovolemia and hemodynamic stability are preserved by administering intravenous crystalloids or colloids solution. The blood lost during surgery is diluted to a lower hematocrit, while the blood with the higher hematocrit that was harvested and stored prior to incision is re-infused at the end of the surgery. The main goal of this strategy is to reduce the need for ABT, defined as a reduction of the number of allogeneic red blood cell units transfused, as well as the number of patients requiring such transfusion. ANH might also help preserve platelet count and coagulation factors by avoiding exposure of the harvested unit to hemodilution and the deleterious effects of CPB on platelet function. The greater the amount of whole blood that can be removed from the patient, the greater the benefit of ANH, with ANH being most effective when blood loss exceeds 20% of estimated blood volume.

The potential benefits of ANH must be weighed against the risks of causing iatrogenic anemia, especially in patients lacking sufficient cardiopulmonary reserve to compensate for the drop in hematocrit. This includes patients with severe ventricular dysfunction, critical aortic stenosis and pediatric patients where the CPB prime includes erythrocytes.

Surgical Factors

Intraoperative blood conservation techniques are crucial in cardiac surgery, and achieving meticulous intraoperative hemostasis is essential. Most surgeons learn these methods during residency, adopting a variety of approaches for opening the chest and controlling bleeding.

Skin Incision

Starting with the skin incision, careful hemostasis is maintained using low-setting electrocautery to minimize thermal injury, crucial for reducing infection risks.

Sternal Incisions

Precise midline sternal incisions and avoiding excessive cauterization are key to preserving sternal vascularization. Attention to detail, such as point cauterizing bleeding sites and carefully treating bone bleeding with bone wax, helps achieve hemostasis without compromising tissue health.

Anterior Mediastinum

In the anterior mediastinum, careful handling of thymic vessels through cauterization or clipping, and preserving thymic tissue, can minimize bleeding from soft tissues and reduce postoperative bleeding. Extra caution is necessary around the innominate vein, especially during reoperations where collateral vessels can pose a problem. Opening the pericardium, a highly vascularized tissue, with cautery or scissors requires caution to prevent excessive bleeding.

Internal Mammary Arteries

When utilizing internal mammary arteries (IMAs) in bypass surgeries, careful dissection is crucial. Proper visualization and gentle handling of the IMA bed and its side branches, using techniques like clipping, tying, or cauterizing, help prevent bleeding. Securing the distal mammary pedicle with double clips or ties is crucial, as this area is a common site for postoperative bleeding. During proximal dissection, avoiding damage to the left subclavian artery or vein is essential.

Endoscopic Saphenous Vein Harvest

During coronary bypass surgeries that require saphenous vein grafts, simultaneous incisions are made on the leg and chest. Precision in hemostasis is achieved using electrocautery, ensuring minimal blood loss during vein extraction. The vein is secured with double ligatures and clips. Leg incisions are sutured promptly, irrespective of heparin administration. In cases of rare coagulopathies, drainage catheters may be employed. Postoperatively, pressure dressings are applied to the legs, aiding in healing and reducing complications. It's important to note that leg bleeding is a frequent source of unrecognized intraoperative blood loss.

Cannulation

Cannulation site selection and handling are vital for effective control and repair, especially in reoperations. Careful placement of the inferior vena cava (IVC) cannula is essential to prevent potentially serious bleeding due to tears. Blood loss during cannulation is managed with cardiotomy sucker or cell saver suction.

Coronary Artery Bypass Grafting (CABG) Surgeries

In CABG surgeries, strategic placement of cardioplegic perfusion catheters and meticulous testing of anastomotic sites are crucial to ensure leak-free anastomosis. Off-pump CABG, an alternative to traditional on bypass surgery avoiding CPB, potentially reduces perioperative bleeding and the need for blood transfusions. Studies have shown off-pump CABG can significantly lower transfusion rates, especially in elective and older patient groups. While some research indicates increased blood loss with off-pump methods, this hasn't consistently led to higher transfusion rates. Overall, recent analyses support off-pump surgery for reduced blood loss and transfusion needs.

Valvular Surgeries

During valvular surgeries, careful incision and suture placement avoid excessive bleeding and facilitate successful closures. Post-bypass, many bleeding sites resolve with heparin reversal, but vigilant observation and control of significant bleeding are necessary.

Closure

Precision in closure techniques is key to avoiding blood pooling and ensuring effective hemostasis. A thorough inspection of wire sites, common areas for postoperative bleeding, is conducted before sternal closure. Additionally, vigilant monitoring of chest tube drainage is crucial to identify and address any significant bleeding promptly.

Perfusion Interventions

MiECC and Microplegia

Reducing hemodilution by reducing CPB circuit size and therefore decreasing prime volume is an important step in blood conservation strategies. Use of a MiECC is a multifaceted method of reducing CBP circuit volume. MiECC is characterized by a closed CPB circuit, shorter lengths of biologically inert (heparin-coated) blood contact surfaces, reduced priming volume (600-750 ml), a centrifugal pump, a membrane oxygenator, a heat exchanger, a cardioplegia system, a venous bubble trap/venous air-removing device, and a shed blood management system. To prevent blood-air contact and activation of the systemic inflammatory response, these systems are closed and thus lack an open venous reservoir. Consequently, there are likely to be more fluctuations in venous return than are seen with an open venous reservoir system.

Another innovative approach in MiECC is the use of microplegia. Standard cardioplegia often involves a blood:crystalloid ratio of 4:1, which can lead to significant hemodilution when large volumes are used to achieve diastolic cardiac arrest. Microplegia, however, uses a highly concentrated mixture of 60 parts blood to one part crystalloid cardioplegia solution. This method effectively reduces the hemodilution effect and prevents wastage of red cell mass in the unused cardioplegia mixture.

Vacuum-Assisted and Kinetic-Assisted Venous Drainage

Reducing the diameter and the length of the venous tubing in CPB circuits to decrease circuit volume can potentially impair gravity-assisted venous return. This is due to increased resistance and reduced height difference between the patient and the venous reservoir. Vacuum-assisted venous drainage (VAVD) improves venous drainage by applying −20 to −40 mmHg pressure to a closed venous reservoir. However, VAVD may cause collapse of the vena cava, impairing venous return and possibly leading to partial or total occlusion of the venous cannula. Another major concern with VAVD is the increased risk of both detected and undetected air microembolism. Despite the use of an arterial filter, significant systemic gaseous microemboli from a venous source may occur. Kinetic-assisted venous drainage (KAVD) utilizes a centrifugal pump interposed in the venous drainage line between the patient and the venous reservoir. Similar to VAAD, KAVD also carries risks of vena cava collapse and microemboli formation.

Ultrafiltration

A. Conventional ultrafiltration (CUF) involves the removal of excess volume in the venous reservoir *during* bypass. An excess venous reservoir volume can be caused by the crystalloid component of cardioplegia, valve testing solution, or simply when a patient has an elevated circulating blood volume. CUF removes excess volume by passing blood, either passively or actively with a roller head, through the ultrafilter.
B. Modified Ultrafiltration

Modified ultrafiltration (MUF) extends ultrafiltration post-CPB, enhancing blood hemoconcentration in both the patient and the bypass circuit. It operates via arteriovenous or venoarterial systems. MUF typically achieves a greater degree of hemoconcentration than can be obtained with CUF alone, especially in small children, and some institutions utilize both CUF and MUF concurrently. However, when a standardized volume of fluid is removed, there is no significant difference in clinical outcome or hemoconcentration between CUF and MUF. For a comprehensive exploration of ultrafiltration techniques, including circuit setup, refer to Chap.19.

Retrograde Autologous Priming (RAP)

RAP is a procedure used to prime the CPB circuit utilizing the patient's own blood. It is intended to decrease hemodilution, as well as exposure to allogeneic blood. It is performed via passive exsanguination into the CPB circuit via the arterial and venous cannulas. The patient's blood is used to displace the crystalloid prime of the CPB retrograde into a collection container, which is discarded. This process can lead to acute hypotension requiring slowing or suspending the RAP process or administration of a vasoconstrictor, such as phenylephrine. Caution should be exerted in patients with physiology that is particularly intolerant of an acute decrease in preload. As with ANH, the greater the volume that is removed, the greater the effectiveness of RAP in reducing blood transfusions.

While the evidence supporting this strategy as regards reducing the need for allogeneic erythrocyte transfusion is inconclusive, the STS/SCA/AmSECT/SABM Update to the Clinical Practice Guidelines on Patient Blood Management recommends that RAP of the CPB circuit should be used wherever possible.

Postoperative Management

Minimizing Iatrogenic Blood Loss

Diagnostic phlebotomy significantly contributes to iatrogenic blood loss, often necessitating increased ABT. To minimize this loss, it is recommended to adopt strategies such as using smaller volume tubes for blood draws in adult patients and considering POC testing (Fig. 18.8). Smaller collection tubes, commonly used for pediatrics, can effectively minimize blood loss in adults, particularly those with anemia, while still providing adequate sample volumes for necessary tests. Replacing standard 3 mL blood gas syringes with 1 mL options can significantly reduce blood draw volume by 60%, without compromising sample integrity. Furthermore, POC testing offers an efficient alternative to conventional laboratory tests, often requiring less than 0.5 mL of blood, further minimizing unnecessary blood draws.

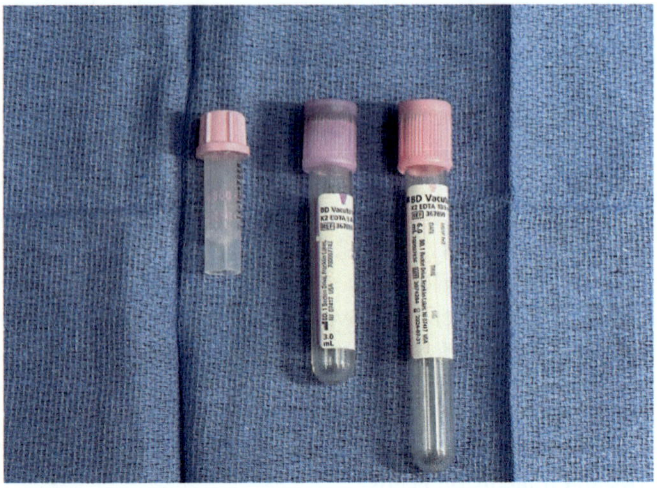

Fig. 18.8 Figure 18.1 Various sizes of test tubes for diagnostic phlebotomy. Emphasizing the importance of minimizing iatrogenic blood loss and the potential need for additional ABT through the strategic use of smaller volume tubes for blood draws in adult patients

Reinfusion of Postoperative Mediastinal Shed Blood

Implementing washed postoperative cell salvage and its effectiveness in possibly reducing ABT remains debated, with mixed evidence from various studies. However, unwashed salvaged blood from surgical drains is high in inflammatory mediators and fibrin split products, which can pose risks for altered coagulation and inflammatory complications. Consequently, the 2021 STS recommendation (Class III, Level of Evidence B) advises against direct reinfusion of mediastinal blood from postoperative chest tubes as a blood conservation strategy. Though currently discouraged, advancements in processing technology may revive this practice in the future.

Iron Replenishment

Continued anemia management with iron supplementation, aimed at replenishing iron stores, potentially improves outcomes. However, there is no clinical evidence from studies to support this conclusively.

Further Reading

Barile L, Fominskiy E, Di Tomasso N, et al. Acute normovolemic hemodilution reduces allogeneic red blood cell transfusion in cardiac surgery: a systematic review and meta-analysis of randomized trials. Anesth Analg. 2017;124(3):743–52. https://doi.org/10.1213/ANE.0000000000001609.

Bracey A, Shander A, Aronson S, et al. The use of topical hemostatic agents in cardiothoracic surgery. Ann Thorac Surg. 2017;104(1):353–60. https://doi.org/10.1016/j.athoracsur.2017.01.096.

Carroll C, Young F. Intraoperative cell salvage. BJA Educ. 2021;21(3):95–101. https://doi.org/10.1016/j.bjae.2020.11.007.

Delaney M, Wendel S, Bercovitz RS, et al. Transfusion reactions: prevention, diagnosis, and treatment. Lancet. 2016;388(10061):2825–36. https://doi.org/10.1016/S0140-6736(15)01313-6

Hare GMT, Mazer CD. Anemia: perioperative risk and treatment opportunity. Anesthesiology. 2021;135(3):520–30. https://doi.org/10.1097/ALN.0000000000003870.

Karkouti K, McCluskey S. Pro: preoperative autologous blood donation has a role in cardiac surgery. J Cardiothorac Vasc Anesth. 2003;17(1):121–5. https://doi.org/10.1053/jcan.2003.23.

Klein AA, Collier TJ, Brar MS, et al. The incidence and importance of anaemia in patients undergoing cardiac surgery in the UK – the first association of cardiothoracic anaesthetists national audit. Anaesthesia. 2016;71(6):627–35. https://doi.org/10.1111/anae.13423.

Lloyd TD, Geneen LJ, Bernhardt K, et al. Cell salvage for minimising perioperative allogeneic blood transfusion in adults undergoing elective surgery. Cochrane Database Syst Rev. 2023;9(9):CD001888. Published 2023 Sep 8. https://doi.org/10.1002/14651858.CD001888.pub5.

Muirhead B. Con: preoperative autologous donation has no role in cardiac surgery. J Cardiothorac Vasc Anesth. 2003;17(1):126–8. https://doi.org/10.1053/jcan.2003.24.

Raphael J, Mazer CD, Subramani S, et al. Society of cardiovascular anesthesiologists clinical practice improvement advisory for management of perioperative bleeding and hemostasis in cardiac surgery patients (published correction appears in Anesth Analg. 2020 Feb;130(2):e44). Anesth Analg. 2019;129(5):1209–21. https://doi.org/10.1213/ANE.0000000000004355.

Sikorski RA, Rizkalla NA, Yang WW, Frank SM. Autologous blood salvage in the era of patient blood management. Vox Sang. 2017;112(6):499–510. https://doi.org/10.1111/vox.12527.

Tibi P, McClure RS, Huang J, Baker RA, Fitzgerald D, Mazer CD, Stone M, Chu D, Stammers AH, Dickinson T, Shore-Lesserson L, Ferraris V, Firestone S, Kissoon K, Moffatt-Bruce S. STS/SCA/AmSECT/SABM update to the clinical practice guidelines on patient blood management. Ann Thorac Surg 2021 Sep;112(3):981–1004. https://doi.org/10.1016/j.athoracsur.2021.03.033. Epub 2021 Jun 30.

Vassallo R, Goldman M, Germain M, Lozano M, Collaborative BEST. Preoperative autologous blood donation: waning indications in an era of improved blood safety. Transfus Med Rev. 2015;29(4):268–75. https://doi.org/10.1016/j.tmrv.2015.04.001.

Warner MA, Shore-Lesserson L, Shander A, Patel SY, Perelman SI, Guinn NR. Perioperative anemia: prevention, diagnosis, and management throughout the Spectrum of perioperative care. Anesth Analg. 2020;130(5):1364–80. https://doi.org/10.1213/ANE.0000000000004727.

Zhou ZF, Jia XP, Sun K, et al. Mild volume acute normovolemic hemodilution is associated with lower intraoperative transfusion and postoperative pulmonary infection in patients undergoing cardiac surgery – a retrospective, propensity matching study. BMC Anesthesiol. 2017;17(1):13. Published 2017 Jan 26. https://doi.org/10.1186/s12871-017-0305-7.

Ultrafiltration and Leukofiltration

19

Levi Mulladzhanov

Introduction

Cardiopulmonary bypass (CPB) serves as an essential component in the majority of cardiac surgical procedures. Its development in the 1950s significantly transformed the landscape of cardiac surgery, enabling a broader range of procedures to be conducted safely and efficiently. Nevertheless, it is important to acknowledge that the CPB circuit and equipment pose notable challenges. There is significant trauma to the body associated with cannulation, exposure of the patient's blood to foreign materials, and the markedly "unphysiologic" nature of CPB. Consequently, numerous studies have been conducted to find ways to mitigate the harmful effects of CPB.

CPB triggers a systemic inflammatory response syndrome (SIRS)-like reaction mediated by various factors, including complement activation, ischemia, the secretion of pro-inflammatory cytokines and endotoxins, and direct trauma to the blood caused by exposure to and contact with CPB components. Other detrimental CPB effects occur due to the significant increase in total body water (TBW). This increase is directly caused by the size of the extracorporeal circuit and its usual priming with a crystalloid volume.

This SIRS-like state predictably affects multiple organ systems. The respiratory system is compromised primarily on account of acute lung injury, interstitial pulmonary edema, and abnormal gas exchange. The central nervous system suffers dysfunction, typically manifesting as postoperative cognitive dysfunction, usually presenting as delirium. The cardiovascular system can suffer as well, ranging from cardiac dysfunction to vasoplegia. The renal system is at high risk on account of significant hemodilution resulting in below-normal levels of oxygen content and thus poor oxygen delivery to sensitive tissues, as well as direct toxicity from exposed hemoglobin molecules because of red blood cell (RBC) trauma upon interfacing with CPB tubing and pumps, and infarction from microemboli.

This brief overview of multi-organ system involvement is not intended to be comprehensive, as these topics and issues are discussed in detail elsewhere; however, it is included to emphasize the significant damage that CPB may inflict on the body. As a result of the plethora of problems introduced by CPB, considerable effort has been directed toward developing different methods to limit these adverse effects. One proposed mechanism for mitigating some of these problems is UF (Fig. 19.1).

Supplementary Information The online version contains supplementary material available at https://doi.org/10.1007/978-3-031-91163-7_19.

L. Mulladzhanov (✉)
Department of Anesthesia, Cooper University Hospital, Camden, NJ, USA
e-mail: mulladzhanov-levi@cooperhealth.edu

A. S. Awad, J. DiNardo (eds.), *Clinical Perfusion for Cardiac Surgery*, https://doi.org/10.1007/978-3-031-91163-7_19

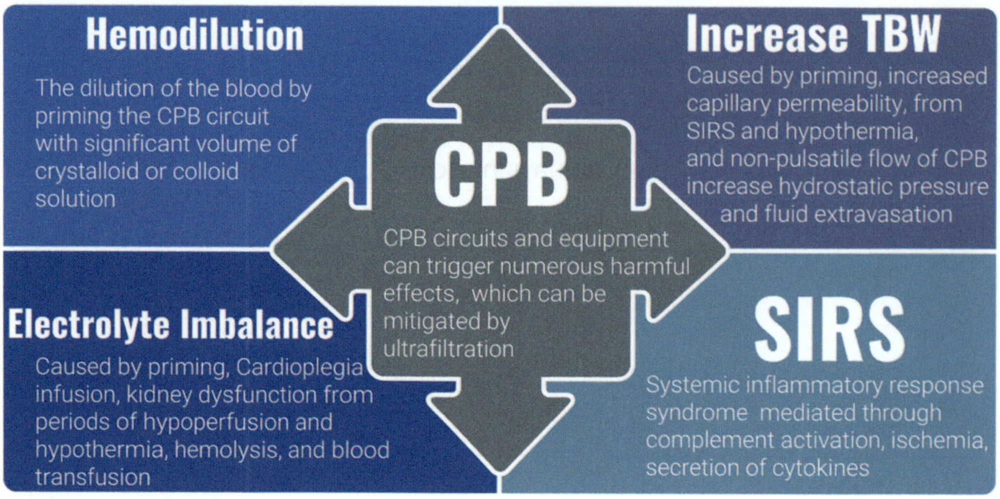

Fig. 19.1 The effects of CPB that can be mitigated by ultrafiltration

The History of Ultrafiltration in Cardiopulmonary Bypass

Ultrafiltration (UF) was first used in CPB in the mid-1970s to treat patients with chronic water retention and pulmonary edema. It was initially used alongside CPB predominantly for patients with preoperative renal issues or edema. However, in the late 1980s and early 1990s, UF began to be used more widely during and after CPB, driven by the hypothesis that postoperative organ dysfunction was caused by tissue edema resulting from TBW accumulation associated with open-heart surgery.

In 1991, Naik et al. pioneered the use of modified ultrafiltration (MUF) in pediatric patients undergoing CPB. They found that MUF reduced the need for blood products and colloids, minimized body fluid volume, and enhanced postoperative cardiac function. These findings have been substantiated by subsequent studies.

Today, UF is a widely used technique in CPB, and it has been shown to improve outcomes for patients with a variety of conditions.

Principles of Ultrafiltration

Before learning about UF, it is important to understand three basic principles: osmosis, diffusion, and convection. Each of these principles describes how solutes and/or solvents can move, and they play a crucial role in how UF works (see Table 19.1).

UF, simply put, is a generic term for the removal of plasma water (the liquid part of the blood, free of cells and colloids) from the blood. This process is called convection, wherein solutes are carried across a semi-permeable membrane by the flow of solvent, which is driven by a transmembrane pressure gradient and is influenced by the membrane's specific sieving coefficient. The rate of UF depends on the pressure gradient across the membrane and the concentration of solutes in the blood. The fluid that is removed is called ultrafiltrate (Fig. 19.2, Table 19.1).

Table 19.1 Principles of ultrafiltration

Property	Osmosis	Diffusion	Convection
Definition	Movement of solvent across a semi-permeable membrane from low to high solute concentration.	Movement of solutes from high to low concentration due to random motion.	Transport of solutes with the bulk flow of solvent, driven by a pressure gradient.
Type of movement	Passive	Passive	Active
Driving force	The concentration gradient of the solvent.	Concentration gradient of the solutes.	Applied pressure gradient.
Role in UF	Counteracted by applying pressure to move solvent against its natural osmotic flow.	Solute separation is based on size and concentration gradient.	It enhances solute removal and mitigates concentration polarization.
Dependency on membrane pore size	It is not applicable, as it primarily involves solvent transport.	This is crucial, as solutes smaller than pore size can diffuse through.	It is important, but solutes can be carried with the solvent bulk flow even if it is slightly larger than the pore size.
Examples	Water moving across the membrane from blood to the dialysate	Solutes moving across the membrane from blood to the dialysate and vice versa	Solutes and water moving across the membrane from the blood by means of pressure to the ultrafiltrate

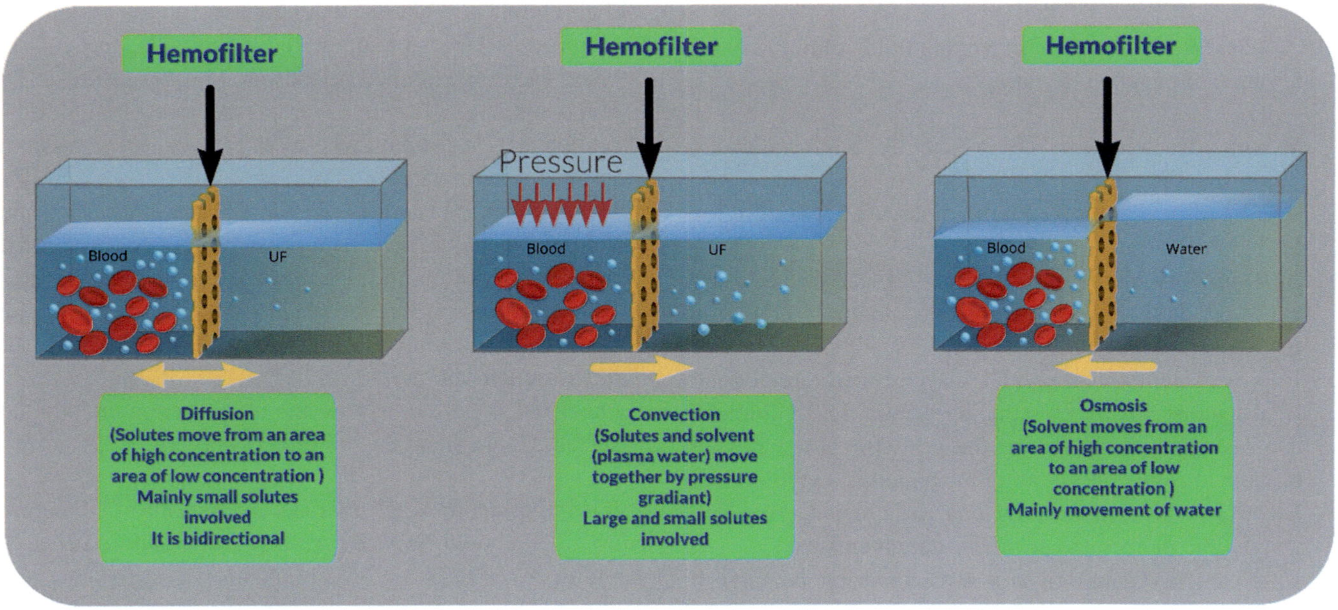

Fig. 19.2 Different mechanisms of ultrafiltration

Ultrafiltration Versus Hemodialysis

UF and hemodialysis are both medical procedures that utilize semi-permeable membranes to mechanically remove fluids and waste products from the blood, although they differ in several key ways (Table 19.2).

Table 19.2 Ultrafiltration vs Hemodialysis

Characteristic	Ultrafiltration	Hemodialysis
Mechanism	Removes excess fluid and smaller solutes via hydrostatic pressure and the process of convection or solute drag.	Removes excess fluid, electrolytes, and other low-molecular-weight toxic substances from the blood through a combination of diffusion and convection, even though diffusion is the primary method of solute removal in standard hemodialysis.
Requirements	No dialysate solution is required.	Dialysate solution is necessary to create a concentration gradient of solutes (waste products) between the blood and the dialysate, which causes the solutes to diffuse from the blood into the dialysate through a semi-permeable membrane.
Clinical context	It is commonly used during CPB to manage hemodilution and can also be utilized in other settings, such as in patients with acute or chronic kidney disease and heart failure.	It is often used in patients with acute or chronic kidney disease (CKD) requiring renal replacement therapy.
Treatment goals	To eliminate excess fluid, enhance oxygen delivery to tissues by elevating hematocrit levels, and improve cardiac and respiratory function.	To remove excess fluid, waste products, and toxins from the blood and maintain electrolyte balance.

Benefits and Risks of Ultrafiltration

UF, a versatile technique for managing fluid volume, offers a wide range of benefits, including:

- Volume Management: UF efficiently removes excess fluid, reducing the risk of fluid overload and edema. Additionally, it helps maintain or increase hematocrit levels by concentrating the blood.
- Inflammatory Mediator Reduction: UF can decrease levels of pro-inflammatory cytokines, potentially mitigating the SIRS seen after CPB.
- Improved Hemodynamics: UF may enhance cardiac function postoperatively by reducing excess fluid volume. It can also potentially reduce the need for blood product transfusions by concentrating the patient's own blood.
- Electrolyte Management: UF can assist in managing electrolyte imbalances and acid/base derangements.
- Improved Oxygen Delivery: By increasing hematocrit, UF may enhance oxygen delivery to tissues.

UF is a safe and effective technique, but it is important to be aware of the potential risks. These risks include:

- Some studies suggest an increased risk of postoperative acute kidney injury (AKI) when more than 32 mL/kg of fluid is removed during UF. This aggressive fluid removal approach may compromise perfusion in vital organs, including the kidneys.
- Altered Drug Concentration: UF can remove certain drugs from the bloodstream, depending on their protein binding and the pore size of the UF membrane. This process can alter the blood levels of these drugs. For instance, protein-bound drugs may exhibit increased blood levels after UF, while non-protein-bound drugs may show decreased levels. As an example, certain cephalosporin antibiotics can be removed by UF, potentially reducing their therapeutic blood concentrations.
- Hemolysis: UF can damage red blood cells, particularly when used for extended periods or at high pressures.
- Hypokalemia: UF can lower plasma potassium levels, particularly in patients who already have low potassium levels before undergoing UF.
- Hemodynamic Instability: While UF can diminish blood volume, potentially causing hemodynamic instability, patients supported on CPB may tolerate higher UF rates without becoming hemodynamically unstable, as the bypass pump controls cardiac output independently of intravascular volume.
- Other risks: UF can expose the blood to non-endothelial surfaces and extend the duration of surgery.

It is important to weigh the risks and benefits of UF before using it. UF should be used carefully and monitored closely to minimize the risks.

Hemoconcentrator (HC) or Hemofilter

Hemoconcentrators are special devices that work like dialysis machines. The main part of a hemoconcentrator is a filter that contains a bundle of hollow microporous fibers. Blood is circulated through the inside of the fibers, and plasma water and solutes are filtered out. A waste bag is connected to the external part of the fibers to collect the filtered substances. The semi-permeable membrane within the HC selectively filters out substances that are smaller than its pore size, including water, electrolytes, some cytokines, and drugs. Everything else, including red blood cells, platelets, and most plasma proteins, stays inside the fibers and is circulated back to the bloodstream (Figs. 19.3 and 19.4)

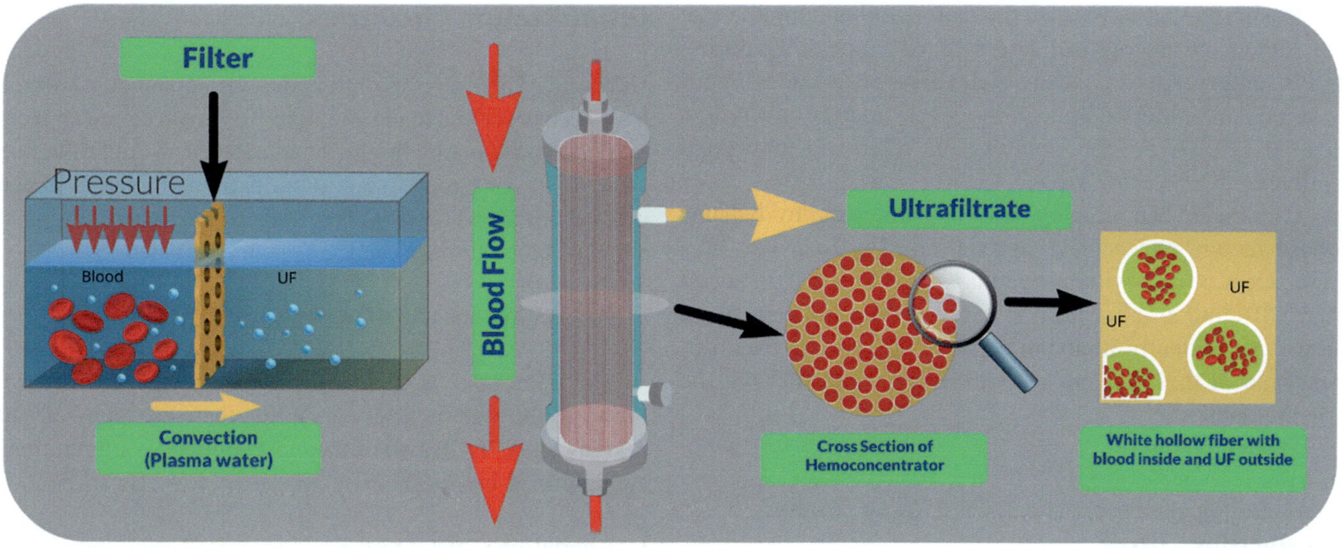

Fig. 19.3 The principles of operation and components of a hemoconcentrator

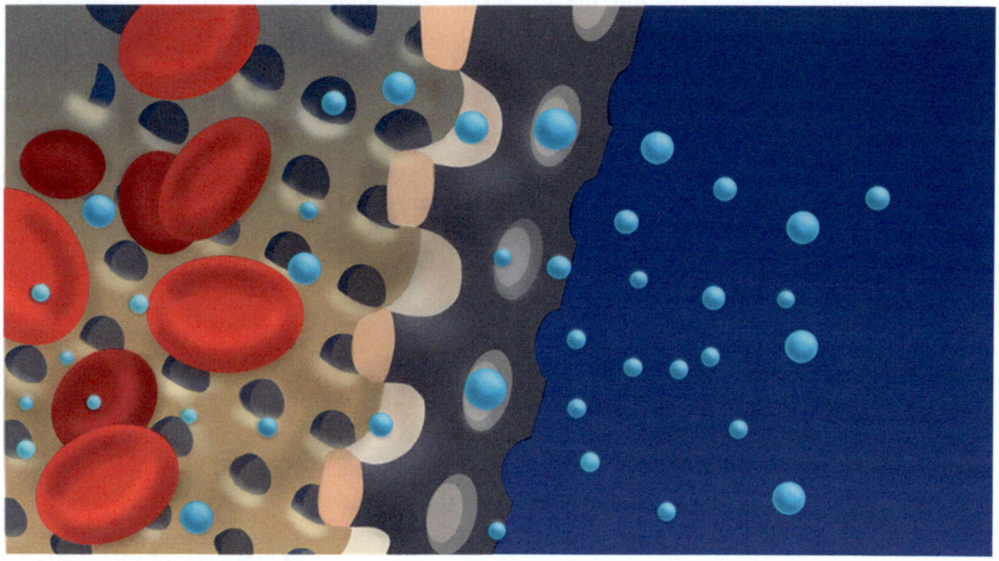

Fig. 19.4 The ultrafiltration process through the hemoconcentrator's semi-permeable membrane

Factors That Affect the Rate of Ultrafiltration

The dynamics of UF involve the crucial influence of several factors that affect the rate of removal, such as:

- Ultrafiltration Coefficient (Kuf): The Kuf measures the permeability of the filter membrane, representing the volume of fluid that can pass through the membrane per unit of pressure over a specific period. A higher Kuf corresponds to a faster UF rate.
- Transmembrane Pressure (TMP): The TMP refers to the pressure difference across the filter membrane and serves as the driving force for UF, pushing fluid through the membrane. A higher TMP results in a faster UF rate.
- Membrane Pore Size: The size of the membrane's pores determines which solutes can pass through the filter. Larger pores permit larger solutes to pass, while smaller pores restrict passage to smaller solutes.
- Hematocrit Level: The hematocrit level is the percentage of red blood cells in the blood. Higher hematocrit levels increase the viscosity of the blood, making filtration more challenging and potentially slowing the rate of UF.
- Rate of Blood Flow: The rate of blood flow through the filter also affects the rate of UF. A higher blood flow results in a faster UF rate.
- Negative Pressure on the Effluent Side (V): Negative pressure on the effluent side of the filter assists in drawing fluid through the membrane, potentially increasing the rate of UF.

It is important to balance the factors influencing the rate of UF to ensure optimal and safe UF, especially during CPB surgery. An excessively high UF rate can lead to hypovolemia and other complications, while an excessively low UF rate may not be effective in removing unwanted solutes.

Clinicians can employ various strategies to balance these factors and achieve optimal UF. For instance, they can select a filter with a specific Kuf and pore size, adjust the TMP, and monitor the rate of blood flow and hematocrit level. Additionally, applying negative pressure on the effluent side of the filter can aid in drawing fluid through the membrane.

Molecular Cutoff

The ultrafiltration devices used during CPB function like a sieve, primarily removing excess fluid and small solutes based on their molecular weight (MW), while retaining larger molecules such as proteins and blood cells. Specifically:

- The MW cutoff is approximately 50,000–65,000 Daltons (Da).
- Most common electrolytes have an MW range of 75–240 Da, meaning they are readily removed.
- Therapeutic drugs typically fall between 6000 and 200,000 Da, and essential blood components are largely retained.

Some studies suggest a relative increase in heparin concentration after UF, possibly due to its negative charge binding to positively charged plasma proteins and altering its filterability during UF. Monitoring heparin levels during and after UF is essential for maintaining appropriate anticoagulation management and adjusting protamine administration as needed.

Types of Ultrafiltration

Various forms of UF have been introduced and evolved from the 1970s through the 1990s, with studies continuing into the 2000s and 2020s. While there are numerous types of UF, this discussion will focus on four main types: Pre-bypass ultrafiltration (PUF or PBUF), conventional ultrafiltration (CUF), modified ultrafiltration (MUF), and zero-balance ultrafiltration (Z-BUF). These four types of UF operate on the same principles but are utilized at different times and for distinct purposes. Additionally, it is possible to combine multiple UF types for the same patient during a single procedure.

Ultrafiltration Circuitries

UF during CPB involves numerous variations, all of which have been described in the literature. Two main circuit connection methods are highlighted: arterio-venous ultrafiltration (A-V UF) and veno-venous ultrafiltration (V-V UF). Each method has a unique setup that utilizes different pathways to circulate blood through the UF system (see Video 19.1).

1. Arterio-Venous Ultrafiltration (A-V UF)

The hemofilter is typically placed between the arterial limb and the venous reservoir. While there are many circuit designs for A-V UF, two of the most common configurations are described below:

- Arterial line (distal to the oxygenator or from the arterial filter purge line) to the venous reservoir (CUF): This is the most commonly used method of CUF. It involves circulating blood from the arterial line to the venous reservoir using the recirculation line—an arterial/venous loop specifically designed to quickly remove air from the CPB circuit.
- Arterial line to venous line (MUF): This is a classical connection method for MUF, where the blood pump is used to regulate the blood flow rate.

2. Veno-venous Ultrafiltration (V-V UF)

The literature exhaustively covers all the possibilities for V-V UF and describes many different techniques. However, the most straightforward method is to connect the venous line to the venous reservoir, incorporating a hemofilter into the circuit.

Methods of Ultrafiltration

Numerous UF methods are used during CPB, each with its own unique advantages and considerations. These methods, including PBUF, CUF, Z-BUF, DUF, MUF, and SMUF, can be differentiated by their timing and specific relationship to the CPB process.

Before CPB

1. Pre-Bypass Ultrafiltration (PUF or PBUF)

In pediatric cardiac surgery involving CPB, the priming solution typically contains a substantial volume of stored blood. Pre-bypass ultrafiltration (PUF or PBUF) is a technique that uses ultrafiltration to filter the stored blood before it is used in CPB. The goal of PUF is to mitigate the deleterious effects and inflammatory cytokine production associated with the use of stored blood.

During CPB

1. Conventional Ultrafiltration (CUF)

CUF is a UF technique employed toward the end of the CPB run, during the rewarming phase, to remove excess fluid and inflammatory mediators from the blood. In terms of setup, the hemofilter is connected to the CPB circuit in parallel, with the inlet of the HC positioned immediately after the oxygenator and the outlet connected to the venous reservoir. This configuration creates a closed and efficient loop for blood circulation and filtration, as illustrated in Figs. 19.5 and 19.7.

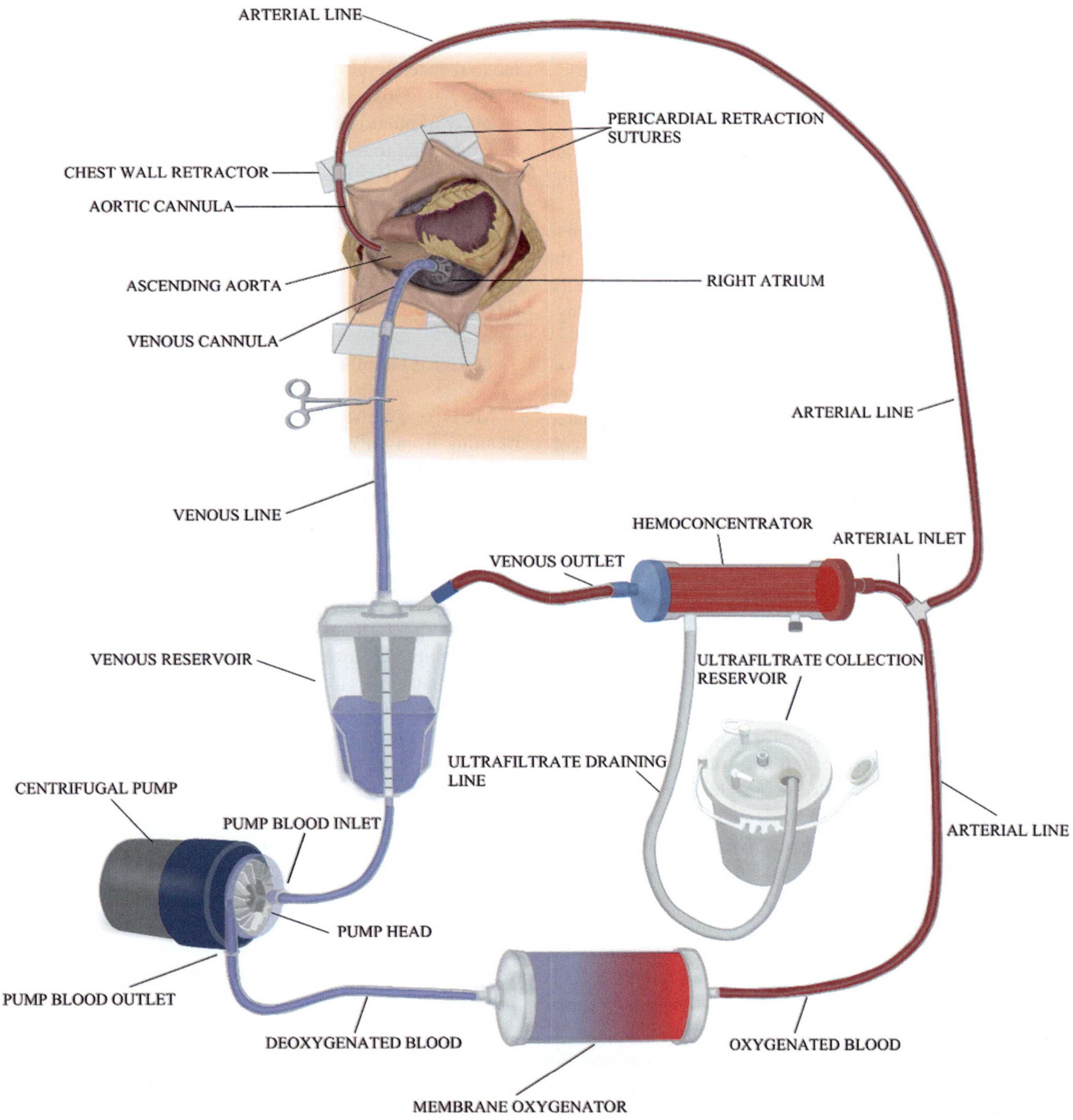

Fig. 19.5 The conventional ultrafiltration circuit (arterio-venous setup). This diagram illustrates the integration of the HC into the system, secured to the arterial line using a Luer-Lok connector positioned immediately after the oxygenator. As a result, a portion of the oxygenated blood is diverted towards the HC, where filtration occurs. Post-filtration, the concentrated blood is channeled towards the venous reservoir. Simultaneously, the fluid separated during filtration is collected in a dedicated waste container, set aside for subsequent disposal

Operational Considerations

A critical consideration when employing CUF is that the HC functions as an arterial-to-venous shunt, diverting blood flow away from the patient. This is especially significant in pediatric cases, where low flow rates could result in the entire blood supply to the patient being diverted through the device.

Integrating the HC into the CPB circuit requires meticulous attention and precision:

- The process begins by noting the arterial pressure prior to engaging the HC.
- Blood is then allowed to begin circulating through the device while the arterial pressure is closely monitored.
- If a decrease in arterial pressure is detected, the flow rate is gradually increased to restore the pressure to its initial level.
- When it is time to discontinue the HC, care must be taken to prevent a possible rise in blood pressure. In this case, the flow should be gradually reduced to allow a return to the original pressure while maintaining hemodynamic stability.

One of the reasons CUF is limited in the amount of volume that can be removed from the patient is that it is conducted while the patient is still being perfused and oxygenated via CPB. CPB requires a certain minimum amount of volume to be left in the venous reservoir to conduct CPB safely. It is challenging for a normal bypass to sustain the liquid level in the oxygenator, which limits the amount of moisture filtered out.

2. Zero-Balance Ultrafiltration (Z-BUF)

Z-BUF is a modification of CUF that is performed while the patient is on CPB. Z-BUF is a technique designed to extract excess fluid from the blood during CPB while preserving the patient's blood volume. In this approach, UF occurs during the rewarming phase, and any volume filtered out is simultaneously replaced with an equivalent volume of crystalloid solution. This practice helps preserve the volume in the reservoir while still enabling ongoing UF. Similar to CUF, the ultrafiltration unit is incorporated in parallel with the CPB circuit, allowing for adjustment of the blood flow rate through the HC to achieve the intended fluid removal rate. Simultaneously, a crystalloid replacement fluid, most commonly a balanced solution like Plasmalyte (refer to Chap. 9, "Prime Solutions for the Circuit"), is infused into the venous reservoir to match the rate of fluid extraction. This parallel process ensures consistency in blood volume throughout the procedure. Z-BUF primarily serves to remove unwanted electrolytes (e.g., potassium) and inflammatory mediators.

While both Z-BUF and CUF effectively remove excess fluid and inflammatory mediators during CPB, some reports suggest that Z-BUF is more effective and has advantages over CUF in scavenging and removing inflammatory mediators. This increased efficiency may stem from Z-BUF's ability to operate without being restricted by the volume in the venous reservoir. Another advantage of Z-BUF over CUF is its ability to maintain blood volume, which contributes to better hemodynamic stability. Some clinical trials have suggested potential improvements in pulmonary function and other postoperative outcomes with the use of Z-BUF, even in cases involving significant lung injury. In pediatric patients, some clinical trials have indicated that Z-BUF may contribute to reduced levels of various cytokines, decreased postoperative blood loss, shorter intubation periods, and improved recovery of pulmonary function. Nonetheless, it is crucial to note that other trials have shown no significant benefits when comparing Z-BUF with CUF. However, these findings are not yet conclusive, and further investigation is required for definitive validation.

After CPB

1. Modified Ultrafiltration (MUF)

MUF is another UF technique employed following weaning from CPB but before the administration of protamine to mitigate the adverse effects associated with the use of CPB, particularly the increase in TBW, capillary leak syndrome, and potential organ dysfunction. Similar to CUF, MUF filters out inflammatory mediators; however, because it is performed after the termination of CPB, a significantly larger volume can be safely removed from the patient without affecting hemodynamic stability. It is conducted within a critical time window immediately post-bypass and prior to the reversal of heparin, typically spanning between 10 and 20 min or until the desired hematocrit (HCT) level is achieved. To calculate the filtrate volume, subtract the ultrafiltrate volume removed during CUF and diuresis volumes from the sum of the priming crystalloid, cardioplegia, any fluid used during valve testing, and crystalloid volumes added during the CPB circuit. MUF, more so than CUF, can hemoconcentrate blood, thereby raising hematocrit.

MUF Can Be Conducted Using Many Different Setups

- A-V MUF Circuit:

First described by Naik and referred to as the Great Ormond Street Hospital method (GOSH method), this is the most commonly used setup. It involves pumping

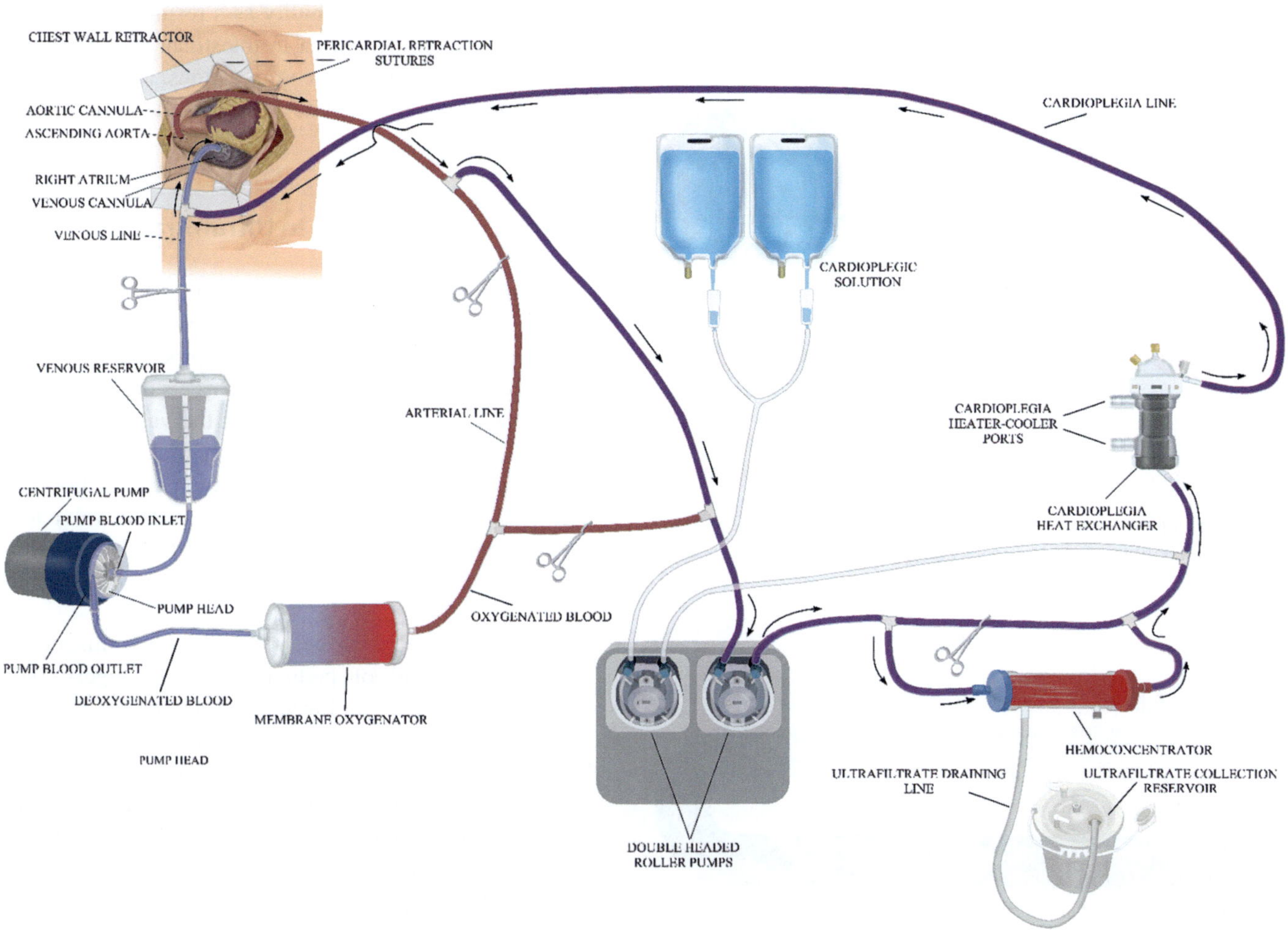

Fig. 19.6 Modified ultrafiltration circuit (arterio-venous setup). This illustrative representation shows the integration of the HC into the cardioplegia delivery system. The circuit demonstrates the reverse flow of blood from the aortic cannula, passing through the HC, where excess water and solutes are meticulously filtered out before being directed back to the right atrium. The integration of the cardioplegia circuit's heat exchanger ensures that the filtrate is warmed to the optimal temperature

blood retrograde from the aortic cannula through the HC and returning it to the right atrium. A modification to this method was created to warm the filtrate using the cardioplegia delivery system and its associated heat exchanger. The HC is connected to the arterial line by means of a connector. When CPB is off, the cardioplegia roller pump is used to drive blood from the aorta and arterial line to the HC, where filtered blood flows into the venous line and returns to the right atrium. In this case, the venous reservoir line is clamped. Filtrate fluid is stored in a separate waste container, to be discarded later, as illustrated in Figs. 19.6 and 19.8 and Video 19.2.

- V-A MUF:
- Also known as simplified modified ultrafiltration (SMUF), it is a relatively new variation of MUF that has been shown to be safe and effective. It is simpler and quicker to perform than A-V MUF, as it does not require reconfiguration of the bypass circuit after weaning from CPB. This makes it ideal for situations where the rapid initiation of ultrafiltration is desired. In this setup, blood is drawn from the venous reservoir, passed through the HC, and the filtered blood is returned to the arterial line.
- V-V MUF:
- This method utilizes a closed-loop circuit that draws blood from the inferior vena cava (IVC) cannula, passes it through an HC, and then returns it to the right atrium.
- Passive MUF:
- In the passive variation of MUF, the patient's pressure drives blood through the HC via the arterial line, and the filtered blood is returned to the IVC, all without the need for a roller pump. This process is facilitated by the pressure gradient between the aorta and the right atrium and is further aided by applying a vacuum of approximately 20 cm H_2O at the ultrafiltrate outlet port of the filter. The operational steps involve meticulous placement and adjustment of the ultrafiltration equipment, followed by a

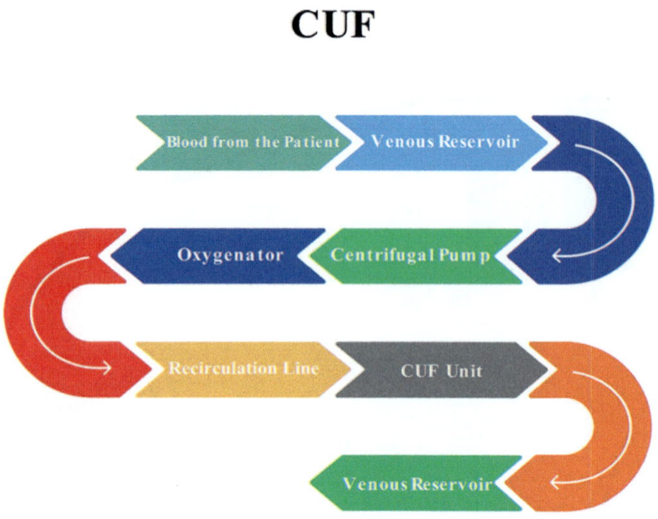

Fig. 19.7 Visual representation of the blood flow in the conventional ultrafiltration circuit (arterio-venous configuration)

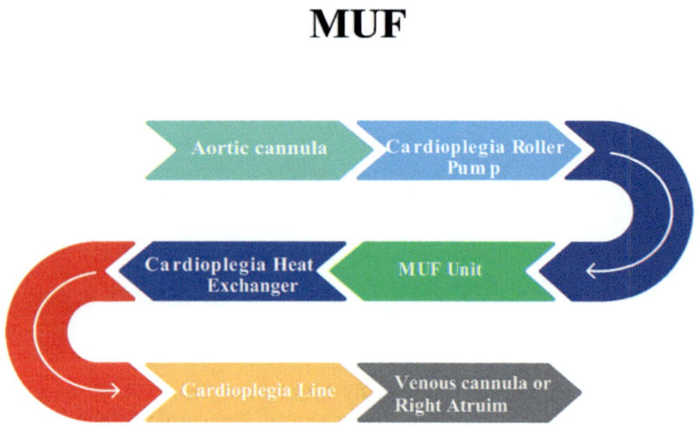

Fig. 19.8 Visual representation of the blood flow in the modified ultrafiltration circuit (arterio-venous configuration)

series of preparatory measures, including clamping, deairing, and warming of the cardioplegia system water bath. These steps ensure the safe and efficient execution of the MUF procedure.

MUF presents a series of advantages, including increased hematocrit levels, conservation of formed elements and clotting factors, and improved overall patient recovery outcomes. Increased hematocrit is directly associated with decreased blood, fresh frozen plasma (FFP), and platelet transfusion after 24 h. There have been studies that show the benefits of MUF in the adult population as well. Indeed, MUF has shown reduced hospital morbidity as a result of lower rates of respiratory, neurological, gastrointestinal, and, to a lesser extent renal and hemorrhagic complications. However, MUF has not been shown to decrease mortality after adult cardiac operations.

Pediatric Considerations in Ultrafiltration

- As previously discussed, PBUF is particularly utilized for neonates when older blood is used to prime the circuit.
- In the majority of pediatric bypass procedures, CUF is employed. This technique chiefly targets the elimination of excess volume accumulating in the venous reservoir during the bypass. This surplus in plasma water can arise from the crystalloid component of the cardioplegia solution, blood products added to the circuit, valve testing solutions, or patients with congestive heart failure (CHF). Additionally, it can help correct high potassium levels.
- In recent years, there has been an increasing utilization of MUF in the field of pediatric cardiac surgery. This technique has been employed as an adjunctive approach to increase hemoconcentration following CPB. The use of MUF often allows for a greater level of hemoconcentration compared to CUF. As a result, numerous pediatric cardiac centers worldwide have incorporated some form of MUF techniques into their practice.
- Many studies support the notion that the aforementioned benefits of CUF and MUF are particularly tangible in the pediatric population, where shifts in TBW are significantly more pronounced than in adults due to their smaller size. Consequently, children are much more susceptible to the associated consequences.
- CUF and MUF combinations have shown consistent benefits for children, as opposed to CUF alone, particularly when considering various early postoperative complications. Studies have demonstrated that pediatric patients who received a combination of CUF and MUF, as opposed to CUF alone, benefited from reduced mechanical ventilation durations and shorter ICU stays. This combination also improved lung function by effectively removing excess body water. Additionally, these patients had a lower need for inotropes and displayed enhanced hemodynamics. The resulting hemoconcentration, characterized by TBW and increased hemoglobin levels, contributed to improved cardiac and pulmonary functions.

Leukofiltration

Leukofiltration is the final concept to consider. The principle of leukofiltration is to remove either activated leukocytes or their byproducts. More specifically, one of the proposed mechanisms of CPB-induced lung damage is the entrapment of activated leukocytes within lung capillaries, where the inflammatory cascade is triggered. Some studies have shown that leukocyte depletion via leukofiltration is associated with reduced heart and lung reperfusion injury mediated by oxygen free radicals. Additionally, they demonstrated significantly better oxygenation indices, lower extravascular lung water scores, and a shorter duration of postoperative mechanical ventilation. Notably, other studies have shown that the benefits of leukofiltration are more significant on the cellular level and play a limited role clinically.

Ultrafiltration and leukofiltration offer several benefits. These stem from removing detrimental inflammatory cytokines and activated neutrophils, decreasing total body water, and reducing the systemic inflammation that results from CPB exposure. Many studies demonstrate varying degrees of benefit from each of these methods; however, some studies indicate that these benefits are limited in their clinical manifestation, particularly in the adult population. In contrast, the CUF/MUF combination is widely recognized for providing significant advantages in the pediatric population. The principle of "do no harm" is particularly relevant here. Fortunately, numerous reviews indicate that there are no significant downsides to using UF and leukofiltration methods in either children or adults. Combined with the potential benefits of these interventions, this supports their integration into clinical practice and encourages ongoing refinement and study to make CPB safer in the future.

Further Reading

Hensley NB, Colao JA, Zorrilla-Vaca et al. Ultrafiltration in cardiac surgery: results of a systematic review and meta-analysis. Perfusion 2023 Feb 16:2676591231157970. https://doi.org/10.1177/02676591231157970. Epub ahead of print.

Lohbusch B, Olson K, Magowan B, Cherichella R, et al. Adult clinical perfusion practice survey: 2020 results. J Extra Corpor Technol 2023 Mar 24;55(1):3–22. https://doi.org/10.1051/ject/2023002. PMID: 37034099; PMCID: PMC10071505.

Padalino MA, Stellin G. Chapter 208–Modified ultrafiltration in pediatric heart surgery in the book critical care nephrology (3rd edn).

Palanzo DA, Wise RK, Myers JL, et al. Safety and utility of modified ultrafiltration in pediatric cardiac surgery. Perfusion 2023 Jan;38(1):150–155. https://doi.org/10.1177/02676591211043697. Epub 2021 Sep 11.

Tibi P, McClure RS, Huang J, Moffatt-Bruce S, et al. STS/SCA/AmSECT/SABM update to the clinical practice guidelines on patient blood management. J Extra Corpor Technol 2021 Jun;53(2):97–124. https://doi.org/10.1182/ject-2100053. PMID: 34194077; PMCID: PMC8220901.

Wahba A, Milojevic M, Boer C, et al. EACTS/EACTA/EBCP committee reviewers. 2019 EACTS/EACTA/EBCP guidelines on cardiopulmonary bypass in adult cardiac surgery. Eur J Cardiothorac Surg. 2020 Feb 1;57(2):210–51. https://doi.org/10.1093/ejcts/ezz267.

Walczak AB, Voss JM, Dreher M, Groom R, et al. International survey of perfusion practice for pediatric and congenital heart surgery: 2021 results. J Extra Corpor Technol 2022 Dec;54(4):291–317. https://doi.org/10.1182/ject-2200012. PMID: 36742024; PMCID: PMC9891471.

Fluid Management During Cardiopulmonary Bypass

20

Emma C. Huang, Ramesh Mariyappa, Siddharth V. Pahwa, and Jiapeng Huang

Introduction

Fluid management during cardiopulmonary bypass (CPB) is challenging, as inadequate volume leads to poor perfusion and ischemia to vital organs, yet too much volume causes hemodilution, fluid extravasation, tissue edema, and coagulopathy. Different types and combinations of crystalloid and colloid solutions have been used. Fluid management is a continuous process before, during, and after CPB. Fluid status at each stage must be evaluated carefully and managed with a holistic approach, not in isolation. In addition, the effects of fluid status on organ perfusion should be monitored continuously to guide fluid management throughout the procedure requiring CPB.

Supplementary Information The online version contains supplementary material available at https://doi.org/10.1007/978-3-031-91163-7_20.

E. C. Huang
Department of Anesthesiology, Duke University, Raleigh, NC, USA
e-mail: emma.huang@duke.edu

R. Mariyappa · J. Huang (✉)
Department of Anesthesiology and Perioperative Medicine, University of Louisville, Louisville, KY, USA
e-mail: ramesh.mariyappa@louisville.edu; jiapeng.huang@louisville.edu

S. V. Pahwa
Department of Cardiovascular and Thoracic Surgery, University of Louisville, Louisville, KY, USA
e-mail: siddharth.pahwa@louisville.edu

General Principles of Fluid Management During CPB

1. Ensure adequate organ perfusion by adjusting fluid status, blood pressure, and pump flow.
2. Maintain normal acid–base homeostasis, glucose levels, and electrolyte balance.
3. Avoid fluid overload causing organ edema and ischemia.
4. Minimize hemodilution.
5. Goal-directed fluid therapy guided by continuous end-organ perfusion measurements.

Many of these principles were discussed in different chapters of the book. We will briefly highlight them and focus on the items that are not covered in other chapters.

Monitoring Fluid Status and End-Organ Perfusion

The 2023 American Society of ExtraCorporeal Technology (AmSECT) Standards and Guidelines for Perfusion Practice outlines key recommendations for monitoring and managing CPB (AmSECT 2023). These recommendations include the continuous monitoring of arterial blood pressure, arterial blood flow, blood gas analyses, venous line occlusion, central venous/pulmonary artery blood pressure, and in-line blood gas monitoring. Additionally, cerebral oximetry monitors cerebral oxygen saturation, and indexed oxygen delivery and consumption calculations are recommended to optimize gas exchange (Bartels 2019; Turro et al. 2020). See Figs. 20.1, 20.2, 20.3, and 20.4 for images of the monitoring devices.

These recommendations aim to maintain MAP between 50 and 70 mmHg, ensure accurate flow delivery, and optimize patient perfusion and oxygenation throughout CPB. Details on the implementation of these guidelines,

A. S. Awad, J. DiNardo (eds.), *Clinical Perfusion for Cardiac Surgery*, https://doi.org/10.1007/978-3-031-91163-7_20

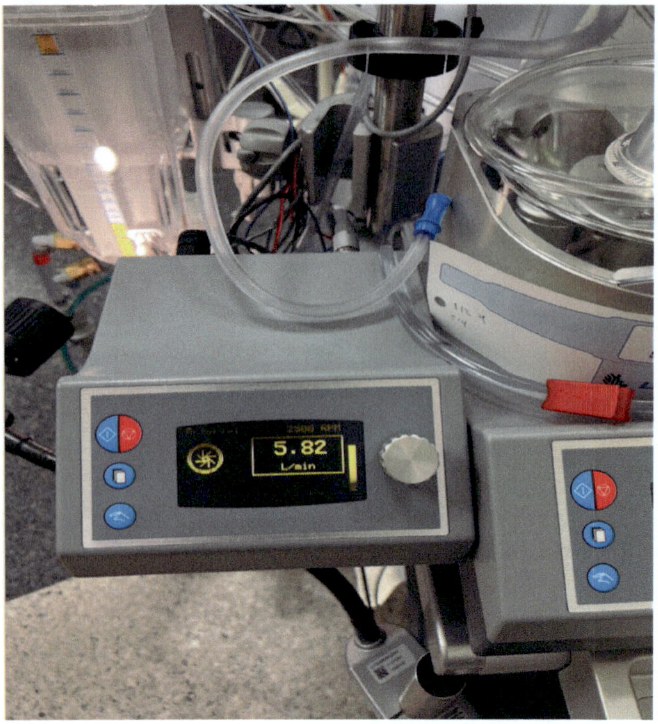

Fig. 20.1 Continuous pump flow measurement on CPB machines

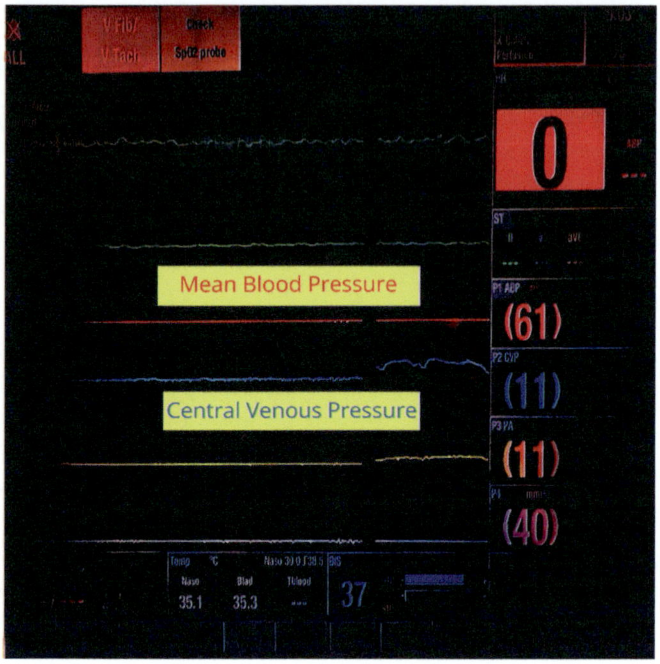

Fig. 20.3 The monitoring screen during CPB displays nonpulsatile MAP in red and CVP in blue, essential for managing patient hemodynamics as recommended by AmSECT while on CPB

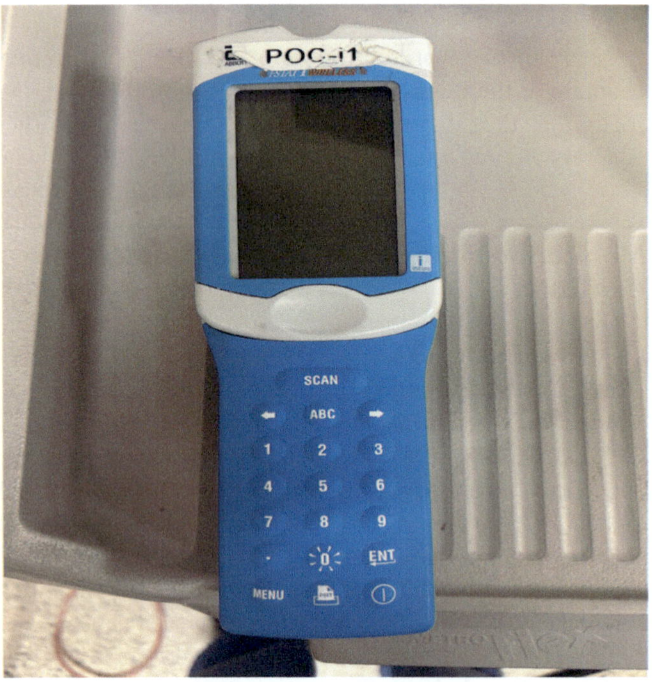

Fig. 20.2 Point of care arterial blood gas analyzer

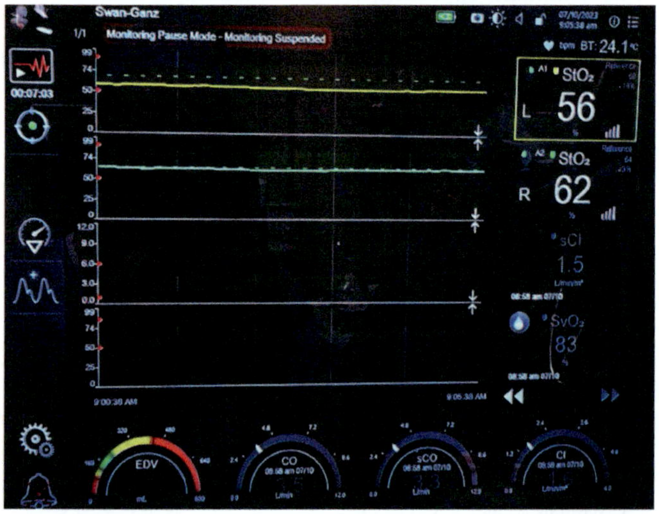

Fig. 20.4 Cerebral oximetry monitoring during CPB. The top right number indicates left cerebral oxygenation, while the number directly below it indicates right cerebral oxygenation. Below these, the cardiac index is displayed, followed by the mixed venous oxygenation value

including specific targets for blood flow rates and considerations for various patient conditions, are discussed in-depth in the corresponding sections of the manual. Please refer to Chaps. 13 and 14 for a detailed discussion on various monitoring techniques and monitoring the adequacy of perfusion during CPB.

Fluid Management Before CPB

The goal of fluid management before CPB is to achieve a delicate balance: aiming to maintain adequate blood pressure and cardiac index to prevent myocardial ischemia while also avoiding fluid overloading the patient, which can lead to further hemodilution and anemia due to the addition of priming fluids to the CPB circuit. Several factors contribute to hemodynamic instability in patients undergoing cardiac surgery before CPB:

1. NPO (nothing by mouth) before surgery causing hypovolemia
2. Congestive heart failure with fluid overload
3. Chronic and/or acute renal insufficiency from cardiac diseases leading to fluid overload
4. Diuretics use or withholding with resultant hyper- or hypovolemia
5. Left ventricular (LV) dysfunction from coronary artery disease (Deidda et al. 2017)
6. LV dysfunction from valvular diseases
7. LV dysfunction from another cardiomyopathy
8. Right ventricular (RV) dysfunction from pulmonary hypertension, LV dysfunction, coronary artery disease (Deidda et al. 2017), valvular diseases, and other causes
9. Myocardial depression from anesthetic drugs and other medications such as beta-blockers
10. Reduced afterload from anesthetic drugs, vasodilators, sepsis, or other causes
11. Arrhythmia such as atrial fibrillation, junctional rhythm, ventricular arrhythmia, and conduction disorders
12. Surgical manipulations

It is prudent to obtain an estimation of the patient's fluid balance from the time of arrival in the operating room until CPB by checking and recording the estimated blood loss, urinary output, and volume of fluids administered by anesthesia personnel. Knowing the patient's estimated blood volume, hematocrit, and circuit priming volume allows for the calculation of an estimated hematocrit after initiation of CPB. This will give the perfusionist and anesthesiologist some indication of CPB fluid or blood requirements.

In this period, hemodynamics should be maintained with judicious fluid administration, inotrope and vasopressor use to maintain adequate blood pressure, cardiac index, and cerebral oxygenation. Fluid amounts administered in this period should be communicated to the perfusionist and considered in the overall CPB fluid management strategy.

Choice of Fluids in Cardiac Surgery

Maintenance of intravascular volume is a common goal for perioperative management in cardiovascular surgery. The merits of specific choices for fluid therapy to replace ongoing fluid loss continue to be debated. Although there may be theoretical advantages to using either colloid or crystalloid for volume replacement, clinical trial data do not definitively support one over the other in terms of mortality outcomes. Both have distinct advantages and disadvantages. More important than the choice of volume replacement is the appropriate volume replacement amount to avoid tissue hypoperfusion (Kaplan 2017).

Saline-based crystalloids usually result in an expansion of the plasma volume by approximately 200–250 mL for each 1 L administered; glucose-based solutions expand the plasma volume by approximately 60–70 mL for each 1 L infused; and colloid solutions result in an expansion of the plasma volume equivalent to the volume infused. Within the semisynthetic colloid solutions, there is variation in the degree of plasma volume expansion and a differential influence on hemostasis and inflammatory processes (Kaplan 2017).

Colloids for volume replacement have issues with hemostasis, adverse reactions, and a greater risk of volume overload. Crystalloids require larger volumes of fluid to achieve volume resuscitation and may lead to tissue edema and a potential reduction in tissue oxygen delivery. It is unclear whether the type of fluid therapy affects the development of pulmonary edema.

Crystalloid solutions commonly used in cardiac surgery are 0.9% (normal) saline and buffered isotonic crystalloid solutions. The use of 0.9% saline may be associated with increased blood transfusion requirements compared with buffered crystalloids in the nonsurgical patient population as well as with a heightened risk of acidosis with high volumes in animal models (Tibi et al. 2021a).

For colloids, albumin has been used extensively in cardiac surgery. The expert consensus on the use of human serum albumin in adult cardiac surgery from the Chinese Association of Cardiovascular Surgeons, the Chinese Society of Thoracic and Cardiovascular Surgery, and the Chinese Society of Cardiothoracic and Vascular Anesthesiology in 2023 recommends the following (Xiang et al. 2023):

- It is reasonable to administer albumin following crystalloid resuscitation in patients who require further volume replacement during and after cardiac surgery to avoid excessive positive fluid balance (Class IIb, Level of Evidence (LOE) B-NR).

- Albumin infusion might be helpful to maintain intravascular volume and arterial pressure when aggressive diuresis is administered to relieve fluid overload and interstitial edema after cardiac surgery. Hypertonic (20% or 25%) albumin is preferred in this setting (Class IIb, LOE C-LD).
- Albumin is not routinely recommended as the first-line choice for fluid resuscitation during and after cardiac surgery (Class III, LOE B-R).
- The use of albumin for fluid resuscitation in patients with hemorrhagic shock and uncontrolled bleeding is not recommended (Class III, LOE C-EO).
- Albumin infusion is reasonable to supplement prior volume and albumin loss in patients with controlled bleeding following a hemorrhagic stroke (Class IIa, LOE C-EO).
- Pump priming with albumin for optimizing blood management might be reasonable (Class IIb, LOE B-NR).
- Pump priming with albumin might be considered in specific cardiac surgical populations, such as those undergoing heart transplantation, pulmonary thromboembolectomy, and deep hypothermia circulatory arrest (Class IIb, LOE C-EO).
- Albumin infusion is reasonable to correct preoperative hypoalbuminemia in normovolemic patients (Class IIb, LOE B-NR).
- Correcting postoperative hypoalbuminemia with albumin infusion in normovolemic patients might be beneficial (Class IIb, LOE C-EO).

The 2021 Update to the Clinical Practice Guidelines on Patient Blood Management by the Society of Thoracic Surgeons (STS), Society of Cardiovascular Anesthesiologists [SCA], the AmSECT, and the Society for the Advancement of Blood Management (SABM) recommends the following:

- Administering human albumin after cardiac surgery is reasonable for intravascular volume replacement and minimizing the need for transfusion (Class IIA, LOE B-R) (Tibi et al. 2021a, b).
- Hydroxyethyl starch (HES), another commonly used colloid solution in cardiac surgery, is not recommended as a volume expander in CPB patients because it may increase the risk of bleeding (Class III: No Benefit, LOE B-R) (Tibi et al. 2021a, b).

Fluid Management During CPB

Priming Volume and Solutions

Please refer to Chap. 9 for detailed information.

Priming Volume The appropriate priming volume for an oxygenator-tubing system is crucial for "safe" priming volume CPB initiation and maintaining adequate flow rates, with the key objective being to avoid air embolism—a serious CPB complication. Priming volume varies with patient and circuit factors and is an integral part of fluid management before, during, and after CPB (Task Force on Patient Blood Management for Adult Cardiac Surgery of the European Association for Cardio-Thoracic Surgery (EACTS), the European Association of Cardiothoracic Anaesthesiology et al. 2018).

Crystalloids versus Colloids There is no consensus upon the best priming solution. Surveys show European centers often prefer crystalloids, typically balanced salt solutions such as lactated Ringers, with or without glucose. Some use colloids, including albumin and gelatin-based solutions. Hemodilution in CPB reduces plasma colloidal oncotic pressure by diluting plasma proteins, potentially driving fluid into the interstitial and intracellular spaces, causing postoperative edema or organ dysfunction. Used solutions include 5% and 25% albumin, dextran, plasma protein fraction, 6% HES (withdrawn in the US by the FDA due to associated complications), along with human plasma.

HES Studies on HES in priming solutions show no significant impact on postoperative blood loss or transfusion requirements, yet a Cochrane review highlights a heightened risk of AKI, discouraging its use. Recently, dextran 40-based priming solutions have been suggested, but their benefits and risks, like reduced fluid balance and allergic reactions, require further large-scale research (Mutter et al. 2013).

Human plasma should be reserved for cases with a clear clinical and laboratory-documented bleeding diathesis. This is particularly relevant for patients undergoing cardiac transplantation or left ventricular assist device (LVAD) implantation, who often have coagulopathy due to a low cardiac output, liver dysfunction, or pharmacologic therapy. Given the difficulty of correcting coagulopathy before CPB in these patients, adding plasma can help mitigate post-CPB coagulopathy.

Mannitol Is added to the priming solution in many centers to reduce the risk of AKI. However, a recent Cochrane review found no evidence to support this notion (Zacharias et al. 2013), noting that the quality of the evidence was not high.

Glucose Hyperglycemia is common during CPB due to the high prevalence of diabetes in cardiac surgery patients, surgery-induced stress, and positive inotrope use. The benefits and risks of tight glycemic control remain controversial. Some studies suggest tighter control offers a lower mortality rate, fewer adverse outcomes (like atrial fibrillation (AF), epicardial pacing need, and prolonged ventilation), and shorter ICU stays (Haga et al. 2011). This has led some centers to eliminate glucose from priming solutions. However, the risk of hypoglycemia, which increases morbidity and mortality, must be considered. Recent guidelines suggest a more liberal strategy for patients with diabetes (up to 180 mg/dL) and tighter control for those without (<140 mg/dL) (Tsai et al. 2016). Conversely, adding glucose to prime raises osmotic pressure, reducing fluid retention, which may be beneficial for certain patients, including those for whom use of blood-derived colloid solutions is restricted (such as members of the Jehovah's Witness faith). However, 2019 EACTS/EACTA/EBCP guidelines advise against modern low-molecular-weight starches in solutions due to bleeding and transfusion risks (Class III, LOE C).

Autologous Priming

Autologous priming, where blood displaces fluid in the circuit for the external reservoir, has gained popularity for reducing priming volume. This technique, often combined with other methods in minimized CPB systems, significantly reduces intraoperative and perioperative transfusion of packed red blood cells (PRBCs), as confirmed by a recent meta-analysis of 10 RCTs (Sun et al. 2013).

Retrograde Autologous Priming [RAP] Displaces 200–600 mL of the circuit's crystalloid solution with the patient's blood before bypass, using a stopcock on the arterial filter or manifold. This procedure demands diligent hemodynamic monitoring to avoid instability and maintain sufficient reservoir volume for pump flows.

Vacuum-Assisted Venous Drainage (VAVD) Enhances venous return and reduces priming volume using a vacuum controller or a centrifugal pump to create negative pressure. This technique can save 400–1000 mL of priming solution before CPB (Gravlee et al. 2016). VAVD allows for smaller cannula usage, improving surgical visibility and reducing priming volume by allowing the reservoir to be closer to the patient. Yet, using VAVD with gravity drainage increases the risk of air embolism and hemolysis (Fig. 20.5).

2019 EACTS/EACTA/EBCP guidelines for adult cardiac surgery recommend:

- Both retrograde and antegrade autologous priming as part of a blood conservation strategies to reduce transfusions (Class I, LOE A)
- Using an approved venous reservoir for VAVD (Class I, LOE C)

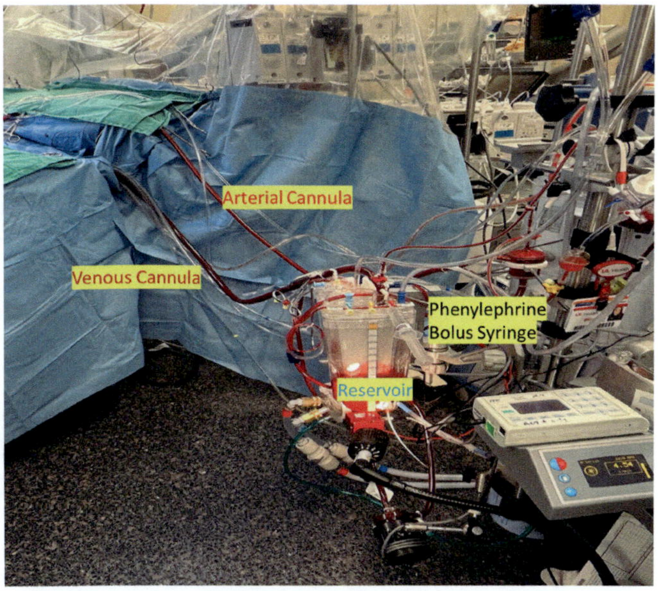

Fig. 20.5 Cardiopulmonary bypass is initiated. Arterial cannula is utilized for RAP before initiation of cardiopulmonary bypass

- Monitoring venous line pressure during VAVD (Class I, LOE C)
- Avoiding excessive negative venous pressures to prevent hemolysis (Class III, LOE B)

Cardioplegia

Cardioplegia aims to protect myocardial function from ischemic damage during CPB, ensuring a quiet and bloodless field via cardiac arrest, typically induced by delivering potassium (8–20 mEq/L) in crystalloid or blood solutions, causing depolarized arrest through fast sodium channels inactivation.

Cardioplegia solutions, either pure crystalloids or blood-crystalloid mixtures, differ in composition: pure crystalloid solutions are categorized by intracellular or extracellular types, and blood cardioplegia is a mix of both crystalloid solution and blood, typically in a ratio (4:1) of 4 parts of blood to 1 part of crystalloid. Del Nido cardioplegia (1:4 blood-to-crystalloid ratio with added lidocaine) and microplegia [which delivers cardioplegia with a minimal crystalloid solution in a ratio of at least 66 parts of blood to 1 part of crystalloid (66:1) or no crystalloid at all].

A recent meta-analysis shows comparable outcomes between blood and crystalloid cardioplegia regarding in-hospital death or perioperative MI (Parke et al. 2015). The 2017 EACTS/EACTA guidelines emphasize limiting hemodilution as a vital part of a blood conservation strategy to

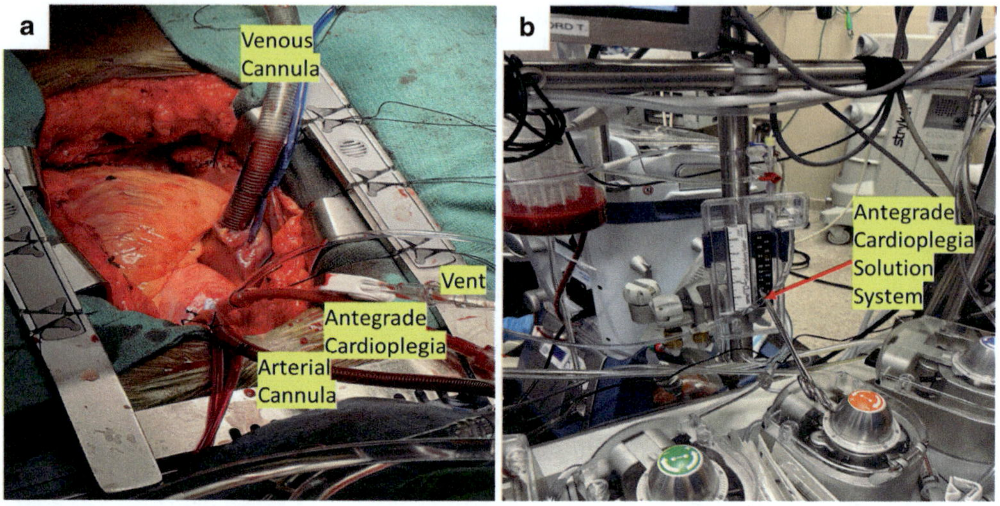

Fig. 20.6 Cardioplegia delivery on cardiopulmonary bypass. (**a**) An antegrade cardioplegia cannula is placed in the ascending aorta. (**b**) Antegrade cardioplegia solution system

reduce perioperative bleeding and transfusion, favoring blood cardioplegia, especially in patients at risk of complications like AKI or bleeding due to anemia, low BSA, chronic kidney disease, or complex surgeries.

Cardioplegia is usually applied antegrade directly into the aortic root or coronary ostia, or retrograde via coronary sinus, often (Fig. 20.6) cold and intermittently every 20–30 minutes, though single-shot techniques may be used in low-risk cases to minimize interruptions during the surgery. While the Del Nido solution has shown benefits in reducing postoperative cardiac enzyme levels, CPB and aortic cross-clamp times, cardioplegia volume, and intraoperative defibrillation needs without affecting mortality, conclusive evidence from RCTs for its superiority remains insufficient (Zhai et al. 2023).

- It is recommended that patient-centered myocardial protective strategies be used based on clinical condition and procedural complexity rather than on the use of a fixed institutional cardioplegic solution (Class I, LOE C).
- Blood cardioplegia should be considered in selected patients to reduce hemodilution, bleeding complications and transfusion requirements (Class IIa, LOE B).

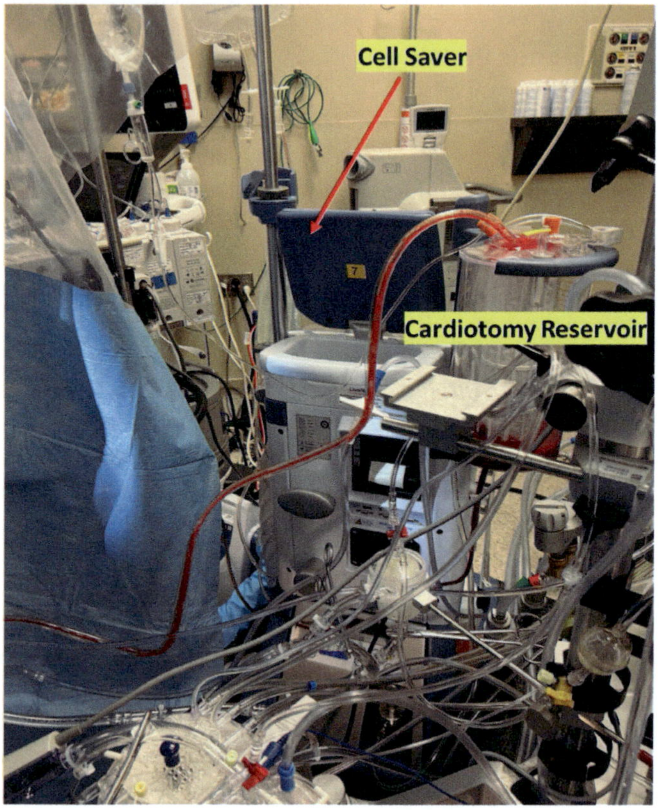

Fig. 20.7 A separate cardiotomy reservoir for shed mediastinal blood

Reservoirs

During CPB, both a venous reservoir to intercept venous drainage and a cardiotomy reservoir for mediastinal and vent lines blood are used, without clear superiority between closed and open venous reservoirs. Open reservoirs have the reputation of being safer and easier to use, while closed reservoirs offer biocompatibility and blood saving benefits. Use of the separated cardiotomy reservoir for shed mediastinal blood is recommended (Fig. 20.7). For more details, see Chap. 7.

2019 EACTS/EACTA/EBCP guidelines on CPB in adult cardiac surgery recommend:

- Considering a separated cardiotomy to mitigate the deleterious effect of shed mediastinal blood (Class IIa, LOE B).
- The potential use of a closed venous reservoir to attenuate the inflammatory response and improve biocompatibility in conjunction with other elements (Class IIb, LOE B).

Type of Circuit

Minimally invasive extracorporeal circulation (MiECC) is designed to improve biocompatibility and minimize hemodilution, as outlined by the minimally invasive extracorporeal technologies International Society's consensus on definitions (Anastasiadis et al. 2016). Essential MiECC components include a closed CPB circuit, coated surfaces, reduced priming volume, a centrifugal pump, membrane oxygenator, heat exchanger, cardioplegia system, venous bubble trap/venous air-removing device, and shed blood management. MiECC has been used in all types of cardiac operations, showing potential benefits such as reduction in blood loss, blood activation, MI, postoperative arrhythmias, cerebrovascular events, and deaths, although, meta-analyses have not consistently confirmed these outcomes in clinical trials (Kowalewski et al. 2015).

The 2019 EACTS/EACTA/EBCP guidelines and the 2021 STS/SCA/AmSECT/SABM Update on CPB and Patient Blood Management recommend:

- Favoring MiECC over standard conventional CPB systems to reduce blood loss, and transfusion needs, and to enhance biocompatibility (Class IIa, LOE B).
- Incorporating MiECC features such as coatings, centrifugal pumps, separated cardiotomy suction, and closed systems for CPB improvement (Class IIa, LOE C).
- MiECC reduced priming volume aims at minimizing hemodilution and supports blood conservation (Class I, LOE B-NR).
- MiECC effectively reduces blood loss and transfusion as part of an integrated blood conservation strategy (Class IIA, LOE B-R).

Acid–Base Homeostasis and Electrolyte Management

Tissue hypoxia or electrolyte imbalances can trigger metabolic acidosis, increasing the risk of injury and organ dysfunction during CPB. Excessive use of normal saline or unbalanced colloids further exacerbates this risk due to their high chloride content. For mild to moderate hypothermia CPB in adults (excluding deep hypothermic circulatory arrest procedures), alpha-stat blood gas management is standard. This means readings taken at 37 °C and interpreted without temperature correction.

Acidosis Moderate acidosis (pH < 7.35) and hyperlactatemia (lactate >4.0 mmol/L) correlate with increased 12-hour chest drainage (Ranucci et al. 2015). The Transfusion Requirements after Cardiac Surgery (TRACS) trial demonstrated that lactate levels >3 mmol/L at 6 hours following surgery increased the odds for major complications (Hajjar et al. 2013). Normal saline and unbalanced colloids can worsen this via hyperchloremic acidosis, highlighting the need for pH management.

Hyperkalemia Commonly associated with CPB due to cardioplegia, but usually self-limiting. Levels above 6.5–7 mmol/L, may require modified ultrafiltration (MUF), calcium, bicarbonate, and/or insulin/dextrose.

Hypocalcemia can occur due to hemodilution and citrated blood transfusions. Its impact on coagulation, cardiac rhythm, positive inotropy, and vascular tone, warrants prompt treatment with calcium chloride or calcium gluconate.

Hypomagnesemia Magnesium might reduce supraventricular arrhythmias post-CPB. Recent comprehensive Scottish recommendations about cardiac arrhythmias in CAD suggest that magnesium may be used for prophylaxis against AF and ventricular arrhythmias (Authors/Task Force Members et al. 2019; Baker et al. 2020; Puis et al. 2020; Wahba et al. 2020).

The 2019 EACTS/EACTA/EBCP guidelines for CPB in adult cardiac surgery recommend:

- Utilizing alpha-stat acid–base management during moderate to mild hypothermia to improve neurological and neurocognitive outcomes (Class IIa, LOE B).
- Maintaining normal pH (7.35–7.45) and preventing hyperchloremic acidosis to reduce the risk of postoperative complications(Class IIa, LOE B).
- Considering perioperative magnesium sulfate for postoperative arrhythmia prophylaxis (Class IIb, LOE B).

Control of Mean Arterial Blood Pressure During CPB

During CPB, it is important to maintain adequate MAP to ensure organ perfusion, especially for the kidneys, brain and gastrointestinal tract. Vasoplegic syndrome during CPB may derive from factors like proinflammatory cytokines, anesthetic drugs, active endocarditis or preoperative use of angiotensin-converting enzyme inhibitors and calcium channel blockers. Conversely, hypertension during CPB may derive from insufficient anesthesia, catecholamine release, or hypothermia-induced vasoconstriction.

- During CPB, MAP should be managed with arterial vasodilators for MAP >80 mmHg or vasoconstrictors for MAP <50 mmHg, ensuring proper anesthesia depth and pump flow (Class I, LOE A).
- Avoid using vasopressors to increase MAP above 80 mmHg (Class III, LOE B).

- It is recommended that vasoplegic syndrome during CPB be treated with alpha-1 adrenergic agonist vasopressors (Class I, LOE C).
- For vasoplegic syndrome refractory to alpha-1-adrenergic agonist vasopressors, consider vasopressin, terlipressin or methylene blue, alone or in combination with alpha-1-agonists (Class IIa, LOE B).
- Hydroxocobalamin may be used to treat vasoplegic syndrome during CPB (Class IIb, LOE C).

Hypotension In managing hypotension, it is crucial to maintain adequate perfusion flow rates. Transient reductions in flow rate may be tolerable, but sustained reductions must be avoided. Once proper flow is confirmed, MAP correction can involve increasing the systemic vascular resistance (SVR) using vasoconstrictors such as phenylephrine (0.5–10 μg/kg/min) or norepinephrine (0.03–0.3 μg/kg/min), with SVR calculated as (MAP − CVP)/effective perfusion flow rate. Due to varying responses to vasoconstrictors during CPB, start with lower doses or less potent agents, adjusting as necessary. Vasopressin (0.01–0.05 units/min) may sometimes be used. Although increasing perfusion flow rate can temporarily address hypotension, (e.g., while vasoconstrictors take effect), it is not an appropriate strategy to correct persistent hypotension.

Hemodilution at CPB start, cardioplegia solution, and reperfusion of the myocardium after release of the aortic cross-clamp commonly reduce SVR, leading to hypotension. Continuous infusions are preferred over intermittent boluses to prevent fluctuating MAP levels.

Hypertension During CPB is usually the result of an increase in SVR due to endogenous sympathetic stimulation or hypothermia. Before using vasodilators like nitroglycerin (0.1–10 μg/kg/min), sodium nitroprusside (0.1–2 μg/kg/min), nicardipine (2–5 mg/h), adequate anesthesia should be ensured, and artifactual hypertension due to aortic cannula malposition should also be excluded. To temporarily manage hypertension, the perfusion flow rate can be reduced (e.g., while vasodilators take effect), but this should not be used to correct persistent hypertension. Hypertension should be avoided during all aortic cross-clamp manipulations, including the application and release of side-biting clamps. Nitroglycerin, with its venous dilation effect, is the first-line drug, followed by sodium nitroprusside for stronger action and nicardipine for a longer duration of action and offset.

Pump Flow Management During CPB

During CPB, perfusion flow rates are initially set around 2.4 L/min/m^2 at 37 °C and approximately 1.5 L/min/m^2 at 28 °C, with the actual pump flow slightly higher to compensate for circuit recirculation (e.g., 200 mL/min filtered and purged from the arterial line to remove microbubbles). Effective perfusion rate is the pump delivery minus this recirculated volume. Inadequate flow results in low venous hemoglobin (Hb) oxygen saturation (monitored continuously in the venous return) and potential metabolic acidosis from anaerobic metabolism. If low venous saturation isn't due to hemodilution, inadequate anesthesia, or excessive rewarming, flow rates should increase. However, even normal venous saturation can't guarantee adequate tissue perfusion due to possible shunting or localized under-perfusion. Conditions with increased metabolic rate (shivering, thyrotoxicosis, or malignant hyperthermia) may also reduce venous saturation despite adequate flow rates (Fig. 20.8).

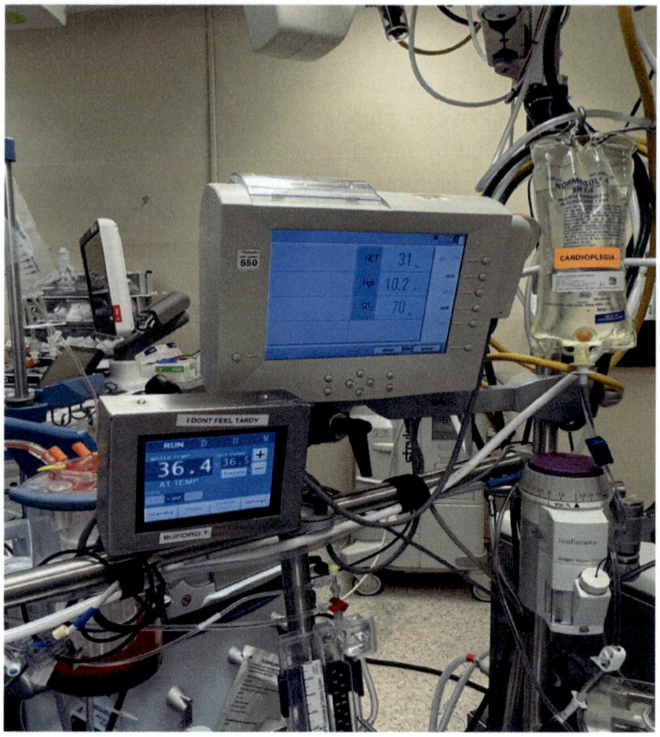

Fig. 20.8 Continuous monitoring of temperature, hemoglobin, hematocrit, and venous hemoglobin saturation on CPB

Guidelines for CPB in adult cardiac surgery advise considering:

- Before initiation of CPB, set the pump flow rate based on BSA and planned temperature (I, LOE: C).
- During CPB, evaluate the pump flow's adequacy using oxygenation and metabolic parameters (SvO2, oxygen extraction ratio, near-infrared spectroscopy (NIRS), CO_2 production, and lactates) (IIa, LOE: B).
- Adjust flow rates to ensure minimal oxygen delivery threshold are met, especially under moderate hypothermia (IIa, LOE: B).

- For obese patients, consider basing flow rates on lean mass (IIb, LOE: B).

Goal-Directed Hemodynamic Therapy

Optimizing the balance between oxygen delivery and oxygen consumption is the cornerstone of managing cardiac surgery patients. Oxygen delivery might be decreased due to factors like myocardial depression, rhythm disturbances, and impaired vascular tone. Goal-directed hemodynamic therapy (GDT) enhances oxygen delivery to tissues by increasing cardiac output through fluids and/or inotropes.

Early implementation (after induction of anesthesia) of GDT, targeting optimal cardiac index, stroke volume variation, and global end-diastolic volume index, has been shown to decrease postoperative complications and shorten ICU stays. Using intravenous fluids, inotropes, and red cell transfusions to maintain a cardiac index of >3.0 L/min/m^2, GDT has been associated with a lower 30-day mortality rate and fewer major postoperative complications. GDT is recommended to reduce the rate of postoperative complications and length of hospital stay (Authors/Task Force Members et al. 2019; Baker et al. 2020; Puis et al. 2020; Schulkens et al. 2014; Wahba et al. 2020).

Management of Shed Blood

Shed blood (from cardiotomy suction, blood spilled into the pleural and pericardial spaces or from the wound) is aspirated back into the CPB machine via cardiotomy suckers and a roller pump. Shed blood is highly activated, potentially leading to thrombin generation, activation of coagulation, fibrinolytic, and inflammatory pathways, increasing transfusion requirements. Its reinfusion may also cause neurological and lung injuries attributed in part to hemolysis and fat content. Separately processing shed blood, such as with a cell saver, before, reinfusion can mitigate these adverse effects, and reduce pathological activation.

While studies on processed shed blood versus unprocessed shed blood offer mixed findings on bleeding, transfusion requirements, and neurological injury, there's a consensus towards avoiding unprocessed shed blood retransfusion. Processing shed blood when reinfusion is necessary is advised to minimize potential harms. It is preferable to first process the shed blood with a cell saver and, thereafter, to filter it.

Shed blood can be collected separately in a cardiotomy reservoir (or integrated cardiotomy reservoir/venous reservoir), a blood transfusion bag or in the reservoir of a cell saver. The best way to deal with shed blood depends on the volume of shed blood and the characteristics (e.g., BSA, preoperative hematocrit, hemoglobin, platelet count) of the patient (Fig. 20.6). For more details, see Chap. 7.

Guidelines for CPB in adult cardiac surgery advise considering:

- Discarding shed blood (Class IIa, LOE B).
- Processing and secondary filtration of red blood cells to decrease the deleterious effects of reinfused shed blood (Class IIa, LOE B).

Monitoring Organ Perfusion on CPB

1. Non-invasive Cerebral Monitoring Adverse cerebral outcomes after cardiac surgery worsen outcomes. Hence, this drives the search for optimal monitoring tools to enable early intervention.

NIRS While early studies suggested that NIRS-based algorithms reduced morbidity and mortality and improved neurocognition (Colak et al. 2015; Kara et al. 2015; Murkin et al. 2007), recent high-quality trials and a meta-analysis showed no clinical benefit of the use of NIRS-based algorithms (Lei et al. 2017; Rogers et al. 2017; Serraino and Murphy 2017) (Fig. 20.4).

Guidelines for CPB in adult cardiac surgery advise considering:

The use of NIRS-guided algorithms to improve clinical outcomes may be considered (Class IIb, LOE B).

Please refer to Chaps. 10 and 14 for a detailed discussion on cerebral monitoring and NIRS-based algorithms.

2. Monitoring the Depth of Anesthesia To prevent the negative psychological effects of intraoperative awareness, processed electroencephalogram (EEG) monitors are widely used. BIS-guided anesthesia has been shown to reduce awareness risk when compared to relying on clinical signs, especially in high-risk patients (Punjasawadwong et al. 2014). These monitors are also instrumental in guiding the administration of inhalational anesthetics, helping to prevent the vasodilation and hypotension that can result from excessive dosages.

Guidelines for CPB in adult cardiac surgery advise considering:

The routine use of processed EEG monitoring to reduce the incidence of intraoperative awareness (Class IIb, LOE B).

Lung Protection During CPB

Modified Ultrafiltration (MUF) involves the removal of fluids and low-molecular-weight substances at the end of

CPB, leading to fewer cases of postoperative respiratory failure and reduced airway resistance (Luciani et al. 2001; Torina et al. 2010).

Pulmonary Artery Perfusion Selective pulsatile pulmonary artery perfusion with oxygenated blood during CPB reduces lung tissue inflammation (evidenced by decreased neutrophilic/lymphocytic alveolar infiltration) and improves postoperative oxygenation and lung compliance. However, its effect on circulating cytokine levels is negligible, and its long-term impact on clinical pulmonary outcomes is uncertain (Santini et al. 2012).

The guidelines for CPB in adult cardiac surgery suggest that considering:

MUF and selective pulmonary artery perfusion could be beneficial for improving postoperative respiratory function (Class IIb, LOE B).

MiECC MiECC, with its essential components detailed earlier, has been associated with shorter durations of postoperative mechanical ventilation and reduced ICU stays, according to a meta-analysis of randomized controlled trials (RCTs). However, the studies varied in their minibypass approaches, and there were no significant longer-term outcomes were reported beyond discharge (Anastasiadis et al. 2013).

Reduce AKI During CPB

Cardiac surgery–associated acute kidney injury (CSA-AKI) affects 15–50% of adults undergoing cardiac surgery, marked by a serum creatinine increase of 0.3 mg/dL or 50% increase from baseline or by oliguria. To decrease the risk of AKI post-cardiac surgery, intraoperative CPB strategies include avoiding hyperthermic perfusion (>37 °C), ensuring adequate oxygen delivery, and employing MiECC techniques. Currently, there is insufficient evidence to endorse the use of heparin-coated circuits, leukocyte filtration, pulsatile flow, intraoperative hemofiltration and ultrafiltration, maintaining relative hypertension during CPB or employing multipass hemoconcentration (as opposed to centrifugation of residual CPB blood) for reducing AKI risk after cardiac surgery, although these strategies may be beneficial for other outcomes (Brown et al. 2023).

The 2023 STS/SCA/AmSECT Clinical Practice Guidelines for the Prevention of Adult Cardiac Surgery–Associated Acute Kidney Injury recommend:

- Avoiding hyperthermic perfusion (>37 °C) in adult cardiac surgery with CPB to reduce the risk of cardiac surgery–associated AKI (Class I, LOE B-R).
- A goal-directed oxygen delivery strategy in adult cardiac surgery with CPB to reduce the risk of cardiac surgery–associated AKI (Class: I, LOE B-R).
- Adopting the kidney disease improving global outcomes (KDIGO) practice guidelines for patients at high-risk of AKI in adult cardiac surgery with CPB to reduce the risk of cardiac surgery–associated AKI (Class IIA, LOE B-R).
- Fenoldopam may be reasonable in adult cardiac surgery with CPB to reduce the risk of cardiac surgery–associated AKI, provided hypotension is avoided (Class IIB, LOE B-R).
- Using MiECC techniques might be reasonable in adult cardiac surgery with CPB to reduce the risk of cardiac surgery–associated AKI (Class IIB, LOE B-R).
- Dopamine infusion alone, during CPB and the perioperative period, is not recommended in adult cardiac surgery with CPB to reduce the risk of cardiac surgery–associated AKI (Class III, No Benefit, LOE A).
- Mannitol is not recommended in adult cardiac surgery with CPB to reduce the risk of cardiac surgery–associated AKI (Class III, No Benefit, LOE B-R).

Postoperative recommendations for high AKI risk patients include:

- Close hemodynamic monitoring and goal-directed volume resuscitation.
- Avoidance of nephrotoxic substances.
- Withholding angiotensin-converting enzyme inhibitors (ACEi)/angiotensin receptor blocker for 48 hours.
- Serial monitoring of serum creatinine and urine output.
- Prevention of hyperglycemia.

Fluid Management at Separation from CPB

Goals of fluid management when separating from CPB are to ensure:

(i) An adequate cardiac index.
(ii) Avoidance of fluid overload.
(iii) Sufficient organ perfusion, achieved through a combination of medications, fluid management, and if necessary, mechanical circulatory support.

Monitoring For weaning from CPB, essential monitoring includes electrocardiogram for the assessment of heart rate, rhythm and myocardial ischemia, alongside hemodynamic monitoring devices like pulmonary artery catheter, minimally invasive pulse contour analysis, and transesophageal echocardiography (TEE). These tools help to assess cardiac performance, including preload, afterload and contractility of left and right ventricles, as well as the quality of the surgical intervention including retained intracardiac air (Authors/

Task Force Members et al. 2019; Baker et al. 2020; Puis et al. 2020; Wahba et al. 2020).

Guidelines for monitoring in CPB cases in adult cardiac surgery:

- Pulmonary artery catheter: May be indicated in selected cases (Class IIb, LOE B).
- Pulse contour analysis for cardiac output: May be indicated in selected cases (Class IIb, LOE B).
- TEE: Should be considered in open-heart and thoracic aortic procedures unless contraindicated (Class IIa, LOE B).

Low cardiac output state in cardiac surgery is a life-threatening complication, particularly during weaning off CPB. It is associated with increased morbidity and both short-term and long-term mortality rates and placing a burden on hospital resources. Reduced cardiac output decreases oxygen delivery to the tissues, causing subsequent tissue hypoxia. Inotropes are usually the first-line therapy to manage this complication and should only be started after correcting potential causes of a low cardiac output state, such as graft dysfunction or hypovolemia. Inotropes such as dobutamine, epinephrine, norepinephrine, phosphodiesterase III inhibitors, and calcium sensitizers are the most used drugs in this setting.

Guidelines for Low Cardiac Output State in Adult Cardiac Surgery:

- Inotropes/Vasopressors: Recommended as first-line treatment to reduce mortality in hemodynamically unstable patients (Class IA, LOE A).
- Phosphodiesterase Inhibitors: Should be considered to increase weaning success (Class IIa, LOE B).
- Prophylactic Levosimendan: Not recommended to adverse events and mortality reduction (Class III, LOE A).
- Therapeutic Levosimendan: May be considered in selected difficult-to-wean patients from CPB (Class IIb, LOE C).
- Levosimendan + Other Support: Not recommended for patients already on inotropes or vasopressors (Class III, LOE B).

Mechanical Circulatory Support (MCS) Represents a well-established and valuable tool for rescuing patients from refractory cardiocirculatory failure (with or without concomitant respiratory dysfunction) in otherwise would almost certainly lead to mortality. These devices improve cardiac output and unloading, helping prevent low cardiac output states and inadequate tissue perfusion.

2020 Expert Consensus (EACTS, ELSO, STS, AATS) Recommendations for Post-Cardiotomy Extracorporeal Life Support (Lorusso et al. 2021):

- Post-cardiotomy support should be initiated prior to end-organ injury or anaerobic metabolism (lactate level <4 mmol/L) if there's a chance of myocardial recovery and uncontrollable bleeding is not present (Class I, LOE B).
- For patients ineligible for transplant or left mechanical support, extracorporeal life support is recommended when native myocardial recovery is unlikely (Class I, LOE C).
- Early extracorporeal life support is recommended after cardiac surgery when a patient with an intra-aortic balloon pump (IABP) and optimal medical therapy fails to wean from CPB or has marginal hemodynamics (Class I, LOE B).

Right Heart Failure Severe RV failure following CPB is serious complication with mortality rates as high as 86%. Several factors can impair RV contractility:

- Poor Myocardial Inotropism: This may be caused by preoperative CAD, myocardial stunning post CPB, inadequate myocardial protection during surgery, or arrhythmias.
- Myocardial Hypoperfusion: Reduced blood flow to the myocardium can occur due to air embolism or thromboembolism in the right coronary artery, kinking of the venous graft after CABG surgery, or a low aorto-coronary pressure gradient caused by LV dysfunction.

After CPB separation, acute RV dysfunction is typically associated with high CVP, reflecting an enlarged RV with depressed contractility. TEE characteristics of RV failure include a tricuspid annular plane systolic excursion below 16 mm and/or an S' wave on Tissue Doppler below 10 cm/s are. Signs of RV enlargement are a right mid-cavity diameter greater than 42 mm and a longitudinal diameter greater than 92 mm. Right fractional area change, assessed in midesophageal four-chambers view on TEE, provides a time-efficient and easy method for evaluating the RV during CPB separation. A right fractional area change below 30% or a reduction of 20% compared to baseline suggests RV dysfunction (Video 20.1).

Managing RV Dysfunction:

1. *Volume Control*: Reduce RV volume by sequestering blood into the reservoir while the venous cannula is in place. Avoid excessive or overzealous transfusion from the CPB machine into the aorta through aortic cannula.
2. *Diuretics*: May help improve function in a failing, dilated RV post-decannulation or perioperatively.
3. *Therapeutic Interventions*:
   (a) Optimize the preload to ensure adequate filling without causing distension.

(b) Reduce afterload to reduce resistance the RV must pump against.
(c) Enhance the contractility to support RV pumping efficiency.
(d) The RV is highly sensitive to increased pulmonary vascular resistance; thus, prevent factors such as hypercarbia, acidosis, pain and light anesthesia, hypoxia, and excessive vasopressors use.

4. *Pharmacological Management*:
   - Dobutamine is preferred for moderate RV dysfunction, characterized by an RV area change of 17–30%, due to its positive inotropic effects without significant increases in pulmonary vascular resistance.
   - Epinephrine is the first-line therapy in case of severe RV failure, especially with hypotension and/or associated LV failure.
   - Selective phosphodiesterase III inhibitor such as milrinone or enoximone may be considered if there is high pulmonary vascular resistance.
   - Inhalational agents such as nitric oxide and iloprost are preferred initial treatments for severe pulmonary hypertension, working to dilate pulmonary vessels and reduce RV afterload.

Left Heart Failure Following CPB separation, acute LV dysfunction is often associated with low blood pressure, indicative of LV diminished contractility. Various factors contribute to this condition. Using the transgastric midpapillary short-axis view on TEE allows for the assessment of LV function and size, crucial for identifying the cause of hypotension. Cavity obliteration, or the "kissing" of the papillary muscles, generally signifies either a very low SVR or hypovolemia. The LV end-diastolic area helps distinguish between these conditions: a large area suggests low SVR, while a small area points to hypovolemia. Additionally, low preload may cause systolic anterior motion (SAM) of the anterior leaflet of the mitral valve, a unique condition of hemodynamic instability that can appear similar to LV dysfunction when TEE is not available. SAM, occurring in 4–8% of all patients after mitral valve repair, can complicate CPB separation and requires specific management strategies (Monaco et al. 2020):

- Intravascular volume expansion
- Decrease of the heart rate to 60–70 beats per minute (e.g., reducing the rate of the pacemaker if the heart is stimulated)
- Stopping epinephrine and /or switching to beta-blockers
- Increasing the afterload with alpha-1 agonists.

LV Diastolic Dysfunction Separation from CPB may be challenged by diastolic dysfunction.

The hallmark of diastolic dysfunction is the inability of the ventricle to accept an adequate volume of blood, despite a normal preload. Diastolic filling abnormalities may become evident after volume overload, tachycardia, ischemia, acute systemic hypertension, AF, conduction abnormalities or electrolyte abnormalities, all of which reflect a reduced cardiac reserve. The diastolic dysfunction is a heterogeneous disease that requires tailored management (Monaco et al. 2020):

- *Impaired relaxation*: Prioritize a longer diastolic time (e.g., relaxation time) and filling time.
- *Dyssynchrony*: Optimize atrioventricular interval with dual chamber pacing.
- *Tachycardia*: Manage with preload optimization, and if systolic function is normal, consider beta-blockers and calcium antagonists.
- *AF*: Prompt cardioversion and/or amiodarone infusion.
- *Phosphodiesterase III Inhibitors and Levosimendan*: Effective options to increase cardiac output and decrease wedge pressure.

The management of diastolic dysfunction in patients with hypertrophic cardiomyopathy, whether idiopathic or secondary to aortic stenosis, is particularly challenging.

- *Fluid Management*: Even minor preload increases can cause high wedge pressure. Balance the need for sufficient stroke volume with the risk of pulmonary edema.
- *Monitoring*: Wedge pressure should guide fluid administration.
- *IABP*: May be useful by improving coronary blood flow in perioperative diastolic dysfunction.

Fluid Management After CPB

Fluid boluses, frequently given for hypotension (65% of cases), contribute significantly to the positive fluid balance observed in patients after cardiac surgery. Crystalloid fluid comprises 65% of these boluses.

Goal-directed fluid therapy (GDFT) can improve outcomes in surgery, particularly cardiac surgery, by guiding clinicians with administering fluids, vasopressors and inotropes using monitoring techniques. While many clinicians informally consider these factors, GDFT uses a standardized algorithm for all patients, targeting metrics, such as blood pressure, cardiac index, systemic venous oxygen saturation, and urine output. Additionally, oxygen consumption, oxygen debt, and lactate levels may augment therapeutic tactics. GDFT trials consistently demonstrate reduced complication rates and length of stay. Consequently, the 2019 Guidelines for Perioperative Care in Cardiac Surgery by the Enhanced

Recovery After Surgery Society endorse GDFT for minimizing postoperative complications (Class I, LOE B-R) (Engelman et al. 2019).

Summary

Optimal fluid management before, during, and after CPB is essential for the safe conduct of CPB and cardiac surgery. The goals of fluid management include ensuring adequate perfusion of vital organs by optimizing hemodynamics, minimizing hemodilution and coagulopathy, and avoiding fluid overload. Large, randomized trials are needed to validate common fluid management strategies in cardiac surgery.

Further Reading

AmSECT. AmSECT standards and guidelines for perfusion practice. 2023. Retrieved from https://www.amsect.org/Portals/0/AmSECT_Perfusion_S%26G_2023%20Ratified%20021023_Digital%20edition.pdf.

Anastasiadis K, Antonitsis P, Haidich AB, Argiriadou H, Deliopoulos A, Papakonstantinou C. Use of minimal extracorporeal circulation improves outcome after heart surgery; a systematic review and meta-analysis of randomized controlled trials. Int J Cardiol. 2013;164(2):158–69. https://doi.org/10.1016/j.ijcard.2012.01.020.

Anastasiadis K, Murkin J, Antonitsis P, Bauer A, Ranucci M, Gygax E, et al. Use of minimal invasive extracorporeal circulation in cardiac surgery: principles, definitions and potential benefits. A position paper from the Minimal invasive Extra-Corporeal Technologies International Society (MiECTiS). Interact Cardiovasc Thorac Surg. 2016;22(5):647–62. https://doi.org/10.1093/icvts/ivv380.

Authors/Task Force Members, Kunst G, Milojevic M, Boer C, De Somer F, Gudbjartsson T, et al. 2019 EACTS/EACTA/EBCP guidelines on cardiopulmonary bypass in adult cardiac surgery. Br J Anaesth. 2019;123(6):713–57. https://doi.org/10.1016/j.bja.2019.09.012.

Baker RA, Nikolic A, Onorati F, Alston RP. 2019 EACTS/EACTA/EBCP guidelines on cardiopulmonary bypass in adult cardiac surgery: a tool to better clinical practice. Eur J Cardiothorac Surg. 2020;57(2):207–9. https://doi.org/10.1093/ejcts/ezz358.

Bartels GPGADSK. Hensley's practical approach to cardiothoracic anesthesia. 6th ed. Wolters Kluwer; 2019.

Brown JR, Baker RA, Shore-Lesserson L, Fox AA, Mongero LB, Lobdell KW, et al. The Society of Thoracic Surgeons/Society of Cardiovascular Anesthesiologists/American Society for Extracorporeal Technology clinical practice guidelines for the prevention of adult cardiac surgery-associated acute kidney injury. Anesth Analg. 2023;136(1):176–84. https://doi.org/10.1213/ANE.0000000000006286.

Colak Z, Borojevic M, Bogovic A, Ivancan V, Biocina B, Majeric-Kogler V. Influence of intraoperative cerebral oximetry monitoring on neurocognitive function after coronary artery bypass surgery: a randomized, prospective study. Eur J Cardiothorac Surg. 2015;47(3):447–54. https://doi.org/10.1093/ejcts/ezu193.

Deidda M, Piras C, Cadeddu Dessalvi C, Locci E, Barberini L, Orofino S, et al. Distinctive metabolomic fingerprint in scleroderma patients with pulmonary arterial hypertension. Int J Cardiol. 2017;241:401–6. https://doi.org/10.1016/j.ijcard.2017.04.024.

Engelman DT, Ben Ali W, Williams JB, Perrault LP, Reddy VS, Arora RC, et al. Guidelines for perioperative care in cardiac surgery: enhanced recovery after surgery society recommendations. JAMA Surg. 2019;154(8):755–66. https://doi.org/10.1001/jamasurg.2019.1153.

Gravlee GP, Davis RF, Hammon JW, Kussman B. Cardiopulmonary bypass and mechanical circulatory support. Wolters Kluwer; 2016.

Haga KK, McClymont KL, Clarke S, Grounds RS, Ng KY, Glyde DW, et al. The effect of tight glycaemic control, during and after cardiac surgery, on patient mortality and morbidity: a systematic review and meta-analysis. J Cardiothorac Surg. 2011;6:3. https://doi.org/10.1186/1749-8090-6-3.

Hajjar LA, Almeida JP, Fukushima JT, Rhodes A, Vincent JL, Osawa EA, Galas FR. High lactate levels are predictors of major complications after cardiac surgery. J Thorac Cardiovasc Surg. 2013;146(2):455–60. https://doi.org/10.1016/j.jtcvs.2013.02.003.

Kaplan JA. kaplan's cardiac anesthesia: for cardiac and noncardiac surgery. 7th ed. Elsevier; 2017.

Kara I, Erkin A, Sacli H, Demirtas M, Percin B, Diler MS, Kirali K. The effects of near-infrared spectroscopy on the neurocognitive functions in the patients undergoing coronary artery bypass grafting with asymptomatic carotid artery disease: a randomized prospective study. Ann Thorac Cardiovasc Surg. 2015;21(6):544–50. https://doi.org/10.5761/atcs.oa.15-00118.

Kowalewski M, Pawliszak W, Kolodziejczak M, Navarese EP, Anisimowicz L. 30-day mortality reduction with miniaturized extracorporeal circulation as compared to conventional cardiopulmonary bypass for coronary revascularization. Meta-analysis of randomized controlled trials. Int J Cardiol. 2015;198:63–5. https://doi.org/10.1016/j.ijcard.2015.06.153.

Lei L, Katznelson R, Fedorko L, Carroll J, Poonawala H, Machina M, et al. Cerebral oximetry and postoperative delirium after cardiac surgery: a randomised, controlled trial. Anaesthesia. 2017;72(12):1456–66. https://doi.org/10.1111/anae.14056.

Lorusso R, Whitman G, Milojevic M, Raffa G, McMullan DM, Boeken U, et al. 2020 EACTS/ELSO/STS/AATS expert consensus on post-cardiotomy extracorporeal life support in adult patients. Eur J Cardiothorac Surg. 2021;59(1):12–53. https://doi.org/10.1093/ejcts/ezaa283.

Luciani GB, Menon T, Vecchi B, Auriemma S, Mazzucco A. Modified ultrafiltration reduces morbidity after adult cardiac operations: a prospective, randomized clinical trial. Circulation. 2001;104(12 Suppl 1):I253–9. https://doi.org/10.1161/hc37t1.094931.

Monaco F, Di Prima AL, Kim JH, Plamondon MJ, Yavorovskiy A, Likhvantsev V, et al. Management of challenging cardiopulmonary bypass separation. J Cardiothorac Vasc Anesth. 2020;34(6):1622–35. https://doi.org/10.1053/j.jvca.2020.02.038.

Murkin JM, Adams SJ, Novick RJ, Quantz M, Bainbridge D, Iglesias I, et al. Monitoring brain oxygen saturation during coronary bypass surgery: a randomized, prospective study. Anesth Analg. 2007;104(1):51–8. https://doi.org/10.1213/01.ane.0000246814.29362.f4.

Mutter TC, Ruth CA, Dart AB. Hydroxyethyl starch (HES) versus other fluid therapies: effects on kidney function. Cochrane Database Syst Rev. 2013;(7):CD007594. https://doi.org/10.1002/14651858.CD007594.pub3.

Parke RL, McGuinness SP, Gilder E, McCarthy LW, Cowdrey KA. A randomised feasibility study to assess a novel strategy to rationalise fluid in patients after cardiac surgery. Br J Anaesth. 2015;115(1):45–52. https://doi.org/10.1093/bja/aev118.

Puis L, Milojevic M, Boer C, De Somer F, Gudbjartsson T, van den Goor J, et al. 2019 EACTS/EACTA/EBCP guidelines on cardiopulmonary bypass in adult cardiac surgery. Interact Cardiovasc Thorac Surg. 2020;30(2):161–202. https://doi.org/10.1093/icvts/ivz251.

Punjasawadwong Y, Phongchiewboon A, Bunchungmongkol N. Bispectral index for improving anaesthetic delivery and postoperative recovery. Cochrane Database Syst Rev. 2014;2014(6):CD003843. https://doi.org/10.1002/14651858.CD003843.pub3.

Ranucci M, Baryshnikova E, Simeone F, Ranucci M, Scolletta S. Moderate-degree acidosis is an independent determinant of postoperative bleeding in cardiac surgery. Minerva Anestesiol. 2015;81(8):885–93. Retrieved from https://www.ncbi.nlm.nih.gov/pubmed/26006154

Rogers CA, Stoica S, Ellis L, Stokes EA, Wordsworth S, Dabner L, et al. Randomized trial of near-infrared spectroscopy for personalized optimization of cerebral tissue oxygenation during cardiac surgery. Br J Anaesth. 2017;119(3):384–93. https://doi.org/10.1093/bja/aex182.

Santini F, Onorati F, Telesca M, Menon T, Mazzi P, Berton G, et al. Selective pulmonary pulsatile perfusion with oxygenated blood during cardiopulmonary bypass attenuates lung tissue inflammation but does not affect circulating cytokine levels. Eur J Cardiothorac Surg. 2012;42(6):942–50. https://doi.org/10.1093/ejcts/ezs199.

Schulkens IA, Castricum KC, Weijers EM, Koolwijk P, Griffioen AW, Thijssen VL. Expression, regulation and function of human metallothioneins in endothelial cells. J Vasc Res. 2014;51(3):231–8. https://doi.org/10.1159/000365550.

Serraino GF, Murphy GJ. Effects of cerebral near-infrared spectroscopy on the outcome of patients undergoing cardiac surgery: a systematic review of randomised trials. BMJ Open. 2017;7(9):e016613. https://doi.org/10.1136/bmjopen-2017-016613.

Sun P, Ji B, Sun Y, Zhu X, Liu J, Long C, Zheng Z. Effects of retrograde autologous priming on blood transfusion and clinical outcomes in adults: a meta-analysis. Perfusion. 2013;28(3):238–43. https://doi.org/10.1177/0267659112474861.

Task Force on Patient Blood Management for Adult Cardiac Surgery of the European Association for Cardio-Thoracic Surgery (EACTS), the European Association of Cardiothoracic Anaesthesiology, Boer C, Meesters MI, Milojevic M, Benedetto U, et al. 2017 EACTS/EACTA Guidelines on patient blood management for adult cardiac surgery. J Cardiothorac Vasc Anesth. 2018;32(1):88–120. https://doi.org/10.1053/j.jvca.2017.06.026.

Tibi P, McClure RS, Huang J, Baker RA, Fitzgerald D, Mazer CD, et al. STS/SCA/AmSECT/SABM update to the clinical practice guidelines on patient blood management. J Cardiothorac Vasc Anesth. 2021a;35(9):2569–91. https://doi.org/10.1053/j.jvca.2021.03.011.

Tibi P, McClure RS, Huang J, Baker RA, Fitzgerald D, Mazer CD, et al. STS/SCA/AmSECT/SABM update to the clinical practice guidelines on patient blood management. Ann Thorac Surg. 2021b;112(3):981–1004. https://doi.org/10.1016/j.athoracsur.2021.03.033.

Torina AG, Petrucci O, Oliveira PP, Severino ES, Vilarinho KA, Lavagnoli CF, et al. The effects of modified ultrafiltration on pulmonary function and transfusion requirements in patients underwent coronary artery bypass graft surgery. Rev Bras Cir Cardiovasc. 2010;25(1):59–65. https://doi.org/10.1590/s0102-76382010000100014.

Tsai LL, Jensen HA, Thourani VH. Intensive glycemic control in cardiac surgery. Curr Diab Rep. 2016;16(4):25. https://doi.org/10.1007/s11892-016-0719-5.

Turro E, Astle WJ, Megy K, Graf S, Greene D, Shamardina O, et al. Whole-genome sequencing of patients with rare diseases in a national health system. Nature. 2020;583(7814):96–102. https://doi.org/10.1038/s41586-020-2434-2.

Wahba A, Milojevic M, Boer C, De Somer F, Gudbjartsson T, van den Goor J, et al. 2019 EACTS/EACTA/EBCP guidelines on cardiopulmonary bypass in adult cardiac surgery. Eur J Cardiothorac Surg. 2020;57(2):210–51. https://doi.org/10.1093/ejcts/ezz267.

Xiang F, Huang F, Huang J, Li X, Dong N, Xiao Y, et al. Expert consensus on the use of human serum albumin in adult cardiac surgery. Chin Med J. 2023;136(10):1135–43. https://doi.org/10.1097/CM9.0000000000002709.

Zacharias M, Mugawar M, Herbison GP, Walker RJ, Hovhannisyan K, Sivalingam P, Conlon NP. Interventions for protecting renal function in the perioperative period. Cochrane Database Syst Rev. 2013;2013(9):CD003590. https://doi.org/10.1002/14651858.CD003590.pub4.

Zhai K, Cheng X, Zhang P, Wei S, Huang J, Wu X, et al. Del Nido cardioplegia for myocardial protection in adult cardiac surgery: a systematic review and update meta-analysis. Perfusion. 2023;38(1):6–17. https://doi.org/10.1177/02676591211031095.

Consideration in Blood Disorders and Cardiopulmonary Bypass

21

Monique L. Roberts, Ragini G. Gupta, and Yuliana Salamanca-Padilla

Introduction

Cardiopulmonary bypass (CPB) is a cornerstone technique in cardiac surgery as a substitute for the heart and lungs to ensure circulatory and respiratory support. However, managing the complexities of CPB becomes more complicated when blood disorders are present. These disorders, ranging from anemias and clotting dysfunctions to more rare genetic conditions, can significantly affect the outcome of surgeries involving CPB. They influence everything from anticoagulation management to the risk of postoperative complications. This chapter delves into the intersection of blood disorders with CPB, emphasizing the importance of a detailed preoperative evaluation and a tailored approach to each patient's unique needs. Understanding these blood disorders is crucial for the multidisciplinary team responsible for planning and executing CPB, aiming to ensure patient safety and optimize surgical outcomes. The challenges and strategies involved in managing patients with blood disorders undergoing CPB are discussed, laying the groundwork for a comprehensive guide designed to enhance clinical practice and patient care in this complex intersection of hematology and cardiac surgery.

M. L. Roberts (✉) · Y. Salamanca-Padilla
Department of Anesthesiology & Perioperative Medicine, Lewis Katz School of Medicine, Temple University, Philadelphia, PA, USA
e-mail: Monique.Roberts@tuhs.temple.edu; Yuliana.Salamanca-Padilla@tuhs.temple.edu

R. G. Gupta
Department of Anesthesiology, Emory School of Medicine, Emory University, Atlanta, GA, USA
e-mail: ragini.grace.gupta@emory.edu

Red Blood Cell (RBC) (Erythrocyte) Disorders

RBC Enzyme Disorders

Enzyme disorders that affect red blood cells (RBCs), including Glucose-6-phosphate dehydrogenase (G6PD) deficiency, Pyruvate Kinase Deficiency, Hexokinase Deficiency, Glutathione Synthetase Deficiency, among others, cause hemolytic anemia by disrupting RBC metabolism and increasing the likelihood of premature cell destruction. Symptoms can vary, encompassing mild to severe hemolytic anemia, jaundice, and splenomegaly. G6PD deficiency, in particular, exemplifies the complexities associated with these conditions. These disorders necessitate meticulous management during cardiac surgeries involving cardiopulmonary bypass (CPB) due to the heightened risk of hemolysis. Thus, a thorough understanding, management of these enzyme deficiencies are vital for ensuring patient safety.

Glucose-6-Phosphate-Dehydrogenase

Glucose-6-phosphate dehydrogenase deficiency (G6PD) stands as the most common enzymatic defect in human red blood cells. G6PD functions to convert glucose-6-phospate into 6-phosphogluconate, facilitating the reduction of NADP to NADPH and replenishing glutathione—a powerful scavenger of reactive oxidative species. Inadequate defense against oxidative stress leads to hemolysis and anemia. However, deficiency of this enzyme alone is not sufficient to cause hemolysis; it requires additional external factors to "trigger" hemolysis. Such factors include the physiologic stress associated with cardiopulmonary bypass (CPB). Conditions like ischemia-reperfusion injury, hypothermia, acidosis, and the mechanical trauma induced by blood flow through the CPB circuit heighten the likelihood of oxidative free radical production and subsequent hemolysis in the presence of inadequate glutathione production.

For patients with G6PD deficiency undergoing cardiac surgery, there is an increased risk of impaired oxygenation, prolonged ventilation, and hemolysis. Thorough perioperative

A. S. Awad, J. DiNardo (eds.), *Clinical Perfusion for Cardiac Surgery*, https://doi.org/10.1007/978-3-031-91163-7_21

assessment and the adoption of hemolysis-reducing strategies are paramount. Effort should be made to shorten the duration of surgery, CPB, and aortic cross-clamp times, as well as to limit the use of occlusive roller pumps. Where possible, maintaining normothermia during bypass and ensuring adequate perfusion pressure are advisable. Additionally, it is crucial for clinicians to avoid administering drugs known to trigger hemolysis:

- Acetazolamide
- Amide local anesthetics (lidocaine, prilocaine)
- Ascorbic acid
- Aspirin
- Diphenhydramine
- Dopamine
- Fluoroquinolones
- Gentamicin
- Methylene blue
- Metoclopramide
- Nitric oxide
- Nitrofurantoin
- Nitroglycerin
- Penicillin
- Sulfonamide antibiotics
- Vitamin K

Early intervention for hypotension, hypoxia, and acidosis is essential in reducing the risk of hemolysis. Clinicians should consider the use of free radical scavengers such as mannitol. Furthermore, ensuring adequate urine output can contribute to lowering morbidity rates.

Hemoglobinopathies

Hemoglobinopathies are genetic disorders affecting red blood cells (RBCs). Mutations in hemoglobin genes disrupt its structure or production, impairing the oxygen-carrying capacity and lifespan of RBCs. These disorders fall into two categories:

- *Structural Hemoglobin Variants* (e.g., sickle cell, Hb C, Hb E): Mutations alter the hemoglobin molecule, making RBCs rigid and prone to deformation, hindering blood flow.
- *Thalassemias* (alpha or beta): Genetic mutations in globin genes impair the production of alpha or beta globin chains, leading to a spectrum of anemia severity.

Sickle Cell Disease (SCD)

Normal adult erythrocytes predominantly contain HbA ($\alpha_2\beta_2$), accounting for 96–98% of their composition, followed by 1.5–3.2% of HbA2 ($\alpha_2\delta_2$) and 0.5–0.8% of HbF ($\alpha_2\gamma_2$). SCD and sickle cell trait (SCT) are hereditary hemoglobinopathies resulting from a mutation in the β-globin gene located on chromosome 11. SCD affects individuals homozygous for hemoglobin S (Hb SS), where HbA is almost absent, and HbS constitutes between 70% and 98% of the hemoglobin (Hb). Hb C-Harlem, characterized by a double amino acid substitution on the *β chain*, results in asymptomatic conditions in patients heterozygous for Hb C. However, patients with heterozygous Hb S as well as Hb C-Harlem tend to have disease similar to those with Hb SS. SCT occurs in patients heterozygous for hemoglobin S (Hb AS), where HbS makes up less than 50% of their hemoglobin, often leading to milder diseases compared to SCD. Additionally, hemoglobinopathies such as Hb SC and Hb S/b-thalassemia exist, with some affected individuals displaying disease severity comparable to those with Hb SS.

When fully oxygenated, HbS doesn't cause issues. However, under conditions of low-oxygen tension, HbS tends to sickle and polymerize. This leads to the red blood cells (RBCs) containing HbS becoming distorted, rigid, and prone to aggregation. The likelihood of sickling is influenced by the duration of exposure to low oxygen, low temperature, and the concentration of HbS. RBCs homozygous for the sickle cell gene require an oxygen concentration below 40 mmHg for 2–4 minutes to exhibit significant distortion, whereas heterozygous RBCs only begin to sickle when oxygen tension falls below 15 mmHg. If reoxygenation occurs early enough, the sickling process can be reversed before extensive polymerization takes place. The clinical manifestations of SCD primarily stem from early hemolysis and the vaso-occlusive events caused by aggregates of sickled RBCs. The specific symptoms experienced by patients are largely determined by which blood vessels are affected.

Patients with SCD undergoing cardiac surgery with CPB are at risk of a potentially fatal sickling crisis triggered by hypothermia, hypoxia, acidosis, or low-flow states. Historically, the strategy was to reduce HbS levels to less than 30%. Current guidelines recommend avoiding anemia and transfusing allogenic erythrocytes to a target hemoglobin level above 8.5–9 g/dL without consideration for the proportion of circulating HbS. Clinicians should aim for total hemoglobin levels exceeding 8.5–9 g/dL before surgery and should provide red cell exchange (RCE) transfusion for patients who require preoperative transfusion but have a high hemoglobin level (>8.5–10 g/dL) that precludes administration of simple transfusion. This strategy is summarized in Fig. 21.1.

RCE during CPB can be accomplished by priming the CPB circuit with Plasmalyte, fresh red blood cells (to reduce K^+ levels), fresh frozen plasma, and albumin. On CPB, two venous reservoirs connected with a Y connector allow the perfusionist to exchange patient blood for fresh red blood

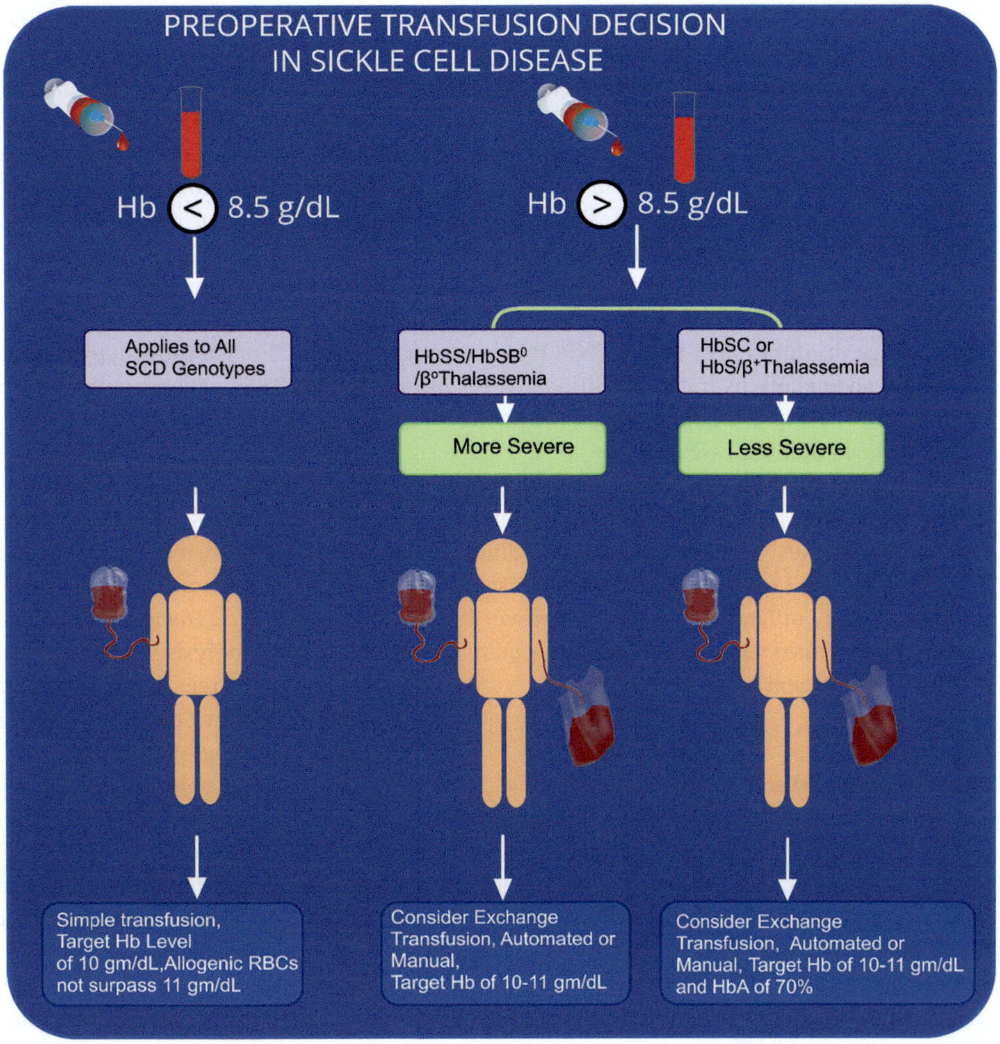

Fig. 21.1 An illustration depicting guidance for preoperative transfusion in sickle cell disease: Decisions regarding preoperative transfusion should involve consultation with a hematologist experienced in SCD management. The use of leukoreduced, sickle trait-free blood is mandatory, following ASH guidelines. For patients with any SCD genotype and an Hb level below 8.5 g/dL, simple transfusions are recommended to raise the Hb level to no more than 11 g/dL after the transfusion, thus minimizing the risk of hyperviscosity. When Hb levels are 8.5 g/dL or higher, an exchange transfusion is advised, with a target post-transfusion Hb between 10 and 11 g/dL. It is important to note that although no specific HbS% target is established for patients with HbSS or HbS/β0-thalassemia, a 70% HbA target is recommended for those with HbSC or HbS/β+-thalassemia

simultaneously ensuring maintenance of hemodynamic stability. Cell saver may be used after exchange transfusion has taken place to reduce HbS collection and reinfusion.

Given the hypothetical risk of inducing sickling and vascular stasis by exposure to decreased temperature, the use of hypothermia during CPB in SCD patients is controversial. While some authors recommend normothermia or mild hypothermia, others have suggested that moderate hypothermia is safe. Nonetheless, both hypothermic CPB and deep hypothermic circulatory arrest have been successfully employed in patients with SCD. The use of cold cardioplegia introduces the risk of inducing sickling within the coronary vasculature. As would be expected, there is a diversity of opinions on the best method to address this issue. Some authors recommend forgoing the use of blood cardioplegia in favor of a crystalloid formulation to reduce the introduction of RBCs that could potentially sickle into the coronary circulation.

Comprehensive Management of SCT and SCD in Cardiac Surgery

Preoperative Considerations

- *Planning*: Engage in early, personalized, and interdisciplinary planning, including consultation with a hematologist experienced in SCD, to assess the necessity for transfusion or exchange transfusion tailored to each patient.
- *Medical History*: Compile a thorough preoperative assessment of the patient's medical history and symptoms related to SCD, focusing on instances of hemolysis, previous transfusions, chronic pain management, and opioid tolerance, to identify perioperative risk factors.
- *Investigations*: Conduct tests to determine blood type and check for antibodies, and assess baseline kidney function, since SCD may affect kidney health, potentially revealing abnormalities even without overt kidney disease. Measure hemoglobin levels and perform hemoglobin

electrophoresis to determine the percentage of HbS. Additionally, an echocardiogram is recommended to screen for pulmonary hypertension (PHTN), a significant complication associated with SCD.

- *Hydration*: Individuals with SCD are at an increased risk of dehydration, particularly during perioperative periods with restricted oral fluid intake. This risk is exacerbated by sickle nephropathy, a condition often developed in early childhood that impairs the kidneys' ability to concentrate urine. It is critical to implement strategies that minimize the duration of fasting (NPO) to ensure patients remain adequately hydrated. Additionally, for those who must be NPO for extended periods, the administration of intravenous fluids is essential.
- *Hydroxyurea Therapy*: Hydroxyurea is a medication that enhances HbF production and thus minimizes sickling and vaso-occlusive events. It also modifies red blood cells, yielding larger cells less prone to sickling, which may lessen inflammation and improve blood flow. Continue hydroxyurea treatment preoperatively if it is part of the patient's current regimen.

Intraoperative Management

- *Sickle Cell Trait*: People with SCT usually don't require the special medical precautions necessary for managing SCD. However, under certain conditions—particularly for those who have a higher percentage of HbS in their blood or who have experienced clinical complications associated with SCT—more proactive strategies may be warranted. These strategies might mirror those used in the management of SCD.
- *Sickle Cell Disease*:
  - *Transfusion*: Depending on the percentage of HbS, thought should be given to allogenic RBCs transfusion or exchange transfusion.
  - *Prevent Sickling Triggers*:
    - *Oxygenation*: 100% O_2 sweep gas, maintain SvO_2 above 80%.
    - *Perfusion*: Avoid low-flow periods and hypoperfusion.
    - *Acidosis*: Take proactive steps to prevent acidosis.
    - *Temperature*: If possible, avoid hypothermia and cold cardioplegia.
    - *Vasoconstrictors*: Use only if absolutely necessary.
  - *Additional Considerations*
    - *Off-Pump Approach*: Consider if feasible.
    - *Cell-Saver*: Avoid cell-salvage systems and minimize cardiotomy suction.
    - *Procedure Duration*: Keep CPB and aortic cross-clamp times as short as possible.
    - *Pain Management*: Ensure effective multimodal analgesia, use anxiolytics.
  - *If Sickle cell Crisis Develop*:
    - *Exchange Transfusion*: Target HbS below 10%.
    - *Blood Pressure*: Maintain MAP above 60 mmHg.
    - *Anticoagulation*: Maintain ACT above 600 s.
    - *Temperature*: Rewarm and correct hypothermia.
    - *Monitor Urine Output*: Aim for 0.5–1 mL/kg/h.
    - *Consider Vasodilators*: Systemic or inhaled vasodilators for elevated peripheral or pulmonary vascular resistance.

For step-by-step management of sickling crises during CPB in patients with sickle cell disease, please refer to Chap. 26.

Postoperative

- *Close Monitoring*: Vigilantly observe for signs of ongoing hemolysis, vaso-occlusive incidents, and organ dysfunction.
- *Track Hemolysis Indicators*: Run repeated labs to detect hemolysis, including measurements of hemoglobin level, cell-free hemoglobin, reticulocyte count, schistocytes, ferritin, bilirubin, haptoglobin, LDH, and urinalysis for hemoglobinuria.
- *Oxygenation*: Prevent hypoxia through oxygen supplementation and promptly address and correct any acidosis.
- *Pain Management*: Ensure effective pain control through the use of comprehensive multimodal analgesia strategies.
- *Coordinate Care*: Engage hematology and critical care specialists to ensure a multidisciplinary approach to post-operative care, enhancing patient recovery, and outcomes.

Thalassemia

Beta-Thalassemia: Causes, Severity, and Cardiac Impact

Beta-thalassemia results from reduced (β+) or absent (β0) synthesis of the hemoglobin's β-globin chains. Disease severity depends mainly on the excess of unmatched α-globin chains. These chains precipitate in the erythrocyte precursors, causing both mechanical and oxidative damage. Phenotype reflects the number and type of α to β globin gene disorders, leading to three forms: β-thalassemia carrier state, thalassemia intermedia, and severe, transfusion-dependent thalassemia major.

Cardiac Complications

Management of severe forms involves regular blood transfusions and chelation therapy; however, over time, these interventions may lead to iron overload. This condition, combined with chronic hemolytic anemia and immune-mediated changes, can result in various cardiac issues, including myocarditis, pericarditis, dilated and restrictive cardiomyopathy, sudden cardiac death, and torsade de pointes.

Surgery in Thalassemia: Challenges and Strategies
Cardiac surgery exacerbates these risks due to stress, use of CPB, hypothermia, and low-flow states. To optimize care:

- *Consider Off-Pump*: If feasible, preferable for patients with hemoglobinopathies.
- *CPB Techniques*: Employ mild hypothermia, warm cardioplegia, centrifugal pumps, erythrocyte priming, and minimize the speed of cardiotomy suction.

Erythrocytosis

Erythrocytosis: Definition and Causes
Erythrocytosis is an excess of red blood cells. It is suspected when Hb and/or hematocrit (Hct) levels are elevated:

- *Men*: Hb > 18 g/dL, Hct > 0.52
- *Women*: Hb > 16.5 g/dL, Hct > 0.47

There are two main types:

- *Relative Erythrocytosis*: Caused by decreased plasma volume (not a true increase in red blood cells).
- *Absolute Erythrocytosis*: An actual increase in red blood cell mass. This can be:
  - *Primary*: Autonomous erythrocyte overproduction as seen in polycythemia vera (PCV).
  - *Secondary*: Stimulated by erythropoietin (EPO), often caused by chronic hypoxia due to conditions such as congenital heart disease (CHD) or chronic obstructive pulmonary disease (COPD).

Key Points for Cardiac Surgery
Understanding the type of erythrocytosis is critical for preoperative evaluation and intraoperative management in the setting of cardiac surgery.

Polycythemia Vera

PCV Overview and Risks
PCV is a chronic bone marrow disorder causing excessive red blood cell production, often also associated with thrombocytosis and leukocytosis. In fact, excessive thrombocytosis (platelet count >800 × 10^9/L) is a common feature of PCV. This substantially increases the risk of thrombosis:

- Arterial thrombosis can lead to cerebrovascular accidents, myocardial infarction, and peripheral vascular events in patients undergoing cardiac surgery.
- Paradoxical bleeding: PCV can also cause bleeding and is likely related to reduced platelet adhesiveness and abnormal platelet aggregation.

PCV Management for Cardiac Surgery

- *Therapeutic Measures*: May include phlebotomy, antiplatelet medications, anticoagulants, hydroxyurea, or interferon alpha.
- *Hematology Consult*: Consultation with hematology is recommended to formulate a comprehensive plan for patients requiring CPB.
- *Platelet Reduction*: In patients with excessive thrombocytosis, therapeutic platelet reduction with plateletpheresis may be necessary.
- *Pre-Bypass Dilution*: Acute normovolemic dilution prior to CPB can be used to effectively reduce Hct in some of these patients.
- *During Bypass*: Given the increased risk of thrombus formation while on bypass monitor ACT closely and monitor for any signs of thrombus formation.

Secondary Erythrocytosis

Thrombotic Risk and CPB Management

- *Thrombosis Risk*: Whether patients with secondary erythrocytosis have an increased risk of thromboembolism remains debated.
- *CPB Management*:
  - *Acute Normovolemic Hemodilution*: This method can be advantageous for such patients by lowering Hct levels during cardiac surgery involving CPB. Lowering the hematocrit helps improve microcirculatory oxygen transport and tissue perfusion in the perioperative period.
  - *Cyanotic CHD*: Children with secondary erythrocytosis due to cyanotic CHD typically experience a reduction in Hct secondary to hemodilution, facilitated by an asanguineous CPB prime.
  - *Considerations for Hemodilution*: It is important to remember that patients with elevated Hct levels have lower plasma volumes. While acute hemodilution may appropriately reduce Hct from 65–70% to the desired level, it also significantly lowers the concentration of coagulation factors within the already diminished plasma volume of 30–35%. Therefore, elective therapeutic phlebotomy with sufficient time for plasma volume normalization, might be a more effective strategy.

Other RBC Disorders

Hemochromatosis

Hereditary hemochromatosis, a common genetic defect in the Caucasian population, leads to progressive iron accumulation in tissues, risking organ damage if untreated. Treatment typically involves chelation and phlebotomy to achieve iron depletion, with the goal of maintaining serum ferritin levels below 50 μg/L and transferrin saturation under 50%. In pediatric patients, the risk of iron overload increases during CPB, suggesting that some form of iron chelation therapy may be advantageous to decrease oxidative stress.

Cold Agglutinins

Chapter 26 covers the topic in more detail and the management of Cold Agglutinins (CAs) crises. Cold agglutinins (CAs), mainly IgM autoantibodies, react with RBCs at temperatures below normal body temperature. Most CAs are benign due to their low thermal amplitude. However, primary chronic cold agglutinin disease (CAD), a rare autoimmune hemolytic anemia, involves CAs that have a higher thermal amplitude, capable of causing agglutination and primarily extravascular complement-mediated hemolysis at temperatures present in peripheral circulation. Managing CAD in CPB requires a nuanced approach due to the variability in CA behavior and disease severity.

Cardiac surgery involving CPB and induced hypothermia poses significant risks to patients with CAs or CAD. Systemic hypothermia and cold cardioplegia can activate CAs, potentially causing microcirculation obstruction and subsequent organ dysfunction. While elevated CA titers greater than 64 are concerning, accurately predicting the risk of hemolysis at lower temperatures is challenging. The clinical severity depends on the titer, the CA's thermal amplitude, and its ability to fix complement.

Management for benign CA includes avoidance of systemic hypothermia and cold cardioplegia, with warm cardioplegia as the alternative. For patients with CAD or surgeries requiring unavoidable hypothermia, a more comprehensive preoperative assessment is necessary. This includes CA titers, thermal amplitude determination and consultation with a hematologist. Medical therapies for CAD or CA may involve plasma exchange, rituximab (for refractory cases), cyclophosphamide, chlorambucil, glucocorticoids, intravenous immunoglobulin, erythropoietin, red blood cell transfusions, and plasma exchange in severe cases. The specific approach should be individualized based on disease severity and the patient's clinical picture.

Malignancies and Myeloproliferative Disorders

Myeloproliferative neoplasms (MPN) such as chronic myelogenous leukemia, polycythemia vera, essential thrombocythemia, and myelofibrosis can have complex effects on blood clotting, increasing both thrombosis and bleeding risks depending on the specific MPN type and severity. On CPB, platelet activation and dysfunction due to contact with artificial surfaces in the oxygenator are major contributors to bleeding. While pre-operative white blood cell count may be linked to ischemic events after surgery, the specific mechanisms are complex and require further investigation.

Inherited Bleeding Disorders

Hemophilia

Hemophilia A and B, the two most common types, are caused by deficiencies in factor VIII (FVIII) and factor IX (FIX), respectively. These X-linked recessive disorders predominantly affect males and lead to significantly increased bleeding risk due to impaired coagulation in the intrinsic pathway. Hemophilia is classified by factor activity level into mild (5–40%), moderate (1–5%), and severe (<1%), each correlating with the clinical bleeding risk. Chronic management typically includes prophylactic plasma-derived or recombinant factor replacement therapy to restore normal coagulation profiles. However, long-term treatment may lead to the development of factor inhibitors such as neutralizing antibodies, reducing the efficacy of transfusions. Immune tolerance therapy reduces this response and limits factor inhibitors.

Patients with hemophilia undergoing cardiac surgery should be assessed by a hematologist and receive perioperative care from a multidisciplinary team. Preoperative factor levels should be elevated to 80–100% normal and maintained through the day of surgery (POD 0). A typical regimen involves administering a 45–50 U/kg before anesthesia and a 2000 U bolus post-CPB, with the goal of maintaining >80% of normal FVIII activity during and after surgery. This regimen usually requires ongoing infusions or intermittent boluses, along with frequent factor level testing. In hemophilia patients, activated partial thromboplastin time (PTT) and ACT are prolonged but should normalize with factor replacement. Viscoelastic tests such as thromboelastography (TEG) or rotational thromboelastometry (ROTEM) can be useful during and after surgery. Standard heparin protocols and ACT targets for CPB anticoagulation and protamine reversal are recommended.

Patients with significant inhibitors may require bypassing agents, such as recombinant activated factor VII (rFVIIa) or factor eight inhibitor bypassing activity (FEIBA), which promote thrombin generation without needing FVIII or FIX. FEIBA is a four-factor (II, VIIa, IX, X) activated prothrombin complex concentrate (aPCC) and is often given at 100 U/kg every 8 hours, while rVIIa is typically 90 mg/kg every 3–4 hours preoperatively and for 48–72 hours after CPB. Antifibrinolytic therapy (aminocaproic, tranexamic acid) is vital during surgery and may be continued up to 24 hours postoperatively. For mild hemophilia A, consider desmopressin acetate (DDAVP), which increases FVIII levels.

Von Willebrand Disease

Von Willebrand disease (vWD) is an inherited or acquired disorder affecting von Willebrand factor (vWF), which is crucial for platelet adhesion and clot stability. Hereditary vWD has three main types: Type 1 (partial deficiency), Type 2 (qualitative defects), and Type 3 (severe deficiency). Acquired vWD (AvWS) can occur due to various diseases such as multiple myeloma, hypothyroidism, aortic stenosis, mitral regurgitation, extracorporeal membrane oxygenation, and ventricular assist devices. Preoperative hematology consultation is crucial.

Treatment options include:

- DDAVP: can be given intravenously (0.3 μg per kilogram of body weight) to increase factor VIII and endogenous von Willebrand factor levels by two to four times. Contraindicated in Type 2B due to thrombocytopenia risk.
- Exogenous vWF (+/− FVIII): Effective for all vWD subtypes, especially Type 2B and Type 3. Consider FVIII supplementation if replacement is close to surgery.
- Antifibrinolytics: Assist in achieving hemostasis and are safe in conjunction with DDAVP or exogenous replacement.
- In AvWS: Treating the underlying cause is key, as high clearance can hinder hemostasis despite factor replacement.

Other (Rare) Factor Deficiencies

Other factor deficiencies, though rare, require individualized treatment with hematologist input and a multidisciplinary approach.

- *Fibrinogen deficiency* (Factor I, Common Pathway): whether quantitative or qualitative, necessitates preoperative fibrinogen normalization for levels below 100–150 mg/dL, usually using plasma-derived fibrinogen concentrate rather than cryoprecipitate.
- *Factor XII Deficiency* (12, Intrinsic Pathway): Manifested by a prolonged PTT and ACT without increased bleeding risk, complicates heparin monitoring during CPB; approaches include empirical dosing or modified ACT tests. Avoid antifibrinolytics.
- *Factor XIII Deficiency* (13, Fibrin Stabilizing Factor): Inhibits fibrinolysis of cross-linked fibrin and requires preoperative factor concentration to be increased to 50–80% using factor concentrate, especially in the setting of hemodilution or significant bleeding. Cryoprecipitate is an alternative.
- *Factor VII Deficiency* (7, Extrinsic Pathway): This vitamin K dependent factor deficiency, whether involving quantitative or qualitative defects, varies in presentation and is treated with recombinant or plasma-derived concentrate to increase perioperative levels; routine prothrombin time (PT)/INR monitoring is affected, while PTT and ACT remain normal. Vitamin K antagonism is not recommended for valvular prophylaxis due to the unpredictability of monitoring.
- *Factor XI Deficiency* (11, Hemophilia C, Intrinsic Pathway): More common in Ashkenazi Jews, this deficiency mildly increases bleeding risk; preoperative correction above 70% is recommended, using antifibrinolytic agents to augment antifibrinolysis. As with hemophiliacs, patients with FXI deficiency may develop inhibitors to replacement therapy, the treatment of which may require preoperative therapeutic plasma exchange.
- *Factor X Deficiency* (10, Common Pathway): This is a vitamin K dependent factor, essential for thrombin generation along with factor V, as part of the intrinsic prothrombinase complex. Clinical bleeding correlates well with factor levels. Levels below 10% are associated with significant bleeding, while levels above 40% are usually symptom free. Perioperative correction of FX levels involves using factor concentrate, fresh frozen plasma (FFP), or prothrombin complex concentrate (PCC), with careful monitoring to avoid overcorrection and increased venous thrombosis risk. FX deficiency prolongs PT and PTT, complicating intraoperative ACT monitoring, and may require preoperative FX levels to be restored prior to surgery or anti-Xa assays for heparin activity monitoring.
- *FV Deficiency* (5, Common Pathway): A rare autosomal recessive condition, FV serves as a cofactor in the prothrombinase complex and is inactivated by activated protein C. Acquired forms of the deficiency may arise from exposure to bovine thrombin. Bleeding risk poorly correlates with FV activity or PT/activated partial thromboplastin time (aPTT) assays, complicating intraoperative ACT and heparin monitoring. With no FV concentrates available, treatment primarily involves FFP or plasma exchange.
- *Factor II Deficiency* (2, Prothrombin, Common Pathway): The deficiency of FII, a Vitamin K-dependent factor, is inherited in an autosomal recessive fashion and ranges from asymptomatic to severe. Levels can be corrected using FFP or PCC. It typically prolongs PT, aPTT, and ACT, complicating intraoperative heparin monitoring. Given its rarity, little is known about factor II replacement, and there are no reported cases of FII-deficient patients and CPB.

Acquired Bleeding Disorders

Vitamin K Deficiency

Vitamin K deficiency increases bleeding risk by impairing the production of factors II, VII, IX and X. Acquired causes include poor dietary intake, warfarin therapy, and conditions such as malabsorption and liver disease. Liver dysfunction is discussed separately.

For urgent reversal of warfarin, use IV vitamin K and 4F-PCC. PCC is superior to FFP for speed, efficacy, and safety. Further, 4F-PCC is preferred over 3F-PCC for improved antagonist reversal as determined by INR and a lower mortality rate. Factor VIIa, while normalizing INR, does not address other factor deficiencies and is not recommended. PCC dosing is complex, relying on bodyweight, INR, and institutional protocols. Note that there is thromboembolic risk associated with PCC utilization, though newer formulations such as Kcentra®, which contain non-activated factors along with Protein C, Protein S, and heparin, may offer a more balanced coagulopathic profile.

Direct-Acting Oral Anticoagulants

Direct-acting oral anticoagulants (DOACs) are increasingly common in cardiac patients, posing new challenges. They offer advantages over warfarin, including fewer drug interactions, less variability, minimal dietary restrictions, reduced need for blood monitoring, and shorter half-lives.

DOAC types include direct factor Xa inhibitors (rivaroxaban, apixaban, edoxaban, and betrixaban), and the direct thrombin inhibitor dabigatran, with dabigatran being the most dependent on renal clearance. For elective surgery, hold DOACs for at least 48 hours (longer for renal dysfunction). Previously, DOAC reversal involved using FFP or aPCC, but specific reversal agents are now available for some DOACs:

Dabigatran Idarucizumab is a monoclonal antibody that irreversibly binds to dabigatran and rapidly neutralizes it. A typical dose is a 5 g bolus or infusion, reversing effects within 15 minutes with a duration of 24 hours. Case reports indicate safe use of idarucizumab prior to CPB, allowing standard heparin and protamine administration following preoperative dosing of idarucizumab. For recent dabigatran ingestion, consider activated charcoal or hemodialysis. If these are unavailable, consider using a PCC.

Factor Xa Inhibitors (Apixaban and rivaroxaban) are reversed by andexanet alfa, a recombinant FXa decoy given IV with dosage based on the last intake. Crucially, andexanet alpha binds ATIII and ATIII-heparin complexes, rendering heparin less effective. Avoid andexanet if the patient may need surgery with heparinization.

For urgent post-andexanet anticoagulation, consider higher heparin doses, ATIII supplementation, or alternative agents (argatroban, bivalirudin). There is no consensus on anticoagulation management for cardiac surgery after andexanet alpha administration. While the Society of Cardiovascular Anesthesiologists recommends ATIII utilization, the manufacturer recommends use of heparin alternatives. Emerging technologies such as CytoSorb, used extracorporeally, may offer additional perioperative DOAC management options, potentially including apixaban reduction.

Antiplatelet Agents

Platelets are essential for coagulation and hemostasis, facilitating primary and secondary hemostasis through sufficient quantities and normal adhesion, activation, and aggregation abilities. Several pathways exist that allow for the manipulation of platelet function. Antiplatelet medications target these specific pathways to modulate platelet function.

Cyclooxygenase Inhibitors

Cyclooxygenase inhibitors target endothelial cell cyclooxygenase, which synthesizes prostaglandins leading to the production of thromboxane A2 and PGI_2. Thromboxane A2, via cyclooxygenase-1 (COX-1), promotes platelet aggregation and vasoconstriction, while PGI_2 via COX-2, inhibits platelet aggregation and induces vasodilation.

- *Aspirin* irreversibly inhibits COX-1, blocking platelet aggregation (TXA2) and vasoconstriction. Aspirin also inhibits COX-2 (PGI_2) at high doses. Hold aspirin 5–7 days pre-surgery due to platelet lifespan.
- *Triflusal* is a similar derivative under investigation.

Adenosine Diphosphate (ADP) Receptor Inhibitors

Adenosine diphosphate (ADP) receptor inhibitors target platelet membrane receptors $P2Y_1$, $P2Y_{12}$ and $P2X_1$. $P2Y_{12}$ is crucial for completing ADP-initiated platelet aggregation, while $P2X_1$ amplifies platelet activation and aggregation. These drugs vary in pharmacokinetics, affecting their efficacy and bleeding risk.

- *Thienopyridines*:
  - *Clopidogrel*: A second-generation thienopyridine prodrug that, once metabolized, irreversibly binds to $P2Y_{12}$ inhibiting platelet activation. Maximum platelet

aggregation inhibition occurs within 6 hours after a loading dose, with complete recovery 7 days after discontinuation.
  - *Prasugrel*: A third-generation thienopyridine prodrug offering advantages over clopidogrel, including less drug–drug interaction and more predictable efficacy due to reduced influence of genetic polymorphisms. However, it carries a higher risk of bleeding.
- *Nonthienopyridines*:
  - *Ticagrelor*: Delivered in its active form, directly and reversibly binds to the $P2Y_{12}$ receptor, offering more potency than thienopyridines and allowing platelet function to recover as drug levels decrease.
  - *Cangrelor*: Reversibly binds to the $P2Y_{12}$ receptor with rapid onset (80% platelet inhibition within 5 minutes) and short duration (complete platelet recovery within 60–90 minutes).

Phosphodiesterase Inhibitors

- *Cilostazol*: Inhibits phosphodiesterase III, altering platelet adhesion. It also uniquely improves endothelial cell function and reduces circulating activated platelets.
- *Dipyridamole*: Reversibly inhibits phosphodiesterase and adenosine deaminase, reducing platelet aggregation, and thrombosis.

Glycoprotein IIB/IIIA Inhibitors

These medications are the most potent class of antiplatelet drugs, blocking the final common pathway of platelet aggregation and achieving >90% inhibition.

- *Abciximab*: A monoclonal Fab molecule, quickly inhibits over >80% of platelet activity. Recovery of platelet function can take up to 48 hours due to slow dissociation, despite its short serum half-life. Its effects can be reversed with platelet transfusion.
- *Eptifibatide*: Achieves over >80% platelet inhibition within 15 minutes and dissociates quickly from platelets, maintaining persistent free drug levels even after discontinuation. Because of this, platelet transfusion is unlikely to reverse its platelet inhibition.
- *Tirofiban*: Is a nonpeptide GP IIb/IIIa receptor antagonist with rapid dissociation, leading to fast reversal of platelet inhibition after stopping the drug.

Others

- *Vorapaxar*: A protease-activated receptor-1 (PAR-1) antagonist, reversibly binds platelet PAR-1 (thrombin) receptors with high affinity, blocking procoagulant release without affecting thrombin-induced fibrin formation. It is active without metabolic transformation and has a long half-life, inhibiting platelets for about 4 weeks after initial and maintenance dosing.

Management of Antiplatelets in Anticipation of CPB

- *Elective Surgery*: Hold clopidogrel for 5 days, prasugrel for 7 days, and ticagrelor for 5 days (some data supports 3 days).
- *Urgent Surgery*: In emergency surgery where antiplatelet therapy cannot be stopped, use point-of-care platelet function testing (TEG with platelet mapping, $P2Y_{12}$ assays) to guide transfusion needs. The extent of platelet inhibition often correlates with the need for transfusions and potential re-exploration for bleeding. The TARGET-CABG study supports platelet inhibition tests for surgical planning over rigid drug discontinuation guidelines.
- *Minimize Blood Loss*: Blood loss can be mitigated by employing acute normovolemic hemodilution, retrograde priming, smaller circuits, cell salvage, and antifibrinolytics (e.g., aminocaproic acid, tranexamic acid).
- *Bridging (if necessary)*: Cangrelor can be used as a bridging therapy to minimize the risk of stent thrombosis when holding antiplatelet therapy may impose unacceptable risk. Glycoprotein IIb/IIIa inhibitors may also serve this purpose.

Inherited Clotting Disorders

Proteins C and S Deficiency

Roles of Protein C and Protein S

Both protein C and protein S function as natural anticoagulants. Protein S is a vitamin K-dependent glycoprotein that serves as a cofactor for activated protein C, which operates in two pathways: inactivation of procoagulant-activated factors V and VIII as well as augmentation of fibrinolysis. Deficiencies of protein C or protein S result in a state of thrombophilia.

Protein S Deficiency: Surgical Considerations

- *Inherited Protein S Deficiency*: Protein S deficiency is inherited in an autosomal dominant pattern and is categorized into three types:
  - *Type 1*: Quantitative and qualitative reduction.
  - *Type 2*: Normal quantity, reduced function.

  - *Type 3*: Selectively reduced free protein S and function.
- *Acquired Protein S Deficiency*: This condition can occur in various states, such as pregnancy, DIC, thrombosis, HIV, and liver or kidney disease, leading to an increased risk of venous thromboembolism (VTE).
- *Management Strategies*:
  - *Acute VTE Treatment*: Typically involves standard anticoagulation for 3–6 months, which may be extended based on the patient's condition.
  - *Preventive Measures*: Asymptomatic patients generally do not require anticoagulation, except in special circumstances such as pregnancy, surgeries involving prolonged immobility, or acute medical illnesses.
  - *Avoidance of Antifibrinolytics*: Substances such as aminocaproic acid and tranexamic acid should be avoided as they can exacerbate the antifibrinolytic state present in protein S deficiency.
  - *Intraoperative Care*: Fresh frozen plasma (FFP) is crucial for prophylaxis and treatment to increase protein S levels. Some protocols recommend priming the CPB circuit with FFP.
  - *Monitoring and Reversal*: Heparin, activated clotting time (ACT) monitoring, and reversal with protamine are safe practices for this population. Clinicians should be vigilant about the potential for thrombophilia in patients with heterozygous genetics, especially if there is early graft failure post-CABG due to thrombosis, suggesting an underlying coagulation disorder.

Protein C Deficiency: Surgical Considerations

Protein C, a zymogen plasma protein synthesized in the liver, is a natural anticoagulant inactivating factors V and VIIIa, and boosting fibrinolysis. Deficiency increases thrombotic risk, worsened by CPB. Inherited types include:

- Type 1—Reduced level and activity
- Type 2—Reduced function only.

Acquired deficiency can occur in DIC, liver disease, infection, uremia, or cancer.

- *Management Strategies*:
  - *Vitamin K Antagonists*: These interfere with protein C production, rendering protein C deficiency workups unreliable in patients recently exposed to warfarin.
  - *Hypercoagulation and Thromboembolic Risks*: Protein C deficiency significantly increases risks, especially during CPB, where the protein is diluted and consumed. Main concerns include VTE and arterial thrombosis.
  - *VTE Anticoagulation Protocol*:
    - *Similar Approach to Non-Deficient Patients*: The management of VTE in patients with protein C deficiency is generally similar to that in patients without the deficiency. However, due to the higher thrombotic risk, these patients may be more likely to require lifelong anticoagulation.
    - *Warfarin Considerations*: Careful use is advised due to increased risk of warfarin-increased skin necrosis; options include DOACs for systemic anticoagulation.
  - *Perioperative Management*:
    - *Preoperative*: Anticoagulation with heparin as usual.
    - *Protein C Level Correction*: Use FFP or concentrate to raise protein C levels, with careful administration of protamine at the conclusion of the case.
    - *Postoperative management*: Early anticoagulation with heparin once bleeding is controlled.
    - *Hematologist Involvement*: Essential for complex decision making in managing protein C deficiency (may need long-term anticoagulation).

Antithrombin Deficiency

Antithrombin-III (ATIII) Deficiency: Surgical Considerations

Antithrombin-III (ATIII) is a plasma protein synthesized by the liver that inhibits thrombin, factor Xa, and other serine proteases, thus potentiating heparin's anticoagulant effect.

Inherited Deficiency Rare autosomal dominant disorder increasing VTE and pregnancy related complications/loss risk:

- Type 1—Reduced level
- Type 2—Reduced function only (various subtypes).

Inherited ATIII deficiency typically does not require long-term systemic anticoagulation in asymptomatic individuals; however, those with a history of VTE will require anticoagulation, the duration of which depends on various factors.

Acquired Deficiency

- Can occur in various conditions, including cirrhosis, nephrotic syndrome, severe trauma, protein-losing enteropathy, sepsis with DIC, burn injuries, CPB/ECMO, and heparinoids such as enoxaparin.
- Causes:
  - Increased loss of ATIII
  - Increased consumption of ATIII
  - Reduced synthesis of ATIII

- The majority of acquired states do not present an increased risk of clotting, except in cases such as asparaginase chemotherapy-induced ATIII deficiency.
- Despite not typically increasing thrombotic risk, acquired deficiencies can lead to intraoperative heparin resistance.
- Diagnosing ATIII deficiency perioperatively can be challenging, especially after recent heparin administration, which can interfere with testing.

ATIII Deficiency and Surgery

Perioperative prophylaxis may require larger heparin doses. ATIII deficiency increases the risk of complications during CPB due to decreased heparin anticoagulation efficacy. ATIII replacement may be achieved through administration of FFP, plasma-derived concentrate, or recombinant ATIII.

Predictors of Deficiency

Predictors of ATIII deficiency include:

- Thrombocytosis >300,000
- Age > 65 years
- Prior heparin exposure

Heparin Resistance Management

- Suspect ATIII deficiency if high heparin doses are needed to achieve target ACT.
- Consider increasing heparin or ATIII replacement.
- Increasing doses of heparin are associated with increased potential for rebound after reversal and thus increased risk of bleeding.
- Replacement can be undertaken utilizing an ATIII product or FFP.
- It's important to remember that heparin resistance can have causes other than ATIII deficiency (e.g., heparin binding to chemokines and growth factors). In those cases, ATIII supplementation won't help.
- If the patient doesn't respond to heparin + ATIII, carefully weigh the risks of proceeding on CPB with insufficient anticoagulation vs. bleeding risk with alternative agents (e.g., bivalirudin, argatroban).

Factor V Leiden

Factor V Leiden (FVL) is a genetic variant causing a hypercoagulable state due to resistance to activated protein C. While common, its clinical severity varies. Patients aren't typically on prophylactic anticoagulation, and VTE treatment duration is individualized.

Key Surgical Considerations

- Increased risk of thromboembolism in the setting of cardiac surgery—especially in the setting of CPB and fresh bypass grafts.
- There is no standard protocol for patients requiring cardiac surgery with a history of FVL.
- Bridge pre-op anticoagulation, often for personal history of VTE, if chronically on warfarin to enoxaparin until day of surgery. Patients are generally at an increased risk of venous thrombosis; therefore, those undergoing CABG are considered to be at particularly high risk. Typical ACT goals and reduced protamine reversal (half or two-thirds of the typical dose) should be utilized with a post reversal goal of ACT around 200 s being reasonable.
- Avoid antifibrinolytic therapy and, if available, utilize TEG to trend the patient profile.
- Postoperatively, if the bleeding risk is low, patients should be started on antiplatelets and a continuous heparin infusion, with a goal PTT of 1.5 times the control.
- Complex cases require a multidisciplinary approach.

Hyperhomocysteinemia

- Homocysteine, an alpha amino acid, requires Vitamins B6 and B12 for its metabolism.
- Elevated levels (hyperhomocysteinemia) can be:
  - *Inherited*: Genetic mutations affecting enzymes (30% heterozygous, 10% homozygous).
  - *Acquired*: Vitamin deficiencies, chronic kidney disease, smoking, or certain medications (fibrates).

Health Risks

- Hyperhomocysteinemia is associated with increased risk of:
  - Cardiovascular disease (coronary artery disease, peripheral arterial disease)
  - Stroke
  - Venous thrombosis
- Co-inheritance of the enzymatic mutation with other genetic risk profiles such as factor V Leiden can further increase the VTE risk.

Cardiac Surgery Considerations

- Perioperative homocysteine testing may be beneficial to identify high-risk patients.
- Current evidence does not support treating elevated levels unless homocystinuria, the autosomal recessive disorder manifested by elevated urine and plasma levels, is confirmed.

- Potential approaches include vitamin supplementation preoperatively, utilization of off-pump techniques when feasible and supplementation of natural anticoagulants such as antithrombin.

Acquired Clotting Disorders

Antiphospholipid Syndrome

Antiphospholipid Syndrome (APS): Key Concepts

Definition: Presence of thrombus (arterial or venous) or pregnancy complications, along with laboratory identification of one of the three specific antiphospholipid antibodies (aPL): lupus anticoagulant (LA), anticardiolipin antibody (aCL), and anti-β_2 glycoprotein I antibody (aβ_2GPI).

Causes: While APS can have a genetic component, it's also linked to environmental triggers, including viral infections (cytomegalovirus (CMV) or parvovirus B19), bacterial infections (E. Coli or leptospirosis) and certain medications (like antiepileptics or oral contraceptives).

Mechanism: APS creates a hypercoagulable state by activating endothelial cells, platelets, and the coagulation cascade. It also inhibits natural anticoagulants such as plasminogen, protein C, and protein S.

Cardiac Risks: Cardiovascular complications of APS include valvular heart disease, coronary artery disease, intracardiac thrombus, pulmonary hypertension, and dilated cardiomyopathy. Valvular disease primarily affects the mitral valve and less frequently involves the aortic and tricuspid valves.

Other Risks in APS: Non-cardiovascular effects include neurologic changes, skin ulcers, and diffuse alveolar hemorrhage. Catastrophic APS can occur acutely, resembling HIT/DIC/SIRS, leading to multiple vascular occlusions, organ failure, and a 50% mortality rate.

APS & Cardiac Surgery: Challenges

- *Pre-Op Concerns*: Increased thrombosis risk when anticoagulation is paused or reversed.
- *Intraoperative Challenges*:
  - *Anticoagulation and Monitoring Difficulties*: Achieving adequate anticoagulation and intraoperative monitoring is complicated by the variability in APS response to standard tests such as aPTT and Kaolin ACT, which may show a hypocoagulable state despite actual hypercoagulability.
  - *Risk of Bleeding*: Patients with APS are also at increased risk of bleeding due to either excessive anticoagulation or clotting factor deficiencies that can occur in APS.
  - *Heparinization Protocols*: No consensus on protocols for CPB; practices vary widely across institutions. Some use standard heparin dosing, while others adjust based on the patient's risk profile (history of thrombosis or thrombocytopenia), potentially doubling usual ACT targets.
  - *Alternative Monitoring Approaches*:
    - Proposals include using anti-Xa concentration (30-minutes turnaround may be impractical for CPB), thrombin time tests (time-consuming), and automated protamine titration to measure heparin concentrations. These methods aim to achieve a target often to double the baseline ACT, using preoperative and intraoperative in vitro heparin-ACT titration curves, or measuring heparin anti factor Xa levels.
    - While standard CPB uses >3 U/mL heparin as a safe threshold, recommendations for APS patients vary widely. Some case reports suggest >3 U/mL is safe for low-risk APS, others recommend >4 U/mL as a standard, and some clinicians advocate for >5 U/mL for high-risk patients.
    - Protamine dosing is also highly variable, from none to half dose, or titration based on bleeding or ACT. The use of TEG is unreliable in APS patients, needing further research.
    - Antifibrinolytics have been reportedly used in patients with APS, but there is no consensus as to whether this is considered safe practice.
    - Key goal: Finding the delicate balance between preventing excessive bleeding and thrombosis (especially catastrophic APS).

Additional/Complex Coagulopathy

Cirrhosis and Liver Disease

Complex Hemostasis

Liver diseases induce complex hemostatic changes in coagulation, including hypercoagulable and prothrombotic tendencies that standard coagulation tests may not accurately capture. This section briefly highlights perioperative considerations. Cirrhotic patients have increased morbidity and mortality due to poor nutrition, infection, and coagulopathy. Preoperative risk assessment is conducted using Child's class or MELD score. Either a Class B or C, or a MELD score of 13–18, is considered an acceptable risk for cardiac surgery. Evidence suggests that liver disease type also impacts prothrombotic versus bleeding risks.

Causes of Prothrombotic Changes

Prohemostatic changes that contribute to a prothrombotic state include:

- High VWF
- High levels of procoagulant factors such as factor VIII
- Reduced plasminogen, decreasing clot breakdown capability

Causes of Coagulopathy

Patients with liver disease are coagulopathic for a variety of reasons.

- Reduced synthesis of anticoagulant factors such as antithrombin and protein C, along with low plasminogen. Antihemostatic changes include low platelet count, decreased levels of procoagulant factors (fibrinogen, factors II, V, VII, IX, X, XI) and reduced plasmin inhibitor.
- Thrombocytopenia is common and often caused by poor nutrition, splenic sequestration and/or bleeding.
- Vitamin K depletion is common in alcohol-associated liver dysfunction. Failure to improve after vitamin K supplementation suggests poor hepatic reserve.

Management Strategies

- *Preoperative*
  Optimize with vitamin K supplementation, though response may be poor. No specific INR or platelet thresholds fully predict procedural risk; therefore, preoperative transfusion of FFP or platelets to "correct" values lacks supporting evidence.
- *Intraoperative*
  - Thromboelastography aids in assessing tendencies toward hyper- and hypo-coagulability both prior to, during and after cardiac surgery.
  - Cryoprecipitate is preferred over FFP for fibrinogen supplementation due to volume concerns.
  - Judicious use of fibrinogen and factor concentrates (PCC) due to thrombosis risk.
  - Antifibrinolytics are generally safe for active bleeding.
  - DDAVP use in liver dysfunction is not evidence-based, even though Von Willebrand factor is often elevated given it is produced from endothelial cells.
- *DIC versus Liver Disease: Factor VIII as a Key Marker*
  New coagulopathy in patients with suspected or known liver disease warrants investigation, as it can mimic disseminated intravascular coagulation (DIC). While factor VIII levels are typically normal or elevated in chronic liver disease due to production by non-hepatic endothelial cells, they are often low in DIC due to consumption.

Disseminated Intravascular Coagulation

DIC is a complex syndrome where both increased thrombosis and bleeding risks are high. DIC occurs when the delicate balance between injury-site coagulation and fibrinolysis to limit coagulation and promote healing is lost.

Characteristic Lab Abnormalities and Differential Diagnosis

Laboratory findings usually show elevated D-dimers, thrombocytopenia, prolonged PT/PTT, and decreased fibrinogen levels. DIC can mimic other conditions, including heparin-induced thrombocytopenia (HIT), thrombotic microangiopathy, cirrhotic bleeding, thrombocytopenic purpura (TTP), hemolytic uremic syndrome (HUS), and various other diseases.

Causes of DIC

DIC can be acute or chronic. Known DIC triggers include sepsis, trauma, liver disease, pancreatitis, malignancies, aortic aneurysm or dissection, drug use, transplant rejection, and obstetrical syndromes like pre-eclampsia, amniotic fluid embolism, and HELLP (hemolysis, elevated liver enzymes, low platelet count) syndrome.

Management Strategies

Management focuses on treating the underlying condition and restoring normal coagulation through transfusions of platelets, FFP, and factor concentrates, along with cautious use of anticoagulants to limit thrombin generation and consumption-induced coagulopathy. Specific targets such as antithrombin III and activated protein C are being studied.

Outside of the operating room, monitor heparin using anti-Xa levels, as aPTT can be unreliable. Antifibrinolytics may be beneficial in early hyperfibrinolytic stages of DIC but could be harmful in later thrombosis stages. While PCC is typically avoided, those with protein C/S and heparin may be less thrombogenic. There is no standard heparin protocol for prolonged ACT. Clinical judgment, considering the DIC stage and bleeding versus thrombosis risks, and consulting hematology are crucial.

Platelet Disorders

Heparin Induced Thrombocytopenia

HIT Overview

Heparin-induced thrombocytopenia (HIT) is an antibody mediated platelet activation disorder causing severe, progressive thrombocytopenia with possible thrombosis (HITT). This is indicated by a platelet count below 100,000/mm^3 or a 30–50% decline from baseline over several days. Onset typically occurs 3–15 days after starting heparin but can happen within hours if there is prior exposure. Unlike other thrombocytopenic disorders, low platelet count in HIT signals an increased risk of thrombosis, not bleeding.

Pathophysiology of HIT

HIT is triggered by immunoglobulin G antibodies that form against complexes of heparin and platelet factor 4 (PF4), binding to the FcγRIIa immunoreceptor on platelets and initiating activation and degranulation. This initiates a cycle of increased release of additional PF4 and subsequent platelet aggregation. Released microparticles enhance thrombin generation, leading to further platelet activation. This cascade of activation, consumption, and sequestration results in acute thrombocytopenia. Platelet aggregation, monocyte tissue factor release, and contributions from endothelial cells and neutrophils all play roles in thrombin production.

Venous thrombosis occurs 3–4 times more frequently than arterial thrombosis. The most common forms are deep venous thrombosis and pulmonary embolism, while arterial thrombosis typically manifests as peripheral arterial embolism, stroke and myocardial infarction, especially after cardiac surgery.

HIT Diagnosis and Lab Abnormalities

HIT diagnosis relies on both clinical suspicion and laboratory confirmation. The 4Ts scoring system is a valuable tool for assessing the likelihood of HIT by evaluating four key factors: the severity of *Thrombocytopenia*, the *Timing* of platelet count decline relative to heparin exposure, the presence of *Thrombosis* or *oTher* complications, and the likelihood of alternative causes for thrombocytopenia. Each factor is scored from 0 to 2, with a total score ranging from 0 to 8. A higher score indicates a greater probability of HIT: 6–8 suggests a high probability, 4–5 indicates intermediate probability, and 0–3 implies a low probability. The 4Ts score helps clinicians determine the need for further testing, such as the heparin-PF4 antibody assay, and guides decisions on heparin cessation and alternative anticoagulation strategies. Laboratory detection primarily utilizes an ELISA to test for specific antibodies, with accuracy depending on the assay's threshold. The diagnostic accuracy of the assay depends on the thresholds. The IgG-specific ELISA achieves 99.6% sensitivity with an optical density of less than 0.7. However, it has over 90% specificity at intermediate optical densities (0.8–1.4). Standard HIT diagnostics include the serotonin release assay and the heparin-induced platelet aggregation assay, both of which assess platelet activation with heparin, patient serum, and donor platelets.

Management Strategies

Treatment involves immediate heparin cessation and switching to an alternative anticoagulant, as thrombosis risk is high. Platelet infusions should be avoided, as they can worsen thrombosis. Antiplatelet therapies that block PF4 release may also be beneficial.

Patients with a history of HIT require special perioperative surgical planning. Table 21.1 below summarizes the classification of HIT based on platelet count and the results of functional and immunoassay assays prior to cardiac surgery and the proposed management.

Antiplatelet Management

Antiplatelet management protocols are often institution specific, requiring interdisciplinary discussions with the hematology, surgical, perfusion, and anesthesiology teams. Please refer to your own institution's protocol. Below are examples of potential management strategies.

Tirofiban (GPIIb/IIIa inhibitor)

- Bolus 10 mcg/kg 10 minutes before heparin administration.
- Infusion of 0.15 mcg/kg/min.
- Stop the infusion 1 hour before ending CPB.

Table. 21.1 Outlining HIT phases, diagnostic criteria, and proposed management approaches for cardiac surgery patients

Outlining HIT phases, diagnostic criteria, and proposed management approaches for cardiac surgery patients			
HIT phase	Platelet count	Assay results	Proposed management
Acute HIT (within 5–10 days of heparin)	Significant drop (e.g., below 50,000/mm^3 or >50% decline)	Both functional and immunoassay positive	Cease heparin immediately. Begin alternative anticoagulant (e.g., argatroban, fondaparinux depending on renal function). Consult hematology
Subacute HIT (after 5–10 days)	Moderate drop, may be recovering	Immunoassay may remain positive, but less strongly, functional assays may be variable	Potential for careful heparin reintroduction IF absolutely needed. Consult hematology, close monitoring, alternative anticoagulants safer. High-risk for recurrence
Remote HIT (weeks to months after episode)	Typically normal	Immunoassay may remain positive for some time, functional assays often negative	Heparin use may be possible with extreme caution. Consult hematology, consider non-heparin alternatives if feasible

Cangrelor ($P2Y_{12}$ inhibitor)

- Bolus 30 mcg/kg approximately 10 minutes before heparin administration.
- Infusion of 4.0 mcg/kg/min.
- Stop the infusion at the end of CPB or when giving protamine.

IV Epoprostenol (alternative)

- Use with heparin before/during the procedure.
- Often requires norepinephrine (0.05–0.1 mcg/kg/min) to manage significant vasodilation.
- Stop after CPB and protamine administration to neutralize heparin anticoagulation.

Immune Thrombocytopenia (ITP)

ITP: Key Concepts

- *Overview*: ITP presents as isolated thrombocytopenia (less than 100,000/m^3 platelets) with normal white blood cell counts and hemoglobin levels, typically alongside a purpuric rash.
- *Etiology*: Primary ITP has no known cause, while secondary ITP is linked to underlying conditions or triggers such as medications (e.g., eptifibatide, heparin, beta-lactam antibiotics) or systemic illnesses. ITP is characterized by autoantibodies targeting platelet membrane glycoprotein complexes, leading to increased platelet clearance by the spleen.
- *Diagnosis*: Evaluation starts with a complete blood count with differential, reticulocyte count, peripheral blood smear, blood type and direct antiglobulin test. Additional tests such as PT and aPTT may be necessary for patients with moderate to severe thrombocytopenia, signs of bleeding, or upcoming invasive procedures.
- *Management*: Treatment depends on the severity of bleeding and the etiology of ITP. Options include immune globulin (IVIG), glucocorticoids, and platelet transfusions. Pre-cardiac surgery management may involve steroids and intraoperative interventions such as platelet transfusions, intravenous immunoglobulin, aprotinin, and the anti-inflammatory agent nafamostat mesylate.

Thrombotic Thrombocytopenic Purpura (TTP)

TTP: Key Concepts

- *Emergency Status*: TTP is a life-threatening condition with an untreated mortality rate of approximately 90%.
- *Clinical Manifestation*: Presents with microangiopathic hemolytic anemia, fever, thrombocytopenia, and renal and neurologic dysfunction.
- *Genetics and Risks*: Caused by a deficiency of ADAMTS13, a protease that cleaves von Willebrand factor, leading to microthrombi and subsequent end-organ damage. Acquired TTP, more common than congenital, can be triggered by antiplatelet drugs, immunosuppressants, and HIV. Congenital TTP often remains asymptomatic until triggered by factors like infection or pregnancy.
- *Diagnosis*: Diagnosed through laboratory findings indicating anemia and thrombocytopenia, alongside signs of active hemolysis such as schistocytes, elevated unconjugated bilirubin, reticulocyte count, and lactate dehydrogenase.
- *Management*: Primary treatment involves plasma exchange and high-dose corticosteroids. Additional treatments may include splenectomy, and medications like cyclosporine, cyclophosphamide, vincristine, and rituximab.

Thrombocytosis

Thrombocytosis: Key Concepts

- *Overview*: Thrombocytosis is a myeloproliferative neoplastic disease marked by elevated platelet count and megakaryocytic hyperplasia in the bone marrow.
- *Genetics and Risks*: About 55% of patients with thrombocytosis have the JAK2 mutation, increasing their risk for vascular events such as thrombosis or hemorrhage and potential progression to the blast phase of myelofibrosis.
- *Diagnostic Evaluation*: Diagnosis involves a complete blood count, bone marrow biopsy showing megakaryocytic proliferation, and genetic testing. Platelet counts must exceed 450,000/mm^3 to be considered thrombocytosis.
- *Differentiation*: Distinguishing essential thrombocytosis from reactive thrombocytosis involves testing for acute phase reactants and obtaining an iron profile.
- *Complications*: Major risks include thrombosis and hemorrhage; leading complications include myocardial infarction, stroke, coronary artery thrombosis, pulmonary embolism, and ventricular fibrillation.

Management Strategies

- *Treatment Focus*: The primary aim is to prevent adverse outcomes.
- *Risk Stratification*: Patient management should be tailored based on risk assessment.
- *Preoperative Management*:
  - Low-risk patients (under 60 years old, no thrombosis history) typically receive aspirin.

- High-risk patients may require systemic anticoagulation, antiplatelet therapy, and cytoreductive therapy such as hydroxyurea.
- *Intraoperative Management*:
  - Patients with mild thrombocytosis generally follow standard CPB protocols.
  - Those with excessive thrombocytosis (platelet count >800 × 10^9/L) may need cytoreduction therapy prior to elective surgeries or plateletpheresis for emergent procedures.
  - Use of cangrelor to reduce thrombosis risk during cardiac surgery has been reported, though no formal recommendations exist.
  - Patients with extreme thrombocytosis and polycythemia vera should be evaluated for acquired von Willebrand syndrome.

Clinical Pearls

- A thorough understanding of the hematological status of cardiac surgical patients is essential prior to surgery. Preoperative optimization and intraoperative plans should be clear and communicated in advance to all team members.
- The coagulation cascade is a delicately balanced process with complex interactions involving multiple factors. Understanding how deviations from the typical profile affect the balance between the bleeding and prothrombotic tendencies, as well as how laboratory guidance is impacted, is crucial for achieving safe anticoagulation for CPB with minimal postoperative bleeding or thrombosis risk.
- In perioperative planning, knowledge of the pharmacokinetics and pharmacodynamics of any given antiplatelet therapy, combined with the results of platelet function assays should guide decisions regarding the timing of surgery and the risk of postoperative coagulopathy.
- Clinical history is important in differentiating thrombocytopenic disorders, as they often present with similar signs, symptoms, and laboratory findings. Accurately identifying the disorder is important in determining the appropriate treatment strategy.
- Strategies to minimize hemolysis during CPB include minimizing the duration of surgery, CPB, and aortic cross-clamp time; maintaining normothermic bypass; avoiding oxidative drugs; maintaining adequate perfusion pressure; promptly addressing hypotension, hypoxia, and acidosis; considering the use of free radical scavengers; minimizing the use of occlusive roller pump; and ensuring good urine output.

Further Reading

Azbell RCG, Lanzkron SM, Desai PC. Current evidence and rationale to guide perioperative management, including transfusion decisions, in patients with sickle cell disease. Anesth Analg. 2023;136(6):1107–14. https://doi.org/10.1213/ANE.0000000000006463. Epub 2023 May 19. PMID: 37205803; PMCID: PMC10171288.

Bolliger D, Lancé MD, Siegemund M. Point-of-care platelet function monitoring: implications for patients with platelet inhibitors in cardiac surgery. J Cardiothorac Vasc Anesth. 2021;35(4):1049–59.

Chou ST, et al. American Society of Hematology 2020 guidelines for sickle cell disease: transfusion support. Blood Adv. 2020;4:327–55.

DeBois W, Liu J, Lee L, Girardi L, Ko W, Tortolani A, Krieger K, Isom OW. Cardiopulmonary bypass in patients with pre-existing coagulopathy. J Extra Corpor Technol. 2005;37(1):15–22. PMID: 15804152; PMCID: PMC4680798.

Farooqui F, et al. Hemoglobinopathies and cardiac surgery. J Cardiothorac Vasc Anesth. 2016;30(5):1409–18.

Finley A, Greenberg C. Review article: heparin sensitivity and resistance: management during cardiopulmonary bypass. Anesth Analg. 2013;116(6):1210–22. https://doi.org/10.1213/ANE.0b013e31827e4e62. Epub 2013 Feb 13. PMID: 23408671.

Lobato E, Bavry A. The patient with coronary stents undergoing noncardiac surgery. In: Kaplan JA, editor. Kaplan's cardiac anesthesia for cardiac and noncardiac surgery. 7th ed. Elsevier; 2017. p. 1472–99.

Smith MM, Renew JR, Nelson JA, Barbara DW. Red blood cell disorders: perioperative considerations for patients undergoing cardiac surgery. J Cardiothorac Vasc Anesth. 2019;33:1393–406.

Spiess BD, Kaplan JA. Transfusion medicine and coagulation disorders. In: Kaplan JA, editor. Kaplan's cardiac anesthesia for cardiac and noncardiac surgery. 7th ed. Elsevier; 2017. p. 1248–90.

Tibi P, McClure RS, Huang J, Baker RA, Fitzgerald D, Mazer CD, Stone M, Chu D, Stammers AH, Dickinson T, Shore-Lesserson L, Ferraris V, Firestone S, Kissoon K, Moffatt-Bruce S. STS/SCA/AmSECT/SABM update to the clinical practice guidelines on patient blood management. J Extra Corpor Technol. 2021;53(2):97–124. https://doi.org/10.1182/ject-2100053. PMID: 34194077; PMCID: PMC8220901.

Uppal V, Rosin M, Marcoux JA, Olson M, Bezaire J, Dalshaug G. Factor V Leiden and cardiopulmonary bypass. J Extra Corpor Technol. 2015;47(4):223–7. PMID: 26834284; PMCID: PMC4730165.

Arterial Blood Gas Interpretation During Cardiopulmonary Bypass

22

William Marion and Dejan Vuckovic

Introduction

Cardiopulmonary bypass (CPB) supports complex cardiac surgeries by providing circulatory and respiratory support when the heart and lungs are inactive. Perfusionists operate the CPB machine, regulating physiological parameters to ensure proper gas exchange. Anesthesiologists monitor anesthesia depth, fluid balance, and patient stability, collaborating with perfusionists to optimize outcomes. These collaborative efforts are crucial in addressing the complexities of CPB, including the management of blood chemistry and temperature, to optimize surgical outcomes.

Arterial blood gas (ABG) monitoring is an indispensable component of patient monitoring during CPB. Blood gas management during CPB is a critical aspect of patient care, as it involves maintaining proper oxygenation, carbon dioxide removal, and acid–base balance while the heart and lungs are excluded from the patients' vascular system. This monitoring facilitates precise adjustments to the CPB machine settings and guides the administration of necessary interventions to maintain these critical physiological variables within optimal ranges. The comprehensive management of ABG during CPB allows the cardiac surgery team to promptly identify and address any deviations in gas exchange or acid–base balance, thereby mitigating the risk of complications. While this chapter primarily focuses on these aspects, the intricate management of hematocrit, electrolytes, glucose levels, and distinct strategies such as alpha-stat and pH-stat will be elaborated upon in detail elsewhere (Chaps. 6, 12, 13, 14, and 16).

Supplementary Information The online version contains supplementary material available at https://doi.org/10.1007/978-3-031-91163-7_22.

W. Marion (✉) · D. Vuckovic
Department of Anesthesiology & Perioperative Medicine, Cardiac Anesthesia, Cooper University Hospital, Camden, NJ, USA
e-mail: marion-william@CooperHealth.edu; Vuckovic-Dejan@cooperhealth.edu

Fundamentals of ABG

Definition and Components of ABG

ABG analysis is a critical diagnostic tool used in medicine, used to a patient's acid–base balance, oxygenation, and carbon dioxide (CO_2) elimination. This analysis quantifies the partial pressures of oxygen (PaO_2) and carbon dioxide ($PaCO_2$) in arterial blood, in conjunction with blood pH, bicarbonate (HCO_3^-) concentration, and oxygen saturation (SaO_2). Modern point-of-care (POC) blood gas analyzers extend beyond these basic ABG parameters to include measurements of oxyhemoglobin saturation (SaO_2), hematocrit (Hct), hemoglobin (Hb), blood glucose, electrolytes, such as sodium (Na^+), potassium (K^+), and chloride (Cl^-), as well as ionized calcium (Ca^+), base excess (BE), anion gap, and lactate levels, offering a comprehensive snapshot of a patient's current metabolic and respiratory status.

Key Parameters Measured

pH

The pH parameter in ABG analysis reflects the acidity or alkalinity of the blood, typically ranging from 7.35 to 7.45. Deviations from this norm can signal significant physiological issues such as acidosis or alkalosis, which are further categorized into metabolic or respiratory types depending on accompanying changes in bicarbonate and carbon dioxide levels.

PaO_2

This component measures the pressure of oxygen dissolved in the blood and indicates the extent to which oxygen is able

A. S. Awad, J. DiNardo (eds.), *Clinical Perfusion for Cardiac Surgery*, https://doi.org/10.1007/978-3-031-91163-7_22

to move from the lungs to the blood or across the membrane oxygenator of the CPB circuit to the blood. Normal values range from 75 to 100 mmHg. Values below this range might indicate issues such as hypoxemia.

$PaCO_2$

This measures the pressure of CO_2 dissolved in arterial blood and reflects how well CO_2 is being eliminated by the lungs or by the membrane oxygenator of the CPB circuit. Normal $PaCO_2$ values are typically between 35 and 45 mmHg. Values outside this range can indicate hypoventilation (if elevated) or hyperventilation (if decreased).

HCO_3^-

Measured indirectly or calculated from the pH and $PaCO_2$, bicarbonate is a component of the buffering system that helps regulate the pH of blood by neutralizing excess acids. Normal plasma bicarbonate levels are usually between 22 and 26 mEq/L.

SaO_2

This is a measure of the percentage of hemoglobin binding sites in the bloodstream occupied by oxygen. Normal SaO_2 values are typically between 95% and 100%. Lower values may indicate an inability of the lungs to adequately oxygenate the blood.

ABG Sampling and Analysis Technology

Techniques for Obtaining ABG Samples During CPB

Traditionally, ABG samples are generally drawn from an indwelling arterial catheter in a peripheral (radial artery) or central (femoral artery) site prior to the start of CPB. During CPB, samples are frequently drawn from the sampling manifold atop the venous reservoir, with regular intervals maintained to closely monitor the patient's blood gases. To prevent contamination and ensure sample purity in both cases, the line is thoroughly flushed, and an initial volume of blood is drawn and discarded before collecting the actual sample for analysis. Prepacked plastic ABG syringes containing 7 IU/mL of spray-dried, calcium-balanced, lyophilized lithium heparin are typically used to prevent clot formation and potential damage to sensitive equipment (Fig. 22.1).

In theory during CPB with full unfractionated heparinization, a standard sterile syringe can be utilized (Fig. 22.2). It is important to recognize that a 0.5 mL sample is of sufficient volume for analysis assuming that enough waste volume is drawn off the sample line to ensure that the sample is pure arterial blood.

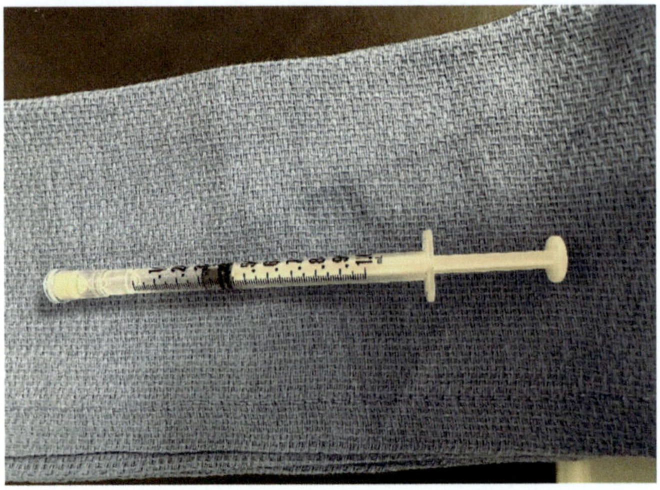

Fig. 22.1 Prepacked plastic ABG syringe. This image shows a prepacked plastic ABG syringe containing 7 IU/mL of spray-dried, calcium-balanced lyophilized lithium heparin, which is used to prevent clot formation

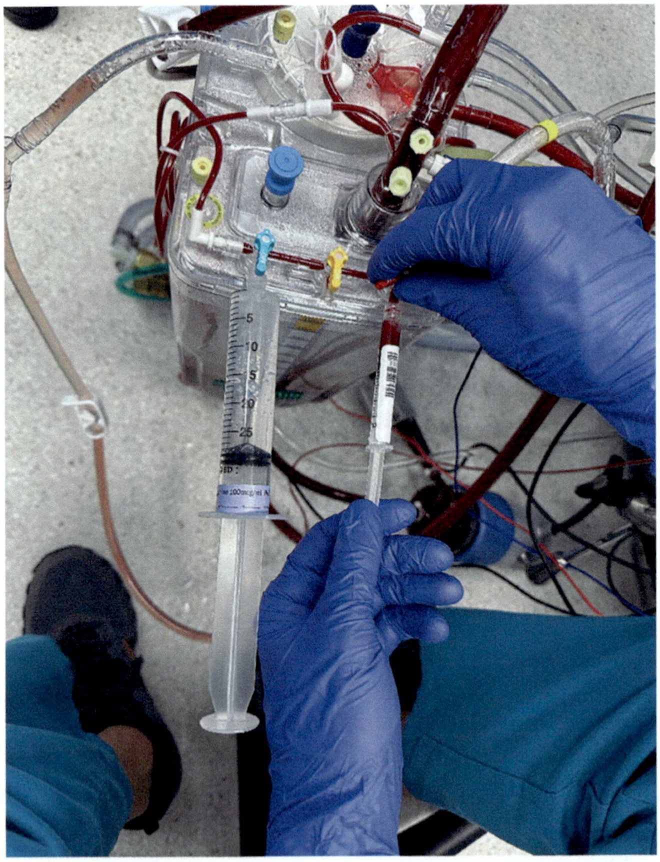

Fig. 22.2 Sampling manifold on top of the venous reservoir. This image illustrates a perfusionist drawing an ABG sample using a standard sterile syringe

Equipment and Analytical Technologies

- *Traditional Electrodes Method*: Traditional blood gas analyzers utilize three fundamental electrodes—pH, PCO_2, and PO_2—each designed to measure a specific component of the ABG, providing accurate assessments of a patient's respiratory and metabolic status. Here's an in-depth look at each type of electrode and how they function:

pH Electrode

Function The pH electrode, often a glass electrode, measures the hydrogen ion (H^+) activity in the blood. Since pH is the negative logarithm of H^+ concentration, a higher H^+ activity translates to a lower pH, indicating increased acidity. Maintaining a tightly regulated pH is vital for optimal enzymatic and biochemical processes in the body.

Design This electrode typically consists of a thin glass bulb containing a specific electrolyte solution. The outer surface of the bulb comes into contact with the blood sample, while the inner surface is connected to an internal reference electrode. The potential difference generated by the H^+ ions diffusing across the specialized glass membrane is measured and then converted into a corresponding pH value (Fig. 22.3).

Significance Vigilant pH monitoring is crucial during procedures such as CPB. Even minor deviations from the normal physiological range (7.35–7.45) can signal significant acid–base disturbances such as acidosis or alkalosis, impacting patient management and potentially leading to adverse outcomes if left unaddressed.

PaO_2 Electrode (Clark Electrode)

Function The PO_2 electrode, also known as the Clark electrode, measures the partial pressure of oxygen (PO_2) in the blood, a vital indicator of a patient's oxygenation status. It operates on the principle of amperometry, wherein oxygen diffuses across a gas-permeable membrane and undergoes a reduction reaction at the cathode surface, generating an electrical current proportional to the oxygen concentration in the blood sample.

Design The electrode typically consists of a platinum cathode and a silver/silver chloride anode submerged in an electrolyte solution. This solution is separated from the blood sample by a thin, gas-permeable membrane. Oxygen molecules diffuse across the membrane and are reduced at the cathode, producing a measurable current. The magnitude of this current is directly proportional to the PO_2 in the blood sample (Fig. 22.4).

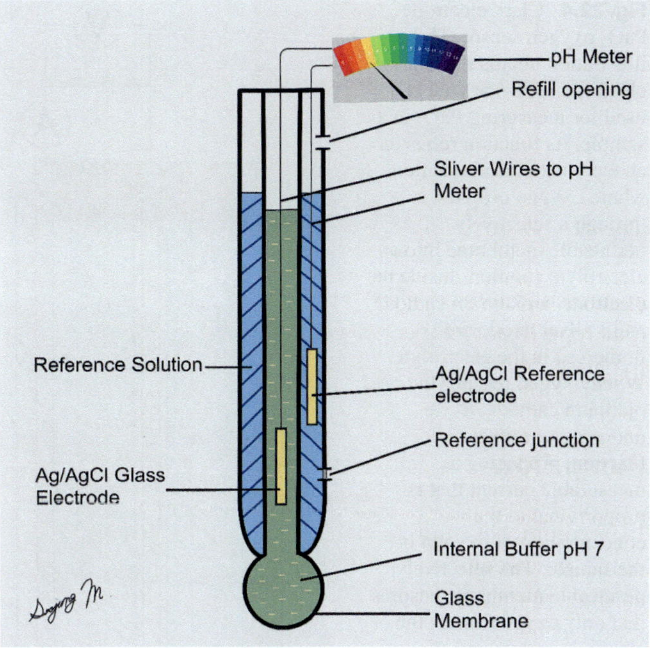

Fig. 22.3 pH electrode. This illustration depicts the detailed structure of a pH glass electrode, highlighting its operational mechanisms. The electrode functions by measuring the electrochemical potential difference between two solutions, similar to a voltmeter. Its core components include a silver/silver chloride (Ag/AgCl) wire, which serves as the primary conductor, and a hydrogen-selective glass membrane that acts as the ion-selective barrier, responding to changes in pH. Additionally, a reference electrolyte solution, typically saturated with potassium chloride (KCl), helps maintain a stable internal environment for accurate readings. Together, these elements generate a measurable voltage that corresponds to the pH of the blood sample

Significance Monitoring PO_2 is essential in critical care and surgical environments to ensure sufficient oxygen delivery to tissues. It is particularly critical during CPB, where the lungs' natural oxygenation function is bypassed, making the PO_2 measurement a key indicator of adequate oxygenation provided by the heart–lung machine.

PCO_2 Electrode (Severinghaus Electrode)

Function The PCO_2 electrode, also known as the Severinghaus electrode, measures the PCO_2 in the blood. It operates on the principle that CO_2 diffuses across a selectively permeable membrane into a bicarbonate solution, where it reacts with water to form carbonic acid (H_2CO_3). This carbonic acid then dissociates into hydrogen ions (H^+) and bicarbonate ions (HCO_3^-), leading to a decrease in pH. The change in pH is detected by a pH-sensitive glass electrode within the PCO_2 electrode assembly.

Design This electrode consists of a pH-sensitive glass membrane situated behind a gas-permeable membrane that is in direct contact with the blood sample. Carbon dioxide

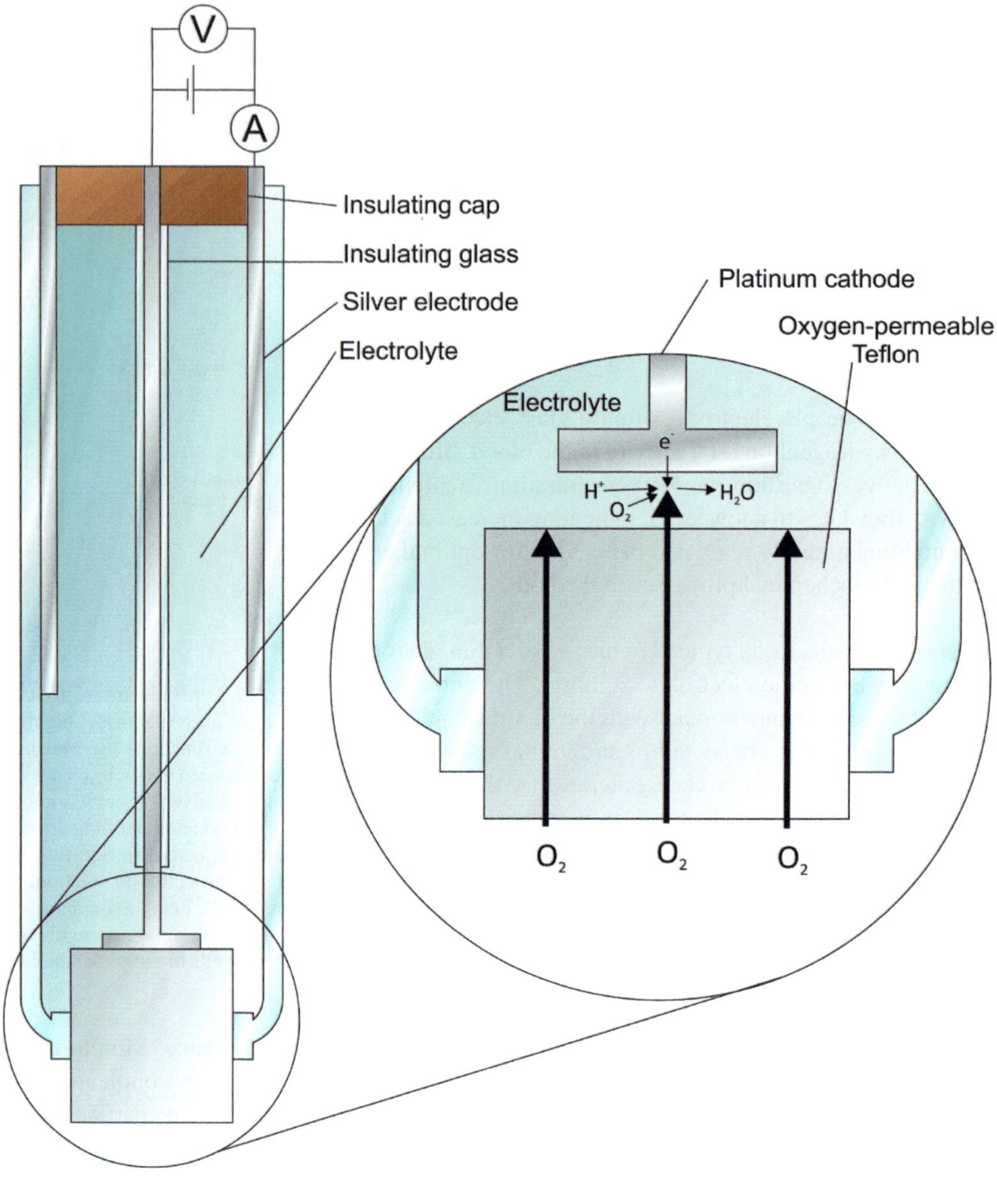

Fig. 22.4 Clark electrode PaO_2 oxygen sensor. This illustration details the Clark electrode, a device widely used for measuring PaO_2 in a sample. Its function relies on an electrochemical reaction, where oxygen diffuses through a selectively permeable membrane into an electrolyte solution. Inside the electrode, a platinum cathode and a silver anode are immersed in the electrolyte. When oxygen reaches the platinum cathode, it undergoes a reduction reaction, producing a measurable current that is proportional to the concentration of oxygen in the sample. The selectively permeable membrane ensures that only oxygen enters the electrode, enhancing accuracy. (Clark Electrode by Larry O'Connell—Own work, CC BY-SA 4.0. https://commons.wikimedia.org/w/index.php?curid=59338426)

from the blood diffuses across the gas-permeable membrane into a bicarbonate buffer solution. The resulting change in pH of the buffer solution, due to the formation of carbonic acid, is measured and used to calculate the PCO_2 of the blood sample (Fig. 22.5).

Significance Accurate PCO_2 measurement is crucial in evaluating respiratory function and ventilation adequacy. It enables healthcare providers to optimize ventilator settings during surgeries and aids in the diagnosis of various respiratory disorders. During procedures like CPB, where the lungs are bypassed, meticulous monitoring of PCO_2 is vital to ensure appropriate CO_2 removal and maintain acid–base balance.

These electrodes are integral to the function of blood gas analyzers, enabling clinicians to rapidly and accurately gauge critical blood gas parameters. Regular maintenance, calibration, and careful handling of these electrodes are essential for their continued accuracy and reliability in clinical settings.

Calculation of HCO_3^- Concentration

Blood gas analyzers utilize the Henderson–Hasselbalch equation to calculate bicarbonate concentration. This equation establishes a relationship between pH, the partial pressure of carbon dioxide ($PaCO_2$), and the bicarbonate concentration in the blood:

$$\mathrm{pH} = \mathrm{pKa} + \log\left(\left[\mathrm{HCO_3^-}\right] / \left(0.03 \times \mathrm{PaCO_2}\right)\right)$$

where:

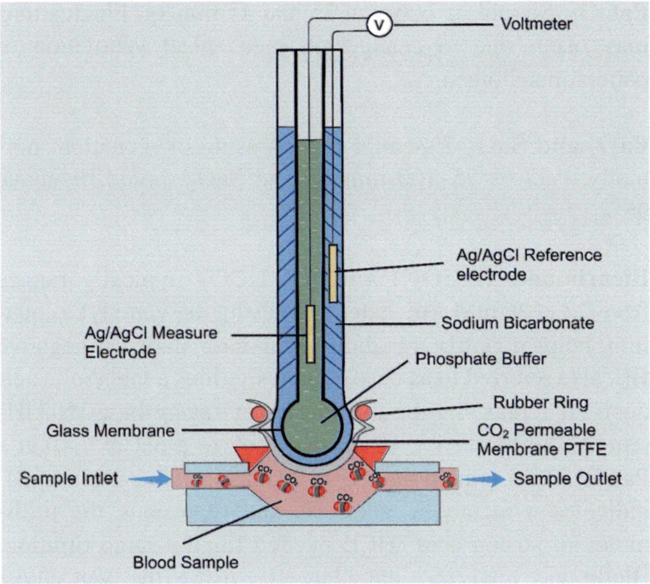

Fig. 22.5 Severinghaus electrode. This illustration details the Severinghaus electrode, a device widely used for measuring $PaCO_2$ in a sample. The electrode operates based on a modified pH electrode. It features a CO_2-permeable membrane that allows carbon dioxide from the blood sample to diffuse into a bicarbonate buffer solution. Once diffused, the CO_2 reacts with water in the buffer, forming carbonic acid (H_2CO_3). This carbonic acid then dissociates, releasing hydrogen ions (H^+), which in turn lower the pH of the buffer. A pH-sensitive glass electrode within the buffer detects this pH change, which is directly proportional to the $PaCO_2$ level in the sample

- pH is the blood's acidity or alkalinity
- pKa is the acid dissociation constant for carbonic acid (approximately 6.1)
- $[HCO_3^-]$ is the bicarbonate concentration
- $PaCO_2$ is the partial pressure of carbon dioxide

By measuring pH and $PaCO_2$, the analyzer can rearrange the equation to solve for $[HCO_3^-]$, giving a quantitative assessment of the metabolic component of acid–base balance.

Measurement of SaO_2

SaO_2 represents the percentage of hemoglobin binding sites occupied by oxygen. It can be measured directly using co-oximetry, a technique that employs absorbance spectroscopy to differentiate various forms of hemoglobin. Alternatively, blood gas analyzers can calculate SaO_2 using algorithms that mimic the oxyhemoglobin dissociation curve, taking into account PaO_2, PCO_2, and pH. One such algorithm is presented:

$$SaO_2 = 100 \times \left(X^3 + 150X\right) / \left(X^3 150X + 23400\right)$$

where $X = PaO_2 \times 10^{\left(0.48(pH-7.4)-0.0013\left(HCO_3^- 25\right)\right)}$

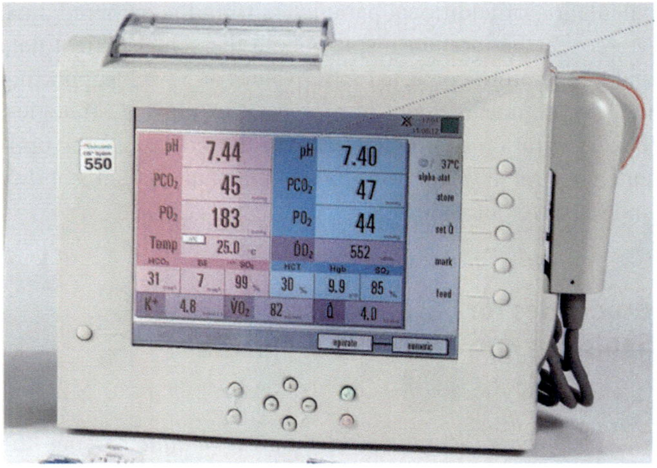

Fig. 22.6 Continuous ABG monitoring during CPB. This image illustrates an example of real-time continuous ABG monitoring during the CPB period using the Terumo CDI® Blood Parameter Monitoring System 550. This advanced system enables the continuous monitoring and analysis of critical parameters such as DO_2, VO_2, CPB flow, Hct, Hb, pH, pCO_2, and pO_2, HCO_3^-, BE, SaO_2, SvO_2, and K^+. This comprehensive monitoring aids in maintaining optimal patient status throughout the CPB process

This calculated SaO_2 provides an indirect estimation of oxygen saturation based on the measured blood gas parameters.

Additional Point
The same techniques used to measure SaO_2 in arterial blood can also be applied to measure SvO_2 (mixed venous oxygen saturation) in venous blood samples. This parameter offers insights into the balance between oxygen delivery and oxygen consumption at the tissue level.

- *Newer Continuous ABG Monitoring Technologies During CPB*

The traditional method of intermittent blood gas sampling has given way to technologies that provide real-time, continuous data on key blood parameters. These advancements enable the continuous monitoring and analysis of crucial parameters such as systemic oxygen delivery (DO_2), systemic oxygen consumption (VO_2), CPB flow, Hct, Hb, pH, pCO_2, pO_2, HCO_3^-, BE, SaO_2, SvO_2, and K^+. This comprehensive monitoring is facilitated by the Terumo CDI® Blood Parameter Monitoring System 550 and similar technologies, state-of-the-art devices that enhance patient management during CPB (Fig. 22.6).

This system employs innovative sensors for real-time data acquisition: a fluorescence sensor integrated into an arterial shunt line measures pH, pCO_2, pO_2, and K^+ while an optical reflectance cuvette in the venous line assesses venous SvO_2, Hct, and Hgb levels. This setup allows for the rapid calculation of additional parameters from the gathered data. Moreover, the monitor displays both the actual patient data and temperature-corrected ABG values at 37 °C, supporting the precise management of alpha-stat or pH-stat strategies. This integration of continuous, real-time data ensures optimal adjustment of CPB settings to maintain patient stability and improve outcomes.

Guidelines for Ensuring Accuracy in ABG Sampling and Analysis During CPB

- *Appropriate Sampling Site and Technique*: Using the technique described above for proper collection to avoid air bubbles or contamination.
- *Equipment Calibration and Maintenance*: Regularly calibrate pH, PCO_2, and PO_2 electrodes and co-oximeters according to manufacturer guidelines.
- *Temperature Corrections*: Apply temperature corrections to ABG readings, especially during hypothermia, to ensure accurate reflection of the patient's metabolic state at normothermia.
- *Frequent Monitoring and Analysis*: Utilize frequent ABG sampling to facilitate immediate adjustments to ventilation and CPB settings.
- *Quality Control Measures*: Implement strict quality control protocols, including routine checks with control solutions, to maintain the accuracy of the analytical system.
- *Staff Training and Competency*: Ensure proper training of medical staff regarding sources of error in ABG measurement, aseptic techniques, and sample handling specifics during CPB.

Adhering to these guidelines will enhance the accuracy of ABG data, enabling optimal management of patient physiology during CPB and improving surgical outcomes.

Interpreting ABG Results and Acid–Base Analysis

CPB-Specific Guidelines for Interpreting ABG Results

Interpreting ABG results during CPB requires a deep understanding of standard physiological ranges and modifications due to CPB specifics. Key parameters include:

pH Normally ranges from 7.35 to 7.45. Deviations may indicate metabolic or respiratory disturbances, influenced by factors such as hypothermia and hemodilution during CPB.

$PaCO_2$ Should be between 35 and 45 mmHg. Fluctuations may occur due to changes in mechanical ventilation or patient metabolism.

PaO_2 and SaO_2 Essential for assessing oxygenation; normally, PaO_2 is 75–100 mmHg, and SaO_2 should be above 95%.

Bicarbonate (HCO_3^-) and BE HCO_3^- typically ranges from 22 to 26 mM. BE, calculated using the Van Slyke equation, helps quantify metabolic acid–base status. A negative BE, also referred to as base deficit, signifies a metabolic acidosis. It represents the millimoles of strong base (NaOH) required to titrate 1 L of plasma back to a pH of 7.40 at a $PaCO_2$ of 40 mmHg and 37 °C. Conversely, a positive BE indicates a metabolic alkalosis and represents the millimoles of strong acid (HCl) needed for the same titration. Blood gas analyzers calculate BE using the Van Slyke equation:

$$BE = \left(HCO_3^- - 24.4\right) + \left(2.3 \times Hb + 7.7\right) \times \left(pH - 7.4\right) \times \left(1 - 0.023 \times Hb\right)$$

One limitation of the BE approach is its potential inaccuracy in patients with low serum albumin, a common scenario in critical illness. In such cases, the reported BE may be more positive than the actual value. This can be corrected using the formula:

$$\text{Base deficit correction} = 0.25\left(4.2 - \text{Serum albumin in g / dL}\right)$$

The corrected base deficit is then added to the reported value.

Three primary methods exist for quantifying acid–base disorders: the physiological approach, the BE approach, and the Stewart method (physicochemical approach). The physiological approach centers on the interplay between renal and pulmonary systems in acid–base regulation, utilizing the Henderson–Hasselbalch equation to describe the carbonic acid-bicarbonate buffer system. The Stewart method focuses on strong ions and pH-dependent changes in weak ions like albumin and phosphate. The BE approach, which quantifies changes in metabolic acid–base status as reported by blood gas analyzers, is the most familiar to anesthesiologists.

Case Studies to Illustrate Typical ABG Scenarios Encountered During CPB

Case studies provide practical examples:

Case Study 1: Metabolic Acidosis during CPB

- *Scenario*: A patient undergoing coronary artery bypass grafting (CABG) on CPB exhibits a gradual decrease in pH and bicarbonate levels (HCO_3^-) with a negative BE (Fig. 22.7).
- *Interpretation*: The lowering pH and HCO_3^- with a negative BE strongly indicate metabolic acidosis. This suggests an excessive accumulation of acid or loss of bicarbonate in the patient's blood during CPB. A closer look for other signs of ischemia and hypoperfusion such as urine output, SvO_2 trend to monitor perfusion of end organ tissues—SvO_2 values above 70% usually adequate for tissue perfusion.

1. *Action*: Increase perfusion rates, adjust temperature settings, or administer bicarbonate.

Case Study 2: Respiratory Alkalosis Post-CPB

2. *Scenario*: A patient undergoing cardiac surgery on CPB exhibits an elevated pH and lowered $PaCO_2$ during CPB (Fig. 22.8).
3. *Interpretation*: The elevated pH and decreased $PaCO_2$ are indicative of respiratory alkalosis. This acid–base imbalance is likely caused by excessive CO_2 elimination, potentially due to an increased gas sweep flow rate during CPB.
4. *Action*: Adjust gas sweep flow by carefully decreasing the gas sweep flow rate to reduce CO_2 elimination and allow $PaCO_2$ to normalize.

Fig. 22.7 Screenshot of ABG results during CPB. This figure displays three ABG results obtained at different times during the CPB period

ARTERIAL BG			
PH ARTERIAL	7.34 ▼	7.37	7.31 ▼
PCO2 ARTERIAL	39	39	46 ▲
PO2 ARTERIAL	416 ▲	372 ▲	372 ▲
HCO3 ARTERIAL	21 ▼	23	22
BE(CALC),ARTERIAL	NEG 5	NEG 2	NEG 3
O2 CONTENT ARTERIAL	11 ▼	13 ▼	12 ▼
TEMP, ARTERIAL	98.6	98.6	98.6
HEMOGLOBIN ARTERIAL	7.3 ▼	8.3 ▼	7.9 ▼
MEAS.O2 SAT.(ART)	>99.4 ▲	>99.4 ▲	>99.4 ▲
TCO2(CALC), ARTERIAL	46 ▲	49 ▲	51 ▲
Fi02 (DATA ON REQ.), ARTERIAL			
VT (DATA ON REQ.), ARTERIAL			
RR (DATA ON REQ.),ARTERIAL			
PEEP (DATA ON REQ.),ARTERIAL			
MODE (DATA ON REQ.) ARTERIAL			
SODIUM WB	135	137	137
POTASSIUM WB	5.1 ▲	5.0	5.1 ▲
CHLORIDE WB	105	107	106
IONIZED CALCIUM (ARTERIAL)	4.3 ▼	4.4 ▼	4.4 ▼
Glucose Arterial Whole Blood	167 ▲	172 ▲	157 ▲
Lactate Arterial Whole Blood	1.5 ▲	0.8	0.8

ARTERIAL BG	
PH ARTERIAL	7.50 ▲
PCO2 ARTERIAL	33 ▼
PO2 ARTERIAL	101 ▲
HCO3 ARTERIAL	27 ▲
BE(CALC),ARTERIAL	2
O2 CONTENT ARTERIAL	13 ▼
TEMP, ARTERIAL	98.6
HEMOGLOBIN ARTERIAL	9.2 ▼
MEAS.O2 SAT.(ART)	98.4
TCO2(CALC), ARTERIAL	23
Fi02 (DATA ON REQ.), ARTERIAL	
VT (DATA ON REQ.), ARTERIAL	
RR (DATA ON REQ.),ARTERIAL	
PEEP (DATA ON REQ.),ARTERIAL	
MODE (DATA ON REQ.) ARTERIAL	
OTHER (DATA ON REQ.),ARTERIAL	
SODIUM WB	131 ▼
POTASSIUM WB	3.8
CHLORIDE WB	104
IONIZED CALCIUM (ARTERIAL)	4.6
Glucose Arterial Whole Blood	107
Lactate Arterial Whole Blood	0.8

Fig. 22.8 Screenshot of ABG results during CPB. This figure displays ABG result obtained during the CPB period

Acid–Base Balance During CPB: Normal Physiology, Abnormalities, and Treatment

Normal Physiology of Acid–Base Balance

The body's buffering system is a crucial component of maintaining acid–base homeostasis, which is essential for normal physiological functions. Buffering systems help minimize pH changes in body fluids by neutralizing added acids or bases. The primary buffers in the human body include bicarbonate, phosphate, and proteins, along with some contribution from hemoglobin in red blood cells.

1. *Bicarbonate Buffer System*:
    - The bicarbonate buffer system is the primary extracellular regulator of blood pH.
    - It operates through a reversible chemical equilibrium between carbon dioxide (CO_2), water (H_2O), carbonic acid (H_2CO_3), bicarbonate ions (HCO_3^-), and hydrogen ions (H^+).
    - The enzyme carbonic anhydrase, primarily found in red blood cells, catalyzes this reaction.
    - This buffer system is tightly regulated by the respiratory system (adjusting CO_2 levels through ventilation) and the kidneys (modulating bicarbonate reabsorption and hydrogen ion excretion).
2. *Phosphate Buffer System*:
    - The phosphate buffer system plays a significant role in the intracellular environment and in the renal tubules.
    - It involves the dihydrogen phosphate ($H_2PO_4^-$) and hydrogen phosphate (HPO_4^{2-}) ions, acting as a weak acid and conjugate base pair, respectively.
    - This buffer is particularly effective in the renal tubules, where the pH can fluctuate more significantly than in other body compartments.
3. *Protein Buffers*:
    - Proteins are the most abundant buffers in both body cells and plasma.
    - Their buffering capacity stems from the amino acids they contain.
        - Carboxyl groups (–COOH) can release H^+ ions (acting as acids).
        - Amino groups (–NH2) can accept H^+ ions (acting as bases).
    - Hemoglobin, a protein within red blood cells, also acts as an important buffer by binding to hydrogen ions produced during CO_2 transport.

Acid–Base Imbalance During CPB: Mechanisms and Implications

During CPB, the impact on acid–base homeostasis is significant and multifaceted, primarily due to the alteration of normal physiological processes and the introduction of artificial mechanisms to maintain circulation and oxygenation.

CPB Effects on Acid–Base Balance

- *Mechanical Nature of CPB*
- CPB utilizes a heart–lung machine to temporarily assume the roles of the heart and lungs during surgical procedures, enabling extracorporeal circulation and oxygenation of the blood. However, this mechanical intervention inherently disrupts the body's natural homeostatic mechanisms:
    - *Blood Flow and Gas Exchange*: The CPB machine maintains systemic blood flow but does so in a nonpulsatile manner, which can affect tissue perfusion and subsequently, cellular metabolism. Additionally, the oxygenators in the CPB system, which replace the gas

exchange function of the lungs, may not mimic the exact physiological conditions of CO_2 removal and O2 uptake, leading to potential imbalances.

- *Impact on Respiratory Acid–Base Control*
  - *CO_2 Removal*: One of the primary functions of the lungs—the regulation of blood carbon dioxide levels through ventilation—is replaced by the oxygenator. The rate of CO_2 removal is controlled by the sweep gas flow through the oxygenator. If not precisely adjusted, this can lead to iatrogenic hypoventilation or hyperventilation, manifesting as respiratory acidosis or alkalosis, respectively.
- *Metabolic Changes*
  - *Non-Physiological Oxygenation*: The artificial nature of oxygenation and the lack of physiological regulatory mechanisms during CPB can lead to abnormal DO_2. This, combined with alterations in blood flow, can cause tissue hypoxia or hyperoxia, each affecting cellular metabolism and potentially leading to metabolic acidosis or alkalosis.
  - *Lactate Production*: Due to potential mismatches in oxygen supply and demand, tissues may rely more on anaerobic glycolysis, leading to increased lactate production (discussed later).
- *Electrolyte and Buffering Changes*
  - *Hemodilution*: The prime solutions used in CPB can lead to hemodilution, which reduces the concentration of bicarbonate and other buffer systems in the blood, diminishing the blood's capacity to neutralize acid loads.
  - *Bicarbonate Levels*: Alterations in bicarbonate handling during CPB, whether from dilution, increased consumption, or altered renal handling due to changes in blood flow, can significantly affect acid–base balance.
- *Temperature Management*
  - *Hypothermia*: CPB often involves the induction of hypothermia to reduce metabolic demands during surgery. Hypothermia can decrease enzymatic rates of both acid production and bicarbonate generation, complicating the management of acid–base balance.

Specific Acid–Base Disorders During CPB

- Metabolic Acidosis

Mild metabolic acidosis is commonly observed during CPB. This condition typically results from a combination of factors, which will be discussed subsequently. Despite its frequency, mild metabolic acidosis is generally manageable within the controlled environment of CPB through careful monitoring and adjustments of the bypass machine. However, severe forms of metabolic acidosis can carry significant risks, including impaired organ function and an increased potential for postoperative complications. Early detection and proactive management are essential to mitigate these risks and improve overall outcomes for patients undergoing CPB.

Factors Contributing to Metabolic Acidosis During CPB

1. *Hypoperfusion and Lactate Accumulation*:

   Physiological Mechanism: During CPB, especially in low-flow states or during periods of inadequate perfusion, tissue oxygen delivery may become insufficient to meet metabolic demands. This leads to a state of tissue hypoxia, forcing cells to shift from aerobic to anaerobic metabolism to generate energy. This metabolic shift causes an accumulation of lactate, a byproduct of anaerobic glycolysis, which in turn increases the acid load in the blood. Anaerobic glycolysis becomes the primary pathway for Adenosine Triphosphate (ATP) production. As glycolysis proceeds much faster than the Krebs cycle under these conditions, pyruvate is diverted to lactate production via lactate dehydrogenase, leading to hyperlactatemia.

   Because glycolysis can continue at several orders of magnitude faster than the Krebs cycle, the pyruvate produced is shunted toward the production of lactate, a weak base, by the enzyme lactate dehydrogenase, resulting in hyperlactatemia. Simultaneously, when excess hydrogen ions are unable to be utilized by aerobic metabolism or neutralized by bicarbonate, lactate, and other body buffer systems, acidosis results. When a reduced pH occurs in association with hyperlactatemia lactic, acidosis is said to be present. Thus, hyperlactatemia is a consequence of cellular acidosis and not a direct cause of acidosis.

   - The CPB machine's reduced capacity to efficiently remove CO_2, a key component of acid–base balance, further exacerbates this acidotic state.
   - *Clinical Implications*: An untreated metabolic acidosis may be associated with refractory hypotension. This is because decreases in pH cause an increase in circulating acetylcholine, which, in turn, increases expression and activity of nitric oxide synthase. Circulating NO and prostacyclin cause endothelial cell hyperpolarization and vascular smooth muscle relaxation. Elevated lactate levels during CPB are a critical clinical marker of underlying tissue hypoxia and inadequate tissue perfusion. Regular monitoring of lactate levels provides essential insights into the adequacy of tissue perfusion and can guide adjustments in CPB management. Prompt identification and correction of tissue hypoxia and perfusion deficits are crucial for optimizing patient outcomes and preventing complications associated with metabolic acidosis. This proactive management

helps in mitigating the effects of metabolic acidosis and improving overall patient outcomes during cardiac surgeries.

- *Management of increased VO_2 and Reduced DO_2*:
  - *Increased VO_2*: Frequently occurring during CPB, increased VO_2 can be due to factors such as light anesthesia or hyperthermia. Every 10 °C increase in organ temperature can be expected to increase VO_2 two–three-fold. Treatment of light anesthesia should be coordinated with the perfusionist to determine the choice of anesthetic agent and the route of delivery while on CPB. Subclinical shivering, which may not be immediately apparent, can also contribute to elevated VO_2. To manage this, clinical strategies include decreasing the patient's body temperature, deepening anesthesia, or administering neuromuscular blocking agents to control shivering.
  - *Reduced DO_2*: Another critical concern during CPB, reduced DO_2 is addressed by assessing the individual components of DO_2 defined as:

$$DO_2 = \text{Pump Flow} \times CaO_2 \times 10$$

Where 10: Conversion factor to change CaO_2 from mL/dL to mL/L, ensuring consistent units.

Where oxygen content equal:

$$CaO_2 = \left(\text{Hgb}\left(\text{gm}/\text{dl}\right) \times 1.34 \times SaO_2 / 100\right) + \left(0.0031 \times PaO_2\right)$$

- *Hb* refers to hemoglobin concentration (usually expressed in grams per deciliter, g/dL).
- *1.34 mL O_2/g Hb* is the oxygen-carrying capacity of hemoglobin, indicating that each gram of hemoglobin can bind approximately 1.34 mL of oxygen.
- *SaO_2* is the percentage of hemoglobin binding sites occupied by oxygen.

Intervening on the components (Hgb, PaO_2, SaO_2, and pump flow) believed to be deficient is warranted.

  - *Bicarbonate Administration*: If treatment of DO_2 and VO_2 fails to correct a negative BE, the administration of sodium bicarbonate ($NaHCO_3$) may be considered. A dose of 0.3 mEq/kg X -BE is generally administered. When a large dose of $NaHCO_3$ is given, it is necessary to monitor Na^+ levels and possibly increase the sweep gas flow rate temporarily to prevent the development of respiratory acidosis as CO_2 is produced.

2. *Hemodilution*:

Physiological Mechanism The dilution of blood components, particularly red blood cells and plasma proteins, during CPB reduces the blood's natural buffering capacity, making it more susceptible to changes in pH.

Clinical Implications Careful management of fluid administration is essential to avoid excessive hemodilution. Monitoring hemoglobin levels and total protein can guide the administration of blood products or colloids to maintain adequate buffering capacity and oxygen-carrying capacity.

3. *Strong Ion Difference (SID) Changes*:
   - *Physiological Mechanism*: SID, the difference between fully dissociated cations and anions in solution, can be altered during CPB by the infusion of chloride-rich fluids or through hemodilution. A decrease in SID leads to a drop in blood pH, contributing to metabolic acidosis.
   - *Clinical Implications*: Managing the type and the quantity of fluids used for priming the CPB circuit and for patient hydration is crucial. Opting for balanced electrolyte solutions can help maintain a stable SID and prevent severe shifts in acid–base balance.
4. *Iatrogenic Factors*:
   - *Physiological Mechanism*: Ringer's lactate solution contains sodium lactate and has an osmolarity of 273 mOsm L^{-1} and a pH of 6.5. The sodium lactate is metabolized into bicarbonate by the liver, which can help correct metabolic acidosis but the low pH is problematic if large volumes are utilized as part of the CPB prime.
5. *Clinical Implications*: Selection of prime solutions and circuit components should be guided by their potential impact on acid–base status.
6. *Biochemical & Physiological Changes*:
   - *Physiological Mechanism*: A patient's underlying conditions, the specific surgical procedures, and the duration of CPB can influence metabolic demand, acid production, and the efficiency of acid clearance.
   - *Clinical Implications*: A thorough preoperative assessment and understanding of the patient's medical history are essential. Adjustments to CPB management, such as the duration of bypass and the specific surgical techniques used, should be considered based on individual risk factors and physiological responses.

By understanding these multifaceted contributors to metabolic acidosis during CPB, cardiac surgery teams can tailor interventions more precisely, aiming to balance DO_2 and VO_2, manage fluid composition and volume, and optimize both metabolic and respiratory factors to stabilize the patient's acid–base status throughout the procedure. This holistic approach ensures that potential complications are minimized, leading to better overall outcomes for patients undergoing CPB.

- *Metabolic Alkalosis During CPB: Causes, Consequences, and Management*
  - *Causes*: Metabolic alkalosis occurs when blood pH rises above the normal range, $PaCO_2$ remains within normal limits, and there is a positive BE. This condition commonly develops during CPB and can result from several factors:
    1. *Excessive Sodium Bicarbonate ($NaHCO_3$) in Priming Solution*: The priming solution used to fill the CPB circuit may contain an excess of $NaHCO_3$, directly contributing to an increase in blood pH.
    2. *Aggressive Diuretic or Ultrafiltration Therapy*: The use of diuretics or ultrafiltration to remove excess fluid during CPB can lead to hypochloremia. This, in turn, can cause a compensatory increase in bicarbonate levels, resulting in metabolic alkalosis.
  - *Consequences of Significant Alkalosis*:
    - *Hypokalemia*: Alkalosis can trigger K^+ to shift into cells in exchange for H^+ via Na^+, K^+-ATPase mediated K^+-H^+ exchange, leading to low K^+ levels in the blood.
    - *Other Potential Effects*: Metabolic alkalosis can also impact cardiovascular function by altering calcium homeostasis.
  - *Management Strategies*:
    - *Addressing Hypochloremia*: If hypochloremia is present, treatment may involve administering potassium chloride (KCl) or normal saline, depending on the patient's potassium level.
    - *Adjusting $NaHCO_3$ Levels*: If the alkalosis is due to excessive $NaHCO_3$ in the priming solution, adjusting the composition of the priming solution can help correct the pH balance.
    - *Other Interventions*: Depending on the severity and underlying causes of alkalosis, additional management strategies may include optimizing gas sweep flow rate, correcting electrolyte imbalances, and addressing any underlying conditions that contributed to the development of alkalosis.
- *Respiratory Acidosis During CPB: Causes, Recognition, and Management*
  - *Causes*: Respiratory acidosis occurs when blood pH falls below the normal range due to an elevated $PaCO_2$, while the BE is within the normal range.
  - During CPB, a respiratory acidosis typically arises from inadequate sweep gas flow across the membrane oxygenator. This insufficient flow fails to match the patient's VCO_2, leading to CO_2 retention and a subsequent decrease in blood pH.
  - *Management*:
  - Fortunately, correcting this imbalance is straightforward. Increasing the sweep gas flow rate effectively enhances CO_2 removal, mirroring the effect of increasing alveolar ventilation in a patient not on CPB. This adjustment helps normalize $PaCO_2$ and restore blood pH to the desired range.
- *Respiratory Alkalosis During CPB: Causes, Recognition, and Management*
  - *Causes*: A respiratory alkalosis occurs when blood pH rises above the normal range due to a decreased $PaCO_2$, is reduced below the normal range, while the BE remains within the normal range. During CPB, a respiratory alkalosis typically arises from excessive sweep gas flow across the membrane oxygenator. This surplus flow removes CO_2 at a rate exceeding the patient's VCO_2, leading to a decrease in $PaCO_2$ and a subsequent increase in blood pH.
  - *Management*:
  - Correcting this imbalance is straightforward. Decreasing the sweep gas flow rate reduces CO_2 removal, allowing $PaCO_2$ to rise and blood pH to normalize. This adjustment is analogous to decreasing alveolar ventilation in a patient not on CPB.

Gas Exchange Abnormalities and Treatment During CPB

Gas exchange abnormalities during CPB, as indicted by abnormal PaO_2 and $PaCO_2$ values, may initially warrant simple adjustments:

- *Low PaO_2*: Increase the fraction of inspired oxygen (FiO_2) to improve oxygen delivery.
- *High $PaCO_2$*: Increase the sweep gas flow rate to enhance CO_2 removal.

However, if these initial adjustments fail to correct the gas exchange abnormalities, it necessitates immediate collaboration between the perfusion and surgical teams to investigate and address potential underlying causes, including:

- *Cannulation-related complications*:
  - Malposition or obstruction of the arterial or venous cannulae can impair systemic oxygen delivery and CO_2 removal.
  - Air embolism or thrombus formation within the circuit can also disrupt gas exchange.
- *Membrane oxygenator dysfunction*:
  - The membrane oxygenator may be failing or experiencing reduced efficiency due to various factors such as clotting, air bubbles, or membrane damage.
- *Impaired gas delivery to the oxygenator*:

– Issues with the gas blender or gas supply lines can lead to inadequate delivery of fresh, blended gas to the oxygenator, compromising gas exchange.

These topics are covered in detail in Chaps. 14, 26, and 27.

Further Reading

Berend K. Diagnostic use of base excess in acid–base disorders. N Engl J Med. 2018;378:1419–28.

Cervantes CE, Menez S, Trujillo JMM, Hanouneh M. Clinical approach to a patient with an acid-base disturbance. Am J Kidney Dis. 2021;77:A9–A11.

Pino RM, Singh J. Appropriate clinical use of lactate measurements. Anesthesiology. 2020;134:637–44.

Seifter JL. Integration of acid–base and electrolyte disorders. N Engl J Med. 2014;371:1821–31.

Story DA. Acid–base analysis in the operating room: a bedside Stewart approach. Anesthesiology. 2023;139:860–7.

Part VI

Pediatrics

Pediatric Cardiopulmonary Bypass

23

William L. Regan and Gregory S. Matte

Introduction to Pediatric Cardiopulmonary Bypass

Pediatric cardiopulmonary bypass (CPB) is fundamentally an extrapolation of adult practice. Many disposables, hardware, and techniques originated in adult cardiac surgery. While the basic tenets of adult CPB hold true for pediatric perfusion, there are several important deviations. This chapter aims to discuss some of those deviations and describe key aspects of pediatric perfusion.

Pediatric CPB commonly refers to perfusion involving primarily pediatric patients who require extracorporeal circulation to repair one or more congenital heart defects and some acquired defects. While this term is accurate, it does not fully capture the role of the pediatric perfusionist. Due to advancements in surgical and perfusion techniques, as well as early intervention in neonates and infants, an increasing number of patients presenting for cardiac surgery are now older children and adults. Furthermore, patients with congenital defects may require multiple interventions and re-repairs, necessitating the highly specialized services offered at congenital heart centers.

The wide variety of patient sizes and ages, coupled with a broad spectrum of anatomical defects, poses significant challenges for pediatric CPB. Developing a comprehensive set of standards and guidelines for perfusion services is key to achieving successful, predictable, and repeatable surgical outcomes. To this end, the American Society of ExtraCorporeal Technology (AmSECT) published a landmark document in 2019 titled "The Standards and Guidelines for Pediatric and Congenital Perfusion Practice" (Standards and Guidelines for Pediatric and Congenital Perfusion Practice 2019). This document has established a series of expectations and recommendations that help ensure patient safety during CPB for congenital heart surgery patients. Every pediatric perfusionist and cardiac surgical program should be familiar with this document. Of the 70 AmSECT standards, the first emphasizes the requirement for programs to develop institutional guidance documents for their perfusion team. These hospital-based documents direct practice and should adhere to the standards set forth by AmSECT. If a program opts not to follow a standard, the reasoning should be detailed in their internal documents. The development of institutional guidance documents (i.e., a policy and procedure manual) that reference the AmSECT standards is a significant but important undertaking for any perfusion team.

The importance of having decided in advance and as a team the factors, goals, and potential problems that could arise during bypass and how to address those problems is crucial. The policy and procedure manual informs practice and ultimately guides the CPB plan. The CPB plan is just one important aspect of the patient's experience in the operating theater (Matte 2015; Matte and DiNardo 2015). The cardiovascular surgery team should conduct a surgical pause prior to skin incision, where the anesthetic plan, invasive lines, surgical plan, bypass plan

W. L. Regan (✉) · G. S. Matte
Department of Cardiac Surgery, Boston Children's Hospital, Boston, MA, USA
e-mail: William.Regan@cardio.chboston.org; Gregory.Matte@cardio.chboston.org

A. S. Awad, J. DiNardo (eds.), *Clinical Perfusion for Cardiac Surgery*, https://doi.org/10.1007/978-3-031-91163-7_23

and any patient-specific concerns are discussed. Key considerations for the CPB plan include the following:

- Patient specifics
- Flow management and monitoring
- Hematocrit management
- Volume management
- Anticoagulation plan
- Blood gas management
- Target patient temperature

These bypass considerations will be discussed after an overview of the heart–lung machine, tubing packs, oxygenators and cannulas.

Heart–Lung Machines (HLMs)

An HLM typically includes five to eight pumps, each serving a defined purpose. Each institution arranges these pumps and ancillary equipment to suit its specific operating room needs. The position of the HLM relative to the surgical field is a primary determinant of the HLM configuration. The desire to minimize circuit line lengths to reduce prime volume is another important consideration. A standard HLMs setup commonly comprises an arterial head, a vent, a cardioplegia delivery system (with one or two pumps), and two field suction heads. Pediatric centers often expand these base systems, adding more heads and features as needed. These may include heads for active ultrafiltration, additional field suctions, and even a secondary head for independent arterial blood flow to a specific region of the body (i.e., selective cerebral perfusion with independent lower body perfusion).

Ancillary devices such as ultrasonic flow probes, pressure monitors, temperature sensors, servoregulating bubble detectors and level sensors, in-line blood gas and hematocrit sensors, and an inhaled anesthetic vaporizer are also commonly added. These devices enhance monitoring and management capabilities for the perfusionist and improve patient safety during critical periods in the operating room.

The evolution of HLMs has significantly improved customization. Modern systems, shown in Fig. 23.1 without disposables attached, allow teams to organize most pump heads closer to the oxygenator-reservoir and to minimize line lengths to the surgical field. This decreases overall prime volume, which influences transfusion requirements, particularly for smaller patients.

The arterial head for pediatric setups is generally a roller head, as opposed to a centrifugal pump. Flow control, especially at very low flow rates required in neonates, is improved with a roller head. The field suction, cardioplegia, and other pumps are typically roller head as well.

Two critical considerations with roller head pumps include their occlusion setting and the verification of output for arterial pumps.

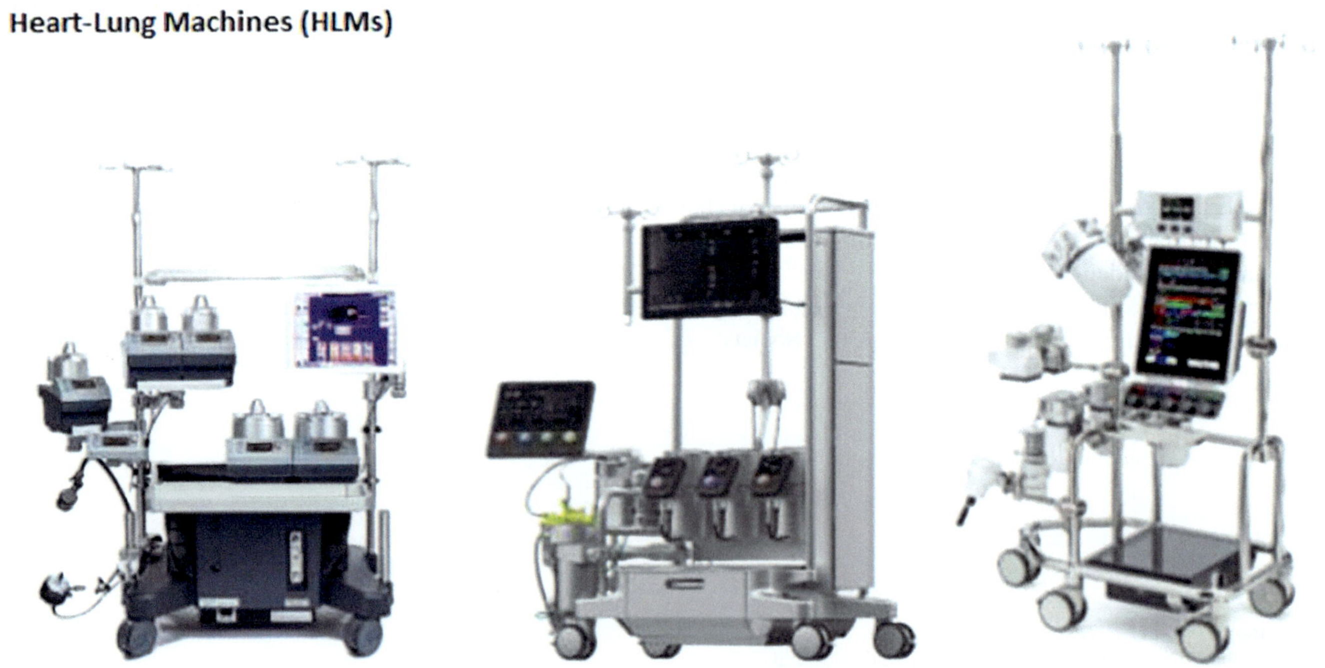

Fig. 23.1 Example of modern HLMs. The Spectrum Medical Quantum HLM. These machines represent the cutting edge of heart–lung technology, facilitating complex cardiac procedures, and improving patient outcomes through precision control and enhanced safety features

Roller Head Pump Occlusion

Occlusion in roller head pumps is defined by how much the rollers compress the tubing within the CPB circuit. Tighter occlusion prevents blood from slipping past the roller during rotation, enhancing flow control. A proper occlusion, especially for the arterial head, is extremely important and should be carefully calibrated during priming. Both under-occlusion and over-occlusion will result in trauma to the blood, tubing, and the arterial head itself.

Excessive occlusion will impart excessive heat and increased mechanical strain on the tubing and blood. Increased spallation of the tubing could result in particulate thrombus generation and potential rupture of the tubing. The increased demand on the equipment could potentially lead to a "pump jam" and/or complete loss of flow. A non-occlusive arterial head could also result in increased hemolysis, due to the excessive rpm's needed to generate forward flow, as well as low or no output to the patient. Proper occlusion of an arterial head is defined as minimally non-occlusive.

Occlusion of the arterial head can be set using one of two main methods:

1. *Fluid Meniscus Drop Rate Technique*:
   - This method involves monitoring the rate at which the fluid level (meniscus) drops in a vertical section of the tubing post arterial head. The meniscus is started at a level 30 cm above the roller head.
   - The objective is to adjust each roller occlusion so that the fluid descends slowly. The generally accepted rate is 1 cm/min.
2. *Pressure Loss Technique*:
   - This technique employs a pressure gauge, digital, or analog, to detect changes in the system pressure within the tubing.
   - The aim is to set a static system pressure and then adjust the roller's occlusion to allow for a minimized pressure loss over time. A commonly used rate is 1 mmHg/s.

Verification of Arterial Blood Flow

According to AmSECT standard 7.3, verifying arterial blood flow to the patient during CPB is mandatory. This ensures that the actual flow matches the set parameters on the arterial pump, guarding against risks such as incorrect tubing size on the pump display or internal shunts within the bypass circuit. An ultrasonic flow probe on the arterial limb of the bypass circuit provides confirmation to the perfusionist that the set flow on the arterial pump is actually being delivered to the patient. Flow probes may also be employed in other locations on the circuit as needed. For example, monitoring venous blood flow may be particularly useful for congenital cardiac surgery patients with aortopulmonary collaterals. A venous flow probe may also help with objective assessment of changes in venous return when drainage issues arise.

Tubing Packs

The perfusionist selects bypass circuit tubing based on the required flow in different parts of the circuit. The goal is to use the smallest tubing possible that will provide the anticipated flow, which helps minimize the prime volume and subsequent hemodilution experienced by the patient once placed on bypass. For neonates, the smallest pediatric circuits may include 3/16″ tubing for the arterial, venous, and boot lines in the pump circuit. The field suctions may also be of this caliber. When a 3/16″ tubing circuit is paired with an infant or neonatal oxygenator, the overall prime volume is typically in the 150–250 mL range.

There is no consensus on how to define circuit prime volume, which is one reason reported prime volumes have a large range. Including the functional reservoir volume and the prime of the hemoconcentrator results in a higher total. Conversely, if one prefers to run their circuit at the lowest reservoir level possible (which is not recommended as a reservoir works in part by dwell time) and excludes the hemoconcentrator prime because that device is not always in the constant blood flow path, then the reported prime volume will be lower. Adult congenital heart surgery patients typically use a circuit consisting of 3/8″ tubing and possibly areas of ½" tubing. These circuits, when paired with an adult oxygenator, will have a prime volume in the 800–1200 mL range. Table 23.1 lists the stroke volume for tubing in the arterial roller head (i.e., the boot line) as well as the typical maximum flow in that position. There is a maximum recommended flow for the boot line with a given tubing size to help ensure the tubing will safely support the patient throughout the bypass run. Excessive RPMs in an arterial boot line and

Table 23.1 Bypass circuit tubing size and specifications

Internal tubing diameter (inches)	3/16	¼	3/8	½
Stroke volume in typical full size arterial pump head (milliliters per revolution)	7.2	12.5	26	44.5
Typical maximum flow for boot (milliliters per minute)	1200	2100	4400	>4400

Table 23.2 Specifications for commonly utilized oxygenators for pediatric perfusion

Manufacturer	Oxygenator	Oxygenator prime volume	Minimum operating level	Manufacturer maximum recommended blood flow range, LPM	Internal arterial filter/pore size/surface area
Sorin	D100	31	10	0.7	No
Terumo	Capiox FX05	43	15	1.5	Yes/32 microns/130 cm²
Sorin	D101	87	30	2.5	No
Medtronic	Affinity Pixie	48	20	2	No
Sorin	Inspire 6F	284	150	6	Yes/38 microns/68 cm²
Terumo	Capiox FX15, 30	144	70	5	Yes/32 microns/360 cm²
Medtronic	Affinity Fusion	260	200	7.00	Yes/25 microns via oxygenator bundle
Terumo	Capiox FX25	260	150	7	Yes/32 microns/600 cm²

extended support times both increase the risk of tubing rupture, which requires circulatory arrest to replace if native cardiopulmonary function cannot be immediately restored.

In addition to prime volume and RPM limitations, an important concept for pediatric perfusion is sizing circuit components for pressure drop and flow characteristics. Using tubing that is too large can result in low velocity flow and low driving pressure, while tubing that is too small can create high shear forces and driving pressures. Furthermore, venous drainage is dependent on the diameter and length of venous line tubing, as well as cannula size and even the venous inlet size on the oxygenator-reservoir.

Oxygenators

Hollow fiber membrane oxygenators are most often employed in the operating room for CPB. These devices have excellent gas exchange and heat exchange properties. The manufacturer of a device typically sets forth a recommended maximum blood flow rate for an oxygenator based primarily on the gas exchange properties, as defined by the American Association of Medical Instrumentation (AAMI) and specifically tested for Food and Drug Administration (FDA) approval (US Department of Health and Human Services 2000). Since modern devices include an integral heat exchanger, cardiotomy, and venous reservoir, and on many models an internal arterial line filter, the perfusionist must consider more than just gas exchange when integrating a device into practice (Matte 2016). A pediatric perfusion program typically requires three or four oxygenators to accommodate the diverse flow requirements of patients with congenital heart defects.

One example that highlights the importance of considering factors beyond manufacturer-defined flow ratings is how a cardiotomy filter functions during the dynamic phases of bypass. Congenital heart surgery patients are more likely to have significant aortopulmonary collaterals (APCs). These APCs return blood to the left atrium during CPB, and this blood may not be captured by a venous cannula. Instead, a field suction sends this blood, mixed with air, to the cardiotomy reservoir for filtration before it is reintegrated into the circuit's constant blood flow path. Another example concerns a patient with significant aortic insufficiency. Retrograde flow across the aortic valve before cross-clamping may require the heart to be vented via the left ventricle. The blood from venting would then be sent to the cardiotomy reservoir for filtration before being reintegrated into the constant blood flow path.

The goal with oxygenator selection, as with tubing packs, is to choose the smallest prime device that will safely support the patient throughout the bypass run (for gas exchange, heat exchange, and cardiotomy filtration). Table 23.2 includes specifications for eight commonly used devices in congenital heart surgery. Note the general progression of an increase in prime volume and minimum operating volume as maximum flow increases. The perfusionist consults the patient's history before selecting which oxygenator to pair with the tubing pack.

Arterial and Venous Cannulae

The perfusionist must understand the cannulation plan when selecting cannula. Congenital cardiac cases can involve four or more separate venous cannula and sometimes two arterial cannulae. The perfusionist selects cannulae based on patient size, anatomy, and flow requirements. These cannulae generally include the arterial, venous, aortic root, vent, and sump. Sizes of cannulae are determined by availability, patient size, and surgeon preference. Below are experience-based charts for arterial and bicaval venous cannulation. Flow capacities will vary by cannula manufacturer. Therefore, Tables 23.3 and 23.4 provide general guidance only.

Table 23.3 Example arterial cannula sizing based on patient weight

Patient weight (kg)	French size	Rated flow (LPM)
<3	6	0.4
3–4.8	8	0.7
4.8–10	10	1.3
10–14	12	2.1
14–28	14	2.8
28–35	16	3.7
35–75	18	4.8
75–100	20	5.7
>100	22	>5.7

Table 23.4 Example venous cannula sizing for bicaval cannulation based on patient weight

Bicaval cannula selection based on patient weight		
Patient weight (kg)	Superior vena cava French size (rated flow)	Inferior vena cava French size (rated flow)
<3	12 (0.8)	12 (0.8)
3–6	12 (0.8)	14 (1.6)
6–8	12 (0.8)	16 (1.9)
8–12	14 (1.6)	16 (1.9)
12–16	14 (1.6)	18 (2.6)
16–22	16 (1.9)	18 (2.6)
22–30	16 (1.9)	20 (3.0)
30–34	18 (2.6)	20 (3.0)
34–46	18 (2.6)/20 (3.0)	22 (4.5)
46–56	20 (3.0)	22 (4.5)
56–70	20 (3.0)/22 (4.5)	24 (5.5)
70–90	22 (4.5)/24 (5.5)	24 (5.5)/28 (>6)
>90	24 (5.5)	28 (>6)

The Patient

Patient pathophysiology has many implications for the pediatric perfusionist (Matte et al. 2024). Specific congenital cardiovascular pathologies are discussed in Chap. 24, which is beyond the scope of this chapter. Chapter 24 covers perfusion techniques, which is also pertinent to patient considerations for the CPB plan.

The most obvious difference between pediatric perfusion and adult perfusion is the patient. Importantly, children are not just small adults. The size and age of the patient and the anatomical abnormalities present unique scenarios not found in adults with acquired heart disease. Some of these anatomical challenges are due to the pathophysiology of their cardiac lesions, immature organ systems, bypass circuit surface area-to-volume ratios, and high metabolic demand. Very often, patients with congenital heart disease (CHD) also suffer from comorbidities. Numerous genetic conditions have a cardiovascular component associated with them. These factors combined into one patient quickly increase the complexity of the anesthetic plan, bypass plan, and surgical approach, making it difficult to establish blanket standards.

Table 23.5 Acyanotic and cyanotic lesion classification for common congenital heart defects

Acyanotic Left-to-right shunting (or no shunting)	*Cyanotic* Right to left-shunting (or insufficient pulmonary blood flow)
Atrial septal defect	Transposition of the great arteries
Ventricular septal defect	Tetralogy of fallot
Atrioventricular canal defects	Truncus arteriosus
Patent ductus arteriosus	Total anomalous pulmonary venous return
	Hypoplastic left heart syndrome
	Tricuspid atresia
	Pulmonary atresia
	Coarctation of the aorta
	Ebstein's anomaly

The basic nature of CHD is that some parts of the anatomy have not developed correctly. The care of these patients is generally aimed at repairing septal wall defects, atretic valves or vessels, redundant or absent vessels, vessels that originate or terminate incorrectly, valve stenosis or insufficiency, or ventricular hypoplasia. These conditions may exist in the setting of dextrocardia or mesocardia.

Generally, patients can be divided into two categories cyanotic and acyanotic. Acyanotic lesions have either no intracardiac shunting or left-to-right shunting (oxygenated pulmonary venous blood is added to pulmonary arterial blood). Cyanotic lesions have limited pulmonary blood flow or right-to-left shunting (deoxygenated systemic venous blood is added to systemic arterial blood). Table 23.5 lists commonly seen defects by typical oxygenation state.

Cyanotic patients can have higher hematocrits and CPB flow requirements, depending on their preoperative state. For example, a neonate with transposition of great arteries (TGA) and a large patent ductus arteriosus (PDA) may present with near-normal hematocrit and cardiac output (Welsh and Hoyle Jr 2021). In contrast, a patient with the same condition diagnosed postnatally weeks later may have erythrocytosis and heart failure. Regardless of specific diagnosis, perfusionists must consider a patient's pump flow requirements, cardiac venting to prevent distention, and hematocrit management.

Pump flow requirements can also change intraoperatively. For instance, a patient with significant aortic regurgitation might initially require high pump flow to compensate for the regurgitant volume flowing retrograde across the aortic valve. This is directed to the left ventricular vent at the initiation of bypass. This higher relative flow compensates for the volume lost to the left ventricle to help ensure adequate effective systemic perfusion. Once the aortic cross-clamp is placed, pump flow can be lowered while still ensuring systemic perfusion flow. However, after the cross-clamp is removed, pump flow may need to be increased again to ensure sufficient coronary blood flow during early myocardial reperfusion, especially in the presence of myocardial hypertrophy.

Pump Flow

It is common to utilize cardiac index (CI) flow to discuss pump flow requirements during CPB. CI is defined as the cardiac output divided by the body surface area and is reported in L/min/m^2. A common target flow for the initiation of CPB is a CI of 2.5–3.0 L/min/m^2. However, the target flow at the initiation of bypass is neither a fixed value nor static. An absolute requirement for setting pump flow is ensuring adequate venous drainage. Therefore, primary communication between the surgeon and perfusionist when going on bypass is verifying that the target pump flow is achievable with adequate venous drainage. For the perfusionist, this typically equates to a stable reservoir level and a central venous pressure at or even below zero (due to gravity drainage to the pump reservoir). For the surgeon, this usually means that the heart and cavae do not appear distended. Once this is established, the perfusionist may begin to cool the patient. The initial target flow may be reduced as the patient is cooled, as metabolic requirements will decrease with reductions in temperature.

It has long been a standard that the safe required CI flow could be estimated by the patient's core temperature, as shown in Table 23.6.

More recently, flow guidance during CPB has largely been driven by indexed systemic oxygen delivery (IDO_2). This development has been supported by adult and pediatric literature linking neurologic and renal outcomes with IDO_2 on bypass (Magruder et al. 2022; Dreher et al. 2023; Garrison 2020; Hayward et al. 2023). It should be noted that guidelines for IDO_2 have been developed during a period when surgeries are increasingly performed at milder levels of hypothermia, often ≥30 °C. There is limited guidance for appropriate IDO_2 during deeper levels of hypothermia. In essence, a common target for IDO_2 in neonates, infants, and small children undergoing CPB is 340–400 mL/min/m^2. In adults, target IDO_2 values may be lower, around 240–300 mL/min/m^2, due to their reduced metabolic demand relative to body surface area. However, these values should be adjusted based on the patient's specific needs and clinical context to ensure adequate systemic perfusion. In CHD patients with conditions like APCs, aortic regurgitation, or other shunts, higher pump flow rates may be needed to achieve adequate systemic flow and IDO_2. Pump flow and hemoglobin concentration are the two main factors influencing IDO_2, highlighting the importance of careful monitoring and adjustment during bypass to ensure optimal oxygen delivery.

Table 23.6 Expected safe CI flow by temperature

Patient temperature °C	>35	32	30	28	26	24	22	20	<20
Expected safe CI flow (L/min/m^2)	2.4–3.5	2.2	2.0	1.8	1.6	1.4	1.2	1.0	0.7

Hematocrit Management in Pediatric CPB

Hemoglobin carries oxygen to the tissues and transports carbon dioxide to the lungs for excretion. Hematocrit represents the percentage of blood that contains red blood cells. During CPB, hematocrit is commonly used as a measure to help ensure adequate oxygen delivery. While patient weight can roughly estimate blood volume with (Table 23.7), those with CHD, particularly cyanotic patients or those with heart failure, may have higher blood volumes.

Understanding a patient's blood volume helps estimate red cell mass and predict hematocrit during CPB. This information can then be used to calculate the hematocrit once the patient's blood mixes with the bypass circuit. The patient's red blood cell mass divided by the estimated total blood volume (patient's blood volume + circuit volume) gives an indication of the hematocrit if the patient were placed on CPB with a clear prime.

$$\frac{\text{PBV}(\text{mL}) \times \text{Patient HCT}(\%)}{\text{PBV}(\text{mL}) + \text{Circuit Volume}(\text{mL})}$$

PBV = patient blood volume
HCT = hematocrit

Very often in pediatrics, adding blood to the prime is necessary to ensure adequate capacity for oxygen delivery (i.e., iDO_2). The ratio of patient blood volume to bypass circuit volume is much smaller in pediatric patients than in adults, resulting in a greater degree of hemodilution once placed on CPB. The perfusionist calculates this dilutional hematocrit and adds red blood cells, with or without plasma, to the bypass circuit as needed to meet standards defined by the cardiovascular team in their policy and procedure manual. An important consideration is that different congenital lesions may require different target values. For example, a cyanotic single ventricle physiology lesion, such as hypoplastic left heart syndrome, may require a hematocrit on bypass in the

Table 23.7 Estimate of patient blood volume by weight

Weight (kg)	Blood Volume (mL/kg)
<10	85
10–20	80
20–30	75
30–40	70
>40	65

30–40% range. However, a patient with an acyanotic lesion, such as a ventricular septal defect, may well tolerate a hematocrit in the mid-20% range. The most comprehensive pediatric study on hematocrit management for congenital heart surgery, published by Boston Children's Hospital, linked hematocrit levels of 24% or higher with improved outcomes in patients with two ventricles (Wypij et al. 2008). This guidance, established in the 1990s and 2000s, is evolving due to advancements in technology, particularly real-time monitoring of iDO_2 during CPB, as previously discussed.

Volume Management in Pediatric CPB

Volume management for the pediatric patient is closely tied to hematocrit management but deserves careful consideration not just for its effect on hematocrit but also its composition. Due to the surface area-to-volume ratio of the patient to the circuit, it is imperative that the perfusionist understands the impact of each solution used. Important considerations for any fluid delivered include the electrolyte profile, oncotic pressure, oxygen-carrying capacity, clotting factors, the amount of the solution needed to achieve the desired effect, and potential hazards of the solution. Much of pediatric perfusion involves paying attention to concentration gradients to avoid overly disrupting the established balance. The electrolyte makeup of a specific solution is probably the most important aspect to consider. Many centers use Plasma-Lyte-A (Baxter International, Deerfield, IL) or a similar electrolyte-balanced solution as the base solution in a bypass circuit prime. The goal is to keep most of the monitored electrolytes within the normal range.

Osmotic pressure is a serious concern for maintaining hydrostatic balance in pediatric patients. In the absence of adding blood products with high oncotic pressure, such as red blood cells, albumin, and fresh frozen plasma, there is a risk that fluid added to the bypass circuit may lead to interstitial or intracellular fluid accumulation. Fluids added during a case, such as valve testing solution, irrigation fluids, and cardioplegia, may be incorporated into the circulating volume during CPB. The total amount of fluids used throughout a pediatric case can easily be 3–4 times the patient's blood volume. This highlights the need to closely monitor the composition and amount. Table 23.8 shows the electrolyte differences for several solutions commonly given during CPB. Smaller patients may be impacted to a greater degree when administering nonphysiologic solutions, but even adults may be affected by electrolyte changes imposed by solutions introduced during a case.

An additional consideration for fluid and volume management during bypass is how these fluids affect myocardial function, particularly during early reperfusion. A majority of congenital heart defects require cardioplegia to arrest the heart in diastole during CPB. Diastolic cardiac arrest offers the surgeon adequate time to perform the operation while simultaneously allowing for recovery of function after cross-clamp removal. While the heart typically starts beating on its own during early reperfusion, function will be depressed to some degree. A key consideration for fluid management, therefore, is to not further insult the myocardium during this period. For example, during early reperfusion, it is not ideal to transfuse fluids with the potential to decrease calcium levels. This is especially important in neonates who are more dependent on exogenous calcium levels for myocardial function. Banked blood products such as packed red blood cells and plasma contain citrate, which binds calcium. Transfusing them into the bypass circuit not only dilutes the circulating calcium level but can also further decrease it due to excess citrate. This citrate-induced hypocalcemia, along with the known storage lesion of blood products, can impact cardiac function in the short term. To avoid this, it is recommended to anticipate and plan transfusions before removing the aortic cross-clamp. Washing a packed red cell unit in a cell saver device for transfusion after cross-clamp removal will improve that blood's profile before transfusion, but it will not make it physiologic. As with many aspects of pediatric perfusion, these considerations become increasingly important in smaller patients.

Table 23.8 Electrolyte values for commonly transfused solutions during bypass

	Plasma-Lyte A 7.4	Lactated ringer's	Normal saline (0.9% NaCl)	Half-normal saline (0.45% NaCl)	Packed red blood cells	Thawed plasma
Sodium (mEq/L)	140	130	154	77	100–140	160
Potassium (mEq/L)	5	4	0	0	10–20	3
Magnesium (mEq/L)	3	0	0	0	0	0
Chloride (mEq/L)	98	109	154	77	80–90	80
Lactate (mEq/L)	0	28	0	0	10–20	2–4
Calcium (mEq/L)	0	1.5–3.0	0	0	0	0
Glucose (mg/dL)	0	0	0	0	500	500
Calculated osmolarity (mOsm/L)	294	273	308	154	300–350	350
pH range	6.5–8.0	6.0–7.5	4.5–7.0	4.5–7.0	6.5–7.0	7.0–7.2

Hemoconcentration and Ultrafiltration in Pediatric CPB

Another essential aspect of volume management for CPB is the use of a hemoconcentrator; please refer to Chap. 19 for more details. In fact, the HLMs could be better described for pediatrics as the heart–lung–kidney machine due to its crucial role in fluid control. In addition to managing overall volume, a hemoconcentrator can adjust the hematocrit, electrolyte, glucose, and lactate profiles of the circulating volume before, during, and after CPB.

- *Pre-CPB*
  AmSECT standards 13.1 and 13.2 direct the perfusionist to correct physiological abnormalities before bypass. Pre-bypass ultrafiltration (PBUF) has long been recognized as a method to achieve this. There is no industry standard for performing PBUF, but numerous techniques have been reported that efficiently improve the profile of a blood-primed circuit before the patient is exposed to it (Standards and Guidelines for Pediatric and Congenital Perfusion Practice 2019; Shimpo et al. 2001; Kohlsaat et al. 2023).
- *During CPB*
  A hemoconcentrator is also commonly used during CPB for conventional ultrafiltration (CUF) to remove excess fluid accumulated during bypass. This excess volume often comes from the crystalloid component of cardioplegia, valve testing solutions, and surgical field irrigation.
  Another technique, zero-balance ultrafiltration (ZBUF), allows for adjusting the electrolyte, glucose, and lactate levels in the circulating volume during CPB. This is typically accomplished by adding a balanced electrolyte solution and then removing an equal amount of fluid through ultrafiltration.
- *Post-CPB*
  Modified ultrafiltration (MUF), another technique utilizing hemofilters, is performed in the post-bypass phase to increase the patient's red cell mass. This is achieved by removing clear fluid and replacing it with residual whole blood left in the bypass circuit.
  All forms of ultrafiltration can potentially remove cytokines and inflammatory mediators (Shimpo et al. 2001). Hemoconcentrators are offered in a variety of sizes, much like oxygenators and tubing packs, to help optimize fluid management for a range of patient sizes.

Anticoagulation Plan

The anticoagulation management strategy for pediatric patients is similar to that for adults in that unfractionated heparin is most often the anticoagulant of choice. A relatively high level of anticoagulation (bolus 300–500 IU/kg heparin) is required pre-bypass because the blood will be activated by exposure to foreign surface area in the bypass circuit as well as by exposure to air. Air exposure occurs with bleeding into the surgical field, subsequent pump sucker use to recover this shed blood, and the air-blood interface in the hardshell venous reservoir. The target for full heparinization on CPB is generally considered anything above 400 to 480 seconds and will depend on the device used to measure the activated clotting time (ACT). The Hemochron Signature Elite (Werfen, Bedford, MA) is a widely used device in pediatrics, and a target ACT of 400 s has been shown to provide appropriate anticoagulation for congenital cardiac patients (Matte et al. 2019). Inadequate anticoagulation places the patient at risk for thromboembolic events and must be avoided.

Anticoagulation with heparin is reversed after the adequacy of surgical repair is assessed and the decision is made that CPB will not have to be reinstituted to address residual lesions. Empiric protamine sulfate dosing, or a dose based on the calculated circulating heparin amount, is given, and a follow-up ACT is then checked. Bleeding after CPB may be multifactorial, with residual circulating heparin as just one possibility. The anesthesia team works to understand ongoing bleeding after protamine dosing. This may include a post-bypass thromboelastography (TEG) or one performed during the rewarm period (Emani et al. 2022). During rewarming, a TEG check typically provides more timely, actionable results for the anesthesia provider to use shortly after separation from CPB. It is common to transfuse platelets immediately after bypass. Cryoprecipitate, plasma, and targeted clotting factors (such as recombinant activated factor VII [rFVIIa]) may also be considered to treat post-bypass coagulopathies.

Blood Gas Management

The perfusionist controls blood oxygen and carbon dioxide levels by adjusting the sweep gas flow through the oxygenator's fiber bundle. Most sweep gas systems for pediatric perfusion allow for adjustments to the oxygen and air mixture (21–100% oxygen) as well as the amount of CO_2 in the sweep gas (commonly quantified in mL/min or L/min). Understanding not only the composition of the sweep gas but also the flow rate relative to the blood flow rate through the device is important. This ratio is referred to as the ventilation-to-perfusion ratio or V/Q ratio. The oxygenator instructions for use (IFU) commonly provides device-specific maximum and minimum values.

A primary consideration for CPB is determining the target levels for oxygen and carbon dioxide.

- *The Oxygenation Strategy*
  First, there is the oxygenation strategy.
  - *Slightly Hyperoxic Technique*: Some programs aim to limit the PaO_2 to a range of 200–300 mmHg, which ensures fully saturated hemoglobin is delivered to the patient. Additional oxygen would increase the PaO_2 but not significantly enhance the overall blood oxygen content. This slightly hyperoxic technique is thought to ameliorate oxygen free radical injury.
  - *Maximal Oxygenation*: An alternate technique provides the patient with 100% oxygen in the sweep gas, which may be diluted slightly with a small amount of CO_2 added to the sweep. This more definitive hyperoxic strategy addresses concerns for tissue oxygenation that may be impaired during the bypass period (den Os et al. 2020). When the patient is transitioned to CPB, blood flow becomes non-pulsatile, which decreases the perfused capillary density and may put some tissue beds at risk.
  - *Target Oxygenation Levels*: Cardiac programs define their oxygenation strategy, and the perfusionist maintains values within the target range using serial blood gas samples and an in-line blood gas monitor, which provides ongoing data in real-time.
- *Carbon Dioxide Management*
  The second consideration for blood gas management is carbon dioxide management. Please refer to Chap. 6. There are two strategies to choose from during hypothermic CPB.
  - *Alpha-stat*: This technique for CO_2 management aims for a $PaCO_2$ of 40 mmHg, as measured at the standardized blood gas analyzer temperature of 37 °C, regardless of the patient's temperature on CPB. Alpha-stat helps preserve intracellular pH and function. From the perspective of the brain, cerebral autoregulation is preserved. This approach may be particularly beneficial in cases with potential embolic phenomena due to a calcified aorta, a condition more prevalent in adults with acquired cardiac disease.
  - *pH-stat*: The alternative carbon dioxide strategy is termed pH-stat. This CO_2 approach also targets a $PaCO_2$ of 40 mmHg, but crucially, this is measured at the patient's actual temperature, not the standardized 37 °C. Since gases, including CO_2, are more soluble at lower temperatures, maintaining a specific partial pressure during hypothermia requires adding more CO_2 to the blood. During CPB, this is achieved by adding CO_2 to the sweep gas, sometimes accompanied by adjustments to the sweep flow rate. While this extra CO_2 elevates the $PaCO_2$ when analyzed at 37 °C, it maintains a normal $PaCO_2$ (~40 mmHg) at the patient's actual temperature. It is important to note that pH-stat does not preserve intracellular pH. Instead, it aims to keep blood pH normal during hypothermia. This helps counteract the leftward shift of the oxyhemoglobin dissociation curve caused by hypothermia, facilitating oxygen release to tissues. However, pH-stat also decouples cerebral autoregulation, making it pressure-passive. This may improve the homogeneity of cerebral cooling and rewarming during CPB. Additionally, a higher $PaCO_2$ can induce pulmonary vasoconstriction, which may be beneficial in patients with APCs by reducing pulmonary blood flow and thus minimizing systemic-to-pulmonary shunting. With the aid of an in-line blood gas monitor, the perfusionist can tightly control the $PaCO_2$ during bypass and seamlessly switch between alpha and pH-stat strategies based on the patient's current temperature.

Temperature Management in Pediatric CPB

Pediatric patients have a higher metabolic rate than adults, necessitating higher CPB flows and IDO_2. Maintaining the same indexed blood flow for pediatric patients as for adults risks not meeting the metabolic requirements during support. Pediatric patients are also more likely to require intracardiac repairs and to experience more left heart return during bypass. Blood flowing into the surgical field can impair the surgeon's ability to perform the planned repair. Therefore, reduced pump flow, and thus reduced runoff into the surgical field, may be necessary. For this reason, pediatric and congenital cardiac patients may be cooled to a greater extent than most adult patients requiring cardiac surgery. Lowering the patient's temperature reduces their metabolic rate and overall pump flow requirements.

Cooling and warming a patient during CPB are relatively straightforward procedures, but there are important considerations to ensure they are done safely. The rate of temperature change is crucial for achieving homogeneous cooling and warming of all organs during nonpulsatile perfusion on CPB. While traditional practice has been to limit the gradient between the venous inlet and arterial outlet blood to 10 °C, more recent literature supports lower gradients. Renal and neurologic outcomes may be improved with gradients in the 4–6 °C range, particularly when the patient is above 30 °C (Engelman et al. 2015). Moreover, the arterial inflow temperature to the patient must be considered a surrogate for brain temperature and should never be hyperthermic (i.e., >37 °C).

Another temperature consideration for pediatric cases involves managing situations requiring cessation of all blood flow for brief or extended periods. The use of circulatory arrest is still required for the repair of some complex congenital heart lesions. While there is no well-defined safe circulatory arrest time, guidance from the 1980s by Kirklin et al. suggests a probable safe circulatory arrest time at 18 °C for about 40 minutes and at 28 °C for about 15 minutes (Kirklin 1985). Surgeons use considerations like these, along with the time spent cooling and the blood gas management strategy, when planning for a technically challenging operation.

Given the ever-present risk of mechanical or disposable product failure, it is common for the surgeon to opt for at least some degree of hypothermia, as it provides a safety margin in case pump flow is interrupted. Regional perfusion strategies that provide selective organ perfusion, particularly of the brain, with or without flow to the lower body, have been developed to mitigate the effects associated with deep hypothermia and circulatory arrest.

Summary

The perfusionist plays a crucial role within the cardiac surgery team, possessing expert knowledge of the hardware and disposables for CPB. Key differences between adult and pediatric patients necessitate tailored bypass plans. Established standards and guidelines exist for perfusion practices in congenital heart surgery, but each perfusion team must develop its own institutional policy and procedure manual to guide practice in accordance with these guidelines. The entire cardiovascular surgery team collaborates to create an individualized CPB plan before initiating support, guided by institutional protocols. Vigilant patient and circuit monitoring, coupled with effective communication, are paramount to ensuring optimal outcomes.

References

den Os MM, van den Brom CE, van Leeuwen ALI, et al. Microcirculatory perfusion disturbances following cardiopulmonary bypass: a systematic review. Crit Care. 2020;24:218.

Dreher M, Min J, Mavroudis C, et al. Indexed oxygen delivery during pediatric cardiopulmonary bypass is a modifiable risk factor for postoperative acute kidney injury. J Extra Corpor Technol. 2023;55(3):112–20.

Emani S, Emani VS, Diallo FB, et al. Comparison of thromboelastography devices TEG®6S point of care device vs. TEG®5000 in pediatric patients undergoing cardiac surgery. J Extra Corpor Technol. 2022;54(1):42–9.

Engelman R, Baker RA, Likosky DS, et al. The Society of Thoracic Surgeons, The Society of Cardiovascular Anesthesiologists, and The American Society of ExtraCorporeal Technology: clinical practice guidelines for cardiopulmonary bypass–temperature management during cardiopulmonary bypass. Ann Thorac Surg. 2015;100(2):748–57.

Garrison L. Cardiopulmonary bypass mean global oxygen delivery may be associated with neurocognitive preservation during hypothermic aortic surgery. J Extra Corpor Technol. 2020;52(4):289–94.

Hayward A, Robertson A, Thiruchelvam T, et al. Oxygen delivery in pediatric cardiac surgery and its association with acute kidney injury using machine learning. J Thorac Cardiovasc Surg. 2023;165(4):1505–16.

Kirklin JK, Kirklin JW, Pacifico AD. Deep hypothermia and total circulatory arrest. In: Arciniegas E, editor. Pediatric cardiac surgery. Chicago: Year Book; 1985. p. 79–85.

Kohlsaat K, Gavreau K, Fynn-Thompson F, et al. Impact of pre-bypass ultrafiltration on prime values and clinical outcomes in neonatal and infant cardiopulmonary bypass. J Extra Corpor Technol. 2023;55(4):175–84.

Magruder JT, Weiss SJ, DeAngelis KG, et al. Correlating oxygen delivery on cardiopulmonary bypass with Society of Thoracic Surgeons outcomes following cardiac surgery. J Thorac Cardiovasc Surg. 2022;164(3):997–1007.

Matte GS. The bypass plan. In: Perfusion for congenital heart surgery: notes on cardiopulmonary bypass for a complex patient population. 1st ed. Hoboken: Wiley-Blackwell; 2015. p. 33–71.

Matte GS. It is time to update membrane oxygenator testing standards and their instructions for use [Letter]. J Extra Corpor Technol. 2016;48:148–51.

Matte GS, DiNardo JA. Pediatric cardiopulmonary bypass. In: Gravlee GP, Davis RF, Hammon JW, Kussman BD, editors. Cardiopulmonary bypass and mechanical support. New York: Wolters Kluwer; 2015. p. 655–81.

Matte GS, Howe RJ, Ibla J, Emani S, Emani SM. Transition from Hemochron Response to Hemochron Signature Elite activated clotting time devices in a congenital cardiac surgery practice. J Extra Corpor Technol. 2019;51(4):221–6.

Matte GS, Quinonez LG, del Nido PJ. Surgical approaches and cardiopulmonary bypass in pediatric cardiac surgery. In: Sellke FW, del Nido PJ, Swanson SJ, editors. Sabiston & Spencer surgery of the chest. 10th ed. Elsevier; 2024. p. 2182–218.

Shimpo H, Shimamoto A, Sawamura Y, et al. Ultrafiltration of the priming blood before cardiopulmonary bypass attenuates inflammatory response and improves postoperative clinical course in pediatric patients. Shock. 2001;16:51–4.

Standards and Guidelines for Pediatric and Congenital Perfusion Practice. 2019. Available at: https://www.amsect.org/policy-practice/amsects-standards-and-guidelines. Accessed 2 Dec 2023.

US Department of Health and Human Services. Guidance for cardiopulmonary bypass oxygenators 510(k) submission; final guidance for industry and FDA staff. Washington, DC: US Department of Health and Human Services Food and Drug Administration Center for Devices and Radiological Health; 2000.

Welsh A, Hoyle JD Jr. A case of delayed presentation of transposition of the great arteries. Pediatr Emerg Care. 2021;37(12):e1753.

Wypij D, Jonas RA, Bellinger DC, et al. The effect of hematocrit during hypothermic cardiopulmonary bypass in infant heart surgery: results from the combined Boston hematocrit trials. J Thorac Cardiovasc Surg. 2008;135(2):355–60.

Congenital Cardiovascular Pathology

24

Jan Friess and Viviane G. Nasr

Introduction

Congenital heart disease (CHD) affects 7–10 per 1000 live births. With advancements in medical and surgical treatment, individuals born with CHD now frequently survive into adulthood. Understanding fetal and neonatal cardiovascular physiology, along with the anatomy and pathophysiology of common cardiac lesions and their progression, is essential for the perioperative care and risk stratification of this patient population. This chapter provides an overview of the physiological and pathophysiological concepts critical to managing CHD, as well as specific considerations for commonly encountered lesions.

Fetal and Postnatal Circulation in CHD

In-Utero Fetal Circulation

Due to the unique physiological features of fetal circulation, severe congenital heart defects in-utero may not become detrimental until ex-utero circulation begins at birth, leading to symptoms, morbidity, and mortality in neonates with CHD.

In the fetus, the placenta serves as the primary source of oxygenation. Oxygenated blood returns from the placenta to the fetus via the umbilical vein to the portal venous system. The *ductus venosus* allows blood to bypass the liver and directly enter the systemic venous system, with 50% of umbilical venous blood entering the systemic circulation without passing through the liver's capillary system. Blood returning from the inferior vena cava (IVC) enters the right atrium (RA) with a higher oxygen content than that from the superior vena cava (SVC). Oxygen-rich blood from the IVC is preferentially diverted through the *foramen ovale* (FO) into the left atrium (LA). Conversely, blood entering the RA from the SVC primarily flows into the right ventricle (RV) and is then ejected into the pulmonary artery (PA). Only 10–15% of this blood reaches the lungs and is delivered into the LA; the vast majority is shunted into the systemic circulation via the *ductus arteriosus*, which connects the PA to the descending aorta. Therefore, the RV contributes significantly to the systemic cardiac output in the fetus. Blood is ejected into the aorta by both the left ventricle (LV) and RV, with blood flow dynamics and shunting at the levels of the ductus venosus, FO, and ductus arteriosus providing the ascending aorta and the coronary and cerebral circulation with the most oxygenated blood (Fig. 24.1).

Fetal Circulation Transition at Birth

At birth, changes in the newborn's circulation initiate the closure of fetal structures that were crucial for in-utero life. The *ductus arteriosus*, maintained open during fetal life by high levels of prostaglandins, begins to close in two stages postbirth. Functional closure typically occurs on the first day of life due to increased oxygen partial pressures and decreased prostaglandin levels, by causing the smooth muscles to contract. Anatomical closure usually follows within 2–3 weeks, leaving the ligamentum arteriosum as a remnant.

The *FO*, a flap-like structure in the fetal heart, allows blood to flow from the higher-pressure RA to lower-pressure LA. At birth, increased pulmonary blood flow and decreased umbilical vein return reverse this pressure gradient, with LA pressures exceeding those in the RA, leading to the functional closure of the FO. While this closure becomes anatomical in many individuals, it remains patent in about 33% of adults.

J. Friess
Department of Anaesthesiology and Pain Medicine, Bern University Hospital, Inselspital, Bern, Switzerland
e-mail: Jan-Oliver.Friess@insel.ch

V. G. Nasr (✉)
Department of Anesthesiology, Critical Care and Pain Medicine, Division of Cardiac Anesthesia, Boston Children's Hospital, Boston, MA, USA
e-mail: viviane.nasr@childrens.harvard.edu

A. S. Awad, J. DiNardo (eds.), *Clinical Perfusion for Cardiac Surgery*, https://doi.org/10.1007/978-3-031-91163-7_24

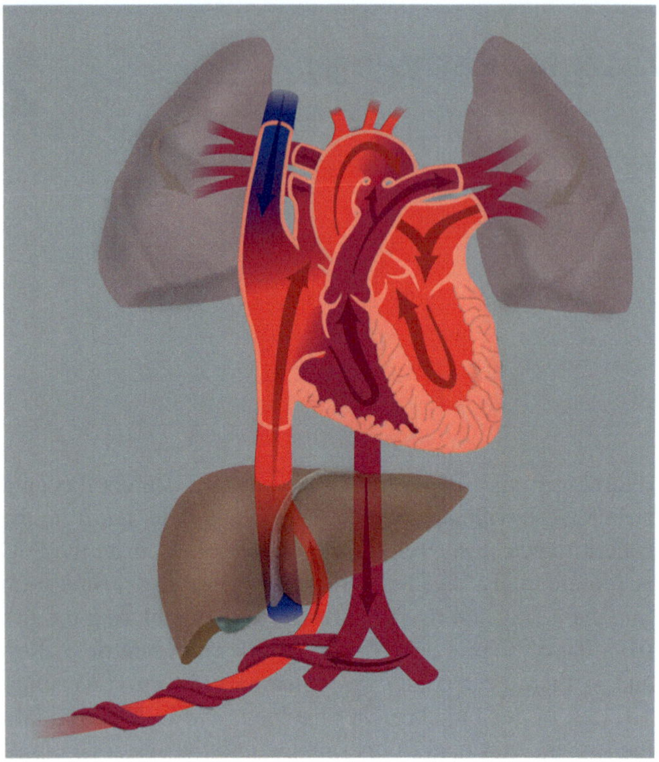

Fig. 24.1 This illustration depicts the fetal circulatory system, highlighting structures vital before birth. Oxygen-rich blood from the placenta travels through the umbilical vein, bypassing the liver via the ductus venosus, and mixes with deoxygenated blood in the IVC. The FO allows blood to bypass the lungs, flowing from the right-to-left atrium. The ductus arteriosus further shunts blood from the PA to the aorta, ensuring oxygen-rich blood reaches the fetal body. Finally, deoxygenated blood returns to the placenta via the umbilical arteries

The *ductus venosus*, which redirects blood from the umbilical vein past the liver, closes passively following the cessation of blood flow from the umbilical vein. Functional closure occurs within the first week of life, with anatomical closure following about 3 months later.

In the fetus, pulmonary vascular resistance (PVR) is high, limiting pulmonary blood flow. After birth, the initiation of breathing reduces the mechanical compression of pulmonary vasculature, and the rise in oxygen partial pressure leads to a significant decrease in PVR. Pulmonary vasculature remodeling continues over the first few months, with near-normal adult PVR values typically reached by 6 months.

However, various factors such as acidosis, hypothermia, hypoxia, and hypercarbia can delay these closures or even cause re-opening of these fetal shunts, leading to persistence of fetal circulation. In some cases, especially in newborns with CHD, maintaining fetal circulation can be beneficial, and re-opening these shunts may be necessary for survival.

Specifically, survival in newborns with "ductal-dependent" CHD lesions depends on the patency of the ductus arteriosus. Functional closure of this duct can be reversed with the administration prostaglandin E1 (PGE1) to reestablish ductal shunting, a critical treatment strategy for critically ill neonates with CHD.

Cardiac Shunts

Physiological shunting occurs when blood is redirected within the same circulation without traversing the usual path through the heart's chambers or lungs. In the systemic circulation, this involves systemic venous blood bypassing the lungs and re-entering the aorta, a process known as a "right-to-left" shunt, where blood remains unoxygenated. Conversely, in the pulmonary circulation, a "left-to-right" shunt recirculates oxygen-rich pulmonary venous blood back into the PA without delivering oxygen to the body's tissues. Effective blood flow measures the volume of blood that successfully transits from the venous system of one circulation to the arterial outflow of the other. Thus, effective systemic blood flow is the amount of pulmonary venous blood reaching the aorta, and effective pulmonary blood flow is the amount of systemic venous blood reaching the PA. Despite complex intracardiac shunts, effective pulmonary and systemic blood flows are invariably equal. Normal cardiac physiology and typical blood flow dynamics without shunting are illustrated in Fig. 24.2.

Anatomic cardiac shunts are physical connections that allow blood to mix from one system to the other. These can occur at the atrial, ventricular, or great vessels levels.

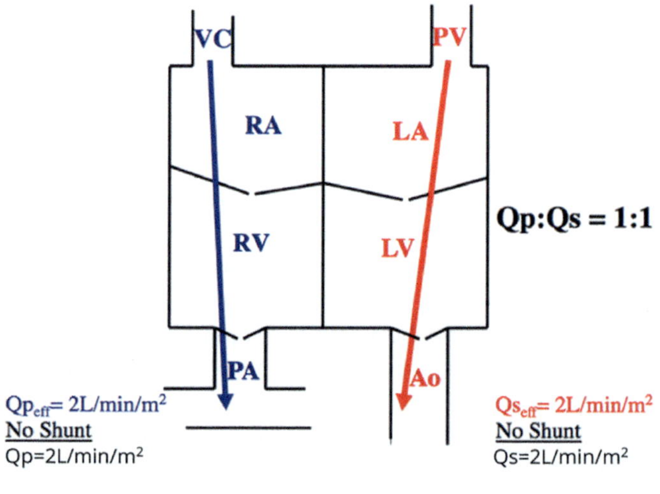

Fig. 24.2 This illustration portrays normal cardiac physiology, emphasizing the typical blood flow dynamics without shunting. Key elements include: Qp (pulmonary blood flow) represents blood volume flowing through the lungs for oxygenation; Qs (systemic blood flow) represents blood volume circulated throughout the body, delivering oxygen and nutrients; Qpeff (effective pulmonary blood flow) represents the portion of Qp actually involved in gas exchange; Qseff (effective systemic blood flow) represents the portion of Qs effectively delivering oxygen to tissues. The diagram illustrates the heart's chambers, major vessels, and blood flow directions in both pulmonary and systemic circuits

Restrictive shunts are shunts of a small anatomic size with a limited amount of blood flow through the shunt. Restrictive shunts have a pressure gradient between the structures they connect. Conversely, *unrestrictive shunts* are larger, permitting substantial blood flow and potential pressure equalization across the shunt. The volume of shunted blood depends on hemodynamic conditions, including the relative systemic and PVR.

Shunts can be classified as *simple*, involving a single direction of flow (only a left-to-right or right-to-left shunt) without affecting ventricular outflow tract dynamics, or *complex* where additional obstructions alter the hemodynamics of one or both ventricles, influencing shunt dynamics. Shunts may also be bidirectional, allowing blood to flow in both directions, though not necessarily in equal volumes.

Specific Lesions

Simple Shunt Lesions

Patent Ductus Arteriosus

Patent ductus arteriosus (PDA) accounts for 10% of all congenital heart defects, with its incidence rising to 20–30% among pre-term infants. The condition shows a female predominance with a male-to-female ratio of 1:3.

Anatomy

PDA is a persistent connection from the fetal circulation that links the main PA to the proximal descending aorta just distal to the left subclavian artery's origin (Fig. 24.3).

Physiology

PDA results in a simple, often nonrestrictive shunt if its diameter is sufficiently large. The direction and magnitude of net flow depend on the relative pressures of the PVR and systemic vascular resistance (SVR). As PVR decreases, a left-to-right shunt forms, necessitating an increase in left ventricular (LV) output to maintain systemic blood flow. This increased volume load can lead to congestive heart failure (CHF). Additionally, the left-to-right shunt boosts pulmonary venous return and left atrial pressure, elevating respiratory effort and potentially leading to recurrent pneumonia. Over time, this can escalate PVR, potentially causing PA hypertension. A significant diastolic run-off from the descending aorta due to the PDA may result in holodiastolic flow reversal in the descending aorta, which is associated with complications such as necrotizing enterocolitis, renal failure, and intraventricular hemorrhage.

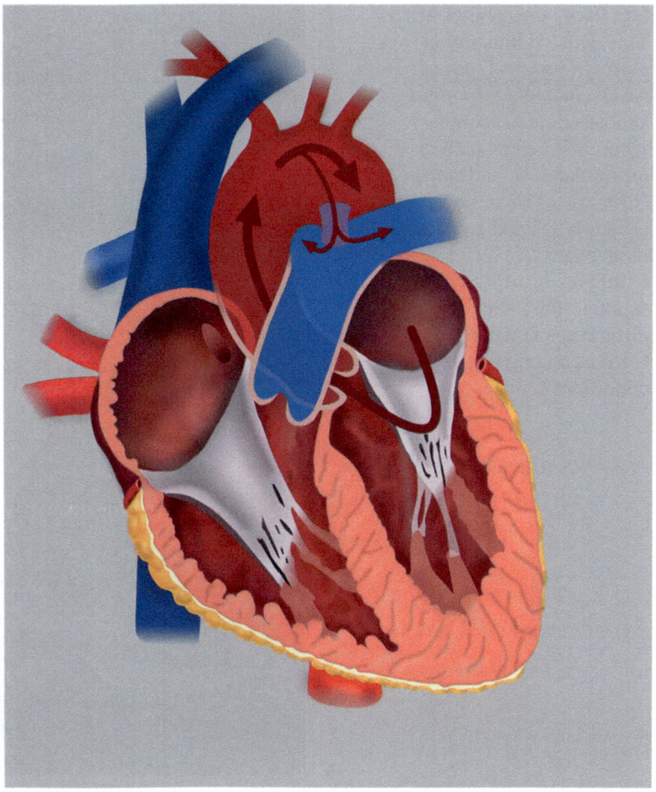

Fig. 24.3 PDA. This illustration shows a PDA, a congenital heart defect where a connection between the aorta and PA remains open after birth. Arrows depict the abnormal blood flow between the aorta and PA, highlighting how the PDA leads to mixing of oxygenated and deoxygenated blood, impacting cardiac function and pulmonary over-circulation

Treatment

The ductus arteriosus may be closed via interventional device closure or surgical ligation, depending on the individual case and the severity of symptoms.

Atrial Septal Defect

Atrial septal defects (ASD) represent the second most common type of CHD, with an incidence of 0.0–0.2%. They occur more frequently in females than males, with a ratio of 2:1.

Anatomy

ASD is a defect in the intra-atrial septum that connects the left and right atria. There are several types of ASDs, classified by their location (Fig. 24.4):

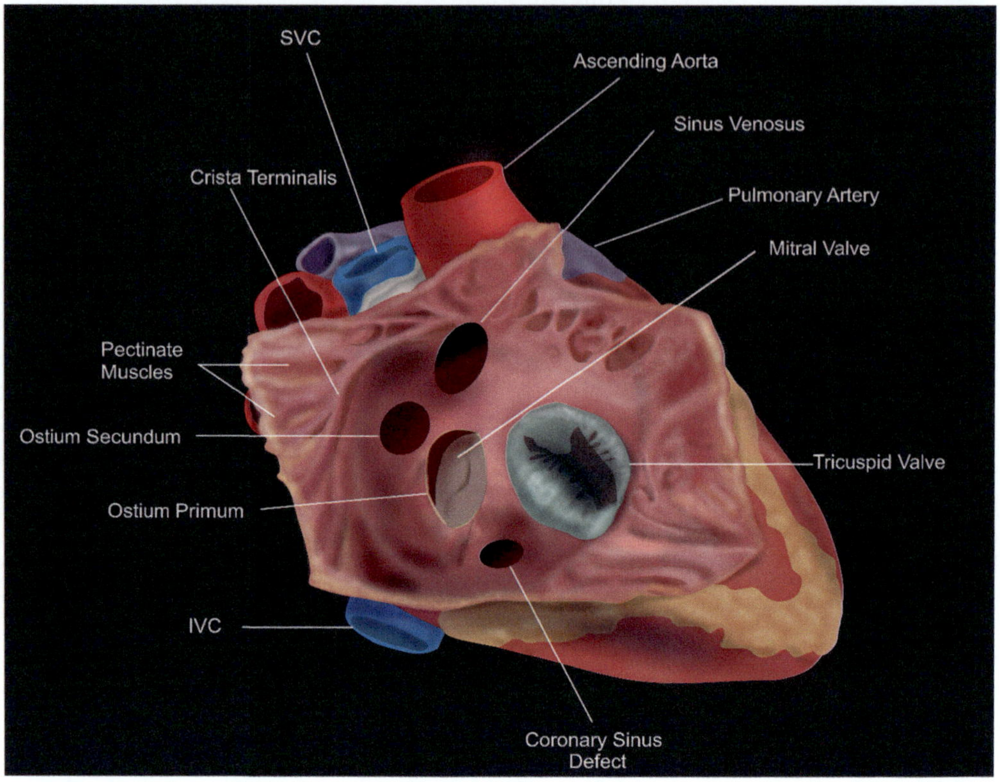

Fig. 24.4 Congenital ASDs. This detailed illustration portrays various types of ASDs, including the sinus venosus defect, ostium secundum defect, ostium primum defect, and sinus coronarius defect. Each defect is clearly labeled and depicted in its respective location within the heart's atrial septum, illustrating the differences in anatomical features among these conditions

1. *Ostium Secundum Defects*: These make up about 80% of ASD cases and occur in the region of the fossa ovalis due to a deficiency in the septum primum.
2. *Ostium Primum Defects*: These are located inferiorly at the level of the atrioventricular valves and may extent from the inferior limbus of the interatrial septum (IAS) to the crest of the interventricular septum. These defects, often associated with a cleft mitral valve and mitral regurgitation, are considered a form of partial atrioventricular canal defect.
3. *Sinus Venosus Defects*: Inferior and superior sinus venosus defects occur at the junctions of the vena cavae (SVC and IVC, respectively) with the RA. These defects are situated within the sinus venosus itself, rather than in the IAS. Both defects are behind the fossa ovalis. Superior sinus venosus defects are more common. These defects often involve a deficiency in the sinus venosus wall, causing right-sided pulmonary veins (either upper or lower) to drain anomalously directly into the vena cava/RA junction. Sinus venosus defects are frequently associated with partially anomalous pulmonary venous return (PAPVR), characterized by a direct anatomical connection between the pulmonary veins and the vena cava.
4. *Coronary Sinus Defect*: Occurs when there's an abnormal communication between the coronary sinus (CS) and the LA, typically due to a partial or complete "unroofing" of the CS where it passes behind the LA. This creates a shunt between the RA and LA, as blood entering the CS from the coronary circulation can now flow directly into the LA. CS defects are often associated with a persistent left superior vena cava (PLSVC).

Physiology

ASDs, being simple shunts, allow blood to flow between the left and right atria. The amount of flow across the defect depends on its size, which can be either restrictive or unrestrictive. The resulting left-to-right shunt primarily occurs during diastole, causing oxygenated blood to recirculate from LA to the RA, RV, and PA before returning to the LA. While the left-to-right shunt produces a volume overload of these structures, the effective (forward) left ventricular outflow is reduced.

Despite increased pulmonary blood flow, PA pressures may remain normal for years, with elevated PVR often not developing until adulthood. Consequently, symptoms of significant ASDs may not manifest until late childhood or later (Fig. 24.5).

Treatment

Some ASDs may decrease in size or even close spontaneously by the age of 4 years. Minimally invasive transluminal catheter-based device closure of secundum ASDs is performed in the catheterization lab. Transesophageal echocardiographic guidance usually requires general anesthesia in children. Specific risks of device closure include air or device

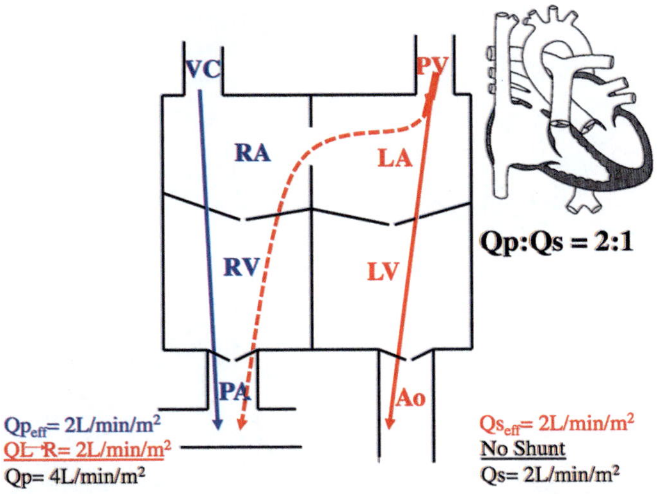

Fig. 24.5 Congenital ASDs. This detailed illustration depicts the blood flow dynamics associated with ASD. It shows both effective systemic and pulmonary blood flows as equal across the lesions, represented by solid lines. Additionally, the shunted flows are indicated with dotted lines. Labels included in the diagram clarify the pulmonary blood flow (Qp), systemic blood flow (Qs), effective pulmonary blood flow (Qpeff), effective systemic blood flow (Qseff), right-to-left physiological shunt (QR -> L), and left-to-right physiological shunt (QL -> R), enhancing understanding of the heart's functional adaptations in ASD

embolization, and transient electrocardiogram changes. Small ASDs can be closed surgically on cardiopulmonary bypass (CPB), while larger defects typically require patching with pericardium. Primum defects often require closure of an associated anterior mitral leaflet cleft as well. If PAPVR is present, additional surgical procedures are necessary to ensure the physiological return of right-sided pulmonary venous blood flow. Surgical repair of the CS ASD depends on whether a LSVC is present. Primary closure of the CS is possible without an LSVC, although this may result in a small right-to-left shunt of the returning coronary sinus blood. If a LSVC is present, its venous return must be surgically diverted before attempting CS closure.

Ventricular Septal Defects

Ventricular septal defects (VDSs) represent the most common CHD. Their incidence ranges from 1.5 to 3 per 1000 live births in term infants and increases to 4.5 to 7 per 1000 in pre-term infants. Spontaneous closure of VSDs occurs in approximately 30–40% of cases.

Anatomy

A VSD is a defect in the ventricular septum that creates a connection between the left and right ventricles. The classification of VSDs is based on their location (Fig. 24.6):

1. *Membranous or Perimembranous VSDs*: These constitute approximately 80% of all VSDs and are located at the membranous septum near the insertion of the septal leaflet of the tricuspid valve (TV). The defect allows communication with the LV just below the aortic valve. Often, partial closure involves TV tissue and membranous septal tissue, giving the septal defect an aneurysmal appearance on imaging studies.
2. *Subpulmonary or Supracristal VSDs*: Located in the infundibular septum below the pulmonary valve, these defects may lead to aortic valve regurgitation due to a lack of structural support of the right coronary cusp of the aortic valve, causing the cusp to prolapse.
3. *Conoventricular VSDs*: These involve the anterior and superior aspects of the membranous septum.
4. *Inlet or Canal Type VSDs*: These are found in the posterior septum close to the atrioventricular valves.
5. *Muscular VSDs*: Located in the lower trabecular septum, muscular VSDs can be further categorized as apical, mid-muscular, anterior, or posterior.

Physiology

VSDs are simple shunts where the magnitude of shunting depends on the defect's size. With unrestrictive defects, the direction and amount of shunted blood flow depend on the relative ratio of SVR and PVR. Initially, infants with large VSD exhibit pulmonary blood flow near-normal values due to the high PVR at birth. By the second week, as PVR decreases, pulmonary flow significantly increases. Patients with large VSDs, characterized by a Qp:Qs ratio above 2:1, typically present with high PA pressures, sometimes reaching systemic levels. This predisposes them to develop pulmonary artery hypertension (PAH) early in life due to the constant exposure of the high flow and pressure in the pulmonary vasculature. To prevent PAH development, early closure of large VSDs is recommended in childhood. Older patients with established PAH and markedly increased PVR are poor candidates for VSD closure, as the RV may struggle to maintain output against such high resistance. Therefore, PVR should be measured in the cardiac catheterization lab prior to any closure or repair decision. Pulmonary overcirculation leads to LA hypertension, causing pulmonary congestion, increased work of breathing, and recurrent pulmonary infections. Large VSDs also result in increased volume load on both the RV and LV, potentially leading to both pulmonary and systemic venous congestion. The timing of surgical intervention is typically dictated by clinical symptoms and failure of medical therapy.

Treatment

Strategies to treat VSDs vary depending on the defect's location. PA banding can be used as a palliative measure to significantly reduce pulmonary blood flow until definitive repair is possible. Surgical patch closure is the standard approach

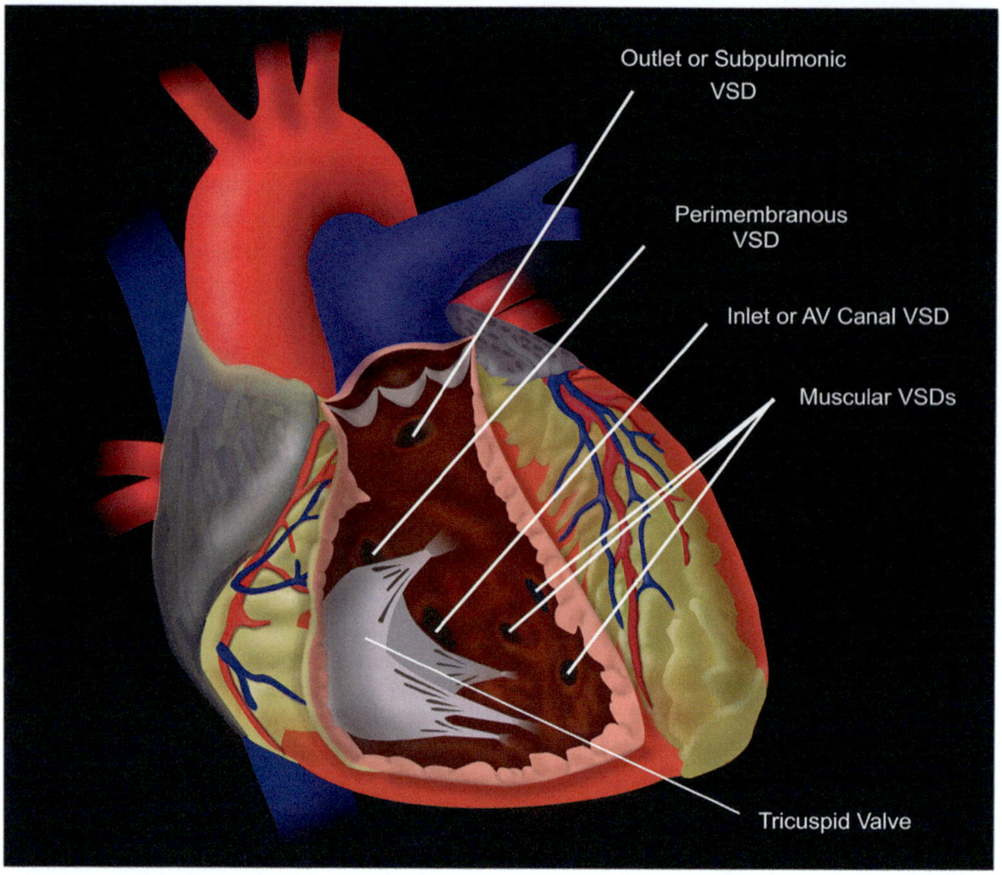

Fig. 24.6 Congenital VSDs. This detailed illustration portrays various types of VSDs, including the anatomical features among perimembranous, muscular, inlet, and outlet defects illustrating the differences in these conditions. Each defect is clearly labeled and depicted in its respective location within the heart's ventricular septum, illustrating the differences in anatomical features among these conditions

for repairing VSDs. Most membranous and conoventricular defects are repaired via an approach that crosses the RA and TV. Although ventriculotomy is generally avoided, it is necessary for repairing subpulmonary or supracristal defects. Muscular VSDs might be amenable for device closure, provided they are remote from any valves.

Aortopulmonary Window

The aortopulmonary window (AP) is a rare congenital heart defect, accounting for less than 0.1% of all CHD cases. It results from the failure of the truncus arteriosus to properly separate into the aorta and PA during cardiac development. AP is often associated with other cardiac abnormalities in 30–50% of cases and can coexist with conditions such as VACTERL, CHARGE, and 22q11.2 deletion syndrome.

Anatomy

AP defects are classified into four types (Fig. 24.7):

1. *Type I (Proximal)*: The defect occurs between the ascending aorta and the main PA.
2. *Type II (Distal)*: The distal ascending aorta connects to the right PA.
3. *Type III (Total)*: Represents a complete absence of the aortopulmonary septum, resulting in the largest defect.
4. *Type IV (Intermediate)*: Features adequate superior and inferior rims.

Physiology

Following birth, the reduction in PVR leads to a significant, unrestrictive left-to-right shunt in patients with AP. This results in high pulmonary blood flow and early onset of CHF.

Treatment

Early surgical intervention is recommended for most patients. The defect is typically repaired with a patch through a median sternotomy, necessitating CPB. In selected cases, such as those with a Type IV defect and normal coronary arteries, percutaneous device closure may be performed in the cardiac catheterization lab.

Right-Sided Lesions

Tetralogy of Fallot

Tetralogy of fallot (TOF) is the most prevalent cyanotic heart defect, occurring in approximately 1 in 3500 live births, and is often linked with chromosomal abnormalities such as trisomy 21 and 22q11.2 microdeletions. TOF manifests in three variants: TOF with pulmonary stenosis (TOF/PS), TOF with pulmonary atresia (TOF/PA), and TOF with absent pulmonary valve (TOF/APV).

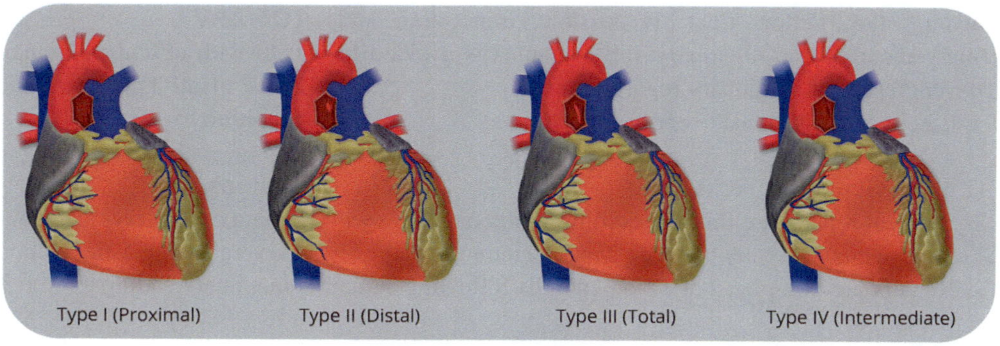

Fig. 24.7 Aortopulmonary window. This detailed illustration portrays various types of aortopulmonarywindow, highlighting their anatomical features and locations. Each type is distinctly shown to demonstrate the differences in how they connect the aorta and PA

TOF/PS

Anatomy

TOF is characterized by four key anatomical features:

1. Underdevelopment of the RV infundibulum.
2. A large, malaligned VSD.
3. An aorta overriding the interventricular septum and the VSD.
4. RV hypertrophy, with thickening of the right ventricle's muscle due to increased workload from pumping against the right ventricular outflow tract (RVOT) obstruction (Fig. 24.8).

Additionally, TOF often presents with varying degrees of infundibular, valvular, or supra-valvular pulmonary stenosis. The pulmonary valve is frequently bicuspid and can exhibit varying degrees of dysplasia, sometimes with near-fusion of the leaflets.

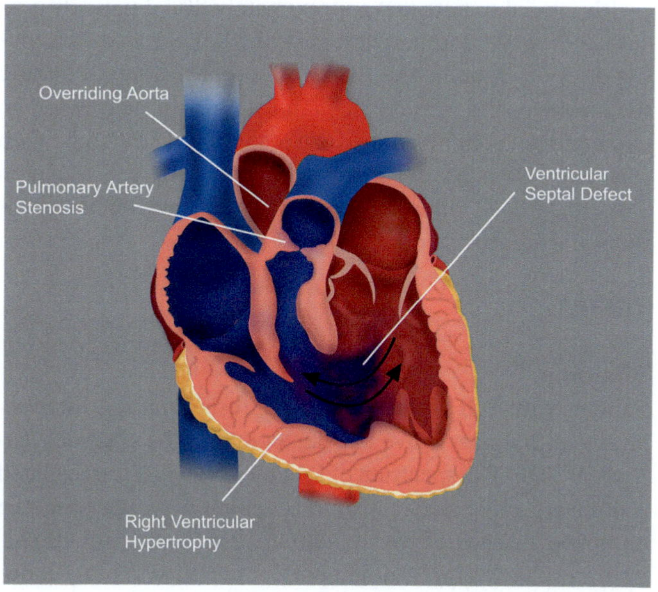

Fig. 24.8 TOF. This detailed illustration showcases a human heart with TOF, highlighting key features such as right ventricular hypertrophy, a large ventricular septal defect, an overriding aorta across the interventricular septum, and various degrees of pulmonary stenosis

Physiology

TOF is classified as a complex shunt lesion, characterized primarily by a VSD and both fixed and dynamic obstructions in the RVOT. The obstructions encompass supra-valvular, valvular, and infundibular regions, with the infundibular segment contributing to the dynamic aspect. This combined obstruction leads to RVOT obstruction (RVOTO), resulting in a right-to-left shunt through the VSD, reduced pulmonary blood flow, and resultant cyanosis.

In a minority of TOF cases, the RVOTO may be minor, allowing near-normal arterial saturations. These patients typically exhibit a left-to-right shunt, characterized by increased pulmonary blood flow, and potential signs of CHF.

Hypoxic Episodes (Tet Spells)

They are acute exacerbations of the right-to-left shunt at the VSD level, often triggered by an increase in the dynamic component of RVOTO due to infundibular constriction. These episodes are frequently precipitated by activities such as crying, defecation, feeding, fever, or awakening. During a spell, the child may appear pale due to diminished cardiac output, and arterial oxygen desaturation occurs. Hypoxia leads to a decrease in SVR, which further amplifies the right-to-left shunt. Additionally, increased venous return enhances RV preload, exacerbating the infundibular obstruction and intensifying the shunt. This escalation in cyanosis can result in severe outcomes such as syncope, convulsions, and potentially death.

Treatment

Palliative shunts are employed surgically to address proximal pulmonary stenosis and enhance pulmonary blood flow. The original Blalock–Taussig shunt (BTS) involved an end-to-side anastomosis between the left or right subclavian artery and the ipsilateral branch PA. The modified Blalock–Thomas–Taussig shunt (mBTTS) utilizes a graft interposed between the innominate artery and the right PA.

Definite repair is aimed to alleviate outflow tract obstruction by resecting hypertrophied myocardial tissue and augmenting the outflow tract. If possible, transection and enlargement of the pulmonary valve annulus is avoided to prevent resultant pulmonary regurgitation.

Based on institutional experience:

1. Neonatal repair is performed.
2. Surgical repairs are timed according to the onset of cyanotic spells, typically between 2 and 10 months of age.
3. Repairs are completed at 12–18 months following shunt palliation.

It's crucial to note that approximately 8% of patients possess a left main coronary artery or the left anterior descending artery as a branch of the right coronary artery, crossing the intended area of surgical augmentation. In such cases, an extracardiac conduit should be considered. Patients with repaired TOF may experience residual disease or develop valve disorders, often managed through catheter interventions and valve replacements.

TOF/PA

Anatomy

Patients with TOF with pulmonary atresia exhibit infundibular and pulmonary valve atresia, alongside the classical features of TOF. The spectrum of PA atresia ranges from isolated pulmonary valve atresia with intact pulmonary arteries to the complete absence of native pulmonary arteries, with all pulmonary blood supply originating from major aortopulmonary collateral vessels (MAPCAs). Echocardiography alone is insufficient to delineate the pulmonary blood supply; thus, cardiac catheterization and/or MRI/CT scans are essential for a comprehensive assessment.

Physiology

TOF/PA typically presents a single-ventricle physiology. Despite this, it often remains amenable to biventricular repair.

Treatment

If the PDA is the primary source of pulmonary blood flow, the pulmonary circulation is considered ductal-dependent. In such cases, administration of PGE1 is initiated while surgical plans are formulated. The definitive repair involves creating a connection between the RV and the PA using a conduit. If the PAs are hypoplastic, PA dilations or stenting may be necessary to encourage PA growth. Coiling of MAPCAs may also be required. In cases where MAPCAs are the sole source of pulmonary circulation, surgical unifocalization is necessary where multiple MAPCAs are connected to create a single, functional PA, allowing for adequate blood flow to the lungs.

TOF/APV

TOF with absent pulmonary valve (TOF/APV) constitutes 2–6% of all TOF cases and presents a rare variant of this condition.

Anatomy

Patients exhibit typical features of TOF/PS, accompanied by a severely dysplastic pulmonary valve that is essentially nonfunctional, leading to both stenotic and regurgitant lesions.

Physiology

The combination of stenosis and regurgitation during development causes dilatation of the RV and both the main and branch pulmonary arteries. At birth, patients may present with compression of the proximal airways by aneurysmatic pulmonary vessels, which can lead to hyperinflation and air-trapping.

Treatment and Periprocedural Considerations

Compromised ventilation may necessitate urgent ventilatory support, and prone positioning may be required to alleviate external airway compression. These patients often require urgent surgical intervention. Surgical repair typically involves reducing PA dilation, closing the VSD, and repairing or replacing the pulmonary valve.

Pulmonary Atresia with Intact Ventricular Septum (PA/IVS)

PA/IVS represents a rare form of CHD, constituting 3% of cases.

Anatomy

In PA/IVS, there is no forward flow from the RV to the PA, and the ventricular septum remains intact. Typically, the RV infundibulum is small yet patent. The pulmonary valve annulus is usually of normal size, but its leaflets are fused into a membrane that blocks flow to the otherwise normal-sized PA. The RV often shows varying degrees of hypoplasia. With a functioning TV, the RV can develop supra-systemic pressures. This leads to the persistence of myocardial sinusoids, which connect the RV to the coronary circulation, acting as a pressure relief mechanism for the ventricle.

Physiology

Blood from the systemic venous systems is shunted through the patent FO (PFO) and completely mixes with pulmonary venous blood in the LA. Subsequently, the left ventricle distributes the mixed blood to the pulmonary and systemic circulation through a PDA. In this context, the PFO and PDA are obligatory shunts, rendering PA/IVS a ductal-dependent, single-ventricle physiology lesion.

The persistence of sinusoids may lead to the development of fistulous connections from the RV cavity to the epicardial right and left coronary arteries. Coronary artery stenoses and ostial atresia may develop, with coronary flow potentially being retrograde, originating from the RV. This situation renders the myocardium distal to any stenoses or atresia dependent on retrograde flow from the RV to the myocardium via ventriculocoronary connections. Right ventricular dependent coronary circulation (RVDCC) is present in 10–20% of cases.

Treatment

Cardiac catheterization is performed on every patient to assess the presence and significance of ventriculocoronary connections and evaluate the status of the coronary circulation before determining the treatment pathway. In the absence of RVDCC, patients may be suitable for biventricular repair if the RV is of adequate size. If RVDCC is present, then single ventricle palliation leading to a Fontan circulation is the only option, as decompressing the RV would lead to myocardial ischemia. For patients without RVDCC, multiple options are available to establish forward flow from the RA to the pulmonary arteries and promote RV growth. Decompression of the RV can be achieved in the catheterization lab by perforating the membrane and dilating the PV or surgically with a trans-annular PA patch. Depending on the degree of RV hypoplasia and subsequent RV growth, the repair options range from single-ventricle palliation in cases of very small RVs to full biventricular repair with an adequately sized RV.

Left-Sided Lesions

Left Ventricular Outflow Tract (LVOT) Obstructions

Obstruction of the LVOT occurs at three distinct levels:

The valvular, sub-valvular, and supra-valvular levels.

Anatomy

A bicuspid aortic valve is the most common cause of LVOT obstruction in young patients. Subaortic stenosis may arise from a membranous ring below the aortic valve or from narrowing of the LVOT caused by fibromuscular tissue or secondary to VSD patch repair. Supra-valvular aortic stenosis (SVAS) is often associated with Williams-Beuren syndrome and an elastin gene deficiency, which typically causes an hourglass-like narrowing at the sinotubular junction. Additionally, many patients with SVAS also experience severe peripheral PA stenoses.

Physiology

Aortic stenosis can result in a small left ventricle and endocardial fibroelastosis. In cases of critical aortic stenosis, systemic perfusion distal to the ductus arteriosus relies on right-to-left shunting through the patent PDA, leading to differential cyanosis with higher oxygen saturations in the upper extremities than in the lower body. When there is no antegrade flow through the aorta, coronary perfusion depends on retrograde flow of deoxygenated blood from the right-to-left shunt at the PDA. In patients with SVAS and Williams-Beuren syndrome, coronary blood flow can be mechanically impaired due to reduced flow at the sinotubular junction.

Treatment

The primary objective of treatment for LVOT obstructions is to surgically alleviate the narrowed regions, which may involve resection of sub-valvular tissue. Other surgical techniques include enlarging the LVOT with a patch or replacing the aortic valve. In some cases, aortic valve stenosis can be addressed through transcatheter aortic valve dilation.

Coarctation of the Aorta (CoA)

CoA is a common congenital heart lesion, more prevalent in males. It is often associated with other cardiac and non-cardiac anomalies, including Turner syndrome.

Anatomy

The coarctation typically manifests as a discrete, posterior invagination of the aortic wall, located just distal to the origin of the left subclavian artery and opposite the ductus arteriosus insertion site (see Fig. 37.2). In some cases, this constriction may be circumferential. Variants include longer segment coarctations and coarctation of the abdominal aorta.

Physiology

CoA leads to left ventricular hypertension and higher blood pressure in the right arm compared to the left arm and lower extremities. Before the ductus arteriosus closes, blood flow through the open duct aids in perfusing the lower body distal to the coarctation, causing differential cyanosis with higher oxygen saturation (SpO_2) in the upper extremities. In cases of severe obstruction, coarctation becomes a ductal-dependent lesion, as the lower body is primarily perfused through the PDA, elevating right ventricular pressures to systemic levels. Ductal closure can cause profound hypoperfusion in the lower body and result in increased pressures in the LV and LA, potentially leading to pulmonary edema. Treatment typically involves initiating PGE1 therapy to reopen the ductus arteriosus, with additional inotropic and ventilatory support as necessary.

Treatment

Surgical repair of CoA is typically performed through a left thoracotomy, employing techniques such as end-to-end anastomosis, patch plasty, or subclavian patch angioplasty. Cross-clamping of the aorta is necessary for all types of surgical repair. For older children and adults, especially those with late-diagnosed lesions, percutaneous stent placement offers an alternative therapeutic option.

Interrupted Aortic Arch

Interrupted aortic arch (IAA) is a rare congenital defect constituting about 1% of CHD and is frequently associated with the 22q11.2 deletion syndrome.

Anatomy

IAA is classified into three types based on the location of the interruption:

- *Type A*: The interruption occurs distal to the left subclavian artery, similar to the location of CoA.
- *Type B*: This most common type (80% of cases) is located between the left carotid artery and the left subclavian artery.
- *Type C*: The rarest type, found between the innominate artery and the right carotid artery. In cases with a biventricular intracardiac morphology, a VSD is invariably present (Fig. 24.9).

Physiology

In IAA, a ductal-dependent lesion, the aortic segment beyond the interruption relies entirely on the ductus arteriosus for blood supply, while the proximal aorta receives blood from the LV and the LVOT. Shunting across the VSD typically occurs from left-to-right, and the PDA shunts from right-to-left, causing differential cyanosis, with higher values of SpO_2, are noted proximal to the interruption and lower values distal to it. The diastolic blood pressure is lower and pulse pressure is wider in the distal aorta due to diastolic run-off into the PA via the ductus arteriosus. Closure of the ductus arteriosus can lead to cardiovascular compromise, necessitating the initiation of PGE_1 therapy.

Treatment

Surgical correction of IAA involves anastomosing the proximal and distal ends of the aorta, sometimes requiring graft material. Division and ligation of the left subclavian artery and occasionally an aberrant right subclavian artery may be necessary. Any associated cardiac defects, such as VSD, are typically repaired concurrently.

Single-Ventricle Lesions

The term "single-ventricle" describes CHDs characterized by a dominant ventricle due to the underdevelopment or absence of the other, resulting in mixed systemic and pulmonary blood flow. Conditions such as hypoplastic left heart syndrome (HLHS), where the left ventricle is underdeveloped, and tricuspid atresia, with an underdeveloped RV, fall into this category. Other examples include double-inlet left ventricle (DILV), common ventricle, univentricular atrioventricular (AV) connection, unbalanced AV septal defect, mitral atresia with a normal aortic root, and certain heterotaxy syndromes.

Physiology

Single-ventricle physiology involves a single-ventricle supporting both pulmonary and systemic circulations, leading to mixed oxygenation and suboptimal systemic oxygen levels.

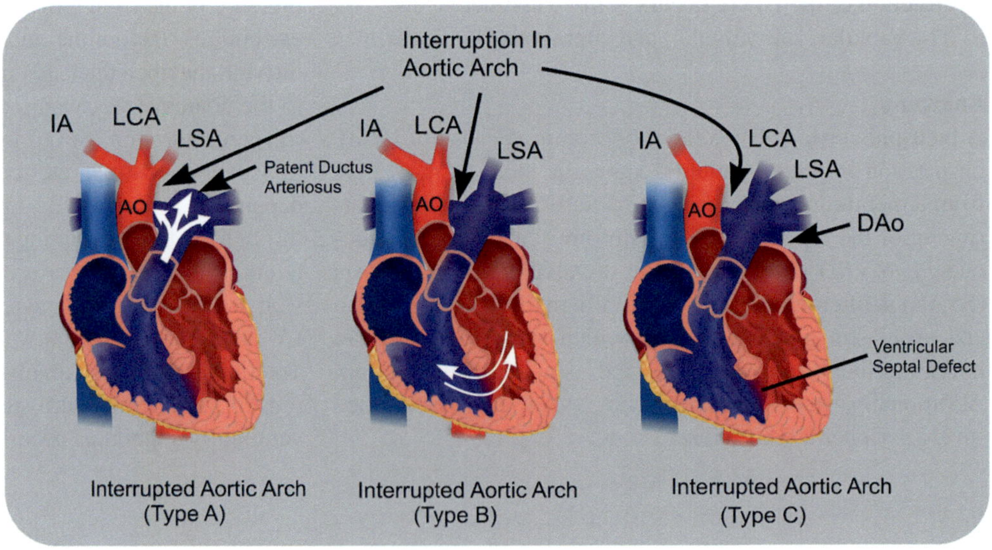

Fig. 24.9 Types of IAA. This detailed illustration depicts the three types of IAA: Type A, located distal to the left subclavian artery; Type B, positioned between the left carotid and left subclavian arteries; and Type C, situated between the innominate and left carotid arteries. LCA Left carotid artery, LSA Left subclavian artery, IA Innominate artery, AO Aorta, DAo Descending aorta

This often necessitates a series of palliative surgeries to improve blood flow and oxygenation.

Key features of single-ventricle physiology are:

1. Complete mixing of systemic and pulmonary venous blood at the atrial and/or ventricular levels.
2. Parallel ventricular output into both systemic and pulmonary systems, with flow distribution dependent on their relative resistances.

Management of Single-Ventricle Physiology

The overall goal in managing patients with single-ventricle physiology is to optimize systemic oxygen delivery. This requires balancing pulmonary (Qp) and systemic (Qs) blood flow, ideally maintaining a ratio close to 1:1. Increased pulmonary circulation may raise pulmonary oxygenation, but due to a fixed cardiac output, systemic blood flow decreases, leading to a net reduction in systemic oxygen delivery. Likewise, with increased systemic blood flow, pulmonary blood flow decreases significantly, to the point where the increased systemic flow cannot compensate for the markedly decreased pulmonary venous return and reduced net systemic oxygen content and delivery.

In scenarios with unrestricted pulmonary blood flow, interventions that influence the Qp:Qs ratio are primarily ventilatory measures affecting PVR. Anesthesia interventions, such as induction of anesthesia, oxygenation, lung recruitment, and inhaled anesthetic agents, can also impact Qp:Qs.

Treatment of Single-Ventricle Lesions: The Staged Surgical Approach

Initial Management: Ensuring Pulmonary Blood Flow

The first treatment step in managing patients with single-ventricle physiology is to ensure adequate pulmonary blood flow. In cases where the ductus arteriosus is the principal source of pulmonary flow (ductal-dependent), urgent administration of PGE1 is initiated to maintain ductal patency. This treatment often results in unrestricted pulmonary blood flow, necessitating further surgical intervention.

Subsequent surgical therapy involves:

- *Shunt Creation*: A surgical shunt, such as an mBTTS or a Sano Shunt (SS), is created from the systemic circulation to the pulmonary circulation. The shunt's size and length determine the degree of controlled pulmonary blood flow.
- *Pulmonary Artery Banding (PAB)*: In *non-ductal-dependent* lesions where there is excessive antegrade pulmonary blood flow, surgical banding of the pulmonary artery (PAB) may be necessary to restrict flow and manage pulmonary pressures effectively.

Second Stage: Bidirectional Glenn Shunt (BDG)

The second surgical stage in the single-ventricle pathway, known as the superior cavopulmonary shunt or bidirectional Glenn, is typically performed when the patient is between 3 and 6 months old. By this time, PVR has decreased sufficiently so that systemic venous pressure alone can drive the pulmonary circulation, providing enough flow and pressure gradient for effective pulmonary blood flow without the need for a systemic-to-PA shunt. During this procedure, the SVC is transected at its entry into the heart, and the cardiac end is oversewn. The SVC is then anastomosed end-to-side to the right PA (RPA). This configuration diverts all blood returning from the upper body and brain directly into the pulmonary arteries. The main PA is oversewn if necessary. This surgery significantly reduces the volume load on the single systemic ventricle by eliminating the recirculation of pulmonary venous blood into the PA through the closure of the systemic-to-PA shunt. Mild arterial hypercarbia is targeted to optimize venous return via the SVC by maintaining cerebral blood flow, as hypocarbia can decrease PVR but also reduce cerebral perfusion. Post-procedure, the expected oxygen saturation (SpO_2) ranges from 75% to 80%.

Final Stage: Fontan Procedure

The Fontan procedure is typically performed when a child is between 2 and 3 years old. As the patient grows, the IVC contributes an increasing proportion of venous blood flow to the total systemic venous return. The surgical creation of a pathway from the IVC directly into the PA allows for a total cavopulmonary connection, thus establishing the Fontan circulation. Following the Fontan procedure, the total systemic venous return now enters the PA directly. Moreover, the circulation is now completely in series: a single systemic ventricle provides the energy to propel blood through the systemic circulation and subsequently through the total cavopulmonary connection (TCPC) to the pulmonary circulation.

The Fontan Procedure: Achieving TCPC

Two main surgical techniques exist to create the Fontan circulation:

- *Lateral Tunnel Fontan*
- *Extracardiac Fontan*

Both techniques aim to connect the IVC to the PA, allowing the single-ventricle to pump blood through both the systemic and pulmonary circulations in series.

Hemodynamic Considerations

- *Increased IVC Pressure*: The Fontan procedure necessitates an increase in IVC pressure to generate the gradient required for blood to flow across the pulmonary vascular bed.

- *Reduced Preload*: This elevated IVC pressure can initially reduce pulmonary venous return and, consequently, lower cardiac output.
- *Fenestration Option*: A surgical fenestration between the Fontan baffle and the atrium can be created to allow some systemic venous blood to augment preload. However, this mixing of oxygenated and deoxygenated blood leads to a decrease in arterial SpO_2, typically to 75–80%.
- *Normal SpO_2*: Without a fenestration, a normal SpO_2 can be expected.

Tricuspid Atresia

Tricuspid atresia (TA) is the third most common cyanotic lesion.

Anatomy

In TA, the RV is hypoplastic. The classification depends on:

1. The alignment of the great vessels, with 70% showing normal relations and 30% displaying transposition.
2. The presence of pulmonary stenosis.
3. The existence and type of VSD.

Physiology

TA features single-ventricle physiology, where systemic and pulmonary circulations mix due to the absence of a functional RV. Key physiological aspects include:

- *Obligatory Atrial Shunt*: Systemic venous blood enters the systemic circulation and mixes with pulmonary venous blood through an atrial shunt, either an ASD or PFO.
- *Pulmonary Blood Flow*: This can be established via a VSD or via an extracardiac pathway by a PDA. In cases with pulmonary atresia, the PDA becomes the sole provider of pulmonary blood flow.
- *Cyanosis*: The degree of pulmonary blood flow typically determines the extent of cyanosis. Patients with a complex shunt involving a VSD and pulmonary stenosis are more likely to exhibit severe cyanosis.
- *Left Ventricular Load*: The LV handles both systemic and pulmonary blood flows in parallel, leading to increased volume load. This elevated pulmonary blood flow typically results in lower levels of cyanosis but increases the risk of CHF symptoms due to the volume strain.

Treatment

TA treatment often requires a staged approach, especially when pulmonary blood flow is ductal-dependent:

1. *Initial Management*
   - *PGE_1*: Urgent administration is necessary [majority of cases (70%)] to keep the ductus arteriosus open and maintain pulmonary blood flow.
2. *Surgical Intervention*

   Depending on the level of pulmonary blood flow, the next step may involve either:
   - *Establishment*: If flow is inadequate, an mBTSS surgically creates a connection to increase pulmonary blood flow.
   - *Restriction*: If flow is excessive, PA banding is performed to limit it and prevent complications.
3. *Progressive Surgical Management*:
   - *Bidirectional Glenn Procedure (BDG)*: This surgery partially separates the systemic and pulmonary circulations, reducing the workload on the single functioning ventricle and improving oxygenation efficiency.
4. *Final Palliation*:
   - The Fontan procedure is typically planned as the long-term solution, establishing a total separation of the circulations and redirecting all systemic venous blood directly into the pulmonary arteries without passing through a ventricle. This step is crucial for improving quality of life and functional status in patients with single-ventricle physiology.

Hypoplastic Left Heart Syndrome

HLHS is a complex congenital defect that is relatively common, occurring in approximately 1 in 10,000 live births.

Anatomy

In patients with HLHS, all left-sided structures of the heart are hypoplastic or atretic, leading to inadequate antegrade blood flow from the left ventricle to the aorta. Consequently, the flow to the proximal aortic arch, and thus the cerebral vascular bed and coronary arteries, is supplied retrograde from the ductus arteriosus.

Physiology

HLHS is a single-ventricle physiology with complex shunting:

- *Atrial Level Shunt*: An obligatory left-to-right shunt through an ASD or PFO and obstruction to left atrial and left ventricular outflow. Complete mixing of blood occurs in the RA.
- *Parallel Circulation*: The RV pumps blood to both the pulmonary and systemic circulations in parallel. Blood flows to the pulmonary and systemic circulation are dependent on their respective vascular resistances.

- *Ductal Dependence*: Systemic blood flow is provided by a PDA. Closure of the PDA leads to cardiovascular collapse, making PGE_1 therapy crucial until definitive surgical interventions are implemented.

Treatment: The Staged Approach

The management of HLHS involves a series of staged surgeries aimed at establishing a single-ventricle circulation (Fontan pathway).

1. *Stage 1- Neonatal Norwood Procedure*: The initial surgery in the neonate has three major goals:
   (a) Establishing sufficient complete mixing with an unrestrictive atrial communication via atrial septectomy.
   (b) Providing pulmonary blood flow with an RV to PA graft (Sano shunt) or with a systemic arterial-to-PA shunt (mBTTs).
   (c) Creating unobstructed antegrade outflow from the systemic ventricle to the aorta. After ligation of the distal main PA, a Damus-Kayne-Stansel anastomosis (DKS) utilizes the pulmonary valve and remaining proximal PA to connect the right systemic ventricle to the ascending aorta in conjunction with a reconstruction of the ascending aorta (Fig. 24.10).

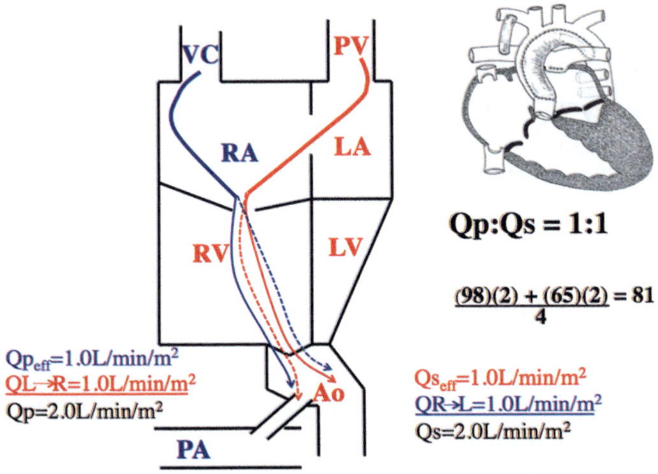

Fig. 24.10 Blood flows and saturations in HLHS with stage 1 palliation. This illustration provides a comprehensive view of the circulatory changes in HLHS following Stage 1 palliation, emphasizing the single-ventricle physiology. Effective pulmonary and systemic blood flows are illustrated with solid lines, depicting the primary circulation paths. In contrast, shunted blood flows, which bypass the normal circulatory route, are depicted with dotted lines. Labels include Qp (pulmonary blood flow), Qs (systemic blood flow), Qpeff (effective pulmonary blood flow), and Qseff (effective systemic blood flow), along with QR -> L (physiologic right-to-left shunt) and QL -> R (physiologic left-to-right shunt). This diagram offers a detailed visualization of the unique circulatory adaptations necessitated by HLHS

2. *Stage 2- Superior Cavopulmonary Connection (Bidirectional Glenn Shunt)*: After the initial Stage 1 procedure, patients undergo a superior cavopulmonary connection. This surgery connects the SVC to the pulmonary arteries, further reducing the volume load on the single-ventricle.
3. *Final Stage (Complete Cavopulmonary Connection—Fontan Procedure)*: This stage connects the IVC to the pulmonary arteries, establishing a TCPC. It creates a series circulation where the single-ventricle efficiently pumps blood through both the body and lungs, as previously described.

Complex Lesions

Transposition of the Great Arteries (TGA)

TGA accounts for 7–8% of CHD lesions, with an incidence of 0.2 per 1000 live births. There is a male predominance, with a male-to-female ratio of 3:1.

Anatomy

The most common TGA anatomy is Dextro-TGA (D-TGA), characterized by atrioventricular concordance but ventriculoarterial disconcordance. The aorta is positioned right-sided and anterior, arising from the RV, while the PA is left-sided and posterior, connected to the LV (Fig. 24.11). This arrangement results in parallel circulatory pathways, unlike the normal sequential circulation.

In TGA, the coronary arteries typically originate from the aortic sinuses facing the PA, with their anatomical position on the aorta being posterior. However, in most cases (70%), the coronary artery associations are normal, with the left coronary artery emerging from the left sinus and the right coronary artery from the right sinus. D-TGA is often associated with PFO, PDA, VSD, and subpulmonic stenosis or LVOT stenosis. Nearly, all patients have a PFO, while true ASDs are rare.

Physiology

Intercirculatory mixing in TGA can occur through intracardiac pathways such as PFO, ASD, or VSD, as well as through extracardiac routes like PDA or bronchopulmonary connections. The effectiveness of blood mixing depends on the number, size, and location of these communication sites. Often, one well-sized communication is more effective than multiple smaller ones.

Significant pulmonary stenosis can lead to hypoxemia in these patients, despite adequate intercirculatory mixing. Anatomic right-to-left shunting typically occurs at the PDA (from the RV to the aorta then to the PA) and, if a VSD is present, between the right and left ventricles to the PA. Conversely, anatomic left-to-right shunting primarily

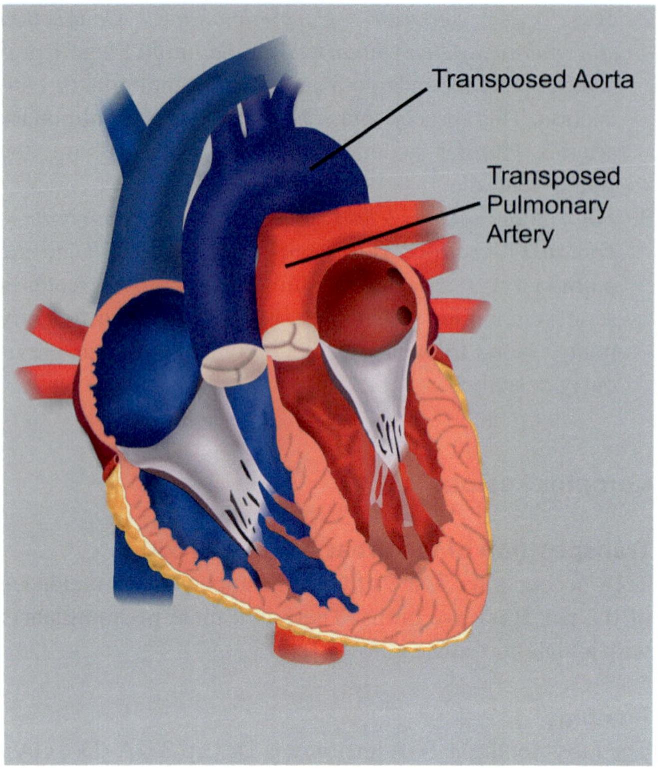

Fig. 24.11 TGA. This illustration provides a comprehensive view of the transposition of the great arteries, showcasing the anatomical misalignment where the aorta arises from the RV and the PA from the left ventricle. It highlights the resulting parallel circulation that impairs normal oxygenation of blood, essential for understanding the pathophysiology of TGA

takes place at the PFO, moving blood from the LA to the RA, then to the RV, and into the aorta.

The dynamics of intercirculatory mixing and shunting, including the direction of shunt, are influenced by various factors such as the size and location of the shunts, the size and compliance of the cardiac structures involved, heart rate, and ventilatory mechanics.

Treatment

In managing patients with TGA, prostaglandin E_1 is administered to maintain the patency of the ductus arteriosus, facilitating essential intercirculatory mixing. If the PFO is restrictive and intercirculatory mixing via the PDA alone proves insufficient, a balloon atrial septostomy (BAS) may be necessary to enhance mixing.

The definitive surgical intervention for TGA is the arterial switch operation (ASO). This procedure corrects the discordant ventriculoarterial connections by realigning the RV with the PA and the LV with the aorta. During ASO, both the PA and aorta are transected just above their respective valves. The coronary arteries are carefully detached from the native aorta with their ostia, and the surrounding tissue defects are meticulously repaired. The coronaries are then reimplanted into the neoaorta, previously the proximal PA.

Following coronary reimplantation, the great arteries are switched; the distal PA, now connected to the RV via the original proximal aorta, is moved anteriorly—a process known as the LeCompte maneuver. Simultaneously, the aorta, positioned posteriorly, is connected to the LV using the former proximal PA. This reconstructive approach ensures the correct routing of blood flow, aligning systemic and pulmonary circulations according to their functional demands.

Total Anomalous Pulmonary Venous Return (TAPVR)

TAPVR, a significant cyanotic CHD, accounts for 0.7–1.5% of all CHD cases with an overall incidence of 0.6–1.2 per 10,000 live births.

Anatomy

In TAPVR, the oxygen-rich blood from the pulmonary veins does not drain into the LA but instead into the systemic venous circulation. There are four types of TAPVR, depending on the drainage route from the pulmonary venous confluence to the systemic venous system:

1. Supracardiac
2. Cardiac
3. Infracardiac
4. Mixed

Physiology

TAPVR creates a left-to-right shunt, mixing systemic (deoxygenated) and pulmonary venous (oxygenated) blood within the RA. A PFO or ASD is crucial for allowing a compensatory right-to-left shunt to sustain blood flow to the LV. Compression or obstruction along the anomalous venous pathway can induce pulmonary venous hypertension, pulmonary edema, and PAH, significantly impairing cardiac output. The length of the venous pathway correlates with an increased risk of compression or stenosis. In severe cases, cardiac output can be significantly suppressed. In severe cases of TAPVR, patients can experience profound hypoxemia with lung edema and impaired oxygenation, intrapulmonary shunting, low pulmonary perfusion due to high PVR, right-to-left shunting via ductus arteriosus, low cardiac output, and high systemic oxygen extraction.

Treatment

- *Maintaining Systemic Circulation*: In patients with high PVR, prostaglandin E_1 therapy may be necessary to keep the ductus arteriosus open and ensure adequate blood flow to the body. However, with sub-systemic PA pressures a PDA will contribute to pulmonary edema.
- *Surgical Repair*: Obstructed TAPVR is a surgical emergency. The procedure involves:

- Creating a direct connection between the LA and the pulmonary venous confluence, typically located behind the LA.
- Closing any existing PFO or ASD.
- Ligating the abnormal connection between the pulmonary veins and the systemic venous system.

Truncus Arteriosus

Truncus arteriosus accounts for about 1–4% of all CHD.

Anatomy

In this condition, a single arterial vessel, known as the truncus, emerges from the heart, supplying blood to the systemic and pulmonary circulations as well as the coronary arteries, instead of the normal two separate vessels. At the base of this vessel sits a truncal valve, which can have four leaflets and may exhibit varying degrees of stenosis and regurgitation. A significant feature of truncus arteriosus is a large VSD located beneath the truncus (Fig. 24.12). The two anatomic classification systems utilize the origin of the pulmonary arteries to define four types of truncus arteriosus.

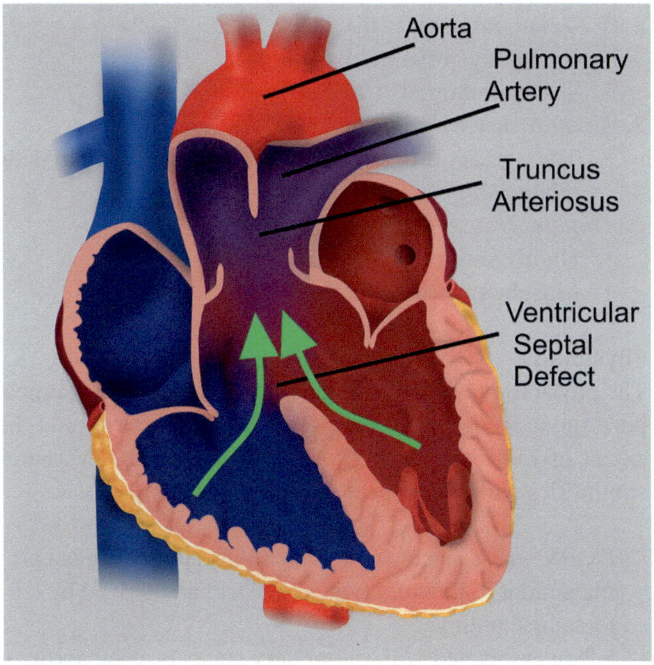

Fig. 24.12 Truncus Arteriosus. This illustration provides a comprehensive view of Truncus Arteriosus, depicting a single arterial vessel emerging from the heart that serves the dual function of supplying blood to both the systemic and pulmonary circuits. The graphic details the common truncal valve and the associated large VSD, highlighting the complex nature of this congenital heart defect and its effects on circulation

Physiology

Truncus arteriosus is characterized by a single-ventricle physiology with complete mixing of blood occurring at the ventricular level through an unrestrictive VSD. In this condition, the systemic and pulmonary circulations operate in parallel, with blood flow distribution dependent on the relative resistances of the pulmonary and systemic vascular beds. After birth, as pulmonary resistance decreases, there is an increased flow to the pulmonary system, potentially compromising systemic circulation. Conversely, if pulmonary hypertension develops, blood flow may preferentially divert to the systemic circulation. The risk of early development of pulmonary hypertension is significant due to the inherently high pulmonary blood flow and pressures associated with this condition.

Treatment

Early surgical repair is essential to prevent the development of pulmonary hypertension. The procedure typically involves the following steps:

1. *Closure of VSD*: A patch is used to close the VSD, preventing mixing of oxygenated and deoxygenated blood.
2. *Creation of RV-PA Conduit*: The pulmonary arteries are detached from the truncus and connected to the right ventricle using a conduit. The connection requires a right ventriculotomy.
3. *Truncal Valve Repair*: If the truncal valve is regurgitant or stenotic, it is repaired or replaced during the same surgery.
4. *Conduit Replacement*: As the child grows, the RV-PA conduit may need to be replaced to accommodate increased blood flow.

Atrioventricular Canal Defects

Atrioventricular canal defects (AVCDs), also known as atrioventricular septal defects or endocardial cushion defects, are congenital heart abnormalities that affect approximately 5% of all CHD and are commonly associated with trisomy 21. These defects affect the center of the heart and are characterized by incomplete development of the structures separating the heart's upper and lower chambers.

Anatomy

There are three primary types of AVCDs (Refer to Fig. 24.13):

- *Partial AVCD*: This type involves a primum ASD and a cleft mitral valve, featuring two distinct AV valves, leading to abnormal blood flow between the left and right atria and accompanied by mitral valve regurgitation.

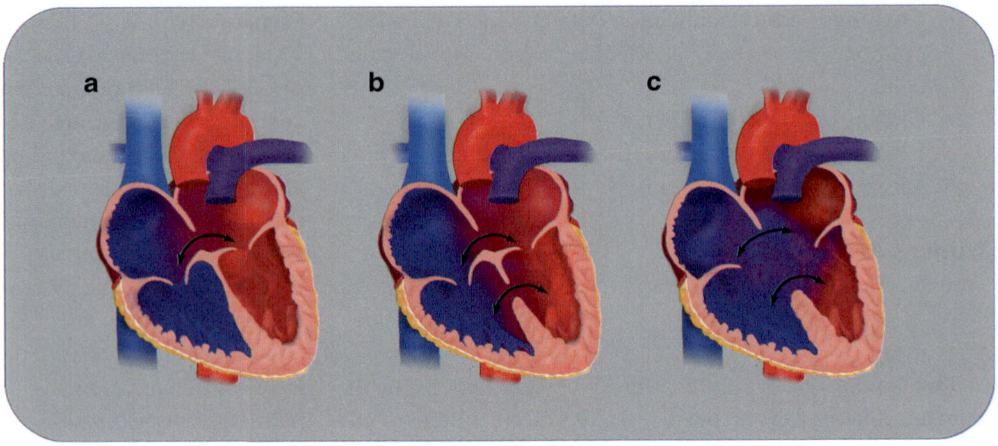

Fig. 24.13 AVCDs. This illustration offers a detailed view of the various types of AVCDs. Image (**a**) displays a Partial AVCD featuring a primum ASD and a cleft mitral valve. Image (**b**) shows a primum ASD along with a common AV valve orifice. Image (**c**) depicts a primum ASD, a common AV valve, and a large VSD

- *Transitional AVCD*: In this type, there is a primum ASD and a common AV valve orifice but functionally separate into two AV valves; the VSD is typically small or absent.
- *Complete AVCs (CAVCs)*: This is the most severe form, characterized by a large primum ASD, a common AV valve, and a large VSD.

Physiology

There is usually shunting between all four chambers due to the septal defects and AV valve regurgitation. The physiology generally follows that of large VSD with simple left-to-right shunting. The increased pulmonary blood flow increases the risk to develop PAH, especially in patients with trisomy 21. The surgical repair needs to be timed before pulmonary hypertension is established and at a time when the AV valve tissue is mature enough to be repaired. The repair is usually performed at around 3 months of age.

Treatment

Complete repair involves closing the ASD and VSD, along with repairing the AV valves. This often requires dividing the single, common AV valve into two separate, functioning valves.

- *Single-patch technique*: A technique exists that addresses the ASD, VSD, and AV valve septation using only one patch.
- *Two-patch technique*: For larger VSDs, a two-patch approach is necessary.

Double Outlet RV (DORV)

DORV has a prevalence of 1–3% among CHDs. It is often associated with genetic conditions such as trisomy 13 and 18.

Anatomy

DORV is a complex CHD where both the aorta and PA arise predominantly from the RV, with a wide range of anatomical variations.

Key features:

1. *VSD*:
   - Present in nearly all cases
   - VSD location distribution:
     - Subaortic: 50%
     - Subpulmonic: 30%
     - Doubly committed: 10%
     - Uncommitted: 10%
2. *Great Artery Relationship*:
   - The great arteries usually have a side-by-side relationship
3. *Outflow Tract and Conal Anatomy*:
   - Highly variable
   - Must be precisely defined

Physiology

The physiology of DORV largely depends on the anatomical positioning of the VSD relative to the great arteries and the extent of LVOT or RVOTO. Each variant of DORV shares similarities with other specific cardiac defects:

- DORV with a subaortic VSD exhibits a physiological profile similar to that of a typical VSD, characterized by left-to-right shunting.
- When associated with pulmonary stenosis, a subaortic or doubly committed VSD in DORV parallels the physiology of TOF, involving right-to-left shunting due to obstruction.
- A subpulmonary VSD in DORV mirrors the physiology seen in transposition of the D-TGA, with predominant

left-to-right shunting affecting systemic and pulmonary blood flow.

Treatment

Treatment strategies for DORV are tailored to the specific anatomical features of each case. A variety of surgical interventions are employed to establish an unobstructed pathway from the LV to the aorta, reconstruct the LVOT, and address the RVOT as needed. In certain cases, where anatomical constraints limit the efficacy of two-ventricle repair strategies, single-ventricle palliation may be considered as a viable alternative.

Please refer to Table 24.1 for a detailed comparison of cardiac shunts, categorized by their complexity and physiological impact.

Please refer to Table 24.2 for a detailed comparison of hemodynamic changes and the frequency of associated problems in various forms of CHD lesions. The table categorizes each condition by key clinical indicators including Hypoxemia, Intracardiac Shunting, Excessive Pulmonary Blood Flow, CHF, Left-Side Obstruction, Coronary Ischemia, Immature Circulation, and Obstruction to Pulmonary Flow.

Table 24.1 Simple and complex shunts

Simple shunts (no obstructive lesions)			*Complex shunts (shunt and obstructive lesions)*	
Restrictive shunts (small communication)	*Nonrestrictive shunts* (large communication)	*Common chambers* (complete mixing)	*Partial outflow obstruction*	*Total outflow obstruction*
Characteristics				
Large pressure gradient	Small pressure gradient	No pressure gradient	Shunt magnitude and direction largely fixed by obstruction	Shunt magnitude and direction totally fixed
Direction and magnitude more independent	Direction and magnitude more dependent on PVR/ SVR	Bidirectional shunting	Shunt depends less on PVR/ SVR	All flow goes through shunt
Less subject to control	More subject to control	Net Qp/Qs totally dependent on PVR/SVR	Orifice and obstruction determine pressure	Pressure gradient depends on orifice
Examples				
Small VSD, small PDA, Blalock shunts, small ASD	Large VSD, large PDA, large Waterston shunts	Single-ventricle, truncus arteriosus, single atrium	TOF, VSD, and pulmonic stenosis, VSD with coarctation	TA, mitral atresia, pulmonary atresia, aortic atresia

PVR Pulmonary vascular resistance, *SVR* Systemic vascular resistance, *VSD* ventricular septal defect

Table 24.2 Hemodynamic changes in CHD lesions

Frequency of hemodynamic problems in various forms of CHD								
Lesion	Hypoxemia	Intracardiac shunting	Excessive pulmonary blood flow	Congestive heart failure	Left-side obstruction	Coronary ischemia	Immature circulation	Obstruction to pulmonary flow
ASD	Rarely	Always (L -> R)	Usually	Rarely	Not seen	Not seen	Not seen	Rarely
PDA	Rarely	Always (L -> R)	Usually	Sometimes	Not seen	Not seen	Sometimes	Rarely
VSD	Rarely	Always (L -> R)	Usually	Often	Not seen	Not seen	Often	Late (PVOD)
Tetralogy of Fallot	Often	Always (L -> R)	Rarely	Sometimes	Not seen	Rare	Occasionally	Usually
Atrioventricular canal (partial or complete)	Rarely	Always (L -> R)	Usually	Often	Not seen	Rare	Often	Late (PVOD)
Transposition of the great arteries	Always	Always (mixing)	Sometimes	Sometimes	Rare	Sometimes	Often	Rarely
Coarctation of the aorta	Not seen	Occasionally (through PDA)	Rarely	Rarely	Always	Occasionally	Sometimes	Not seen
Interrupted aortic arch	Always (in lower body half)	Always (through PDA)	Rarely	Rarely	Always	Rarely	Usually	Not seen
Pulmonary atresia	Always	Always) (R -> L)	Sometimes	Sometimes	Rare	Occasionally	Usually	Always

(continued)

Table 24.2 (continued)

Frequency of hemodynamic problems in various forms of CHD								
Lesion	Hypoxemia	Intracardiac shunting	Excessive pulmonary blood flow	Congestive heart failure	Left-side obstruction	Coronary ischemia	Immature circulation	Obstruction to pulmonary flow
Truncus arteriosus	Usually	Always (mixing)	Usually	Often	Rare	Sometimes	Usually	Late (PVOD)
Anomalous origin of coronary arteries	Not seen	Not seen	Not seen	Often	Not seen	Always	Occasionally	Not seen
Single-ventricle	Usually	Always (mixing)	Often	Often	Occasionally	Sometimes	Usually	Occasionally
Aortic stenosis	Not seen	Not seen	Not seen	Occasionally	Always	Not seen	Occasionally	Sometimes
Critical aortic stenosis	Sometimes in lower body	Usually (PDA)	Not seen	Usually	Always	Usually	Frequently	Occasionally
Pulmonic stenosis	Occasionally	Not seen	Not seen	Occasionally	Not seen	Always	Not seen	Always
Critical pulmonary stenosis	Always	Usually (PDA)	Not seen	Usually	Not seen	Always	Not seen	Always
Tricuspid atresia	Always	Always	Frequently	Occasionally	Not seen	Always	Rarely	Frequently
Total anomalous pulmonary venous return	Always	Always	Sometimes	Frequently	Not seen	Frequently	Rarely	Always

L Left, *PDA* Patent ductus arteriosus, *PVOD* pulmonary vascular obstructive disease, *R* right

Further Reading

Jonas RA. Comprehensive surgical management of congenital heart disease. CRC Press; 2014.

Matte GS. Perfusion for congenital heart surgery: notes on cardiopulmonary bypass for a complex patient population. Wiley; 2015.

Nasr VG, DiNardo JA. The pediatric cardiac anesthesia handbook. Wiley; 2017.

Advanced Perfusion Strategies for Complex Pediatric Cardiac Surgery

25

Hugo Clifford, Ron Angona, and Ahmed Zaky

Introduction

Complex congenital cardiac surgery is increasingly common, thanks to advances in diagnosis, surgical techniques, medical management, and intensive care unit management, all contributing to improved outcomes and a broader range of pathologies now deemed operable. This chapter offers a detailed examination of advanced pediatric perfusion strategies for complex congenital cardiac surgery, highlighting the unique challenges of using cardiopulmonary bypass (CPB) in managing congenital heart defects in children. It underscores the importance of understanding cardiac anomalies and adapting perfusion methods specifically for pediatric patients, who differ significantly from adults in both anatomy and physiology. The role of the perfusionist is critical in pediatric cardiac surgery, as each congenital heart defect brings unique challenges related to the anomaly's complexity and the distinct physiological nuances of a developing child. The role of perfusion in making these cases possible cannot be overstated, as advances in monitoring and techniques have enabled smaller and sicker children to undergo bypass runs.

Building upon the valuable foundation laid by the American Society of ExtraCorporeal Technology (AmSECT) in their 2019 Standards and Guidelines for Pediatric and Congenital Perfusion Practice, this chapter is aims to equip perfusionists with the knowledge and tools to deliver safe and efficient extracorporeal support. While the AmSECT document provides a structured framework, each individual case presents a unique challenge, demanding a customized approach, tailored to meet individual challenges.

In this chapter, we will explore various congenital anomalies and their effects on cardiac function and blood flow. Additionally, we will review key physiologic considerations. Our focus will include strategies such as minimizing volume administration and reducing blood transfusions to optimize patient outcomes and minimize postoperative complications in the repair of complex cardiac defects.

Understanding and Classification of Congenital Heart Defects

Congenital heart defects are a diverse group of anomalies in the structure and function of the heart, present at birth. These defects range in complexity, requiring varied surgical approaches, and presenting unique challenges for perfusionists and demanding a customized CPB strategy.

1. Complexity:
   - Complex congenital defects are defects are those that may necessitate complex multistage surgeries, novel cannulation strategies, additional heart and pulmonary isolation, unusual coronary perfusion or prolonged cross-clamp times to facilitate extensive surgical repairs.
   - Non-complex congenital heart defects include simple atrial (ASD) or ventricular septal defects (VSD), partial anomalous pulmonary venous return, and most valve repair or replacement surgeries.
2. Cyanotic vs. non-cyanotic:

   They can broadly be described as either cyanotic or non-cyanotic.
   - Cyanotic defects are defects where deoxygenated systemic venous blood is delivered into the systemic cir-

H. Clifford
Department of Anesthesiology and Perioperative Medicine, University of Rochester School of Medicine and Dentistry, Rochester, NY, USA
e-mail: Hugo_Clifford@urmc.rochester.edu

R. Angona
Department of Surgery, Cardiovascular Perfusion, University of Rochester School of Medicine and Dentistry, Rochester, NY, USA
e-mail: Ron_Angona@urmc.rochester.edu

A. Zaky (✉)
Department of Anesthesiology and Perioperative Medicine, University of Alabama at Birmingham, Birmingham, AL, USA
e-mail: azaky@uabmc.edu

A. S. Awad, J. DiNardo (eds.), *Clinical Perfusion for Cardiac Surgery*, https://doi.org/10.1007/978-3-031-91163-7_25

culation, resulting in reduced oxygen saturation of arterial blood and cyanosis.
  - Non-cyanotic defects are those where the pulmonary and systemic systems are either isolated, preventing right to left physiologic shunting, or defects involving communications with predominantly left to right physiologic shunts.

Spectrum of Congenital Heart Defects

Please refer to Chap. 24 for a more comprehensive understanding of the spectrum of CHD pathologies.

- Septal defects: Abnormalities in the walls separating the heart chambers, allowing abnormal blood flow between them. Examples include ASD and VSD.
- Valve abnormalities: Defects affecting the function of the heart valves, leading to stenosis or regurgitation. Examples include tetralogy of Fallot (TOF) with pulmonary stenosis and aortic valve regurgitation.
- Single ventricle physiology: In patients with single ventricle physiology lesions wherein complete mixing of pulmonary venous and systemic venous blood occurs at the atrial or ventricular level and the ventricle(s) then distribute output to both the systemic and pulmonary beds in parallel. With these lesions it is possible for excessive pulmonary blood (PBF) or "pulmonary overcirculation" to steal flow from the systemic system, resulting in high output heart failure and low systemic blood pressure despite high arterial oxygen saturations. While management challenges posed by intracardiac shunting are often ameliorated while on bypass, extracardiac sources of shunting such as patent ductus arteriosus (PDA) and major aortopulmonary collateral arteries (MAPCAs) necessitate additional attention from the perfusion and surgical teams.
- *Extracardiac Shunting*
  The most common extracardiac source of shunting is a PDA. In some instances, this is an unrelated defect to the primary pathology and can be closed without substantial alteration to the patient's physiology. In other cases, however, it is an important source of pulmonary or systemic blood flow. In cases involving a hypoplastic arch, blood flow from the pulmonary artery through the duct is often necessary for lower body perfusion, and in cases of severe aortic stenosis or atresia retrograde flow to the proximal arch and root provides coronary circulation. In cases of pulmonic stenosis or atresia, flow from the distal arch through the duct provides an important source of pulmonary blood flow. In all these instances, PDA patency must be maintained with either a prostaglandin E_1 (PGE_1) infusion or a PDA stent.
- MAPCAs are collateral vessel communications between the aorta and the pulmonary vasculature that are a major or solitary source of PBF. They typically occur in conjunction with pulmonary atresia (PA); the most common lesion being TOF with PA. They vary in size, departure point from the aorta, course and number. Computerized tomography angiography (CTA) and cardiac catheterization, alone or in combination, are necessary to delineate their origins, course, and physiologic significance prior to operative intervention. Because they emerge from the aorta, they are a potential source of excessive PBF while on bypass. To ensure adequate systemic flow while on pump and to prevent large volumes of blood from returning to the left atrium via the pulmonary veins, their origins need to be dissected out and the surgical team must be ready to isolate them upon initiation of bypass. Definitive surgical therapy involves either unifocalization of the MAPCAs that are an important source of segmental lung perfusion to a central pulmonary artery, RV to pulmonary artery conduit creation, and VSD closure. Alternatively, as part of a staged palliative procedure, the unifocalized MAPCAs can be connected to aorta with a shunt appropriately sized to regulate PBF in preparation for further palliation or definitive repair.

General Principles Guiding Perfusion Practice in CHDs

- Minimizing CPB Time: Avoiding prolonged exposure to CPB is crucial to minimize potential complications.
- Maintaining Adequate Perfusion: Optimizing pump flow and oxygen delivery is essential for ensuring adequate organ perfusion and tissue oxygenation to meet the metabolic demands of the patient.
- Customized Prime Solutions: In pediatric patients, the volume of the prime solution can have a substantial impact due to their small blood volume. The prime is customized by adjusting electrolytes, adding medications, and possibly including blood products to ensure it is as physiologically close as possible.
- Custom Flow Rates: The flow rate during CPB is critical and is adjusted based on the patient's size, age, and specific cardiac condition. Pediatric patients require different flow rates compared to adults. For example, if the patient's weight is less than 3 kg, the desired CPB flow rate is typically between 150 and 200 mL/kg/min.
- Implementing a High-Flow, Low-Pressure Perfusion Approach: During CHD, surgeries are practiced in certain institutions, such as Texas Children's Hospital, where the flow rate is calculated as the patient's weight in kg multi-

plied by 150 mL/kg/min for patients weighing less than 10 kg.

- Preventing Blood Loss and Transfusion: Minimizing blood loss during surgery and reducing the need for blood transfusions are crucial for improving patient outcomes.
- Maintaining Temperature Control: Avoiding hypothermia and ensuring stable body temperature are essential for optimal physiologic function.
- Acid-Base Strategy of Arterial Blood Gas (ABG) Management: pH stat aims to maintain a normal pH level (7.4) throughout CPB. This strategy is preferred for most CHDs and can help prevent acidemia and its associated complications.

Advanced Techniques Guiding Perfusion Practice in CHDs

Advanced perfusion techniques necessitate meticulous planning and execution of CPB strategies, each tailored to the unique anatomical and physiological needs of individual patients. A key aspect of these techniques is the use of individualized CPB circuits, which significantly reduce prime volume and blood-product exposure. Also, cannulation strategy and regional perfusion. Additionally, advanced monitoring systems, including near-infrared spectroscopy (NIRS), flow rate monitoring, and continuous blood gas analysis, provide real-time data, enabling precise adjustments during surgery. Temperature management, particularly hypothermia, plays a significant role in protecting neurological function during complex procedures. Furthermore, the use of blood conservation techniques such as ultrafiltration. These advanced techniques, combined with a multidisciplinary team approach, ensure that perfusion practices in CHD surgeries are safe, efficient, and patient-centered.

Individualized Circuit Design

Pediatric patients vary greatly in size and weight, especially when comparing neonates to older children. Therefore, the CPB circuit is often customized for each patient. This involves selecting appropriate tubing sizes, oxygenator types, and other components that are proportionate to the patient's size with the goal toward reducing the prime volume, particularly for neonates and infants, thus decreasing hemodilution. One effective method to achieve this reduction is using smaller diameter tubing. This not only decreases the prime volume but also reduces the overall surface area, thereby lowering the volume required for effective perfusion. For children weighing less than 7 kg, CPB circuits can typically be primed with as little as 220 mL. Another method to further reduce the prime volume is by excluding the arterial filter, which can decrease the prime volume to 180 mL. This technique has been effectively used in bloodless surgeries. For children weighing between 7 and 12 kg, circuits with a 270 mL prime volume are suitable. In the case of children weighing between 15 and 30 kg, specific A-V loops and pediatric oxygenators are used. However, in the high-flow, low-pressure technique, a minimum of 350 mL of priming is required for children weighing less than 7 kg. This is because it requires arterial and venous cannulae that are usually larger in size to accommodate the necessary flow.

Cannulation Strategy and Regional Perfusion

1. Repair of intracardiac defects requires isolation of the surgical field during bypass and aortic cross-clamping. This is generally achieved with a bicaval cannulation technique to capture venous return through the superior and inferior vena cava. A left ventricular vent is placed to capture any return through the pulmonary veins and to assist in deairing prior to separation from bypass. For non-complex repairs such as straightforward atrial and VSD or valve repairs or replacements, this, along with single or multiple dose cardioplegia delivered through the aortic root, is generally sufficient. More complex pathologies require additional techniques.
   - When a persistent left superior vena cava is present, this venous blood return is often captured with an additional venous cannula.
   - Alterations in coronary anatomy, or surgeries requiring reimplantation of the coronaries, may require cardioplegia to be delivered retrograde or directly into the individual coronary arteries.
   - Coronary sinusoids present a unique challenge for myocardial perfusion while on bypass, and may be a contraindication to heart isolation entirely, as retrograde coronary perfusion is dependent on ventricular filling and pressurization.
2. Patients with defects of the aortic arch present challenges for perfusion. Alterations in cannula placement, size, or number, as well as specialized techniques such as regional perfusion or deep hypothermic circulatory arrest may be utilized. When considering the approach to arch defects, it is important to bear in mind the purpose of CPB, which is the delivery of sufficient oxygenated blood to the tissues to meet metabolic requirements. In particular, the perfusion strategy must be designed to minimize disruption of perfusion of the myocardium and brain via the coronary and carotid arteries, respectively, as these organs are highly susceptible to ischemic injury.

- In patients with normal aortic arch anatomy, the proximal ascending aorta can be cannulated. This allows antegrade flow through the arch, up the carotids, and down to the descending aorta, as well as flow back to the aortic root and coronary arteries until a cross-clamp is applied.
  - In patients with arch defects, such placement is often impractical. Flow through the arch during bypass makes opening the aorta to achieve a repair impossible, and in cases of interrupted aortic arch, an arterial cannula in the ascending aorta will not provide flow to the descending aorta or the left carotid and subclavian arteries. These surgical exposure and perfusion issues can be managed using either deep hypothermic circulatory arrest or regional perfusion. In deep hypothermic circulatory arrest, the patient is placed on bypass in the normal fashion, then cooled to 18–22 °C in order to reduce their metabolic demand total body oxygen consumption (VO_2). A PDA, if present, must be ligated prior to cooling. If an interrupted aortic arch (IAA) is present, a second arterial cannula Y-ed off the primary arterial cannula is placed through the PDA to achieve lower body perfusion and cooling. Once the target temperature is achieved, flow perfusion is then stopped to provide a dry field while the surgeon opens the aorta and performs the repair. Meticulous surgery planning is necessary to minimize circulatory arrest time and must be kept as short as possible to reduce the risk of ischemic brain injury.
  - Antegrade cerebral perfusion (ACP) allows for selective perfusion of the brain, while allowing termination of flow into the surgical field for surgery on the ascending aorta, aortic arch, and proximal descending aorta. Typically, an arterial cannula is placed through a chimney graft that is sewn onto the base of the innominate artery. Once the patient is placed on CPB through this graft, antegrade flow is provided through the artery to the right subclavian and carotid, and retrograde flow is provided into the aortic arch. The patient is cooled to reduce VO_2, and then a clamp is applied proximal to the chimney graft. Flow is then delivered solely down the right subclavian artery and up the right carotid artery. In the presence of an intact circle of Willis, it is generally acknowledged that the entire brain is perfused. The quantity of flow delivered through the cannula is reduced to approximately 30—70 mL/kg/min, given that only the brain, with reduced metabolic demand due to hypothermia, is being perfused (Fig. 25.1).

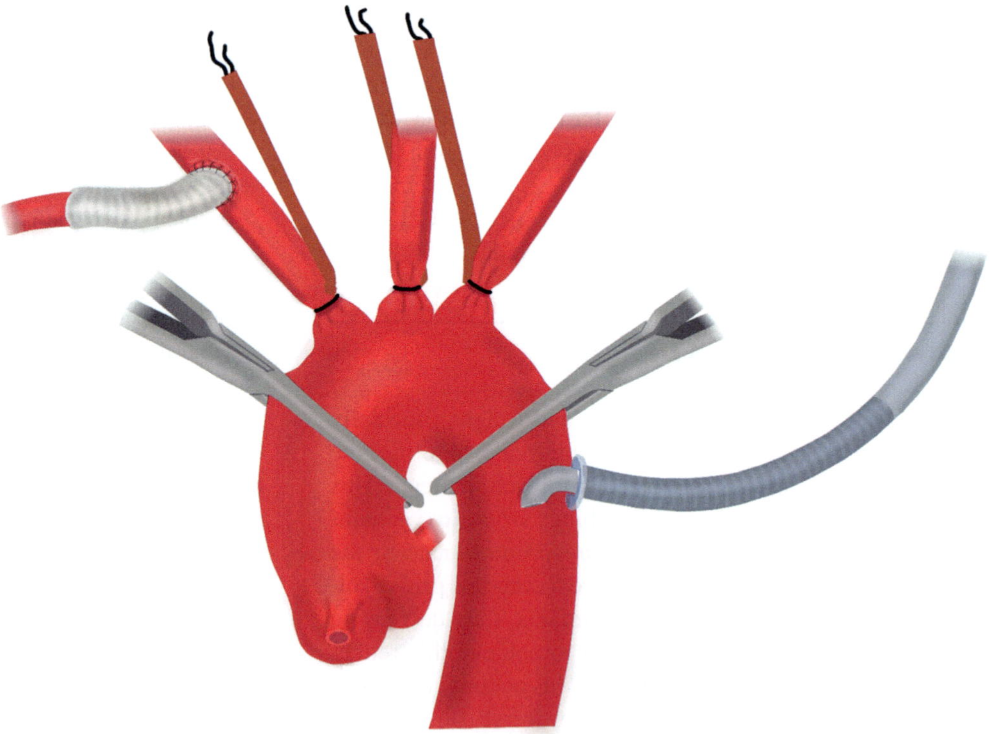

Fig. 25.1 This illustration demonstrates aortic arch reconstruction using ACP, a technique that ensures cerebral protection during surgery by providing direct blood flow to the brain. Arterial inflow is channeled through a cannulated polytetrafluoroethylene graft after anastomosis to the innominate artery. Snares on the arch arteries are used to maintain a bloodless surgical field, while a clamp on the descending aorta isolates the arch. Distal aortic perfusion is maintained using an aortic cannula

Continuous Gas Monitoring

The ability to monitor arterial and venous blood gases at the point-of-care is essential to delivery of modern pediatric cardiac surgical care. Historically, blood samples had to be sent to a central lab for blood gas analysis, resulting in an unavoidable delay in obtaining results. The development of reliable, validated point-of-care blood gas systems has greatly reduced (or eliminated) this delay by allowing practitioners to perform their own testing, typically right in the operating room. This is particularly critical in pediatric cardiac surgery where decisions need to be made on a moment-to-moment basis. However, while samples can be run serially, it is burdensome and impractical to do this while performing clinical practice and a benchtop point-of-care blood gas analyzers provide only intermittent, point in time data. Therefore, continuous gas monitoring systems have been developed in the past 20 years that provide a stream of data that can be viewed in addition to performing traditional point-of-care blood gas analysis. The use of continuous gas monitoring devices has become a standard in modern pediatric perfusion.

- Continuous gas monitoring systems take advantage of the unique properties of CPB, the presence of continuous blood flow through extracorporeal tubing.

Continuous gas monitoring systems are generally categorized into two categories: In-line gas monitors where sensors are inserted into the blood path within the CPB circuit, and external monitors that utilize "clip-on" probes attached to the cardiopulmonary bypass circuit tubing. While there are differences in functionality, both systems provide perfusionists with real-time blood gas data. Both systems also have alarm capabilities that alert clinicians if a particular parameter falls outside a predetermined range.

- *In-line gas monitors* utilize a cuvette-based system generally placed within a shunt line in the bypass circuit. Blood passes through the cuvette, which is attached to a sensor. Utilizing optical fluorescence technology, data is collected and displayed on the attached screen. The cuvettes are disposable and are discarded at the end of each case. Prior to use, a two-point, in vitro calibration is performed.
- *External systems* utilize probes that clip around the PVC tubing of the CPB circuit. Readings are gathered using ultrasonic technology and transit time. The probes are reusable, and therefore the only expense associated with the system is the purchase of the hardware. There is nothing in the physical blood path of the circuit. External systems also provide the advantage of being able to detect gaseous microemboli (GME).

Depending on the platform used, currently available continuous gas monitoring systems measure or calculate data such as pH, pO_2, pCO_2, Hemoglobin/Hematocrit, temperature, saturation, and electrolytes such as K^+ and Ca^+. Some systems can monitor both arterial and venous blood gases. When connected to the CPB machine and incorporating bypass flow rates, variables such as oxygen delivery (DO_2) and consumption (VO_2) can be calculated and displayed.

In comparison to traditional time-based performance of arterial and venous blood gases during pediatric open heart surgery, the use of continuous gas monitoring provides limitless opportunities for data collection.

- Typical continuous gas monitoring systems collect a data point every 1–6 seconds.

This can allow for comparison of this data against hemodynamic parameters, CPB pump flows, and other variables. Commercially available continuous gas monitoring systems interface with almost all major electronic medical record (EMR) platforms, as well as bypass charting systems available from perfusion product manufacturers. Practitioners are continuing to find new ways to utilize the data collected to improve practice. Much of the currently available literature centers around standardization of practice and adherence to accepted ranges for various parameters. Users are more quickly alerted to changes in patient status than with traditional blood gas monitoring devices. In 2019, AmSECT, in the Pediatric Standards and Guidelines document, which, was mentioned earlier, recommends the use of continuous blood gas monitoring in pediatric cardiac surgery, based on available literature at the time. These standards were then published in peer reviewed journals supported by pediatric cardiac surgery and pediatric cardiac anesthesia societies.

- There are limitations that exist with utilization of current continuous gas monitoring systems.

Despite the ease of performing the required calibration prior to use, some of the current systems exhibit a significant drift of values over time, requiring additional in-vivo calibration. If significant enough, this drift can present practitioners with inaccurate data which if acted upon could have clinical significance. There is a significant cost associated with incorporating the system into practice. Additionally, current regulatory limitations do not allow continuous gas monitoring systems to replace existing point-of-care blood gas monitoring devices. They are only approved for use as a "trending device" to assist with clinical practice. Blood gas analysis on traditional benchtop models still needs to be performed according to institutional protocols.

Flow Rate Monitoring

The accurate measurement of flow (volume/time) within a bypass circuit is an essential monitoring component across all patient populations. In pediatric patients particularly the smallest and those with complex anatomy, it becomes even more critical. While the most commonly reported flow within a bypass circuit is the arterial flow, flows in the venous line, cardioplegia system, and cardiotomy suctions and vents are also important in making clinical decisions.

- In roller-pump based CPB circuits, as are typically used in the pediatric population, arterial flow is measured at the location of the pump boot or raceway.

The flow is calculated from the direct measurement of pump revolutions per minute (RPMs) multiplied by the volume of fluid within the pump head raceway. The volume of fluid within the pump head raceway is determined by the tubing diameter within the raceway and the raceway size. Output is reported in liters or milliliters per minute. In systems where a centrifugal-based arterial pump is used, flow is measured via an external probe that clips around the bypass tubing. Flow is directly measured and displayed using ultrasonic technology, with the probes calibrated to the type and size of tubing. Flow measurements obtained by both methods are generally captured and documented in the EMR.

- A limitation of arterial flow monitoring at the location of the raceway is that it may not accurately reflect the net flow delivered to the patient due to the presence of multiple *shunts* within the bypass circuit that are distal to the flow monitoring location.

These shunts recirculate some of the pump output away from the patient to a location prior to the raceway such as the venous reservoir.

- In a situation where a shunt—or multiple shunts—is present, the actual flow delivered to the patient might be significantly less than what is displayed on the output screen.

Typical shunts within a bypass circuit can include a sampling manifold, oxygenator recirculation lines, continuous gas monitoring, or ultrafiltration systems.

- Despite other hemodynamic and laboratory measurements being present during bypass, inaccurate flow monitoring still risks organ hypoperfusion and can have deleterious effects.

Shunt flow should be compensated for while on CPB by increasing arterial blood flow by an amount equivalent that is diverted through shunts. This can be achieved by altering arterial flow to keep arterial line pressure constant. Unfortunately, this method is only valid if it is assumed that patient systemic vascular resistance (SVR) is constant. In addition, this method is relatively insensitive to acute changes in shunt flow. For these reasons, the guidelines for pediatric perfusion practice by AmSECT recommend the use of an external flow monitoring device at the most distal point in the bypass circuit, to ensure accurate measurement and documentation of net patient arterial flow. This guideline is based on literature demonstrating that shunt flow becomes more and more relevant as patient size decreases, to a point where in the smallest children a clinically significant percentage of proximally measured arterial flow might not be reaching the patient. Inaccurate flow measurement in this situation can have catastrophic consequences, particularly when there are shunts open. This is made worse as patient size decreases, with the very smallest patients being most at risk for injury.

- One unique situation where accurate measurement of arterial flow is magnified in importance is during the conduct of ACP. Because typical ACP flows are 30–70 mL/kg/min, very small changes (often, just 1 RPM) in arterial pump speed can significantly alter the flow being delivered.

Another less frequently used location for flow monitoring during bypass, is on the venous side of the circuit utilizing external flow probes. This technology is particularly useful in children with MAPCAs. MAPCAs represent another location for "recirculation"—wherein arterial flow does not get delivered to the patient. However, unlike in circuit shunt flow, this loss of flow through collaterals would not be identified with a distal external flow probe on the arterial line. Using a flow probe on the venous line, a flow mismatch could be identified that will alert the clinician to the presence of collateral blood flow, and the potential need to modify practice accordingly. Frequently this can be visually identified by the surgeon first through excessive return to the left heart requiring the use of left heart venting.

As in arterial flow monitoring, venous flow monitoring can be uniquely useful during ACP. The use of a venous flow probe can identify potential problems during ACP, by identifying a mismatch with blood flow from the arterial line.

Nearly all bypass systems incorporate flow monitoring in the cardioplegia systems. As with arterial flow monitoring, cardioplegia flow is measured at the level of the pump head. However, there are typically no shunts present in the cardioplegia system, so measurement of flow at this location is sufficient. Flow monitoring is essential to quantify not just the rate of cardioplegia administration but also the volume of solution delivered. Additionally, many centers utilize the cardioplegia system to perform modified ultrafiltration (MUF) as well. Here it is even more essential to accurately quantify flow as the flow delivered to the MUF circuit is a set percentage of arterial flow, and the inaccurate measurement of flow could create a safety concern.

A frequently used technique in pediatric cardiac surgery is aortic venting, used to decompress the aorta during the cross-clamp period and de-air the heart prior to and after removal of the aortic cross-clamp. A catheter is placed directly in the base of the aortic root and connected to a line that returns blood to the cardiotomy reservoir via a roller pump. Flow monitoring occurs at the roller pump.

- Prior to and after removal of the aortic cross-clamp, any blood being pulled through the aortic sump decreases the amount of output coming from the arterial cannula.

This puts the patient at risk of coronary steal or hypoperfusion if this sump flow rate is too high. An aortic sump flow rate of less than 10% of the arterial flow is generally agreed to be safe within the pediatric perfusion community.

Managing Drainage Problems

Children requiring CPB for cardiac surgery encounter the same spectrum of problems with venous drainage experienced in the adult population. However, there are elements of congenital anatomy and physiology which present unique situations where modifications to traditional venous cannulation and drainage strategies are required.

Ideally, adequate venous drainage can be achieved utilizing appropriately sized and placed venous cannulas and gravity alone. In general, bi-caval or dual cannulation is more frequently utilized in pediatric practice than in adults. Assessment of adequate venous drainage during bypass should occur at the onset of CPB but also throughout the bypass run, as changes to heart position and other variables can impact drainage. Pulmonary artery catheters are rarely utilized during pediatric cardiac surgery, so a central venous catheter in the superior vena cava (SVC) is likely to be the only hemodynamic monitor capable of detecting elevated right heart and SVC pressures. However, in the presence of an SVC caval snare, the tip of the central venous catheter may be located distal to the snare. In this case, direct visualization of a distended SVC would be indicative of impaired SVC drainage. In this situation the patient's head must be inspected for evidence of SVC syndrome. Cerebral NIRS, utilized by many centers, may be useful in identifying cannula malposition and/or inadequate drainage. A precipitous decrease in a stable NIRS value should raise concern about such issues. As with adult patients, cannula repositioning or replacement of an existing cannula with a larger cannula may be necessary.

Despite adequate venous drainage, there can continue to be left heart distension on CPB with left ventricle (LV) ejection if the heart is not arrested. Blood flow to the left heart during CPB arises from several sources. The Thebesian veins drain a very small portion of the coronary circulation into the left atrium and ventricle. This flow will cease when the aortic cross-clamp terminates coronary blood flow. The bronchial veins drain into the pulmonary veins and subsequently into the left atrium and ventricle. The bronchial circulation may be very large in patients with cyanotic heart disease. In some patients, a large portion of pulmonary blood flow may be supplied by anatomic (PDA, MAPCAs) or surgical systemic-to-pulmonary artery communications (Blalock-Thomas-Taussig, Waterston, Potts, or central shunts). If these communications are not ligated or controlled before initiating CPB, the blood return to the pulmonary artery—and subsequently to the left atrium and left ventricle—may be substantial. In this circumstance, venting will relieve left heart distension. However, unless CPB flow rate is increased by an amount equal to the vented blood systemic oxygen delivery to the patient will be compromised. Flow return to the left ventricle also may result from an incompetent aortic valve. In this instance, retrograde filling of the left ventricle with blood from the aortic cannula will occur until the aortic cross-clamp is applied.

In some congenital defects surgical exposure to an extended portion of the SVC may be necessary to complete the surgical repair. For example, in patients undergoing a superior cavopulmonary anastomosis (bidirectional Glenn procedure) it may be necessary to cannulate the innominate vein, often with a downsized cannula, to facilitate surgical exposure and drain the upper body. A similar strategy may be necessary in repair of sinus venosus defects with anomalous drainage of the right pulmonary veins to the SVC.

A commonly encountered systemic venous anomaly encountered in children with congenital heart defects is a persistent left superior vena cava (LSVC). Management of the LSVC on CPB depends on several factors:

- proposed procedure and desired exposure
- size of the vessel
- drainage site into the coronary sinus or directly into the atrium
- presence or absence of a bridging vein connecting the LSVC to right superior vena cava (RSVC)

Based on these variables, a decision must be made as to whether the LSVC drainage can be managed with cannulation of the RSVC, separate cannulation of both SVC, or with continuous cardiotomy suction at the site of LSVC drainage once the heart is opened.

Many children with heterotaxy syndrome have an inferior vena cava (IVC) that is interrupted between the kidneys and the liver. These patients have direct drainage of the hepatic veins into the floor of the atrium and drainage of the IVC below the interruption to the SVC via an azygos or a hemiazygous vein. As with management of an LSVC, interrupted IVC can be managed with separate cannulation that is then Y-ed into the main venous drainage line.

Venous drainage during CPB typically occurs by gravity. The height difference between the heart and the venous reservoir, coupled with a "siphon" effect in the system enables drainage adequate enough for most patients. In congenital heart disease, however, many of the issues discussed above prohibit gravity alone from providing adequate venous drainage.

Vacuum-assisted venous drainage (VAVD) is one method that can be utilized to augment venous return to the bypass circuit. Modern hard-shell venous reservoirs for cardiac surgery are open to the atmosphere. VAVD involves "sealing" the reservoir to the outside by closing tubing connection ports and then applying regulated vacuum to the reservoir. By generating a larger negative pressure gradient, VAVD can be used to augment venous drainage beyond what would be expected from gravity alone for a venous cannula and venous line of a given size., Consequently, the use of VAVD is very effective in enabling the miniaturization of the CPB circuit by allowing for much shorter and smaller diameter tubing. Additionally, VAVD can be utilized in cases where significant venous air, or even an air lock, is present to maintain the venous drainage. VAVD is not typically successful in correcting drainage from a poorly positioned venous cannula.

When utilizing VAVD, certain safety considerations should be adhered to prevent adverse events. The range of negative pressure generally utilized for VAVD is −40–60 mmHg, although some centers will utilize pressures as low as −100 mmHg. A primary concern is the potential for negative pressure to cause lysis of erythrocytes leading to high levels of plasma-free hemoglobin. An additional safety concern is the potential for VAVD to pressurize the venous line and cause retrograde flow up the venous line, putting the patient at risk for systemic air embolism. Used cautiously and with appropriate safety equipment and monitoring, VAVD can be a very useful technique in pediatric cardiac surgery.

Autologous Priming Techniques

Autologous priming techniques are a family of CPB techniques utilized to decrease the dilutional effect of the circuitry prime volume. Originally developed in adult cardiac surgery, all of the techniques are now selectively utilized in the conduct of pediatric cardiac surgery to mitigate the hemodilution effects of a large CPB prime volume relative to patient blood volume.

- Retrograde autologous priming (RAP), while relatively common in adult practice, is infrequently utilized in the conduct of pediatric cardiac surgery.

After heparinization and arterial cannulation, retrograde flow is permitted down the arterial line. This displaces the crystalloid "prime" solution of the bypass circuit with the patients' own (autologous) blood. The crystalloid is collected in a bag or a reservoir. The effect is a net decrease in the overall crystalloid volume that is interfaced with the patients' blood volume, and therefore less hemodilution. Frequently cited benefits of RAP include a reduction in the use of homologous blood products, as well as a higher Hct while on CPB.

RAP takes advantage of the fact that most patients have excess blood volume that is not needed to maintain cardiac preload and mean arterial pressure. Volume removal during RAP cannot be done indiscriminately or too quickly.

- RAP requires an attentive operator to prevent adverse events. Attention must be paid to the mean arterial pressure and cardiac rhythm during performance of the technique, and clear communication should exist between the perfusion, anesthesia, and surgical teams prior to the initiation of RAP and while it is being conducted.

RAP can be discontinued at any time if the patient experiences any hemodynamic compromise. Hemodynamic instability occurs more frequently in patients with critical aortic stenosis, patients of small size, and single ventricle patients, who are often more preload dependent.

The conduct of RAP should be undertaken gradually to ensure that excessive negative pressure is not created, which could potentially entrain air through an aortic purse string and into the arterial line. Constant vigilance by the perfusionist to the arterial line is essential, as is the slow, gradual removal of volume.

Venous autologous priming (VAP) utilizes volume removed from the venous line to displace circuit crystalloid circuit volume. VAP begins after placement of one or both of the venous cannulae. Unlike RAP, VAP involves the FORWARD flow of volume down the venous line and into a collection bag. Depending on institutional preference, the collection site can be sited either before or after the venous reservoir. Typically, the venous line is partially unclamped to begin slow drainage of crystalloid out of the circuit. Much like RAP, VAP needs to be undertaken in a slow, controlled manner to ensure there is no compromise of hemodynamic stability.

Acute normovolemic hemodilution (ANH) is a blood conservation technique that involves the pre-bypass removal of whole blood from the patient into collection bags prior to systemic anticoagulation. ANH can be undertaken at any time after induction of anesthesia and is usually accomplished by draining patient blood out of a large-bore central venous catheter into collection bags that contain a predetermined quantity of citrate as an anticoagulant. As blood is drained into the storage bags euvolemia is maintained with simultaneous infusion of a balanced crystalloid solution. Much like RAP and VAP, ANH can be discontinued at any time if the patient exhibits hemodynamic instability. Following ANH, any blood lost during the surgical procedure will have a reduced red cell mass as compared to the collected blood, and consequently erythrocyte loss will be reduced. In addition, because whole blood is withdrawn from the patient, reinfusion of the collected blood will provide a plasma transfusion as well as a transfusion of platelets that have not been exposed to the CPB circuit. Reinfusion is undertaken after termination of CPB and protamine administration.

Ultrafiltration Techniques

Ultrafiltrators are devices commonly added to the CPB circuit to remove excess fluid and produce hemoconcentration. When used in conjunction with CPB, these devices produce an ultrafiltrate that occurs as the result of a hydrostatic pressure gradient across a semipermeable membrane. These are the same devices that can be used for hemodialysis when they are used in conjunction with a dialysate. When used during CPB, they are commonly called hemoconcentrators, as they produce an increase in hematocrit by removing excess fluid. Please refer to Chap. 19 for a more comprehensive understanding of ultrafiltration techniques.

Further Reading

Chai P, Kussman BD. Myocardial protection and preservation for neonates and infants. In: Gravlee GP, Davis RF, Hammon JW, Kussman BD, editors. Cardiopulmonary bypass principles and practice. 4th ed. Philadelphia: Lippincott Williams and Wilkins; 2016.

Mascio CE, Gaynor JW. Brain injury and neuroprotective strategies in pediatric cardiac surgery. In: Gravlee GP, Davis RF, Hammon JW, Kussman BD, editors. Cardiopulmonary bypass principles and practice. 4th ed. Philadelphia: Lippincott Williams and Wilkins; 2016.

Matte GS. Perfusion for congenital heart surgery: notes on cardiopulmonary bypass for a complex patient population. 1st ed. Hoboken: Wiley-Blackwell; 2015.

Matte GS, DiNardo JA. Pediatric cardiopulmonary bypass. In: Gravlee GP, Davis RF, Hammon JW, Kussman BD, editors. Cardiopulmonary bypass principles and practice. 4th ed. Philadelphia: Lippincott Williams and Wilkins; 2016.

Oldeen ME, Angona RE, Hodge A, Klein T. American Society of ExtraCorporeal Technology: development of standards and guidelines for pediatric and congenital perfusion practice (2019). J Extra Corpor Technol. 2020;52(4):319–26. https://doi.org/10.1182/ject-2000045. PMID: 33343035; PMCID: PMC7728496.

Ungerleider RM, Meliones JN, McMillan KN, Cooper DS, Jacobs JP, editors. Critical heart disease in infants and children. 3rd ed. Philadelphia: Elsevier; 2019.

Part VII

Clinical Problems and Complications During Cardiopulmonary Bypass

Mechanical Complications of Cardiopulmonary Bypass

26

Brian J. Kinsman, Naomi Hood, and Michael G. Fitzsimons

Introduction

Cardiopulmonary bypass (CPB) is a critical tool to successfully perform open cardiac surgery, but not without significant risk. Despite 70 years of clinical application with ongoing improvements in safety measures, mechanical complications of cardiopulmonary bypass occur with incidence rates of approximately 1:1400 with injury and 1:4600 with mortality.

National surveys of cardiopulmonary bypass performed in the 1990s–2000s highlighted the most common and morbid complications of CPB. However, resources for the identification and management of these complications are limited. This chapter aims to provide a guide that identifies the most morbid and common mechanical complications of CPB, the risk to the patient, etiology, clinical presentation, and management for mechanical complications of cardiopulmonary bypass along each component of the CPB circuit.

The perfusion team plays a central role in the safe conduct of CPB, although all perioperative team members, including surgeons, anesthesiologists, and nurses, share responsibility for comprehensive patient safety. Therefore, we consider each of these complications in the context of a coordinated, team-based response to intraoperative cardiopulmonary bypass emergencies. A standardized intraoperative emergency event response protocol should be activated that includes (1) a clear announcement of the complication in question to all care teams to re-focus attention toward emergency management, (2) call for additional human and equipment resources including additional perfusionist, anesthesiologist and surgeon if possible, (3) a discussion and decision of the viability to wean off CPB until resolution of the emergency if indicated, (4) a clear announcement when the emergency is resolved, (5) discussion of the impact of the complication on remainder of the operation and patient care needs, and (6) postoperative debrief that includes all team members involved with a focus on quality improvement rather than assigning blame.

Iatrogenic Aortic Dissection

Central cannulation for CPB is typically performed at the distal ascending aorta. Peripheral cannulation may include access via the femoral, axillary, or subclavian arteries. Complications of aortic cannulation include aortic dissection, intramural hematoma, and cannula malposition. Aortic dissection, while a relatively rare complication (1: 1700 cases), is associated with high rates of neurologic morbidity and mortality. Aortic dissection is posited to be caused by intimal injury with subsequent pressurized propagation and extension of this subintimal space (Fig. 26.1). Aortic dissection can happen at any stage during CPB, including postoperatively, but it most frequently occurs shortly after the initiation of CPB. Most cases of iatrogenic aortic dissection (IAD), classified as Stanford Type A, typically originate from the aortic cannula site. However, other potential origins include the site of the aortic cross-clamp or partial occluding clamp, the site of proximal vein anastomosis, and the cardioplegia cannula insertion point.

B. J. Kinsman · M. G. Fitzsimons (✉)
Department of Anesthesia, Critical Care, and Pain Medicine, Massachusetts General Hospital, Boston, MA, USA
e-mail: BKINSMAN@mgh.harvard.edu; MFITZSIMONS@mgh.harvard.edu

N. Hood
Cardiac Surgery, Department of Surgery, Massachusetts General Hospital, Boston, MA, USA
e-mail: NHOOD1@mgh.harvard.edu

A. S. Awad, J. DiNardo (eds.), *Clinical Perfusion for Cardiac Surgery*, https://doi.org/10.1007/978-3-031-91163-7_26

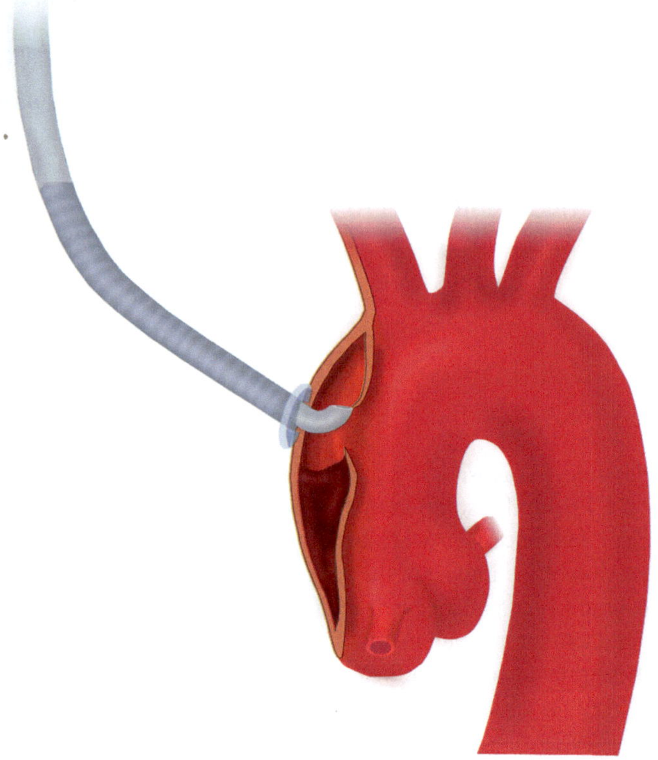

Fig. 26.1 Improper central cannulation at the distal ascending aorta leading to IAD

Initially, an aortic dissection may manifest as a change in the coloration near the site where the arterial cannula is inserted into the aorta, resembling an aortic hematoma. This discoloration can quickly extend toward the aortic arch and descend along the aorta. Signs of aortic dissection noted by the perfusion team include high arterial bypass line pressures, unexplained reduction in venous return, and reduced patient oxygen saturations. This is likely to be accompanied by progressive and persistent hypotension in patient arterial line blood pressures. However, it's important to distinguish this from the hypotension typically observed at the onset of CPB, which is often attributed to relatively benign causes. Therefore, before fully committing to CPB, it's essential to exclude aortic dissection as a potential cause of the observed hypotension. In the setting of a roller pump, circuit flow rates and reservoir volumes will not be impacted, but if a centrifugal pump circuit is employed, then decreasing pump flow rates accompanied by increasing reservoir volumes may be observed. Additional signs may include ST-elevation on the electrocardiogram (EKG) associated with coronary artery involvement.

Summary of Signs of Iatrogenic Aortic Dissection

- High arterial bypass line pressure that is significantly higher than the systemic arterial pressure reading.
- Unexplained reduction in venous return.
- Progressive systemic hypotension.
- Decreased cerebral oxygen saturation levels detected by cerebral oximetry.
- Reduced amplitude and dampening of the radial artery waveform.
- Discoloration of the ascending aorta at the cannula insertion site.
- Elevation of the ST segment on the EKG, indicative of myocardial ischemia.
- Impaired urine output.
- Asymmetry of facial features due to an intimal flap obstructing arterial blood flow to one side of the neck vessel.

Early recognition and communication of rising arterial bypass line pressures to the cardiac surgeon and anesthesiologist are vital to mitigate morbidity. Simultaneously, the perfusion team may evaluate for alternative causes of high line pressures. Potential causes of high arterial line pressure include systemic arterial hypertension, arterial cannula placement in a branch vessel (like the innominate, left carotid, or left subclavian artery), intramural cannula placement, aortic dissection, the cannula tip pressing against the aortic wall, arterial line kinking, an unremoved clamp on the line, an undersized arterial cannula, blockage in the arterial microfilter or bubble trap, or excessive cannula flow due to calibration or pump function errors. The surgeon will meanwhile evaluate the appearance of the aorta and cannula position to assess for the presence of discoloration and/or a tense aortic hematoma. If possible, weaning from bypass may help to avoid extension of the dissection and facilitate clearer evaluation of the aorta. Transesophageal echocardiographic evaluation of the ascending aorta in mid-esophageal views by the cardiac anesthesiologist may expedite identification of an aortic dissection or intramural hematoma. Furthermore, the anesthesiologist may provide additional resuscitative support with vasoactive medications or blood products as guided by hypotension, active bleeding, and emergent laboratory testing. If an aortic dissection is discovered and weaning from CPB is not viable, the injurious arterial cannula line and venous line are clamped off, a peripheral cannulation strategy is emergently pursued, and preparations are made to facilitate repair of the dissection under deep hypothermic circulatory arrest (DHCA).

Summary of Intraoperative Management of IAD

- Evaluate the scope of the IAD through direct surgical inspection, TEE, or epiaortic ultrasound.
- Evaluate and monitor cerebral and myocardial perfusion, and aortic regurgitation severity using TEE, epi-aortic scanning, cerebral oximetry, and EEG.
- In the event of an aortic dissection occurring during the initiation of CPB, swiftly lower the flow rate and consider immediate termination of CPB if feasible.
- In instances where cardioplegia has been administered and cardiac arrest ensues, promptly reduce the pump flow and lower blood pressure to minimize the risk of dissection extension.
- Initiate cooling and induce deep hypothermia, with consideration for head cooling, in preparation for deep hypothermic circulatory arrest.
- Relocate the aortic cross-clamp as distally as possible, ensuring maintained flow to the innominate artery and reinitiate CPB if feasible.
- Otherwise, the surgeon should evaluate and select alternative sites for cannulation, transferring the arterial inflow cannula to an alternate location such as the femoral artery, the far distal ascending aorta, or the arch. It is crucial to avoid cannulating the false lumen, which can be ensured by epi-aortic ultrasound and TEE.
- Perform an aortic incision and evaluate the extent and type of the injury.
- Devise a perfusion strategy tailored to the surgical repair, which may vary from simple plication to a full arch replacement.
- Regularly assess lactate levels and blood gas analysis to detect metabolic acidosis or hypoxia.

Measures to minimizing aortic cannulation dissection in CPB:

1. Epiaortic ultrasound for cannulation site: Using epiaortic ultrasound helps locate a safe cannulation area, avoiding atherosclerotic and thinned aortic regions.
2. Hypotension induction before cannulation: Lowering blood pressure pre-cannulation reduces stress on the aortic wall, decreasing dissection chances.
3. Aortic line pulsatility check: The perfusionist ensures that the aortic line is pulsatile and it correlates with systemic arterial pressure prior to commencing CPB.
4. Pressure testing with minimal fluid: Injecting a small fluid amount of 100–200 mL into the aortic cannula to test pressure responses helps detect obstructions or leaks early.
5. Careful cross-clamp use at low flow: Gentle handling of the X-clamp at low flow rates during cannulation and decannulation minimizes aortic damage.
6. During retrograde arterial priming, blood is withdrawn from the aortic cannula into a reservoir bag. If there is no return of blood or if the flow rate is less than 500 mL/min, this indicates that the cannula may be incorrectly placed, kinked, or blocked.
7. Identifying High-Risk Patients: Recognizing patients with increased risk and allows for tailored preventive measures. These patients include those with:

   - Atherosclerosis or a thin, dilated ascending aorta.
   - Genetic/congenital disorders such as Marfan syndrome or Turner's syndrome.
   - Family history of aortic aneurysm or dissection.
   - Bicuspid aortic valve.
   - Coarctation of aorta.
   - Hypertension.
   - Intra-aortic balloon pump.
   - Cocaine use.
   - History of trauma.

These strategies significantly lower the likelihood of complications during aortic cannulation, enhancing the safety of cardiac surgeries.

Arterial Cannula Displacement

Arterial cannula displacement occurs with an incidence of 1:650 to 1:4000 cases depending on the survey and is more common than aortic dissection but associated with less morbidity, with serious injury or death occurring in 4–7% of reported cases (Gerstein et al. 2022). The aortic cannula should be positioned to direct flow toward the aortic arch, ensuring perfusion of the innominate artery, left common carotid artery, and left subclavian artery. Aortic cannula displacement resulting in malposition may result in perfusion jet biased toward any one of the arteries branching off the aortic arch (Fig. 26.2) and consequently result in unilateral cerebral ischemia and potential neurological complications, including stroke. While collateral cerebral circulation may offer some protection, it is

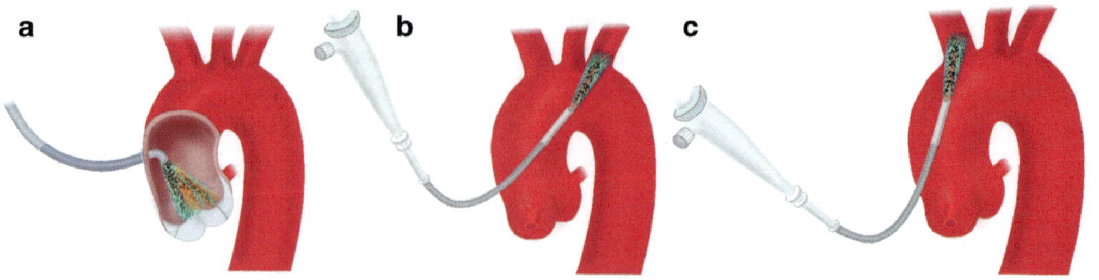

Fig. 26.2 Illustrations highlighting potential cannula malposition during central cannulation in CPB. The jet is directed toward the aortic valve (**a**), the jet is directed toward the left subclavian artery (**b**), the jet is directed toward the innominate artery (**c**)

not always adequate to prevent damage. If the perfusion jet is directed toward the left subclavian artery, it can lead to ischemia in the right upper extremity and also compromise bilateral cerebral circulation. Aortic cannula displacement toward the aortic valve may precipitate acute aortic regurgitation and potentially cause rupture of the arterial tubing. This risk of arterial tubing rupture is reduced when using a centrifugal pump as opposed to a roller pump. However, acute aortic regurgitation is typically unlikely, as the aortic valve is usually protected by the aortic cross-clamp.

Signs of arterial cannula displacement are largely indices of end-organ hypoperfusion and possibly elevated arterial bypass line pressures. Unilateral reductions in cerebral oximetry and increased burst suppression or slow-delta waveforms in a processed electroencephalogram (EEG) spectrograph may reflect cerebral hypoperfusion. Whereas acute dampening in the patient's upper extremity invasive blood pressure waveform may indicate limb hypoperfusion. Other indices of hypoperfusion, such as a rising lactate, decreased mixed venous oxygen saturation, and low urine output, may also be present.

Similar to managing IAD, the first step in addressing suspected cannula dislodgement is to alert all perioperative teams, whether the issue is identified by the perfusionist or anesthesiologist based on monitoring evidence. Transesophageal echocardiogram (TEE) evaluations of the ascending aorta, left ventricular outflow tract, aortic valve, and left ventricle can help assess for cannula misdirection, aortic perfusion jet flow asymmetries, new aortic regurgitation, or the development of an aortic dissection. Ultimately, the cardiac surgeon will assess the cannula and aorta, adjust positioning, and re-secure operatively as needed. If significant evidence of hypoperfusion is observed during monitoring, the postoperative care team should maintain heightened clinical vigilance for the emergence of new neurologic deficits.

Arterial Cannula Extrication or Arterial Limb Tubing Disconnection

An exceedingly rare and extreme circumstance of arterial cannula dislodgement may occur if either the entire arterial cannula were extricated from the aorta or the arterial limb tubing became suddenly disconnected from the cannula. Risk factors for such an emergency include unsecured high-pressure connections and an over-pressurized arterial bypass line (>350 mmHg). An arterial limb circuit disconnection would be marked by a sudden drop in bypass arterial line pressures, rapid depletion of the hard-shell venous reservoir volume, and patient hypotension caused by ongoing exsanguination from the arterial cannula. Pumped blood from the arterial limb may either be flooding the thorax (salvageable) or pooling on the OR floor (unsalvageable).

Within seconds, all teams must be immediately alerted to the situation, pump flow must be stopped, and venous and arterial lines clamped. Early extrication prior to cross-clamp placement and cardioplegia administration may allow rapid weaning from bypass. Extrication after administration of cardioplegia may require resumption of ventilation and open cardiac massage until alternative arterial access is established. New tubing must be acquired, primed, and attached to the bypass circuit. The cardiac surgeon may need to repair an existing aortotomy and recannulate while assisting to bring the CPB circuit back into continuity. The anesthesiology team may assist in TEE-guided assessment of aortic injury and repairs, resuscitation with additional vasoactive support, and acquisition and transfusion of emergency blood products until CPB can be restored.

Tubing Fracture or Leakage

Tubing fracture, leakage, or disconnection are reported to occur at incidences ranging from 1:461–1:4294 cases of CPB (Jenkins et al. 1997; Mejak et al. 2000; Charrière et al. n.d.; Groenenberg et al. 2010) and are associated with a related morbidity and mortality rate of 3.1% (Mejak et al. 2000). Tubing fracture or leakage are potential causes of patient blood loss, mechanical hemolysis, embolism of microplastics, and gaseous emboli. Causes may include an over-pressurized arterial bypass line (>350 mmHg), over-occluded pump heads, inappropriate tubing material use, and prolonged bypass times resulting in tubing wear, particularly from roller pumps. Clinical signs may include visible blood leakage from the circuit, a sudden drop in bypass arterial line pressures, progressive patient hypotension on invasive blood pressures, progressive decline in venous reservoir blood levels, and potentially even hematuria in the setting of significant hemolysis. Management involves activating the intraoperative emergency response, temporary shutting off the pump to clamp venous and arterial lines, isolating the affected tubing segment, promptly replacing it, de-airing the circuit, and resuming CPB.

Venous Cannula Malposition

Venous cannulation is an essential component of CPB, ensuring proper blood circulation during the procedure. Various techniques are employed, including a single atrial cannula, a cavoatrial cannula, or a bicaval cannulation approach. Each technique uses either a single-stage cannula (angled or straight) or a two-stage cannula. However, malposition of the venous cannula can lead to various complications. If the cannula is inserted too far into the inferior vena cava or into hepatic veins, it can cause liver congestion, potentially leading to liver injury. Conversely, if inserted too high in the superior vena cava, it may result in an elevation of intracranial pressure and a reduction in cerebral perfusion pressure. Additionally, it is important to note that the insertion of the cannula into the azygous vein can potentially lead to cerebral and upper extremity congestion. Each of these malpositions can have significant clinical consequences, underscoring the importance of accurate cannula placement during surgery. TEE is a valuable tool for confirming the appropriate location of venous cannulas before initiating CPB. Additionally, a sudden decrease in cerebral oximetry, or uneven readings between the brain hemispheres, can indicate an obstruction in the superior vena cava cannula drainage.

Venous Air Lock

Venous air lock in the bypass circuit may occur when air is entrained in the venous cannula or circuit that prevents blood drainage into the venous reservoir. The incidence of such an event is not documented, but limited case reports document the event in the setting of vacuum-assisted venous drainage (Burch and Locke 2012) or inferior vena cava tear introducing an air lock. Ultimately, a venous air lock is marked by inadequate venous drainage to the reservoir, resulting in a progressive decrease in reservoir volume, and is associated with elevated and rising patient central venous pressures or evidence of distention of the heart due to filling with blood. An obvious accumulation of air may be visible in the circuit if located in extracorporeal tubing.

Management of a venous air lock includes alerting the surgical and anesthesiology teams of the suspicion and attempting to identify the airlock on gross inspection. Meanwhile, CPB flows should be reduced, and blood products or crystalloid added to the bypass circuit to provide supplemental reservoir volume. The surgeon should disconnect the venous tubing from the venous cannula while the perfusionist re-primes the venous line to walk the airlock out of the tubing onto the field or venous reservoir before resuming CPB.

Iatrogenic Inferior Vena Cava Injury

Much like an IAD, an intraoperative inferior vena cava (IVC) injury can be a catastrophic complication during CPB. The incidence of IVC injury on CPB is not well-published only highlighted by limited case reports. The primary risks to the patient are rapid exsanguination, venous air lock, and massive air embolism with CPB circuit shutdown if not recognized early. Signs heralding this complication include a patient's systemic hypotension, unexplained rapid reduction in venous return and dark, venous blood flooding the surgical field. The venous cannula is the most commonly described source of injury, often precipitated by manual cardiac manipulation. Management involves intraoperative emergency response protocol activation; the venous cannula should be advanced beyond the site of the tear, the IVC then clamped, and repair may be performed under DHCA if needed. Primary suture closure and endovascular IVC tube grafting have been reported as surgical repair options (Narayan et al. 2015; Güney et al. 2001).

Chattering Phenomenon

This condition arises from the collapse of the right atrium around the venous cannula, potentially diminishing venous return. It happens when the rate of venous drainage surpasses that of blood return, causing the vena cava and atrium to intermittently collapse against the cannula. This collapse alternates quickly with the atria refilling with blood, creating a fluttering effect. To address this issue, the perfusionist can decrease venous drainage by modifying the clamp or occlusion on the venous line, thereby increasing resistance. This adjustment helps alleviate the chattering phenomenon and enhances venous return.

Left Ventricle (LV) Distension During CPB

LV distension during CPB is a critical issue requiring immediate attention and specific interventions to mitigate potential complications, as it increases LV wall stress and myocardial oxygen demand, potentially leading to subendocardial ischemia. It is typically evident either by direct visual inspection or through the use of TEE. The causes of LV distension can vary, including aortic incompetence, an incompletely closed aortic cross-clamp, undetected persistent ductus arteriosus, atypical persistent left superior vena cava opening in the left atruim, inadequate venous drainage, suboptimal venting strategy, and abnormal shunts from the right to the left heart, such as atrial or ventricular septal defects. The first step in managing LV distension is to ensure the venting system is functioning properly. This includes checking that the vent tubing is not inverted, verifying the patency of the vent tip, and confirming the correct placement of the venting catheter. Simultaneously, reduce the flow and assess if the venous return is adequate. Additionally, the surgeon may perform manual compression of the heart to alleviate the distension.

Systemic Gaseous Emboli

Massive systemic gas embolism is a rare complication that carries a high rate of neurologic morbidity and mortality (Gerstein et al. 2022). Gas emboli may cause arterial occlusion with diameters as small as 30–60 μm. However, arterial line filters and in-line bubble detectors typically prevent this. The formation of gas bubbles exceeding 40 μm per minute per body surface area may lead to a significant risk of massive gas embolism. Massive gas embolism represents an urgent medical emergency, and its management is comprehensively discussed in Chap. 27, "Accidents and Crisis Management of Cardiopulmonary Bypass." Gaseous emboli can unintentionally be introduced into the bypass circuit from the surgical field or through actions undertaken by the perfusionist. Potential sources from the surgical field include air entrainment in the venous line from loosely secured venous or coronary sinus catheters, the presence of an atrial or ventricular septal defect when a left heart chamber is open, laceration of the vena cava, and displacement of the venous cannula leading to exposure of its holes to the atmosphere. Risks are also present at aortic cannulation sites or during the placement of left atrial or left ventricular vent cannulas. Sources from the CPB circuit may occur in the setting of a runaway pump, left ventricular vent reversal, low venous reservoir volumes, oxygenator malfunction, inadequate air clearance from the arterial circuit, or a pressurized cardiotomy circuit. Microbubble alarms and low reservoir alarms herald high-risk conditions for gas embolism formation, but it is rare and devastating for gas emboli to be grossly visible in the arterial circuit.

In the event of detecting gaseous emboli within the CPB circuit, immediate and careful management is crucial. The first step is to allow the reservoir level to rise. This step is particularly important because venous air is not fully removed in open hard-shell venous reservoirs, and a lower reservoir level can increase the number of microbubble passages. Simultaneously, the gas sweep blend should be turned to 100% O_2, increasing oxygenation and decreasing decavitation. Pump flow must be reduced to 2.2 L/m^2/min, a critical adjustment to decrease the likelihood of further gas entrainment. Inspecting the venous line for visible air and immediately notifying the surgeon is crucial, as it helps identify the source or severity of the embolic event. Additionally, it's important to decrease vacuum-assisted venous drainage, which, while typically used to enhance venous drainage during bypass, can increase the likelihood of gaseous emboli entering the circuit. Flow rates for cardiotomy and vent suction should be decreased to avoid introducing additional air into the system. Temporarily separating the cardiotomy reservoir from the main reservoir permits the aspirated blood to release trapped gas bubbles. Minimize temperature gradients to less than 10 degrees, as rapid rewarming, which can cause soluble nitrogen bubbles in the CPB circuit to become insoluble, leads to gaseous emboli.

If a massive gas embolism is detected, activate the CPB emergency response. Detailed protocols are available in Chap. 27.

Circuit Thrombus Formation

Thrombus formation in the CPB circuit occurs at an estimated incidence of 1:350–1:4400 and causes significant morbidity in 2.5–3% of cases (Jenkins et al. 1997; Mejak et al. 2000; Charrière et al. n.d.; Groenenberg et al. 2010). The primary risk factor for coagulation in the bypass circuit is inadequate heparinization, either iatrogenic (e.g., delay in interval heparin administration), due to patient heparin resistance (Levy and Connors 2021) (e.g., antithrombin III deficiency, heparin-binding proteins), cryoglobulinemia, sickle cell disease with crisis, or premature protamine administration. Visible thrombus in the venous reservoir or arterial circuit and rising arterial bypass line pressures, such as in the arterial line filter, suggests thrombus formation in the circuit. Prompt recognition and a low threshold for suspicion of coagulation in the circuit are critical to prevent massive thrombus formation causing disseminated extracorporeal thrombosis resulting in CPB collapse and intravascular thromboembolic morbidity.

A pre-bypass checklist ensuring adequate anticoagulation with Activated Clotting Time (ACT) at least above 400 s is the first step toward preventing circuit coagulation along with regular ACT checks while on CPB. If ACT is inadequate, additional heparin should be administered as indicated. If heparin resistance is a concern, then also check partial thromboplastin time (PTT), anti-Xa levels, antithrombin III (ATIII) levels, and consider viscoelastic testing (Levy and Connors 2021). Heparin resistance can be treated with products such as synthetic ATIII or fresh frozen plasma (FFP) as indicated. Conversely, if a thrombus is already present in either the venous reservoir or clogging a filter or identified by TEE in the ascending aorta or cardiac chambers, immediate intervention is crucial. Management strategies include heparin redosing, circuit adjustments, and potential circuit replacement. Detailed discussion of these strategies, along with an example of an intraoperative management protocol for a CPB circuit clot, can be found in Chap. 27.

Reservoir Overflow

Overflow of the venous reservoir is an uncommon complication of CPB not well described in the literature, in part because it is more likely a sign of another mechanical problem. In isolation, the primary risk associated with reservoir overflow is the loss of patient blood. This may be caused by iatrogenic reservoir overfilling with crystalloid, blood, or field suction, particularly if there is uncommunicated addition of significant volume to the circuit and patient simultaneously. Alternative causes may include pump malfunction or partial obstruction of a downstream filter or membrane oxygenator by thrombus. The latter of which would be associated with high arterial line pressures. To manage venous reservoir overflow, one approach is to divert blood away from the reservoir into a citrate phosphate dextrose bag. If the overflow is due to dilution, hemoconcentration may be employed. Additionally, addressing the underlying mechanical issue is crucial for resolving the overflow.

Reservoir Depletion

Venous reservoir depletion, much like reservoir overfilling, often indicates an underlying mechanical issue in the CPB circuit. The consequences of reservoir depletion are potentially more serious and severe, causing either unexpected termination of pump flow with activation of the low-flow shutoff valve fail-safe and/or causing massive air embolism, if air is entrained from a low-volume reservoir (Nielsen et al. 2008). Hence, management is primarily determined by identification of the underlying mechanical compromise, which may include venous airlock, venous cannula malposition, circuit tubing leak or disconnect, or hypovolemia/hemorrhage in the surgical field. Intervention begins promptly with alerting all intraoperative teams to identify the underlying etiology, initiating vacuum-assisted drainage to prevent reservoir depletion, and replenishing blood volume with crystalloid or blood products into the circuit, and the patient. In the event of air entrainment into the circuit, the situation should be managed accordingly, whether venous air lock or high-risk air embolism, as discussed above, with the goal of expeditiously resuming CPB.

Runaway Pump

Runaway pump-head refers to uncontrolled, spontaneous acceleration of an arterial pump-head. This is a greater risk with CPB driven by roller pumps, as opposed to centrifugal pumps, due to the insensitivity of roller pumps to arterial line pressure. Overall incidence of pump failure during CPB is reported as 1:2514 CPB cases (Mejak et al. 2000). Runaway pump is a rare type of pump failure with an undocumented incidence that is associated with an increased risk of massive gas embolism (Kurusz et al. 1979). Causes include manufacturing defects, lack of preventive maintenance, or electrical malfunction caused by fluid spillage into the pump. Signs of a runaway pump include systemic hypertension in the patient, elevated arterial line pressures, and progressive venous reservoir depletion. In the event of a runaway pump, all intraoperative teams should be alerted. The affected pump should be immediately unplugged from the electric outlet, and the pump may then be operated by hand-crank. Vacuum-assisted drainage should be temporarily activated to restore patient euvolemia. Meanwhile, other members of the perfusion team should assist with hand-crank operation and setup a backup pump that can be integrated into the circuit to restore automatic CPB pump function.

Pump Electrical Malfunction or Power Failure

CPB pump failure due to arterial pump electrical malfunction or hospital-wide power failure are reported at incidences of 1:1695–1:7833 and 1:560–1:30512, respectively, with only one related mortality across perfusion incident surveys (Jenkins et al. 1997; Mejak et al. 2000; Charrière et al. n.d.; Groenenberg et al. 2010). This rare associated morbidity and mortality can be attributed to multiple safety measures, including the use of isolated electrical circuit power sources to prevent circuit overload, activation of backup battery power in case of hospital power failure, and fail-safe manual hand-crank operation of the pump (Fig. 26.3).

Management of pump electrical failure is primarily focused on prevention, as discussed above, which includes contingency planning for backup OR generators and regular testing of the pump's battery back-up function. Nevertheless, in case of a pump power failure, the intraoperative emergency response should be activated, and the pump should be transitioned to back-up battery power or a manual hand-crank operation. If there is concern about the pump being plugged into a non-isolated power supply, it is advisable to attempt resetting the circuit breaker. Ultimately the goal is to either exchange the pump if an isolated equipment electrical failure or provide a temporary power source to continue CPB until it can be safely weaned. For a more detailed discussion

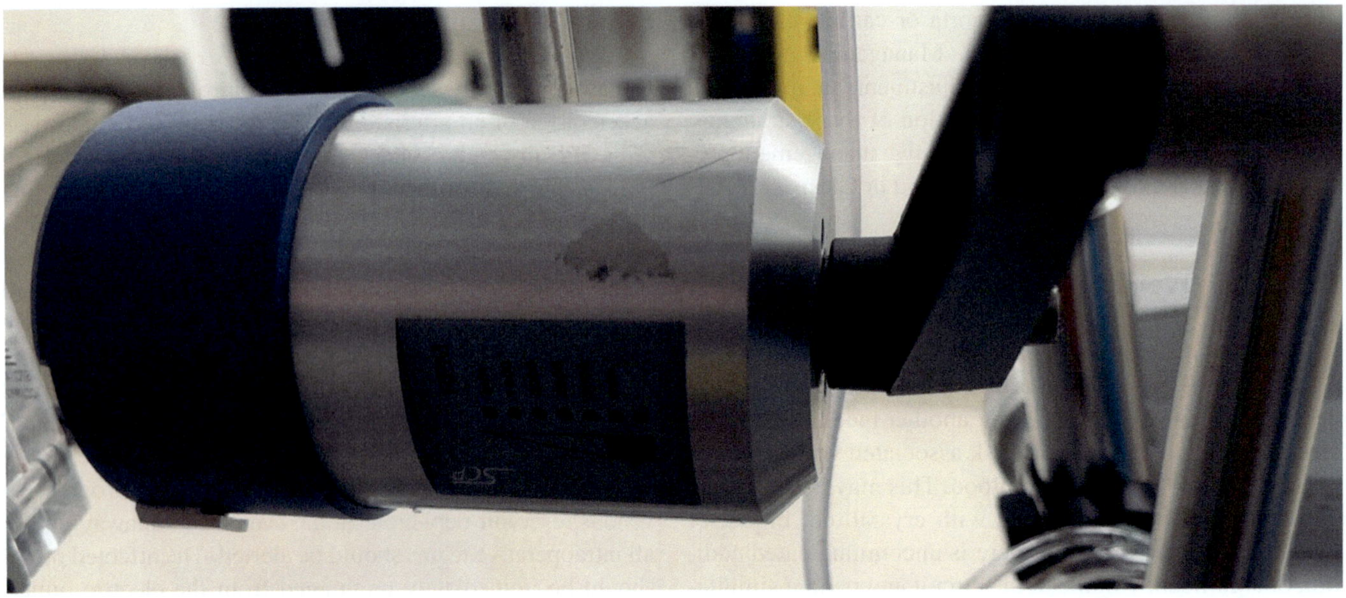

Fig. 26.3 Manual hand-crank: A reliable backup for emergencies in cardiopulmonary bypass procedures

and an example of intraoperative management protocol of power outage in the cardiac operating room during CPB, please refer to Chap. 27.

Arterial Filter Fracture

Arterial filters are critical components of the bypass circuit that remove potentially injurious particulate and air microemboli >40 μm with a bubble trap and filter. Fractures of arterial filters are reported to occur at an incidence of 1:1175–1:3380 cases without significant morbidity (Jenkins et al. 1997; Groenenberg et al. 2010). The primary patient risk associated with filter fracture is blood loss leading to end-organ hypoperfusion due to blood leaking from the filter. Signs of blood loss from the arterial limb of the bypass circuit include a progressive decline in patient invasive arterial blood pressures, along with reduced arterial bypass line pressures and flows. Damage to the arterial filter may be a consequence of manufacturing errors or damage incurred to the filter during circuit priming. Early identification of arterial filter leaks during circuit setup is the first step in harm prevention.

Management of arterial filter fracture involves intraoperative emergency response activation. The anesthesiologist may assist by providing vasopressor support and administering fluids or blood products to correct patient hypotension and support end organ perfusion in the setting of bypass circuit blood loss. The ultimate intervention is the replacement of the arterial filter. This can be achieved by either stopping the pump, clamping arterial and venous lines, and double clamp to exclude the arterial filter, or using a bypass loop around the arterial filter to shunt blood around the fractured filter and facilitate retrograde priming of the new filter (Hawkins et al. n.d.). However, this latter approach is associated with increased risk of microembolism of platelet aggregates present in the normally stagnant arterial filter bypass loop. CPB may be resumed after the new arterial filter is primed, de-aired, and the circuit is placed back into continuity.

Oxygenator Dysfunction

Oxygenator failure during CPB can be fatal, yet it is among the more common disposable equipment failures during CPB, with an incidence of membrane oxygenator failure requiring replacement in 1:773 to 1:2394 CPB cases (Jenkins et al. 1997; Mejak et al. 2000; Groenenberg et al. 2010). The primary risk of membrane oxygenator failure to the patient is hypoxia, which can cause ischemia to vital end organs, including the brain, heart, kidney, and liver. Dark deoxygenated blood distal to the oxygenator, such as in the arterial cannula or the surgical field, may be the first visible sign of oxygenator failure. On patient monitors, this may manifest as evidence of coronary ischemia, reduced cerebral oximetry, new isoelectric patterns on processed EEG, and/or hypotension. Labs drawn off the arterial bypass limb after the oxygenator may show elevated $PaCO_2$, low PaO_2, acidosis, and elevated lactate levels, consistent with failed gas diffusion and systemic hypoperfusion. Causes include thrombosis, membrane leak, housing leak, inappropriate oxygenator size, and disruptions in gas flow, such as a broken gas line adapter or incorrect gas filling from the hospital's oxygen supply.

Management of membrane oxygenator failure primarily involves activating the intraoperative emergency response and requesting an emergency replacement oxygenator. The anesthesiologist may assist with resuscitation, including providing vasopressor support and deepening the depth of anesthesia and muscle relaxation. The perfusionist may temporize the situation by maximizing inspired oxygen concentration, lowering inflow temperature to 20 °C and increasing sweep gas flows and blood flows to the oxygenator. Identifying the cause of failed oxygenation requires confirming secure tubing connections at each adapter from the gas supply to the oxygenator inlet port, ensuring that adequate gas flow is present, checking for the absence of leaks or cracks, and verifying that pump flows are within normal limits (Gerstein et al. 2022). The arterial pump should be stopped, and the arterial and venous lines should be clamped. Additionally, the oxygenator inflow and outflow lines should be double clamped to exclude and remove the failed oxygenator (Soo et al. n.d.). The new oxygenator may then be integrated into the circuit by connecting the gas line, followed by the inlet and recirculation lines to prime the new oxygenator. Residual air may be removed via the purge line in the bypass arterial filter, and CPB can be resumed.

Sweep Gas Supply Failure

Sweep gas supply failure, much like oxygenator failure, is another potentially catastrophic cause of patient hypoxemia. The incidence of gas supply failure, as reported in perfusion incident surveys, varies significantly, ranging from as high as 1:300 to as low as 1:13831 CPB cases (Charrière et al. n.d.; Groenenberg et al. 2010). As previously mentioned in the context of membrane oxygenator failure, the morbid risks and clinical presentations, including hypoxemia, hypercarbia, acidosis, and hypoperfusion, are similar. Cases of gas supply failure can arise from multiple causes, including hospital gas supply failure, gas blender or anesthetic vaporizer malfunction, and disconnection of tubing from the gas source outlet, blender, gas flow meter, anesthetic vaporizer, or membrane oxygenator inflow.

Initial steps in managing sweep gas supply failure, as with oxygenator failure, focus on activating emergency response and temporarily stabilizing patient hypoxemia and hypoperfusion. To identify the cause of failed oxygenation, it's necessary to confirm that tubing connections at each adapter from the gas supply to the oxygenator inlet port are secure, ensure that there is adequate gas flow, check for the absence of leaks or cracks, and verify that pump flows are within normal limits (Gerstein et al. 2022). If a gas supply failure is identified proximal to the membrane oxygenator inlet, management should focus on emergent actions such as replacing or reconnecting tubing, replacing the vaporizer or blender, or in the case of hospital gas supply failure, switching to a backup oxygen tank supply and alerting facility maintenance about the failure.

Heater–Cooler Unit Failure

Core temperature management on CPB is managed primarily with the heater-cooler unit (HCU). The HCU plays a crucial role in ensuring safe CPB by facilitating hypothermia, which reduces postoperative neurologic morbidity by lowering the cerebral metabolic rate of oxygen consumption. Additionally, during rewarming, it aids in neurologic and cardiac recovery, mitigates coagulopathy, and helps prevent shivering, among other benefits. HCU failure, while being the most common equipment failure during CPB, has incidences ranging from 1:314 to 1:1761 CPB cases, with no reported serious complications or mortality. The primary indicator of HCU failure is the inability to achieve the target core temperature, either by overshooting or undershooting the desired value. Other signs include visible leaks between the water and blood compartments of the HCU, as well as gross contamination or microbial colonization in the water compartment.

Management of HCU failure first involves activation of the intraoperative emergency response. Intraoperative teams should assess for alternative causes of temperature mismanagement, especially in the case of unanticipated hyperthermia. The room temperature and assistive warming or cooling devices may be employed to aid in temperature management. Topical application of either warmed saline or ice may be applied. A makeshift countercurrent warming pump can be created by using a spare pump head to circulate water from an external heated water bath into the heat exchanger's water inlet, allowing it then drain back into the same water bath. The ultimate goal is to expeditiously exclude the faulty HCU from the circuit and replace it with a functional HCU.

Further Reading

Blauth CI. Macroemboli and microemboli during cardiopulmonary bypass. Ann Thorac Surg. 1995;59:1300–3.

Burch TM, Locke AQ. Air lock and embolism upon attempted initiation of cardiopulmonary bypass while using vacuum-assisted venous drainage. J Cardiothorac Vasc Anesth. 2012;26:468–70.

Charrière J-M, Pouard P, de Riberolles C, et al., Survey: retrospective survey of monitoring/safety devices and incidents of cardiopulmonary bypass for cardiac surgery in France, n.d.

Gerstein NS, Panikkath PV, Mirrakhimov AE, et al. Cardiopulmonary bypass emergencies and intraoperative issues. J Cardiothorac Vasc Anesth. 2022;36:4505–22.

Groenenberg I, Weerwind PW, Everts PA, et al. Dutch perfusion incident survey. Perfusion. 2010;25:329–36.

Güney MR, Aksoy N, Sezerman Ö. Repair of lacerated inferior vena cava with the intravascular tube graft in redo cardiac surgery. J Thorac Cardiovasc Surg. 2001;121:187–8.
Hawkins JL, Myers GJ, Légaré J-F, et al., Arterial filter bypass loop: what occurs in this area during cardiopulmonary bypass and are there potential patient implications, n.d.
Jenkins OF, Morris R, Simpson JM. Australasian perfusion incident survey. Perfusion. 1997;12:279–88.
Kurusz M, Shaffer CW, Christman EW, et al. Runaway pump head: new cause of gas embolism during cardiopulmonary bypass. J Thorac Cardiovasc Surg. 1979;77:792–5.
Levy JH, Connors JM. Heparin resistance – clinical perspectives and management strategies. Longo DL (ed). N Engl J Med. 2021;385:826–32.
Matte GS, Connor KR, Liu H, et al., Arterial limb microemboli during cardiopulmonary bypass: observations from a congenital cardiac surgery practice, n.d.
Mejak BL, Stammers A, Rauch E, et al. A retrospective study on perfusion incidents and safety devices. Perfusion. 2000;15:51–61.
Narayan P, Das D, Saha A, et al. Successful repair of iatrogenic inferior vena cava injury during cardiac surgery. Perfusion. 2015;30:166–8.
Nielsen P, Funder J, Jensen M, et al. Influence of venous reservoir level on microbubbles in cardiopulmonary bypass. Perfusion. 2008;23:347–53.
Ram H, Dwarakanath S, Green AE, et al. Iatrogenic aortic dissection associated with cardiac surgery: a narrative review. J Cardiothorac Vasc Anesth. 2021;35:3050–66.
Soo A, Booth K, Parissis H, Successful management of membrane oxygenator failure during cardiopulmonary bypass – the importance of safety algorithm and simulation drills, n.d.

Accidents and Crisis Management of Cardiopulmonary Bypass

27

Yang Gu and Karen Jones

Introduction

Since the invention of cardiopulmonary bypass (CPB) by John Gibbons Jr., considerable improvements have been undertaken to ensure its safety and efficacy in clinical use. Despite its widespread use and significant advancements in technology and techniques, CPB can occasionally be associated with unpredictable crises that demand immediate attention and intervention. Accidents are unfortunate incidents that happen unexpectedly and unintentionally and can occur even in a system with redundant safety features (Charriere et al. 2007; Kunst et al. 2019).

Acute CPB crises present formidable challenges to the surgical team, requiring prompt recognition, decisive action, and effective management. These crises include complications that can arise during CPB, including hemorrhage, thromboembolism, air embolism, hypothermia-related incidents, and many others (Williams et al. 2010; Mills and Ochsner 1980). Each crisis carries the potential for severe morbidity and mortality if not promptly and appropriately addressed.

Successfully managing acute CPB crises requires a comprehensive understanding of the underlying pathophysiology, vigilant monitoring, and a proactive approach to patient care. This chapter focuses on managing acute CPB crises, aiming to provide an understanding of the various complications that can occur during CPB, and the strategies employed to mitigate their impact. It outlines the principles and interventions critical in managing these crisis, emphasizing the importance of a multidisciplinary approach and effective communication among the surgical team, perfusionists, anesthesiologists, and other healthcare providers while other complications related to CPB are discussed in Chap. 25, this chapter centers on catastrophic events. The most important aspects of effective crisis management include teamwork, effective communication, and the immediate implementation of readily established protocols.

Y. Gu (✉)
Department of Anesthesiology & Perioperative Medicine, University of Rochester, Rochester, NY, USA
e-mail: Yang_Gu@URMC.Rochester.edu

K. Jones
Department of Cardiology- Adult Perfusion, University of Rochester, Rochester, NY, USA
e-mail: KarenL_Jones@URMC.Rochester.edu

Navigating a CPB Crisis

In the face of a CPB crisis, the cardiac team's calm expertise becomes their most potent weapon. This roadmap guides you through navigating these turbulent waters:

- Embrace Calmness: The team should avoid panic. Every member should take a moment to breathe, evaluate the situation clearly, and focus on the primary issue.
- The team should identify the root cause: Understanding where the issue originates is essential for effective intervention.
- The team should maintain clear communication: Continuous and effective updates with the whole cardiac team are essential for coordinated efforts.
- Follow Established Protocols: The team should activate proven crisis management procedures and maintain vigilant patient monitoring.
- Act Decisively: Time is precious. Based on the identified problem, the perfusionist must adjust flow rates, administer necessary medications, or replace equipment swiftly and flawlessly. All while maintaining clear communication with the cardiac surgeon, anesthesia provider, and OR nurse.
- Focus on the patient: Never Lose Sight: Constantly monitor the patient's vital signs and blood gases. These indicators are crucial for evaluating the effectiveness of the team's actions and the patient's response to the crisis.
- Be Prepared for Emergencies: Anticipate the need for emergency measures such as manual pump operation or emergency surgical interventions.

A. S. Awad, J. DiNardo (eds.), *Clinical Perfusion for Cardiac Surgery*, https://doi.org/10.1007/978-3-031-91163-7_27

- Document Thoroughly: After resolving the crisis, record all events and actions. This documentation is invaluable for future reference and improvement.
- Reflect and Learn: The team should use each crisis as a learning opportunity. Discussing the event between members of the team to analyze it and identify areas for future enhancement is crucial.
- Commit to Ongoing Education: The team should stay current on the latest developments in CPB techniques and crisis management. Engaging in consistent training sessions, attending workshops, and participating in simulation exercises are crucial for sustaining and improving the team's ability to manage complex scenarios effectively.

Hemorrhage-Related Accidents

Hemorrhage-related accidents can pose significant risks during the CPB procedures. These accidents involve bleeding from various sources, including the cannulation site, vascular access points, and pump- or circuit-related leaks.

Cannulation Site Bleeding

One potential hemorrhage-related accident is bleeding from the cannulation site. Improper cannula placement or inadequate securing resulting in dislodgement or rupture of the vascular access point can lead to bleeding at the cannulation site (Williams et al. 2010; Mills and Ochsner 1980; Kurusz et al. 2002; Winiszewski et al. 2018). This can result in blood loss, hemodynamic instability, and compromise the effectiveness of the bypass procedure. The connection between the patient's blood vessels and the bypass circuit needs to be secure and leak-free. Close monitoring and proper placement of cannulas, along with meticulous surgical techniques, are essential to prevent cannulation site bleeding accidents. Constant monitoring of the line pressure within the circuit will prevent excessive pressures that increase the risk of dislodgement of the vascular access point and disconnections. For a comprehensive discussion on other cannulation site complications, please refer to Chap. 25.

Massive Hemorrhage: Crisis Management

In the event of massive hemorrhage, which usually occurs during redo-sternotomy procedures, the inherent challenges are significantly magnified. Redo sternotomies frequently involve navigating through dense adhesions formed from previous surgeries. These adhesions can obscure the surgical field, making the identification and preservation of vital structures exceedingly difficult. This complexity significantly increases the risk of inadvertent vascular injury, including the potential for injury to the aorta upon sternal re-entry, the right atrium, or the right ventricle—common sites of trauma in such procedures due to their anterior position. Such injuries can lead to rapid, substantial blood loss.

The following steps should be taken simultaneously with collaboration between the surgical team, perfusionists, and anesthesia providers:

1. *Oxygenation*: Administer 100% oxygen to the patient.
2. *Fluid Replacement*: Aggressively transfuse fluids using a rapid infusion device, such as Belmont or Level 1, to maintain adequate circulation, and blood pressure, and to achieve rapid reversal of shock.
3. *Massive Transfusion Protocol Activation*: Immediately contact Blood Bank and activate the Massive Transfusion Protocol to ensure a readily available blood supply.
4. *Vasopressor Administration*: Utilize vasopressors only as needed to sustain vital organ perfusion.
5. *Anticoagulation*: In cases of overwhelming blood loss, and in preparation to go on to CPB, administer 400 IU/kg of intravenous heparin. Add 400 IU/kg of heparin to the pump reservoir. If circulation is insufficient for heparin redistribution, initiate cardiotomy suction.
6. *Transfusion of Salvaged Blood*: Transfuse salvaged blood through a peripheral to replenish blood volume.
7. *Bleeding Control*: The primary objective is to control bleeding, initiate CPB, and reduce body temperature to cease circulation, thereby enabling the dissection and subsequent repair of the tear.
8. *Placement of the Arterial Cannula*: CPB can be established through cannulation at various sites, including the ascending aorta or peripheral vessels such as the femoral or right axillary arteries. However, in the case of ("crash") bypass, transapical aortic cannulation can be performed by retrogradely inserting a cannula from the apex of the heart across the aortic valve. If the sternum is not fully limiting access, the surgeon may manually approximate the sternal edges to temporarily halt bleeding to allow the surgeon to carry out groin cannulation.
9. *Roller Pump Vent Repurposing*: Consider using the roller pump vent as a secondary cardiotomy suction if the primary suction proves inadequate.
10. *Crash (Suckers) Bypass Establishment*: Initiate bypass using suckers either as the venous limb to draw blood from the chest cavity or by placing the sucker in the right atrium, along with the aortic cannula, for blood recirculation as soon as conditions permit, in order to restore normal circulation and oxygenation.

Precautions taken in high-risk patients for hemorrhage that are associated with redo-sternotomy:

- Conduct preoperative CT scan to check for adhesions and the distance between the sternum and the anterior cardiac surface, and to assess the proximity of the ascending aorta or bypass grafts to the sternum.

- Secure two large-caliber peripheral IVs for rapid volume resuscitation.
- Ensure cross-matched blood is available in the OR and cross-checked before performing the sternotomy.
- External defibrillator pads are placed on every patient.
- Ensure primed and divided CPB lines for rapid initiation of bypass if needed.
- Keep a cell saver readily available to maximize blood salvage.
- Lower the central venous pressure, especially in patients with right atrial or ventricular dilation due to severe tricuspid regurgitation or dilated cardiomyopathy, by using the reversed Trendelenburg position prior to sternotomy. Or cannulate the peripheral vessels and initiate CPB prior to sternotomy. The decision to perform a cut down and expose or place wires in the femoral vessels is individualized, based on the anticipated risk of cardiac injury.
- Utilize an oscillating saw for sternotomy: In redo-sternotomy, especially for complex cases, an oscillating saw offers precise, controlled cutting, minimizing injury risk to heart and vessels, crucial for patients with altered cardiac anatomy. Some surgeons prefer using high-speed craniotome drill.

Thromboembolic Accidents

Thromboembolic accidents are a significant concern during CPB procedures, and they involve the formation of blood clots that can potentially lead to blockages in vessels or organs. The use of foreign surfaces and contact between blood and non-endothelialized materials in the bypass circuit can trigger hemostatic activation, yielding thrombotic deposition. These clots can potentially obstruct the flow within the cardiopulmonary bypass circuit and compromise the effectiveness of CPB. Regular monitoring of the circuit, including the filters and oxygenator, as well as appropriate anticoagulation management, can help prevent the formation of clots and minimize the risk of thromboembolic accidents. An ACT greater than 480 s should be achieved from the initial heparin bolus for safe initiation of CPB. ACT should be rechecked at regular intervals to maintain therapeutic range once on CPB.

Stroke or neurologic complications are particularly concerning thromboembolic accidents during CPB. Proper anticoagulation management and vigilant monitoring of perfusion pressures and cerebral oxygenation are crucial to minimize the risk of neurologic complications. Additionally, interventions such as using filters in the CPB circuit or specialized monitoring techniques like cerebral oximeters or transcranial Doppler can aid in the early detection of cerebral embolic events during CPB.

Regular monitoring of clotting factors, platelet counts, and coagulation profiles helps optimize anticoagulation and prevent clot formation. The strongest preventive strategy to mitigate the risk of thromboembolic accidents during CPB is proper anticoagulation management.

CPB Circuit Clot: Crisis Management

1. *Assess Clot*: Determine the extent and potential embolization risk. TEE can be invaluable.
2. *Wean Off CPB*: If clinically appropriate and if the situation permits, wean as soon as possible.
3. *Heparin*: If weaning from CPB is not possible, administer an additional 10,000 IU. Check ACT afterward.
4. *Oxygenation*: Switch Fio2 to 100%.
5. *Investigate All Potential Causes*: Consider the presence of cold agglutinins, inadequate anticoagulation, heparin-induced thrombocytopenia and thrombosis syndrome (HITTS), etc.
6. *Alternative Anticoagulants*: Switch to different anticoagulants in instances of HITTS.
7. *Hemodilution for Hypercoagulability*: Achieved by administering 5% albumin, preferred for both diluting blood and coating the circuit, thereby preventing fibrinogen adsorption and platelet aggregation, key in reducing clot risks. Alternatively, plasmalyte can be used for hemodilution.
8. *Cooling*: Initiate rapid cooling to prepare for potential circuit change.
9. *Cell Salvage*: Redirect cardiotomy blood for cell salvage.
10. *Oxygenator Change*: Indicated for oxygenator failure (PaO2 < 100 mmHg or SvO2 < 50%) or if the clot is primarily in the oxygenator.
11. *Full Circuit Change*: May be needed for extensive clotting. If a backup machine is not ready, assign someone to perform the set up using the emergency pump setup protocols.
12. *Post-op Anticoagulation*: If there is suspicion of systemic embolization following surgery, it becomes crucial to implement an effective anticoagulation strategy.

Several factors can contribute to the formation of clots during CPB procedures:

- Inadequate Anticoagulation: Often leads to clot formation especially in areas of low blood flow. Also extended times of low-flow.
- Heparin Reversal: Persisting with cardiotomy suction after the administration of protamine or recombinant activated factor VII (rFVIIa) might contribute to the risk of clot formation.

- Procoagulant Application: Topical hemostatic agents or procoagulants used surgically in the operative field can inadvertently enter circulation and reach the CPB circuit. This significantly increases the risk of clot formation. Examples include fibrin sealants, thrombin, and gelatin- or collagen-based agents.
- Cold Agglutinins: Clots forming in colder regions of the circuit may suggest the presence of cold agglutinins, requiring modifications to maintain temperature balance.
- HITTS: In cases where patients have been exposed to heparin 5–14 days prior and present with thrombocytopenia, HITTS should be considered, necessitating the use of different anticoagulation strategies.
- Conditions Associated with Hypercoagulable State:
  - *Polycythemia*: An increase in red blood cells that elevates blood viscosity, thereby raising the risk of clot formation.
  - *Protein C/S Deficiencies*: Lack of these proteins, which regulate clotting, increases clot risk.
  - *Thrombocytosis*: Elevated platelet counts enhance clotting ability.
  - *Factor V Leiden Mutation*: A genetic mutation that makes blood more prone to clot. It causes resistance to the anticoagulant action of activated protein C, increasing the risk of clotting.
  - *Oral Contraceptive Use*: Hormonal birth control can increase the risk of blood clots, particularly in women with other risk factors for thrombosis.
  - *Antiphospholipid Syndrome*: An autoimmune disorder characterized by the presence of antiphospholipid antibodies in the blood, leading to an increased risk of clot formation.
  - *Malignancies*: Certain cancers can produce substances that increase clotting.
  - *Antithrombin III Deficiency*: A deficiency in antithrombin III Lack of this protein impairs clot regulation and heparin response.
  - *Hyperfibrinogenemia*: High fibrinogen levels promote clotting.

Air-Related Accidents

Introduction of air bubbles into the CPB circuit can potentially cause an air embolism (Sahu et al. 2006). Air entrainment can occur from inattention to oxygenator blood level, reversal of the left ventricular vent flow, or unexpected resumption of cardiac ejection in a previously opened heart. If air bubbles enter the arterial circulation and reach the brain or coronary arteries, they can cause significant neurologic or cardiac complications. These complications include stroke (from air embolism in the brain) and myocardial ischemia or infarction (from air embolism in the coronary arteries). Close monitoring of the CPB circuit, vigilant de-airing techniques, and meticulous attention to detail during setup and management are critical to preventing air embolism accidents. Early recognition of symptoms such as sudden neurologic changes or hemodynamic instability is crucial to initiate prompt interventions, including discontinuing CPB, positioning the patient appropriately, administering mild hypertension therapy, and administering 100% oxygen.

Airlocks

Significant air accumulation in the venous line, blocking venous drainage, is known as an airlock. This is another potential air-related accident during CPB. Possible causes for this accident include lacerated right atrium (RA) or vena cavae, dislodged venous cannula due to inadequate securing of the cannula can allow air entry if the cannula holes are exposed to air, or open left atrium communication with RA cannula. The consequences of an airlock are serious:

- Cessation of venous return drainage: An airlock blocks the drainage of blood from the right side of the heart.
- Depletion of the venous reservoir: As the pump continues to move blood along the arterial line without adequate venous return, the reservoir collecting venous blood rapidly empties.
- Interruption of Bypass: Without timely intervention, these conditions can lead to a forced halt of the bypass.

Airlocks Management Strategies

- Reposition the Venous Cannula: Ensure proper cannula position. If considerably displaced, reposition it.
- Chase the Air: Sequentially lifting each section of the venous line, guiding the air back into the venous reservoir.
- Re-prime Venous Line: If necessary, the surgeon should refill the line from the surgical field with fluids.
- Vacuum-Assisted Venous Drainage (VAVD): Significant air entry during periods of low-flow can lead to airlocks. By applying vacuum, VAVD substantially reduces airlock risks.

Proper de-airing techniques, meticulous attention during weaning from CPB, and careful monitoring of cardiac function are essential to prevent and manage airlock incidents. Microbubbles are classified as air bubbles with a diameter less than 1000 micrometers (μm). In current CPB systems, arterial line filters are employed to intercept gas microemboli exceeding 40 μm in size. However, smaller microbubbles can potentially merge into larger bubbles, depending on the circuit's flow rates (Gerstein et al. 2022).

To minimize the risk of air-related accidents during CPB, follow these essential steps:

- Meticulously de-air the CPB circuit before initiation, ensuring proper priming with blood or crystalloid solutions.
- Utilize specialized filters or bubble detectors in the circuit and cardioplegia line.
- Regularly monitor for air in the circuit.
- Continuously assess arterial and central venous pressures.
- Remain vigilant for signs of air embolism throughout the CPB procedure.

Massive Air Embolism Crisis Management

Immediate Interventions: Air Embolism During CPB

1. *Cease CPB*: Cease CPB immediately to prevent additional air entry, clamp arterial and venous lines, and notify the team.
2. *Aspirate Air*: Attempt to aspirate as much gas as possible.
3. *Trendelenburg Positioning*: Place the patient in step Trendelenburg position.
4. *Ventilation*: Provide 100% oxygen.
5. *Cooling*: Adjust the heater-cooler temperature setting to 20 °C.
6. *Vent Suction*: Once correct positioning in race verified, suction on vents and evacuate pulmonary venous air.
7. *Bilateral Carotid Occlusion*: Consider this maneuver to reduce airflow to the brain.
8. *Address Source*: Locate and correct the air entry source, then re-prime the circuit.
9. *Small Air Volume (<20 mL)*: To eliminate air from the arterial perfusion line, the surgeon first removes the arterial cannula and purge it with blood. Next, air is aspirated from the heart and aorta before restarting the CPB.
10. *Large Air Volume (>20 mL)*: The surgeon connects the arterial cannula to the venous line, recirculates, and primes the circuit. Consider retrograde cerebral perfusion.

Re-establishing CPB: Hypothermia Strategies for Air Embolism Management

1. *Cooling*: Maintain hypothermic bypass at 25° for 45 min. This enhances gas bubble solubility and facilitate the clearance of air emboli.
2. *Supportive Measures*: Alongside hypothermia, implement the following:
   (a) Oxygenation: Administer 100% O_2.
   (b) Hemodilution: Achieve a target Hct 25%.
   (c) Increased Flow: Aim for a flow rate of 2.6 L/min/m^2.
   (d) Moderate Hypertension: Maintain a mean arterial pressure of 70 mmHg.

After Resuming CPB

1. *Hypothermia*: Maintain deep hypothermia, carefully clear gas from the coronary circulation using a combination of massage and needle venting before attempting to wean off CPB.
2. *Hypertension*: Use moderate hypertension to help clear air emboli from circulation.
3. *Hyperbaric Oxygen Therapy*: Contact the nearest hyperbaric chamber facility.
4. *Antiseizure Prophylaxis*: Consider administering anticonvulsant medication to prevent seizure.

A detailed example of a pre-defined emergency protocol for managing massive air embolism can be found in Fig. 27.1.

For information on sources of massive air embolism, please refer to Table 27.1 provided earlier.

Retrograde Cerebral Perfusion (RCP)

1. *Criteria for Initiating RCP*:
   - *Indications*
     – Aspiration of air from the ascending aorta and aortic root.
     – Estimated air embolic volume to be over 20 mL.
     – Sudden decline in cerebral oximetry values.
     – Detection of regional wall motion abnormalities (RWMAs) or air visualized on TEE.
     – Evidence of air in the coronaries (visualized by the surgeon).
2. *Preparation Steps*:
   - *Cannulation Process*:
     – *Manage Existing Venous Cannulation*:
       - In cases of bicaval cannulation, clamp the IVC line to isolate the superior vena cava (SVC) for retrograde perfusion (Fig. 27.2).
       - With a single venous cannula setup, it is necessary for the surgeon to adjust the placement of the venous cannula into the SVC to enable retrograde flow.
       - Shift the recirculation shunt line towards the venous line, which may require installing a Luer port connector close to the reservoir. Ensure that a clamp is placed at the proximal venous line.
       - Clamp the arterial line.
     – *Establish SVC Cannulation (if no pre-existing arterial-venous shunt)*:
       - *Option 1*: The surgeon cuts into the arterial tubing and attaches the line to the SVC. Ensure the arterial line is air-free.
       - *Option 2*: Alternatively, after removing the aortic cannula, reposition it in the SVC above the azygos vein and secure it with a snare or clamp below.

University of Rochester
Strong Memorial Hospital
Protocols an Guidelines of Cardiovascular Perfusion

Air Embolism

Air has Reached the Patient

1. Stop the pump. Clamp venous and arterial lines.
2. Notifiy surgeon
3. Note time.

- **Perfusion**
  1. Find the source of air and correct.
  2. Reciruclate through the recirculation line.
  3. Reciruclate through the AV loop (when surgeon has the lines connected), inverting arterial line filter (ALF).
  4. If ALF is completely deprimed, clamp it out and bypass it completely.
  5. Stop pump. Clamp lines.
  6. Ask surgeon to recannulate.
  7. Initiate bypass.
  8. Document events and times.
  9. Correct blood gases.
- **Anesthesia**
  1. Deep Trendelenburg
  2. Carotid Occlusion
- **Surgeon**
  1. Disconnect arterial and venous line from cannulae. Connect to each other to allow recirculating.
  2. Purge aorta and arterial cannula of air
  3. Flood field with cold saline.

Gravelee, pgs 732-733; Manual of Clinical Perfusion, page 105
Page 1 of 2 10/17/18

Fig. 27.1 Example of an established emergency response plan to air embolism

University of Rochester
Strong Memorial Hospital
Protocols and Guidelines of Cardiovascular Perfusion

Air in the Line

1. Stop the arterial pump and clamp the venous and arterial lines.
2. Notify surgeon.
3. Note time.
4. Find the source of air and correct (See possible sources.)
5. Open the recirculation line and purge air from the line.
6. Clamp distal to the arterial line filter (ALF) and purge the air out through the arterial filter.
7. Remove the arterial filter from its holder and invert, Check for air in filter outlet:
    - **If there is no air**, remount ALF and clamp the proximal arterial line. Uncalmp the distal arterial line. Turn pump off and clamp the recirulation line. Transfuse slowly, Intiate bypass, Note and document events and times. Correct blood chemistry
    - **If there is air**, unclamp ALF bypass line. Debubble through the bypass line and through the ALF purge line. Manipulate air through the purge line while slowly turning the arterial pump head, and forcing blood through the filter. When fully debubbled, reclamp ALF bypass and proximal arterial line. Unclamp the distal arterial line. Transfuse slowly before initating bypass. Note time and document events and times. Correct blood chemistry

Consider

1. Steroids to decrease brain swelling.
2. Phenobarbital for barbiturate coma.
3. Pack the head in ice.
4. Retrograde cerebral perfusion (RCP)
    - Surgeon must decannulate aorta to pur aortic cannula into venous cannula.
    - Surgeon must reposition venous cannula into the SVC.
    - Begin RCP at low flow while venting air from aorta for 1 to 2 minutes.
    - Discontinue RCP and reinstitute bypass with 100% FIO_2 and high perfusion pressures.
    - Document even and times.

Hyperbaric chamber within 48 hours.

Gravelee, pgs 732-33; Manual of Clinical Perfusion, page 105
Page 2 of 2 10/17/18

Fig. 27.1 (continued)

- *Ensure Lines are Air-Free*:
  - Thoroughly remove all air from the venous cannula and lines, either by draining back or flushing forward into a basin.

3. *Initiating RCP*:
   - *Begin Flow*: Reinitiate bypass with cooled retrograde flow at a rate of 1–2 L/min for 1–2 min or until the surgeon observes air being released from the aorta or chooses to cease the RCP.

Table 27.1 Sources of gas embolism during CPB

Sources of gas embolism during CPB	Potential causes
Surgical field openings	Direct air entry into open heart or vessels
Flow reversal errors in venting cannula	Air drawn into the venous circuit
Reductions in venous reservoir volume	Air pulled through when reservoir blood level drops
Oxygenator malfunctions	Break in filter/housing, low oxygenator blood level introduces air
Inadequate clearance of air from arterial circuit or intracardiac air	Air remaining after priming or during procedures
Unexpected cardiac activity when heart or aorta is open to air	Air entrainment with blood flow
ASD or VSD	Open right heart chamber with these defects

   - *Monitor Pressure*: Carefully monitor SVC pressure to prevent over-pressurization of the cerebral venous system (target below 25 mmHg).
   - *Carotid Occlusions*: Once air release from the aorta stops, begin intermittent (1–2 min) carotid artery occlusion to purge the vertebral artery system.
   - *Blood Recovery*: Use a pump sucker to capture blood expelled from the aorta back into the circuit.

4. *Weaning from RCP*:
   - *Assessment*: Consider using TEE to evaluate for residual air.
   - *Gradual Weaning*: Slowly reduce RCP flow.
   - *Recannulation*: Return the circuit and cannulas to original configuration.
   - *Establish Systemic CPB*: Transitioning back to antegrade systemic CPB flow.
   - *Hypothermia*: Maintain systemic hypothermia at 20–25 °C for 45 min.
   - *Higher Flows and Pressure*: Use higher flows and pressures to push bubbles out of vasculature.
   - *Slow Rewarming*: Rewarm the patient slowly to avoid temperature gradients exceeding 10 °C, which can cause air to transition from a soluble state in the blood to forming bubbles.

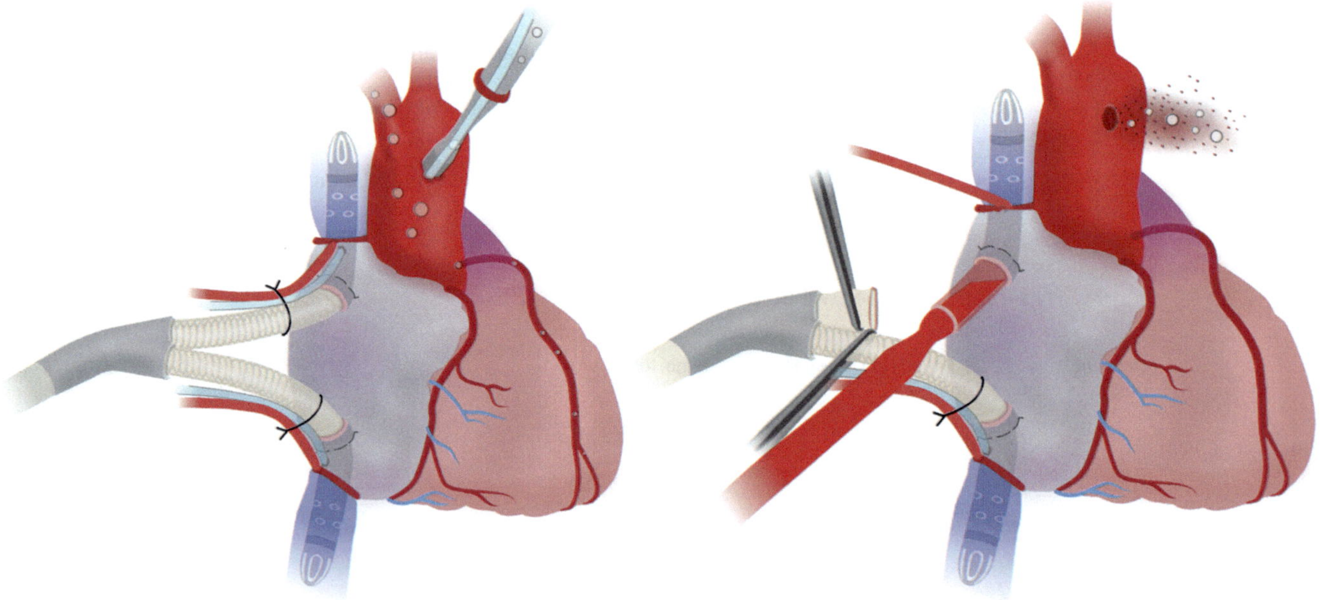

Fig. 27.2 Illustration of RCP in managing massive air embolism during CPB: Highlighting the procedure's indications, including air aspiration from the ascending aorta and aortic root, air embolic volume exceeding 20 mL, rapid drops in cerebral oximetry, RWMAs or air detected on TEE, and visible air in the coronaries. The left side displays air presence in the coronaries and aortic root (indicated by circles), while the right demonstrates the application of bicaval venous cannulation with the IVC line clamped, cutting into the arterial tubing, and connecting the line to the snared SVC cannula for RCP

Important Considerations

- *Teamwork*: RCP requires close coordination between the surgeon, perfusionist, and anesthesiologist.
- *Institutional Protocols*: Ensure all steps and specific flow rates align with your institution's guidelines.
- *Risks*: RCP carries risks, including cerebral edema and hemorrhage. Careful assessment is crucial before and during its use.
- *Additional Therapeutic Measures*:
  - Steroids: Employing high-dose steroids, such as 2 g of Methylprednisolone or 20 mg of Dexamethasone, could be beneficial for mitigating cerebral edema.
  - Mannitol: Administering 25 g of Mannitol may aid in reducing tissue edema.
  - Barbiturate Coma: A barbiturate-induced coma can be used aimed at lowering metabolic demand and protecting the brain.

Temperature-Related Accidents

Hypothermia is widely used to protect vital organs during cardiac surgery; however, managing body temperature improperly can result in various complications and adverse events. Thus, meticulous monitoring and regulation of body temperature are crucial to avoid hypothermia-related issues and ensure patient safety during CPB.

Hypothermia is commonly induced during CPB to reduce metabolic demands and protect the patient's organs. However, excessive lowering of the patient's body temperature or significant temperature fluctuations can lead to adverse outcomes, including cardiac arrhythmias, coagulopathies, impaired oxygenation, and increased susceptibility to infection. As the body temperature decreases, the electrical conductivity of the heart can be affected, potentially causing rhythm disturbances, such as bradycardia, atrial fibrillation, and ventricular fibrillation. Continuous electrocardiogram monitoring, vigilant observation, and employing appropriate temperature management techniques, such as rewarming protocols, can help prevent and manage hypothermia-induced arrhythmias (refer to Fig. 27.3). The use of temperature monitoring devices such as bladder or esophageal probes along with arterial and venous circuit temperature probes facilitates accurate temperature assessment.

Prolonged exposure to cold temperatures can impair platelet function and clotting factors, increasing the risk of excessive bleeding or inadequate hemostasis.

Cold agglutinins (CAs) are a rare form of autoimmune hemolytic anemia characterized by the production of cold agglutinins—typically IgM antibodies targeting antigens on the red blood cells. These antibodies become active at lower temperatures, causing red blood cells to clump together (hemagglutination), leading to their premature destruction and hemolysis on rewarming, driven by complement fixation (Fig. 27.4). Cold agglutinin titer refers to the concentration of CAs in the blood, while thermal amplitude is the highest temperature at which these CAs can still cause red blood cells to agglutinate. Both measures are crucial in the diagnosis and assessment of cold agglutinin disease. A higher cold agglutinin titer (such as 1:64) indicates a greater concentration of CAs compared to the typical 1:16 seen in healthy individuals. This suggests a potentially more severe form of the disease. CAs with a low thermal amplitude are only active at lower temperatures and may

Temperature Management

A. Cool or drift per surgeon's request.

B. Flows may be decreased as the patient's temperature is decreased. Flow rates may be interpolated between temperatures as needed or warranted.

C. Rewarming
Do not exceed a 10°C gradient between heater temperature and venous line.
Do not exceed a 10°C gradient between arterial line and bladder temperature.
Do not exceed a 10°C gradient between arterial line and venous line.
The arterial line temperature should not exceed 37°C.

D. See circulatory arrest protocol: Circulatory Arrest on Bypass

Temperature	37°C	32°C	28°C
Cardiac Index	≥2.4	≥2.0	≥1.6

Fig. 27.3 Example of a standardized protocol for temperature management

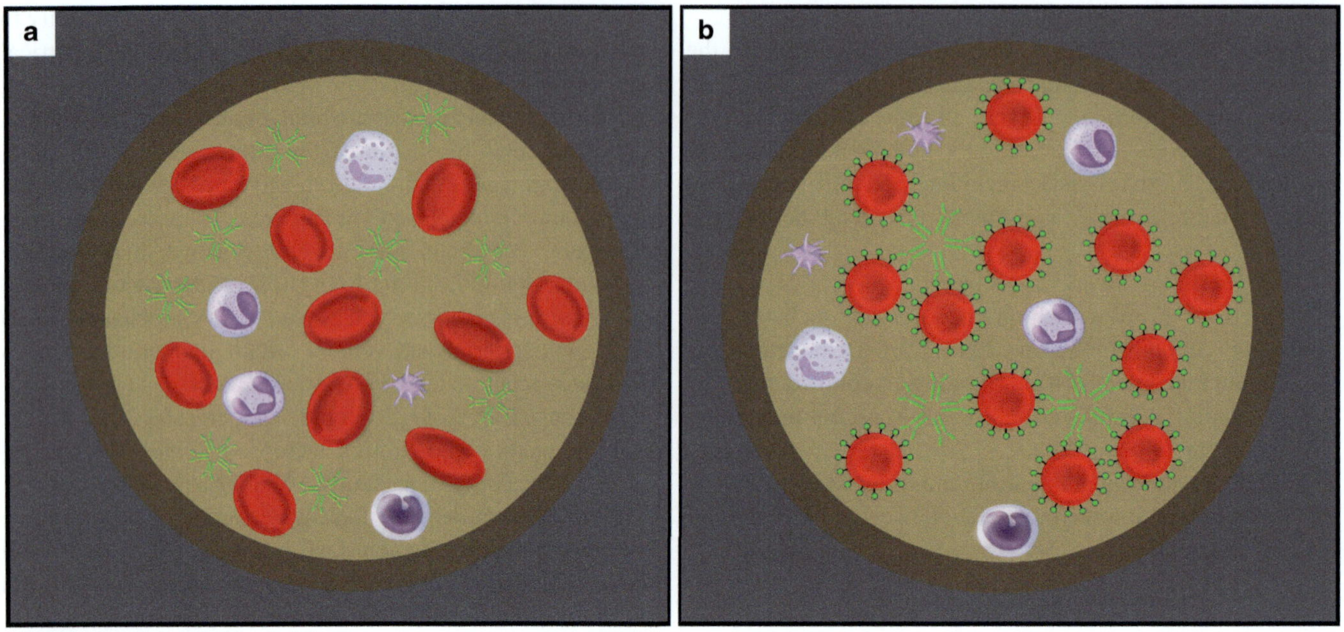

Fig. 27.4 Panel (**a**) shows red blood cells and inactive CAs at body temperature. Panel (**b**) shows red blood cells at a low temperature with activated CAs bound to their surface receptors. In this image, IgM antibodies are depicted in green, highlighting their pentameric structure, which enables them to attach to multiple red blood cells, causing hemagglutination

pose less of a risk. If CAs are detected preoperatively, involvement of a hematologist is required. Additional therapeutic strategies may include Rituximab, a monoclonal antibody that targets CD20 on B cells, effectively depleting these immune cells and reducing autoantibody production. This approach is particularly beneficial for treating CAs, where autoantibodies lead to hemolysis. Plasmapheresis, or therapeutic plasma exchange, removes plasma containing harmful IgM cold agglutinin antibodies from the blood. This rapid reduction of antibodies can potentially prevent complications related to CAs. It is important to discuss warm CPB techniques and implement strategies that minimize the patient's exposure to cold, as well as to have a protocol in place for the immediate treatment of any hemolytic or hypothermic events during CPB. Hypothermia-induced coagulopathies may manifest as prolonged bleeding after surgery, increased transfusion requirements, or excessive postoperative blood loss.

Cold Agglutinin: Crisis Management

Immediate Actions

1. *Stop Cooling, Start Warming*: Immediately stop cooling and rewarm to 37 °C.
2. *Check Oxygenator*: Evaluate the oxygenator for any signs of malfunction.
3. *Address Cardioplegia (CPL) Line*:
   - Detach the CPL line at the operating table and flush it with warm blood or lukewarm crystalloid solution to remove any blockages.
   - Should the CPL line continue to be blocked, it should be replaced or alternatively, switch to administering lukewarm crystalloid cardioplegia delivered via a pressurized, bubble-free intravenous IV line.

Additional Considerations

- *Postpone DHCA*: If feasible, Postpone DHCA or opt for higher temperatures during arrest.
- *CPL Strategy*:
  – Use continuous warm blood cardioplegia.
  – Use warm wash out followed by cold crystalloid cardioplegia.
  – Consider performing the procedure off-pump and at normothermic conditions to avoid the need for cardioplegia entirely.
- *Assess for Hemolysis*: Send a blood sample for thermal amplitude and titer testing. Be ready to identify and manage hemolysis.
- *Retrograde CPL*: Employ retrograde CPL before weaning from bypass to flush out red blood cells aggregates.

Malignant Hyperthermia (MH)

MH is a rare but life-threatening pharmacogenetic disorder triggered during various medical procedures by exposure to certain anesthetic agents, most notably volatile inhalational anesthetics and the muscle relaxant succinylcholine.

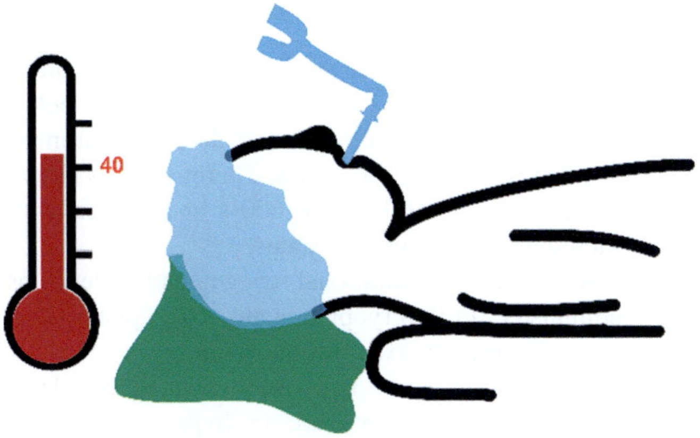

MH can result in a rapid and dangerous increase in body temperature, extreme muscle rigidity, acidosis, and elevated carbon dioxide levels. MH can quickly worsen into a life-threatening emergency, potentially causing cardiac arrest, multi-organ failure, and death without immediate intervention. During cardiac surgery involving CPB, MH poses unique challenges; the hypermetabolic response characteristic of MH may be intensified. Furthermore, because CPB diverts the patient's blood away from the heart and lungs to an external circuit, bypassing natural temperature regulation mechanisms, recognizing a hyperthermic state becomes significantly more difficult.

In the context of CPB, early identification of MH is paramount. Both anesthesiologists and perfusionists must be vigilant in monitoring for signs such as an unexplained rise in end-tidal carbon dioxide (ETCO2), decrease SvO_2, tachycardia, muscle rigidity, metabolic acidosis, increase lactate levels, dark urine, and rapid increases in body temperature. Immediate cessation of trigger agents and the initiation of therapeutic interventions are crucial steps. Dantrolene, a Ryanodine receptor antagonist that inhibits calcium release from the sarcoplasmic reticulum, is recognized as the definitive treatment for MH.

MH: Crisis Management

1. *Alert Team*: Immediately notify the surgical team to stop the procedure and call for additional help.
2. *Discontinue Triggers*: Cease all potential triggering agents (volatile anesthetics).
3. *Switch Anesthesia*: Maintain anesthesia with total intravenous anesthesia (TIVA).
4. *Ventilation*: Set FiO_2 at 100% oxygen.
5. *Active Cooling*: Stop rewarming and initiate active cooling measures.
6. *Purge Anesthetic*: Remove volatile anesthetic agents from the circuit. Attempts to decontaminate gas supply and oxygenator from volatile anesthetic.
7. *Assess Surgery*: If feasible, cancel or postpone the surgery.
8. *Dantrolene*: Administer IV dantrolene 2.5 mg/kg quickly via central line, if feasible. Continue dosing as often as necessary until signs of improvement are observed, such as reduced ETCO2, decreased muscle rigidity, or a decrease in heart rate. For cases of ongoing contractures or stiffness, higher doses exceeding 10 mg/kg may be essential.
9. *Dantrolene Alternative*: administer Ryanodex (lyophilized dantrolene) at 250 mg diluted in 5 mL of water, with subsequent doses of 1 mg/kg every 6 h as needed.
10. *Expert Advice*: Call the MH hotline at 1-800-644-9737 for further resources and assistance.
11. *Bypass Support*: Maintain CPB until response to therapy.
12. *Manage Complications*: Manage any arising complications like hyperkalemia, acidosis, and arrhythmias.
13. *Hydration*: Ensure adequate hydration, aim for a urine output greater than 2 mL/kg/h, using IV fluids and diuretics like furosemide as necessary.
14. *Monitoring*: Closely track the patient's temperature, blood chemistry, coagulation status, and arterial blood gases.

Sickle Cell Crisis Management Protocol During CPB

Sickle cell disease (SCD) and trait were thoroughly explored in Chap. 21. In this section, we will provide a concise overview of perioperative management and concentrate specifically on crisis management strategies for sickling events that occur during CPB.

A. *Preparation and Preoperative Care*:
   - *Exchange Transfusion*: Target HbS <30% preoperatively. Aim for <10% if time permits.
   - *Hydration and Anxiolysis*: Minimize fasting, ensure adequate IV fluids, and provide effective anxiolysis to mitigate crisis risk.

- *Hydroxyurea*: Important for long-term management but less helpful in urgent scenarios due to its delayed effect.
- *CPB Setup*:

B. *Intraoperative Goals*:
- *Prevent Sickling Triggers*: maintain O_2 sweep gas 100% and SvO2 over 80%. Perfusion must be adequate to avoid low-flow and hypoperfusion. Prevention of acidosis, hypothermia, and cold cardioplegia reduces sickling. Limit use vasoconstrictors to prevent blood flow decrease and sickle cell crises.
- *HbS Dilution*: Maintain HbS <30%, ideally <10%, throughout the procedure.
- *Controlled Hemodilution*: Target hematocrit (Hct) of 20–30%.
- *Exchange Transfusion on Bypass*: When intentionally inducing hypothermia during CPB, it is recommended to carry out exchange transfusions. Perform once to precisely achieve desired HbS level.
- *Oxygenation*: Ensure PaO2 > 100 mmHg, SpO2 > 95% to prevent sickling and provide a safety margin.
- *CPB Flow and Suction*: Increase flow rates gradually and minimize suction to reduce red blood cells (RBC) trauma.

Sickle Cell: Crisis Management

The following steps should be taken:

1. *Immediate Action*: Initiate partial exchange transfusion or red cell depletion/apheresis (if technology permits) to rapidly reduce HbS to below 5%. The optimal strategy depends on the available technology and patient severity:
   - *Pre-Bypass Removal*: To reduce the HbS percentage before initiating CPB, a calculated volume, as recommended by a hematologist, of the patient's blood is removed into the cell saver machine. A matching volume of allogeneic donor blood is then transfused. The collected blood in the cell saver is processed with minimal fluid wash ("emergency mode") to separate plasma, platelets, and RBCs. Subsequently, only the plasma and platelets are reinfused, while the RBCs are discarded.
   - *Priming Volume & Exchange on Bypass*:
     1. *Priming*: Use primarily allogeneic blood in the CPB priming volume.
     2. *Exchange*: After initiating CPB, the patient's venous blood is diverted into an autologous transfusion bag, while warmed donor allogeneic blood from the priming volume is simultaneously administered to the patient. The patient's blood collected in the autologous transfusion bag then sent to the cell saver machine and processed as above.
2. *Manage Hemolysis*: Address complications such as hyperkalemia and metabolic acidosis while closely monitoring electrolytes and acid-base balance.
3. *Coagulation Management*:
   - Patients with SCD are prone to a hypercoagulable state and face risks of thromboembolic events, including stroke, myocardial infarction, deep vein thrombosis, and pulmonary embolism. Therefore, it is crucial to maintain an ACT above 600 s and to frequently monitor their coagulation status.
   - During CPB, if dilutional coagulopathy develops, administer FFP, cryoprecipitate, and platelets as needed to prevent excessive bleeding.
   - Viscoelastic tests are particularly valuable for identifying whether patients are in hypercoagulable or hypocoagulable states.
4. *Vaso-occlusion Management*: Treat according to presentation, consider using vasodilatory agents, and rewarm.
5. *Renal Protection*:
   - *Aggressive Hydration*: Promote urine flow to dilute free hemoglobin with a target urine output of 0.5–1 mL/kg/h.
   - *Urine alkalinization*: Use IV bicarbonate to prevent free hemoglobin aggregation in acidic urine.
   - *Diuresis*: Use furosemide or mannitol to increase urine output, aiding in the clearance of free hemoglobin.
   - *Haptoglobin*: Bind free hemoglobin released during hemolysis to prevent kidney damage; note that haptoglobin is not available in the US due to concerns about potential disease transmission.

A. *During-Bypass Management*
1. *Expedited Separation*: Minimize suction, avoid roller pump over-occlusion.
2. *Frequent Monitoring*: ACT, transmembrane pressure, circuit inspection for clotting or abnormal noise.
3. *Hemolysis Vigilance*: Check for tea-colored urine, plasma hemoglobin >10 mg/dL.

B. *Postoperative Care*
1. *Hyperbilirubinemia Monitoring*: Early elevation may indicate poor prognosis.
2. *Renal Protection Continued*: Adjust as needed based on renal function.
3. *Viscosity and Organ Damage*: Be alert for signs of increased blood viscosity and microvascular constriction (especially acute kidney injury).

Additional Considerations

1. *Hematology Consult*: Involve hematologist urgently.
2. *Individualization*: patient factors may necessitate adjustments to this protocol.

Circuit Integrity and Sterility Accidents

Blood-to-water and water-to-blood leaks are concerning complications during CPB. Such leaks might occur at various circuit points, including tubing connections or within the heat exchangers. A blood leaks into the surrounding environment can cause several problems. Primarily, it leads to blood volume loss, potentially resulting in inadequate tissue perfusion and oxygenation. Additionally, blood leaks may allow air to enter the CPB circuit, creating a risk of air embolism.

Conversely, water entering the blood circuit can have severe consequences, including hemolysis, air emboli, and life-threatening infections. This issue may be indicated by an unexpected increase in circuit volume, which should be distinguished from the uptake of irrigation solutions or the unintentional infusion of crystalloid solutions. Indicators of water entry include a decline in pH, reduced hematocrit, disturbances in electrolyte levels, and hemolysis manifesting as hemoglobinuria. Furthermore, water leaks can negatively affect the accuracy of monitoring equipment and impair temperature regulation.

Conducting routine inspections and upkeep of the circuit both before and throughout the surgery can facilitate the early identification of potential problems. It's crucial for the surgical team to be equipped for immediate action in case of a leak, which entails having backup components such as replacement tubing or oxygenators on hand, along with established clear communication channels and emergency protocols.

Circuit Leak: Crisis Management

1. *Reduce Flow*: Lower the flow rate.
2. *Check the Source*: Identify the leak's source.
3. *Assess Severity*: If possible, maintain CPB operation during the troubleshooting process. In cases of significant leaks, or when circumstances allow, wean from CPB to address the problem.
4. *Maintain Reservoir Volume*: Ensure the reservoir level stays more than 500 ml above the sensor by adding volume.
5. *Address the leak*: Evaluate the rate of leaking and apply corrective measures based on the compromised component.
6. *Low-pressure Component*: Components located before the pump (reservoir crack, pump head inflow tubing, etc.) attempt to patch with bone wax for a temporary fix or consider replacing components.
7. *High-pressure Component*: Components located after the pump (oxygenator, pump head, aortic line, etc.) replace the affected high-pressure component.
8. *Cardioplegia Circuit*: Examine and replace if required.
9. *Resume Bypass*: Restore normal CPB flow.

Additional Considerations for Leak Management

Typical leak origins can be traced back to issues such as cracked reservoirs, filters, pump heads inflow tubing, or within the cardioplegia circuit. Leaks occurring in low-pressure sections pose a risk of air being drawn into the system, while leaks in high-pressure areas present a danger of rapid blood loss. Temporary application of bone wax may be employed to repair hard plastic components until the cessation of the CPB. In patients who are adequately warmed, on ventilatory support, and have a beating heart, weaning from CPB will immediately solve this problem. To mitigate the risks associated with leaks, maintaining extra volume in the reservoir is advised as a protective strategy against potential losses during component exchange or due to leaks. Always have essential supplies such as connectors for joining tubing segments, alcohol wipes for sterilization, scissors for cutting or adjusting tubing, and sterile caps are readily available.

Failed Oxygenator

Conditions requiring immediate oxygenator replacement include:

1. *Inadequate Oxygenation*: Signaled by the appearance of dark arterial blood despite administering FiO_2 at 100% oxygen. Confirmation with ABGs is recommended.
2. *Oxygenator Leaking*: Replace immediately.
3. *Heat Exchanger Leak*: Water entering the blood circuit necessitates replacement.
4. *High Inlet Pressure*: Persistent high pressure impeding perfusion signals the need for replacement.
5. *Clotting*: Notable clot formation within the oxygenator obstructing flow requires replacement.

The process of substituting a malfunctioning oxygenator during CPB requires detailed planning and careful execution to minimize potential risks. Two primary methods exist for replacing a defective oxygenator: the direct swap technique and the parallel replacement technique, known as the PRONTO procedure, for failing oxygenators.

Oxygenator Swap During CPB: Crisis Management

When it becomes necessary to replace an oxygenator during CPB, a structured approach is essential to minimize potential complications. Here's a step-by-step guide for executing an oxygenator swap effectively:

Preparation

1. *Assess and Communicate*:
   - Diagnose the oxygenator failure (e.g., low oxygenation, leak).
   - Notify the team and request assistance.
2. *Patient Temperature Management*:
   - If feasible, rewarm the patient for weaning from CPB.
   - If weaning from CPB is not feasible, cool to 20 °C for circulatory arrest (approx. 20 min safe). Administer neuroprotective pharmacological agents if needed.
3. *Oxygen and Gas Checks*: Verify the oxygen source and switch to an oxygen tank if needed. Set the sweep gas to 100% O_2.
4. *Check Blood Gases*: Review the patient's blood gases in anticipation of discontinuing CPB.
5. *Collect Supplies*:
   - Replacement oxygenator (custom unit or cut from a new integrated circuit).
   - Connectors (3/8 & 1/4), clamps, scissors, alcohol wipes, cable ties, and a towel.
   - IV pole and holder for the new oxygenator.
6. *Replenish Reservoir*: Increase the reservoir's volume with additional priming fluid to ensure air is not entrained while priming the new oxygenator.

Replacement Process

1. *Position New Oxygenator*
   - Place it next to the failed unit, ensuring correct flow direction.
   - Attach to an IV pole or secure on towels.
   - Leave the failed oxygenator in place for reference and line stability.
2. *Disconnecting Failed Unit*
   - Pronounce separation from CPB.
   - Stop the pump.
   - Clamp arterial and venous lines.
   - Securely double clamp the recirculation, inlet, and outlet lines of the malfunctioning oxygenator, positioning the clamps close to the unit while ensuring enough space between to facilitate cutting and subsequent reconnection to the new oxygenator.
   - Sterilize the lines between the clamps using alcohol swabs, then use sterile scissors to cut between the clamps.
3. *Connecting New Oxygenator*
   - Attach the circuit to the replacement oxygenator's inlet and outlet using connectors. Then, detach the gas line from the old oxygenator and reattach it to the new one.
   - Connect the recirculation line of the replacement oxygenator to the reservoir.
   - Unclamp the inlet line of the replacement oxygenator to allow for filling by gravity.
4. *De-airing and Re-priming*
   - Increase pump flow to de-air the replacement oxygenator. Remaining air can be eliminated through the purge line.
   - De-air the arterial line.
   - Connect the cardioplegia line to the new unit.
   - Recirculate and de-air the cardioplegia line.
5. *Final Checks and Transfer Remaining Components*
   - Ensure complete de-airing.
   - Reclamp the recirculation line and reattach the bubble alarm.
   - Ensure adequate reservoir volume.
   - Transfer sampling manifold, temperature probe, heater–cooler lines, and gas scavenging line.
   - Secure all connections with cable ties.
6. *Re-establish Bypass*
   - Pronounce that the procedure is complete, and the CPB is ready to resume.

Important Considerations
- *Safety First*: Prioritize patient safety throughout.
- *Teamwork*: This requires coordinated effort from multiple team members.
- *Time*: Work efficiently, especially if relying on circulatory arrest.

PRONTO Technique: Parallel Oxygenator Replacement
The PRONTO technique allows for swift oxygenator replacement during CPB without interrupting blood flow. Here's how it works:

Circuit Prep
- During standard CPB setup, insert a shunt (10″ tubing of 3/8-inch with connectors) between the oxygenator's inlet and outlet. This includes a Luer-lock connector, which is placed midway along the shunt for arterial line pressure monitoring and allows for pre- and post-membrane pressure measurements by clamping the shunt either side of the Luer-lock.

Equipment Needed

- For a change-out, you'll need: a clamp, scissors, alcohol swab, and a primed replacement oxygenator.

Procedure Steps

1. *Increase Volume*: Add volume to the reservoir equivalent to the priming volume of the new oxygenator.
2. *Clamp*: Secure the shunt line with a clamp near the distal "Y" connector.
3. *Cut and Connect*: Sterilize and cut the tubing midway between the Luer-lock and the distal "Y." Attach the new oxygenator to the cut ends.
4. *Prime New Unit*: Attach the recirculation line from the new oxygenator to the cardiotomy reservoir, leaving it open. Open the recirculation line to the reservoir, then unclamp the oxygenator inlet. Tap gently to de-air.
5. *Transfer Gas & Recirc*: After confirming no air, transfer the gas line, close the recirculation line, and move the clamp to isolate the failed oxygenator.
6. *Monitor & Reconnect*: Ensure adequate oxygenation, then connect the heat exchanger as needed (Fig. 27.5).

Key Points

- Safety devices like air bubble detectors and low-level alarms remain functional during the process.
- You can monitor pre-membrane pressure and calculate transmembrane pressure if desired.
- This process usually requires only a few minutes to complete.
- Some perfusionists advise against this technique due to concerns about blood stagnation in the shunt positioned between the oxygenator's inlet and outlet between the two clamps.

Inadvertent Drug Administration During CPB

Careful medication management is crucial during CPB to achieve specific therapeutic goals and to ensure the safety of the patient. Inadvertent drug administration during CPB is a rare but potentially serious complication. These can range from the improper loading dose when priming the CPB circuit to more critical mistakes, such as the unintentional premature administration of protamine while the patient is still on CPB (Nielsen et al. 2017). Such incidents might introduce unsuitable drugs into the patient's system, potentially causing adverse effects, allergic reactions, or negative interactions with other medications being administered during the procedure. The impact of inadvertent drug administration largely depends on the specific medication involved, its dosage, and the patient's individual response.

To mitigate the risk of such errors, stringent safety measures and protocols are essential. This includes meticulous verification of medication labels, proper labeling of syringes and infusion lines, and a collaborative approach to double-checking drug administration. Any discrepancies or potential issues should be promptly identified and corrected. Effective communication among the surgical team members, including anesthesiologists, perfusionists, and nurses, is essential to ensure that everyone is aware of the medications being used and their intended purposes.

In addition to direct medication errors, CPB complications can arise from a variety of factors related to drug administration, leading to equipment malfunctions. These include:

- *Filter Blockages*: Blockages in the filters of venous or cardiotomy reservoirs may occur due to the crystallization of medications such as calcium chloride, furosemide, or mannitol. To reduce the risk of such crystallization and ensuing filter blockages in CPB circuits, adherence to proper mixing guidelines, storage conditions, and usage of drugs within their stability periods is essential.
- *Electrical Faults*: Medications like potassium chloride, magnesium sulfate, calcium chloride, sodium bicarbonate, and lidocaine can, when dissolved in saline, form electrolyte solutions capable of conducting electricity. If these solutions come into contact with the CPB circuit's electrical components, such as sensors or electronic modules of the pump, they pose a risk of causing electrical hazards.

In the event that adverse medication or transfusion reaction leads to malfunction of the oxygenator due to accumulation of blood clots or clogged with high lipid solution administration, an oxygenator change-out may be needed.

Emergency Pump Change-Out Procedure

1. *Isolate Faulty Pump*:
   - Clamp the venous line.
   - Shut off any shunts.
2. *Assess Raceway*: Ensure the raceway is intact and free of obstructions.
3. *Attempt Reboot*:
   - Turn the faulty pump's RPM to zero.
   - Reboot the pump to see if the issue is resolved.
4. *Transition to Backup*:
   - If the reboot fails, immediately bring in the backup pump.
   - While powering up the new pump, hand-crank the faulty pump to maintain flow.

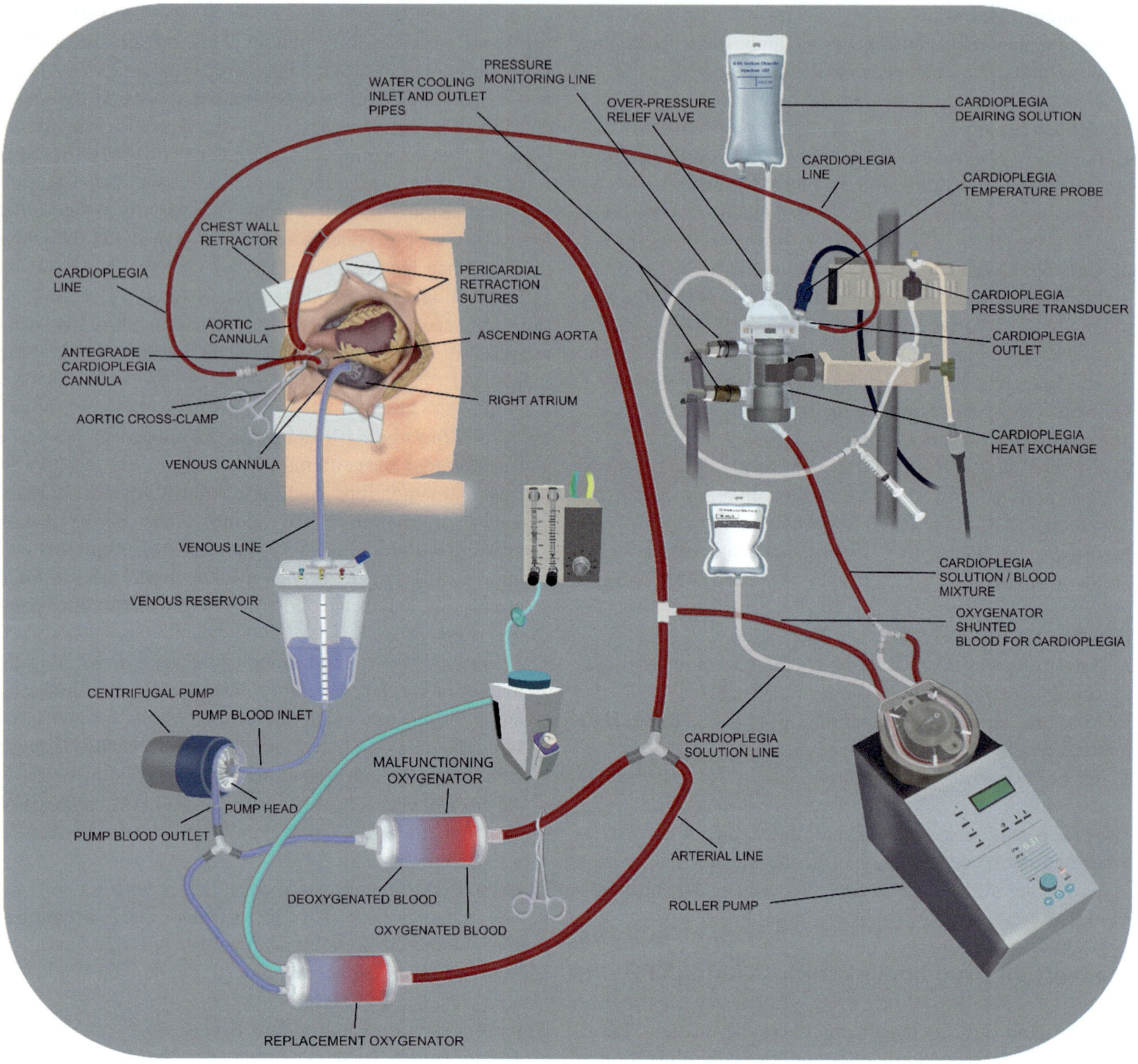

Fig. 27.5 An illustration showing the PRONTO technique that allows for swift oxygenator replacement during CPB without interrupting blood flow

- Once the backup pump has power, stop hand-cranking, transfer tubing to the new pump, and re-establish flow.

Important Considerations

- *Teamwork*: This procedure requires coordinated action.
- *Safety*: Prioritize patient safety throughout the process.

Accidents During CPB: Prevention, Response, and Preparedness

Although uncommon, accidents like pump failure, electrical failure, and the risk of fire in the operating room represent rare but potentially catastrophic complications. These emergencies require prompt action and a coordinated response from the entire surgical team to mitigate risks and ensure patient safety (Hargrove et al. 2002; Kolff et al. 1996).

- *Fire Risk*: The combination of oxygen-enriched environments in the operating room and the use of flammable substances, such as alcohol-based skin prep solutions, increases the risk of fire. Oxygen fuels combustion, and the introduction of a spark or open flame in such an environment can ignite a fire. Although the occurrence of fires during CPB is extremely rare, they are considered high-risk due to potentially catastrophic consequences. To prevent such incidents, it's essential to establish a "fire-safe" environment by minimizing the use of flammable substances and ensuring that electrical devices and surgical drapes are in good condition, well-maintained, and properly grounded. In the event of a fire, immediate actions, including stopping oxygen flow and deploying fire extinguishers, are crucial for suppressing the fire and safeguarding the patient.

The Power of Teamwork
A skilled, experienced team is the most potent safeguard against accidents. This includes the surgeon, perfusionist, anesthesiologist, and support staff, ensuring smooth operation and vigilance through clear communication, defined roles, and adherence to protocols.

Emergency Response
A pre-defined emergency response plan for CPB accidents is essential. Clear roles, communication protocols, and a systematic approach allow for rapid troubleshooting and resolution, protecting the patient. For further details, please refer to the previously discussed section titled "Navigating a CPB Crisis."

Monitoring and Surveillance
Continuous monitoring of vital signs and specialized devices (arterial/venous pressure, TEE, cerebral oximetry) enables early detection of complications. Timely intervention can prevent adverse events.

Simulation Training
Simulation prepares teams for real-life CPB emergencies (pump failure, circuit rupture, etc.). It builds technical skills, decision-making, and communication, leading to better outcomes in this high-stakes environment.

Further Reading

Charriere JM, Pelissie J, Verd C, Leger P, Pouard P, Riberolles C. Analysis of incidents, monitoring and safety devices of cardiopulmonary bypass for cardiac surgery for the year 2005 in France. Ann Fr Anesth Reanim. 2007;26:e19–31. https://doi.org/10.1016/j.annfar.2007.09.025.

Gerstein NS, Panikkath PV, Mirrakhimov AE, Lewis AE, Ram H. Cardiopulmonary bypass emergencies and intraoperative issues. J Cardiothorac Vasc Anesth. 2022;36(12):4505–22. https://doi.org/10.1053/j.jvca.2022.07.011.

Hargrove M, Ramish B, O'Donnell A, Aherne T. Electrical failure during cardiopulmonary bypass: an evaluation of incidence, causes, management and guidelines for preventative measures. Perfusion. 2002;17(5):369–72.

Kolff J, Ankney RN, Wurzel D, Devineni R. Centrifugal pump failures. J Extra Corpor Technol. 1996;28(3):118–22.

Kunst G, Milojevic M, Boer C, De Somer F, Gudbjartsson T, Task Force Members, et al. EACTS/EACTA/EBCP guidelines on cardiopulmonary bypass in adult cardiac surgery. Br J Anaesth. 2019;123(6):718–98. https://doi.org/10.1016/j.bja.2019.09.009.

Kurusz M, Girouard MK, Brown PS. Coronary sinus rupture with retrograde cardioplegia. Perfusion. 2002;17(5):343–6. https://doi.org/10.1191/0267659102pf534cr.

Mills NL, Ochsner JL. Massive air embolism during cardiopulmonary bypass. Causes, prevention, and management. J Thorac Cardiovasc Surg. 1980;80(5):708–17.

Nielsen VG, Paidy SR, Meek CA, Thornton TK, Lick SD. Survival after intravenous thrombin prior to cardiopulmonary bypass. Int J Legal Med. 2017;131(5):1315–7.

Niyibizi E, Kembi GE, Lae C, Pignel R, Sologashvili T. Delayed hyperbaric oxygen therapy for air emboli after open heart surgery: case report and review of a success story. J Cardiothorac Surg. 2016;11(3):167. https://doi.org/10.1186/s13019-015-0380-7.

Sahu MK, Ingole PR, Bisoi AK, Venugopal P. Successful management of a case of massive air embolism from cardiopulmonary bypass with retrograde cerebral perfusion in a child. J Cardiothorac Vasc Anesth. 2006;20(1):80–1.

Stammers AH, Mejak BL. An update on perfusion safety: does the type of perfusion practice affect the rate of incidents related to cardiopulmonary bypass? Perfusion. 2001;16(3):189–98.

Williams ML, Sheng S, Gammie JS, Rankin JS, Smith PK, Hughes GC, et al. Aortic dissection as a complication of cardiac surgery: report from the Society of Thoracic Surgeons database. Ann Thorac Surg. 2010;90(6):1812–6; discussion 6–7.

Winiszewski H, Perrotti A, Chocron S, Capellier G, Piton G. Malposition of the extracorporeal membrane oxygenation venous cannula in an accessory hepatic vein. J Extra Corpor Technol. 2018;50(2):98–9.

Part VIII

Organ Protection During Cardiopulmonary Bypass

Strategies of Myocardial Protection During Cardiopulmonary Bypass

28

Quoc-Sy Nguyen and Dalia Banks

Introduction

Techniques for myocardial preservation are a critical component of modern cardiac surgery. By reducing metabolic demand and maintaining myocardial cell viability during the operative procedure, these techniques allow surgeons sufficient time to perform complex cardiac repairs with precision and safety. Early cardiac surgery presented substantial challenges: even after technically successful surgeries, patients frequently had postoperative myocardial failure as a result of extensive damage sustained during the operation. At first, surgeons tried to perform procedures on hearts under various conditions, including normothermic and hypothermic empty, beating, or fibrillating hearts. These conditions not only offered inadequate operative exposure but also resulted in myocardial necrosis. Aortic cross-clamping eventually emerged as the preferred method to isolate the heart from circulation, greatly enhancing surgical exposure by establishing a bloodless field. While this method provides a bloodless field, it also cuts off vital myocardial perfusion. The heart must withstand this period of ischemia (cross-clamp interval) without sustaining damage. Myocardial preservation strategies have advanced to offer optimal protection of the heart during aortic cross-clamping and in the subsequent reperfusion phase after cross-clamp release. This chapter examines perioperative myocardial preservation strategies, with a particular focus on the CPB interval, especially aortic cross-clamping and the immediate reperfusion period.

Myocardial Preservation in Cardiac Surgery

There are four key phases for myocardial preservation during cardiac surgery, with strategies tailored to patient pathophysiology and surgical technique:

1. *Preoperative*: Strategies in medical therapy focus on optimizing the balance between oxygen supply and demand. Nitrates are administered to enhance coronary flow, anticoagulants are used to minimize thromboembolic risks, and an intra-aortic balloon pump may be employed if medical therapy is insufficient.
2. *Pre-CPB*: Managed primarily by the anesthesia provider, strategies focus on increasing myocardial blood supply and reducing demand. Key measures include controlling pain, tachycardia, and severe hypertension—which increase afterload and wall stress—during high-demand moments such as incision, sternotomy, and aortic manipulation, thereby maximizing protection against myocardial ischemia.

Q.-S. Nguyen · D. Banks (✉)
Department of Anesthesiology & Perioperative Medicine, UC San Diego Health, La Jolla, CA, USA
e-mail: q6nguyen@ucsd.edu; dabanks@ucsd.edu

A. S. Awad, J. DiNardo (eds.), *Clinical Perfusion for Cardiac Surgery*, https://doi.org/10.1007/978-3-031-91163-7_28

3. *Bypass and Aortic Cross-Clamping*: The myocardium sustains its greatest injury during this period. Cardioplegia stands as a key tool for myocardial protection. This chapter will provide a comprehensive overview of available protective strategies for this critical phase.
4. *Pre-Weaning from CPB*: Specific strategies taken during rewarming and weaning can help prevent myocardial damage.

CPB and Aortic Cross-Clamping: Pathophysiology and Myocardial Injury

As an obligate aerobe, the heart requires a constant supply of oxygen, with most myocardial oxygen consumption (MVO2) dedicated to contractile activity and baseline metabolism. Its high oxygen extraction rate (75%) makes the heart especially vulnerable to reductions in coronary flow. Normally, the heart's energy is derived from mitochondrial oxidation of fatty acids, which is the primary energy source. CPB presents significant risks to myocardial viability due to the pathophysiology of injury associated with the technique, creating a significant mismatch between oxygen supply and demand. Consequently, this mismatch triggers ischemia in cardiomyocytes, characterized by the depletion of high-energy phosphate substrates adenosine triphosphate (ATP) and creatine phosphate (CP), increased intracellular calcium, and a shift to less efficient anaerobic energy metabolism. Aortic cross-clamping further compounds the problem by completely isolating the coronary circulation, leading to global myocardial ischemia unless protective measures are in place. This halted perfusion results in several metabolic disturbances: cessation of oxidative phosphorylation, further depletion of ATP and CP, initiation of anaerobic metabolism, inhibition of free fatty acid oxidation, depletion of the adenine nucleotide pool, impairment of calcium homeostasis, and disruption of cellular architecture. Consequently, glycolytic byproducts accumulate, causing severe intracellular acidosis that compromises contractile function, enzyme activity, and cell membrane stability. The duration of aortic cross-clamping is directly linked to the risk of ischemic injury. The longer the clamping period, the greater the potential for damage.

Furthermore, the subsequent release of the aortic clamp introduces another peril: reperfusion injury. This phase is characterized by the onslaught of free radicals and reactive oxygen species that induce oxidative stress, cellular edema, and overload of intracellular calcium, compounding the injury to cardiomyocytes. Additionally, embolic events, such as fat, air, or thrombus, may occur post-clamp release, exacerbating the risk and complicating recovery.

Understanding these mechanisms is crucial for implementing strategies that mitigate risks associated with aortic cross-clamping and CPB, aiming to preserve myocardial function through careful management of ischemic and reperfusion phases.

Identifying High-Risk Patients for CPB-Related Myocardial Damage

Several patient-specific factors increase the risk of myocardial injury during CPB. Pre-existing conditions like poor left ventricular function and left ventricular hypertrophy make the myocardium more vulnerable to damage. Additionally, severe and widespread coronary artery disease significantly heightens the risk of injury during the procedure.

Strategies for Myocardial Preservation During CPB

During cardiac surgery, the interruption of natural blood flow to the heart necessitates the implementation of myocardial preservation strategies to minimize myocardial damage. These strategies include cardioplegia, which involves delivering a solution that arrests the heart in a controlled manner to protect against ischemia. Left ventricular venting reduces distension within the left ventricle chamber, alleviating increased myocardial wall tension and protecting against subendocardial ischemia. Additionally, systemic hypothermia lowers body temperature, thereby decreasing metabolic demands and further protecting the heart against ischemic injury. Figure 28.1 provides insight into the pathophysiology of perioperative myocardial injury and potential protective strategies.

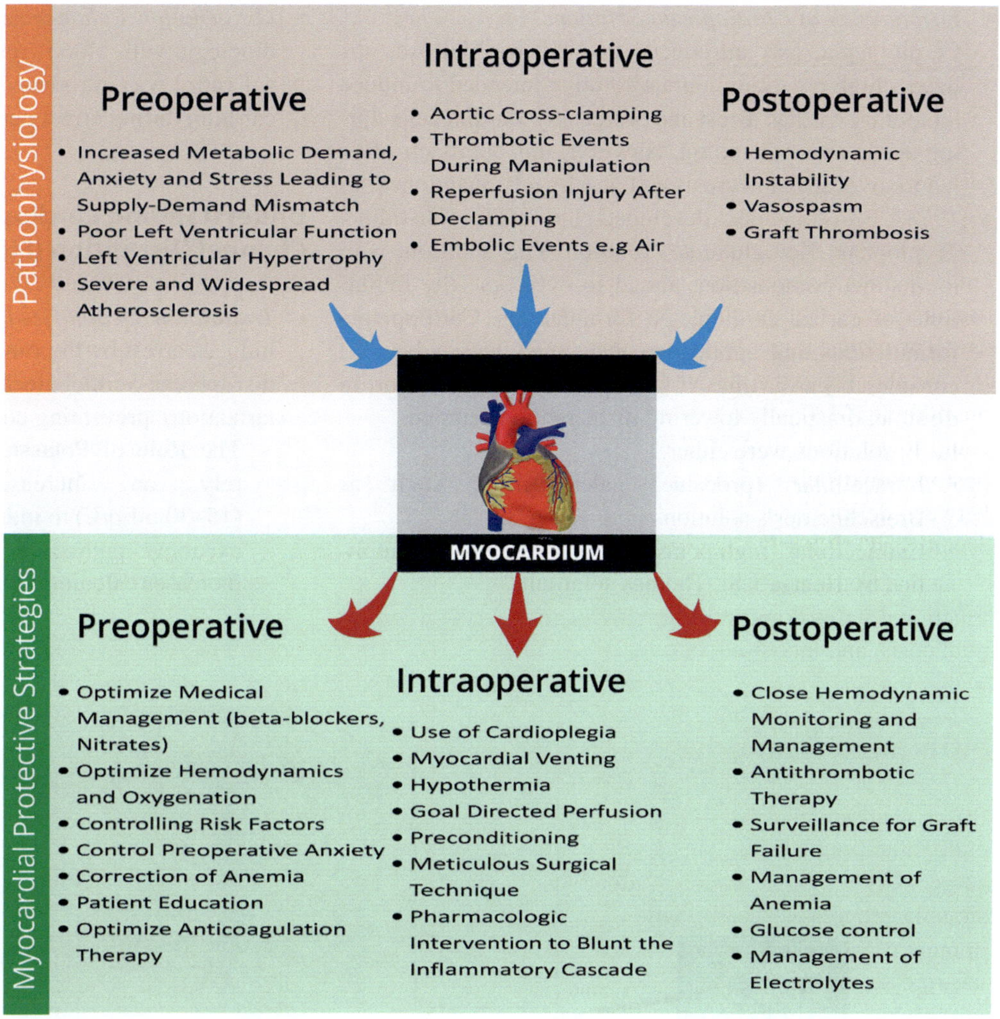

Fig. 28.1 Overview of pathophysiological features and myocardial protective strategies during the perioperative period—this diagram outlines the pathophysiology of cardiac ischemia during the perioperative period and highlights the myocardial protective strategies used to minimize damage and preserve heart function throughout the surgical process

Cardioplegia: The Cornerstone of Myocardial Protection

Definition

The term "cardioplegia" is derived from the combination of "cardio" (heart) and "plegia" (paralysis). This reflects its primary purpose: to induce temporary cardiac arrest, creating a still and flaccid heart for surgical procedures. The overarching goal of cardioplegia is myocardial preservation during periods of ischemia, ensuring a functional heart at the conclusion of the operation.

History of Myocardial Protection Strategies

- *Early Techniques and Limitations*: In the 1960s, normothermic ischemic arrest (Fast Operators) was predominant. While effective for short procedures, prolonged ischemia often led to "stone heart" syndrome due to depletion of high-energy phosphate molecules (primarily ATP) within myocardial cells.
- *Developments in Cardioplegia and Cross-Clamping*:
  - *Intermittent Aortic Cross-Clamping (XC)*: This technique, involving 15-min cross-clamp intervals with 5-min reperfusion periods, minimized ischemic damage. While still used for short cross-clamp times and good ventricular function, its complexity limits broader adoption.
  - *Fibrillatory Arrest without XC*: While effective in select cases, this approach risked subendocardial ischemia and was primarily used for coronary surgery.
  - *Continuous Coronary Perfusion*: This method, though cumbersome and sometimes necessitating interruptions, has demonstrated success with skilled surgeons for both coronary and valvular procedures. Potential risks include coronary injury.
  - *Topical Hypothermia*: Employing cold jackets to cool the heart, this method faced challenges due to rewarming by surrounding tissues.

- *Introduction of Cardioplegia Solutions.*
  Cardioplegia, first introduced in 1955 by Melrose, utilized a high potassium citrate solution intended to induce temporary cardiac arrest and protect myocardial cells during aortic cross-clamping. However, this approach often led to myocardial necrosis and was largely abandoned. In 1973, Bretschneider developed the HTK (Histidine, Tryptophan, Ketoglutarate) solution. This solution, with its distinct composition, aimed to overcome the limitations of earlier cardioplegia formulations. Cardioplegia formulations and application techniques have advanced considerably over time. It works by arresting the heart in diastole, drastically lowering its metabolic demand.
  Early solutions were either:
  - Intracellular (procaine, calcium-free), such as Bretschneider's solution.
  - Extracellular (high potassium, low calcium), exemplified by Hearse's St. Thomas solution.
- *Oxygenation Enhancement*: The practice of mixing cardioplegia with blood from the arterial circuit (often in a 4:1 ratio) was introduced to provide oxygen to the myocardium during arrest periods.

Understanding Cardioplegia Mechanisms: Ion Channel Disruption (Fig. 28.2)

- *Traditional Depolarized Arrest*: The standard approach induces arrest by flooding the heart with potassium. This disrupts the normal electrical balance within cells (depolarization), preventing contractions.
  – The Role of Potassium Most cardioplegia solutions rely on increased extracellular potassium (15–30 mEq/L) to induce depolarized arrest. However, excessive potassium (>40 mEq/L) is harmful as it increases calcium influx, damaging the ischemic heart.

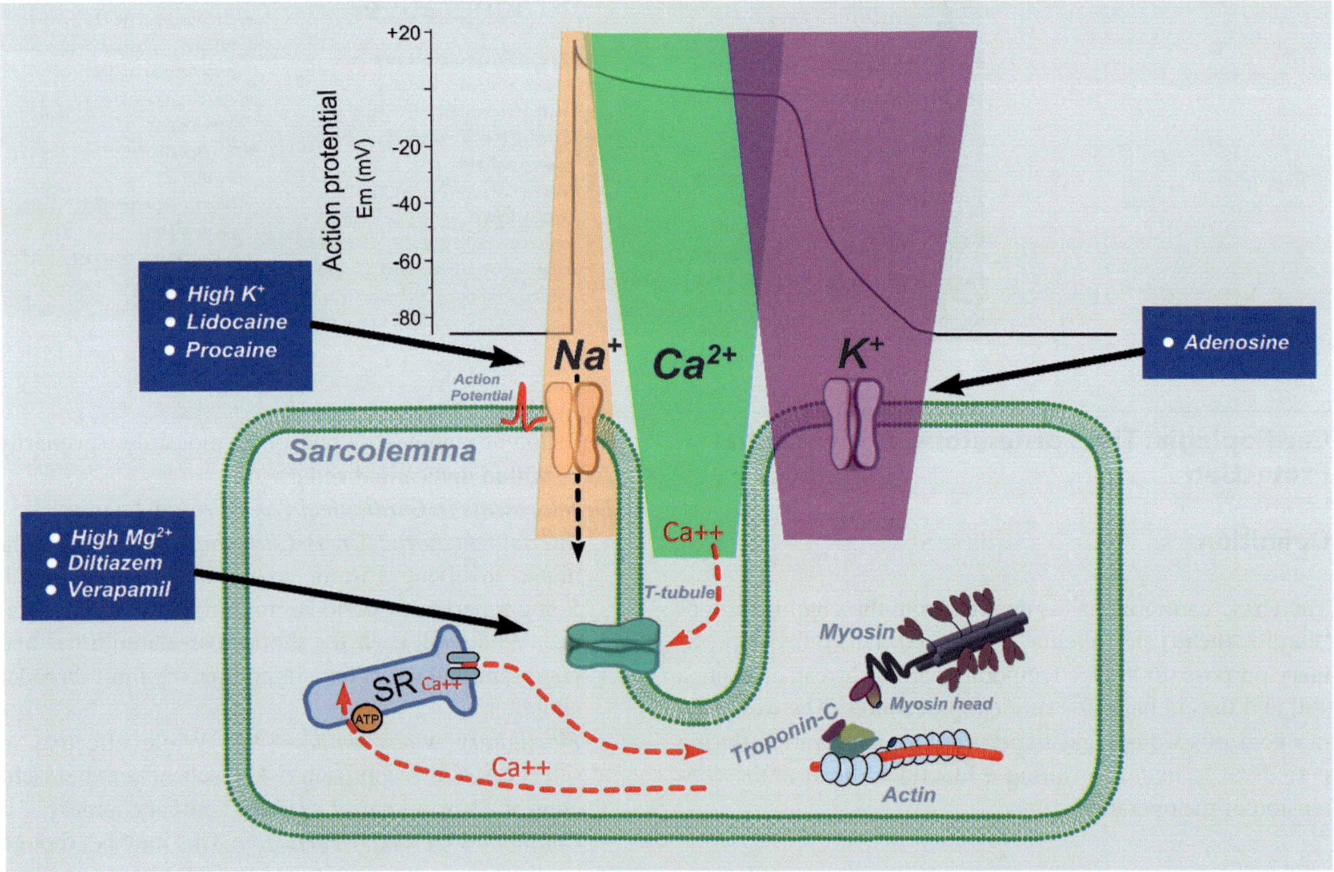

Fig. 28.2 This illustration demonstrates how cardioplegic arrest is achieved by targeting key cellular components within the cardiac action potential. Drugs targeting specific ion channels (e.g., sodium and calcium channels) or cellular processes (e.g., potassium efflux) can manipulate the action potential at various points to halt cardiac activity during surgery, inducing either depolarized or polarized arrest. Understanding these mechanisms is crucial for developing and optimizing cardioplegic solutions for cardiac protection during CPB

- *Alternative Approaches*: Newer techniques are being explored to enhance myocardial protection, including:
  - *Polarized Arrest*: These agents maintain the cell's membrane potential close to its resting state. This approach aims to minimize the energy-depleting side effects of depolarization. Common agents include potassium channel openers like adenosine and sodium channel blockers such as lidocaine.
  - *Calcium Modulation*: This strategy targets calcium regulation within heart cells to avoid ischemic and reperfusion calcium overload. Agents used include calcium channel blockers (diltiazem, verapamil), which limit calcium entry, and compounds like 2,3-butanedione monoxime that inhibit calcium-induced contractions.
  - *Combination Approaches*: Potential for synergistic protection when combining different strategies, such as polarized arrest with calcium modulation, to enhance myocardial protection.

  The goal of these alternative approaches is to rapidly arrest the heart while minimizing the harmful effects of ischemia and reperfusion, ultimately improving cardiac recovery post-surgery.

Fundamental Components of Cardioplegia Solutions

Cardioplegia solutions, administered immediately upon cross-clamp application, rapidly reduce myocardial oxygen consumption. While crucial for myocardial protection, cardioplegia alone is not sufficient. Addressing the consequences of surgically induced ischemia requires additional strategies, including (Table 28.1):

1. *Buffering and Acidosis Management*: Ischemia leads to a buildup of acids within heart cells. Cardioplegia solutions contain buffers to neutralize this acidity. Common buffers include bicarbonate, histidine, tris (hydroxymethyl) aminomethane (THAM), amino sulfonic acid, and phosphate. Maintaining a pH of 6.8 or higher is important for adequate protection.
2. *Maintaining Metabolic Substrates*: To support anaerobic metabolism during ischemia and facilitate recovery upon reperfusion, cardioplegia solutions may include substrates such as glucose (with or without insulin), aspartate, glutamate, among others. This ensures that pre-ischemic energy stores are not depleted and supports cellular energy needs and homeostasis.
3. *Osmotic Regulation for Edema Prevention*: Edema buildup in the myocardial cells, a detrimental effect of ischemia, can be controlled by maintaining cardioplegia solutions at an isotonic level between 290–330 mOsm/L. Agents used to achieve this osmolarity include inert sugars (mannitol and sorbitol), metabolizable sugars (glucose, dextrose), and oncotic agents like albumin.

Cardiac arrest drastically reduces the heart's energy needs, as electromechanical work constitutes most of its oxygen consumption. In this arrested state, the heart mainly needs to meet basal metabolic demands. Cardioplegia solutions facilitate this through periodic substrate replenishment and metabolite washout, allowing aerobic and anaerobic metabolism to produce enough energy.

Although cardioplegia formulations vary widely across institutions, there are essential properties shared by all: inducing prompt diastolic arrest, incorporating hypothermia, providing sufficient substrates, buffering against acidosis, increasing osmolarity to prevent cellular edema, providing membrane stabilization, all while being safe for comprehensive myocardial delivery without adverse effects.

The primary mechanism for achieving electromechanical arrest in most cardioplegia solutions involves increasing extracellular potassium levels, typically ranging from 15 to 30 mEq/L, to ensure prompt cardiac arrest. However,

Table 28.1 Essential components of cardioplegia solutions and their functions

Basic element	Agents	Mechanisms	Purpose
Depolarized arrest	Potassium, lidocaine.	Depolarized arrest by sodium channel blockers	Stops cardiac contractions quickly, conserving energy
Polarized arrest	Adenosine, procaine, lidocaine	Polarized arrest by potassium channel openers or by sodium channel blockers	Reduce myocardial demand
Calcium modulation arrest	Calcium Channel blockers (diltiazem, verapamil), elevated magnesium	Calcium regulation in the myocardial cells to avoid ischemic and reperfusion calcium overload	Minimize myocardial work by inhibiting calcium-induced contractions
Buffering	Bicarbonate, phosphate, Aminosulfonic acid, THAM, histidine	Neutralize harmful hydrogen ions buildup due to ischemia	Prevent acidosis
Supplemental metabolic substrates	Glucose, insulin, aspartate, glutamate, dextrose	Provide energy	Support anaerobic metabolism during ischemia, aid in recovery
Isotonic solution	Mannitol, sorbitol, glucose, dextrose, albumin	Increase oncotic pressure	Prevent myocardial swelling (edema)

potassium levels above 40 mEq/L are detrimental, as they increase calcium influx, exacerbating ischemic damage and elevating myocardial oxygen demands.

Types of Cardioplegic Solution

Cardioplegia solutions are available as crystalloid-based, blood-based, or a combination of both. While no definitive evidence favors one type over another, combined solutions are predominantly used in the United States. Both solutions can be temperature-regulated and administered cool, tepid, or warm.

Cold Crystalloid Cardioplegic Solutions

Crystalloid cardioplegic solutions are broadly categorized based on their electrolyte content and how closely they mimic cellular environments:

- *Extracellular Based Solutions*: These are formulated to mirror the external cellular environment, featuring higher concentrations of sodium, calcium, and magnesium, along with additional potassium and bicarbonate. An example is St. Thomas' Hospital II solution (Plegisol, Pfizer, Inc.), which has a sodium level of 110 mEq/L.
- *Intracellular Based Solutions*: Formulated to resemble the electrolyte composition within the cells, containing low or no sodium and calcium. A prominent example is Custodiol, also known as HTK or Brettschneider's solution, with a sodium concentration of only 15 mEq/L.

Blood Cardioplegia

Blood cardioplegia offers several advantages over crystalloid cardioplegic solutions: it enhances oxygen delivery through the oxygen-carrying capacity of red blood cells, provides superior buffering capabilities via histidine and carbonic anhydrase in red blood cells, and helps mitigate ischemic damage by scavenging free radicals present in red blood cells and plasma components. Additionally, blood's natural composition maintains optimal oncotic pressure, crucial for tissue integrity. However, concerns with cold blood cardioplegia include a hypothermic shift in the oxyhemoglobin curve, which reduces oxygen release to tissues, and the risk of blood sludging and red cell rouleaux formation due to hypothermia. Blood cardioplegia can be delivered in warm, tepid, or cold states.

- *Cold blood cardioplegia.*
  Cold blood cardioplegia uses a potassium-rich solution and is typically diluted to minimize microcirculatory sludging. Oxygenated autologous blood drawn from the CPB circuit's oxygenator is then diluted and mixed with a crystalloid cardioplegia solution to induce electromechanical arrest (see Fig. 7.6). The blood-to-crystalloid ratio can be adjusted, and the mixture is circulated through a roller pump to a heat-exchanger where it is either warmed or cooled prior to administration. Both the line pressure and temperature of the cardioplegia solution are closely monitored. For more details on the cardioplegia delivery system setup, please refer to Chap. 7. The solution is usually maintained at temperatures between 4 and 12 °C. The Buckberg solution is mixed at a blood-to-crystalloid ratio of 4:1 or 8:1, while the del Nido solution uses a 1:4 ratio.
- *Additional Techniques.*
  - *Warm blood cardioplegia*: is typically administered as an additional "hot shot"—a single dose given just before the aorta is declamped—to recover myocardial enzymes essential for energy production, enhance oxygen delivery by shifting the oxygen dissociation curve back to the right, and provide metabolic substrates to replenish energy stores, supporting heart recovery post-CPB. It is administered at 37 °C.
  - *Tepid blood cardioplegia*: typically, at 29 °C but ranging from 25 to 32 °C, seeks to optimize the metabolic benefits of hypothermia while minimizing issues like impaired oxygen release. It is used either alone or in conjunction with other cardioplegic techniques.

While many types of cardioplegic solutions exist, Del Nido, Bretschneider, and Buckberg will be focused on (see Table 28.2).

Table 28.2 Comparison of cardioplegic solutions contents

Solution	Basic solution	Type	Na^{++} mEq/L	K^{+} mEq/L	Mg^{++} mEq/L	Ca^{++} mEq/L	pH	Glucose (mg/dL)	Other key components	Effective protection time per dose
Del Nido	Plasma-Lyte A	Extracellular based	130–140	20–30	6	0.4	7.4	–	Lidocaine 130 mg, mannitol 14.5 mmol/L	90 min
Buckberg (modified buckberg)	D5 ¼ NS	Extracellular based	110–120	10–20	16	0–0.1	7.5–7.7	100–200	CPD 225, lidocaine 27 mg/L tromethamine 225, amino acids: Aspartate 13, glutamate 13	20 min
HTK (bretschneider)		Intracellular based	15	9	4	0.015	7.4	–	Mannitol 30, histidine 198, tryptophan 2, ketoglutarate 1	0–120 min Enables up to 240 min preservation of allograft

Del Nido Cardioplegia (DNC) Origins and Key Characteristics

Adult cardiac surgery has grown more complex, with patients often requiring multiple grafts, emergency procedures, and dealing with comorbidities like diabetes and heart failure. There's also a rise in minimally invasive valve surgeries. These complexities increase challenges such as prolonged cross-clamp times—a significant risk factor—and necessitate frequent or continuous cardioplegia administration. Most available cardioplegic need to be readministered every 10 to 30 min or infused continuously for myocardial protection.

Developed by Dr. Pedro del Nido in the 1990s at Boston Children's Hospital, DNC was designed specifically for the unique needs of immature myocytes in pediatric cardiac surgery. Key features include:

- *Classification*: DNC cardioplegia solution, classified as a modified depolarizing arrest cardioplegia, is an extracellular solution mixed with autologous blood.
- *Composition*: DNC cardioplegia solution uses Plasma-Lyte A (Baxter Healthcare Corp., Deerfield, IL, USA) as its glucose-free crystalloid base.
  This solution is supplemented with (Fig. 28.3):
  - Potassium chloride (26 mEq/L).
  - Lidocaine (1%, 13 mL).
  - Mannitol (20%, 3.2 g/L).
  - Magnesium sulfate (50%, 2 g).
  - Sodium bicarbonate (13 mEq/L).

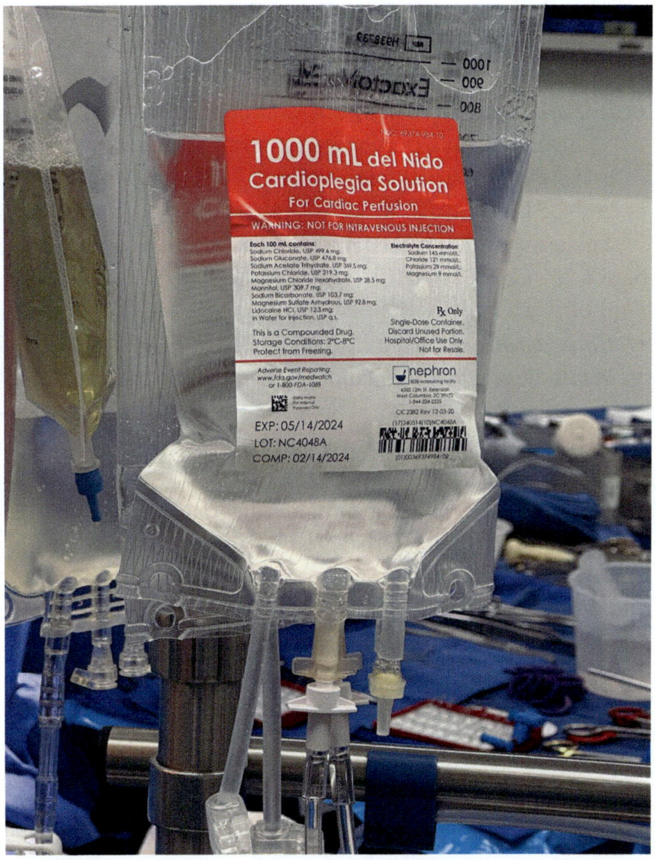

Fig. 28.3 An image of the DNC solution: This single-dose solution is specifically formulated to extend myocardial protection during cardiac surgeries, reducing the need for multiple dosages and streamlining the surgical process

- *Rationale*:
  - Neonatal myocytes are more tolerant of ischemia than adult cells but highly susceptible to calcium influx.
  - Magnesium reduces calcium entry during reperfusion and inhibits myocyte contraction.
  - Lidocaine stabilizes membranes (prolonging arrest) and blocks sodium-calcium channels (decreasing calcium influx), thus preventing intracellular calcium buildup during ischemia.
- *Administration*: This cardioplegia formulation allows for extended intervals between infusions, up to 90 minutes, using a 1:4 blood cardioplegia ratio (1 part oxygenated patient blood to 4 parts cardioplegia solution). A single antegrade dose of 20 mL/kg is administered through the cardioplegia delivery system at temperatures between 4–12 °C. However, some surgeons prefer an alternative two-dose strategy for enhanced effect:
  - *Initial Arresting Dose*: Administered once the aorta is clamped, this dose consists of about two-thirds of the total volume planned.
  - *Supplemental Dose:* An additional 200–400 mL is given shortly after the initial dose, just before the activation of the root vent.

The goal remains achieving a myocardial temperature below 15 °C.

- *Considerations for Adult Use*.
  While developed for pediatric hearts, del Nido cardioplegia's simplicity makes it appealing for adult use, particularly in minimally invasive procedures. However, caution is advised as:
  - It was designed for immature hearts with distinct biochemical characteristics and higher reliance on glucose metabolism.
  - Its safety in adults with diseased ventricles or diffuse coronary artery disease is uncertain.
- *When might DNC be considered in adults?*
  - Short cross-clamp times anticipated.
  - Good ventricular function.
  - Minimally invasive surgeries where complex cardioplegia administration is less desirable.

Buckberg and Modified Buckberg Cardioplegia: Composition, Administration, and Benefits

The Buckberg cardioplegia, developed by Dr. Gerald Buckberg, is a blood-based solution primarily designed for extended myocardial protection. It contains a dextrose-based solution in normal saline, alongside potassium chloride for magnesium to reduce ischemic damage, and procaine as a membrane stabilizer. Buckberg solution is typically given in multiple cold doses, sometimes with a warm reperfusion dose for metabolic recovery. Buckberg cardioplegia contains a dextrose-based solution in normal saline, alongside potassium chloride for depolarization, tromethamine for buffering, and citrate phosphate double dextrose to chelate calcium. This solution is mixed with oxygenated patient blood at a 4:1 (blood: crystalloid) ratio. Modified Buckberg cardioplegia varies across institutions. Common modifications include replacing procaine with lidocaine for longer-lasting effects, using tromethamine (THAM) as a buffer, and adjusting blood-to-crystalloid ratios. These adaptations aim to improve stability and metabolic support during cardiac arrest and reperfusion. It is strategically administered in three phases:

- Induction: The initial dose, delivered at 4 °C, induces cardiac arrest.
- Maintenance: Follow-up doses are given approximately every 15–20 min, also at 4 °C, to maintain cardiac arrest and provide oxygen and nutrients.
- Reperfusion ("Hot Shot"): Just before the aortic cross-clamp is removed, a reperfusion dose at 37 °C delivers a surge of glutamate and aspartate, essential nutrients that support the heart as it resumes its beating function.

Key Characteristics and Benefits

- *Intermittent Delivery*: Antegrade and retrograde administration as above.
- *Hypothermia*: Reduces metabolic demands, preserving myocardial function.
- *Controlled Reperfusion*: Lasting 3–5 min before the release of the cross-clamp, this phase is designed to:
  - Low calcium CPD (citrate phosphate dextrose) to aid the resumption of electrical activity.
  - Low potassium supports consistent electrical activity.
  - Keep reperfusion pressure below 50 mmHg to reduce endothelial damage.
  - Employ slight hyperosmolarity (360–400 mOsm) helps prevent myocardial edema.
- *Amino Acid Enhancement*:
  - Substrate Enhancement: The addition of glutamate and aspartate, critical intermediates in the Krebs cycle, enhances post-ischemic contractility. This is especially beneficial for hearts that are energy-depleted.
  - Enhanced Recovery: The benefits are particularly pronounced in hearts suffering from prior ischemia or cardiogenic shock. Incorporating glutamate and aspartate in a warm induction solution before cardiac arrest can further enhance myocardial protection.

Histidine–Tryptophan–Ketoglutarate (HTK) Solution (Custodiol/Bretschneider)

Developed by Dr. Bretschneider in Germany. Key features include:

- *Classification*: Bretschneider cardioplegia solution, classified as a hyperpolarization diastolic arrest cardioplegia, is an intracellular solution with low sodium and a high histidine concentration.
- *Composition*: Bretschneider's solution utilizes a specific crystalloid base, typically Plasma-lyte A. Its key components include:
  This solution is supplemented with:
  - *Potassium chloride*: At a lower concentration compared to other cardioplegia solutions, it helps in inducing diastolic arrest.
  - *Histidine*: A key amino acid, serving as a buffering agent and free radical scavenger. It provides substrate for ATP production.
  - *Tryptophan*: Functions as a membrane stabilizer.
  - *Ketoglutarate*: An intermediate in the Krebs cycle, aiding in ATP production during reperfusion.
  - *Mannitol*: An osmotic diuretic is included to help reduce myocardial edema.
  - *Magnesium sulfate*: Stabilizes cell membranes and reduces calcium influx, which can damage cells.
- *Benefits*:
  - Extended protection (up to several hours) with a single dose.
  - Technical ease, especially valuable for complex or minimally invasive surgeries.
  - Reduced ischemia-reperfusion injury (theoretically, due to composition).
  - Suitable for organ preservation during transplant.

Considerations

- May cause electrolyte disturbances (hyponatremia), though these are typically manageable.
- Controversies exist regarding the potential increased risk of postoperative cardiac enzyme elevation and myocardial edema in certain cases.

Less ideal for patients with severe multi-vessel disease or significant left ventricular hypertrophy due to the potential for uneven distribution.

Methods of Administering Cardioplegia

Optimal delivery of cardioplegia must be tailored to the operative procedure and operative technique. Several methods are available for cardioplegia delivery. Delivery may be via the arterial system (antegrade) or via the venous system (retrograde). Figure 2.1 illustrates these two methods.

Antegrade Cardioplegia Infusion

Antegrade Infusion into the Aortic Root

This technique involves inserting a cannula into the aortic root, positioned between the aortic cross-clamp on one side, the aortic valve, and coronary ostia on the other side. A dual-lumen cannula is commonly used, with one lumen designated for delivering cardioplegia and the other for venting or monitoring pressure. This setup enables the measurement of aortic root pressure during the administration of cardioplegia. However, for the technique to be effective, the aortic valve must be competent. If it is not competent, the cardioplegia solution will flow back into the left ventricle, causing ventricular distension and preventing adequate distribution of cardioplegia through the coronary arteries.

Cardioplegia Administration into the Grafts

During coronary artery bypass grafting (CABG) procedures, a cardioplegic solution is infused directly into the free end of each saphenous vein graft after the surgeon completes the distal anastomosis. This is typically performed using a syringe attached to the free end of the graft. While this traditional method is highly effective, its protection is limited to the specific artery being bypassed.

Direct Cardioplegia Infusion into the Coronary Ostia

This method is used when the aortic valve is incompetent (preventing delivery of cardioplegia into the aortic root) or when surgery requires opening the aortic root (e.g., aortic valve replacement). The surgeon must precisely locate the coronary ostia and insert specially designed catheters for cardioplegia infusion. Catheters are carefully sized to prevent damage to the ostia (Fig. 28.4).

- Potential Complications:
  Direct ostial cardioplegia delivery presents several potential complications.
  - *Incomplete Perfusion*:
    If the catheter tip extends beyond the bifurcation of the left main coronary artery, only the territories of the left anterior descending or circumflex artery territory might receive protection. This is especially risky in patients with bicuspid aortic valves due to their shorter left main coronary artery.
  - *Conus Artery Exclusion*: In approximately 50% of patients, the right ventricle's conus artery branches separately from the aortic sinus and won't be protected by cannulating the right coronary ostium.

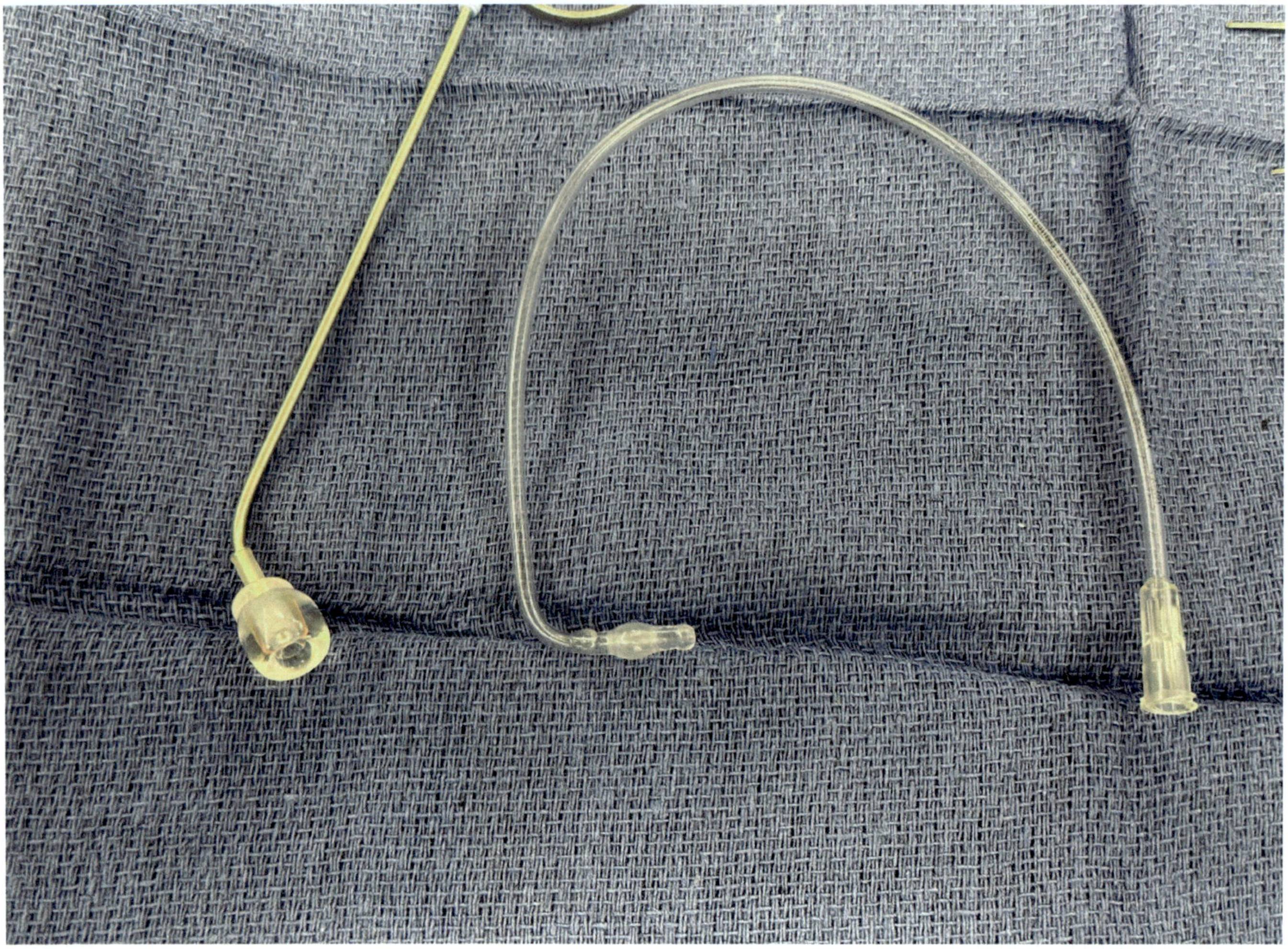

Fig. 28.4 Image of two types of catheters that enable targeted infusion of cardioplegic solution directly into the coronary ostia. This provides myocardial protection during specific cardiac surgeries, such as those involving a malfunctioning aortic valve or requiring access to the aortic root

- *Ostial Stenosis*: Directly cannulating the ostia carries a risk of damaging them, potentially leading to later stenosis.

For any antegrade delivery methods, infusion pressure should not exceed 150 mmHg to prevent complications.

Retrograde Coronary Sinus Perfusion

- *Understanding Coronary Drainage.*
  Approximately 70% of coronary blood drains through the small, middle, oblique, and great cardiac veins into the coronary sinus (CS), which then empties into the right atrium (RA). The remaining 30% drains directly into the RA via the anterior cardiac veins, or into the right ventricle via Thebesian veins.
- *Retrograde coronary sinus perfusion (RCSP).*
  RCSP involves infusing cardioplegia into the CS, from where it flows in a retrograde fashion into the great and small cardiac veins. This method's extensive venous network, typically free of atherosclerosis, allows for protection of the entire myocardium (Fig. 28.5).
- *Procedure.*
  - A balloon -tipped catheter secures placement in the CS, preventing backflow. Cardioplegia delivery begins after aortic cross-clamping.
  - Venting (via the aortic root or left ventricle) Most of the retrograde perfusion drains via the Thebesian veins, but either the aortic root or the left ventricle is usually vented during cardioplegia infusion to allow egress of the solution.
  - A central lumen in the CS catheter monitors pressure during cardioplegia infusion to prevent injury to the coronary venous system. The acceptable range for retrograde perfusion is 30–50 mmHg.

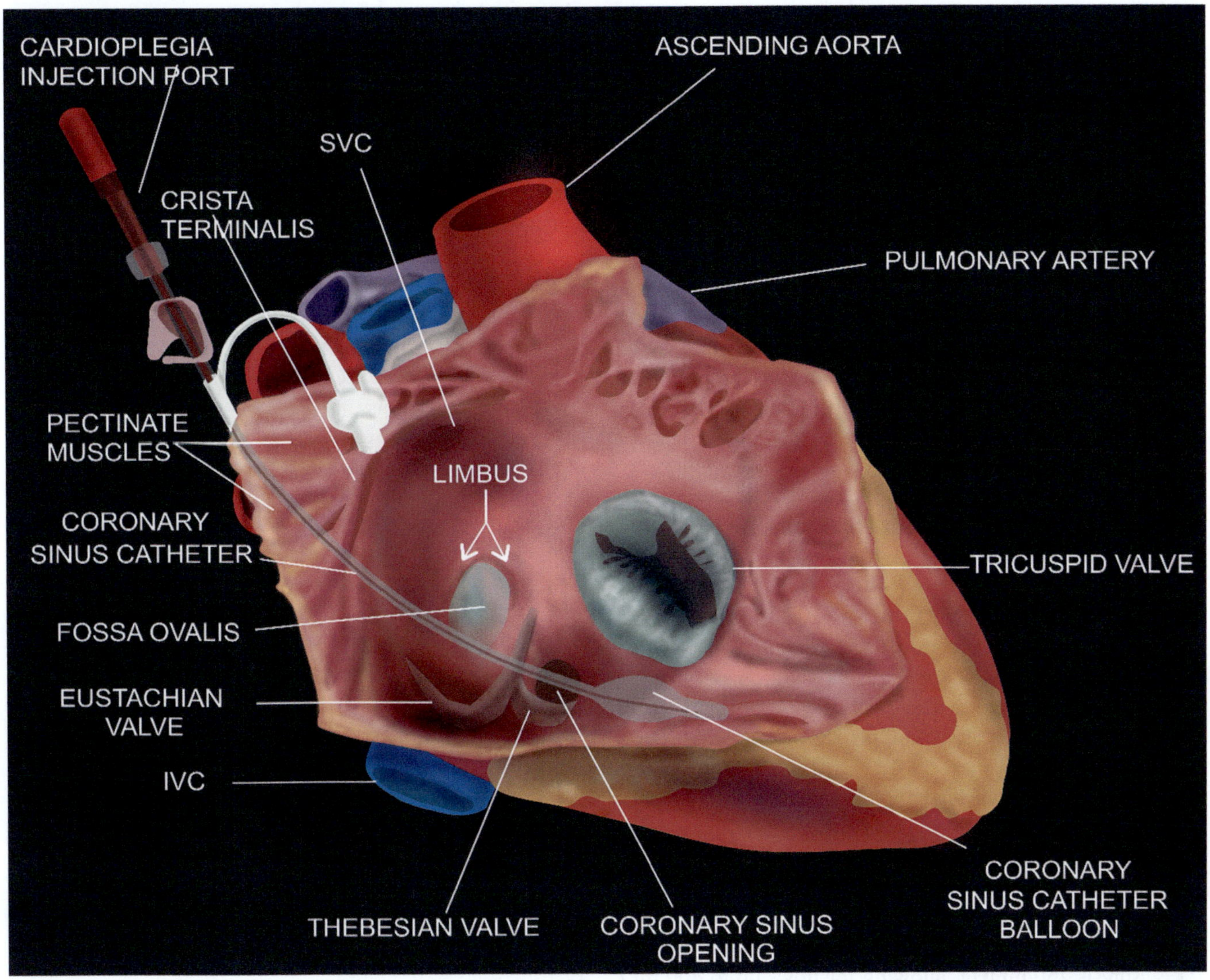

Fig. 28.5 This illustration shows the internal structure of an opened RA and features a retrograde cardioplegia cannula used for delivering cardioplegic solutions through the CS. The cannula is equipped with either a self-inflating or manually inflating balloon. In the self-inflating version, the cardioplegia solution inflates the soft polyurethane balloon through the primary lumen, automatically sealing and securing the cannula tip within the CS. The manual version includes a third lumen for balloon inflation. Pressure at the cannula tip can be continuously monitored through a dedicated measuring lumen. A flexible or rigid stylet aids in guiding the cannula's insertion and positioning

- Benefits of Retrograde Cardioplegia.
  Retrograde cardioplegia is useful in several circumstances.
  - *Aortic Valve Surgeries*: Ideal for aortic valve replacement, avoiding direct ostial cannulation ostia. Also superior to aortic root perfusion when aortic incompetence is present.
  - *Coronary Stenosis*: Retrograde cardioplegia provides a more uniform distribution compared to antegrade delivery when coronary stenoses are present. This improved distribution is likely due to the large venous network that is free from atherosclerotic disease.
  - *Reoperations*: Retrograde perfusion proves beneficial in redo surgeries for patients with patent left internal mammary artery (LIMA) grafts. During LIMA occlusion, retrograde perfusion facilitates the delivery of cardioplegia to the myocardium supplied by the patent graft.
  - *Continuous Delivery*: Retrograde perfusion enables to continuously infuse cardioplegia or re-dosing without interrupting the surgery. This feature is particularly advantageous during aortic valve/root or mitral valve (MV) surgeries. Additionally, it can aid in removing air and flushing debris from the coronary arteries during aortic valve operations.
- *Contraindications and Considerations.*
  - *Persistent Left Superior Vena Cava (PLSVC)*: A major contraindications for retrograde delivery of cardioplegia is the presence of a PLSVC that drains into the CS,

as illustrated in Fig. 28.6. This anomaly impedes the pressurization of the CS, leading to the systemic delivery of cardioplegia rather than targeted delivery.

- *RV and Septum Protection*: RCSP offers limited protection for the RV and posterior septum due to venovenous shunting through arteriosinusoidal and Thebesian vessels directly into the RV. Consequently, only 30–70% of the retrograde cardioplegia administered actually reaches the myocardial tissue.
- *Variable distribution*: Due to venous anatomy differences, retrograde delivery can be uneven, especially in hypertrophied or ischemic hearts.
- *Combined Approach*: Many institutions employ both antegrade and retrograde cardioplegia to achieve optimal myocardial protection in a single patient.

Key Cardioplegia Parameters: Flow Rate and Delivery Pressure

After beginning cardioplegia, the surgeon and perfusionist must collaborate to ensure proper line pressure and adequate flow. The initial dose of cardioplegia solution is typically between 1 and 1.2 liters. Maintaining appropriate pressure throughout delivery is crucial (Table 28.3):

- *High pressure*: Can lead to dissection of the coronary arteries.
- *Low pressure*: Indicates inadequate delivery, potentially compromising myocardial protection.

1. *Aortic Antegrade Cannulation*: Maximum pump pressure is 250 mmHg, allowing for flows up to 400 mL/min. Typical aortic root pressure is 50–60 mmHg.
2. *Retrograde Cannulation*: Target flow of 200–400 mL/min with a CS pressure of 20–45 mmHg.

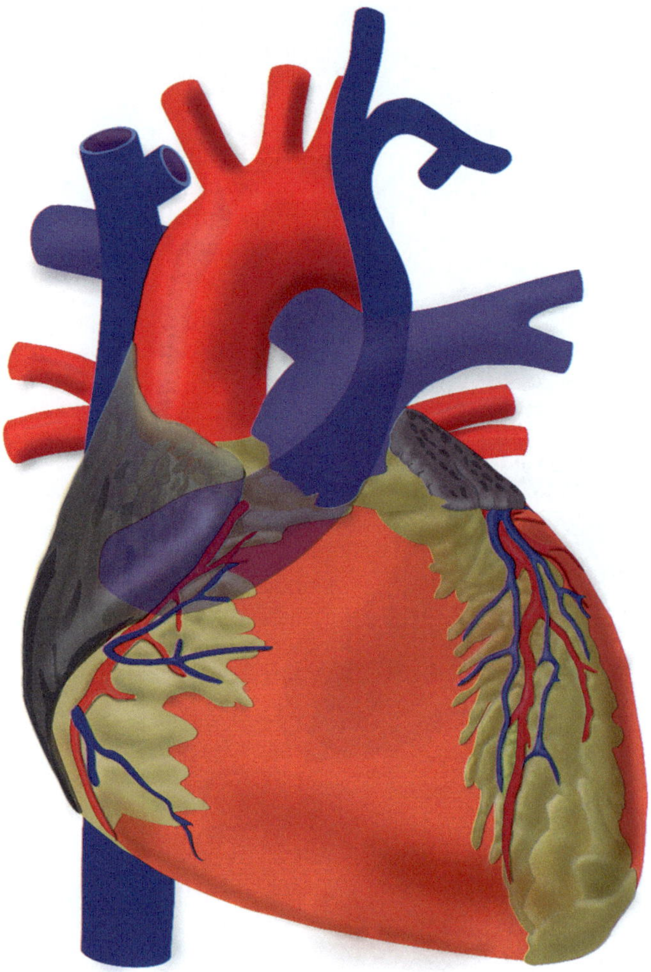

Fig. 28.6 Illustration of a human heart showing PLSVC: This anatomical anomaly, when present, poses a significant contraindication for retrograde cardioplegia delivery. With PLSVC draining into the CS, as shown here, pressurizing the CS for cardioplegia delivery becomes ineffective. This can lead to unintended systemic delivery of the cardioplegic solution instead of the targeted coronary circulation

Table 28.3 Key cardioplegia parameters: flow rate and delivery pressure

Cardioplegic route	Target flow rate (mL/min)	Pressure limit (mmHg)
Aortic antegrade cannulation	Up to 500 mL/min	Max pump pressure: 250 mmHg typical aortic root pressure: 50–60 mmHg
Retrograde	200–400	CS pressure: 20–45 mmHg
Direct coronary cannulation (right coronary artery)	25–100	Max pump pressure: 200 mmHg
Direct coronary cannulation (left coronary artery)	25–150	Max pump pressure: 200 mmHg

3. *Direct Coronary Cannulation*: Limit pump pressure to 200 mmHg, allowing for flows of 50–250 mL/min.

Factors Contributing to Persistent Cardiac Activity Despite Cardioplegia

Even with ideal technique, electrical activity can sometimes persist after cardioplegia is administered. Here are common causes:

Inadequate Cardioplegia Delivery

1. *Right Coronary Artery Lesion*: A proximal blockage in this artery can impede the delivery of cardioplegia to the sinoatrial (SA) node. This continued lack of cardioplegic arrest in the SA node allows it to maintain electrical activity and initiate heartbeats.
2. *Aortic Insufficiency*: Blood backflow can fill and distend the left ventricle, diluting the cardioplegia and reducing flow to the coronary arteries.
3. *Incomplete Aortic Cross-Clamping*: The cross-clamp is not fully occlusive, and leakage of blood past the clamp can dilute the cardioplegia solution.

Other Factors:

1. *Defective Cardioplegia Solution*: Problems with composition or incorrect preparation can render the cardioplegia ineffective.
2. *Insufficient Cooling*: Cardioplegia must be sufficiently cooled to function optimally.
3. *Inadequate Venous Drainage*: Incomplete heart drainage can limit the removal of blood that dilutes the cardioplegia.

Optimizing CPB and Aortic Cross-Clamp Time for Myocardial Protection

Cardioplegia and its various delivery methods have enabled surgeons to perform increasingly complex cardiac surgical procedures. Consequently, CPB duration and aortic cross-clamp time have progressively increased to meet this demand. However, minimizing both CPB and aortic cross-clamp times is crucial, as prolonged periods can negatively impact cardiac function.

CPB Duration

The duration of CPB and the blood's exposure to the artificial bypass circuit surfaces significantly influence systemic inflammatory response syndrome (SIRs). Specifically, there is a positive correlation between CPB duration and the magnitude of the interleukin (IL)-6 response. Chapter 6 explores the detailed impact of this inflammatory response on myocardial function.

Aortic Cross-Clamp Time

Aortic cross-clamp time by itself is an independent predictor of morbidity and mortality in cardiac surgical patients. Cross-clamp times exceeding 90 min are associated with significantly increased in-hospital mortality when compared to under 60 min. They also correlate with low cardiac output and prolonged postoperative ventilation.

Upon aortic cross-clamp release, the heart is reperfused with immunologically primed blood. Continuous blood flow through the non-endothelialized bypass circuit triggers an inflammatory cascade involving neutrophil recruitment and activation. This generates excess reactive oxygen species (free radicals) that activate proinflammatory and apoptotic pathways, ultimately impacting postoperative cardiac function. Chapter 6 delves into the triggers, pathways, and mitigation strategies for the inflammatory response induced by CPB.

Other Myocardial Protection Strategies in Addition to Cardioplegia

Cardioplegia is a cornerstone of myocardial protection, but it's not the only strategy. Other myocardial protection strategies are employed, including left ventricular venting to prevent blood accumulation and ventricular distension during CPB, systemic hypothermia (which significantly lowers metabolic demand and oxygen consumption), and off-pump CABG to minimize ischemic time altogether. Further strategies like intermittent cross-clamp fibrillation on bypass, ischemic preconditioning, pump-assisted beating heart procedures, and deep hypothermic circulatory arrest enrich the toolkit for preserving heart function during surgery. These diverse approaches ensure a comprehensive protection strategy for optimal myocardial preservation.

Left Ventricular Venting During CPB

During CPB, blood can accumulate in the left ventricle from sources like aortic insufficiency, Thebesian veins, and bronchial circulation. If this blood is not expelled, the ventricle can distend, increasing its diameter, myocardial wall tension, and temperature. This elevation in wall tension not only increases the oxygen demand of the heart tissues but also impedes subendocardial blood flow. Left ventricular venting alleviates this by diverting accumulated blood to the CPB reservoir, thereby decompressing the ventricle, enhancing surgical visibility and access, which facilitates faster and more precise procedures, reduces ischemic time, and promotes myocardial protection. Venting also minimizes blood contact with the septum, preventing excessive rewarming of the septum during this critical stage, and helps evacuate air from the ventricle.

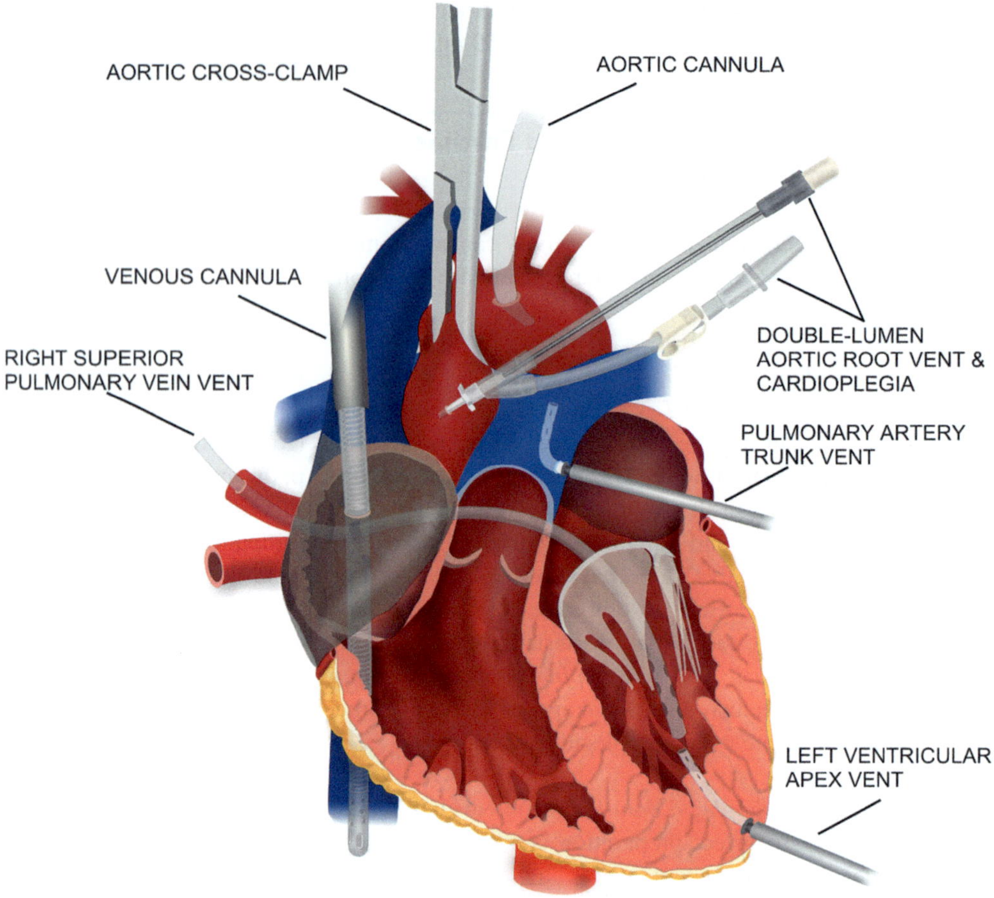

Fig. 28.7 The illustration depicts various strategies for venting blood from the left ventricle during cardiac surgery. These methods include cannulation of the aortic root, left ventricular apex, or routing the catheter through the right superior pulmonary vein to access the left atrium, then across the MV into the left ventricle, and finally, placement within the pulmonary trunk

The most common venting locations are (Fig. 28.7):

- *Left Ventricular Venting*:
  - *Right Superior Pulmonary Vein*: This is indeed the most common site for left ventricular venting during CPB. A multi-holed catheter is inserted into the right upper pulmonary vein and then passes across the MV into the left ventricle to drain accumulated blood. This technique is particularly employed in patients with inadequate left ventricular function and during aortic and MV surgery, specifically when aortic regurgitation is present (see Fig. 7.7).
  - *Left Ventricular Apex Venting*: The LV apex can be an effective venting site for decompressing the LV and clearing trapped air in the ventricular cavity, particularly when other approaches are not feasible. However, it is seldom used today due to the risk of bleeding after removal, and is primarily considered for venting the LV in reoperations where the risk of sternotomy is high.
- *Aortic Root Venting*: It is the predominant technique employed during CABG surgery. It facilitates drainage of blood from the left ventricle by creating suction at the aortic root, which indirectly decompresses the ventricle. However, it's effective only under specific conditions: a clamped aorta, no antegrade cardioplegia being infused, and a closed aortic root (see Fig. 7.8).
- *Pulmonary Artery Trunk Venting*: Left ventricular venting via the pulmonary artery although used in the past seldom used today due to its limitations. Specifically, this technique does not consistently ensure effective decompression of the LV when aortic regurgitation is present. Additionally, closing the incision in the pulmonary artery may pose significant challenges in patients with pulmonary hypertension.

Please refer to Chap. 7, 'Fundamentals of Cardiopulmonary Bypass Machine Equipment,' for more details on the venting system setup and circuit.

Systemic Hypothermia

Inducing systemic hypothermia offers protective benefits to the heart and brain by reducing the metabolic breakdown of energy stores. This protection occurs during surgically induced ischemia caused by reduced perfusion. For a detailed exploration of the protective mechanisms of systemic hypothermia, refer to Chap. 6, "Physiologic Changes and Inflammatory Response to Cardiopulmonary Bypass," and Chap. 12, "Metabolic Derangements During Cardiopulmonary Bypass."

Systemic hypothermia induction can be either active or passive:

- *Active Cooling*: This involves using the CPB circuit's heat-exchanger system (refer to Chap. 7, Fig. 7.19).
- *Passive Cooling*: Methods include applying ice slush directly to the thoracic cavity and using cold cardioplegia as discussed above.

Deep Hypothermic Circulatory Arrest (DHCA)

DHCA offers an alternative for cardiac and brain protection when aortic clamping is impossible. This method is particularly valuable in cases where conditions like porcelain aorta preclude the use of aortic clamping.

Ischemic Preconditioning.

- *During CPB*: Ischemic preconditioning (IPC), as initially described by Murry and colleagues, is a phenomenon where short, controlled periods of ischemia followed by reperfusion several times help protect the heart against subsequent prolonged ischemic episodes. This "preconditioning" helps the heart withstand the longer blockage by preservation of key cellular energy molecules like ATP and CP, stabilization of cell pH, and reduced cellular structural damage.

  IPC has two phases:

- Early phase: Offers short-term protection, lasting up to 2 h.
- Late phase: Provides weaker protection that kicks in 24–96 h after preconditioning.

While ischemic preconditioning created by clamping and declamping the ascending aorta in two three-minute episodes provides myocardial protection, it also increases the risk of neurological complications due to potential embolic events; consequently, this practice fell out of favor.

- *During Off-Pump*: The efficacy of IPC in off-pump heart bypass surgery is still under debate. Research by Laurikka et al., which involved occluding the left anterior descending coronary artery using silicon tape for two cycles of 2-minute occlusions followed by 3-minute reperfusions, showed improvements in heart function and reduced damage. However, other studies have not reported any significant benefits from IPC in similar surgical settings.
- *Remote Ischemic Preconditioning (RIPC) for Cardiac Surgery*: RIPC is a technique where briefly restricting blood flow in one area of the body can protect distant organs from damage caused by ischemic injury, typically achieved by inflating and deflating a cuff on a lower limb through several short cycles. Although RIPC has demonstrated promise in minimizing postoperative myocardial injury, extensive studies are required to conclusively establish its benefits in clinical practice.

Off-Pump

CPB and aortic cross-clamp is often necessary, therefore, it is crucial to limit the duration even though there is technically no upper limit. Any procedure on interior cardiac structures (e.g., valves, ventricular/atrial septal defects) and great vessels require aortic cross-clamping, with cardiac arrest to provide a motionless and bloodless field for the surgeon. However, to avoid CPB, aortic cross-clamping/diastolic arrest altogether it is feasible to perform some cardiac surgical procedures either off-pump or on-pump beating. Off-pump cardiac surgery is typically limited to procedures on the exterior heart, specifically CABG, as illustrated in Fig. 28.8. However, this approach can be difficult if the patient has a low left ventricular ejection fraction with potential for significant hemodynamic instability during manipulation of the heart.

Pump-Assisted Beating Heart (PABH)

Beating heart and non-cardioplegic CABG without cross-clamping provides an alternative for coronary patients by utilizing CPB to offer hemodynamic support during cardiac procedures. This method keeps the heart normothermically beating and the coronaries perfused, thus avoiding both cardiac arrest and aortic cross-clamping. PABH procedures have a wide range of applications, and clinical evidence has demonstrated especially positive outcomes in certain patient groups who might not tolerate cardioplegic arrest well. These include patients with renal failure, patients considered to be high-risk, and those suffering from poor left ventricular function. The primary benefits of the PABH technique include achieving complete revascularization while maintaining hemodynamic stability, and it is associated with low morbidity and mortality rates, particularly in patients with poor left ventricular function.

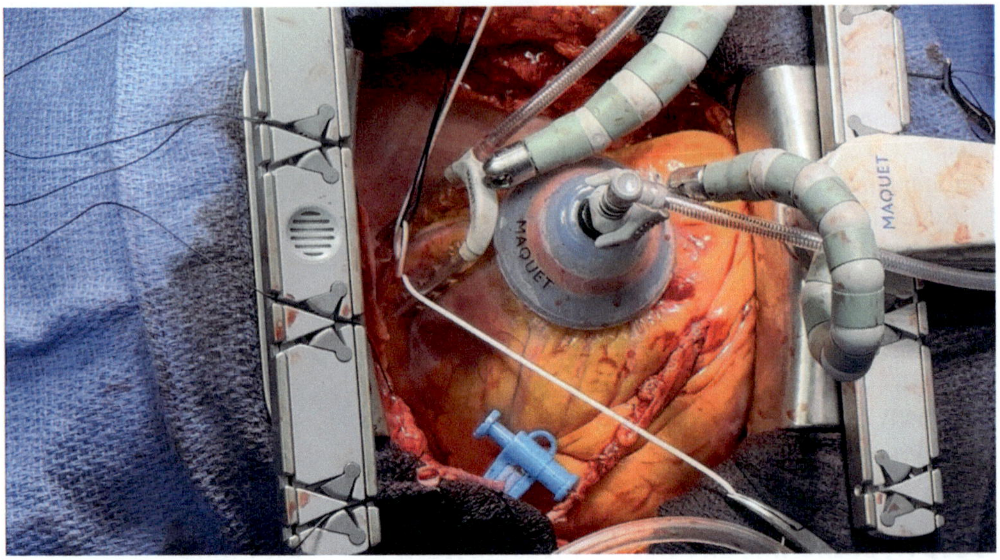

Fig. 28.8 An image of off-pump CABG with myocardial stabilizer. This approach avoids aortic cross-clamping and the associated need for cardiac arrest

Indicators of Suboptimal Myocardial Preservation

Assessing myocardial preservation effectively during CPB presents significant challenges, as the cessation of heart activity precludes the use of electrocardiography and transesophageal echocardiography. Consequently, the evaluation of myocardial function is predominantly undertaken once cardiac activity has been resumed. Here are key indicators of suboptimal preservation:

1. *Reduced Cardiac Output*: Low cardiac output is confirmed by TEE and Swan values, often accompanied by global wall motion abnormalities.
2. *Hemodynamic instability*: The need for significant pharmacological support or mechanical assist devices suggests suboptimal myocardial preservation.
3. *Arrhythmias*: Recurrent fibrillation requiring multiple electrical therapies is a concerning sign of potential myocardial damage.

Further Reading

Matte GS, del Nido PJ. History and use of del Nido cardioplegia solution at Boston Children's Hospital. J Extra Corpor Technol. 2012;44:98–103.

UpToDate.

Vaidya Y, et al. Myocardial stunning and hibernation. StatPearls [Internet]. 2022;

Velez A, et al. A novel, clinically useful definition of myocardial stunning after cardiac surgery. J Am Coll Cardiol. 2022;79(9_Supplement):1042.

Whittaker A, Aboughdir M, Mahbub S, Ahmed A, Harky A. Myocardial protection in cardiac surgery: how limited are the options? A comprehensive literature review. Perfusion. 2021;36(4):338–51.

29 Strategies of Neurological Protection During Cardiopulmonary Bypass

Julie Wyrobek

Introduction

Neurological injury after cardiac surgery is a common, multifactorial, and incompletely understood complication (Table 29.1). It can significantly worsen recovery, prolong hospital stays, and reduce quality of life. Stroke, seizures, delirium, and cognitive decline have overlapping features and etiologies, which have led to viewing these conditions as a continuum of pathophysiological processes. This chapter will explore the incidence and risk factors for these conditions, delve into the current understanding of neurological injury etiology, and discuss the latest studies and recommendations for mitigating neurological complications during cardiopulmonary bypass (CPB).

Table 29.1 Neurological complications after cardiac surgery

Category	Complications
Brain injury	Silent cerebral infarcts, intracranial hemorrhage, delirium, postoperative neurocognitive dysfunction, seizures, coma
Ophthalmologic	Retinal infarctions, supranuclear gaze palsy
Movement disorders	Chorea
Nerve injury	Peripheral neuropathy, brachial plexus injury, phrenic nerve injury, intercostal nerve injury

Types of Neurological Injury

In cardiac surgery, central nervous system (CNS) outcomes are categorized into two types according to the Multicenter Study of Perioperative Ischemia (McSPI) group:

- Type I: Overt and clinically significant neurological damage such as stroke or coma.
- Type II: Subtle cognitive and functional impairments like memory problems or confusion.

Definitions

Before exploring the main types of neurological injuries that can occur during perioperative cardiac surgery, here are some key definitions. These will assist in distinguishing each type of injury, which is crucial given their often overlapping characteristics.

Stroke: The clinical definition of a stroke is the rapid onset of a new focal neurological deficit. It can also be defined radiologically based on criteria assessed by neuroimaging techniques.

J. Wyrobek (✉)
Department of Anesthesiology & Perioperative Medicine, Strong Memorial Hospital, University of Rochester, Rochester, NY, USA
e-mail: Julie_Wyrobek@urmc.rochester.edu

A. S. Awad, J. DiNardo (eds.), *Clinical Perfusion for Cardiac Surgery*, https://doi.org/10.1007/978-3-031-91163-7_29

Transient Ischemic Attack (TIA): A temporary episode of neurological dysfunction resolving within 24 h without lasting damage.

Delirium: A transient, acute state of confusion marked by disturbances in attention, awareness, and cognition, often fluctuating in consciousness and possibly including hallucinations, delusions, and agitation.

Postoperative Encephalopathy: It refers to a syndrome of global brain dysfunction occurring after surgery. It encompasses various neurological and psychiatric manifestations, including delirium, but it also covers a wider range of neurological impairments such as seizures, focal neurological deficits, and coma.

Postoperative Neurocognitive Dysfunction: A condition characterized by a measurable decline in cognitive functions, assessed through formal neuropsychological testing conducted before and after surgery.

Seizure: A seizure is a sudden, uncontrolled electrical disturbance in the brain that can manifest as convulsive or nonconvulsive episodes. It may result from direct brain injury, temporary biochemical imbalances, or side effects of medications.

Stroke

Variability in Stroke Incidence Following Cardiac Surgery: Analysis and Implications

The incidence of stroke after cardiac surgery varies depending on the procedure. The incidence of clinically apparent strokes after cardiac surgery ranges from 1.2% to 6%, while silent (covert) strokes may affect up to 50% of patients. The overall stroke rate is approximately 1–3%, but for closed-chamber procedures, it is closer to 1%. This rate increases to 1.6% for isolated valve surgeries and 2.9% for combined coronary artery bypass graft (CABG) and valve procedures, according to data from the Society of Thoracic Surgeons database. Perioperative strokes can be classified as early, apparent upon emergence from anesthesia, delayed, developing more than 24 h postoperatively, or late, occurring over 30 days later, with significant implications for identifying causative factors like intraoperative events or the progression of underlying diseases.

Silent Brain Infarcts

Clinically silent brain infarcts, detectable on neuroimaging without accompanying stroke symptoms, occur in approximately 20% of low-risk and 50% of high-risk cardiac surgery patients. These lesions, often small and multiple, are primarily located in the frontal and watershed regions of the brain—areas vulnerable to damage due to low blood flow or blockages, as they are situated furthest from the major arterial supplies. Their presence in both on- and off-pump surgeries suggests that they may not result solely from embolic events. The incidence of new infarcts, detected within two weeks post-op via DWI-MRI, varies depending on the timing of the MRI and patient factors such as age and preexisting cerebrovascular disease. The impact of these infarcts remains uncertain; some studies suggest they may lead to early brain dysfunction or cognitive decline, while others find no clear association.

Identifying High-Risk Patients for Stroke Prior to Cardiac Surgery

Understanding the risk factors associated with stroke before cardiac surgery is crucial for identifying at-risk patients and developing preventative strategies. Here's a breakdown of the key risk factors:

- Increasing age.
- Female gender.
- Prior cerebrovascular disease.
- Preoperative atrial fibrillation increases the risk of both early and late stroke following cardiac surgery.
- Postoperative atrial fibrillation is primarily associated with strokes occurring in the later postoperative period.
- Lower ejection fraction.
- Diabetes.
- Longer CPB and cross-clamp times.
- Carotid artery stenosis.
- Atherosclerosis.
- Peripheral arterial disease.
- Urgent or emergent surgery.
- The use of deep hypothermic cardiac arrest.

Postoperative Stroke After CABG: Risks, Types, and Prediction

Stroke after CABG is associated with an increase in 30-day mortality and a threefold increase in ten-year mortality. Strokes can either be focal, thought to result from emboli, or more diffuse, likely from hypoperfusion. Incidence, or diagnosis, of postoperative stroke peaks at 40 h post-surgery. Perioperative stroke has been divided into early, occurring less than 48 h after surgery, versus late, occurring within 2 years of surgery. While the incidence is similar, early strokes have a greater mortality risk, are associated with intraoperative aortic manipulation and emboli, and have a decreased incidence during CABGs done without CPB. Approximately 5% of strokes will lead to hemorrhagic transformation. Late strokes are associated with postoperative atrial fibrillation and cerebrovascular disease. The STS risk calculator is a commonly used tool to evaluate a patient's permanent stroke risk. A CHADS score of two or higher can also be used to predict postoperative stroke.

Seizure

Diagnosing seizure activity after cardiac surgery is challenging without continuous electroencephalogram (EEG) monitoring or formal evaluation by a specialist. Postoperative movements, such as myoclonus, shivering, stroke, or dystonia, can be mistakenly identified as seizures, and nonconvulsive seizures often go unrecognized and underreported. The incidence of seizures during the postoperative period, depending on the surgery and patient risk factors, ranges from 0.5 to 3%, with half of the seizures occurring within 24 h of surgery. Risk factors identified include deep hypothermic cardiac arrest, aortic calcification or atheroma, critical preoperative states, use of tranexamic acid, preoperative cardiac arrest, existing neurological disease, valve and CABG combined procedures, CPB longer than 159 min, and previous cardiac surgery. Seizures are associated with a fivefold increase in mortality and complication rate, although the type of seizure does not influence the outcome. Recurrent seizures, occurring at a rate of 0.5%, are associated with higher preoperative creatinine levels, thoracic aortic surgery, and early onset (<4 h after surgery) but do not necessarily lead to worse outcomes compared to an isolated seizure.

Post-cardiac surgery patients, particularly older individuals (65+) undergoing open-chamber procedures with prolonged CPB times exceeding 120 min, or those with renal dysfunction and receiving high doses of tranexamic acid (TXA), are at increased risk for electroencephalographically detected seizures due to impaired GABAergic neurotransmission.

Coma

Coma rarely occurs after cardiac surgery and is typically caused by widespread anoxic damage, massive strokes, intracerebral hemorrhages, seizures, or severe metabolic imbalances. When coma results from anoxic or structural brain injuries, the prognosis is generally very poor, often accompanied by post-anoxic myoclonus and seizures. Hypoxic cerebral injury can result from perioperative cardiac arrest caused by malignant dysrhythmias, cardiac tamponade, or other related complications.

Cardiac Arrest and Therapeutic Hypothermia

Cardiac arrest during surgery can lead to hypoxic brain injury. While therapeutic hypothermia is established for out-of-hospital cardiac arrest, its specific benefits for post-cardiac surgery patients are less clear. In cases of suspected brain injury due to poor perfusion, targeted temperature management (mild hypothermia or controlled normothermia) should be considered, with particular attention to preventing fever.

Therapeutic Hypothermia Challenges and Considerations

Coagulopathy and immunosuppression are potential risks of therapeutic hypothermia. Current guidelines recommend monitoring comatose post-arrest patients for fever and preventing temperatures above 37.7 °C for at least 72 h. More research is needed on the role of specific temperature targets (32–36 °C) and early cooling for post-arrest care.

Delirium

Delirium is an acute neuropsychiatric condition marked by impaired attention, fluctuating consciousness, and disorganized thinking, as outlined in the Diagnostic and Statistical Manual, fifth edition (DSM-5). Delirium commonly occurs after cardiac surgery, affecting approximately 5–10% of patients; however, it is often underdiagnosed and typically requires formal assessment, such as the Confusion Assessment Method, for accurate detection.

Risk Factors and Consequences

Risk factors for delirium include older age, preexisting cognitive issues, existing medical conditions such as cerebrovascular disease, diabetes, and low ejection fraction, as well as urgent surgery, high transfusion requirements, and advanced age. The management of mean arterial pressure (MAP) during surgery might also influence delirium incidence, as maintaining MAP within the patient's autoregulation range could lower the risk. While there's an association between postoperative delirium and preexisting dementia, the link between delirium and later development of dementia is less established.

Delirium after cardiac surgery is correlated with decreased functional status, long-term cognitive decline, increased hospital costs, and increased long-term mortality.

Intracranial Hemorrhage

Primary intracranial hemorrhage, often secondary to ischemic infarction, is a rare but serious complication of cardiac surgery. Although perioperative ischemic strokes may occasionally progress to hemorrhagic transformation, the development of major hemorrhages with space-occupying effects is a rare occurrence. Major risk factors for substantial bleeding following a stroke include the presence of large infarcts, a history of prior hemorrhagic infarcts, and early administration of anticoagulant medication within 12 h of the stroke. Patients with a history of cerebral hemorrhage require prompt neurological evaluation after surgery to identify any signs of deterioration that could necessitate neurosurgical intervention. In situations where sedation precludes a thorough neurological assessment, an early postoperative noncontrast CT scan serves as an alternative assessment for hemodynamically stable patients. During CPB, patients diagnosed with endocarditis and mycotic aneurysms face an elevated susceptibility to experiencing cerebral hemorrhage when administered anticoagulant medication. It is recommended to postpone surgery for a period of 4 to 6 weeks to conclude antibiotic treatment, mitigating the risk of cerebral hemorrhage. A heparin-bonded circuit may be considered to decrease the required heparin dose, potentially lowering the bleeding risk.

Cognitive Dysfunction

Postoperative cognitive dysfunction (POCD), a concept first introduced by Bedford in 1955, is the most common neurological sequelae after cardiac surgery, affecting up to 60% of patients in the postoperative period. The actual occurrence may be higher given the lack of routine in-depth neurological testing postoperatively and the higher proportion of patients having the subtype of hypoactive delirium, which is clinically harder to diagnose. It involves a decline from baseline cognitive functions such as attention, memory, and executive skills, detected through neuropsychological assessments by trained examiners, comparing pre- and postoperative cognitive abilities. Despite controversy over its significance, the evidence largely acknowledges POCD's existence, underpinned by consistent detection across studies and its association with adverse outcomes like prolonged hospital stays and decreased quality of life.

Neuropsychological Tests for Diagnosing POCD

Commonly employed neuropsychological tests for diagnosing POCD include the Trail-Making Test, Letter-Digit Coding Test, Boston Naming Test, Stroop-Word Interference Test, and several others focusing on memory and psychomotor speed. The criteria for diagnosing POCD often involve a significant percentage decline in several tests or a decrease beyond a specific standard deviation from baseline scores.

Risk Factors

POCD is a significant concern following both cardiac and noncardiac surgeries, influenced by factors beyond CPB such as patient age, preexisting conditions, surgical methods, and anesthesia. It's increasingly recognized that POCD may exacerbate underlying neurodegenerative diseases in susceptible patients. Risk factors, including age >65 years, carotid artery stenosis, female gender, preoperative depression, diabetes, aortic atherosclerosis, hypertension, and preexisting cerebrovascular disease, are associated with POCD. Alarmingly, Cognitive dysfunction may affect up to 40% of patients 5 years after surgery. Factors associated with cognitive decline include older age, lower education level, higher baseline cognitive function, and evidence of cognitive decline at discharge. Understanding these risk factors is crucial for mitigating long-term cognitive impairments in surgical patients.

Cerebral Dynamics in Cardiac Surgery: Metabolism and Blood Flow Regulation

Cerebral Metabolism and Blood Flow

The human brain, consuming 20% of the body's oxygen, primarily uses 60% of this for ATP generation to support electrophysiological function, while the remaining 40% is used for cellular integrity (Fig. 29.1). Cerebral metabolic rate (CMR) in adults averages 3.5 mL/100 g/min, predominantly in the gray matter. The brain's high oxygen use, coupled with minimal reserves, means even brief interruptions in perfusion can cause rapid unconsciousness and potential irreversible damage after just a few minutes. Glucose is the primary

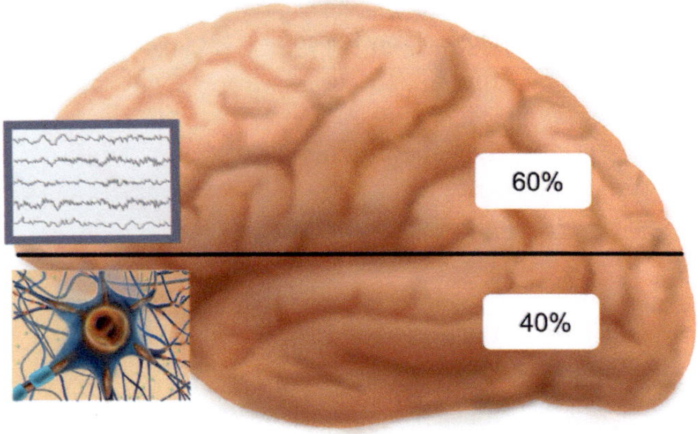

Fig. 29.1 An illustration of the brain, depicting that 60% of its energy is dedicated to ATP generation for electrophysiological functions, while the remaining 40% supports cellular integrity

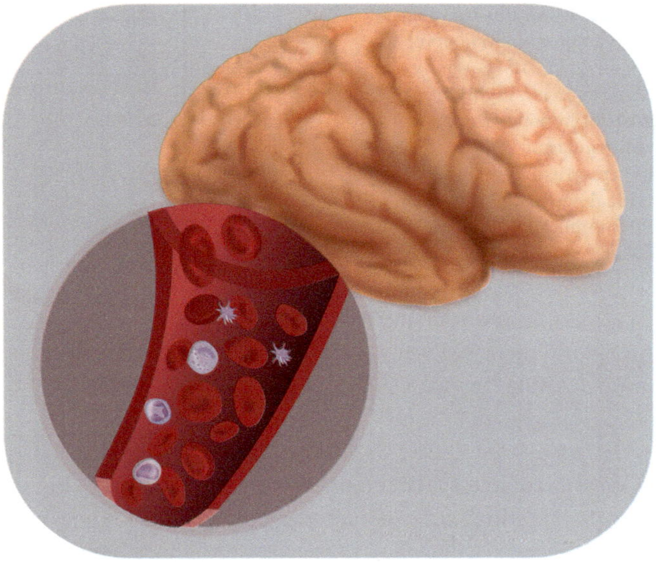

Fig. 29.2 An illustration of the brain, depicting CBF, which represents 15–20% of cardiac output. Compromised blood flow can inevitably lead to neurological damage

energy source for the brain, with over 90% metabolized aerobically. Alternative substrates like ketone bodies and lactate can also be utilized under certain conditions. Both acute hypoglycemia and hyperglycemia can be detrimental, influencing management strategies during ischemic episodes to balance glucose levels carefully.

Cerebral Blood Flow (CBF)

CBF, which is tightly linked to metabolic activity, can be measured through techniques like PET, CT, and SPECT, but these are not suited for real-time bedside monitoring. Flow varies significantly across different brain regions based on activity, with gray matter having a higher flow than white matter. Total adult CBF averages 750 mL/min, representing 15–20% of cardiac output. A flow below 20–25 mL/100 g/min is associated with neurological damage. CBF is often estimated indirectly through methods like transcranial Doppler, which measures blood flow velocity, or near-infrared spectroscopy that reflects venous oxygen saturation (Fig. 29.2).

Regulation of CBF

CBF is vital for brain function and is influenced by several factors:

1. *Cerebral Perfusion Pressure (CPP)*
   - CPP is determined by MAP minus the higher of intracranial pressure (ICP) or central venous pressure (CVP).
   - Normally, CPP ranges from 80 to 100 mmHg and is primarily dependent on MAP.
   - Elevated CVP (e.g., from partial SVC obstruction during CPB) can cause cerebral hypoperfusion even if MAP appears normal. This can lead to cerebral venous hypertension, edema, and ischemia, especially with single two-stage venous cannulas.
   - Surgical manipulation of the heart can also raise SVC pressure and reduce CBF, despite stable MAP and pump flow. This unrecognized cerebral venous hypertension can contribute to postoperative neurological complications.
   - CPP <50 mmHg is associated with EEG slowing, while CPP <25 mmHg can lead to a flat EEG and potential permanent brain injury.
2. *Autoregulation*

   Cerebral autoregulation is the brain's ability to maintain stable CBF despite changes in MAP. This mechanism works most effectively around 30 °C and is strongly influenced by $PaCO_2$ levels. CBF becomes pressure-dependent outside the autoregulatory range (60–160 mmHg) (Fig. 29.3). This risks ischemia below 23 mmHg and microemboli above 58 mmHg due to doubled CBF. Autoregulation weakens at lower temperatures, making CBF more vulnerable to blood pressure fluctuations. Chronic hypertension shifts the autoregulatory curve rightward. Myogenic (smooth

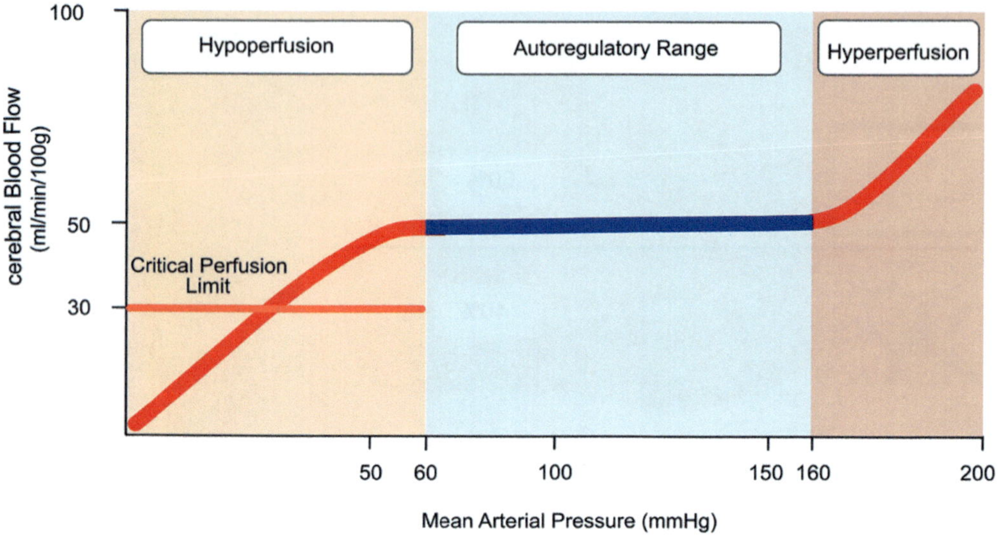

Fig. 29.3 An illustration of CBF autoregulation curve: displaying CBF (y-axis) vs. MAP (x-axis), highlighting areas of hypoperfusion, autoregulation range, hyperperfusion, and the critical perfusion limit at 30 ml/min/100 g

muscle) and metabolic (tissue demand) mechanisms contribute to this process.

3. *Extrinsic Factors*
   - *Respiratory Gas Tensions.*
     $PaCO_2$ is directly proportional to CBF within a specific range (20–80 mmHg). Hypocapnia and hypercapnia effects lessen over time due to cerebrospinal fluid (CSF) compensation. Acute metabolic acidosis has minimal impact due to the blood–brain barrier, but severe hypoxemia ($PaO_2 < 50$ mmHg) increases CBF.
   - *Temperature*:
     CBF and CMR adjust by 5% to 7% for each 1 °C change in temperature. Hypothermia reduces both CMR and CBF, while hyperthermia increases them. Specifically, a 10 °C rise in temperature increases the CMR two folds, while a 10 °C decrease cuts it by half. For example, cooling the brain from 37 °C to 27 °C halves the CMR, and a further reduction to 17 °C halves it again. At 20 °C, the EEG becomes isoelectric, indicating minimal brain activity. In contrast, extreme hyperthermia, above 42 °C, can cause neuronal damage (Fig. 29.4).
   - *Viscosity.*
     Blood viscosity is a critical factor influencing CBF. The primary determinant of blood viscosity is hematocrit (Hct). Lowering Hct, as seen in anemia or hemodilution, decreases viscosity, allowing blood to flow more easily through the cerebral vasculature and potentially improving CBF. However, this reduction in Hct also comes with a trade-off: decreased oxygen-carrying capacity. Conversely, a high Hct, often observed in polycythemia, increases viscosity and can lead to sluggish blood flow, thereby reducing CBF. Striking the right balance between viscosity and oxygen-carrying capacity is crucial in optimizing cerebral perfusion, particularly during conditions like CPB where deliberate hemodilution is employed.
   - *Autonomic Influences.*
     The autonomic nervous system, comprised of the sympathetic and parasympathetic branches, plays a significant role in modulating CBF. Sympathetic stimulation triggers vasoconstriction. In contrast, parasympathetic stimulation induces vasodilation. This dynamic interplay allows for fine-tuning of cerebral perfusion to meet the brain's metabolic demands under varying physiological conditions. Notably, disruptions in autonomic innervation have been implicated in the development of vasospasm following traumatic brain injury or stroke, contributing to secondary ischemic damage.

Source and Etiology of Neurological Injury

Neurological complications after cardiac surgery, such as stroke, encephalopathy, and neurocognitive dysfunction, are thought to stem from a similar etiology, with the specific nature and severity of each condition determined by the location and extent of brain injury. Key factors contributing to neurological complications during CPB include cerebral embolization, hypoperfusion, and inflammatory responses.

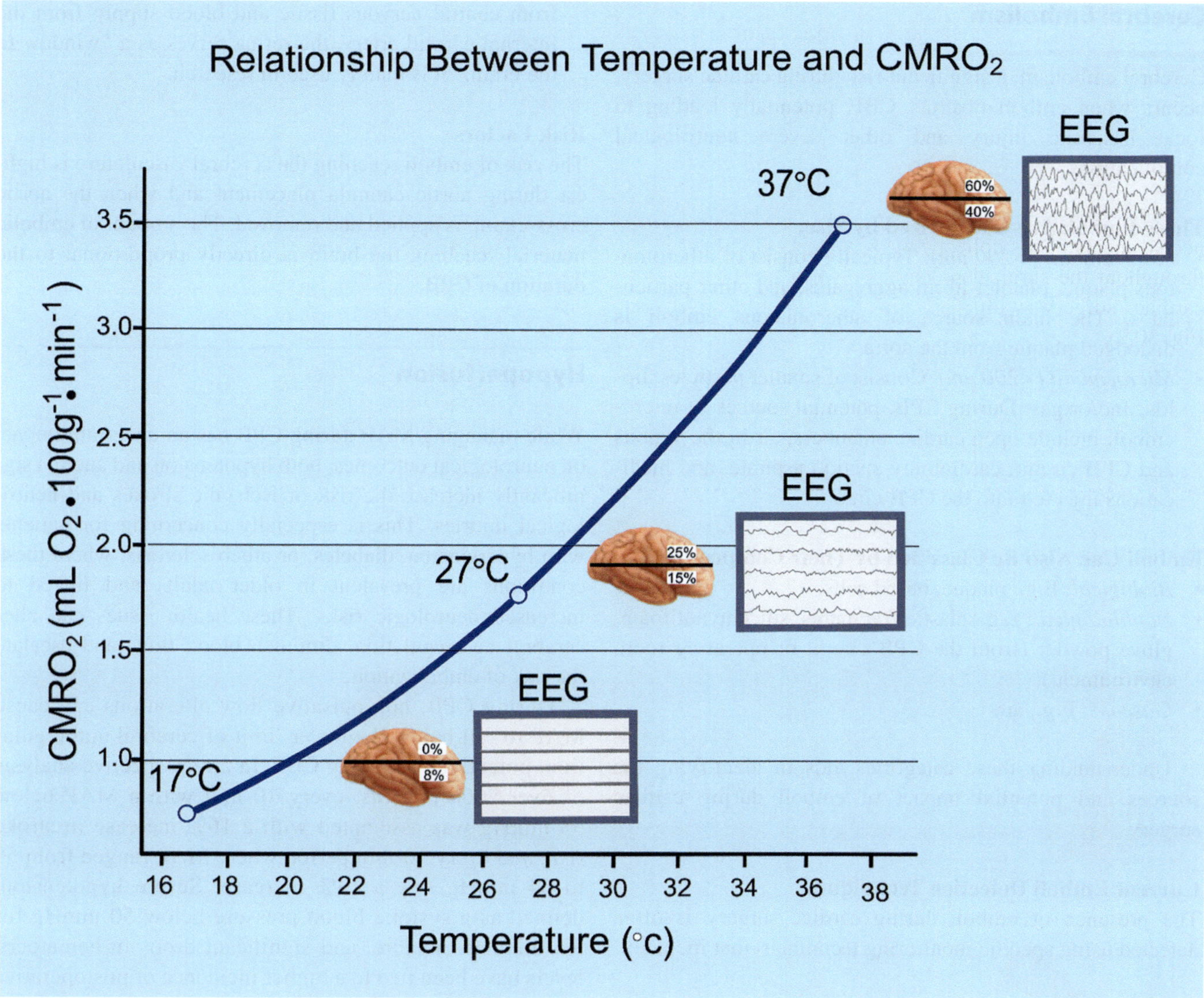

Fig. 29.4 The figure illustrates the relationship between temperature and cerebral metabolic rate of oxygen (CMRO2). An illustration of the impact of hypothermia on the cerebral metabolic rate of oxygen (CMRO2) is illustrated, showing reductions in both neuronal electrical activity ("Function") and cellular maintenance ("Integrity") components at different temperatures. Unlike anesthetics, which primarily affect only the functional component, hypothermia affects both. The illustration displays CMRO2 and EEG screens at three different temperatures: 37 °C, 27 °C, and 17 °C

Cerebral Embolism

Cerebral embolism, a significant risk during cardiac surgery, occurs when emboli obstruct CBF, potentially leading to focal ischemic injury and other severe neurological complications.

These Emboli Are Categorized by Size:

- *Macroemboli (>200 μm)*: Typically consist of atheromatous plaque, platelet-fibrin aggregates, and other particulates. The main source of atheromatous emboli is dislodged plaque from the aorta.
- *Microemboli (<200 μm)*: Consist of smaller particles, lipids, and/or gas. During CPB, potential sources of microemboli include open cardiac chambers, air in the venous and CPB circuit, cardiotomy suction aspirate, and medications injected into the CPB circuit.

Emboli Can Also Be Classified by Their Composition:

- *Biological*: E.g., plaque, blood cells.
- *Nonbiological*: E.g., plastic fragments, silicone antifoam, glove powder (from the CPB circuit or operating room environment).
- *Gaseous*: E.g., air.

Understanding these categories aids in identifying the sources and potential impact of emboli during cardiac surgery.

Current Emboli Detection Techniques.
The presence of emboli during cardiac surgery is often detected using specific monitoring techniques that include:

- *Transcranial Doppler (TCD)*: This tool utilizes the Doppler effect to detect and quantify emboli during cardiac surgery, providing real-time insights into cerebral embolic load. Advanced technology allows for estimation of emboli number and size. Probe placement on the temporal bone, focusing on the middle cerebral artery, is traditional, but positioning over the common carotid artery enables broader monitoring. While TCD cannot directly measure CBF, it reveals relative changes through velocity fluctuations. This non-invasive tool aids in identifying risk factors and refining surgical techniques to minimize cerebral injury.
- *Transesophageal Echocardiography (TEE)*: Identifies intracardiac air, though it may not reflect the total cerebral embolic load. It allows visualization of the heart and great vessels and can be instrumental in assessing and adjusting surgical strategies to minimize air entry, helping with de-airing prior to weaning off bypass.
- *Retinal fluorescein angiography (RFA)*: This tool can detect microemboli events during CPB. Given its origin from central nervous tissue and blood supply from the internal carotid artery, the retina serves as a "window to the brain." It is mainly used in research.

Risk Factors
The risk of emboli reaching the cerebral vasculature is highest during aortic cannula placement and when the aortic cross-clamp is applied and removed. The amount of embolic material reaching the brain is directly proportional to the duration of CPB.

Hypoperfusion

While managing MAP during CPB has an uncertain impact on neurological outcomes, both hypotension and anemia significantly increase the risk of ischemic strokes and neurological injuries. This is especially concerning for patients with hypertension, diabetes, or atherosclerosis, where these conditions are prevalent in older adults and linked to increased neurologic risks. These health issues can alter cerebral autoregulation, diminish blood flow, and escalate the risk of embolization.

During CPB, non-pulsative flow alterations can cause MAP to fall below the lower limit of cerebral autoregulation, potentially reducing CBF. In a retrospective analysis of over 7000 patients, every 10 min with a MAP below 55 mmHg was associated with a 16% increase in stroke risk, and every 10-min period where MAP ranged from 55 to 64 mmHg saw a 13% increase. Severe hypotension, defined as a systolic blood pressure below 50 mmHg for ten minutes or more, and significant drops in hematocrit levels have been tied to a higher incidence of postoperative complications.

Furthermore, CBF can be compromised by any reduction in cardiac output or systemic vascular resistance, including effects from general anesthesia. Certain brain areas, such as the CA1 and CA4 areas of the hippocampus, cerebellar Purkinje cells, thalamic reticular nucleus, and cortical layers II, V, and VI, are particularly vulnerable to damage during global ischemia. Given that cerebral autoregulation, often altered in patients with chronic hypertension, deviations from baseline blood pressure and hematocrit levels could be strong predictors of stroke risk post-surgery. Thus, managing regional hypoperfusion—whether resulting from preexisting conditions or intraoperative events like embolization—is crucial to prevent cerebral ischemia, particularly in populations vulnerable to these changes. The exact impact of less severe hypoperfusion relative to a patient's baseline conditions, however, remains less clear, emphasizing the need for vigilant monitoring and management during cardiac surgeries.

Inflammation

Understanding brain injury after cardiac surgery has expanded beyond just vascular obstruction and hypoperfusion. CPB-induced ischemia and reperfusion injuries trigger a multiphase systemic inflammatory response, activating leukocytes and compromising vascular integrity through mechanisms like capillary plugging and the release of damaging free radicals and enzymes. Additionally, contact with the CPB circuit activates platelets, monocytes, and neutrophils, potentially overwhelming the endothelium's natural defenses. Elevated levels of interleukin-1, interleukin-6, tumor necrosis factor, fibrinolysis markers, and platelet activation markers have been observed during CPB. For detailed information about this inflammatory response, please refer to Chap. 6, "Physiologic Changes and Inflammatory Response to Cardiopulmonary Bypass."

Inflammation has been shown to be neurotoxic and associated with delirium and dementia. Recent studies have shown that CPB alone can cause significant endothelial dysfunction in the CNS, as evidenced by disruptions in the blood–brain barrier and increased inflammatory markers. This broader understanding of CPB's impact on inflammation and endothelial dysfunction underscores the complexity of managing neurological outcomes after surgery. The degree to which the inflammatory response during CPB directly or indirectly causes neurological damage remains unclear.

Pharmacologic Agents

Several medications commonly used during cardiac surgery can lower the seizure threshold, including volatile anesthetics, propofol, ketamine, and etomidate. While benzodiazepines and opioids are thought to increase the risk of delirium, there is no definitive evidence that supports eliminating their use during the perioperative period. TXA, an antifibrinolytic and lysine analog, crosses the blood–brain barrier and can act as a competitive inhibitor of glycine receptors. High doses of TXA have been linked to postoperative seizures. Since TXA is renally excreted, dosages should be adjusted downward for patients with impaired renal function to reduce seizure risk.

Strategies to Minimize Neurological Injury in Cardiac Surgery

Strategies to minimize neurological complications following cardiac surgery encompass a variety of measures, including preoperative assessments, intraoperative neuromonitoring, maintaining cerebral perfusion pressure by targeting optimal MAP levels, and utilizing hypothermic circulatory arrest with options for either selective antegrade or retrograde cerebral perfusion. Efforts also focus on sustaining CBF through autoregulation monitoring and employing both pharmacological and non-pharmacological approaches, such as nerve blocks for pain management and reduced reliance on opiates. Understanding the limitations and potential drawbacks of these strategies is crucial to enhance their effectiveness and mitigate adverse effects.

These approaches are categorized into (Fig. 29.5):

Preoperative: Identifying high-risk patients and customizing surgical and anesthesia plans accordingly.

Intraoperative: This stage involves optimizing surgical techniques, regulating physiological parameters, managing CPB circuits, and implementing specific anesthesia approaches, including the use of neuromonitoring and pharmacologic interventions.

Postoperative: Implementing pharmacologic measures and cognitive rehabilitation strategies to support recovery.

Preoperative Strategies for Neurological Protection

Preoperative Assessment for Stroke Risk Reduction in Cardiac Surgery

A comprehensive preoperative evaluation is crucial for minimizing neurological complications in cardiac surgery by identifying and managing preexisting risk factors and facilitating tailored surgical and anesthesia strategies. While routine preoperative cognitive screening is recommended in cardiac surgery settings, it is not commonly performed for most patients due to the priority of cardiac issues and the costs in time and money, which stem from the need for specialized neuropsychologists and the time-consuming nature of neurocognitive test batteries.

Cerebrovascular Disease Assessment and Management of Carotid Stenosis

Older patients are prone to preexisting cerebrovascular disease, significantly increasing stroke risk. In these patients, carotid duplex imaging is recommended if they have a history of stroke, TIA, or audible bruit. When significant carotid disease is present, a multidisciplinary team should determine the timing and method of revascularization, often prioritizing carotid endarterectomy (CEA).

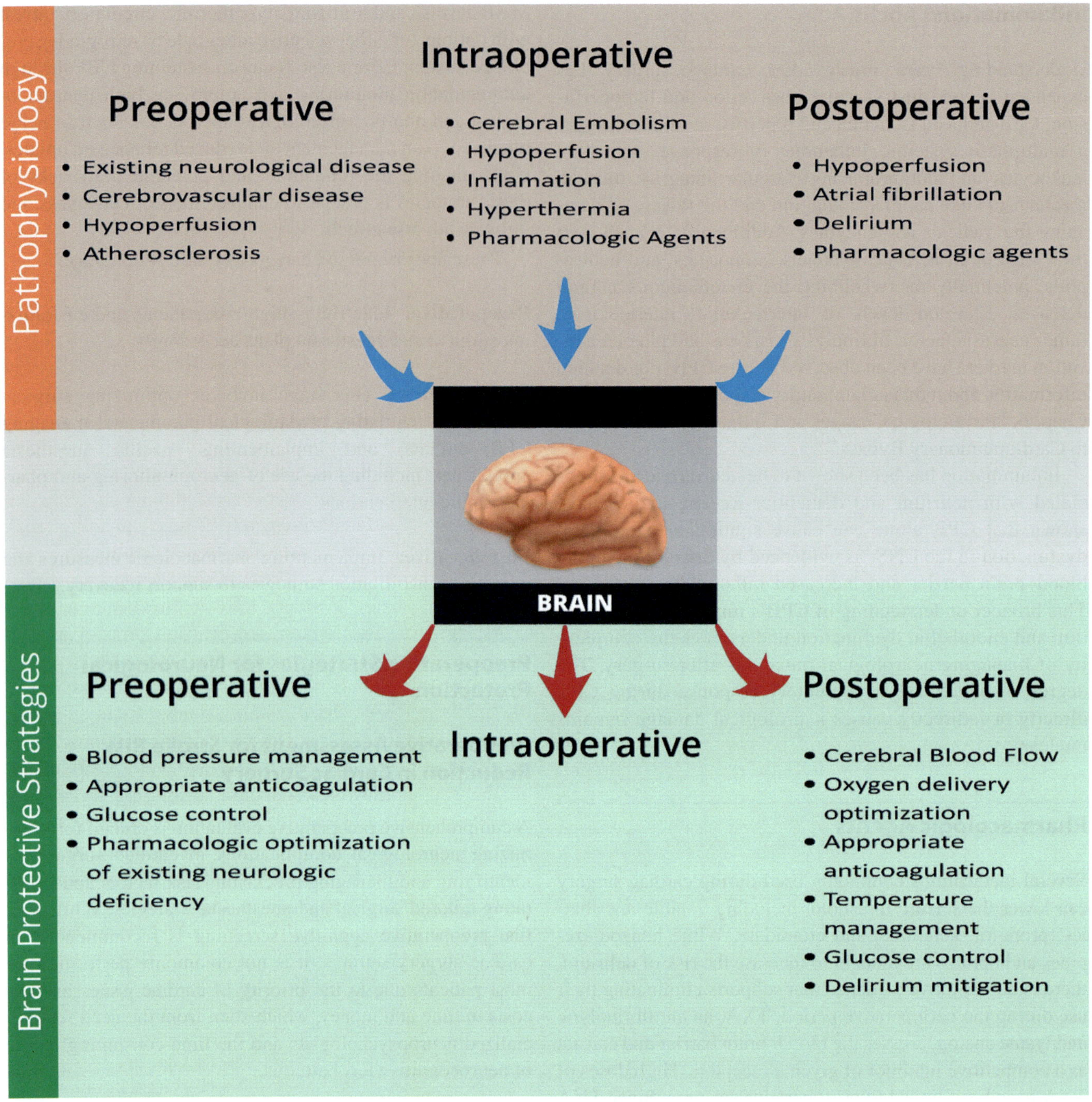

Fig. 29.5 Preventing Neurological Complications in Cardiac Surgery: This diagram outlines the multifaceted factors that contribute to neurological injury during cardiac surgery and highlights targeted strategies to mitigate these risks. The strategies are categorized into preoperative, intraoperative, and postoperative periods to provide a comprehensive approach to enhancing patient outcomes

Intracranial and Aortic Atherosclerosis

Reviewing prior brain imaging for signs of intracranial atherosclerosis and silent infarcts is crucial, as these also increase stroke risk. Additionally, aortic atherosclerosis assessment via CT, TEE, or MRI is essential when planning aortic manipulation to guide surgical modifications that may mitigate stroke risk.

Preoperative Decision-Making in Patients with Cardiac Embolic Sources

The presence of a large left ventricular aneurysm with thrombus or left atrial thrombus in patients with atrial fibrillation necessitates meticulous preoperative planning and careful operative handling to prevent embolization during surgery. Additionally, for patients with left-sided endocarditis, brain imaging is required to detect intracranial mycotic aneurysms or strokes, which might necessitate delayed surgery for antibiotic management as discussed above.

Collaborative Decision-Making

A "heart team" approach, involving cardiac surgeons, cardiac anesthesiologists, and cardiologists, is recommended to determine the optimal surgical strategy. The choice of procedure should be individualized based on surgical expertise, the patient's vascular anatomy, their specific risk factors, and available interventional options. For example, in high-risk patients, balancing the benefits of off-pump CABG (OPCAB) with its potential limitations is crucial. Hybrid procedures combining CABG with percutaneous coronary intervention (PCI) may be considered when OPCAB alone is insufficient or overly risky.

Intraoperative Strategies for Neurological Protection

Intraoperative Assessment

Techniques such as TEE and epiaortic ultrasonography are crucial for preoperative assessments, detecting aortic atherosclerosis, and guiding surgical decisions. While TEE offers broad insights, it is limited in evaluating the mid and distal ascending aorta due to the air-filled left main bronchus obstructing the view. Epiaortic ultrasonography, however, excels at identifying atherosclerotic lesions and is considered the gold standard for aortic assessment. Detecting large or mobile atheromas is critical as they significantly increase the risk of embolic stroke.

During surgery, TEE remains invaluable for identifying potential complications like patent foramen ovale, left atrial thrombus, and retained intracardiac air. It also aids in strategically positioning aortic cross-clamps and cannulas to minimize atheroma disruption and the subsequent risk of embolization. Epiaortic ultrasound complements TEE by precisely locating atheromatous plaques, allowing surgeons to adjust their techniques to avoid plaque disruption and potential embolization.

Modifications of Surgical and Technical Interventions

Aorta Management

Manipulation of the ascending aorta during cannulation and cross-clamp placement is a significant known source of atherosclerotic emboli in cardiac surgery. To mitigate this risk, various strategies have been adopted to minimize aortic manipulation, such as the use of epiaortic ultrasound as discussed above guide the placement of aortic cannulas and cross-clamps. Techniques to minimize aortic manipulation include the use of single cross-clamps. Also, the use of longer cannulas or those with dispersing tips creates lower exit velocities. This reduces the "sandblasting" effect of the perfusion jet on the aortic wall and minimizes plaque disruption. Additionally, alternative cannulation sites, such as the right innominate or axillary artery, can provide greater surgical flexibility and reduce the need for direct manipulation of the ascending aorta. Additionally, intra-aortic cannula filters capture embolic material and decrease TCD-detected embolic signals. However, these methods can extend surgical time and potentially increase aortic manipulation. Off-pump CABG entirely avoids aortic manipulation, significantly reducing stroke risk with a no-touch technique. For heavily calcified aortas, hybrid procedures that combine CABG with delayed PCI provide an effective strategy to achieve revascularization while minimizing extensive aortic manipulation.

Air Embolism Risk Reduction Strategy

To minimize the risk of air embolism during cardiac surgery, several strategies can be employed:

1. *Trendelenburg Position*:
   - Before weaning patients from CPB, placing them in the Trendelenburg position helps to retain air in the

cardiac chambers to be vented through the ventricular vent. Additionally, it allows air in the aorta to rise and collect within the aortic root, facilitating effective venting before the ventricle starts ejecting.

2. *Surgical De-airing.*
   - The surgeon and perfusionist will perform de-airing procedures under TEE guidance. TEE allows for real-time visualization of air bubbles and ensures thorough removal from the cardiac chambers and aorta, significantly reducing the risk of air embolism.

MAP and CBF

Optimal blood pressure management during CPB remains a complex issue. it is still unclear what ranges should be targeted to mitigate or prevent perioperative neurologic dysfunction. Both hypotension and hypertension can lead to neurological complications. Severe hypotension can lead to tissue hypoxia, whereas hypertension can lead to hyperemia, edema, and delirium. The ideal MAP target during CPB is still under debate, commonly ranging from 50–80 mmHg based on Class I recommendations. However, there is growing evidence that maintaining MAP within a patient-specific autoregulation range (Fig. 29.3) could optimize CBF. The upper and lower limits of cerebral autoregulation in the population at large are broad and altered in patients with hypertension, prior neurological injury, and diabetes. Recent evidence suggests that the duration of time a patient's MAP is less than the lower cerebral autoregulation limit predicts morbidity and mortality. It is also very likely that the duration and magnitude of deviations from the lower cerebral autoregulation will be a strong predictor of adverse outcomes. There is not yet a widely available method of determining a patient's individualized autoregulation-determined MAP goals during clinical care, but The use of advanced monitoring technologies such as the mean velocity index (Mx) and cerebral oximeter index (Cx) is promising for tailoring perfusion pressures more accurately to individual needs. Additionally, while CPB traditionally employs non-pulsatile flow, pulsatile flow has been suggested to improve end-organ perfusion and neurological outcomes.

Flow rates during CPB are typically indexed to body surface area, ranging from 2.2 to 2.8 L/min/m^2. However, flow should ideally be determined by measuring systemic oxygen delivery (DO_2) which is pump flow X blood oxygen-carrying capacity with adjustments made for the reduced systemic oxygen consumption (VO_2) associated with reduced temperature.

Neuromonitoring

While advancements in intraoperative CNS monitoring hold the promise of early detection and prevention of brain injuries during cardiac and complex aortic surgeries, their broad applicability remains a subject of ongoing research. Nonetheless, several techniques are available to assess CBF, cortical electrical activity, and spinal cord integrity.

The two primary techniques currently used for neuromonitoring are processed EEG (pEEG) and regional cerebral oxygen saturation monitored by near-infrared spectroscopy (NIRS rScO2).

EEG

While EEG can sometimes detect cerebral ischemia in specific scenarios (stable anesthesia, abrupt insult, normal pre-op EEG), it mainly monitors the superficial cortex, missing deeper areas. Its sensitivity is limited by anesthesia, hypothermia, medications, electrical noise, and preexisting conditions. This means strokes can occur without EEG changes, and not all changes signify a stroke. Raw EEG monitoring is complex and not universally used in cardiac surgery due to its limitations in ischemia detection.

Processed EEG (pEEG)

Processed EEG monitors, like bispectral index monitor (BIS; Medtronic, Inc., Minneapolis, MN) and the patient state index (Masimo Corporation, Irvine, CA), have become popular because of their user-friendly interface. These monitors display a numerical value representing brain activity, with 0 indicating no activity and 100 representing an awake state. While easy to use, processed EEG has limitations in sensitivity and specificity for detecting ischemia and anesthesia depth. The efficacy of pEEG for improving neurological outcomes remains inconclusive.

NIRS

Cerebral oximetry is a non-invasive monitor for measuring regional oxygen delivery utilizing NIRS. Adhesive strips are applied to the forehead, emitting infrared light that penetrates the skin, skull, and underlying issue. Oxygenated and deoxygenated tissues absorb light at different wavelengths, which is then reflected back to the oximetry sensors. A desaturation is defined as a decrease of more than 20% from base-

Table 29.2 Overview of neuromonitoring modalities for cardiac surgery, including advantages and disadvantages

Neuromonitoring modality	Advantages	Disadvantages
EEG (electroencephalography)	Detects global changes in brain activity, useful for monitoring depth of anesthesia and detecting ischemia	Sensitive to interference from other electrical equipment, may not identify small, localized ischemic events. Technically demanding and complex to interpret
Processed EEG (e.g., BIS)	User-friendly, continuous monitoring of brain activity. Useful for adjusting anesthetic depth	May not always correlate with actual brain activity, less specific for detecting ischemia compared to raw EEG
NIRS	Non-invasive, continuous monitoring of regional cerebral oxygen saturation. Can detect trends and potential ischemia earlier than other methods	Affected by extracranial factors (e.g., skin pigmentation, scalp edema), may not reflect deeper brain regions
Jugular Bulb Venous Oxygen Saturation (SjVO2) Monitoring	Directly assesses global cerebral oxygen extraction and balance. Can detect early signs of cerebral ischemia	Invasive procedure, requires technical expertise for placement of the jugular bulb catheter
Transcranial Doppler (TCD)	Non-invasive assessment of CBF velocity. Can detect emboli and monitor changes in blood flow patterns	Operator-dependent, requires specialized training, and may not be feasible in all patients due to anatomical variations that make it difficult to identify suitable acoustic windows

line, which is obtained prior to sedation and supplemental oxygenation. Treatment algorithms (see Fig. 14.4 for examples of managing unilateral and bilateral cerebral desaturation) have been proposed to address desaturation events. These strategies include repositioning CPB cannulas, treating hypotension, increasing PaO_2, optimizing hemoglobin, lowering body temperature, increasing CPB flow, and deepening anesthetic. These interventions aim to either increase oxygen supply to the brain or decrease oxygen demand. While NIRS is considered a non-invasive, low-risk tool for optimizing intraoperative care, its impact on improving outcomes remains unclear. NIRS assesses cerebral oxygenation and reflects the balance between oxygen supply and demand. Studies on NIRS-guided care have yielded mixed results, often due to methodological issues like small sample sizes, limited follow-up, and inconsistent definitions. A comprehensive discussion of these modalities is available in Chap. 14.

Table 29.2 summarizes these neuromonitoring methods, highlighting the advantages and disadvantages of each (see Fig. 14.2).

Regulating Physiological Parameters

During cardiac surgery with CPB, CBF and oxygenation can be significantly impacted by various physiological parameters, including hemoglobin concentration, pH, PaO_2, $PaCO_2$, hypothermia, anesthetic drugs, and CPB circuit design. Proper regulation of these parameters can potentially improve neurological outcomes.

Hemoglobin Levels and Hemodilution

Maintaining appropriate hemoglobin levels during CPB is critical to reducing the risk of stroke and other neurological complications. Extreme hemodilution (hematocrit <18%) during CPB, previously used to reduce transfusion risks, is now avoided due to links with decreased brain oxygenation, increased stroke risk, and cognitive decline. Current guidelines recommend a target hemoglobin of at least 6 g/dl during CPB. Techniques such as retrograde autologous priming and appropriate CPB circuit sizing can help minimize hemodilution.

A recent randomized controlled trial (RCT) found no difference in stroke rates between restrictive transfusion levels (<7.5 g/dl) and more liberal levels of (9.5 g/dl), though other neurological outcomes were not examined. Another RCT indicated that patients with Hct levels above 25% had better neurological outcomes than those with Hct levels between 21 and 25%. European guidelines suggest maintaining Hct between 18–24% with a target DO_2 of 273 mL/min/m^2 (class IIb recommendation). Maintaining hemoglobin levels of at least 7 g/dL postoperatively is recommended, with individual adjustments as needed.

Blood Gas Management

Temperature and Blood Gases

Managing blood gas measurements during cardiac surgery when blood is cooled presents a unique challenge. As temperature decreases, CO_2 is more soluble, and blood becomes more alkalotic. Two primary strategies are used to manage blood gases during hypothermia:

- *pH-Stat Strategy*:
  This approach aims to maintain a pH of 7.4 and a CO_2 level of 40 mmHg, regardless of patient's body temperature. To achieve this, the increased solubility of CO_2 in blood during hypothermia is counteracted by adding CO_2. This can be done by reducing sweep gas flow to the membrane oxygenator or by directly adding CO_2 to the sweep gas during cooling.
- *Alpha-Stat Strategy*:
  Based on the theory of acid-base neutrality, this method allows pH and $PaCO_2$ to become progressively more alkalotic as body temperature decreases. When a blood sample drawn at patient's temperature is warmed to 37 °C, it should exhibit a pH 7.4 and a $PaCO_2$ of 40 mmHg. This approach respects the body's natural compensatory mechanisms, allowing it to self-regulate as it normally would at its natural temperature.

Neuroprotection and CBF

The main difference in the two strategies during CPB relates to the change in CBF. The pH-stat method effectively leads to a higher $PaCO_2$, cerebral vasodilation, and increased CBF during CPB. In children, this can be beneficial if brain cooling prior to circulatory arrest is desired. Given the concern for embolic load during CPB in the adult population, the increase in CBF associated with pH-stat during hypothermia may be detrimental. Consequently, the use of alpha-stat management in adults is currently a Class IIa recommendation.

Temperature Management

Temperature significantly influences cerebral physiology and pathophysiology, especially during cardiac surgery with CPB.

Clinical Evidence and Practice

Hypothermia, defined as a core body temperature less than 35 °C (Table 6.1), reduces cerebral metabolic rate of oxygen ($CMRO_2$) and anesthetic requirements, while also decreasing the release of excitatory neurotransmitters (glutamate, aspartate, etc.). This reduced metabolic oxygen demand allows for lower CPB flow rates and DO_2. Historically, hypothermia was used during CPB to protect against neurological events. However, recent meta-analysis and systemic reviews of high-quality RCTS have shown no difference in neurocognitive outcomes between hypothermic and normothermic patients. In fact, some studies suggest hypothermia might increase cardiac injury and mortality. Despite the lack of conclusive evidence for neuroprotection, mild hypothermia (32 °C) is commonly used for closed-chamber cardiac procedures requiring CPB, while moderate hypothermia (28 °C) is standard for open-chamber procedures.

Two theories explain why hypothermia has not shown clear neurological benefits.

1. First, during high-risk periods for macroemboli (aortic cross-clamping and removal), brain temperature is often near normothermia.
2. Second, the detrimental effects of rewarming might outweigh any benefits of hypothermia.

Rewarming Practices

During CPB, arterial blood temperature is a reasonable surrogate for cerebral temperature, though it may underestimate brain temperature during rewarming. When rewarming, it is essential to keep a less than 10 °C the temperature gradient between the arterial and venous cannula below 10 °C to minimize the risk of dissolved gases coming out of the blood and forming gas emboli. Slow rewarming (<0.5 °C/min when the patient's temperature exceeds 30 °C) is recommended to reduce the risk of neurological injury. While it is debatable as to whether hypothermia is a neuroprotective agent, the literature strongly suggests that hyperthermia, defined as 37 °C or higher at the oxygenator's arterial outlet blood temperature, leads to significantly worse neurological outcomes. To mitigate the risk of cerebral hyperthermia, some surgeons prefer to wean patients off CPB with mild core hypothermia. However, this practice can lead to a continuous fall in core temperature postoperatively due to uneven rewarming and continual heat dissipation. Hyperthermia can lead to cytoskeletal protein damage, tissue injury, and increased tissue metabolic demands. It has been associated with cognitive dysfunction 4–6 weeks after surgery.

Sites for Temperature Monitoring

During weaning and the post-bypass period, a pulmonary artery catheter or a nasopharyngeal temperature probe can estimate cerebral temperature. While venous jugular bulb temperature is considered the gold standard surrogate measure of cerebral temperature, it is not often used clinically. Bladder temperature can be as much as 4 °C lower than cerebral temperature during rewarming.

Guidelines

According to current STS guidelines, the oxygenator's arterial outlet blood temperature should be used as an analog for brain temperature (class I, level C). During the process of rewarming, it should be assumed that the oxygenator's arterial outlet blood temperature is lower than the brain perfusate temperature. Perfusionists should restrict the oxygenator's arterial outlet blood temperature to under 37 °C in order to prevent high brain temperatures (class 1, Level c).

Carbon Dioxide

CO_2 plays a crucial role in the responsiveness of the cerebral vasculature, with hypercapnia causing vasodilation and hypocapnia leading to vasoconstriction. As previously discussed, air emboli are a potential source of neurological injury and CO_2, being denser than air and 25 times more soluble, can help mitigate this risk. Insufflating CO_2 in open-chamber procedures displaces air, reducing the burden and lifespan of potential vessel occlusions. Studies have shown that CO_2 insufflation can decrease the amount of intracavitary air detected by TEE after aortic cross-clamp removal. For instance, Svenarud et al. found a 78% reduction in emboli in the ascending aorta with CO_2 insufflation. Martens et al. observed improved auditory-evoked potentials but no differences in neuropsychological outcomes. While CO_2 flooding has been effective in reducing the amount and duration of cerebral gaseous emboli, it can increase systemic pCO_2 levels if administered for too long. Therefore, it is recommended to limit CO_2 insufflation to a few minutes before releasing the aortic cross-clamp to reduce intracavitary air as detected by TEE. Despite these potential benefits, two recent meta-analyses have not demonstrated significant differences in neurological outcomes with CO_2 use.

Glucose Management

Glucose control during cardiac surgery is critical due to its significant impact on morbidity and mortality. Preoperative hemoglobin A1c levels above 6.5% correlate with postoperative glucose fluctuations, leading to adverse outcomes, including stroke. Factors such as hypothermia and inflammation can lead to insulin resistance during cardiac surgery. Conditions like diabetes, intraoperative hyperglycemia, and even mild hypoglycemia are associated with an increased risk of postoperative delirium. Insulin, the mainstay therapy in controlling glucose during cardiac surgery, is also believed to have anti-inflammatory properties. Current guidelines recommend maintaining glucose levels at or below 180 mg/dL during the perioperative period (Class I recommendation). However, tight glycemic control (target glucose 80–110 mg/dL) may increase the risk of postoperative delirium. It is common practice to maintain patients on an insulin infusion during surgery to achieve optimum glucose levels. For patients requiring prolonged ICU care (e.g., ventilation, inotropes, dialysis), continuous insulin infusion is recommended to keep blood glucose below 150 mg/dL, regardless of diabetes history.

Pharmacologic Intervention

Preventing neurological complications in cardiac surgery is often more effective than treating them. The use of pharmacologic interventions to prevent postoperative neurological complications is an active area of research.

Intravenous and Inhalational Anesthetics

The risk-benefit profile of each anesthetic must be carefully evaluated, as many can modulate CBF, neurotransmitter levels, and brain electrical activity. For example, propofol decreases $CMRO_2$ and CBF, while volatile anesthetics uncouple the $CMRO_2$ and CBF relationship, causing an increase in CBF but a decrease in $CMRO_2$. In contrast, ketamine, a noncompetitive N-methyl-D-aspartic acid receptor antagonist, increases both CBF and $CMRO_2$. Although opioids may not directly affect cognitive decline, they can contribute to postoperative delirium. The α_2 adrenoceptor agonist dexmedetomidine, often used for its sedative properties, may reduce the risk of postoperative delirium in cardiac surgery patients, but evidence for broader neurological benefits remains inconclusive. While some intravenous anesthetic adjuvants like lidocaine show promise in specific scenarios, such as in non-diabetic patients or those receiving a 48-h infusion, their neuroprotective effects remain unproven.

Other Pharmacological Therapies

Several other classes of drugs have been investigated for their neuroprotective potential, including free radical scavengers, antifibrinolytic agents, magnesium, mannitol, receptor antagonists, growth factors, ionic pump modulators (such as Na+/K+-ATPase inhibitors), statins, ischemic pathway inhibitors (such as edaravone), calcium channel blockers, antiadhesion agents, hormones (such as estrogen and progesterone), and antineutrophil and antiplatelet agents. However, despite encouraging results in non-clinical studies, these benefits have not consistently translated to human trials.

Anti-Inflammatory Agents

Anti-inflammatory strategies, such as steroid use, may suppress systemic inflammation during CPB, but their impact on neurological outcomes requires further study.

Conclusion

Despite extensive research, no single medication has been definitively proven to prevent postoperative delirium, seizures, or other neurological complications during cardiac surgery with CPB.

CPB Circuit Design

While John Gibbons' groundbreaking CPB circuit revolutionized cardiac surgery, it also introduced neurological risks ranging from cognitive decline to stroke and coma. These complications are primarily attributed to cerebral embolization, hypoperfusion, and inflammatory responses. Although extensive research has explored the role of microemboli and cognitive impairment post-CPB, recent studies challenge their direct connection, particularly in comparison to non-CPB procedures. Nonetheless, enhancing CPB to reduce these complications is critical. Ongoing efforts aim to refine CPB equipment, reducing cerebral embolization and improving patient outcomes, affirming CPB's essential role in modern cardiac surgery. There have been several changes and new technologies added to the CPB circuit intended to improve neurological outcomes. These changes center around decreasing the micro and macro-emboli load to the patient and decreasing the inflammatory response from contact with the CPB circuit.

Filters

Arterial line filters have been crucial in reducing cerebral injury during CPB by significantly decreasing emboli, particularly with smaller filters (25 mm), although smaller pore sizes may increase the risk of hemolysis. While leukocyte-depleting filters are designed to filter inflammatory proteins, their use during CPB has produced mixed results in studies, with no clear consensus on their overall benefits. Conversely, dynamic bubble traps have been effective in reducing gaseous microemboli.

Oxygenators

A significant advancement in CPB technology was the replacement of bubble oxygenators with membrane oxygenators. Bubble oxygenators, despite defoaming agents, posed risks of cerebral embolization and blood trauma. In contrast, microporous hollow fiber membrane oxygenators are superior in managing emboli and reducing inflammation, leading to their widespread adoption in cardiac surgery.

Cardiotomy Suction vs Cell-Saver

Cardiotomy suction, effective in minimizing blood loss during CPB, is considered a significant source of emboli. It can introduce air, fat, and cellular debris into the bloodstream, potentially leading to cerebral emboli. Several studies have shown that using a cell-saver device, which processes shed blood before reinfusion, can significantly reduce these emboli compared to direct cardiotomy suction. as an alternative. However, this approach may worsen postoperative bleeding by removing coagulation factors and platelets, and its ability to improve neurological outcomes has not been uniformly demonstrated.

Vacuum-Assisted Venous Drainage

Venous return during CPB can be achieved through gravity or vacuum-assisted venous drainage (VAVD). VAVD, developed for use with smaller cannulas in minimally invasive procedures, may increase emboli risk if air is introduced or suction pressure is excessive. However, studies suggest VAVD is likely safe when used cautiously, avoiding air entrainment and high negative pressures.

Pumps

The use of centrifugal pumps may offer some advantages in terms of neurological protection compared to roller pumps. Purported advantages include decreases in shearing forces, microemboli transmission, and a reduced systemic inflammatory response. However, a conclusive difference in neurological outcomes between these two types of pumps has not been demonstrated.

Cannulas

Numerous arterial cannula types exist for CPB, though clinical studies haven't shown a clear reduction in cerebral emboli with those designed for lower blood flow velocities and less turbulence. Cerebral embolization during cardiac surgery can be reduced by employing a meticulous aortic cannulation technique, with particular attention to de-airing the cannula using a side stopcock before initiating flow.

Circuit Tubing

Efforts to ameliorate the systemic inflammatory response have included the use of biocompatible CPB circuitry coatings, the most common of which is a heparin-bonded coating, to potentially minimize neurological damage during CPB. However, there is no conclusive evidence that there is a direct correlation between the use of circuit coatings, including heparin bonding, and better neurological outcomes.

Iatrogenic Sources of Emboli

Surgical and perfusion-related activities during cardiac surgery are known to generate cerebral emboli. During cardiac surgery, activities such as starting or stopping CPB, applying and removing aortic clamps, and inserting or removing the cardioplegia vent are associated with a higher risk of cerebral embolization. The use of partial occluding clamps during CABG for proximal anastomosis, in particular, has been linked to increased rates of neuropsychological deficits compared to single clamping. Furthermore, perfusionist activities, such as injecting drugs or sampling blood during CPB, significantly raise the likelihood of cerebral emboli due to the introduction of gaseous emboli into the circuit. Measures such as meticulous de-airing of the CPB circuit, removing air from the venous line before starting CPB, and insufflating the surgical field with carbon dioxide have proven effective in reducing cerebral emboli.

Postoperative Strategies for Neurological Protection

Postoperative strategies for reducing neurologic complications focus on maintaining hemodynamic stability to preserve CBF and oxygen delivery. Addressing factors like hypoxia, anemia, and hyperglycemia can improve neurological outcomes. Current guidelines recommend maintaining hemoglobin levels above 7.5 g/dL (or 8.5 g/dL for patients over 70) and blood glucose levels less than 180 mg/dL.

Pharmacological interventions play a role in neuroprotection. Early aspirin administration is standard, while statins, ideally used in conjunction with beta-blockers, reduce stroke and non-neurological complications. For persistent postoperative atrial fibrillation, anticoagulation is recommended to mitigate stroke risk. Beta-blockers and amiodarone can help prevent atrial fibrillation, but their use should be weighed against side effects.

Despite research, optimal strategies for certain interventions remain unclear. For example, the timing and duration of oral anticoagulant use for postoperative atrial fibrillation warrant further investigation due to increasing awareness of long-term stroke risk.

Enhancing Neurocognitive Recovery After Cardiac Surgery

Harnessing the brain's natural adaptability (neuroplasticity) is a promising strategy to counter cognitive decline after cardiac surgery. In the acute phase, focusing on good sleep may help prevent early cognitive disruptions. Mid- to long-term, increasing activities of daily living and social engagement can contribute to cognitive recovery, especially when combined with preexisting higher education and cognitive baseline.

Conclusion

Protecting the brain during CPB necessitates a multimodal, multidisciplinary plan combined with active diligence and attention to detail. At a minimum, efforts to reduce embolic load and to maintain cerebral perfusion throughout the perioperative period should be undertaken. While there is a spectrum of neurological deficits observed in conjunction with CPB, a comprehensive understanding of the individual pathologic processes involved, particularly for postoperative altered mental status and cognitive decline, is lacking.

Further Reading

Abbasciano RG, Koulouroudias M, Chad T, et al. Role of hypothermia in adult cardiac surgery patients: a systematic review and meta-analysis. J Cardiothorac Vasc Anesth. 2022;36(7):1883–90.

Augoustides JG. The inflammatory response to cardiac surgery with cardiopulmonary bypass: should steroid prophylaxis be routine? J Cardiothorac Vasc Anesth. 2012;26(5):952–8.

Banbury MK, Kouchoukos NT, Allen KB, et al. Emboli capture using the Embol-X intraaortic filter in cardiac surgery: a multi-centered randomized trial of 1,289 patients. Ann Thorac Surg. 2003;76(2):508–15. discussion 515

Benedetto U, Caputo M, Guida G, et al. Carbon dioxide insufflation during cardiac surgery: a meta-analysis of randomized controlled trials. Semin Thorac Cardiovasc Surg. 2017;29(3):301–10.

Biancari F, Santini F, Tauriainen T, et al. Epiaortic ultrasound to prevent stroke in coronary artery bypass grafting. Ann Thorac Surg. 2020;109(1):294–301.

Blessing JM, Riley JB. Lean flow: optimizing cardiopulmonary bypass equipment and flow for obese patients-a technique article. J Extra Corpor Technol. 2017;49(1):30–5.

Bonser RS, Pagano D, Haverich A. Brain protection in cardiac. Surgery. 2011; https://doi.org/10.1007/978-1-84996-293-3.

Boodram S, Evans E. Use of leukocyte-depleting filters during cardiac surgery with cardiopulmonary bypass: a review. J Extra Corpor Technol. 2008;40(1):27–42.

Brown CH. Delirium in the cardiac surgical ICU. Curr Opin Anaesthesiol. 2014;27(2):117–22.

Chen H, Mo L, Hu H, Ou Y, Luo J. Risk factors of postoperative delirium after cardiac surgery: a meta-analysis. J Cardiothorac Surg. 2021;16(1):113.

Choi H, Park CS, Huh J, et al. Intraoperative glycemic variability and mean glucose are predictors for postoperative delirium after cardiac surgery: a retrospective cohort study. Clin Interv Aging. 2022;17:79–95.

Clark RE, Brillman J, Davis DA, Lovell MR, Price TR, Magovern GJ. Microemboli during coronary artery bypass grafting. Genesis and effect on outcome. J Thorac Cardiovasc Surg. 1995;109(2):249–57. discussion 257–248

Dacey LJ, Likosky DS, Leavitt BJ, et al. Perioperative stroke and long-term survival after coronary bypass graft surgery. Ann Thorac Surg. 2005;79(2):532–6. discussion 537

Djaiani G, Fedorko L, Borger MA, et al. Continuous-flow cell saver reduces cognitive decline in elderly patients after coronary bypass surgery. Circulation. 2007;116(17):1888–95.

Engelman R, Baker RA, Likosky DS, et al. The Society of Thoracic Surgeons, The Society of Cardiovascular Anesthesiologists, and The American Society of ExtraCorporeal Technology: clinical practice guidelines for cardiopulmonary bypass – temperature management during cardiopulmonary bypass. J Extra Corpor Technol. 2015;47(3):145–54.

Gaudino M, Rahouma M, Di Mauro M, et al. Early versus delayed stroke after cardiac surgery: a systematic review and meta-analysis. J Am Heart Assoc. 2019;8(13):e012447.

Gilbey T, Milne B, de Somer F, Kunst G. Neurologic complications after cardiopulmonary bypass – a narrative review. Perfusion. 2022;2676591221119312:1545.

Goldstone AB, Bronster DJ, Anyanwu AC, et al. Predictors and outcomes of seizures after cardiac surgery: a multivariable analysis of 2,578 patients. Ann Thorac Surg. 2011;91(2):514–8.

Grocott HP, Mackensen GB, Grigore AM, et al. Postoperative hyperthermia is associated with cognitive dysfunction after coronary artery bypass graft surgery. Stroke. 2002;33(2):537–41.

Ho KM, Tan JA. Benefits and risks of maintaining normothermia during cardiopulmonary bypass in adult cardiac surgery: a systematic review. Cardiovasc Ther. 2011;29(4):260–79.

Hogue CW Jr, Palin CA, Arrowsmith JE. Cardiopulmonary bypass management and neurologic outcomes: an evidence-based appraisal of current practices. Anesth Analg. 2006;103(1):21–37.

Hogue CW, Brown CHT, Hori D, et al. Personalized blood pressure management during cardiac surgery with cerebral autoregulation monitoring: a randomized trial. Semin Thorac Cardiovasc Surg. 2021;33(2):429–38.

Hori D, Nomura Y, Ono M, et al. Optimal blood pressure during cardiopulmonary bypass defined by cerebral autoregulation monitoring. J Thorac Cardiovasc Surg. 2017;154(5):1590–1598 e1592.

Hunter GR, Young GB. Seizures after cardiac surgery. J Cardiothorac Vasc Anesth. 2011;25(2):299–305.

Jovin DG, Katlaps KG, Ellis BK, Dharmaraj B. Neuroprotection against stroke and encephalopathy after cardiac surgery. Interv Med Appl Sci. 2019;11(1):27–37.

Kadoi Y. Pharmacological neuroprotection during cardiac surgery. Asian Cardiovasc Thorac Ann. 2007;15(2):167–77.

Karkouti K, Djaiani G, Borger MA, et al. Low hematocrit during cardiopulmonary bypass is associated with increased risk of perioperative stroke in cardiac surgery. Ann Thorac Surg. 2005;80(4):1381–7.

Kazmierski J, Kowman M, Banach M, et al. Incidence and predictors of delirium after cardiac surgery: results from the IPDACS study. J Psychosom Res. 2010;69(2):179–85.

Kim KM, Arghami A, Habib R, et al. The Society of Thoracic Surgeons adult cardiac surgery database: 2022 update on outcomes and research. Ann Thorac Surg. 2023;115(3):566–74.

Lazar HL, McDonnell M, Chipkin SR, et al. The Society of Thoracic Surgeons practice guideline series: blood glucose management during adult cardiac surgery. Ann Thorac Surg. 2009;87(2):663–9.

Lin Z, Xiaoyi Z. Tranexamic acid-associated seizures: a meta-analysis. Seizure. 2016;36:70–3.

Low A, Mak E, Rowe JB, Markus HS, O'Brien JT. Inflammation and cerebral small vessel disease: a systematic review. Ageing Res Rev. 2019;53:100916.

Manji RA, Grocott HP, Leake J, et al. Seizures following cardiac surgery: the impact of tranexamic acid and other risk factors. Can J Anaesth. 2012;59(1):6–13.

Manji RA, Grocott HP, Manji JS, Menkis AH, Jacobsohn E. Recurrent seizures following cardiac surgery: risk factors and outcomes in a historical cohort study. J Cardiothorac Vasc Anesth. 2015;29(5):1206–11.

Mazer CD, Whitlock RP, Fergusson DA, et al. Six-month outcomes after restrictive or liberal transfusion for cardiac surgery. N Engl J Med. 2018;379(13):1224–33.

Mlejnsky F, Klein AA, Lindner J, et al. A randomised controlled trial of roller versus centrifugal cardiopulmonary bypass pumps in patients undergoing pulmonary endarterectomy. Perfusion. 2015;30(7):520–8.

Murkin JM, Adams SJ, Novick RJ, et al. Monitoring brain oxygen saturation during coronary bypass surgery: a randomized, prospective study. Anesth Analg. 2007;104(1):51–8.

Newman MF, Kirchner JL, Phillips-Bute B, et al. Longitudinal assessment of neurocognitive function after coronary-artery bypass surgery. N Engl J Med. 2001;344(6):395–402.

Noah AM, Almghairbi D, Evley R, Moppett IK. Preoperative inflammatory mediators and postoperative delirium: systematic review and meta-analysis. Br J Anaesth. 2021;127(3):424–34.

Nyman J, Svenarud P, van der Linden J. Carbon dioxide de-airing in minimal invasive cardiac surgery, a new effective device. J Cardiothorac Surg. 2019;14(1):12.

Pataraia E, Jung R, Aull-Watschinger S, Skhirtladze-Dworschak K, Dworschak M. Seizures after adult cardiac surgery and interventional cardiac procedures. J Cardiothorac Vasc Anesth. 2018;32(5):2323–9.

Rubens FD, Boodhwani M, Mesana T, et al. The cardiotomy trial: a randomized, double-blind study to assess the effect of processing of shed blood during cardiopulmonary bypass on transfusion and neurocognitive function. Circulation. 2007;116(11 Suppl):I89–97.

Saager L, Duncan AE, Yared JP, et al. Intraoperative tight glucose control using hyperinsulinemic normoglycemia increases delirium after cardiac surgery. Anesthesiology. 2015;122(6):1214–23.

Saczkowski R, Maklin M, Mesana T, Boodhwani M, Ruel M. Centrifugal pump and roller pump in adult cardiac surgery: a meta-analysis of randomized controlled trials. Artif Organs. 2012;36(8):668–76.

Scott DA, Evered LA, Silbert BS. Cardiac surgery, the brain, and inflammation. J Extra Corpor Technol. 2014;46(1):15–22.

Shaaban Ali M, Harmer M, Kirkham F. Cardiopulmonary bypass temperature and brain function. Anaesthesia. 2005;60(4):365–72.

Soliman R, Saad D, Abukhudair W, Abdeldayem S. The neurocognitive outcomes of hemodilution in adult patients undergoing coronary artery bypass grafting using cardiopulmonary bypass. Ann Card Anaesth. 2022;25(2):133–40.

Sultan I, Bianco V, Kilic A, et al. Predictors and outcomes of ischemic stroke after cardiac surgery. Ann Thorac Surg. 2020;110(2):448–56.

Sun Y, Ji B, Zhu X, Zheng Z. Efficacy of carbon dioxide insufflation for cerebral and cardiac protection during open heart surgery: a systematic review and meta-analysis. Artif Organs. 2013;37(5):439–46.

Sun LY, Chung AM, Farkouh ME, et al. Defining an intraoperative hypotension threshold in association with stroke in cardiac surgery. Anesthesiology. 2018;129(3):440–7.

Tarakji KG, Sabik JF 3rd, Bhudia SK, Batizy LH, Blackstone EH. Temporal onset, risk factors, and outcomes associated with stroke after coronary artery bypass grafting. JAMA. 2011;305(4):381–90.

Task Force M, Kunst G, Milojevic M, et al. 2019 EACTS/EACTA/EBCP guidelines on cardiopulmonary bypass in adult cardiac surgery. Br J Anaesth. 2019;123(6):713–57.

Whitaker DC, Newman SP, Stygall J, Hope-Wynne C, Harrison MJ, Walesby RK. The effect of leucocyte-depleting arterial line filters on cerebral microemboli and neuropsychological outcome following coronary artery bypass surgery. Eur J Cardiothorac Surg. 2004;25(2):267–74.

Whitlock R, Healey JS, Connolly SJ, et al. Predictors of early and late stroke following cardiac surgery. CMAJ. 2014;186(12):905–11.

Zhao DF, Edelman JJ, Seco M, et al. Coronary artery bypass grafting with and without manipulation of the ascending aorta: a network meta-analysis. J Am Coll Cardiol. 2017;69(8):924–36.

Strategies of Kidney Protection During Cardiopulmonary Bypass

30

Marie Caruso

Introduction

Acute kidney injury (AKI) is a common and serious complication that can arise after cardiac surgery, particularly in cases where cardiopulmonary bypass (CPB) is used. Defined by the abrupt deterioration in renal function, AKI can manifest as increased serum creatinine levels, reduced urine output, or the need for renal replacement therapy in severe cases. The significance of AKI in the context of cardiac surgery is profound. It can result in numerous adverse consequences and various short- and long-term complications. Short-term complications include volume overload and electrolyte imbalances, extended intensive care unit (ICU) and hospital stays, increased risk of infections, and cardiovascular complications. Severe AKI significantly increases the risk of mortality, with an associated odds ratio of three to eight, emphasizing the critical need for effective prevention and management strategies. Long-term consequences may include the progression to or onset of chronic kidney disease, potentially necessitating hemodialysis, increased costs associated with long-term healthcare, long-term health challenges, overall deterioration of the patient's quality of life, and mortality.

This chapter provides definitions of AKI and reviews risk stratification for its development. It explores the complex nature of AKI pathophysiology in the setting of CPB, focusing on the significant roles played by hemodynamic shifts, the inflammatory cascade, oxidative stress, and microemboli formation. The importance of a comprehensive approach to renal protection during CPB is emphasized. Strategies to ensure optimal perfusion, judicious temperature management, and reduction in inflammation and oxidative stress are critical. Additionally, the potential benefits of filtration techniques, such as ultrafiltration and the role of intraoperative pharmacological agents, will be discussed.

Implications and Clinical Significance of AKI

Recognizing and preventing cardiac surgery-associated acute kidney injury (CSA-AKI) is paramount. A significant proportion (20–70%) of cardiac surgery patients will develop AKI, and mortality rates can reach up to 50% for those requiring renal replacement therapy. When AKI occurs after cardiac surgery, mortality can climb to 60%, compared to just 1.3% in CABG patients who do not experience AKI. Even transient postoperative creatinine elevations are associated with risks of chronic renal insufficiency, end-stage renal disease, postoperative cardiovascular events, and mortality. For patients with preexisting end-stage renal disease requiring dialysis, undergoing cardiac surgery carries a 10–15% mortality rate.

Beyond the alarming mortality rates, the cost of care escalates dramatically with postoperative AKI due to extended ICU and hospital stays and the need for renal replacement therapy. These factors underscore the critical importance of implementing meticulous preventive measures and effective treatment strategies for CSA-AKI in cardiac surgery patients.

Definition and Diagnosis of AKI

Three classifications for the diagnosis and staging of AKI are currently widely employed: Risk, Injury, and Failure (RIFLE), Acute Kidney Injury Network (AKIN), and Kidney Disease: Improving Global Outcomes (KDIGO). They are summarized in Table 30.1.

There are limitations to the use of these three criteria in diagnosing AKI. These include a delay in diagnosis as oligu-

Supplementary Information The online version contains supplementary material available at https://doi.org/10.1007/978-3-031-91163-7_30.

M. Caruso (✉)
Department of Anesthesiology, Cooper Medical School of Rowan University, Camden, NJ, USA
e-mail: carusozatorski-marie@cooperhealth.edu

A. S. Awad, J. DiNardo (eds.), *Clinical Perfusion for Cardiac Surgery*, https://doi.org/10.1007/978-3-031-91163-7_30

Table 30.1 Diagnostic criteria for AKI

Classification system	Severity level (class/stage)	Serum creatinine criteria	Urine output criteria
RIFLE	Risk	Serum creatinine increase by 1.5 times baseline OR glomerular filtration rate (GFR) decrease ≥25%	Urine output <0.5 mL/kg/h for ≥6 h
	Injury	Serum creatinine increase by 2 times baseline OR GFR decrease ≥50%	Urine output <0.5 mL/kg/h for ≥12 h
	Failure	Serum creatinine increase by 3 times baseline OR increase by ≥0.5 to ≥4.0 mg/dL OR GFR decrease ≥75% OR initiation of renal replacement therapy (RRT)	Urine output <0.3 mL/kg/h for ≥24 h OR anuria for ≥12 h
	Loss	Loss of kidney function for >4 weeks	–
	End-stage	Loss of kidney function for >3 months	–
AKIN	Stage 1	Serum creatinine increase by ≥0.3 mg/dL within 48 h OR serum creatinine increase by 1.5–2 times baseline within 48 h	Urine output <0.5 mL/kg/h for ≥6 h
	Stage 2	Serum creatinine increase to ≥2 times baseline within 48 h	Urine output <0.5 mL/kg/h for ≥12 h
	Stage 3	Serum creatinine increase by >3 times baseline OR increase by ≥0.5 to ≥4.0 mg/dL OR initiation of RRT	Urine output <0.3 mL/kg/h for ≥24 h OR anuria for ≥12 h
KDIGO	Stage 1	Serum creatinine increase by ≥0.3 mg/dL within 48 h OR serum creatinine increase by 1.5–1.9 times baseline within 7 days	Urine output <0.5 mL/kg/h for ≥6 h
	Stage 2	Serum creatinine increase by 2.0–2.9 times baseline	Urine output <0.5 mL/kg/h for ≥12 h
	Stage 3	Serum creatinine increase by >3 times baseline OR increase by ≥0.5 to ≥4.0 mg/dL OR initiation of RRT OR anuria for ≥12 h OR a decrease in eGFR to <35 mL/min/1.73 m^2 in children	Urine output <0.3 mL/kg/h for ≥24 h OR anuria for ≥12 h

ria and elevated creatinine are often not seen post surgically for 48 h to 7 days after the initial preoperative or intraoperative insult because serum creatinine level may be normal even if GFR is decreased and because serum creatinine levels are affected by other factors including age, sex, muscle mass, diet, volume status, independent of kidney function. Therefore, initiation of treatments and interventions may be delayed due to delayed recognition of AKI. In addition, these criteria do not aid in the diagnosis of the etiology of the AKI, whether it be ischemic, embolic, nephrotoxic, or a combination of multiple insults.

Biomarkers for Diagnosis and Prediction

The most accurate biomarkers for AKI are those that facilitate early detection, offer high sensitivity and specificity, and provide valuable information regarding the severity or progression of kidney damage. Blood and urine biomarkers that enable earlier detection and prediction of CSA-AKI have been identified. These biomarkers either originate from the kidneys in response to ischemic injury or reflect changes in glomerular filtration rate (GFR). Summarized in Table 30.2 and Fig. 30.1, these biomarkers can be detected in blood or urine within 2–6 h post-injury, providing clinicians with crucial information to guide timely intervention.

Pathophysiology of Kidney Injury During CPB

The development of AKI during CPB is driven by a complex combination of factors, including hemodynamic disturbances, inflammatory responses, hemolysis, red cell transfusions, oxidative damage, genetic predisposition, nephrotoxic medications, and microemboli formation. These intercon-

Table 30.2 Blood and urine biomarkers for early detection and risk stratification of CS AKI

Biomarker	Location	Mechanism of action	Clinical application	Constraints
Cystatin C	Detected in blood	A functional biomarker that exhibits reduced clearance during AKI	Allows early identification of AKI, independent of muscle mass and dietary choices	Several studies demonstrated lower predictive value compared to other markers
Neutrophil gelatinase-associated lipocalin (NGAL)	Found in blood and urine	Expressed at higher levels in the proximal tubules following ischemia or nephrotoxic damage	Allows early identification of AKI	Demonstrates higher specificity in pediatric and adult populations in the absence of underlying chronic kidney disease
Kidney injury molecule-1 (KIM-1)	Detected in urine	Quickly upregulated in the cells of the proximal tubules following ischemia injury	Allows early identification of AKI	Peaks 2–3 days after injury, limiting its utility for early diagnosis
C-C motif chemokine ligand 14 (CCL14)	Detected in urine	Implicated in proximal tubule inflammation damage	Predicting the progression of AKI and the likelihood of requiring renal replacement therapy	Does not allow early identification of AKI
Interleukin-18 (IL-18)	Detected in urine	A pro-inflammatory cytokine implicated in ischemic and inflammatory damage to the proximal tubules	Allows early identification of AKI	Predictive value may be lower in certain studies
[Tissue inhibitor of metalloproteinase-2] × [insulin-like growth factor-binding protein 7] [TIMP-2] × [IGFBP7]	Detected in urine	Triggers cell cycle inhibition within the renal tubular cells	Allows early identification of AKI	May show reduced specificity in some research findings

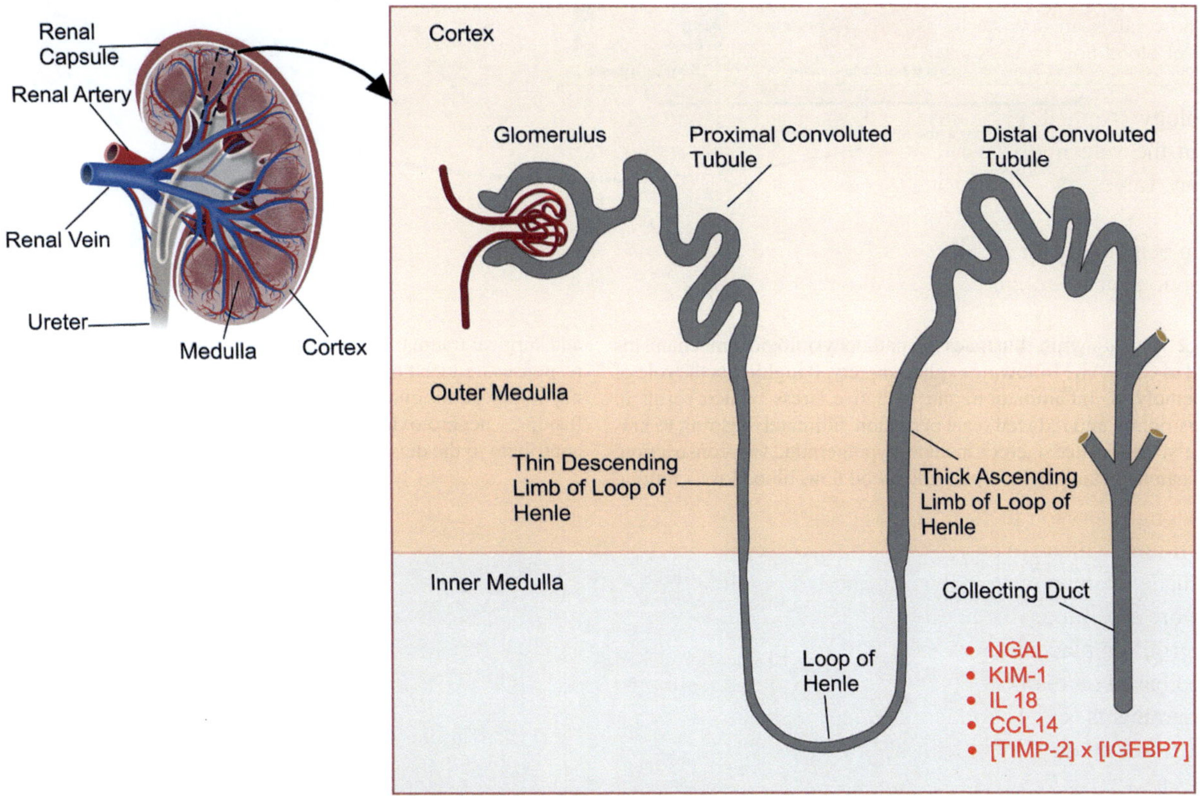

Fig. 30.1 This illustration depicts a cross-section of the kidney, focusing on magnified structures involved in urine production within the tubules. The process of urine formation is traced, highlighting key biomarkers used for the diagnosis of CSA-AKI. These biomarkers, indicated in red text, include NGAL (Neutrophil Gelatinase-Associated Lipocalin), an early marker of tubular injury, and KIM-1 (Kidney Injury Molecule-1), which is rapidly expressed in proximal tubular cells after ischemic damage. IL-18 (Interleukin-18) is another important marker, mediating ischemic and inflammatory kidney injury. CCL14 (C-C Motif Chemokine Ligand 14) is associated with predicting persistent AKI and progression to RRT, while the combination of [TIMP-2] × [IGFBP7] indicates cell cycle arrest in renal tubular cells and is commonly used to assess AKI risk. These biomarkers are crucial for the early detection and monitoring of CSA-AKI

nected mechanisms collectively contribute to kidney injury throughout the surgical process. The etiology of AKI after cardiac surgery with CPB is thus multifactorial (see Fig. 30.2).

Hemodynamic Instability and Hypoperfusion

CPB and non-pulsatile flow induce significant hemodynamic alterations, leading to substantial variations in renal perfusion pressure. This instability reduces blood flow to the kidneys, particularly in vulnerable areas like the renal medulla,

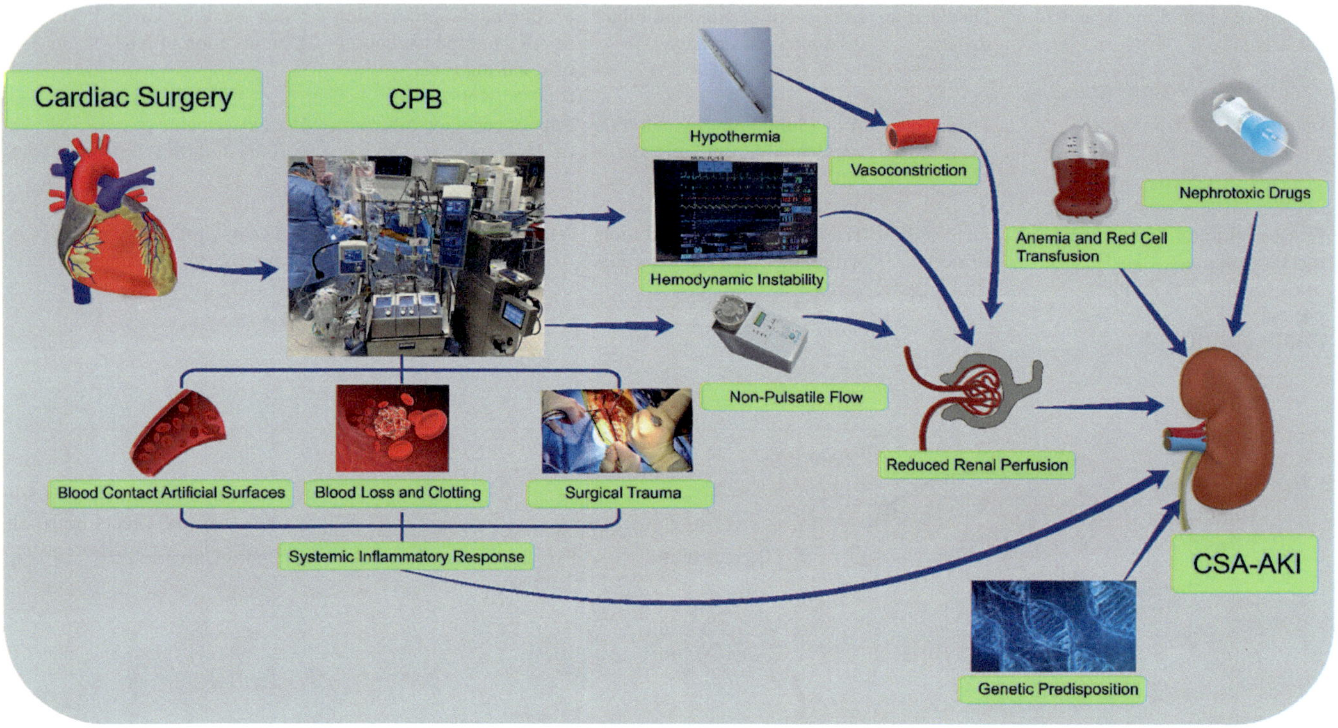

Fig. 30.2 This diagram illustrates the pathophysiological mechanisms that lead to CSA-AKI following cardiac surgery. It highlights the role of CPB, hemolysis, inflammation, and oxidative stress, which result in vasoconstriction and reduced renal perfusion, ultimately leading to kidney injury. Associated factors include hypothermia, vasoconstriction, hemodynamic instability, non-pulsatile blood flow, blood loss, clotting, and surgical trauma. These factors contribute to systemic inflammatory responses, reduced renal perfusion, and increased susceptibility to kidney injury. Additional risk factors, such as anemia, red blood cell transfusions, nephrotoxic drugs, and genetic predisposition, further contribute to the development of CSA-AKI

resulting in ischemia and depriving kidney tissues of essential oxygen and nutrients. The hypoperfusion during CPB, often exacerbated by episodes of hypotension, increases the risk of renal ischemia and reperfusion injury once normal blood circulation is restored. Additionally, renal ischemia is mediated by sympathetic activation and the renin-angiotensin-aldosterone system (RAAS), which is triggered by the non-pulsatile flow during CPB and low renal perfusion pressure (RPP). Renin, released by the juxtaglomerular cells in the kidney in response to low RPP (as seen in Fig. 30.3), is converted to angiotensin II, a potent vasoconstrictor, which constricts the renal arteries and afferent arterioles, further reducing oxygen (O_2) delivery to the kidneys and intensifying hypoperfusion. Together, these mechanisms significantly increase the likelihood of AKI during and after CPB.

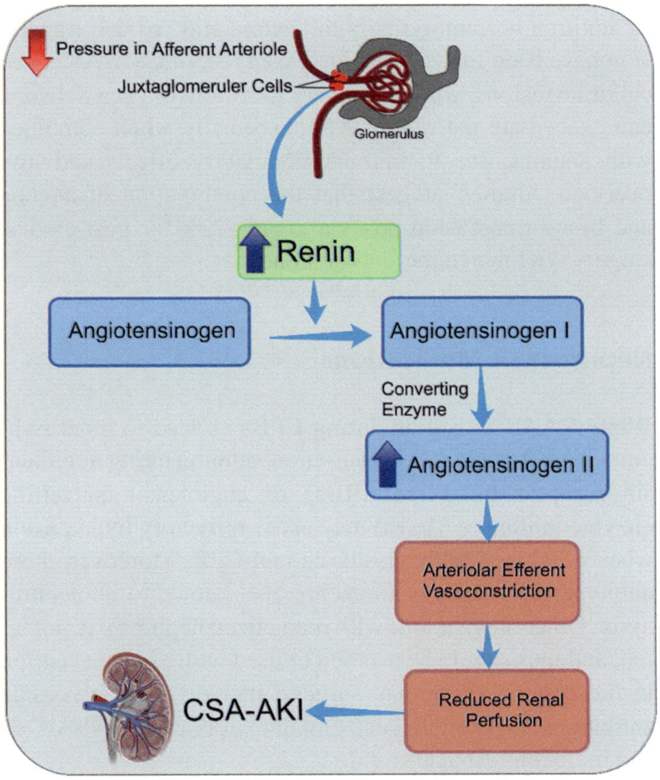

Fig. 30.3 This illustration demonstrates the role of the RAAS in the development of CSA-AKI. Hypotension during CPB triggers afferent arteriole vasoconstriction, leading to reduced renal blood flow. In response, renin is released from the juxtaglomerular cells, converting angiotensinogen to angiotensin I, which is then converted to angiotensin II. Angiotensin II, a potent vasoconstrictor, further reduces renal perfusion, ultimately contributing to the onset of CSA-AKI

Systemic Inflammatory Response (SIRS) and Oxidative Stress

CPB initiates SIRS when blood interacts with the artificial surfaces of the bypass circuit, leading to the release of pro-inflammatory cytokines such as tumor necrosis factor-alpha (TNF-alpha), interleukin-6 (IL-6), and interleukin-8 (IL-8). Please refer to Chap. 6 for more information. These cytokines, along with oxidative stress mediators, contribute significantly to renal tissue damage and systemic inflammation, impairing circulatory autoregulation and reducing renal perfusion (see Fig. 30.4). Prolonged CPB time and aortic cross-clamping further exacerbate this pro-inflammatory state, increasing the production of reactive oxygen species (ROS), which intensifies ischemia and leads to direct cellular injury in the kidneys. The ischemia-reperfusion process triggers oxidative stress, a key factor in kidney injury. The overproduction of ROS damages cellular structures by targeting lipids, proteins, and DNA within kidney tissues, further compounding the injury. Despite heparinization, patients remain in a hypercoagulable state due to widespread inflammation and clotting dysregulation, increasing the risk of embolic events. Peripheral vasodilation caused by SIRS also worsens renal hypoperfusion, while the combination of ROS and inflammatory pathways accelerates cell damage and death. Together, these factors make the inflammatory response and SIRS key contributors to AKI during and after CPB (Fig. 30.4).

Hemolysis

Red cell hemolysis is a known consequence of CPB, caused by mechanical trauma and shear forces from the flow through

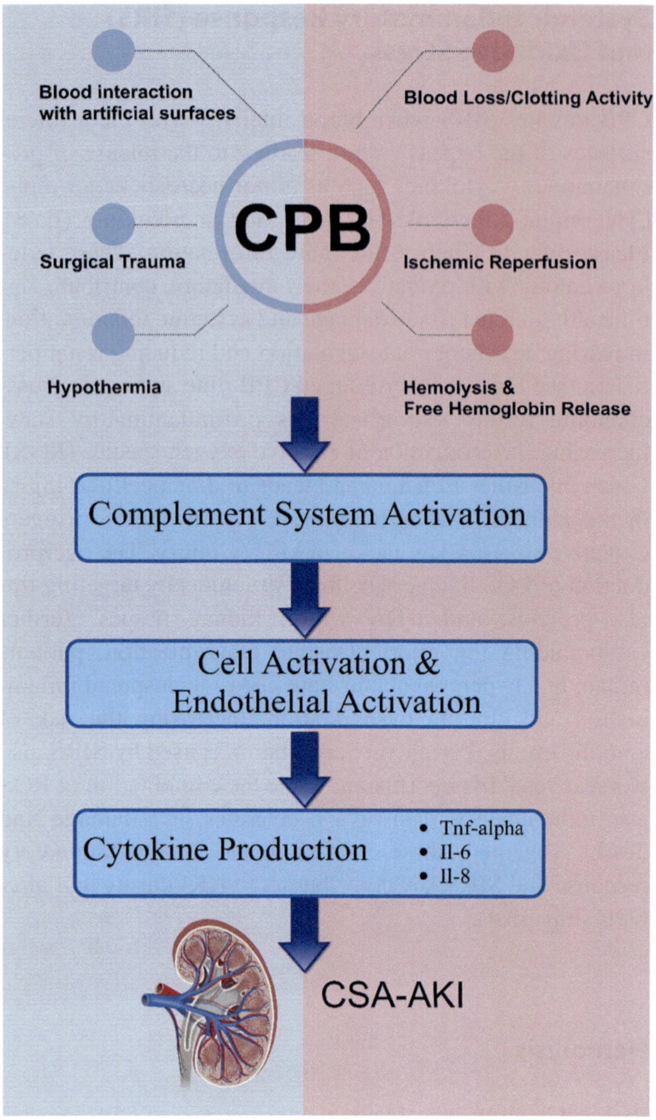

Fig. 30.4 This diagram illustrates SIRS and oxidative stress during CPB, which contributes to AKI. At the center, CPB is shown to initiate key effects: blood interaction with artificial surfaces, hypothermia, Hemolysis and free hemoglobin release, surgical trauma, ischemic reperfusion, and blood loss/clotting activity. These events trigger the complement system, leading to cell and endothelial activation, and the release of pro-inflammatory cytokines such as TNF-alpha, IL-6, and IL-8. The cytokine storm impairs circulatory autoregulation, reduces renal perfusion, and, along with prolonged CPB time and cross-clamping, increases ROS, resulting in ischemia and direct kidney injury Peripheral vasodilation exacerbates renal hypoperfusion, while oxidative stress and a hypercoagulable state increase the risk of embolic events, ultimately leading to CSA-AKI

the CPB circuit, turbulence in the oxygenator, cardiotomy suction, LV venting, and the use of the cell saver apparatus. Hemolysis releases free iron and hemoglobin, which induce oxidative stress, inflammation, and tissue damage. Under normal conditions, free hemoglobin is bound by haptoglobin, forming hemoglobin-haptoglobin complexes that are processed by macrophages in the reticuloendothelial system. However, when free hemoglobin exceeds the body's haptoglobin stores, it becomes toxic. Excess free hemoglobin, not bound by haptoglobin, is filtered and excreted by the kidneys, where it acts as a potent vasoconstrictor, reducing renal perfusion and contributing to ischemia. In addition, free hemoglobin binds nitric oxide, a vasodilator produced by endothelial cells, further promoting vasoconstriction, ischemia, endothelial dysfunction, and the generation of free radicals that cascade into cell injury and death.

Anemia and Red Cell Transfusion

In addition to hemolysis, both anemia and red cell transfusion have been linked to an increased risk of CSA-AKI. Red cell transfusions, while necessary to restore oxygen delivery, can exacerbate the risk of AKI, especially when combined with anemia, due to immunomodulatory effects and iron overload. Studies suggest that the combination of anemia and blood transfusion poses a greater risk for post-cardiac surgery AKI than either factor alone.

Nephrotoxic Medications

While RAAS activation during CPB can lead to renal ischemia mediated via vasoconstriction, administering angiotensin receptor blockers (ARBs) or angiotensin-converting enzyme inhibitors (ACEi) may cause refractory hypotension when combined with anesthesia and CPB. Moreover, these antihypertensive medications are also known to be nephrotoxic. Other medications with recognized nephrotoxic potential, and thus should be avoided or used with extreme caution in the context of cardiac surgery, include aminoglycoside antibiotics, nonsteroidal anti-inflammatory drugs (NSAIDs), and radiocontrast agents.

Metformin, although not directly nephrotoxic, should be withheld prior to cardiac surgery due to its association with an increased risk of lactic acidosis, particularly in the setting of reduced renal function that may occur during or after CPB. Similarly, Sodium–glucose cotransporter-2 (SGLT2) inhibitors, including canagliflozin, dapagliflozin, and empagliflozin, can induce diabetic ketoacidosis and should also be withheld prior to cardiac surgery to mitigate these potential complications.

Genetics

Genetics may play a role in predisposition to AKI, as patient populations respond differently to oxidative stress and inflammation. For example, certain alleles of Apolipoprotein E, a lipoprotein involved in tissue repair and immunomodulation, have been shown to be protective against AKI. The presence of these alleles has been linked to a reduced incidence of AKI following cardiac surgery.

Microemboli

The generation of microemboli during CPB plays a crucial role in the onset of AKI. These microemboli, which consist of fibrin, platelet clumps, cellular debris, fat, and air bubbles, can obstruct the renal microcirculation, resulting in localized ischemia and tissue necrosis within the renal parenchyma. This blockage of blood flow further worsens renal ischemia, significantly raising the risk of developing AKI.

Perioperative Management Strategies to Prevent AKI in Cardiac Surgery

To mitigate the risk of CSA-AKI, comprehensive perioperative management strategies are essential. These strategies span the preoperative, intraoperative (during CPB), and postoperative phases, addressing modifiable risk factors and optimizing renal protection. The Society of Thoracic Surgeons (STS), the Society of Cardiovascular Anesthesiologists (SCA), and the American Society of Extracorporeal Technology (AmSECT) have collaboratively developed clinical practice guidelines aimed at preventing CSA-AKI.

Preoperative Strategies for Kidney Protection

In patients undergoing cardiac surgery with CPB, especially those at high risk for AKI, implementing preoperative strategies to optimize kidney function is crucial. These strategies focus on risk stratification, renal function optimization, and avoidance of factors that could worsen renal injury. Their recommendations for perioperative prevention are as follows:

1. Risk Stratification and Prediction of CSA-AKI

   Identifying patients at high risk for CSA-AKI is the first step in developing a targeted strategy for kidney protection and initiating timely interventions to mitigate patient risk throughout the perioperative period. An ideal risk prediction model helps identify modifiable risk factors, enabling clinicians to implement preventive measures effectively. Three widely used clinical prediction models that assess the risk of developing CSA-AKI, particularly stage 3 AKI, include the Cleveland Clinic Score, Mehta Score, and the Simplified Renal Index. These models utilize preoperative variables to predict AKI risk. The Cleveland Clinic Score assigns points based on factors such as female gender, congestive heart failure, left ventricular ejection fraction below 35%, and the use of a preoperative intra-aortic balloon pump, among others. The Mehta Score, developed from a large cohort of over 449,000 patients, incorporates additional variables such as age ≥55, non-White race, preoperative serum creatinine levels, and cardiogenic shock, allowing for a broader assessment of patient risk. The Simplified Renal Index uses fewer variables, such as preoperative GFR, diabetes, and the urgency of surgery, making it a more streamlined model for AKI prediction. Collectively, these models help clinicians stratify patients' risk for AKI and guide perioperative management to reduce the likelihood of postoperative kidney injury. A summary of clinical prediction models is summarized in Table 30.3.
2. Renal Function Optimization
   - *Blood Pressure and Glucose Control*: Ensuring optimal management of blood pressure and glucose levels is critical to preserving kidney function. Hypertension and hyperglycemia increase the risk of renal injury, so maintaining these within recommended limits preoperatively can reduce the likelihood of AKI.
   - *Avoidance of Nephrotoxic Drugs*: Medications such as NSAIDs, ACE inhibitors, ARBs, and radiocontrast agents should be avoided in the preoperative period.

Table 30.3 Summary of clinical prediction models for AKI after cardiac surgery

Model name	Derivation cohort	Validation cohort	Scoring variables		Score range
Cleveland clinic score risk factors	15,838 patients (Single U.S. Center, 1993–2002)	17,379 patients (Same center and time period)	*Gender*: Female	1 point	0–17 points
			Heart Failure: Presence of congestive heart failure	1 point	
			Cardiac Function: Left ventricular ejection fraction below 35%	1 point	
			Support Device: Use of a preoperative intra-aortic balloon pump	2 points	
			Lung Disease: Chronic obstructive pulmonary disease (COPD)	1 point	
			Diabetes: Insulin-dependent	1 point	
			Surgery Type: Depending on complexity	2 points	
			Emergency Surgery:	2 points	
			Prior cardiac surgery: Redo	1 point	
			Kidney Function: Preoperative serum creatinine level	0–5 points	
Mehta score risk factors	449,524 patients (Database of >600 centers, 2002–2004)	86,009 patients (Same database, 2005)	*Age*: 55 or older	2 points	0–85 points
			Ethnicity: Non-white	1 point	
			Kidney function: Preoperative serum creatinine	5–40 points	
			Heart failure severity: New York Heart Association (NYHA) Class IV heart failure	3 points	
			Diabetes: Managed with oral medications	2 points	
			Diabetes: Insulin-dependent	5 points	
			Lung Disease: COPD	1 point	
			Recent myocardial infarction	3 points	
			Prior cardiac surgery: Redo	2 points	
			Cardiogenic shock:	7 points	
			Surgery type: Depending on complexity	3 points	
Simplified renal index risk factors	10,751 patients (Single Canadian Center, 1999–2004)	9380 patients (Two Canadian centers, 1999–2003)	*Kidney function*: Preoperative GFR	1–2 points	0–8 points
			Diabetes: Requiring medications	1 point	
			Cardiac function: Left ventricular ejection fraction ≤40%	1 point	
			Prior cardiac surgery: Redo	1 point	
			Support device: Preoperative intra-aortic balloon pump	1 point	
			Urgent or emergency surgery: Nonelective surgery	1 point	
			Surgery type: Depending on complexity	0–1 point	

These drugs are associated with increased kidney injury and should be discontinued or replaced with safer alternatives in high-risk patients.

- *Preoperative Hydration*: Proper hydration before surgery helps improve renal perfusion and reduce the risk of ischemia during CPB. Hydration strategies should be carefully monitored to avoid volume overload.
- *Management of Anemia*: Preoperative anemia is associated with an increased risk of AKI. The use of erythropoietin and iron supplementation in anemic patients can help optimize red blood cell levels, improving oxygen delivery to the kidneys and reducing the risk of injury.

By carefully assessing risk and implementing these preoperative measures, healthcare providers can significantly improve the protection of renal function in patients undergoing cardiac surgery, ultimately reducing the incidence of CSA-AKI and improving overall patient outcomes.

Intraoperative Strategies for Reducing CSA-AKI Risk and Enhancing Renal Protection During CPB

In adult cardiac surgery with CPB, various intraoperative strategies have been identified to reduce the risk of CSA-AKI. These strategies focus on optimizing perfusion, temperature management, oxygen delivery, and the use of pharmacological agents. Below are the key recommendations:

1. *Temperature Management*
   - *Avoidance of Hyperthermic Perfusion*: In adult cardiac surgery with CPB, avoiding hyperthermic perfusion (>37 °C) is recommended to reduce the risk of CSA-AKI. Hyperthermia can exacerbate ischemia-reperfusion injury and increase the risk of kidney damage. This recommendation is supported by a Class I, Level, with moderate evidence (Class of Recommendation I, Level of Evidence B-R).
2. *Oxygen Delivery and Perfusion Optimization*

   Ensuring adequate oxygen delivery (DO2) and maintaining proper perfusion during CPB are essential strategies to reduce the risk of CSA-AKI. These strategies involve goal-directed perfusion to prevent renal hypoxia and ischemia, which are key contributors to AKI.
   - *Goal-Directed DO_2*: Maintaining a goal-directed strategy for DO2 during CPB is critical to preventing renal injury. Adequate oxygen delivery helps avert renal hypoxia and ischemia, which are leading causes of AKI. This strategy is supported by strong evidence (Class of Recommendation: I, Level of Evidence: B-R). Traditionally, some institutions target a cardiac index (CI) of >2.4 L/min/m^2 based on body surface area; however, this approach does not factor in the oxygen content of the patient's blood. A more refined goal-directed perfusion strategy maintains DO2 above a prespecified threshold, typically 280–350 mL/min/m^2 for patients undergoing moderately hypothermic CPB (>32 °C). This method has been shown to reduce CPB-associated AKI. DO2 is maintained by adjusting CPB arterial flow in accordance with hematocrit values. If DO2 falls below the target and venous oxygen saturation (SvO2) drops below 68% or the oxygen extraction rate exceeds 40%, a unit of red blood cells is transfused to enhance oxygen delivery. In theory, lower DO2 thresholds could be targeted at lower CPB temperatures due to temperature-induced reductions in oxygen consumption (VO2).
   - *Maintaining Adequate Mean Arterial Pressure (MAP)*: Maintaining an adequate MAP of >70 mmHg during CPB is crucial for ensuring proper renal perfusion, helping to prevent hypoperfusion and ischemia, which are major contributors to AKI. Although it is generally recommended to maintain a MAP ≥65 mmHg due to impaired renal autoregulation during CPB, especially in patients with baseline hypertension, recent studies suggest this threshold should be interpreted with caution. For example, an association has been demonstrated between MAP <65 mmHg for 10 min or more after CPB and the need for post-operative RRT. Additionally, every 10-min episode of hypotension (MAP <65 mmHg) before, during, or after CPB has been linked with increased odds of a composite outcome of stroke, AKI, or death. However, when analyzing hypotension specifically during CPB, independent of pre- and post-CPB periods, no direct association was found with these adverse outcomes.
   - *Use of Pulsatile Flow*: The use of pulsatile flow during CPB may further improve microcirculatory perfusion and oxygen delivery to the kidneys compared to non-pulsatile flow. Pulsatile flow mimics the natural rhythm of the heart, promoting better organ perfusion and reducing the risk of ischemic injury to the kidneys.
3. *CPB Circuitry and Technological Innovations*
   - *Biocompatible Circuit Coatings*:
   - Researchers have developed circuits coated with heparin or phosphorylcholine to create a more physiologically compatible surface. These coatings aim to:
   1. Minimize the risk of hemolysis
   2. Reduce the activation of pro-inflammatory pathways
   3. Decrease oxidative stress
   - Studies examining these biocompatible coatings have yielded promising results, including:
     - Decreased need for blood transfusions
     - Shorter hospital stays
     - Lower postoperative creatinine levels
     - Potential renal protective effects

   Recent European guidelines have acknowledged the potential benefits of these coatings, granting them a Class IIa recommendation. This classification indicates that while evidence may be conflicting, the overall weight of data supports their clinical utility.
   - *Miniaturized CPB Systems*: They are compact versions of traditional CPB machines designed to reduce the surface area of extracorporeal circuits and minimize blood contact with artificial surfaces. This reduction decreases the inflammatory response during surgery. By limiting hemodilution, contact activation, and exposure to foreign surfaces, these systems may lower the risk of CSA-AKI.
   - *Minimally Invasive Extracorporeal Circulation (MiECC) Techniques*: MiECC represents an advanced evolution of miniaturized CPB systems designed to minimize the physiological impact of traditional

CPB. Key components of MiECC include biocompatible coatings, integrated suction systems, and leukocyte filters. These features incorporate heparin-coated circuits to reduce the activation of coagulation and inflammatory pathways, a smaller priming volume to limit hemodilution, a closed-loop system to prevent air embolism and contamination, a centrifugal pump for gentler blood handling, and the elimination of a venous reservoir to reduce blood trauma and inflammatory responses. By integrating these innovations, MiECC aims to lower the risks of hemolysis, SIRS, and organ dysfunction, particularly AKI. Studies suggest that MiECC offers improved clinical outcomes, including reduced transfusion requirements, lower postoperative inflammation, and enhanced renal protection compared to conventional CPB techniques. This approach marks significant progress in patient safety and complication reduction in cardiac surgery. While MiECC techniques show promise in reducing the risk of CSA-AKI, the supporting evidence remains moderate (Class of Recommendation IIB, Level of Evidence B-R).

4. *Pharmacological Agents and Techniques*
   - *Dopamine Infusion*: Dopamine infusion alone during CPB and in the perioperative period is not recommended for reducing the risk of CSA-AKI. Studies have shown no significant benefit of dopamine in protecting renal function in this context (Class of Recommendation III: No Benefit, Level of Evidence A).
   - *Fenoldopam*: Fenoldopam, a selective dopamine 1 receptor agonist, promotes renal perfusion and helps maintain GFR. It may be reasonable to use fenoldopam to reduce the risk of CSA-AKI, provided that hypotension, a common side effect, is carefully managed. This treatment may be particularly beneficial in patients with preexisting serum creatinine levels >1.4 mg/dL, offering some kidney protection (Class of Recommendation IIB, Level of Evidence B-R).
   - *Mannitol*: The use of mannitol, an osmotic diuretic, is not recommended for preventing CSA-AKI. There is no demonstrated benefit in using mannitol for renal protection in patients undergoing cardiac surgery with CPB (Class of Recommendation III: No Benefit, Level of Evidence B-R).
   - In addition to the core recommendations from the STS, the SCA, and the AmSECT, other pharmacological agents and techniques have been proposed to further optimize perfusion and protect renal function in patients undergoing cardiac surgery with CPB.
   - *Volatile Anesthetics*: Volatile anesthetics, such as sevoflurane and isoflurane, may offer some degree of renal protection due to their anti-inflammatory properties and ability to reduce ischemia-reperfusion injury. Their use in combination with CPB has been associated with better postoperative renal function.
   - *Natriuretic Peptides*: The use of natriuretic peptides, such as atrial natriuretic peptide (ANP), has been studied for their potential to improve renal perfusion and protect against AKI. These agents may reduce renal vasoconstriction and promote diuresis, helping to maintain kidney function during surgery.
   - *Nitric Oxide (NO)*: Nitric oxide plays a key role in maintaining vascular tone and preventing vasoconstriction in the renal vasculature. The administration of NO or NO donors during CPB may help improve renal blood flow and reduce the risk of AKI.
   - *Dexmedetomidine*: Dexmedetomidine, a selective alpha-2 adrenergic agonist, has sedative and analgesic properties that may provide renal protection during cardiac surgery by reducing sympathetic outflow and preserving renal perfusion. It decreases renin release, mitigates vasoconstriction, and lowers norepinephrine and cortisol levels post-surgery. Although some evidence suggests that dexmedetomidine may reduce the incidence of AKI in cardiac surgery patients, conflicting and inconsistent data prevent its routine recommendation for AKI prevention.
5. *KDIGO Guidelines*:
   - *KDIGO Bundle of Care*: In adult cardiac surgery with CPB, it is reasonable to adopt the KDIGO practice guidelines ("KDIGO bundle of care") as outlined in the STS/SCA/AmSECT Clinical Practice Guidelines by Brown et al. for patients at high-risk of AKI to reduce the risk of CSA-AKI (Class of Recommendation IIA; Level of Evidence B-R). Key measures include:
     – Avoidance of nephrotoxic agents
     – Discontinuation of ACEi, and ARB during the first 48 h after surgery
     – Avoidance of hydroxyethyl starch (HES), gelatine, and chloride rich solutions (including 0.9% saline)
     – Monitoring of serum creatinine every 12 h
     – Monitoring of fluid balance and urine output hourly
     – Managing fluid balance and avoiding hyperglycemia (defined as blood glucose levels >150 mg/dL for >3 h) in the first 72 h after surgery
     – Using alternatives to radiocontrast agents when possible
     – Close hemodynamic monitoring should utilize functional hemodynamic tools, such as a pulse index continuous cardiac output (PiCCO) monitor, to track stroke volume variation (SVV) and CI. This approach helps guide the administration of fluids and inotropes, optimizing volume status and hemodynamic parameters based on a prespecified algorithm, as outlined below:

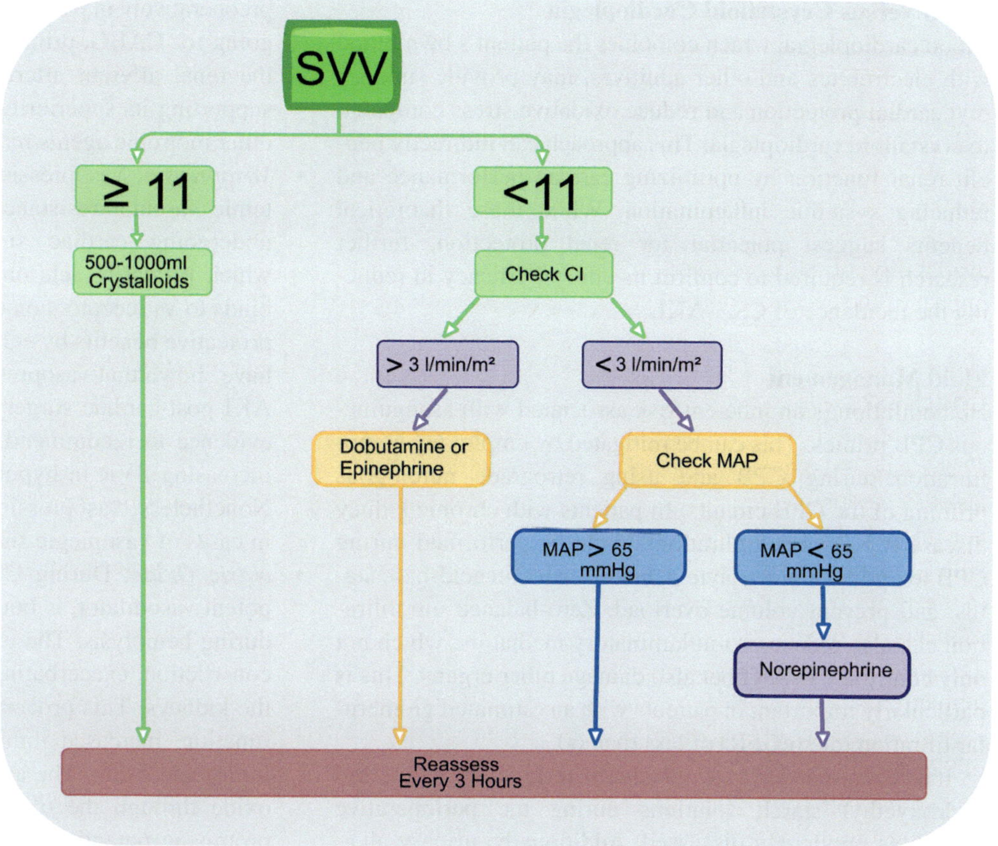

Fig. 30.5 This diagram illustrates a structured algorithm for hemodynamic optimization during cardiac surgery, implemented as part of the KDIGO bundle. It utilizes SVV, CI, and MAP as key parameters. The algorithm guides fluid administration and inotropic support to maintain optimal volume status and hemodynamic stability. When SVV is ≥11, crystalloids are administered. If SVV is <11, CI is evaluated. If CI is below 3 L/min/m², Dobutamine or Epinephrine is administered to improve cardiac output. MAP is then assessed, with Norepinephrine administered if MAP is below 65 mmHg. Reassessment is performed every 3 h to ensure therapeutic goals are achieved, reducing the risk of CSA-AKI

- *SVV ≥ 11*: Administer 500–1000 mL of crystalloids.
- *SVV < 11*: Check the CI.
- If *CI > 3 L/min/m²*, assess MAP.
- If *CI < 3 L/min/m²*, administer *Dobutamine/Epinephrine* to improve cardiac output.
- *MAP*: If MAP is <65 mmHg, administer *Norepinephrine* to maintain MAP >65 mmHg.
- Reassess every 3 h for up to 12 h after randomization to ensure the goal is achieved.

This structured algorithm effectively guides hemodynamic optimization using SVV, CI, and MAP as key parameters (Fig. 30.5). Notably, sub-analysis has shown that Dobutamine may help reduce the risk of CSA-AKI when implemented as part of the KDIGO bundle.

In addition to the core recommendations from the STS, SCA, and AmSECT, several other strategies can be employed to protect the kidneys during the intraoperative period.

Mitigation of Hemolysis-Related Nephrotoxins

Hemolysis during CPB is a significant contributor to CSA-AKI. To reduce hemolysis caused by shear forces on red cells and the subsequent release of free hemoglobin and iron, efforts should focus on minimizing red blood cell trauma. Key strategies include reducing the time on CPB, avoiding high-pressure cardiotomy suction and intracardiac vents, and utilizing a cell saver to remove hemolysis products. Although the Cytosorb filter, designed to capture mid-molecular weight inflammatory mediators, has not proven effective in removing cell-free hemoglobin. Another theoretical approach involves the administration of exogenous haptoglobin to reduce free hemoglobin. This binds to free hemoglobin when endogenous haptoglobin stores are depleted. However, this is an experimental treatment that carries risks such as high cost and potential anaphylactic reactions, and it is not currently approved in the United States. Furthermore, hemolysis can be mitigated by avoiding the transfusion of older red blood cells, which are more susceptible to shear-induced lysis as they near expiration.

Antioxidant Supplementation

Adding antioxidants like glutathione, N-acetylcysteine (see below), or mannitol (see above) to the cardioplegia solution may help scavenge free radicals and mitigate oxidative damage to the kidneys during reperfusion. While this approach offers theoretical benefits for renal protection, further research is needed to establish its clinical efficacy in reducing CSA-AKI.

Blood Versus Crystalloid Cardioplegia

Blood cardioplegia, which combines the patient's own blood with electrolytes and other additives, may provide superior myocardial protection and reduce oxidative stress compared to crystalloid cardioplegia. This approach can indirectly benefit renal function by optimizing cardiac performance and reducing systemic inflammation. While these theoretical benefits suggest potential for renal protection, further research is required to confirm its clinical efficacy in reducing the incidence of CSA-AKI.

Fluid Management

Hemodilution is an inherent risk associated with asanguineous CPB primes. This can be mitigated by employing hemofiltration during CPB and using retrograde autologous priming of the CPB circuits. In patients with chronic kidney disease (CKD), hemofiltration should be performed during CPB to optimize electrolyte balance, maintain acid-base status, and prevent volume overload. Zero-balance ultrafiltration can also reduce pro-inflammatory mediators, which not only contribute to AKI but also damage other organs. This is particularly important in patients with an estimated glomerular filtration rate (eGFR) of less than 60.

It is recommended to avoid administering 0.9% saline and hydroxyethyl starch solutions during the perioperative period, as previously discussed. Additionally, urinary alkalinization with sodium bicarbonate has not been proven to prevent CSA-AKI, nor has the use of 4% albumin in the CPB prime or for intraoperative fluid replacement.

Adjuvant Therapies

Several additional medications, not previously discussed, have shown potential in reducing the incidence of AKI during CPB:

- *Antifibrinolytics*: The lysine analogues, such as aminocaproic acid and tranexamic acid, are commonly used antifibrinolytic agents during CPB. These medications help reduce perioperative bleeding, thereby indirectly lowering the risk of AKI by reducing the need for blood transfusions. Since both agents are renally excreted, their dosages must be adjusted in patients with renal dysfunction.
- *Human Atrial Natriuretic Peptides (hANP) and Nesiritide*: These agents, including hANP and nesiritide (recombinant human B-type natriuretic peptide), enhance kidney perfusion by dilating afferent arterioles and inhibiting the RAAS system. By promoting diuresis and preventing vasoconstriction, they help maintain renal perfusion, thereby preventing ischemia and kidney injury.
- *Levosimendan*: Levosimendan is a calcium sensitizer used to improve contractility in patients with heart failure. It has demonstrated reno-protective effects when administered preoperatively in patients with low ejection fraction undergoing for CABG, primarily by promoting vasodilation of the renal afferent arteriole. However, reliable evidence supporting its superiority as a reno-protective agent over other inotropic agents remains limited.
- *Vasopressin*: Vasopressin is valuable for increasing systemic vascular resistance (SVR) in vasoplegic patients undergoing cardiac surgery. Unlike norepinephrine, which primarily acts on afferent arterioles, vasopressin binds to V_1 receptors on efferent arterioles, offering reno-protective benefits by enhancing renal blood flow. Studies have shown that vasopressin may reduce the incidence of AKI post-cardiac surgery. However, there is insufficient evidence to recommend its use as a first-line agent for increasing SVR in hypotensive cardiac surgery patients. Nonetheless, vasopressin should be strongly considered in cases of vasoplegic shock.
- *Nitric Oxide*: During CPB, endogenous nitric oxide, a potent vasodilator, is bound by free hemoglobin released during hemolysis. The loss of nitric oxide leads to vasoconstriction, exacerbating ischemia-reperfusion injury in the kidneys. This process contributes to endothelial dysfunction, increased inflammation, and eventual cellular injury and death. The administration of exogenous nitric oxide through the oxygenator during CPB has shown promising potential in reducing the incidence of AKI in cardiac surgery patients.
- *N-Acetylcysteine and Acetaminophen*: Both N-acetylcysteine and acetaminophen possess anti-inflammatory and antioxidative properties. Acetaminophen, in particular, acts as a lipid peroxidation inhibitor, preventing conversion of free iron into its more toxic form, which may help reduce the incidence of AKI. While both agents theoretically offer protection against AKI by reducing inflammation and oxygen free radicals, there is currently no definitive evidence to support their routine use in cardiac surgery patients for AKI prevention.

Postoperative Strategies for Reducing CSA-AKI

Following cardiac surgery with CPB, patients remain at significant risk of developing AKI. Proactive post-operative management is crucial in mitigating this risk. Evidence from randomized controlled trials indicates that implementing the KDIGO bundle can significantly reduce AKI incidence after cardiac surgery. An effective management strategy includes a multifaceted approach: close monitoring of renal function, appropriate use of pharmacological interventions, and, when necessary, timely initiation of RRT. The following sections outline the key strategies for managing post-operative AKI, including monitoring, KDIGO bundle implementation, pharmacological treatments, and early initiation of RRT.

1. *Monitoring*:
   - *Biomarkers for Early Detection of AKI*: Continuous monitoring of biomarkers is crucial in the postoperative period for early detection of AKI. Key biomarkers include serum creatinine, NGAL, and Cystatin C. As discussed in the intraoperative section, these biomarkers provide valuable insights into kidney function, often before significant clinical signs appear.
   - *Urine Output and Other Clinical Indicators*: Regular monitoring of urine output remains a vital indicator of renal function. A reduction in urine output, along with changes in other clinical parameters such as fluid balance, may signal the onset of AKI and requires prompt intervention.
2. *Pharmacological Agents*:
   - *Diuretics*: Diuretics may be used postoperatively to manage fluid balance and reduce fluid overload, but they must be administered carefully to avoid compromising renal perfusion, particularly in patients at risk of AKI.
   - *Other Agents*: Agents such as fenoldopam, dopamine, and N-acetylcysteine, previously discussed, have been investigated for their potential reno-protective effects during the post-operative period.
3. *RRT*:

   To address post-operative strategies for reducing CSA-AKI, RRT is a critical intervention for managing severe cases of CSA-AKI when conservative measures fail. Early initiation of RRT, specifically within 8 h of a KDIGO stage 2 AKI diagnosis, has been shown to lead to better patient outcomes (Fig. 30.6). These benefits include a reduced mortality rate, shorter RRT duration, decreased duration of mechanical ventilation, and reduced hospital stay. Additionally, early RRT use resulted in higher rates of renal recovery when compared to delayed RRT initiation after cardiac surgery.
   - *Indications and Timing*: RRT is indicated in severe cases of AKI when conservative measures fail to manage fluid overload, electrolyte imbalances, or uremia. Early initiation of RRT in patients with worsening renal function can improve outcomes and prevent further complications.
   - *Different RRT Modalities*: Post-operative RRT used post-operatively primarily encompasses Continuous Renal Replacement Therapy (CRRT), conventional Intermittent Hemodialysis (IHD), Extended Daily Dialysis (EDD), and Peritoneal Dialysis (PD).

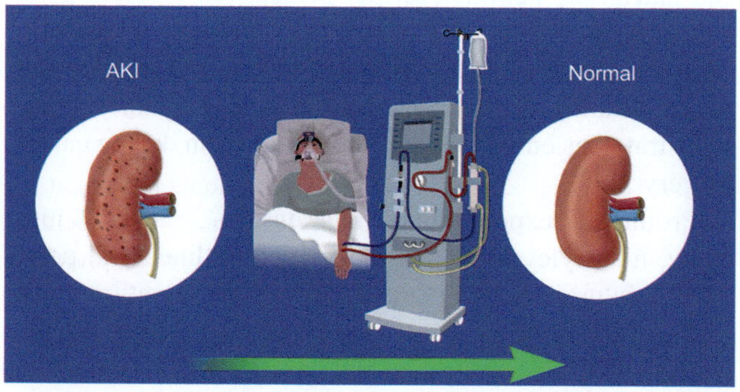

Fig. 30.6 This illustration demonstrates that initiating RRT early, specifically within 8 h of a post-operative KDIGO stage 2 AKI diagnosis, has been shown to improve patient outcomes. RRT is effective in managing CPB-associated AKI

1. *CRRT*: According to KDIGO guidelines (Grade 2B), CRRT is recommended for hemodynamically unstable patients after cardiac surgery due to its slower and more controlled fluid removal, which enhances tolerance.
2. *IHD*: Suitable for stable patients who can tolerate larger and more rapid fluid shifts during shorter treatment sessions.
3. *EDD*: A hybrid approach combining aspects of CRRT and IHD, offering longer sessions than IHD but not continuous like CRRT. It may be beneficial for certain patient populations, balancing hemodynamic stability and solute clearance.
4. *PD*: In high-risk pediatric patients, particularly neonates and infants, the early initiation of PD after cardiac surgery has been associated with improved fluid balance and a reduction in postoperative complications.
   - The choice of modality should be tailored to the patient's clinical status, hemodynamic stability, and specific needs in the postoperative period. Clinicians should consider transitioning between modalities as the patient's condition evolves.

These strategies, implemented postoperatively, are essential for managing AKI and improving outcomes in cardiac surgery patients, ensuring early detection, appropriate pharmacological intervention, and timely initiation of renal support when necessary.

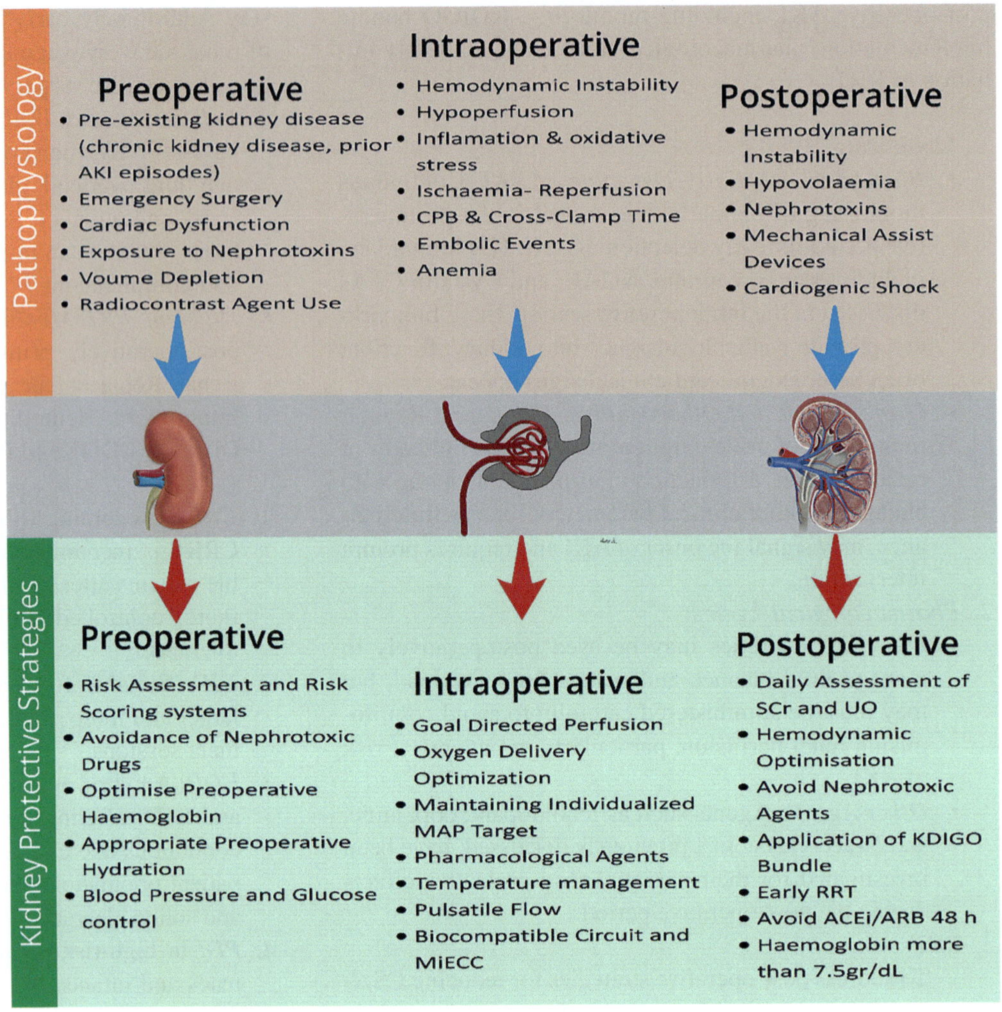

Fig. 30.7 This diagram provides an overview of the complex pathophysiology and contributing factors leading to AKI during cardiac surgery, highlighting current strategies for renal protection

Conclusion

Preventing CSA-AKI requires a multifaceted approach to CPB management, focusing on minimizing renal injury. Understanding the complex pathophysiology of AKI during CPB is crucial. While genetic predisposition plays a role, renal ischemia emerges as a major contributor. This ischemia stems from factors such as decreased RPP and non-pulsatile flow during CPB, further exacerbated by the activation of the RAAS system. Inflammatory responses triggered by CPB, including hemolysis-induced oxidative stress and inflammation, also significantly impact renal function.

Transfusion, while necessary to maintain adequate hemoglobin levels, presents a delicate balance, as excessive transfusions can increase the risk of AKI. Identifying high-risk patients based on pre-existing conditions like renal dysfunction, advanced age, and comorbidities is crucial for targeted interventions. Preoperative optimization through careful fluid management, acid–base control, medication adjustments, and potential surgical delay is paramount in preventing AKI.

Intraoperative strategies such as maintaining optimal hemodynamics, minimizing hemolysis, and employing goal-directed perfusion and hemofiltration are essential for reducing AKI risk.

Additionally, avoiding nephrotoxic medications and utilizing adjunct therapies like antifibrinolytics, fenoldopam, and natriuretic peptides further protect renal function during surgery. Figure 30.7 provides a comprehensive overview of the complex pathophysiology and contributing factors leading to AKI during cardiac surgery and the current strategies employed for renal protection during cardiac surgery.

Promising experimental interventions, such as nitric oxide, n-acetylcysteine, and dexmedetomidine, hold potential for future advancements in kidney preservation during cardiac surgery. Continued research and development in this area are vital to further refine and improve the prevention and management of CSA-AKI.

Further Reading

Brown JR, Baker RA, Shore-Lesserson L, et al. The Society of Thoracic Surgeons/Society of Cardiovascular Anesthesiologists/ American Society for Extracorporeal Technology Clinical Practice Guidelines for the Prevention of Adult Cardiac surgery-associated acute kidney injury. Anesth Analg. 2023;136(1):176–84.

Cheruku SR, Raphael J, Neyra JA, Fox AA. Acute kidney injury after cardiac surgery: prediction, prevention, and management. Anesthesiology. 2023;139:880–98.

Dasta JF, Kane-Gill SL, Durtschi AJ, Pathak DS, Kellum JA. Costs and outcomes of acute kidney injury (AKI) following cardiac surgery. Nephrol Dial Transplant. 2008;23:1970–4.

de la Hoz MA, et al. Intraoperative hypotension and acute kidney injury, stroke, and mortality during and outside cardiopulmonary bypass: a retrospective observational cohort study. Anesthesiology. 2022;136:927–39.

Fujii Y. Evaluation of inflammation caused by cardiopulmonary bypass in a small animal model. Biology. 2020;9(4):81.

Kidney Disease: Improving Global Outcomes (KDIGO) Acute Kidney Injury Work Group. KDIGO clinical practice guideline for acute kidney injury. Kidney Int Suppl. 2012;2:1–138.

Meersch M, et al. Prevention of cardiac surgery-associated AKI by implementing the KDIGO guidelines in high risk patients identified by biomarkers: the PrevAKI randomized controlled trial. Intensive Care Med. 2017;43:1551–61.

Milne B, Gilbey T, Kunst G. Perioperative management of the patient at high-risk for cardiac surgery-associated acute kidney injury. J Cardiothorac Vasc Anesth. 2022;36(12):4460–82. https://doi.org/10.1053/j.jvca.2022.08.016. Epub 2022 Aug 28.

Ngu JMC, et al. Defining an intraoperative hypotension threshold in association with de novo renal replacement therapy after cardiac surgery. Anesthesiology. 2020;132:1447–57.

Palmer BF. Disturbances in renal autoregulation and the susceptibility to hypertension-induced chronic kidney disease. Am J Med Sci. 2004;328(6):330–43.

Peng K, McIlroy DR, Bollen BA, Billings FT, Zarbock A, Popescu WM, Fox AA, Shore-Lesserson L, Zhou S, Geube MA, Ji F, Bhatia M, Schwann NM, Shaw AD, Liu H. Society of Cardiovascular Anesthesiologists Clinical Practice Update for Management of Acute Kidney Injury Associated with Cardiac Surgery. Anesth Analg. 2022;135(4):744–56.

Rasmussen SB, Boyko Y, Ranucci M, de Somer F, Ravn HB. Cardiac surgery-associated acute kidney injury – a narrative review. Perfusion. 2024;39(8):1516–30. https://doi.org/10.1177/02676591231211503.

Taylor KM, Morton IJ, Brown JJ, Bain WH, Caves PK. Hypertension and the renin-angiotensin system following open-heart surgery. J Thorac Cardiovasc Surg. 1977;74(6):840–5.

Vives M. Cardiac surgery-associated acute kidney injury. In: Vives M, Hernandez A, editors. Cardiac anesthesia and post-operative care in the 21st century. Cham: Springer; 2022.

Wang Y, Bellomo R. Cardiac surgery-associated acute kidney injury: risk factors, pathophysiology and treatment. Nat Rev Nephrol. 2017;13:697–711.

Zou C, et al. Advances in the study of subclinical AKI biomarkers. Front Physiol. 2022;13:960059.

Part IX

Safety During Cardiopulmonary Bypass

Safeguards and Checklists During Cardiac Surgery

31

David C. Wang, Joe Catricala, and Michael G. Fitzsimons

Introduction

Cardiac surgery is one of the most complex medical undertakings a team of medical providers will navigate. It involves multiple highly skilled care providers, procedural interventions, physiologic transitions, and exposure to many different medications via variable systems for administration leading to a scenario where the risk for error is high. The American Society of Anesthesiologists (ASA) Closed Claims study revealed in 1994 that 3% of cases reported were for injuries associated with cardiac surgery. Equipment malfunction or misuse was responsible for 37% of events compared with only 9% for noncardiac claims.

Cardiac surgery consists of a series of critical procedures, each of which, if improperly performed and not identified early or managed immediately, can lead to immediate or long-term consequences. The evolution of cardiac surgery and cardiopulmonary bypass (CPB) has included multiple innovations to improve patient safety. Technological advancements have included incorporating safety devices into the CPB machine, which prevent system failures or facilitate early identification of potential issues. System innovations that have improved safety include structured team interactions. These occur at established points in the operative and perioperative period, facilitating open exchange of system or patient-specific information among multiple team members. We will explore some of these safeguards and checklists below.

Dr. Wang died prior publication of this work. The chapter is dedicated to his memory.

D. C. Wang (Deceased) · M. G. Fitzsimons (✉)
Department of Anesthesia, Critical Care, and Pain Medicine, Massachusetts General Hospital, Boston, MA, USA
e-mail: DWANG@mgh.harvard.edu; MFITZSIMONS@mgh.harvard.edu

J. Catricala
Cardiac Surgery, Department of Surgery, Massachusetts General Hospital, Boston, MA, USA
e-mail: jcatricala@mgh.org

Key Alarms and Safety Devices on the CPB Machine

Perfusionists, as the primary line of defense in CPB procedures, heavily rely on a variety of safety and monitoring devices within the CPB system. A safety device is a component within the CPB system that protects against inadvertent acts (such as power failure) or provider-associated errors. In contrast, a monitoring device within the CPB system continuously tracks and reports key operational parameters like blood flow rates, pressure, temperature, and oxygen levels, ensuring the CPB system operates within safe and effective thresholds for patient care during surgery. These devices are detailed in Chap. 13. From the first use of the CPB in the early 1950s until today, perfusion circuits have incorporated intelligent multilevel safety devices and complex feedback loops. Safety devices may include system additions that are capable of acting, while monitoring devices can aid in quickly identifying a problem. It is crucial that perfusionists understand the common safeguards in CPB. While alarms play a vital role in alerting the perfusionist to potential problems, their effectiveness hinges on the attentiveness and actions of the operator. Safety devices can be divided into invasive or non-invasive, which refers to whether the component is part of the disposable machinery or reusable.

Invasive

Invasive safety devices are disposable components that contact the patient's blood. These may include:

One-Way Valves One-way valves prevent unintended reversal (retrograde) of blood flow by only permitting the flow of fluids in one direction (see Fig. 31.1). One-way valves may be incorporated into the construction of the circuit or added afterwards to improve safety. Examples include a one-way valve in a shunt line from the arterial-line filter to the venous reservoir. According to the American Society of ExtraCorporeal

A. S. Awad, J. DiNardo (eds.), *Clinical Perfusion for Cardiac Surgery*, https://doi.org/10.1007/978-3-031-91163-7_31

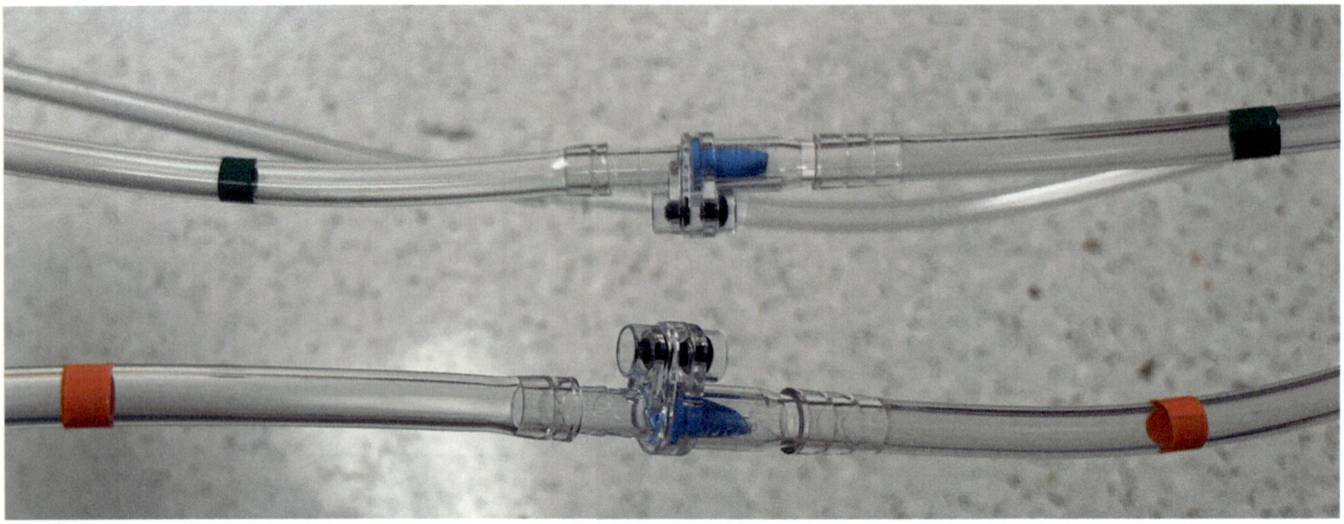

Fig. 31.1 This image depicts examples of one-way valves in CPB circuits. These valves are specifically designed to prevent the unintended reversal of blood flow by allowing fluid to flow in only one direction. They can be either integrated into the circuit's construction or added later to enhance safety measures

Technology (AmSECT) Standard 6.6, the use of a one-way valve in the vent line is mandatory during CPB procedures. One-way valves may also be incorporated into a cardiotomy suction line that will be used for intracardiac vents to prevent air from being pumped into the vascular system if a roller head malfunctions or the tubing is loaded into the pump incorrectly.

Bubble Traps and Filters Filters and bubble traps are devices within the CPB circuit that facilitate trapping of microemboli, air, or other debris. There are two primary types of microfilters. Depth filters, now considered obsolete and traditionally made of Dacron wool, work by creating a path among fibers to mechanically trap particles. In contrast, screen filters, which are currently the standard type, are typically made from woven polyester mesh or nylon thread. Their pore size ranges from 20 to 40 μm. The primary sites for microfilter placement in the CPB circuit are carefully selected based on the flow of blood and the potential sources of contaminants. Here are the different types of filters that are integrated in the CPB circuit:

1. Arterial-Line Filter: One key location is downstream from the oxygenator unit, the arterial-line filter, just before the blood enters the systemic circulation. The new-generation screen arterial-line filters are incorporated directly into membrane oxygenators (see Fig. 31.2), eliminating the need for a separate external arterial-line filter and thus reducing the required priming volume. In accordance with AmSECT Standard 6.5, the use of an arterial-line filter, whether external or integrated, is required during CPB procedures.
2. Venous Reservoirs Filter: A screen micropore filter is integrated in the hard-shell venous reservoir.

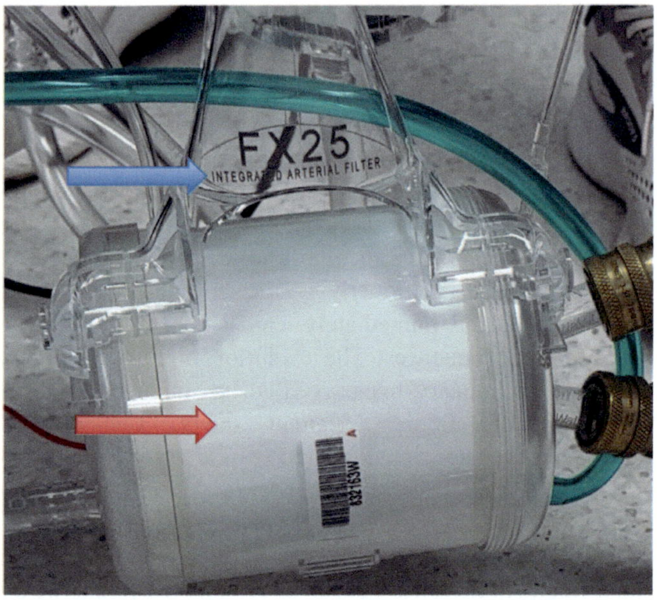

Fig. 31.2 This image shows an example of the new-generation screen arterial-line filter, which is directly incorporated into a membrane oxygenator (indicated by the red arrow). The blue arrow points to the labeling that indicates an integrated arterial filter

3. Cardiotomy Reservoirs Filter: Currently, the majority of commercial cardiotomy reservoirs come equipped with integrated screen micropore filters. In the latest generation of these reservoirs, they are typically integrated into the venous reservoir, positioned above and behind it, and each is equipped with its own screen micropore filter coated with a defoaming chemical agent (see Fig. 31.3). This defoamer works by altering the surface tension of bubbles, effectively causing them to dissipate and thereby eliminating foam.

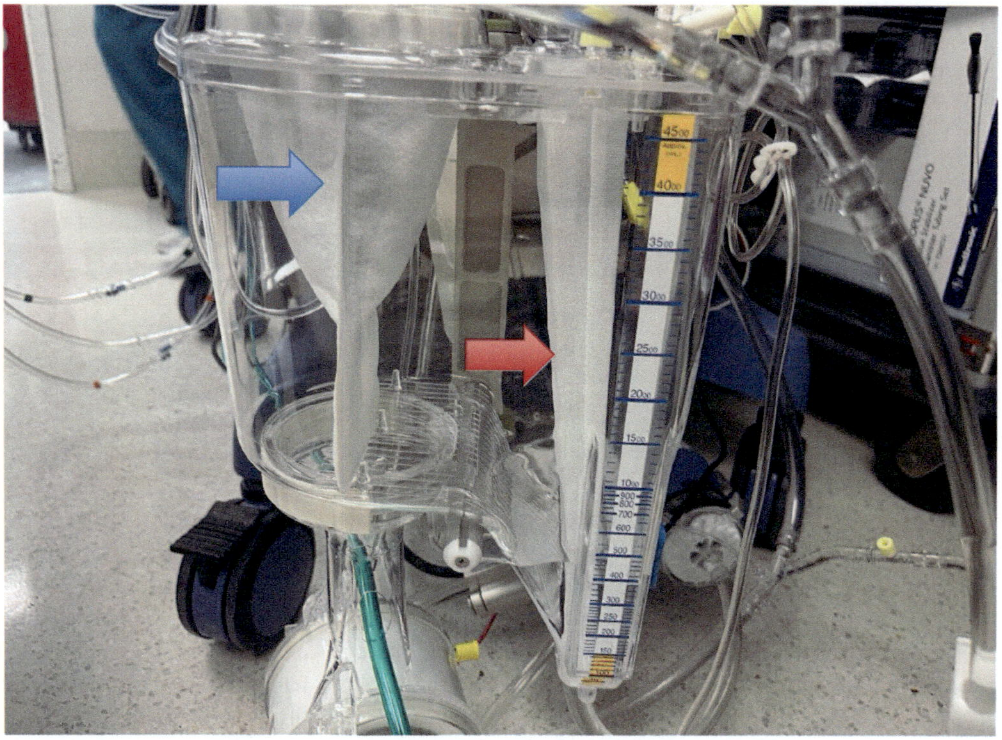

Fig. 31.3 This image depicts a cardiotomy reservoir integrated into the venous reservoir, positioned above and behind it. Each reservoir is equipped with its own screen micropore filter (blue arrow pointing to the cardiotomy reservoir filter, and red arrow pointing to the venous reservoir filter), each coated with a defoaming chemical agent

A shunt line can be added to a filter to increase the effectiveness of the filter by directing blood to repeat circulation through the filter. Bubble traps are able to contain a small volume of air, allowing the perfusionist time to react and manage a potential crisis. Bubble traps are typically found in cardioplegia delivery systems but may also be integrated into arterial-line filters.

Other filters can be integrated with CPB to provide specific functions such as:

1. Priming Filter: Throughout the de-airing and priming process of the CPB circuit, a 0.2 μm filter is utilized to remove unintended particulate matter and any potential microbial contaminants (see Fig. 31.4). These filters must be removed initiating cardiopulmonary bypass due to the pore size being smaller than the size of a red blood cell.
2. Gas Flow Line Filter: Placed in the gas line that is connected to the oxygenator, this filter helps remove bacteria found in the gas stream, thus reducing the risk of contamination between the patient and the CPB machine (see Fig. 31.5).
3. Blood Transfusion Filter: In cases where allogeneic blood transfusion is needed, a blood filter is employed to eliminate blood clots and other debris formed in stored blood, thus preventing embolization.
4. Leukocyte Depletion Filters: Given the significant role of neutrophils in the damage caused by the inflammatory response, leukocyte-depleting filters can be used to attenuate the systemic inflammatory response. These filters

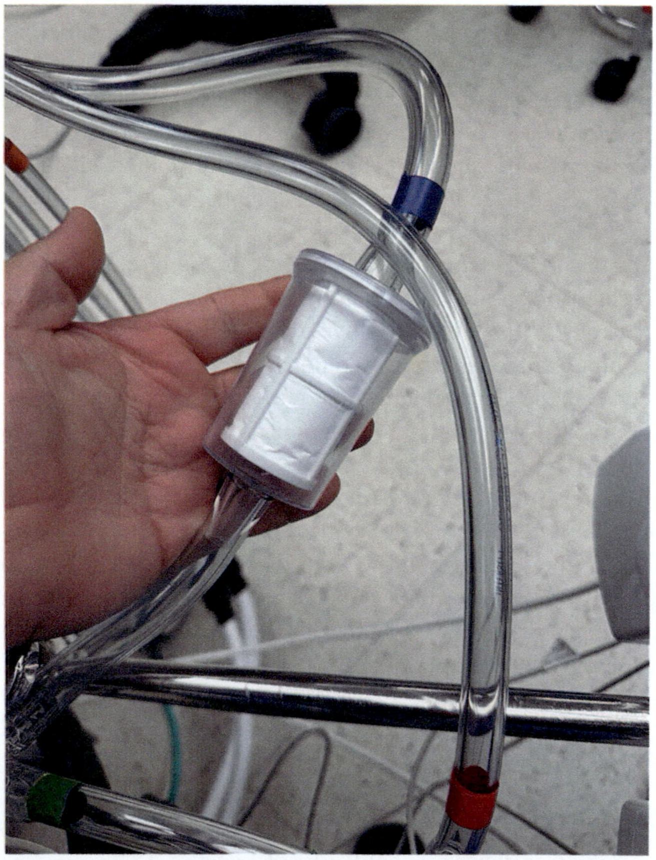

Fig. 31.4 This image displays a priming prebypass filter

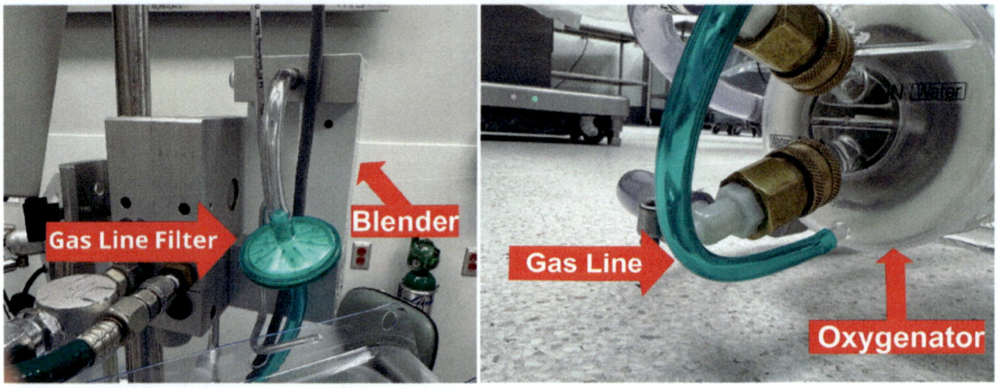

Fig. 31.5 Left image: Gas line emerging from the blender, featuring a gas flow filter connected to the line. Right image: Gas line as it connects to the oxygenator

effectively reduce the number of activated leukocytes in the systemic circulation during CPB. In lung transplant cases, modifications to the circuit are necessary to accommodate these filters.

Centrifugal Pump Heads Centrifugal pump heads, being preload dependent and after-load sensitive, are unable to move blood if a critical volume of air enters the pump head. Additionally, centrifugal pumps are limited in the amount of flow that can be generated if elevated vascular resistance is encountered.

Collapsible-Bag Venous Reservoir Collapsible-bag venous reservoirs collect blood without the degree of air–blood interface found in a hard-shell reservoir. This design may reduce air entry into the CPB system. The heparin level of the patient can be reduced due to the limited air-blood interface, thus reducing bleeding complications.

Reservoir Pressure Relief Valve A pressure relief valve is located on the top of a hard-shell venous reservoir and is activated by excessive positive or negative pressure that may build up in the reservoir. Additionally, a pressure relief valve can be added to the guide path of the perfusion circuit, these are typically found in the cardioplegia circuit.

Temperature Out of Range Monitoring of the Arterial Outflow Per AmSECT Standard 6.4, temperature monitoring of the arterial outflow from the oxygenator is required during CPB procedures. The temperature sensor must be equipped with both audible and visual alarms to prevent excessively high arterial outlet temperatures.

Non-invasive

Non-invasive devices, in comparison to invasive devices, do not contact the patient's blood and are reused from case to case. Non-invasive safety devices include:

Bubble Detector

Neurological complications in CPB procedures, a significant cause of morbidity, often arise from microemboli, which can be air or particulate matter such as clots, calcium, or fat emboli. Air emboli may enter the system through membrane oxygenators or leaks, while particulate material can originate from blood products, calcium fractures, existing thrombi, or lipid breakdown. Importantly, the embolic load has the potential to rise substantially with every extra hour of CPB run.

Air can enter the CPB system from various sources, each posing a risk that must be vigilantly managed for patient safety. Common entry points include cannula insertion and removal, especially if not meticulously de-aired or securely lodged, present obvious entry points. Loose connections or inadequate seals tubing junctions, filters, and even within the oxygenator itself (due to improper priming or membrane defects) can become dangerous entry points. In the venous reservoir, low blood levels or leaks can lead to air entry. Cardiotomy suction, used to remove blood and debris from the surgical field, can entrain air into the system. Additionally, air can be inadvertently introduced during the infusion of fluids or medications if the containers or syringes contain air. The patient's own venous system, especially in cases of open veins or surgical incisions, is another source. To mitigate the risk of air embolism, perfusionists employ a combination of de-airing techniques, precise placement and sealing of arterial and venous cannulae, and careful monitoring. The use of devices such as bubble detectors, de-airing filters, and filtration systems is critical in detecting and removing air and microemboli. Ensuring proper setup and a prompt response to any air detected in the system are essential steps in maintaining patient safety during procedures. According to the AmSECT Standard 6.2, employing a bubble detector is required during CPB procedures. This device, commonly known as a gross/macro bubble detector, plays a crucial role in potentially interrupting arterial blood flow when necessary. To maximize efficacy and safety, the detector is equipped with both audible and visual alarms. Smaller bubbles are indicated as microbubble activity, prompting the perfusionist to investigate and mitigate their cause. Larger bubbles trigger immediate cessation of the arterial pump, necessitating prompt removal of the bubble before resuming bypass. The bubble detector alarms when air is detected at certain points in the CPB system. Currently, bubble detectors are categorized into two types: capacitive and piezoelectric ultrasonic transducers. Capacitive bubble detectors operate on the principle of capacitance change, where electrodes forming a capacitor detect changes in the dielectric constant caused by a bubble passing between them. Piezoelectric ultrasonic transducers, on the other hand, use high-frequency sound waves that reflect off bubbles to signal their presence. These transducers are highly sensitive, particularly to small bubbles. For optimal performance, piezoelectric ultrasonic transducers typically require gel application and may be sensitive to external noise. The optimal placement of these detectors is a subject of debate. The most common sites for bubble detectors are illustrated in (see Fig. 31.6).

Level Detector

This alarm system safeguards against air embolism, a potentially life-threatening complication in CPB. It employs an electronic probe, which is located on the hard-shell venous reservoir and is wired to connect with the CPB machine's control system. The level detector is affixed to the reservoir at a specific minimum level and triggered by depletion of venous blood in the reservoir below that level (150–200 mL) (Fig. 31.7). According to AmSECT Standard 6.3, CPB machines employing hard-shell reservoirs must utilize a level sensor for precise arterial blood flow regulation. It possesses the capability to interrupt arterial blood flow if necessary. To ensure maximum efficacy and safety, the level sensor is equipped with both audible and visual alarms. These alarms must be positioned in accordance with the manufacturer's guidelines to guarantee optimal performance and adherence to safety protocols. The majority of current detectors rely on the capacitance principle, detecting the presence of fluid through the reservoir's plastic. When the fluid level reaches the preset limit, the CPB machine sounds an alarm, alerting the clinical perfusionist to a possible problem and causing the arterial pump to slow down. At this point, the clinical perfusionist should investigate the cause of the drop in the reser-

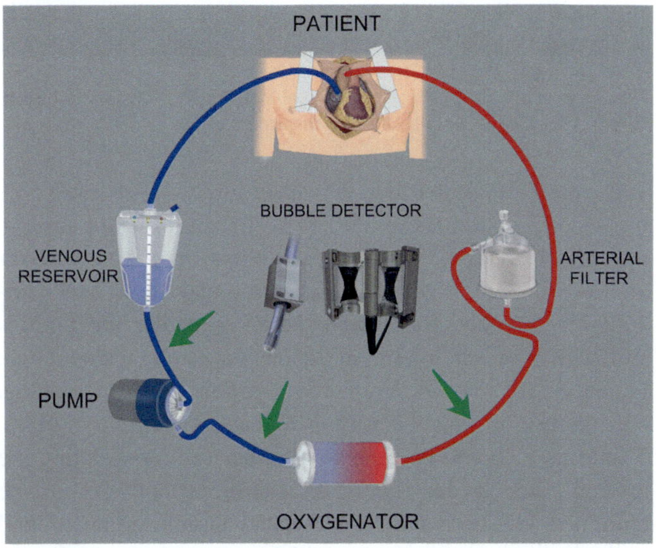

Fig. 31.6 This illustration presents a simplified drawing of a CPB circuit, highlighting the bubble detector device. On the left, the device is shown engaged with the circuit tubing, while on the right, it appears in the open position without the tubing. The most common sites for bubble detector insertions are indicated by the green arrows

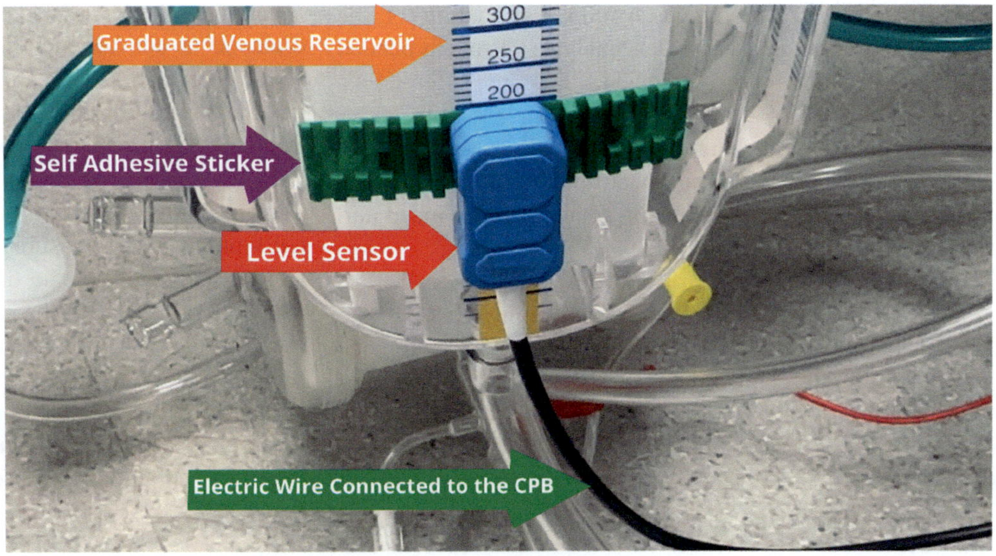

Fig. 31.7 This image: hard-shell venous reservoir, graduated for blood volume measurement (orange arrow), featuring a self-adhesive sticker (purple arrow) and a blue level detector device indicated by a red arrow. A black electric wire, highlighted by a green arrow, connects the level detector device to the CPB control panel

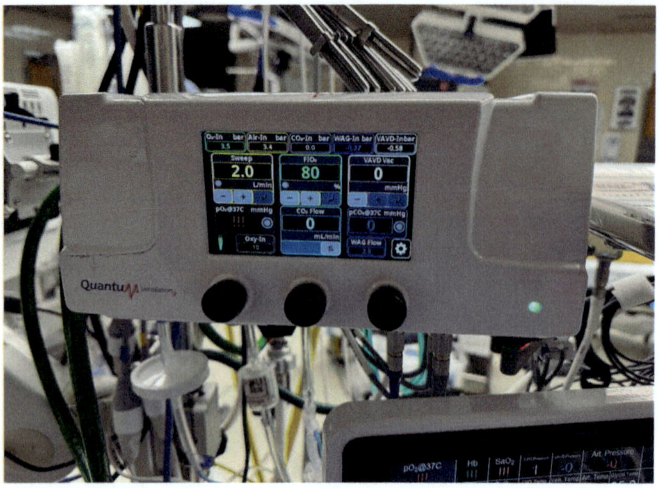

Fig. 31.8 This image shows an O2 analyzer, a device designed to measure the fractional concentration of inspired oxygen

voir's blood level and address it accordingly. If the reservoir's blood level continues to fall below the set limit, the arterial pump will stop to prevent complete emptying of the reservoir and air from entering the arterial pump and the patient's circulation. Notably, the audible alarm signaling the pump's stoppage differs in tone from the one indicating a slowdown. However, for soft-shell reservoirs, per AmSECT Guideline 6.2, the use of a level sensor is advised in CPB procedures. This sensor should be capable of either servo-regulating the arterial pump or interrupting arterial blood flow. It must be equipped with both audible and visual alarms and positioned as per the manufacturer's guidelines to ensure a timely response and maintain a safe operational volume. Additionally, an air bubble detector placed distal to the outlet of the reservoir can serve as an alternative level detector.

O_2 Analyzer The O2 analyzer measures fractional inspired oxygen concentration (FiO_2) emerging from the blender to the artificial lung. According to AmSECT Guideline 6.1, the use of a ventilating gas oxygen analyzer is recommended during CPB procedures (see Fig. 31.8).

Anesthetic Gas Scavenge Line According to AmSECT Standard 6.8, CPB machines must utilize an anesthetic gas scavenge line whenever inhalation agents are introduced into the circuit during CPB procedures.

Electrical Remote-Controlled Tubing Clamp (ERC) The ERC is a crucial safety device in the CPB circuit, automatically and rapidly clamps the arterial-line tubing under specific conditions (such as low blood level, bubble detection, or retrograde flow). This immediate response minimizes the risk of air embolism (Fig. 31.9).

Roller Pump Lid Opening of the transparent roller pump lid results in the pump immediately ceasing to flow.

Power Loss Alarm The Power Loss Alarm will sound if the electrical power supply ceases and back-up battery power is activated. Per AmSECT Standard 6.11, the CPB machine must be equipped with a backup power source to ensure an uninterrupted power supply throughout CPB procedures.

Hand Cranks Per AmSECT Standard 6.9, Hand cranks must be easily accessible and available for use during CPB procedures. The manual hand crank allows an individual to generate blood flow via a roller or centrifugal pump. Hand cranking for roller pumps is usually a one-to-one crank to Revolutions Per Minute (RPM) ratio. The hand crank for centrifugal pump heads is typically geared to provide a mechanical advantage due to the high levels of RPMs needed (typically 2500–4000 RPM).

Hand Crank Alarm The manual hand crank alarm sounds when the pump is cranked in the wrong direction. Hand cranks for centrifugal pump heads typically have a mechanical limit or will not operate when cranked in the wrong direction.

In-Line Pressure Monitoring and Pressure Regulation In-line pressure monitors are in direct contact with the machinery, so they are considered invasive, while pressure control is not. These monitoring safety devices allow continuous pressure sampling. Pressure regulators are computer-controlled controls that the bypass pump can monitor pressure and limit and/or stop RPMs based on high-pressure limits that are set by users. There is also typically a pressure monitor on a hard-shell venous reservoir to ensure that there is little to no positive pressure buildup and that the negative pressure applied during vacuum-assisted venous drainage is not beyond the manufacturer's recommended level. There can also be a pressure line with both minimum and maximum limits on the cardioplegia circuit. These help to protect the circuit from pulling air from the solution and from exceeding the manufacturer's recommendation for pressure limits. According to AmSECT Standard 6.1, during CPB procedures, pressure monitoring is essential for the arterial line, cardioplegia delivery systems, and the venous reservoir, particularly when augmented venous drainage is in use. The pressure monitor used should be capable of either servo regulation to manage the arterial/cardioplegia pump or to facilitate the interruption of arterial/cardioplegia flow. Additionally, this monitor must be equipped with both audible and visual alarms for effective alerting.

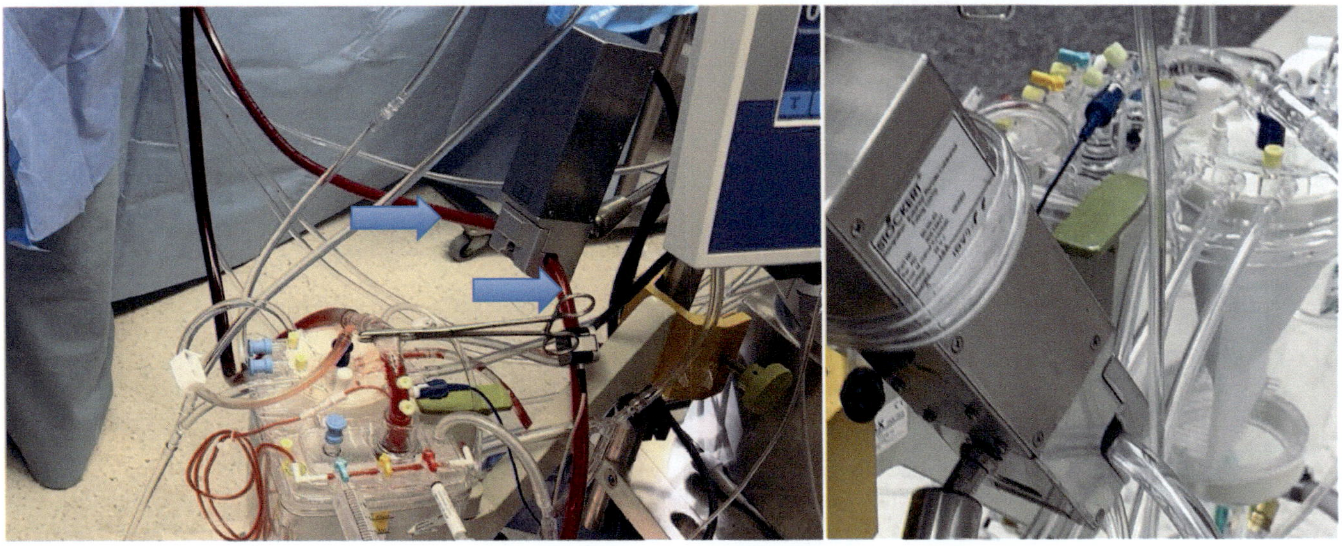

Fig. 31.9 These two photos showcase the ERC device. The left image, indicated by two blue arrows, shows the position of the ERC in the arterial line during a CPB run, both before and after the ERC's location. The right image provides a zoomed-in view of the device itself

Back-Up Gas Supply As stipulated by AmSECT Standard 6.10, a back-up gas supply must be accessible and ready for use during CPB procedures.

Additional Flow Probes Adding additional flow tubing may result in the need for other flow probes to allow assessment of individual flows.

Physiological Parameter Alarms With newer perfusion technology, most physiological parameters can be associated with alarms to warn the user when they deviate from the user-set physiological norm.

Critical Team Interactions

The care of the cardiac surgery patient is a dynamic and fluid interaction between various medical professionals, including operating room (OR) nursing personnel, intensive care unit team members, cardiac surgeons, anesthesia providers, OR technicians, and perfusion staff. Cardiac surgery cannot proceed if any team member is absent, and each role may have crucial information that may affect the efficiency, safety, or outcome of the procedure. Communication interaction at predetermined periods reduces the risk of communication failures. The primary types of critical team interactions in surgery are divided into briefings, debriefings, huddles, time-outs, and handoffs (Table 31.1). These interactions are often accompanied by the use of formal written checklists to ensure that no important components are omitted. Additional critical team interactions may also include inter-procedure "stops" which will also be discussed below.

Team Huddle

A huddle often refers to a team meeting less focused on specific details of an individual case but on service specifics. Huddles involve a meeting among representatives from each team (surgery, nursing, perfusion, anesthesia, critical care). This may take place at the beginning of a shift, at regular intervals throughout the day, or as needed in response to changing circumstances. The goal of a huddle is to ensure that team representatives are aware of the planned cases and durations, anticipated changes or updates since scheduling or the last huddle, availability of ICU beds, and personnel issues. Huddles promote shared understanding of service goals and limitations and help identify potential problems before they become more significant. A team huddle promotes a culture of teamwork and collaboration by providing an opportunity for all representative team members to contribute to the discussion and share their perspectives.

Table 31.1 Critical team interactions, explained further below

Critical team interaction	Timing	General intention
Team huddle	Prior to beginning procedural day or later	Service planning, replanning, information exchange, safety information
Pre-procedure briefing	Prior to induction of anesthesia	Case-specific planning and preparation, team member introduction, individual team member input
Time-out	After surgical preparation and prior to incision, or at an unplanned change in surgical direction requiring a different team	Final confirmation of correct patient, procedure, laterality, and other issues
Post-procedure debriefing	After completion of surgery	Learning, improvement, quality assurance, exchange of identified safety issues
Handoff	During any transition of care (i.e. provider change, transfer to intensive care unit (ICU)).	Ensuring safe continuity of care, exchange of information critical to further management (medications, lab values, recent study results, upcoming interventions)
Inter-procedure time-out	After a set period of time (i.e., 4 h), at a change in procedure, addition of another team, or when a critical event occurs that alters the planned course of the procedure	Refocus

Pre-procedure Briefings

Briefings are discussions held prior to a single patient's surgical procedure that involve all members of the assigned OR team. The purpose is to confirm and define the procedure to be performed, including changes in the procedure that may have arisen since initial scheduling. All members of the team are introduced by name and role. Surgical team members can clarify equipment and other needs. Perfusion team members outline the extracorporeal support strategy needed including cannulation, myocardial protection, and target parameters for blood pressure and flows. The anesthesiology team defines monitoring, airway management, and other concerns such as antifibrinolytics or weaning strategy. Separate measures such as blood management strategy or adherence to quality measures may be defined for the team. The process and content of briefing often differs between institutions, and one should consider referencing internal guidelines and protocols, specifically for unusual circumstances.

Strict hierarchies in the cardiac surgery theater may inhibit trainees and support staff from raising concerns or questioning procedural plans. Several surveys have indicated that among OR personnel, a large percentage has trouble speaking up, even if they believe patient safety may be compromised. Briefings improve the teamwork climate and are associated with greater team satisfaction. All members of the team assume equal hierarchy in terms of raising concerns and identifying vulnerabilities during a briefing because the briefing provides a safe environment for sharing needs and expectations. Briefings often employ checklists to guarantee that all aspects and phases of the procedure are addressed prior to the induction of anesthesia. By clarifying these points immediately prior to the procedure, preoperative briefings can reduce unexpected delays in surgical procedures by identifying missing equipment or personnel.

Time-Out

In 2003, The Joint Commission implemented a practice known as a "time-out" as part of the Universal Protocol for Preventing Wrong Site, Wrong Procedure, and Wrong Person Surgery. The Joint Commission defines a time-out as an immediate pause prior to incision by the entire surgical team to ensure accuracy in patient identification, procedure confirmation, and surgical site verification. This protocol applies to all accredited hospitals, ambulatory care centers, and office-based surgery facilities.

As per the protocol requirements, healthcare organizations are obligated to conduct a time-out prior to commencing any surgical procedure. During this designated time, the entire OR team gathers to review essential information, including the patient's identity, the planned procedure, and the specific surgical site. This serves as an opportunity for team members to voice any concerns regarding patient safety or the procedure at hand.

Table 31.2 AmSECT's patient handoff tool for perfusionist

I pass the clamp off		
I	Isolation precautions	Contact, droplet, airborne
P	Patient name/procedure	Surgical approach, cannulation, back-up plan
A	Age/allergies	Medications, adverse reactions, and associated risks
S	Stage of the procedure	Preoperative, perioperative, postoperative, surgical status
S	Status of temperature	Target temperatures, current temperatures, rewarming rate
T	Transfusion	Blood type, targets, product use, availability
H	History	Symptoms, risk factors, diagnosis, prior procedures, preoperative medications
E	Equipment condition	Mechanical concerns or issues
C	Circuit	Oxygenator, tubing size and coating, cardioplegia, shunts, hemoconcentrator, accessories
L	Lab values and targets	Hematocrit, blood gasses, electrolytes, enzymes, targets
A	Anticoagulation	Status, targets, heparin use, alternative anticoagulants, blood components
M	Medications	Vasoconstrictors, vasodilators, cardioplegia, electrolytes, antiarrhythmics, colloids
P	Pump settings	FiO2, sweep, blood flow, vacuum, RPMs, timers, shunts
O	Other conditions or concerns	Jehovah's witness, sickle cell anemia, pregnancy, sepsis, DIC
F	Fluid status	I/Os, crystalloid use, ultrafiltrate amount and rate, urine
F	Final thoughts	

Adapted from https://www.amsect.org/Portals/0/AmSECT%20Documents/I%20PASS%20THE%20CLAMP%20OFF%20(1).pdf

Post-procedure Debriefings

Debriefings are critical team interactions that occur upon completion of a surgical procedure and prior to departure from the room. Debriefings provide an opportunity for the OR team to reflect on the procedure and discuss lessons learned or safety factors identified. Debriefings differ in terms of timing, content, and purpose. The postoperative debriefing is used to ensure that all necessary steps were completed, to identify underappreciated hazards, to reflect upon mistakes or near-misses, and to suggest improvements moving forward. Identification of errors and near-misses during a debriefing is useful to implement changes to reduce risk, assuming that critical points identified are funneled to the quality assurance/quality improvement system. Debriefings may also include discussions of the plan for transition from the OR to the ICU.

Handoffs

Handoffs are critical team interactions that are performed when any transition of patient care occurs. Handoffs ensure that critical information is formally passed between care providers or teams. Such transitions of care can occur at multiple stages in the perioperative process, including handoff to another perfusionist in the OR and eventual patient transport with monitoring to a separate physical location such as the post-anesthesia care unit (PACU) or ICU. Formal standardized handoff protocols for both verbal and written communication are used during the transfer of patient care from one individual or team to another. It has been repeatedly demonstrated over multiple studies that a structured interdisciplinary handover from the OR to the ICU after cardiac surgery results in less adverse events and is associated with improved provider satisfaction, increased compliance with process measures such as efficiency in transfer of equipment, and successful transfer of critical information compared with unstructured handoffs. The AmSECT has established a handoff tool based on a mnemonic, "I PASS THE CLAMP OFF" (Table 31.2).

Interprocedure Time-out

An interprocedure time-out is a critical team interaction that occurs when a significant event occurs or when the complexity of the procedure unexpectedly changes. Events may include vascular injury or abdominal compartment syndrome, requiring an additional team to assist with management. Some institutions mandate an intra-procedure stop at a certain case duration. Components of a stop may include defining how the procedure has changed, ensuring the availability of blood components, or a discussion of the impact of the event on subsequent scheduled procedures.

Checklists

Checklists are standardized lists of specific information or tasks to be completed or addressed to ensure that steps are not missed. The aviation industry was the first industry to widely adopt and use checklists, which were first developed in the 1930s by psychologists and pilots, after a preventable sequence of events caused a B17 bomber aircraft to crash. The development of checklists was further driven by the human factors movement, which emerged in 1979 after the largest air disaster in United States history, claiming the lives of 273 people. These checklists were designed to help highly trained pilots perform safety-critical tasks consistently, even under operational stress.

Routine use of a printed algorithmic approach to clinical medicine situations eliminates potential human error associated with reliance upon recall while improving focus on the task. The concept of using checklists takes into account neurophysiological knowledge that suggests that during periods of excessive acute stress, hypoperfusion of specific areas of the brain can result in increased amygdala and brain stem survival activity. This can negatively impact the memory and decision-making abilities of even highly trained individuals in their field of expertise. In simpler terms, experts may experience reduced cognitive ability during periods of high stress.

Checklists are successfully incorporated into clinical medicine when several practices are followed: (1) The checklist is an expected component of care and provides valuable information, (2) the checklist is printed and visible, (3) the information is understandable. Checklists are common during pre-procedure briefings, procedural time-outs, post-procedural debriefings, and handoffs. In the context of CPB, checklists can be used prior to critical phases such as initiation or weaning to ensure the proper steps are followed. The WHO Surgical Safety Checklist is a notable example of this, with systematic reviews and meta-analyses demonstrating significant reductions in mortality, morbidity, surgical site infections, pneumonia, unplanned return to the OR, urinary tract infections, blood loss requiring transfusion, unplanned intubation, and sepsis with its routine use.

Checklists in CPB

As previously mentioned, checklists play a crucial role in multiple stages of CPB procedures, including pump preparation before bypass, initiation and weaning from bypass, and during practices that are not a routine part of all procedures involving cardiopulmonary bypass, such as the implementation of deep hypothermic circulatory arrest (DHCA). Although these checklists are brief, they are essential. The perfusionist, who is responsible for operating the heart–lung machine during the procedure, must ensure that all team members are aware of the critical event, acknowledge the checklist components, and agree to follow them. An example of checklists is shown here in Fig. 31.10.

Emergency Manuals

Emergency checklists can also be activated during critical events like cardiopulmonary arrest. These checklists are often accessible through an emergency manual that can be accessed quickly in moments of crisis. Research has demonstrated the effectiveness of checklists during crises, as the use of emergency manuals can lead to a decrease in missed critical steps. Simulation training can be important in this context because it provides a safe and controlled environment for healthcare professionals to practice and develop their skills without putting real patients at risk. Simulation training may use computer-based virtual reality scenarios or simulated clinical environments to replicate medical procedures, emergencies, or complex clinical situations. This has been shown to improve patient safety and reduce medical errors.

COOPER UNIVERSITY HOSPITAL
PERFUSION PRE/POST BYPASS CHECKLIST

PATIENT
- ☐ Procedure verified
- ☐ Chart reviewed

STERILITY
- ☐ Components checked for package integrity/ expiration dates

LIVANOVA HEART LUNG MACHINE: UNIT S5
- ☐ Speed controls/ pumps operational
- ☐ Occlusions set
- ☐ Flow sensor in correct direction and calibrated
- ☐ Holders secure

ELECTRICAL
- ☐ All power cords secure
- ☐ ACT controls complete

GAS SUPPLY
- ☐ Gas lines secure
- ☐ Blender flow meter operational
- ☐ Hose leak free
- ☐ Gas exhaust unobstructed
- ☐ Vacuum operational

LINES/ PUMP TUBING
- ☐ Connections secure
- ☐ Tubing direction traced and correct
- ☐ No kinks
- ☐ Circuit debubbled/ leak free

CARDIOPLEGIA
- ☐ Patent arterial line
- ☐ Retrograde pressure alarm set
- ☐ System debubbled
- ☐ Temperature probes connected
- ☐ Water lines attached and leak free

SAFTEY MECHANISM-MONITORS
- ☐ Level sensor positioned correctly
- ☐ Bubble sensor positioned correctly
- ☐ Cardiotomy reservoir vented
- ☐ Pressure monitors calibrated

TEMPERATURE
- ☐ Heater/Cooler connected and operational
- ☐ Ice checked/available

SUPPLIES
- ☐ Tubing clamps Available (6)
- ☐ Drugs available
- ☐ Blood available
- ☐ Syringes available (3, 10, 30, 60cc)
- ☐ 18 gauge needles available
- ☐ Pacemaker
- ☐ Spare O2 tank

BACK-UP
- ☐ Hand Crank
- ☐ Duplicate circuit assembled

TAVR
- ☐ A/V, central cannulas (patient size determined)
- ☐ A/V femoral cannulas (patient size determined)
- ☐ PIC-A kit and or Medtronic dilator kit
- ☐ Pump sucker
- ☐ 3/8 tubing, 3/8 x ½ connector

COMMENTS: ______________________________
____
____

Pre bypass Signature:______________________________

Date:__________________ Time:__________________

POST CPB CLEANING CHECKLIST:
- ☐ wipe down heart lung machine (Purple Wipes)
- ☐ wipe down heater cooler machine (purple wipes)
- ☐ wipe down perfusion cart in room (purple wipes)
- ☐ wipe down the Hemochron machine (purple
- ☐ wipes) wipe down the 6 clamps w/purple wipes and return to Instrument tray before sending to sterile processing
- ☐ LivaNova Cell Saver: Unit # ______
- ☐ wipe down cell saver machine (purple wipes)

Signature:______________________________

Date:__________________ Time:__________________

Fig. 31.10 Example of a perfusion checklist: pre and post bypass—this checklist outlines the essential steps and considerations for perfusionists before initiating bypass and after bypass

Closed-Loop Communication

Critical information is continually verbalized in the cardiac OR to ensure that all team members are aware of important details. Communication breakdowns are a significant contributor to adverse events during cardiac procedures. Such breakdowns can occur when messages are not clearly enunciated, when the intended audience is not reached, or when critical information is omitted. Closed-loop communication is a two-way exchange of information where a message is transmitted and the receiver verbally confirms that they have heard and understand the information. This approach is especially important in critical situations where errors can have a devastating impact, or when the action results in a significant change in the sequence, such as the administration of heparin or protamine, aortic cannulation, or adjustments in cardiopulmonary bypass flow rates.

Here is an example of closed-loop communication during a delicate time, preparing for CPB initiation that may occur in the OR:

Surgeon: "Okay, we're ready to start cannulation of the aorta. Anesthesiologist, please lower the patient's blood pressure."

Anesthesiologist: "Ok, I raised the head of the bed and gave some Nitroglycerine. Systolic Blood pressure is now at 90 mmHg."

Surgeon: "Great. Now I am placing the venous cannula. Anesthesiologist, I am mugging the heart, please drop the lungs and update me on the blood pressure."

Anesthesiologist: "Blood pressure is stable and no arrhythmia."

Surgeon: "Great. Perfusionist, are you ready to initiate the bypass?"

Anesthesiologist: "Perfusionist, what is the final activated clotting time (ACT)?"

Perfusionist: "ACT is 450, and we added an extra 10,000 units of heparin in the pump."

Surgeon: "If ACT is good, Perfusionist, are you ready to initiate the bypass?"

Perfusionist: "We finished RAP (Retrograde autologous priming) and ACT is good. Yes, we are ready to initiate bypass."

Surgeon: "Okay, please initiate bypass. Anesthesiologist, please turn the ventilator off?"

Anesthesiologist: "Perfusionist, are we full flow yet?"

Perfusionist: "Yes, we are now."

Anesthesiologist: "Thank you, Perfusionist. I've turned the ventilator off, surgeon."

Surgeon: "Thank you. Perfusionist, can you confirm that you're maintaining adequate flow and pressure?"

Perfusionist: "Yes, Flow is stable at 4 liters per minute, and arterial pressure is 70 mmHg."

Surgeon: "Great. Anesthesiologist, can you continue to monitor the patient's vital signs and please check the transesophageal echocardiography (TEE) for left ventricular distension (LV)?"

Anesthesiologist: "Absolutely, surgeon. There is no LV distension; the A line tracing is flat with no ejection, and the mean blood pressure is 70."

By maintaining this closed-loop communication, the surgical team can work together effectively to ensure the patient's safety and optimize the outcome of the procedure. See Fig. 31.11.

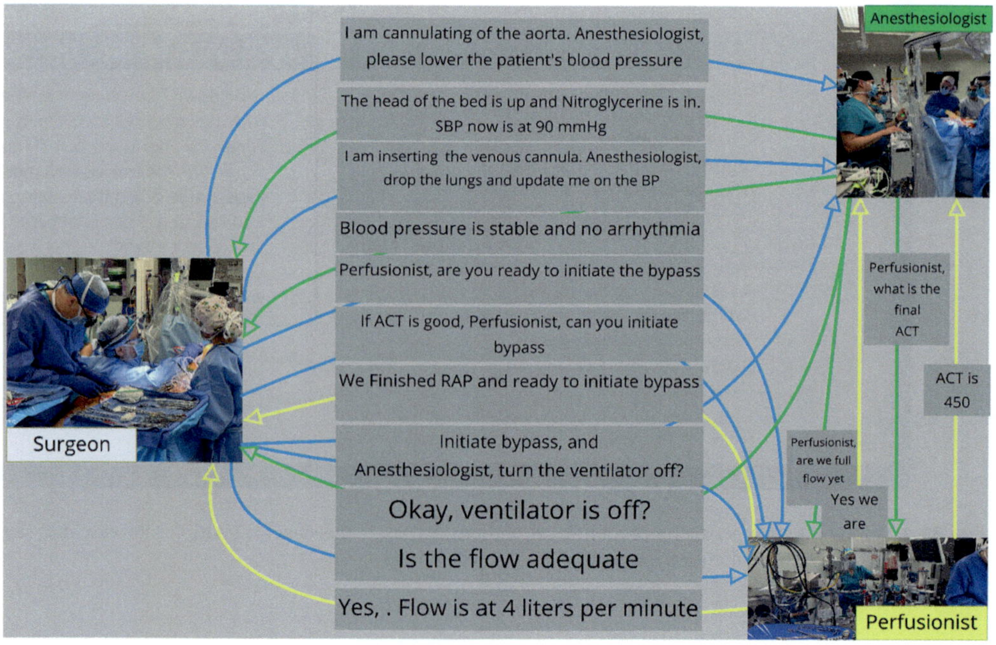

Fig. 31.11 Example of closed-loop communication: This diagram illustrates a critical moment of teamwork among the perfusionist, anesthesia provider, and cardiac surgeon, engaging in precise and confirmatory communication just prior to the initiation of CPB, ensuring clarity and coordination for patient safety

Conclusion

The safety of CPB procedures has been significantly improved by advancements in safety devices and system-level processes. Invasive safety devices that have been incorporated into the design of CPB help to reduce the likelihood of potentially catastrophic events occurring. Non-invasive safety devices also play an important role in enhancing the ability of the perfusionist to ensure the safe performance of the procedure. Furthermore, formalizing critical team interactions and utilizing checklists at fixed, consistent points has been found to reduce the occurrence of human error during CPB procedures. Checklists also improve consistency, clarity, and communication between team members, ultimately leading to safer and more efficient procedures.

Further Reading

Agency for Healthcare Research and Quality. Optimize briefings and debriefings: facilitator notes. [Internet]. [cited 2024 Aug 10]. Available from: https://www.ahrq.gov/hai/tools/surgery/modules/implementation/opt-briefings-fac-notes.html.

AmSECT. Patient handoff tool. [Internet]. [cited 2024 Aug 10]. Available from: https://www.amsect.org/Portals/0/AmSECT%20Documents/I%20PASS%20THE%20CLAMP%20OFF%20(1).pdf.

Boeing. The role of human factors in improving aviation safety. [Internet]. [cited 2024 Aug 10]. Available from: http://www.boeing.com/commercial/aeromagazine/aero_08/human_textonly.html.

Flight Safety Australia. One thing at a time: a brief history of the checklist. [Internet]. 2018 Nov [cited 2024 Aug 10]. Available from: https://www.flightsafetyaustralia.com/2018/11/one-thing-at-a-time-a-brief-history-of-the-checklist/.

Freundlich RE, Bulka CM, Wanderer JP, Rothman BS, Sandberg WS, Ehrenfeld JM. Prospective investigation of the operating room time-out process. Anesth Analg. 2020;130(3):725–9. https://doi.org/10.1213/ANE.0000000000004661.

Kaplan JA. Kaplan's cardiac anesthesia. 5th ed. Philadelphia: Elsevier Saunders; 2006.

Sotto KT, Burian BK, Brindle ME. Impact of the WHO surgical safety checklist relative to its design and intended use: a systematic review and meta-meta-analysis. J Am Coll Surg. 2021;233(6):794–809.e8. https://doi.org/10.1016/j.jamcollsurg.2021.06.014.

Part X

Mechanical Circulatory Support

Intra-Aortic Balloon Pump

32

Ramesh Mariyappa, Emma C. Huang, and Jiapeng Huang

Introduction

Intra-Aortic Balloon Pump (IABP) is a type of mechanical circulatory support (MCS) device used to provide temporary circulatory support for patients with severe cardiac dysfunction. Developed in the 1960s and clinical use since the early 1970s, the IABP has proven its efficacy over decades. Despite the advent of newer MCS devices—such as Impella, TandemHeart, ECMO (Extracorporeal Membrane Oxygenation), and VAD (Ventricular Assist Device)—which offer full circulatory support for failing hearts, the IABP remains the most commonly used MCS device due to its widespread availability and ease of placement. The primary goal of the IABP is to both increase cardiac output and improve cardiac oxygen supply-demand balance by increasing the myocardial oxygen supply while simultaneously reducing its demand.

Background

Over the past five decades, IABP has been extensively utilized in various clinical scenarios:

- Management of cardiogenic shock and acute myocardial infarction (MI).
- Peri-procedural support for patients with high-grade coronary artery stenosis undergoing percutaneous coronary interventions (PCI) and surgical revascularization.
- Facilitating separation from cardiopulmonary bypass (CPB) after cardiac surgery.

R. Mariyappa (✉) · J. Huang
Department of Anesthesiology and Perioperative Medicine, University of Louisville, Louisville, KY, USA
e-mail: ramesh.mariyappa@louisville.edu; jiapeng.huang@louisville.edu

E. C. Huang
Department of Anesthesiology, Duke University, Raleigh, NC, USA
e-mail: emma.huang@duke.edu

While the IABP-SHOCK II trial did not demonstrate a reduction in mortality in cardiogenic shock following acute MI, it did provide short-term hemodynamic improvement. IABP was associated with improved outcomes when used in conjunction with thrombolysis and high-risk PCIs; however, long-term data suggested no significant improvement in mortality. Despite the lack of definitive proof of improved clinical outcomes, IABP is still widely used. It delivers beneficial physiological effects (increased myocardial perfusion and decreased afterload) to patients with myocardial ischemia and cardiogenic shock in a relatively simple, low-risk manner.

Physiological Effects of IABP

The intra-aortic balloon is a balloon-tipped catheter positioned in the descending thoracic aorta, distal to the origin of the left subclavian artery. It operates through counterpulsation, inflating during diastole and deflating during systole.

- *Diastolic Augmentation*: Balloon inflation during diastole increases pressure in the proximal aorta. This boosts blood flow to the coronary arteries through retrograde displacement, enhancing myocardial oxygen supply.
- *Systolic Unloading*: Deflation of the balloon during early systole reduces end-diastolic pressure, thus decreasing the afterload through a vacuum effect.

These combined actions result in:

- Increased diastolic coronary perfusion
- Decreased left ventricular (LV) end-diastolic pressure and volume
- Improved LV stroke volume and cardiac output
- Enhanced organ perfusion
- Better myocardial oxygen supply-demand balance.

A. S. Awad, J. DiNardo (eds.), *Clinical Perfusion for Cardiac Surgery*, https://doi.org/10.1007/978-3-031-91163-7_32

Though most of the afterload reduction benefits LV contraction, the improved ejection of LV reduces left atrial and pulmonary wedge pressure and thus can also improve right ventricular (RV) ejection.

This favorable condition is utilized to provide time for a failing heart to recover or used as a bridge to a definitive treatment.

Balloon Augmentation Ratio

Balloon inflation and deflation frequencies are adjustable relative to the cardiac cycle.

- *1:1 Support*: The balloon inflates and deflates with every cardiac cycle. After the initial placement of IABP, counterpulsation is started at a 1:1 frequency to provide maximum support to the heart.
- *1:2 Support*: Following the improvement of the patient's hemodynamics, the ratio may be decreased to 1:2. In this mode, the balloon assists every other cardiac cycle, providing moderate support.
- *1:3 Support*: This ratio is typically used during IABP weaning when the patient's condition is further stabilized. It is important to note that prolonged use at this ratio increases thromboembolism risk without anticoagulation (Fig. 32.1).

Components of IABP

The IABP consists of two main components:

1. *Dual Lumen Catheter*: This flexible catheter is equipped with a long sausage-shaped polyurethane balloon at the distal end.
   - *Inner Lumen*: Used for guidewire insertion, blood flushing or aspiration, and monitoring aortic blood pressure. Fiberoptic-tipped catheters can provide arterial waveforms for triggering balloon inflation.
   - *Outer Lumen*: Dedicated to delivering helium gas for balloon inflation and deflation.
2. *Mobile Console*: This unit houses the helium delivery system, pump, and computer controller that governs the balloon's inflation and deflation cycles.

Helium: The Gas of Choice

Helium is preferred for IABP balloons due to its properties:

- *Low-Density*: Allows for rapid inflation and deflation, crucial for precise timing with the cardiac cycle.
- *Low Turbulent Flow*: Minimizes the risk of hemolysis.
- *Safe Absorption*: There is also a lower risk of harmful embolism in case of a leak or rupture of the balloon, as helium is rapidly absorbed by the bloodstream (Figs. 32.2 and 32.3).

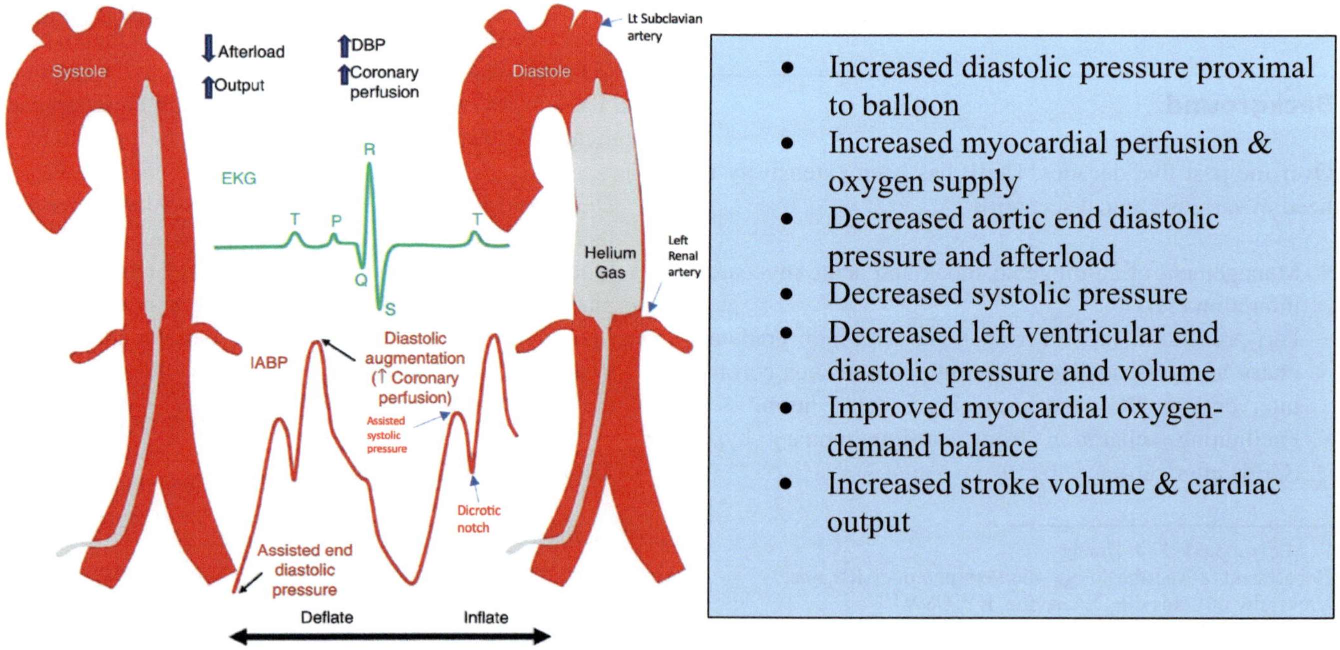

Fig. 32.1 Mechanism of action of an IABP: the device inflates during diastole and deflates during systole. The inset shows the timing of the inflation and deflation as ascertained by the arterial line tracing with respect to the EKG. (Reproduced with permission from Springer Nature: Notarianni A, Tickoo M, Bardia A. Mechanical cardiac circulatory support: an overview of the challenges for the anesthetist. Curr Anesthesiol Rep. 2021;11:421–8)

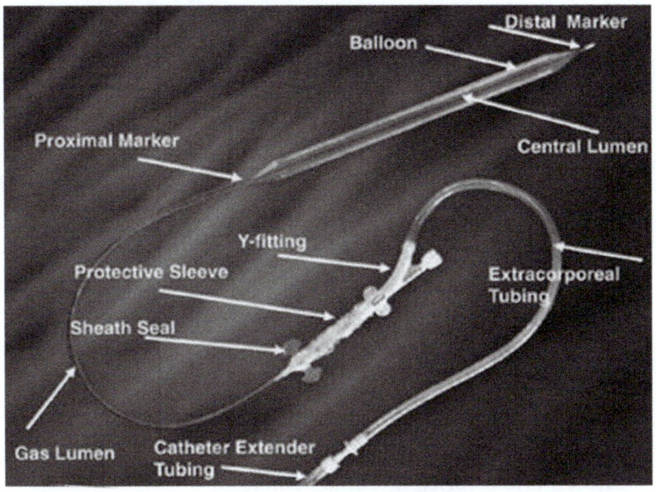

Fig. 32.2 Intra-aortic balloon pump catheter. (Reproduced with permission from Springer Nature: Briggs et al. 2021)

IABP Indications

- Cardiogenic shock
- Acute MI
- Refractory unstable angina
- Failure to wean from CPB machine after cardiac surgery
- Support during high-risk percutaneous angioplasty or coronary stent placement
- High-grade coronary artery stenosis (especially left main) with low ejection fraction while waiting for definitive treatment
- Mechanical complications from ischemia, such as a ventricular septal defect or severe mitral regurgitation, while waiting for surgery
- Post myocardial contusion with expected recovery
- Bridge to therapy for refractory ventricular arrhythmias or heart failure

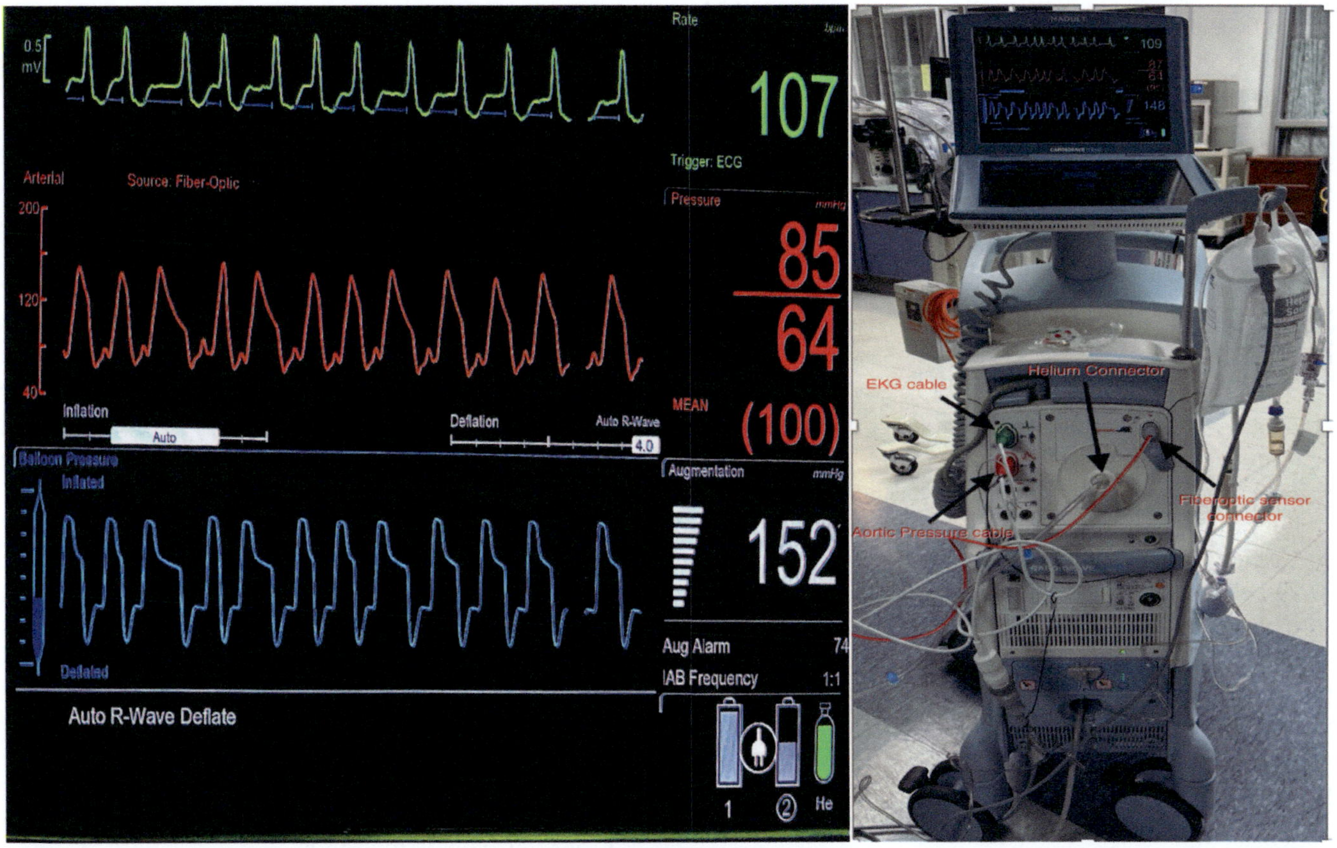

Fig. 32.3 Intra-aortic balloon pump console with monitor showing EKG, IABP balloon (blue), and arterial blood pressure waveforms (red)

IABP Contraindications

Absolute Contraindications

- Severe aortic regurgitation: diminishes diastolic augmentation, worsens regurgitation, increases LV end-diastolic volume/pressure, and wall tension.
- Aortic dissection: Risk of catheter placement in the false lumen, worsening the dissection or causing rupture during catheter insertion and balloon inflation.

Relative Contraindications

- Severe aorto-iliac atherosclerotic and/or occlusive disease: Increased risk for thrombo-embolism, vascular injury, and ischemia.
- Prosthetic vascular graft in the aorta: Increased risk of graft disruption.
- Aortic aneurysm: Risk of rupture due to mechanical stress from balloon inflation and during placement of the IABP catheter.
- Severe sepsis: Increased risk of infection from catheter placement (foreign body).
- Severe coagulopathy: Increased risk for excessive bleeding at the insertion site, retroperitoneal space, and hematoma formation.

Complications

- *Bleeding, hematoma formation*: Can be local or remote (retroperitoneal).
- *Infection*: Can cause or worsen local and/or systemic infection.
- *Vascular injury*: More common in patients with severe vascular disease, and during catheter insertion/removal. Includes damage to femoral/iliac arteries, aortic dissection or tear, pseudoaneurysm at access site.
- *Thromboembolism*: Disruption of atherosclerotic plaque can cause emboli to the brain, limbs, bowel, viscera, and/or kidneys, leading to ischemia.
- *Timing errors*: Incorrect timing of balloon inflation/deflation can cause hemodynamic instability.
- *Thrombocytopenia and anemia*: Shearing effects of balloon inflation and deflation damage blood cells.
- *Balloon rupture*: Rupture of the IABP balloon can cause gas embolism. Suspect this if augmentation is lost or blood is seen in the gas tubing. The patient should be immediately placed in the Trendelenburg position to reduce the risk of cerebral helium embolism, although this is unlikely due to rapid absorption of helium by the blood. The ruptured balloon should be removed and replaced as soon as possible to prevent thrombus formation on the balloon.
- *Limb ischemia*:
  - *Lower extremity*: Due to thromboembolism and/or compromised distal arterial flow from catheter placement.
  - *Left upper extremity*: Due to thromboembolism and/or occlusion of the ostium of the left subclavian artery by malposition of the intra-aortic balloon.
- *Mesenteric ischemia*: Caused by thromboembolism, misplaced balloon, or improperly sized balloon occluding mesenteric arteries or celiac trunk.
- *Renal insufficiency*: Due to occlusion of renal arteries from balloon misplacement.

Intra-Aortic Balloon Placement

IABP catheters are available in many sizes, from 2.5 to 50 mL, and are selected based on the height of the patient. Using the Seldinger technique, the catheter is inserted through the common femoral artery and advanced into the descending thoracic aorta under fluoroscopic or transesophageal echocardiography (TEE) guidance.

- *Optimal Positioning*: The ideal balloon position is as close to the aortic root as possible to maximize diastolic augmentation and myocardial perfusion. However, the distal tip of the catheter should be positioned about 1–2 cm distal to the origin of the left subclavian artery to avoid occluding major head vessels.
- *Avoiding Renal Arteries Obstructions*: The base of the IABP catheter should be positioned above the renal arteries to prevent obstruction of renal blood flow.
- *Imaging Confirmation*: Chest X-ray or fluoroscopy typically shows the catheter tip in the second/third intercostal space, near the carina, and about 2 cm below the aortic bulb. (Fig. 32.4).
- *Left Subclavian Insertion*: In rare cases, the IABP catheter may be inserted via the left subclavian/axillary artery. In this instance, the base of the catheter should be distal to the left subclavian. (Fig. 32.5).
- *Inflation and Deflation Control*: Inflation and deflation of the balloon are controlled by the console with input from the patient's EKG or aortic blood pressure waveform, and rarely from pacemaker spikes.

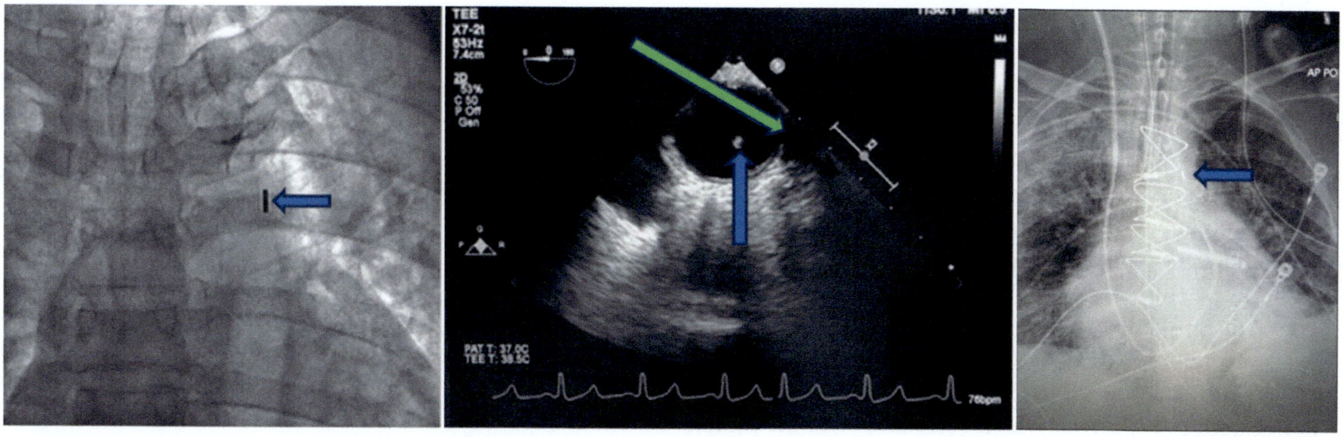

Fig. 32.4 Confirmation of intra-aortic balloon placement by: (**a**) fluoroscopy, (**b**) transesophageal echocardiography (green arrow denotes takeoff of left subclavian artery from the aorta), (**c**) chest X-ray. The blue arrows mark the tip of balloon. (Reproduced with permission from Springer Nature: Fleischman F, Cleveland JD. Intra-aortic balloon pump insertion and management, 2018)

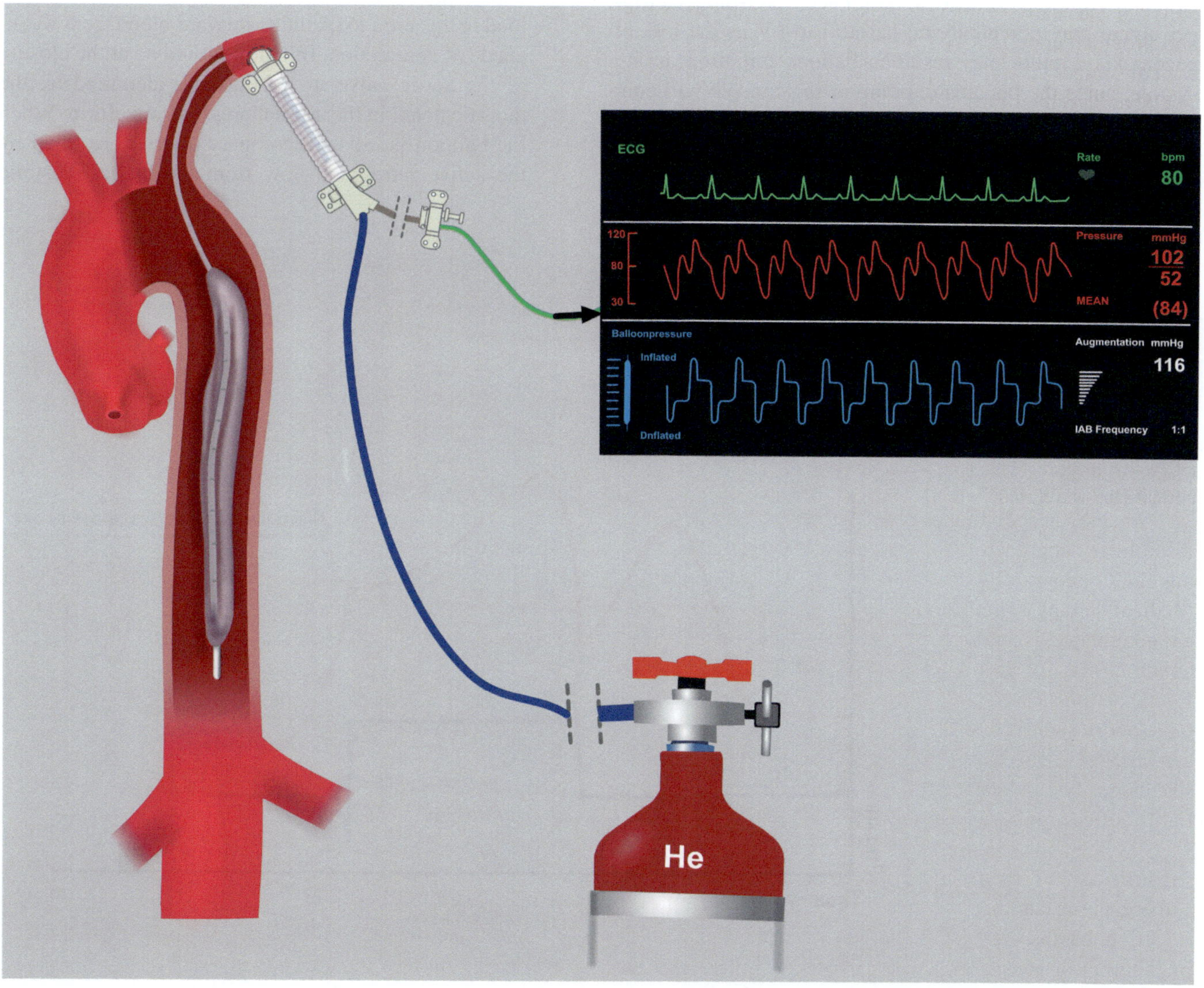

Fig. 32.5 Illustration of IABP placement: the thoracic aorta and arch are shown with the IABP inserted via the left axillary/subclavian artery. The balloon is depicted in the deflated mode, connected to the IABP console, which displays the monitoring screen and helium tank connection

IABP Triggering and Timing: Optimizing Myocardial Support

The optimal benefits of IABP depend on the triggering and timing of the intra-aortic balloon inflation and deflation. Triggering refers to the physiologic sign that identifies the beginning of a new cardiac cycle. Timing refers to the inflation and deflation of the intra-aortic balloon to the patient's cardiac cycle (Fig. 32.6).

The most reliable and common trigger signal is the R-wave from the EKG, which denotes systole and the onset of a new cardiac cycle. Inflation of the balloon is triggered by the beginning of diastole, which correlates with the middle of the T wave. The balloon is timed to deflate at the very end of the diastole. This correlates with the R-wave on the EKG. Other trigger signals that are used include the aortic pressure waveform obtained from tip of the fiberoptic catheter, and seldom pacemaker spikes. Pacemaker-induced trigger signal may potentially be harmful to LV as the loss of pacemaker capture may result in balloon initiation during systole, since the pneumatic pump in the console will continue to inflate at the pacing rate rather than the true signal from ventricular contraction. Irregular heart rhythms present challenging conditions for using IABP.

- *Irregular Rhythms*
  Irregular heart rhythms present challenging conditions for using IABP. In atrial fibrillation, the EKG trigger is timed to deflate on the R-wave as usual, but the R-R interval varies. The best way to manage these conditions is to convert arrhythmias into a regular rhythm for optimal IABP benefits.
  During ventricular systole, there is higher resistance for coronary arterial blood flow due to myocardial contraction. Hence, most of the myocardial perfusion occurs during diastole, where the myocardium is relaxed, and coronary arteries are filled with passive diastolic blood flow.
- *Optimal Timing*
  - *Inflation*:
    The goal of the IABP is to inflate the balloon during diastole to increase the coronary blood flow and to deflate immediately before systole to reduce the afterload in the aorta to facilitate forward blood from weakened LV contraction. Inflation should be at the closure of the aortic valve in the diastole, identified by the dicrotic notch in the arterial pressure waveform. When the balloon is inflated, coronary arteries are filled by the active retrograde flow from the higher diastolic

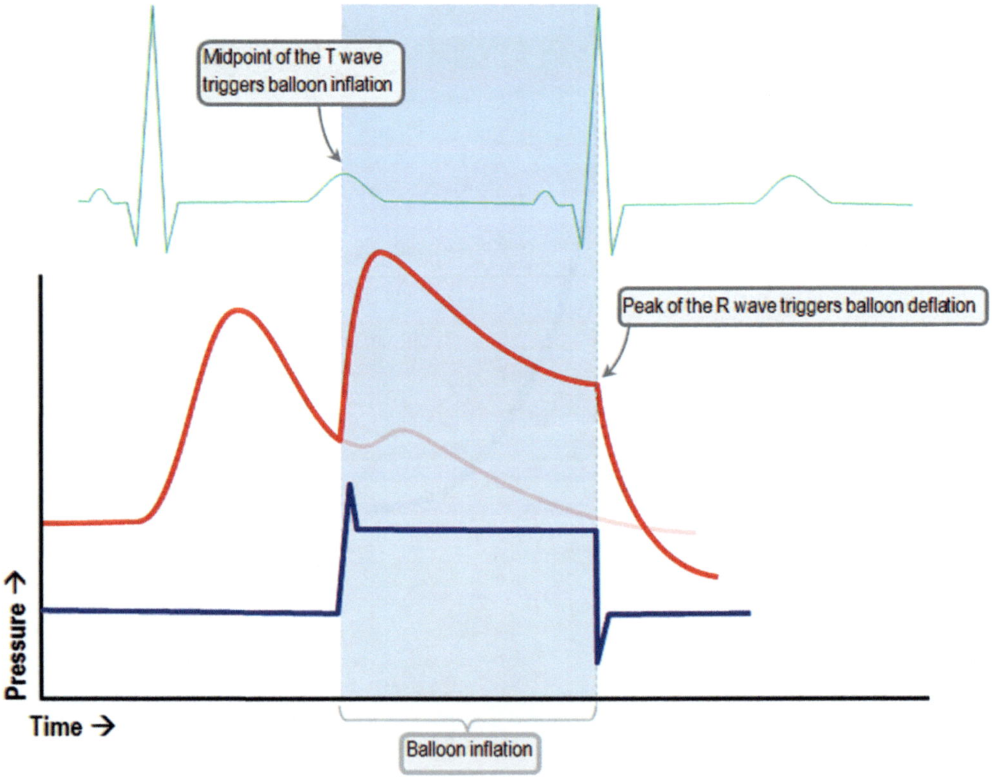

Fig. 32.6 Illustration of IABP triggering from EKG with aortic blood pressure (red) and balloon (blue) waveforms. (Reused with permission from https://derangedphysiology.com/main/required-reading/cardiothoracic-intensive-care/Chapter%20634/normal-iabp-waveform)

pressure proximal to the balloon, enhancing myocardial perfusion. The sharp V-shaped dicrotic notch indicates the correct timing of the balloon inflation.

- *Deflation*:
  Balloon deflation should occur at the onset of systole during the isovolumetric phase. Rapid deflation of the balloon causes a vacuum effect, creating lower pressure in the aorta and thus lowering the afterload just before LV ejection. This action increases LV emptying with reduced workload. With correct timing, the end-diastolic pressure is lower than the unassisted end-diastolic pressure and is displayed as such in the arterial waveform.

• *Timing Errors*
- *Early Inflation*:
  Early inflation of balloon causes forced closure of aortic valve during systole and increased afterload for LV contraction, leading to increased workload and increased myocardial oxygen demand. The resulting shortened systole and increased afterload lead to decreased stroke volume and cardiac output.
- *Late Inflation*:
  Late inflation of the balloon reduces the diastolic augmentation and its benefits. If inflation occurs after the closure of aortic valve (after the dicrotic notch), it is displayed on the arterial waveform as a W shape, indicating suboptimal timing for coronary perfusion.
- *Early Deflation*:
  In early deflation, the waveform will display a sharp drop (cliff shape) following diastolic augmentation. The following end-diastolic pressure may not be lower than the unassisted end-diastolic pressure. This results in reduced beneficial effects of afterload reduction on LV contraction. The negative pressure created by early balloon deflation before LV ejection may cause coronary steal.
- *Late Deflation*:
  In late deflation, the balloon remains inflated when the LV is contracting, leading to increased LV workload, impaired oxygen supply-demand balance, and reduced cardiac output. The pressure waveform will have a higher end-diastolic pressure compared to the unassisted cycle's end-diastolic pressure.

• *Manual Adjustments*
  Manual adjustments may be needed if balloon inflation and deflation are found to be incorrect.
  (Refer to Figs. 32.7, 32.8, 32.9, 32.10, 32.11 and Table 32.1 for detailed waveforms and guidelines)

Inadequate Diastolic Augmentation: Causes and Management

Inadequate diastolic augmentation leads to reduced benefits, and it may be due to several factors:

• *Pump Factors*: Errors in the timing of triggering of balloon inflation and deflation. Ensure proper timing with the dicrotic notch on the arterial waveform.

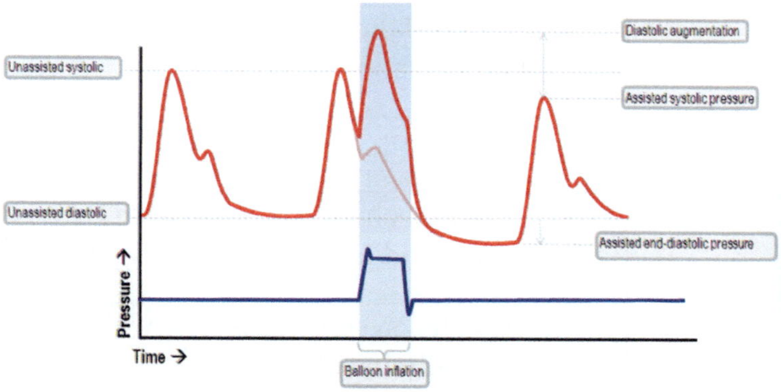

- Augmented diastolic pressure is higher than unassisted systolic pressure
- Reduced assisted end-diastolic pressure
- Reduced assisted systolic pressure
- Sharp V appearance at dicrotic notch

Fig. 32.7 Normal IABP balloon (blue) and aortic blood pressure (red) waveforms. (Reused with permission from https://derangedphysiology.com/main/required-reading/cardiothoracic-intensive-care/Chapter%20634/normal-iabp-waveform)

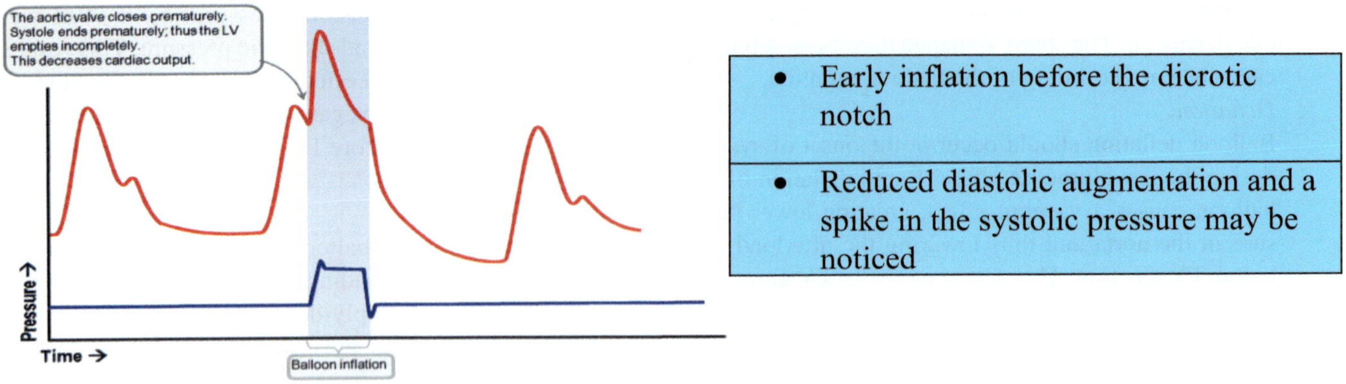

Fig. 32.8 Early balloon inflation. (Reused with permission from https://derangedphysiology.com/main/required-reading/cardiothoracic-intensive-care/Chapter%206342/pathophysiology-abnormal-iabp-arterial-waveforms)

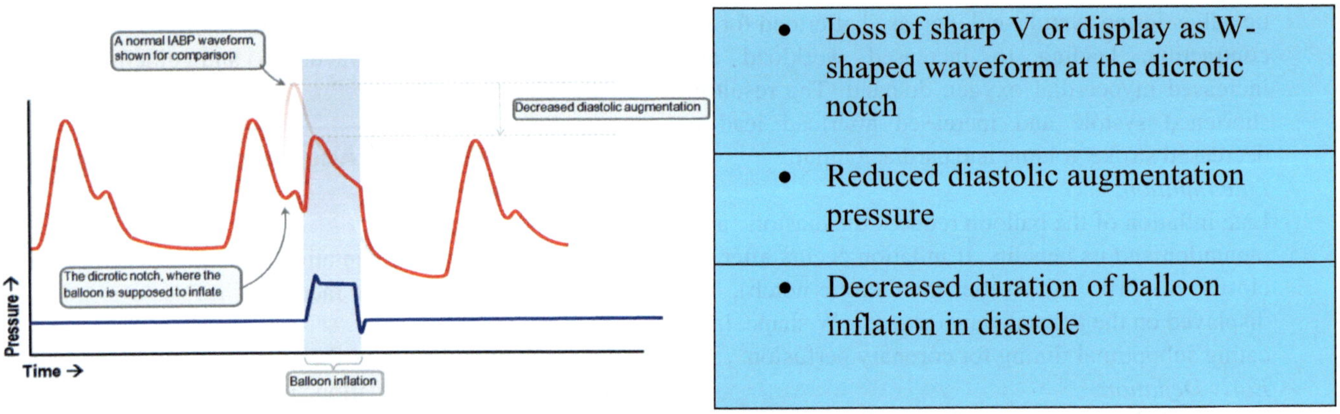

Fig. 32.9 Late balloon inflation. (Reused with permission from https://derangedphysiology.com/main/required-reading/cardiothoracic-intensive-care/Chapter%206342/pathophysiology-abnormal-iabp-arterial-waveforms)

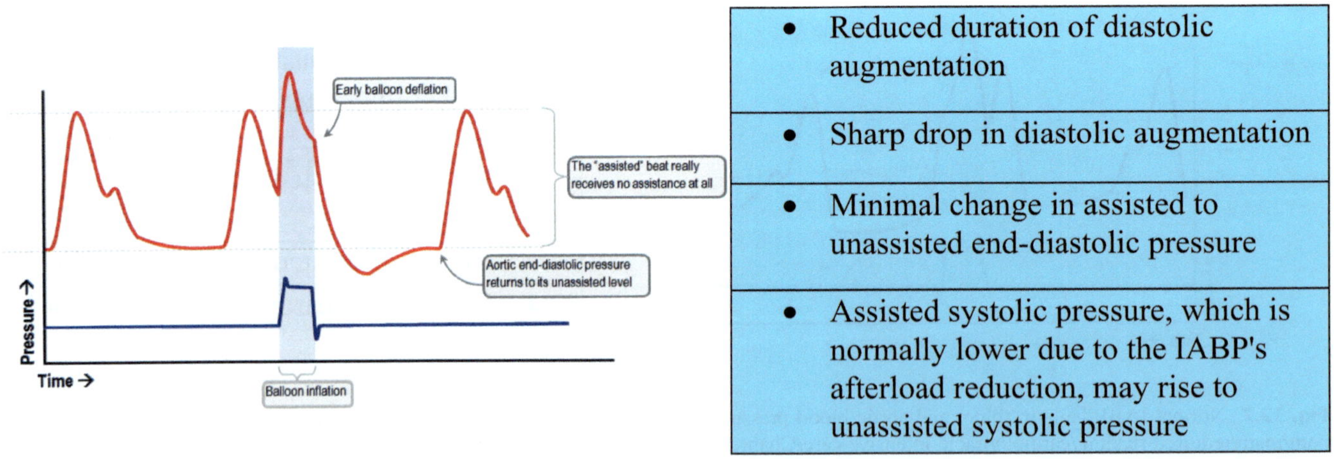

Fig. 32.10 Early balloon deflation. (Reused with permission from https://derangedphysiology.com/main/required-reading/cardiothoracic-intensive-care/Chapter%206342/pathophysiology-abnormal-iabp-arterial-waveforms)

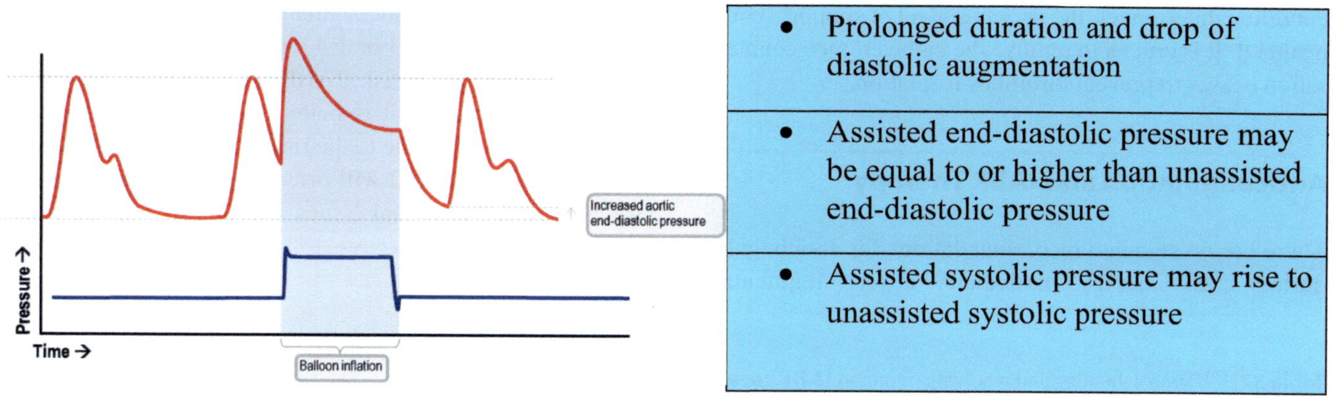

Fig. 32.11 Late balloon deflation. (Reused with permission from https://derangedphysiology.com/main/required-reading/cardiothoracic-intensive-care/Chapter%206342/pathophysiology-abnormal-iabp-arterial-waveforms)

Table 32.1 Changes associated with timing of intra-aortic balloon inflation and deflation

Timing of balloon inflation & deflation	Physiologic changes
Correct inflation	Augmentation of diastolic pressure & flow Increased myocardial perfusion Increased myocardial oxygen supply.
Early inflation	Premature closure of aortic valve Decreased stroke volume & cardiac output Increased LV volume, pressure & wall tension Increased afterload Increased myocardial oxygen demand
Late inflation	Decreased duration & amount of diastolic augmentation Suboptimal myocardial perfusion & oxygen supply
Correct deflation	Lower aortic end-diastolic pressure Lower after load Reduced myocardial workload & lower oxygen demand Increased stroke volume and cardiac output Increased peripheral and vital organ perfusion
Early deflation	Decreased duration of diastolic augmentation Suboptimal myocardial perfusion & oxygen supply Reduced drop in aortic end-diastolic pressure Suboptimal reduction in afterload and myocardial workload Reduced stroke volume and cardiac output Suboptimal increase in myocardial oxygen demand ratio May cause coronary steal
Late deflation	LV contraction against an inflated balloon Increased afterload Increased LV end-diastolic volume, pressure & wall tension Increased myocardial workload & increased myocardial oxygen demand Minimal, if any reduction in assisted end-diastolic pressure Decreased stroke volume & cardiac output

LV left ventricle

- *Patient factors*:
  - *Tachycardia/Arrhythmias*: Shortened diastolic filling time reduces the effectiveness of augmentation. Aim for rate control.
  - *Hypovolemia and Hypotension*: Low blood volume or pressure limits the balloon's ability to displace blood and augment coronary flow. Optimize fluid status and consider vasopressors.
  - *Poor Ventricular Function*: Reduced LV contractility decreases stroke volume and diastolic augmentation. Consider inotropic support.
- *Catheter Issues*:
  - *Distal Placement*: The IABP catheter is positioned too far distally in the descending aorta (further away from the left subclavian artery).
  - *Small Size or Low Volume*: An undersized or underinflated balloon may not displace enough blood to achieve optimal augmentation.
  - *Rupture*: Suspect balloon rupture if augmentation is lost or blood appears in the gas tubing. Promptly remove and replace the balloon to prevent complications, including cerebral embolism.

IABP Weaning

Once treatment goals are met (e.g., minimal ionotropic requirement, improved ventricular function, hemodynamic stability, resolution of the primary problem, or preparation for definitive therapy), IABP weaning should be initiated. This involves gradually reducing the augmentation ratio over several hours (e.g., from 1:1 to 1:2 to 1:3) or gradually decreasing the balloon inflation volume (e.g., by 10% every hour). If the patient tolerates a filling volume of 20 mL or a 1:3 setting for 1–6 h, the device can be removed. However, if the patient's condition deteriorates, the previous level of support should be resumed. It is crucial to remove the catheter once counterpulsation ceases to prevent thrombus formation.

Anticoagulation and IABP Therapy

There are no standard recommendations for anticoagulation during IABP therapy, particularly at 1:1 augmentation. However, systemic anticoagulation is recommended when weaning the IABP (1:3 or 1:4 ratio) for extended periods to minimize thrombosis risk. IABP should never be placed in standby mode unless it is being removed or the patient is fully anticoagulated due to the risk of thrombus formation on the balloon. Table 32.2 will provide a comprehensive guide for addressing technical issues and alarms that may arise during IABP therapy.

Table 32.2 Troubleshooting and resolving common IABP console problems and alarms

Problem	Causes	Interventions
Inadequate augmentation	Patient hemodynamic instability factors: 1. Low cardiac output 2. Hypotension 3. Decreased systemic vascular resistance	Administer necessary treatment. 1. Inotropes 2. Vasopressors
	Small balloon	Remove and replace with correctly sized balloon if needed
	Too high of an alarm threshold	Decrease the alarm limit
	Timing issues	Correct synchronization with the cardiac cycle
Sudden depletion of helium	There is IABP circuit leakage	Inspect the extension tubing: For any holes or leaks. The presence of blood in the tube indicates a balloon rupture, which necessitates the removal of the balloon
Unable to trigger	Failure to sense trigger	Inspect and reattach the EKG/pressure cable. Change to a different mode
IABP disconnection	The IABP extension gas tubing has been detached	Check and re-establish the connection of the gas tubing Refill IAB with gas or change the helium cylinder Then reactivate IABP
Assess IAB catheter for: potential issues	IAB catheter/tubing twisted or kinked	Untwist and resolve any kinks
	IAB Catheter Migration.	Verify IAB markings to ensure it is properly positioned.
	Tip location	Adjust balloon position
	The balloon is partially inflated	Make sure that the full augmentation is enabled Attempt manually inflating and deflating the balloon
IABP malfunction	Failure of the internal IABP console/computer	Verify that there are no electrical failures or presence of blood in the condensers
Insufficient helium	Level of helium is extremely low	Change the helium cylinder Verify that the yoke is securely fastened

Summary

IABP is the most widely used mechanical circulatory support device since its introduction in the 1960s. It is commonly placed percutaneously through the femoral artery in critical care settings involving cardiogenic shock, acute MI, cardiac surgery, and high-risk PCI. By increasing coronary perfusion through augmented diastolic pressure and decreasing afterload, IABP improves the myocardial oxygen supply-demand balance, for a failing heart to recover or provide more time to institute a definitive treatment.

Further Reading

Ali JM, Abu-Omar Y. Intra-aortic balloon pump and other methods of mechanical circulatory support. Surgery (Oxford). 2018;36(2):68–74.

Briggs K, Najarro G, Mirza O. Intra-aortic balloon pump counterpulsation. In: Interventional critical care—a manual for advanced practice providers. 2nd ed. Cham: Springer; 2021.

Gonzalez LS, Chaney MA. Intraaortic balloon pump counterpulsation, part I: history, technical aspects, physiologic effects, contraindications, medical applications/outcomes. Anesth Analg. 2020a;131(3):776–91.

Gonzalez LS, Chaney MA. Balloon pump counterpulsation part II: peri-operative henodynamic support and new directions. Anesth Analg. 2020b;131(3):792–807.

Helwani MA, Srinivasan JD. Chapter 23: Intra-aortic balloon pump. In: Data interpretation in anesthesia: a clinical guide. Cham: Springer; 2017. p. 125–30.

Parissis H, Graham V, et al. IABP: history-evolution-pathophysiology-indications: what we need to know. J Cardiothorac Surg. 2016;11:122.

Yartsev A. Anatomy of the intra aortic balloon pump. In: Deranged physiology. Cardiovascular Intensive Care; 2015. https://derangedphysiology.com/main/required-reading/cardiothoracic-intensive-care/Chapter%20630/anatomy-intra-aortic-balloon-pump.

Ventricular Assist Devices

33

Muhammad Talha Mustafa, Jiapeng Huang, and Siddharth V. Pahwa

Introduction

Heart failure (HF) is a condition where the heart is unable to pump blood at a rate sufficient to meet the metabolic demands of the body's tissues and organs. The American College of Cardiology Foundation (ACCF) and the American Heart Association (AHA) have created an HF staging system, where stage D represents advanced HF that is unresponsive to medical therapy. Stage D HF carries an extremely dismal prognosis even with the most aggressive medical management and cardiac synchronization therapy, which may include inotropes, pulmonary vasodilators, vasopressors, diuretics, biventricular pacing, and/or AICD placement. Table 33.1 outlines the four stages of HF.

Heart failure is categorized based on left ventricular (LV) function into two main groups: those with preserved ejection fraction (HFpEF) and those with reduced ejection fraction (HFrEF).

According to the 2024 AHA Heart Disease and Stroke Statistics Update, about 6.7 million Americans over 20 years of age currently have HF. In patients with HF, the prevalence of stage D is reported as high as 13% in some studies. Despite the growing number of heart transplants in the US (over 4000 in 2023), demand still outpaces supply due to the lack of donor organs.

Advanced HF unresponsive to standard medical therapies requires specialized interventions, including heart transplantation, long-term mechanical circulatory support (MCS), or continuous inotropic therapy. While heart transplantation offers the best outcomes, donor organ scarcity and recipient eligibility limit its availability. Inotropic therapy may improve symptoms but does not prolong survival.

Table 33.1 ACCF/AHA sages of heart failure (Hunt et al. Circulation. 2009)

Stage	ACCF/AHA stages of HF description
A	High-risk for HF, asymptomatic with normal cardiac structure
B	Asymptomatic structural heart disease
C	Symptomatic structural heart disease prior or current
D	Advanced HF unresponsive to standard therapies requiring advanced intervention

ACCF American College of Cardiology Foundation, *AHA* American Heart Association, *HF* heart failure

MCS Devices

MCS devices, initially intended as a bridge to transplantation (BTT) for end-stage HF patients, LVADs have since become a viable "destination therapy" (DT) for non-transplant candidates. This shift was driven by the exceptional results demonstrated in trials like REMATCH and INTrEPID, showcasing significant improvements in survival and quality of life compared to medical management alone.

MCS is a versatile tool in the treatment of advanced HF, with applications ranging from acute interventions to long-term solutions. In the chronic setting, MCS devices, often ventricular assist devices (VADs), can be used as a BTT or as DT for patients ineligible for transplant, significantly improving their quality of life and survival. DT has become the most common indication for LVAD, especially since a 2018 UNOS policy change broadened heart allocation criteria. Conversely, in acute situations, MCS serves as a critical bridge-to-recovery (BTR) for patients with cardiogenic shock, or as a bridge-to-decision (BTD), buying time while a long-term treatment plan is formulated. This approach is particularly crucial in cases of acute myocardial infarction, myocarditis, or post-operative cardiac complications.

M. T. Mustafa · S. V. Pahwa (✉)
Department of Cardiovascular and Thoracic Surgery, University of Louisville, Louisville, KY, USA
e-mail: muhammad.mustafa@louisville.edu; siddharth.pahwa@louisville.edu

J. Huang
Department of Anesthesiology and Perioperative Medicine, University of Louisville, Louisville, KY, USA
e-mail: jiapeng.huang@louisville.edu

A. S. Awad, J. DiNardo (eds.), *Clinical Perfusion for Cardiac Surgery*, https://doi.org/10.1007/978-3-031-91163-7_33

For patients requiring biventricular support who are not suitable for isolated LVAD, a total artificial heart (TAH) is a viable option. This is particularly relevant for those with advanced biventricular systolic dysfunction, refractory arrhythmias, restrictive/hypertrophic cardiomyopathies, congenital heart disease, or other intracardiac defects.

Temporary MCS Devices (<14 Days)

Various devices can provide temporary perioperative MCS, including the intra-aortic balloon pump (IABP), continuous miniature axial flow pumps (Impella®), and extracorporeal systems (TandemHeart®, ECMO). The optimal choice depends on factors like the required duration of support and the urgency of the clinical situation. By enhancing vital organ perfusion and reducing cardiac filling pressures and LV workload, these devices help to improve the balance of myocardial oxygen supply and demand. IABP and ECMO will be discussed in greater detail in their respective chapters (32 & 34).

Specific Devices

Left Ventricle to Aorta Assist Device

Impella 5.5 The Impella system (Abiomed, Danvers, MA) is a miniature axial flow ventricular assist device designed for temporary LV assistance by pumping blood directly from the left ventricle to the ascending aorta. It has a flow capacity of up to 6.0 L/min and two insertion options:

- *Direct aortic insertion*: Through the ascending aorta into the left ventricle.
- *Axillary artery insertion*: Via the axillary artery through a surgical cutdown.

Left-Atrium-to-Aorta Assist Device

The TandemHeart (CardiacAssist, Inc.) is a percutaneous LV assist device used primarily in the cardiac catheterization lab to provide short-term support for patients with severely impaired LV function. It pumps blood from the left atrium, via a transseptal cannula and the femoral vein, to the descending aorta through the iliofemoral artery. Its flow rate can reach 3.5-5 L/min, depending on cannula size. An external controller regulates the pump.

Temporary Assist Devices for Isolated Right Ventricular Failure

Impella RP Flex This right ventricular support system pumps blood from the vena cava to the pulmonary artery using a microaxial pump mounted on the catheter tip. It is inserted via the internal jugular vein (IJ), femoral vein, or superior vena cava to provide right ventricular support.

Long-Term Mechanical Circulatory Support and TAH

LVADs are surgically implanted electromechanical pumps that support or replace the function of a failing left ventricle (LV) to maintain sufficient cardiac output and, consequently, adequate oxygenation to the body. They form an external circulatory system, bypassing the dysfunctional LV.

Anatomy of the LVADs

LVADs are usually implanted during an open-heart surgery, and the main components include the following:

- *Inflow Cannula*: Drains blood passively from the LV apex.
- *Pump*: Actively propels blood through the system.
- *Outflow Cannula*: Delivers blood to the ascending aorta.
- *Driveline*: Connects the internal pump to the external controller.
- *External Controller*: Regulates pump function and houses the battery. The electrical controller is carried by the patient on a belt, and the batteries are worn on shoulder straps.

Current LVADs use either axial flow or centrifugal flow pumps.

Physiological Changes

Implanting an LVAD and restoring circulation rapidly improves end-organ function, as reflected in normalized serum kidney and liver markers. Initially, LV unloading reduces its size, slightly improves ejection fraction (EF), and lowers wall tension, enhancing myocardial energetics.

While first-generation VADs used pulsatile pumps, second- and third-generation devices are continuous-flow, resulting in a non-palpable pulse. However, third-generation LVADs, like the HeartMate 3, incorporate technology to generate a subtle pulsatile flow. Blood flow in these devices is determined by ventricular loading and estimated via power consumption.

In essence, the right ventricle fills the left ventricle, whose output is then augmented by the LVAD. This interconnectedness highlights the importance of considering both ventricles in VAD management.

History and Development

The development of LVAD was driven by the prevalence of advanced-stage left-sided HF and the shortage of heart transplantation, as discussed earlier. The first LVAD, developed by Dr. Domingo Liotta in the 1960s, was a paracorporeal pneumatically powered pulsatile pump, connecting the left atrium to the right axillary artery. The first successful implantation of this device was performed by Dr. Michael DeBakey on a female patient in postcardiotomy shock following aortic valve replacement. She received a heart transplant ten days later.

The first generation of the electronically powered LVADs, introduced in the 1980s, included the Novacor left ventricular assist system (LVAS) (World Heart Corporation, CA, USA) (Fig. 33.1) and the HeartMate I pump (Thoratec Corporation, CA, USA.) (Fig. 33.2). The Novacor LVAS featured bioprosthetic (pericardial) inflow and outflow tissue valves with dual pusher-plates. The dual pusher plates provided continuous flow throughout the device to minimize thrombus formation. In contrast, the HeartMate I pump utilized a single pusher plate. Both pumps generated pulsatile blood flow. Despite these advancements, significant challenges persisted:

1. Limited portability due to short battery life (5 hours).
2. Potential for total system failure due to interdependent impeller components.
3. The risks of infection, hemorrhage, and thrombus formation.

Second-generation LVADs were developed to address the concerns associated with the earlier devices. This generation included Jarvik 2000 (Figs. 33.3 and 33.4) and HeartMate II (Fig. 33.5), among others. These models incorporated a single axial rotatory motor pump for continuous blood flow, minimizing the risk of malfunctioning by eliminating the need for bioprosthetic valves and compliance chambers. To combat thrombosis, HeartMate II featured a textured interior surface that reduced the number of thromboembolic events despite minimal anticoagulation. These innovative LVADs

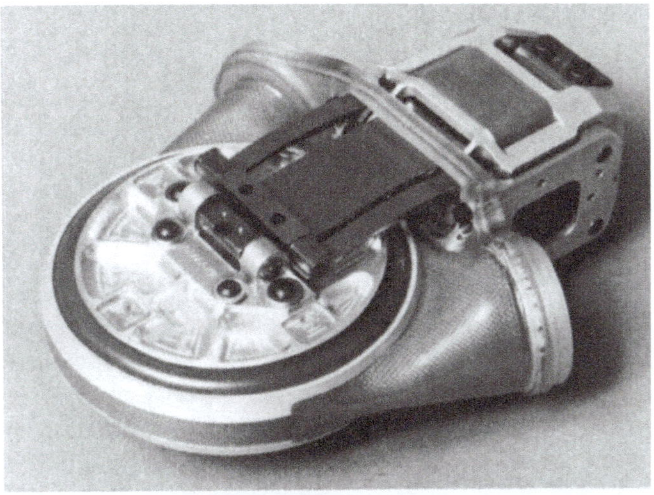

Fig. 33.1 Assembled Novacor LVAD with inflow and outflow fittings for biologic valves (Starnes et al. 1988)

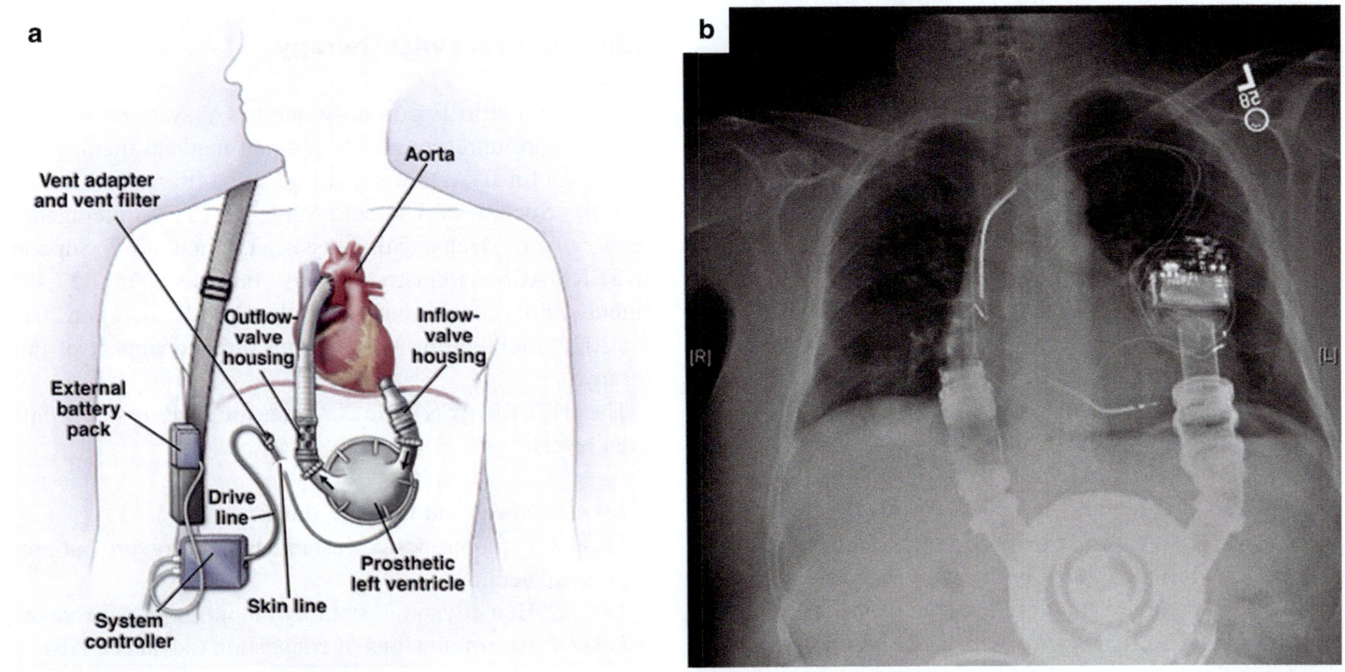

Fig. 33.2 (**a**) Labeled diagram highlighting the parts of an implanted HeartMate I (**b**) X-ray of an implanted HeartMate I (Rodriguez et al. 2013)

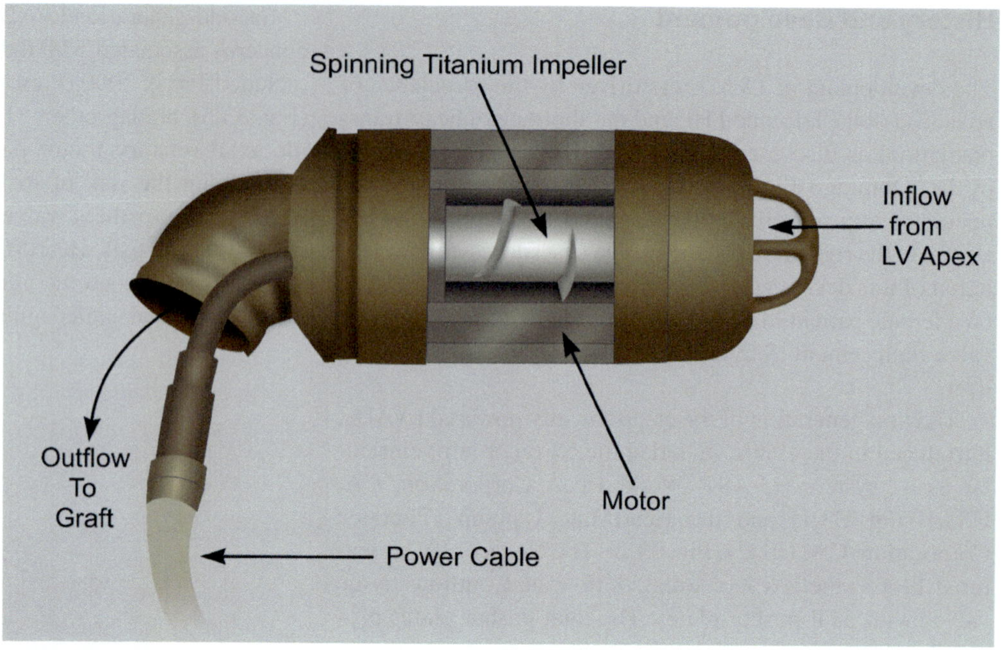

Fig. 33.3 The Jarvik 2000, an LVAD, is designed to support heart function in patients with advanced heart failure. This illustration reveals the internal structure and key components of the device, including the inflow port that draws blood from the LV apex and pumps it through the outflow tract, which connects to the conduit graft. Notable internal components, such as the motor and the spinning titanium impeller that provides continuous blood flow, are also visible

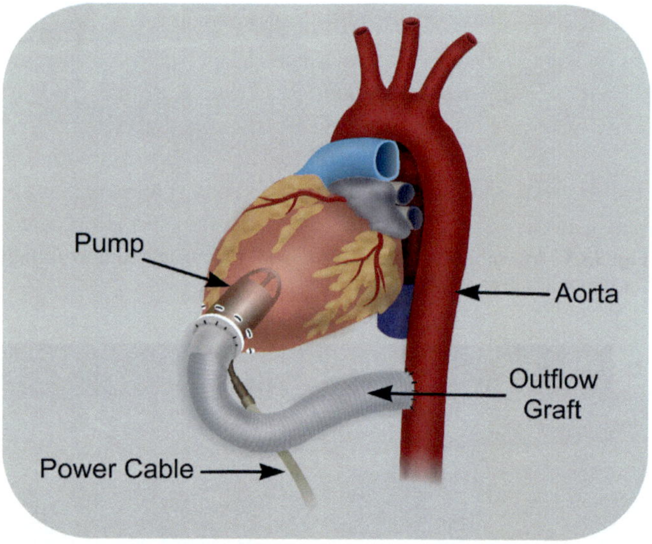

Fig. 33.4 This illustration shows the Jarvik 2000 LVAD implanted in a patient with advanced heart failure. The device is positioned in the left ventricular apex and connected to the aorta via an outflow graft, providing circulatory support

enhanced survival rates among patients by 15% and provided a self-reported improvement in quality of life.

The third-generation LVAD has been further improved to decrease reoperations and thrombotic events. The HeartMate III (Abbott, Lake Bluff, IL) (Fig. 33.6), in particular, uses a centrifugal continuous-flow pump with magnetic levitation and rotor balancing to enable a non-contact mechanism with the flowing blood. Combined with large blood-filled gaps, this technology decreases heat formation, friction, reducing the possibility of thrombus formation. Additionally, oscillations in the speed of the blood flow are used to produce an artificial pulse rate of 30 beats per minute. Another third-generation LVAD enrolled in non-inferior trials to HeartMate III is the EVAHEART 2 (Sun Medical Technology Research, Nagano, Japan) (Fig. 33.7). It features a centrifugal pump with a hydraulically levitated impeller and a Double Cuff Tipless (DCT) inflow cannula. The goal of this design is to decrease thrombotic events and allow for broader angles of insertion into the LV.

Indications for LVAD Therapy

Patients with HFrEF, primarily due to LV systolic dysfunction, who are unresponsive to optimal medical therapy, are candidates for LVAD implantation. The 14th Annual Report from the Society of Thoracic Surgeons (STS) Interagency Registry for Mechanically Assisted Circulatory Support (INTERMACS) Registry details outcomes for 27,493 patients who received continuous-flow LVADs between 2013 and 2022, highlighting the growing use and impact of this therapy.

The INTERMACS scale classifies the severity of HF into seven levels:

1. *Level 1*: Severe cardiogenic shock.
2. *Level 2*: On inotropes with stable blood pressure but progressive decline.
3. *Level 3*: Hemodynamic stability but inotrope-dependent.
4. *Level 4*: Recurrent signs of congestion (advanced HF).
5. *Level 5*: Exertion intolerant and complete cessation of physical activity.

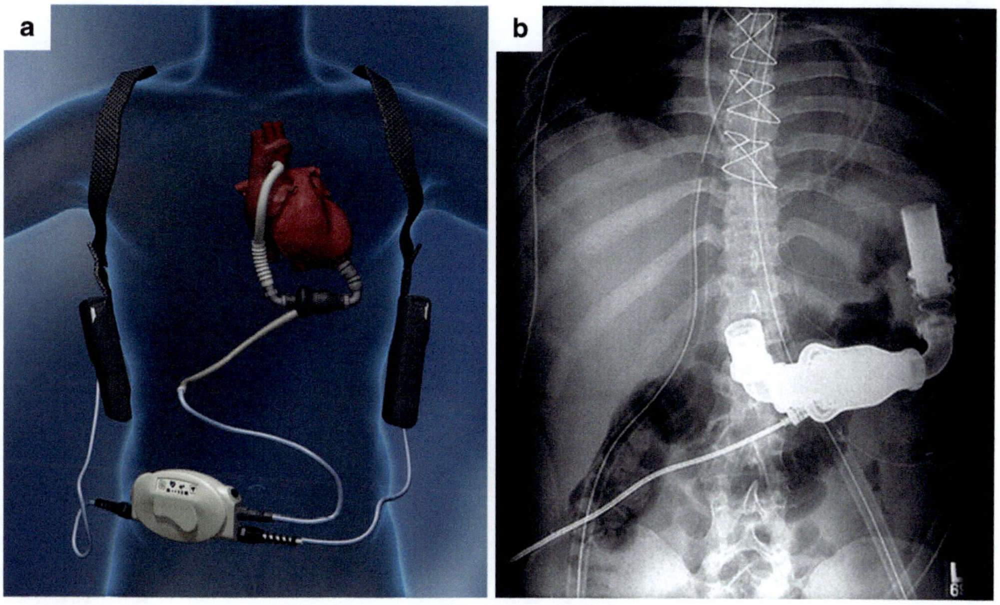

Fig. 33.5 (**a**) Diagram highlighting the parts of an implanted HeartMate II (**b**) X-ray of an implanted HeartMate II (Rodriguez et al. 2013)

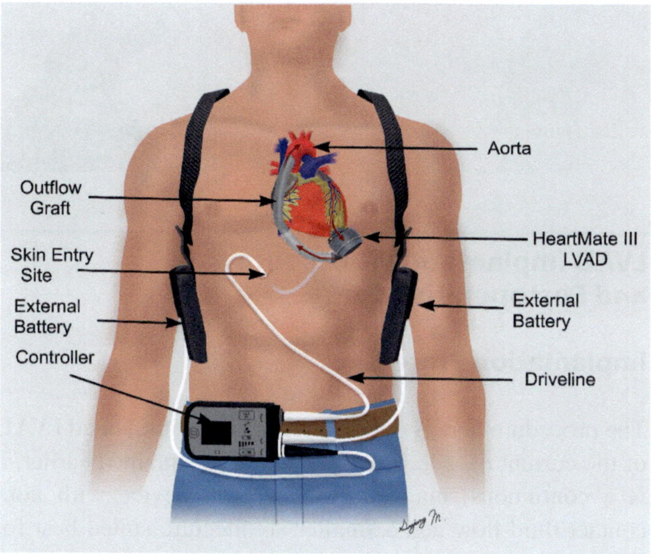

Fig. 33.6 This diagram illustrates the key components of an implanted HeartMate III LVAD system. Highlighted parts include the controller, driveline, and external battery, which provide power and control to the device. The LVAD itself is connected to the left ventricle (LV) with an outflow graft attached to the aorta for blood flow support. Also shown is the percutaneous cable with its skin entry site, which connects the internal and external components

6. *Level 6*: Limitation on physical activity.
7. *Level 7*: Recompensated HF, no current or recent signs of congestion.

The INTERMACS scale, classifying HF severity from 1 (most critical) to 7, guides MCS decisions. Generally, levels 1–4, corresponding to NYHA Class IV, are considered indications for MCS. The choice between LVAD or biventricular support (BVAD or TAH) depends on the specific type and severity of HF:

- *Severe Cardiogenic Shock (INTERMACS Level 1)*: Requires BVAD or TAH.
- *Primary Left Ventricular Failure (INTERMACS Levels 2–4)*: LVAD is usually sufficient.
- *Imminent Right Ventricular (RV) Failure*: May require additional temporary or permanent RV support, potentially with an implantable BVAD.

Purposes for LVAD Implantation

- *BTT*: For patients who are eligible for a heart transplant, but a compatible heart is unavailable, while the heart function continues to worsen, resulting in end-organ hypoperfusion and subsequent hypoxic damage.
- *BTR*: Less common practice where a patient receiving extended MCS via an LVAD implantation has shown improvements in myocyte histology and biochemistry, as well as LV morphology, physiology, and hemodynamics.
- *BTD*: Temporary support while evaluating a patient's suitability for longer term therapies like transplantation or assessing potential for heart recovery. It can also be used to address transplant contraindications like renal hypoperfusion, pulmonary hypertension, or nutritional deficiencies.
- *DT*: This is a permanent solution for patients who are not eligible for a heart transplant due to absolute contraindications.

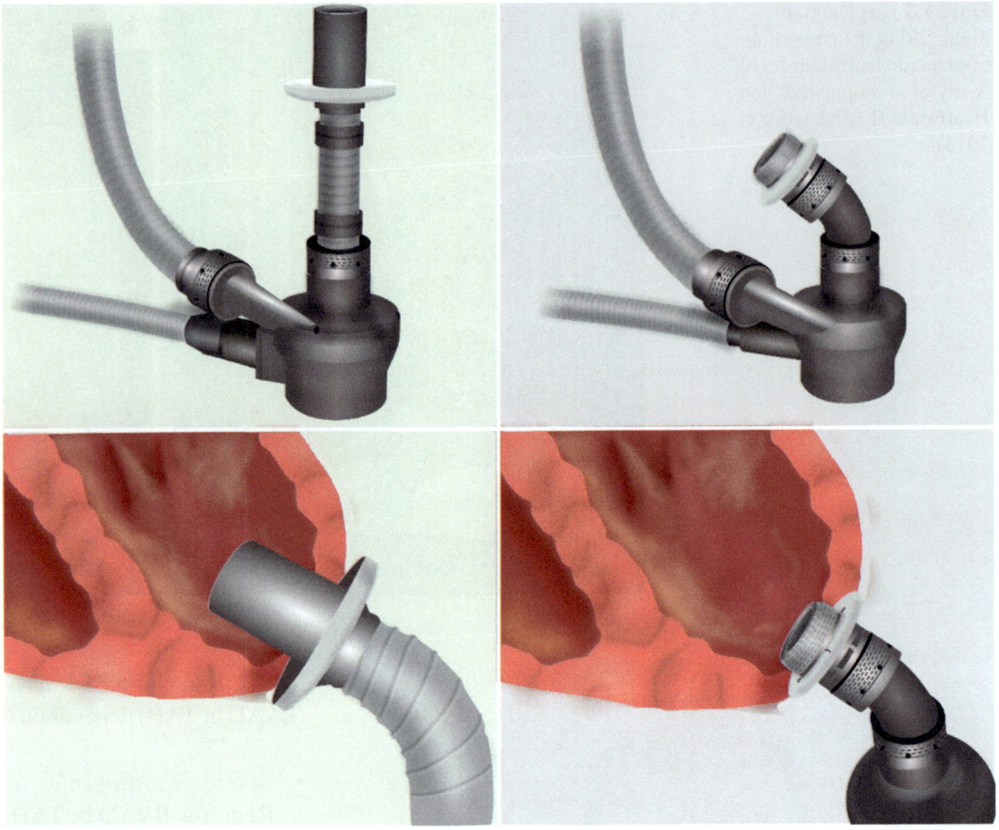

Fig. 33.7 This figure illustrates a side-by-side comparison of the EVAHEART 1 (left) and EVAHEART 2 (right) LVADs. The most notable difference is the redesigned inflow cannula in EVAHEART 2, which features a DCT design. This innovative feature offers advantages by reducing thrombotic events and allowing for broader angles of insertion into the LV

Patient Selection for LVAD Implantation

Patients with advanced HF, characterized by LV EF of less than 25%, New York Heart Association functional class IIIB-IV, on continuous inotropic or vasopressor medications, end-organ hypoperfusion, or with temporary MCS devices, are eligible for an LVAD as discussed earlier.

Preoperative measures for LVADs are as important as the implantation itself. The patient must be involved in their care around the clock, so patient candidacy is determined with input from the patient, family members, and a multidisciplinary healthcare team. This team includes, but is not limited to, surgeons, HF cardiologists, cardiac anesthesiologists, perfusionists, advanced nurse practitioners, pharmacists, nutritionists, social workers, and consulting physicians. Once eligibility is established, education and counseling sessions are held with the patient and family to assess their willingness and ability to contribute to the postoperative success of the implantation. The patient needs to be monitored for infections at the driveline exit site, worsening HF, and emergency situations.

LVAD Implantation Procedure and Postoperative Care

Implantation Procedure

The procedure here is outlined for the most implanted LVAD of the current decade, HeartMate III. As explained earlier, it is a continuous, magnetically levitated device with non-contact fluid flow and a smaller architecture suited best for intrapericardial implantations.

Exposure and Preparation

- The exposure of the LV is achieved traditionally via a medial sternotomy.
- The pericardium is cleared of fat and adventitial tissue, then excised infero-laterally around the apex of the heart. The pericardium on the right is used to cover the outflow graft for potential sternal re-entry for eventual transplant.
- The pericardium is generously divided to avoid any device constriction by its margin, and the left pleural space is

also accessed for eventual seating of the pump. Device assembly is being conducted simultaneously by a perfusionist team, and the device is handed to the surgeons wrapped in two antibiotic-laden pads.

Driveline Tunneling

- Before heparinization, an incision is made in the posterior rectus sheath, a few centimeters away from the midline towards the left for tunneling of the driveline into the pericardium. The distance from midline helps establish safer re-entry for future heart transplant and allows for minimization of tension on the line as it leaves the pericardium.
- The cutaneous exit is about 3 cm below the right costal margin, medial to the axillary line. This enables the patient to wear the device without interference and effectively monitor and disinfect the driveline site.
- A circular knife is utilized to make an incision on the skin, and a tunneling device is passed through to the pericardium. The driveline is screwed onto it allowing the gentle withdrawal to outside the skin.

Heparinization

Heparin is initially avoided to prevent rectus sheath hematomas and is administered once the driveline site is ready.

CPB Establishment

- CPB is established via aortic and right atrial appendage cannulation.
- Bicaval venous cannulation is undertaken if tricuspid or mitral valve surgery is required or if a patent foramen ovale needs to be repaired.
- Non-pledgetted polypropylene sutures are used to reduce adhesions and prepare for potential future access, and CPB is initiated after the activated clotting time is satisfactory.
- Immediately after commencing CPB, the left atrial appendage (LAA) is occluded via a clip or ligation to prevent strokes, with apixaban given post-operatively for anticoagulation. LAA occlusion has proven to be an effective way to prevent strokes in cardiac surgery patients.

Inflow Cannula Preparation

- Multiple lap pads are placed under the heart and marque structures, such as the left anterior descending (LAD) artery and the true LV apex, are identified to choose the best site for the inflow cannula placement.
- The inflow cannula needs to be positioned at the LV apex, directed towards the mitral valve annulus, and be parallel to the interventricular septum to prevent the inflow cannula from acting as a nidus for thrombus formation. Approximation of this site is usually 2.5 cm above the cardiac apex and 2.5 cm lateral to the LAD.
- An apical cuff is sewn onto the LV before coring is performed, using 2–0 Ethibond sutures with large pledgets in an interrupted, horizontal mattress fashion. Initially, four sutures are placed in a clockwise manner, 90 degrees apart from each other, and then 1–2 additional sutures are placed in each quadrant, ensuring a proper seal. Full-thickness bites, along with a gentle technique following the curve of the suture needle, are needed to prevent unnecessary bleeding. Sutures are now passed through the outer half of the apical cuff to prevent piling of the cuff onto the heart tissue. Interrupted pledgetted technique is sufficient to provide complete hemostasis, thus removing the need for a second continuous suture layer.
- A heavy silk suture is placed in the center of the apical cuff to serve as the handle to lift the muscle as the coring device performs its function. This avoids losing the muscle inside the ventricle. Prior to coring, the patient is positioned in Trendelenburg, and the perfusionist empties the heart incompletely (Fig. 33.8).

Pump and Outflow Graft Placement

- The pump with the outflow graft is de-aired using normal saline. The inflow cannula is positioned onto the apical cuff while the outflow graft and driveline are placed inferior to the acute margin of the heart to ensure appropriate pump mechanics and safer access to the heart for the future (Fig. 33.9).
- Lap pads are now removed to return the heart to its anatomical position, and a transesophageal echocardiogram (TEE) is used to verify the position of the inflow cannula.
- The outflow graft is sized accurately to avoid right ventricle constriction or injury during reoperation, if too short, and prevent kinking or LVAD dysfunction, if too long. This is achieved by partial filling of the LV. Distal vascular clamp is applied to the graft while a side-biting clamp is applied to the greater curvature of the ascending aorta. An aortotomy is performed to accommodate the 14 mm diameter outflow graft of the HeartMate III graft, to aorta anastomosis is completed in an end-to-side manner using running 5-0 polypropylene. Vascular clamp on the graft and side-biting clamp on the aorta are released and reapplied to de-air the construct.

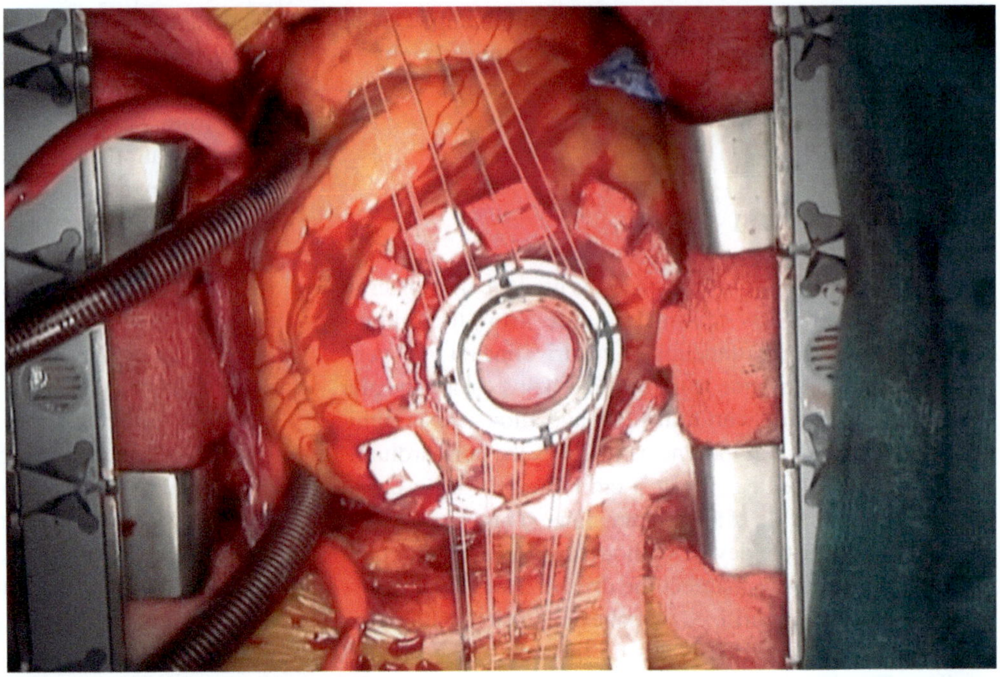

Fig. 33.8 Sewing ring of the HeartMate III on the LV apex

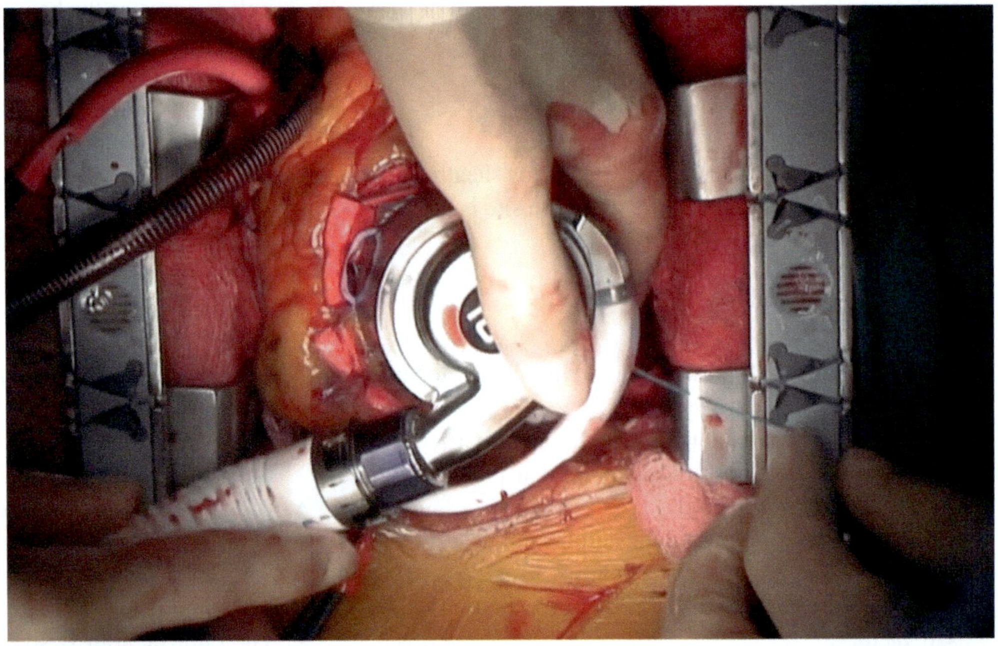

Fig. 33.9 HeartMate III pump secured to the sewing ring

Intra-Operative Management, De-Airing and Wean from CPB

The intra-operative management of LVAD patients follows a structured protocol to support hemodynamic stability and optimize RV function.

- *De-airing and weaning from CPB*: Initiate de-airing and weaning by placing an aortic root vent in the ascending aorta and inserting an 18-gauge needle in the outflow graft, just proximal to the vascular clamp.
- *Inhaled Pulmonary Vasodilators*: Inhaled epoprostenol or nitric oxide is administered in all cases to support pulmonary vasodilation.
- *Inopressors*: Intravenous (IV) infusion of dobutamine, levophed, milrinone, and vasopressin are the preferred inopressors. Dobutamine is favored over epinephrine to avoid lactate buildup, thus preventing unnecessary volume resuscitation. Epinephrine is avoided where possible to reduce potential increases in pulmonary vascular resistance (PVR), especially at high doses. Typically, a dose of 5 μg/kg/min of dobutamine suffices for most patients.

- *LVAD Activation*: The driveline is connected to the LVAD device, and the pump is initiated at its lowest speed of 3000 revolutions per minute (rpm). This facilitates de-airing, and the process continues till complete separation from CPB. The speed is then sequentially increased in 200–400 rpm increments until the LVAD achieves a flow rate of 4.6–5.0 liters per minute.
- *Mean Arterial Pressure (MAP)*: Maintain MAP at 80 mmHg during CPB separation to promote LVAD flow and prevent left ventricular outflow tract (LVOT) collapse and septal shift, which may lead to RV failure. After verifying hemodynamic stability and absence of air via TEE, the aortic root vent is removed, and the patient is decannulated. Protamine is given to reverse heparinization.
  - *Vasoplegia Management*: Routinely administer methylene blue and Cyano-Kit (B12) to manage post-pump vasoplegia.
- *Pacing*: For patients with an ICD or permanent pacemaker (PPM), cardiology should interrogate and adjust pacing to 90 bpm to support the RV. Otherwise, place a temporary pacing wire.
- *Ventilation management*: During CPB, continue low tidal volume ventilation to decrease PVR and reduce afterload on the RV when separating from CPB. After separation from bypass, aim for a $PaCO_2$ level below 40 mmHg to alleviate RV strain.
- *RV TEE Evaluation*: Use a transgastric short-axis echocardiographic view to confirm a circular septal shape. Avoid "D-shaped" septal flattening or LV bowing, which indicates RV pressure/volume overload. This overload can lead to acute RV failure, and compression of the LV cavity may impede diastolic filling and result in systemic hypotension and hemodynamic instability.
- *Temperature Management*: Maintain normothermia to reduce bleeding risks. Use upper and lower body warming devices and warm the operating room.
- *Diuretics*: Administer Lasix or Bumex intraoperatively or shortly after CPB separation to manage RV preload.
- *Decannulation and Heparin Reversal*: After confirming hemodynamic stability and the absence of air via TEE, remove the aortic root vent, decannulate the patient, and administer protamine to reverse heparinization.

Final Steps

- The bend relief portion of the outflow tract is wrapped in a Gore-Tex membrane to minimize adhesions to the right ventricle and the sternum. Loose application of the membrane is needed to prevent seroma formation between the graft and Gore-Tex. Sutures are placed to fixate the driveline in its intended position.
- Three chest tubes are placed: left pleural space, retrocardiac, and retrosternal. The cut pericardium is draped over the outflow graft and driveline.
- The sternum is closed, and a 5-0 subcuticular polypropylene suture is used in a purse-string fashion to cause skin apposition. Further anchoring is achieved 6–8 cm beyond the driveline exit with 3-0 polypropylene sutures to decrease jerking at the exit site.

Postoperative Care

- Given the RV's sensitivity to positive pressure and sedation-related vasodilation, aim to extubate patients the same day as surgery whenever possible.
- Post-operative monitoring includes checking for infections at the driveline exit site, managing HF symptoms, and preparing for emergencies.
- Education and counseling sessions are provided to the patient and family to ensure their understanding and commitment to post-operative care.

Management of Complications Associated with LVAD Implantation

Post-LVAD implantations can result in certain complications that can be classified as early (within 30 days) or late (beyond 30 days), with higher frequencies noted in pulsatile compared to continuous-flow devices. This section will highlight the most prevalent complications.

Early Complications

Bleeding

Bleeding is the most common complication following LVAD implantation. It is monitored by evaluating hemodynamic variables, hemoglobin levels, and chest tube output (>200 cc per hour). With the improvement in technology of continuous-flow LVADs, bleeding events are declining, but still occur. Management depends on whether the bleeding is surgical or due to coagulopathy, monitored via PT, PTT, platelet counts/function, and thromboelastogram. Treatment includes red cells, platelets, fresh frozen plasma, cryoprecipitate, or prothrombin complex concentrates.

Neurological Complications

While uncommon, both hemorrhagic and ischemic strokes are devastating complications in VAD patients. Hemorrhagic strokes are often linked to aggressive anticoagulation, while ischemic strokes arise from thromboembolic events. The

LVAD's artificial surfaces and turbulent flow can promote clot formation, further exacerbated by suboptimal blood pressure control and inadequate anticoagulation. Notably, stroke rates are similar between pulsatile and continuous-flow LVADs.

For managing hemorrhagic stroke, immediately address the bleeding source, reverse anticoagulation, monitor neurological status, and use imaging to assess the extent of bleeding.

For ischemic stroke, evaluate thrombolysis eligibility, consider alternative anticoagulants or antiplatelet therapies, and provide supportive care with closely monitoring neurological status.

Preventive measures include optimizing anticoagulation to balance bleeding and thrombotic risks, regular monitoring of blood pressure and coagulation parameters, and educating patients to recognize stroke symptoms and seek immediate medical attention.

Cardiac Arrhythmias

Cardiac arrhythmias, both atrial (e.g., atrial fibrillation, flutter) and ventricular (e.g., ventricular tachycardia, fibrillation), are common in patients with VADs. While ventricular arrhythmias may not always be fatal, they can strain the right ventricle, which can further exacerbate arrhythmias. Syncope (fainting) can also be a concerning symptom of underlying ventricular arrhythmia.

Managing arrhythmias in LVAD patients requires a multidisciplinary approach. Early identification through continuous ECG monitoring and clinical assessment is critical. Medical therapy optimization, including antiarrhythmics and anticoagulants, is tailored to the patient's condition. Catheter ablation may correct certain arrhythmias, and adjusting LVAD settings can improve hemodynamics. Right ventricular support, such as inotropes or temporary RVADs, is necessary for related dysfunction. Addressing underlying causes like electrolyte imbalances, ischemia, or infections is essential for effective management.

Infections

Infections are another common morbidity. Commonly, the infection begins at the driveline site and can progress to pneumonia or sepsis. Pocket infections and pump internal infections are rare occurrences. Skin organisms, such as Staphylococcus, Corynebacterium, Pseudomonas, Enterobacteriaceae, and Candida, are the most frequent culprits. Recommended prophylactic antibiotic therapy includes the use of a beta-lactam or vancomycin, along with topical mupirocin and antifungal gels at the driveline sites post-operation. If early signs of infection, such as inflammation or drainage, are detected, more rigorous empiric antibiotic therapy should be started. Although no standard therapy is established, a 10-day regiment of ciprofloxacin 500 mg BID and doxycycline 100 mg PO BID has been used successfully. Additionally, the driveline site should be cultured to modulate antibiotic therapy.

Suction Events in LVADs

Suction events occur when the LV wall gets "sucked" onto the inflow cannula of the LVAD, triggering an alarm and reduced pump speed. This is usually caused by low LV volume due to factors like right ventricular failure or tamponade. Suction events can lead to reduced LVAD flow and ventricular arrhythmias. It's crucial to address the underlying cause and optimize LV filling to prevent these events.

End-Organ Failure

Despite often improving after VAD implantation, renal and hepatic failure can occur in patients with underlying organ dysfunction, right ventricular failure, malnutrition, infection, or exposure to nephrotoxic and hepatotoxic drugs. These complications negatively impact outcomes in VAD-supported patients.

Managing end-organ failure in VAD patients requires a comprehensive approach. It involves identifying and addressing underlying causes, like infections and optimizing right ventricular function. Nutritional support with adequate caloric and protein intake is essential. Medication adjustments to minimize nephrotoxic or hepatotoxic exposure are crucial. For severe renal dysfunction, diuretics or renal replacement therapy may be necessary. A multidisciplinary team, including nephrologists, hepatologists, and dieticians, ensures comprehensive care. Early intervention and a collaborative approach are vital for improving patient outcomes.

Late Complications

Gastrointestinal (GI) Bleeding

GI bleeding can occur due to angiodysplasia from increased intraluminal pressure and sheer stress, or acquired von Willebrand syndrome (AvWS). AvWS results from the LVAD pump's mechanics, causing cleavage of von Willebrand factor (vWF) into smaller non-functional multimers, impairing platelet adhesion and clot formation. Using a high-pulsatile index can reduce non-surgical bleeding instances.

Thrombotic Events

Thrombotic events are usually due to device-related factors. Second-generation LVADs, which use axial flow pumps, produce higher shear stress and hemolysis than centrifugal rotors, leading to thrombus formation on the rotor or inflow bearing. Heat generated by the fast-moving rotors can also contribute to thrombus formation. Third-generation LVADs have fewer contact points because they utilize magnetically levitated rotors that spin centrifugally to achieve the same physiological cardiac flow, thereby reducing the incidence of thrombotic events.

Aortic Valve Degeneration

In patients with continuous-flow LVADs, the aortic valve often remains closed, exposing it to continuous high pressure. This can accelerate valve degeneration and lead to aortic regurgitation. Management strategies include regular echocardiograms are essential to assess valve function. For severe aortic regurgitation, surgical intervention such as aortic valve replacement (bioprosthetic or mechanical) is recommended if the patient is a suitable candidate. For high-risk surgical patients, Transcatheter Aortic Valve Replacement (TAVR) is a less invasive option. Emerging therapies are also being researched to develop new, minimally invasive approaches for valve replacement in LVAD patients.

Outcomes and Long-Term Survival with LVADs

The MOMENTUM 3 study demonstrated that superior outcomes with HeartMate III implantation compared to HeartMate II, including a lower incidence of disabling strokes or reoperation to replace/remove the device at the 2-year mark. Additionally, higher survival rates were reported in patients with HeartMate III at the 2-year mark and beyond. Patients also reported substantial improvements in their quality of life because they experienced reduced HF symptoms and an enhanced ability to perform activities of daily living (ADLs). Conclusively, HeartMate III has proven to be the most effective iteration of the LVAD so far.

Further Reading

Acharya MN, Som R, Tsui S. What is the optimum antibiotic prophylaxis in patients undergoing implantation of a left ventricular assist device? Interact Cardiovasc Thorac Surg. 2012;14(2):209–14. https://doi.org/10.1093/icvts/ivr054.

Birks EJ. Left ventricular assist devices. Heart. 2010;96(1):63–71. https://doi.org/10.1136/hrt.2007.130740.

Birks EJ. Molecular changes after left ventricular assist device support for heart failure. Circ Res. 2013;113(6):777–91. https://doi.org/10.1161/CIRCRESAHA.113.301413.

Birschmann I, Dittrich M, Eller T, Wiegmann B, Reininger AJ, Budde U, et al. Ambient hemolysis and activation of coagulation is different between HeartMate II and HeartWare left ventricular assist devices. J Heart Lung Transplant. 2014;33(1):80–7. https://doi.org/10.1016/j.healun.2013.11.010.

Capoccia M. Mechanical circulatory support for advanced heart failure: are we about to witness a new "gold standard"? J Cardiovasc Dev Dis. 2016;3(4) https://doi.org/10.3390/jcdd3040035.

Chatterjee A, Feldmann C, Hanke JS, Ricklefs M, Shrestha M, Dogan G, et al. The momentum of HeartMate 3: a novel active magnetically levitated centrifugal left ventricular assist device (LVAD). J Thorac Dis. 2018;10(Suppl 15):S1790–S3. https://doi.org/10.21037/jtd.2017.10.124.

DeBakey ME. Left ventricular bypass pump for cardiac assistance. Clinical experience. Am J Cardiol. 1971;27(1):3–11. https://doi.org/10.1016/0002-9149(71)90076-2.

Englert JA 3rd, Davis JA, Krim SR. Mechanical circulatory support for the failing heart: continuous-flow left ventricular assist devices. Ochsner J. 2016;16(3):263–9.

Fang P, Du J, Boraschi A, Bozzi S, Redaelli A, Schmid Daners M, et al. Insights into the low rate of in-pump thrombosis with the HeartMate 3: does the artificial pulse improve washout? Front Cardiovasc Med. 2022;9:775780. https://doi.org/10.3389/fcvm.2022.775780.

Frazier OH, Myers TJ, Gregoric ID, Khan T, Delgado R, Croitoru M, et al. Initial clinical experience with the Jarvik 2000 implantable axial-flow left ventricular assist system. Circulation. 2002;105(24):2855–60. https://doi.org/10.1161/01.cir.0000018167.47314.af.

Haglund NA, Davis ME, Tricarico NM, Keebler ME, Maltais S. Readmissions after continuous flow left ventricular assist device implantation: differences observed between two contemporary device types. ASAIO J. 2015;61(4):410–6. https://doi.org/10.1097/MAT.0000000000000218.

Hall JL, Fermin DR, Birks EJ, Barton PJ, Slaughter M, Eckman P, et al. Clinical, molecular, and genomic changes in response to a left ventricular assist device. J Am Coll Cardiol. 2011;57(6):641–52. https://doi.org/10.1016/j.jacc.2010.11.010.

Health Quality O. Left ventricular assist devices for destination therapy: a Health technology assessment. Ont Health Technol Assess Ser. 2016;16(3):1–60.

Holley CT, Harvey L, John R. Left ventricular assist devices as a bridge to cardiac transplantation. J Thorac Dis. 2014;6(8):1110–9. https://doi.org/10.3978/j.issn.2072-1439.2014.06.46.

Kannojiya V, Das AK, Das PK. Comparative assessment of different versions of axial and centrifugal LVADs: a review. Artif Organs. 2021;45(7):665–81. https://doi.org/10.1111/aor.13914.

Kato N, Jaarsma T, Ben Gal T. Learning self-care after left ventricular assist device implantation. Curr Heart Fail Rep. 2014;11(3):290–8. https://doi.org/10.1007/s11897-014-0201-0.

Kato NP, Melnikov S, Denfeld QE, Casida J, Stromberg A, Ben-Gal T, et al. Validity and reliability of the left ventricular assist device self-care behaviour scale. PLoS One. 2023;18(2):e0275465. https://doi.org/10.1371/journal.pone.0275465.

Leuck AM. Left ventricular assist device driveline infections: recent advances and future goals. J Thorac Dis. 2015;7(12):2151–7. https://doi.org/10.3978/j.issn.2072-1439.2015.11.06.

Liotta D. Early clinical application of assisted circulation. Tex Heart Inst J. 2002;29(3):229–30.

Loforte A, Gliozzi G, Mariani C, Cavalli GG, Martin-Suarez S, Pacini D. Ventricular assist devices implantation: surgical assessment and technical strategies. Cardiovasc Diagn Ther. 2021;11(1):277–91. https://doi.org/10.21037/cdt-20-325.

May-Newman K, Montes R, Campos J, Marquez-Maya N, Vu V, Zebrowski E, et al. Reducing regional flow stasis and improving intraventricular hemodynamics with a tipless inflow cannula design: an in vitro flow visualization study using the EVAHEART LVAD. Artif Organs. 2019;43(9):834–48. https://doi.org/10.1111/aor.13477.

Mehra MR, Uriel N, Naka Y, Cleveland JC Jr, Yuzefpolskaya M, Salerno CT, et al. A fully magnetically levitated left ventricular assist device – final report. N Engl J Med. 2019;380(17):1618–27. https://doi.org/10.1056/NEJMoa1900486.

Molina EJ, Shah P, Kiernan MS, Cornwell WK 3rd, Copeland H, Takeda K, et al. The Society of Thoracic Surgeons Intermacs 2020 annual report. Ann Thorac Surg. 2021;111(3):778–92. https://doi.org/10.1016/j.athoracsur.2020.12.038.

Patel SR, Vukelic S, Chinnadurai T, Madan S, Sibinga N, Kwah J, et al. Gastrointestinal angiodysplasia in heart failure and during

CF LVAD support. J Heart Lung Transplant. 2022;41(2):129–32. https://doi.org/10.1016/j.healun.2021.11.009.

Potapov EV, Antonides C, Crespo-Leiro MG, Combes A, Farber G, Hannan MM, et al. 2019 EACTS expert consensus on long-term mechanical circulatory support. Eur J Cardiothorac Surg. 2019;56(2):230–70. https://doi.org/10.1093/ejcts/ezz098.

Rauch A, Susen S, Zieger B. Acquired von Willebrand syndrome in patients with ventricular assist device. Front Med (Lausanne). 2019;6:7. https://doi.org/10.3389/fmed.2019.00007.

Rodriguez LE, Suarez EE, Loebe M, Bruckner BA. General surgery considerations in the era of mechanical circulatory assist devices. Surg Clin North Am. 2013;93(6):1343–57. https://doi.org/10.1016/j.suc.2013.08.004.

Rose EA, Gelijns AC, Moskowitz AJ, Heitjan DF, Stevenson LW, Dembitsky W, et al. Long-term use of a left ventricular assist device for end-stage heart failure. N Engl J Med. 2001;345(20):1435–43. https://doi.org/10.1056/NEJMoa012175.

Slater JP, Rose EA, Levin HR, Frazier OH, Roberts JK, Weinberg AD, et al. Low thromboembolic risk without anticoagulation using advanced-design left ventricular assist devices. Ann Thorac Surg. 1996;62(5):1321–7.; discussion 8. https://doi.org/10.1016/0003-4975(96)00750-3.

Slaughter MS, Rogers JG, Milano CA, Russell SD, Conte JV, Feldman D, et al. Advanced heart failure treated with continuous-flow left ventricular assist device. N Engl J Med. 2009;361(23):2241–51. https://doi.org/10.1056/NEJMoa0909938.

Starnes VA, Oyer PE, Portner PM, Ramasamy N, Miller PJ, Stinson EB, et al. Isolated left ventricular assist as bridge to cardiac transplantation. J Thorac Cardiovasc Surg. 1988;96(1):62–71.

Symalla T, Jeevanandam V. Choosing the appropriate left ventricular assist device for your patient. Indian J Thorac Cardiovasc Surg. 2020;36(Suppl 2):256–64. https://doi.org/10.1007/s12055-019-00890-3.

Takayama H, Soni L, Kalesan B, Truby LK, Ota T, Cedola S, et al. Bridge-to-decision therapy with a continuous-flow external ventricular assist device in refractory cardiogenic shock of various causes. Circ Heart Fail. 2014;7(5):799–806. https://doi.org/10.1161/CIRCHEARTFAILURE.113.000271.

Uriel N, Han J, Morrison KA, Nahumi N, Yuzefpolskaya M, Garan AR, et al. Device thrombosis in HeartMate II continuous-flow left ventricular assist devices: a multifactorial phenomenon. J Heart Lung Transplant. 2014;33(1):51–9. https://doi.org/10.1016/j.healun.2013.10.005.

Wever-Pinzon O, Selzman CH, Drakos SG, Saidi A, Stoddard GJ, Gilbert EM, et al. Pulsatility and the risk of nonsurgical bleeding in patients supported with the continuous-flow left ventricular assist device HeartMate II. Circ Heart Fail. 2013;6(3):517–26. https://doi.org/10.1161/CIRCHEARTFAILURE.112.000206.

Whitlock RP, Belley-Cote EP, Paparella D, Healey JS, Brady K, Sharma M, et al. Left atrial appendage occlusion during cardiac surgery to prevent stroke. N Engl J Med. 2021;384(22):2081–91. https://doi.org/10.1056/NEJMoa2101897.

Extracorporeal Membrane Oxygenation

34

Aneeta Bhatia, Aaron Buckley, and Jiapeng Huang

"We are there to throw them a lifeline."

A rescue story about ECMO on University of Minnesota's series on 'Where Discovery Creates Hope.'

Introduction

Extracorporeal membrane oxygenation (ECMO) has grown exponentially as the mainstream modality for advanced life support in patients with severe respiratory failure or refractory cardiogenic shock. Technological advances in circuit design, ease of cannulation, and the ability to deploy ECMO in emergencies have paved the way for its widespread use. More recently, a new era is unfolding with the novel use of perioperative ECMO for complex thoracic and cardiac procedures, allowing patients who were previously relegated to conservative management an opportunity for a surgical option toward a better outcome. According to the Extracorporeal Life Support Organization (ELSO) registry, through 2023, ECMO has been utilized on 219,301 patients, including 50,070 neonates, 39,094 children, and 130,137 adults (Fig. 34.1).

A. Bhatia (✉)
Department of Anesthesiology and Perioperative Medicine, University of Louisville Health, Louisville, KY, USA
e-mail: aneeta.bhatia@uoflhealth.org

A. Buckley
School of Medicine, University of Louisville, Louisville, KY, USA
e-mail: aaron.buckley@louisville.edu

J. Huang
Department of Anesthesiology and Perioperative Medicine, University of Louisville, Louisville, KY, USA
e-mail: jiapeng.huang@louisville.edu

A. S. Awad, J. DiNardo (eds.), *Clinical Perfusion for Cardiac Surgery*, https://doi.org/10.1007/978-3-031-91163-7_34

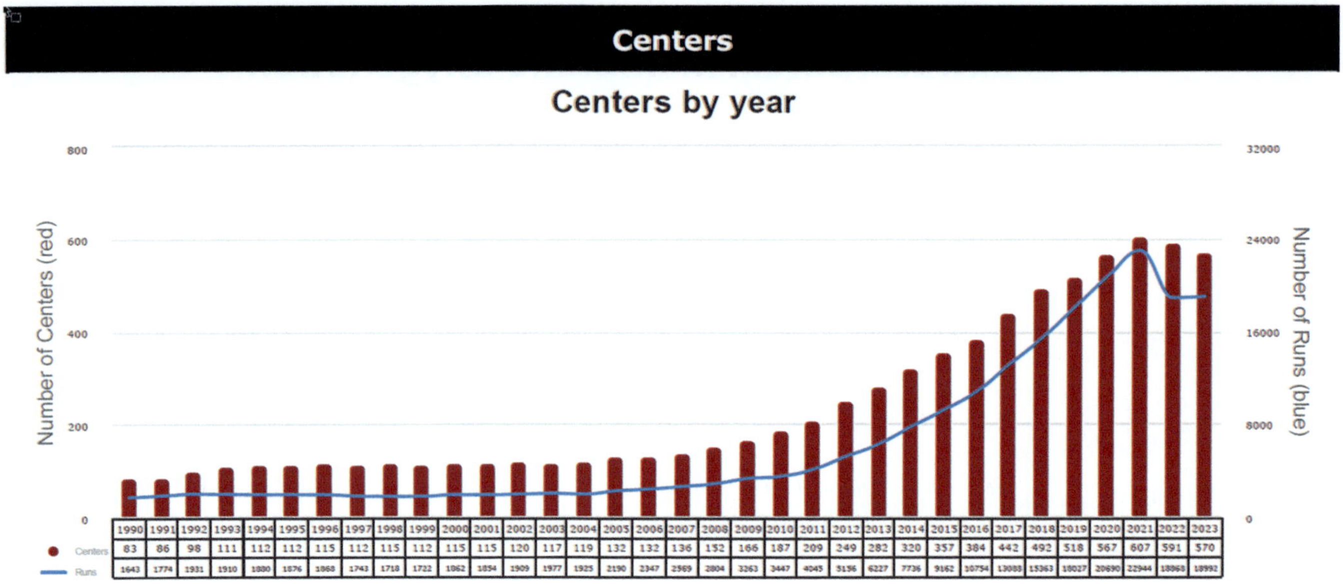

Fig. 34.1 Extracorporeal Life Support Organization's (ELSO) centers and runs of Extracorporeal Membrane Oxygenation per year up to 2023 in the ELSO Registry

History of ECMO

Almost 50 years ago, Robert Bartlett, known as the "Father of ECMO," developed a prototype heart-lung machine. In 1976, the Bartlett team reported the first successful neonatal ECMO survivor, a patient who received 3 days of ECMO support for respiratory failure secondary to meconium aspiration. The CESAR trial (conventional ventilator support vs Extracorporeal Membrane Oxygenation for severe adult respiratory failure) demonstrated a great benefit of ECMO for treating adult respiratory distress syndrome (ARDS) in adults. In 2000, Bartlett reported the world's largest single-institution series of 1000 consecutive patients successfully treated with extracorporeal life support (ECLS) between 1980 and 1998. Despite these successes, challenges remained in the early days of ECMO regarding pump and oxygenator design, activation of coagulation factors, and biocompatibility of tubing circuitry. Decades of innovations, coupled with publicized successful outcomes, have propelled ECMO to the forefront, not only as a first-line rescue option for severe cardiopulmonary disease but also as a successful perioperative option for hemodynamic and/or airway support during complex, high-risk surgical procedures.

Principles of ECMO

The primary objective of ECMO is to serve as a bridge, providing temporary circulatory and/or respiratory support during refractory cardiopulmonary failure. ECMO does not address and treat the underlying causes of the patient's condition, but instead, provides a temporary solution until recovery or a decision regarding long-term support options, such as a durable left ventricular assist device (LVAD). In cases of end-stage heart or lung disease, ECMO can bridge patients to transplantation decisions. While not a destination therapy in itself, ECMO's use is expanding to include perioperative support for complex cardiac and thoracic surgeries. By providing hemodynamic stability and acting as an artificial lung, ECMO allows surgeons to undertake procedures previously considered high-risk or even impossible.

Components of the ECMO Circuit

An ECMO circuit consists of several key components: cannulae, tubing, a membrane oxygenator, a heat exchanger, a gas blender, and a centrifugal pump (Fig. 34.2). The circuit operates by draining deoxygenated blood from the venous system, pumping it through the oxygenator, and then returning it to the patient's circulation.

Cannulation Plastic cannulae are placed in large veins or arteries in the groins, neck, or chest cavity of the patient. ECMO cannulae are named based on their relationship to the pump rather than to the patient. "Inflow" cannulae transport blood toward the pump, while "outflow" cannulae carry blood away from the pump. In simpler terms, the inflow cannula draws venous blood with high carbon dioxide (CO_2) and low oxygen (O_2) content into the circuit, and the outflow cannula returns oxygenated blood to the patient.

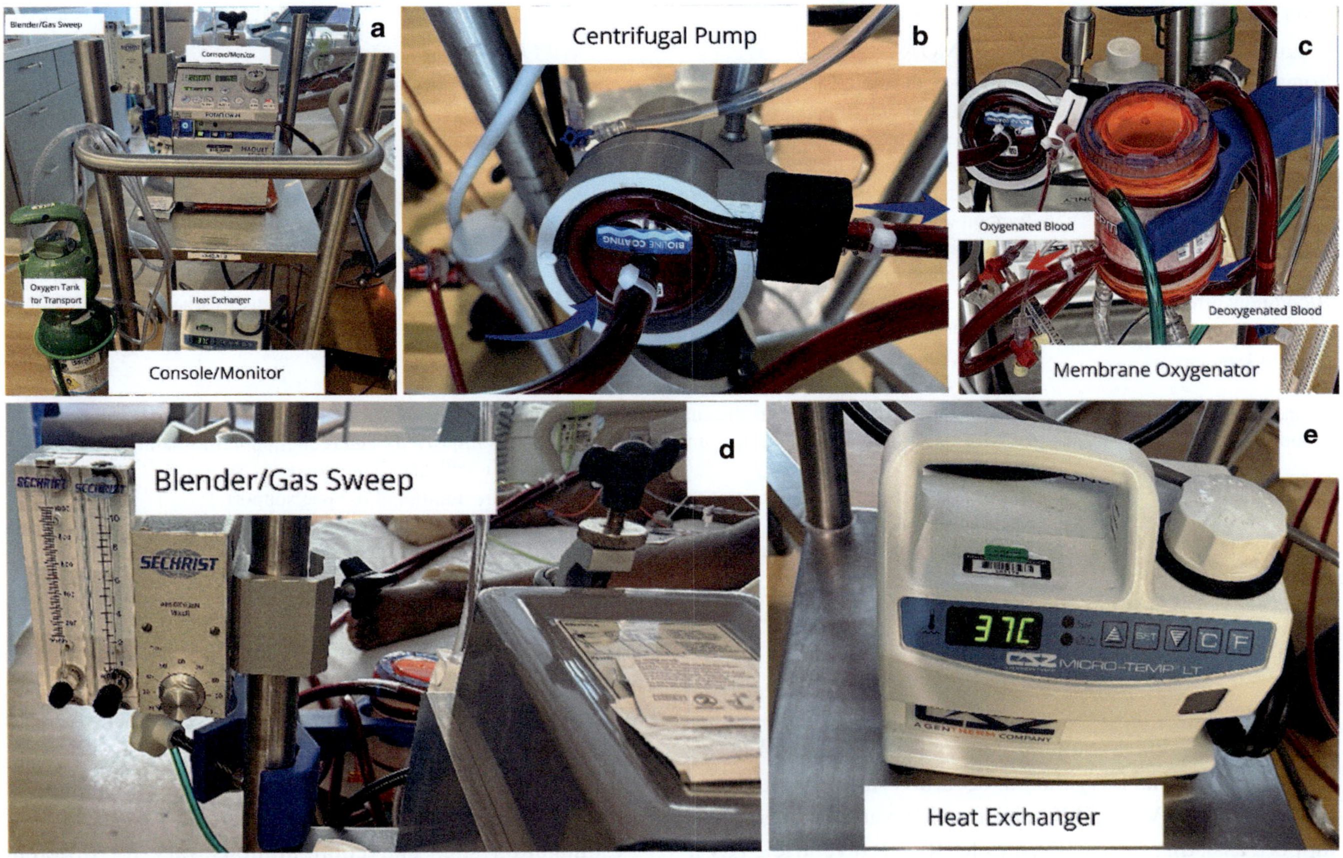

Fig. 34.2 Essential components of an ECMO system. (**a**) Console, which controls and monitors functions. (**b**) Centrifugal pump, which circulates blood. A curved arrow indicates blood coming in, and a straight arrow indicates blood being pumped out. (**c**) Membrane oxygenator, which facilitates gas exchange. A blue arrow shows deoxygenated blood entering, and a red arrow shows oxygenated blood exiting. (**d**) Gas blender. (**e**) Heat exchanger, which regulates the temperature of the circulating blood

Pump There are several types of pumps used in ECMO circuits, including centrifugal, roller, and peristaltic pumps. Unlike the cardiopulmonary bypass circuit, the ECMO circuit does not include a reservoir.

Oxygenation and CO_2 Removal The blood is then pumped through a membrane oxygenator made of polymethylpentene (PMP) functioning as an artificial lung. A blended mix of air and oxygen flows through the hollow fibers of the oxygenator. Oxygen leaves the fibers and replaces CO_2 in the blood. A "sweep gas" with little or no CO_2 runs along the opposite side of the membrane, creating a diffusion gradient that promotes CO_2 removal. CO_2 entering the fibers is then expelled in the exhaust gas. Oxygenated, decarboxylated blood flows through the return outflow cannula back to the patient.

Managing ECMO Parameters Blood flow, oxygenation, and CO_2 removal are precisely controlled by adjusting pump speed, delivered oxygen, (F_DO_2), and sweep gas flow. Sweep gas is the gas that flows through the oxygenator in liters per minute. The sweep gas flow is typically equal to the blood flow rate.

Configurations of ECMO

The two main configurations of ECMO are veno-arterial (V-A) ECMO and veno-venous (V-V) ECMO. Depending upon its configuration, ECMO can deliver respiratory support alone, respiratory support with cardiac assistance, or full cardiopulmonary support. A less common configuration is veno-pulmonary arterial (V-P) ECMO, which supports both the lungs and a failing right ventricle. This configuration is becoming more feasible with the availability of percutaneous dual-lumen cannulas. In ECMO terminology, the letter before the hyphen indicates the blood vessel from which blood is drained, and the letter after the hyphen indicates where the blood is returned.

Table 34.1 The key differences between V-A and V-V ECMO

Feature	V-A ECMO	V-V ECMO
Primary function	Provides both respiratory and circulatory support (heart and lungs)	Provides primarily respiratory support (lungs)
Indications	Cardiogenic shock, cardiac arrest, and respiratory failure with cardiac dysfunction	Respiratory failure (ARDS, pneumonia, etc.)
Cannulation sites	Venous cannula: Typically inserted into the femoral or internal jugular vein Arterial cannula: Typically inserted into the femoral artery	Venous cannula: Typically inserted into the femoral or internal jugular vein Return cannula: Typically inserted into the femoral vein
Blood flow direction	The circuit drains venous blood and delivers it to the arterial side after oxygenation	Circuit drains venous blood and delivers it to the venous side after oxygenation
Support type	Provides respiratory support with cardiac support, or full cardiopulmonary support	Provides respiratory support
Impact on heart and systemic blood flow	Systemic arterial blood flow is the sum of the ECMO circuit flow and ejection from the LV	No direct support of cardiac function, however cardiac function is improved from reduction in mechanical ventilation and oxygen delivery to the heart
Additional considerations	Requires anticoagulation, potential for left ventricular distension Works in parallel with the heart and lungs	May require additional oxygen support Works in series, with both drainage and return cannula being placed in systemic large veins

Veno-Arterial V-A-ECMO

A V-A-ECMO circuit drains deoxygenated venous blood through the drainage cannula, passes it through the ECMO circuit, and returns oxygenated, decarboxylated blood to the arterial system. VA-ECMO can provide varying degrees of support, assisting the right ventricle (RV), left ventricle (LV), or both, and can bypass both the circulatory and respiratory systems. Blood flow through the ECMO circuit can be complete or partial, depending on the patient's native heart and lung function. VA-ECMO serves as a bridge:

- *To Recovery*: For acute but potentially reversible heart and/or lung conditions.
- *To Decision/Therapy*: For patients with acute cardiogenic shock or combined cardiorespiratory failure until transition to a durable LVAD or heart transplant.
- *Perioperative support*: For patients at high-risk therapeutic procedure, VA-ECMO can provide temporary cardiopulmonary support during risky procedures.

Veno-Venous V-V-ECMO

In V-V-ECMO, both drainage and return cannula are placed in large systemic veins. Typically, the circuit drains deoxygenated blood from either the femoral vein or inferior vena cava (IVC) and pumps it through the ECMO circuit to the right atrium (RA). This setup bypasses the native lungs, providing respiratory gas exchange through the ECMO membrane oxygenator. Blood pumped into the RA by the return cannula has a higher oxygen and lower CO_2 content. V-V ECMO can bridge the native lungs to recovery, or in eligible patients with ESLD, to lung transplant. V-V-ECMO can also enable extensive airway or thoracic surgery by bypassing the native airway and lungs, making it a new perioperative tool for complex thoracic procedures.

Important Considerations

- Cannulation sites and configurations vary for different ECMO types.
- Peripheral V-A ECMO, central post-cardiotomy V-A ECMO, and V-V ECMO all have distinct cannulation strategies.
- Refer to the ELSO Registry and (Table 34.1) for specific details.

Cannulation Sites and Techniques for ECMO

Cannulation sites for V-A ECMO can either be central or peripheral (Figs. 34.3 and 34.4).

Central V-A ECMO Cannulation

- Used for post-cardiotomy shock following failure to wean from CPB after cardiac surgery.
- The sternum remains open, and the heart and vessels are already exposed, allowing the use of existing cannulae for CPB.
- Drainage cannula in the RA, return cannula in the ascending aorta.
- Advantages: large-bore cannulae, lower risk of peripheral vessel injury.

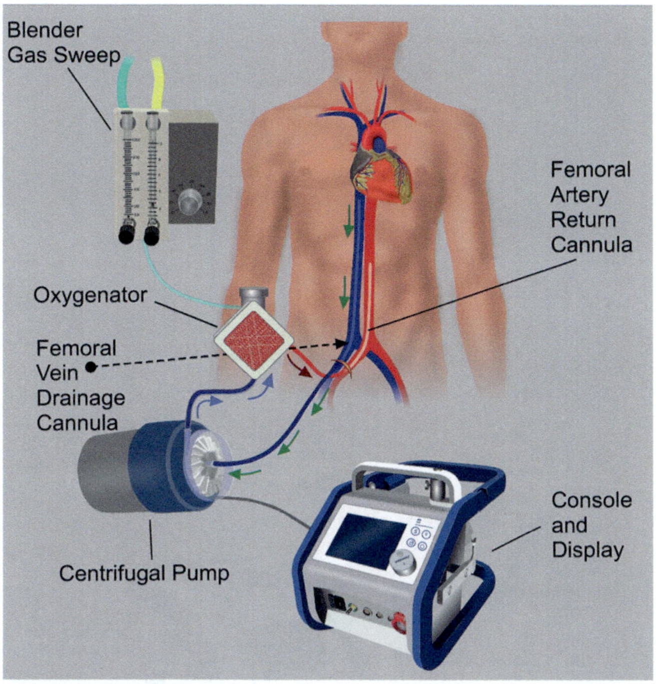

Fig. 34.3 Peripheral veno-arterial ECMO configuration. This diagram illustrates the placement of cannulas in peripheral veno-arterial ECMO. The drainage cannula is located in the right femoral vein with its tip extending into the IVC, while the return cannula is positioned in the femoral artery, facilitating effective circulatory support

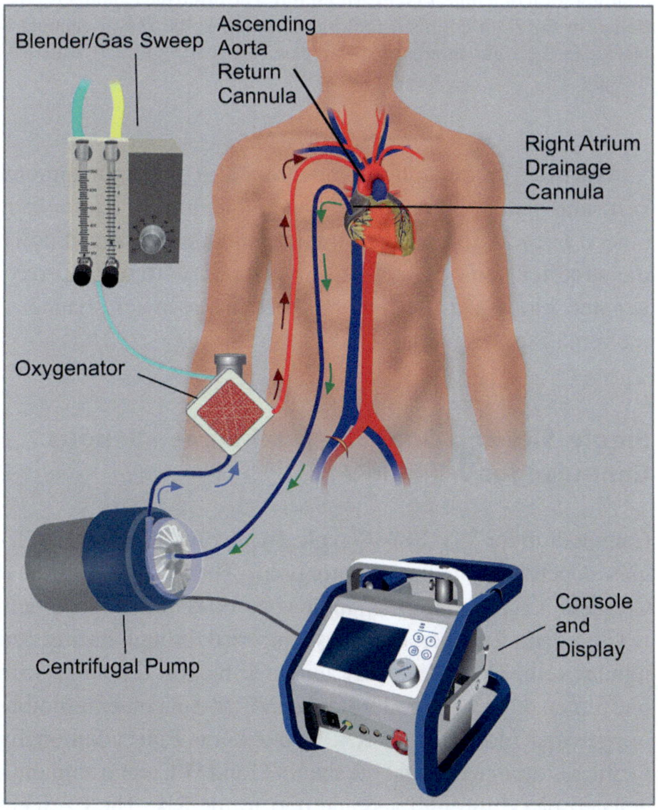

Fig. 34.4 Central veno-arterial ECMO setup. This illustration depicts a central veno-arterial ECMO configuration. The drainage cannula is strategically positioned in the RA, while the return cannula is placed directly in the aorta, highlighting their roles in effective cardiac and circulatory support

- Disadvantages: Increased bleeding risk from residual CPB anticoagulation.
- RV Assistance: Oxygenated blood can be infused into the pulmonary artery to bypass the RV if needed.

Peripheral V-A ECMO Cannulation

- Blood is drained from a femoral vein, with a cannula advanced percutaneously to the RA.
- Return cannula in the femoral or axillary artery.
- V-A ECMO provides both hemodynamic and respiratory support.
- Risks: Vascular injury, differential hypoxia ("North-South syndrome").
- North-South Syndrome: Oxygenated blood, delivered retrogradely to the aorta from the ECMO circuit, perfuses the lower body, while deoxygenated blood from the LV circulates in the upper body. North-South syndrome, also known as Harlequin syndrome, is common when the native LV has recovered its ejection and has blood circulating through it. Retrograde blood flow can also increase afterload, diminish stroke volume from LV, and cause LV distention, potentially leading to pulmonary edema.
- LV Distension Management: If LV distension occurs, an additional device or drainage cannula may be necessary. Pressurized blood return into the aorta, whether ascending or descending, can worsen LV function by increasing afterload and reducing ejection. Inotropic support may be used to enhance LV ejection and prevent clot formation. Close monitoring and fine adjustment of the flows are required with an advanced configuration employing three cannulas.
  - Other strategies (Fig. 34.5) for unloading the LV during V-A ECMO support includes the following:
    - *Placement of an Intra-Aortic Balloon Pump (IABP)*: This method is widely used for LV unloading in conjunction with VA-ECMO. IABP helps reduce the heart's workload (afterload) and enhances blood flow to the coronary arteries. Clinical observation suggests that IABP plus VA-ECMO improves cardiac performance, facilitates weaning from support, and enhances survival rates.
    - *ECPELLA (ECMO + Impella)*: This strategy involves the use of an Impella device alongside VA-ECMO to more effectively reduce the pressure and volume in the LV, which can improve the chances of recovery and survival. ECPELLA can unload the LV providing significant cardiac decompression. Despite potential risks such as increased bleeding, vascular issues, and stroke, recent research suggests that these risks are not significantly higher than when using VA-ECMO alone.
    - *Surgical or Percutaneous Left Atrial Decompression*: These methods involve directly removing blood

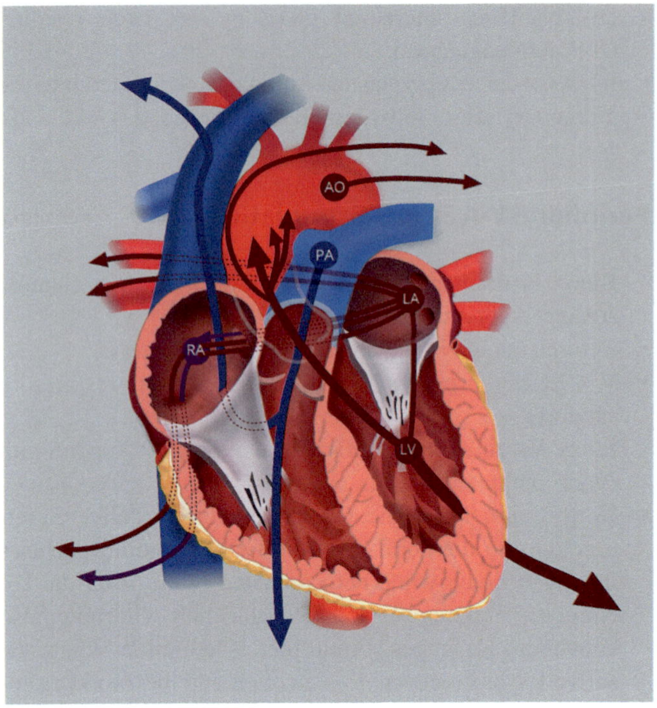

Fig. 34.5 Medical illustration depicting various modalities of LV unloading strategies during VA-ECMO, including IABP, ECPELLA (ECMO + Impella) setup, surgical or percutaneous left atrial decompression, and enhanced right-side drainage

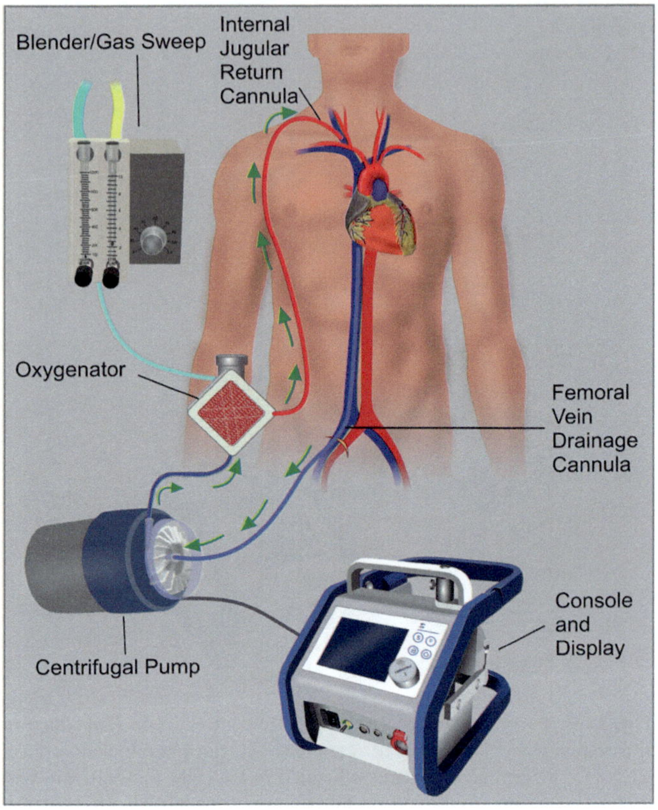

Fig. 34.6 Dual veno-venous ECMO setup. This illustration shows the configuration of a dual V-V ECMO setup. The drainage cannula is positioned in the right common femoral vein, while the return cannula is placed in the right internal jugular vein, facilitating effective ECMO therapy

from the left atrium to decrease pressure and volume in the LV.
  - *Direct LV Decompression*: This can be achieved through techniques that directly remove blood from the left ventricle.
  - *Enhanced Right-Side Drainage*: Increasing the extraction of blood from the right-side of the heart indirectly reduces the amount of blood entering the LV, thereby easing its workload.
- Limb Ischemia: Can occur due to partial femoral artery occlusion. Managed with a reperfusion cannula inserted into the femoral artery distal to the original cannula or by cannulating the tibial artery.

V-V ECMO Cannulation Techniques

V-V ECMO configuration can involve percutaneous insertion of a single dual-lumen cannula through the internal jugular vein or a double cannula set up. (ELSO Registry).

The ideal setup involves two cannulae:

1. *Inflow Cannula*: draining blood from the femoral vein into the ECMO circuit and oxygenator.
2. *Outflow Cannula*: Returns oxygenated blood to either the contralateral femoral vein or RA.

With the inflow cannula positioned in the right femoral vein and extending into the IVC, the outflow cannula is placed in the right internal jugular vein and advanced down the superior vena cava (SVC) into the RA. Returning oxygenated blood via the femoral vein has a lower chance of recirculation. (Fig. 34.6).

Single-Site and Dual-Site Dual-Lumen Venous Cannulae for V-V ECMO

Cannulation for V-V ECMO typically involves different strategies depending on the system used. The Avalon Elite and Crescent Cannula use a single-site, dual-lumen approach, where a cannula is percutaneously inserted through the internal jugular vein. These cannulas allow for bicaval drainage, with one lumen draining blood from the IVC and the other returning oxygenated blood to the RA. The Avalon Elite additionally facilitates drainage from both the SVC and IVC, returning oxygenated blood through a single port to the RA. The Crescent Cannula, similar to the Avalon Elite, features a unique crescent-shaped tip to enhance blood flow and reduce recirculation.

Conversely, the Bio-Medicus system requires dual-site cannulation using separate single-lumen cannulae for blood drainage and return, adaptable for femoral venous, arterial, or jugular venous configurations for either V-V or V-A ECMO. Choosing the appropriate cannula involves considering patient anatomy, institutional preferences, and specific case needs such as the potential for recirculation or patient ambulation. Consulting with the medical team to select the most suitable cannula based on these factors is essential.

Advantages and Challenges

The advantage of a single venous cannula is that it allows for patient ambulation after extubation. However, this setup is more sensitive to blood flow changes with movement. Transesophageal echocardiography (TEE) or fluoroscopic guidance is essential to ensure proper positioning of both SVC and IVC lumens to prevent recirculation of the newly oxygenated blood.

Preventing and Detecting Recirculation

Recirculation occurs when oxygenated blood from the return cannula flows directly back into the drainage cannula instead of mixing with the systemic venous blood.

To prevent recirculation:

- Ensure the return cannula tip is directed toward the tricuspid valve.
- Maintain a distance greater than 8 cm between the two lumens.

Recirculation can be detected by observing:

- Blood Color: Bright red blood in both drainage and return cannulae indicates recirculation.
- Venous Blood Gas: A PO2 of 30–40 mmHg is normal; higher values suggest recirculation (Fig. 34.7a, b).

Cannulation Guidance

Radiopaque markers are crucial for accurately positioning the catheter, identifying drainage sites, the infusion port, the catheter tip, and the axial orientation of the port. The return cannula should ideally be directed toward the tricuspid valve. To prevent recirculation and maintain effective ECMO support, the two lumens should be positioned at least 8 cm apart. Transitioning from V-V ECMO to V-A ECMO can also help correct recirculation. Cannulation for peripheral ECMO may be performed under fluoroscopic guidance, TEE guidance, or both.

Recirculation reduces the delivery of oxygenated blood to the pulmonary artery, leading to a reduction in mixed venous oxygen saturation (SvO_2). In the absence of significant recirculation, ECMO circuit flow is the most important determinant of arterial oxygen saturation (SaO_2). SaO_2 is determined by the combination of oxygen saturation of blood entering the lungs, SvO_2, and additional oxygenation of blood occurring within the lungs. SvO_2 is determined by contributions from the oxygenated blood from the ECMO return cannula and the systemic venous deoxygenated blood returning to the lungs. In the absence of effective pulmonary function, SvO_2 behaves similarly to SaO_2.

Other Hybrid Extracorporeal Membrane Oxygenator Circuit Configurations

- *Venoveno-arterial (VV-A) ECMO*: A hybrid variant of V-A ECMO, where patients receiving V-V ECMO may have an arterial reinfusion cannula placed when additional cardiac support is needed, particularly if inadequate venous drainage leads to excessive shunting of deoxygenated blood through the lungs. VV-A ECMO utilizes two drainage cannulae—typically one placed in the IVC and another in the right atrium—connected by a Y-shaped connector, alongside a return cannula in the femoral

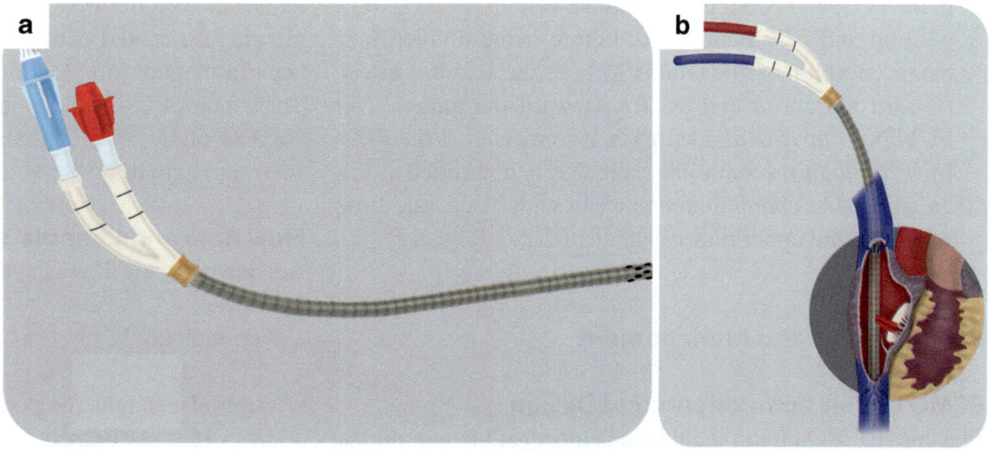

Fig. 34.7 (**a**) The top illustration displays a Crescent Single Jugular Double Lumen Catheter designed for VV-ECMO. (**b**) The bottom illustration shows the catheter inserted through the superior vena cava into the right atrium, with deoxygenated blood flowing into the venous side and oxygenated blood flowing out through the other lumen

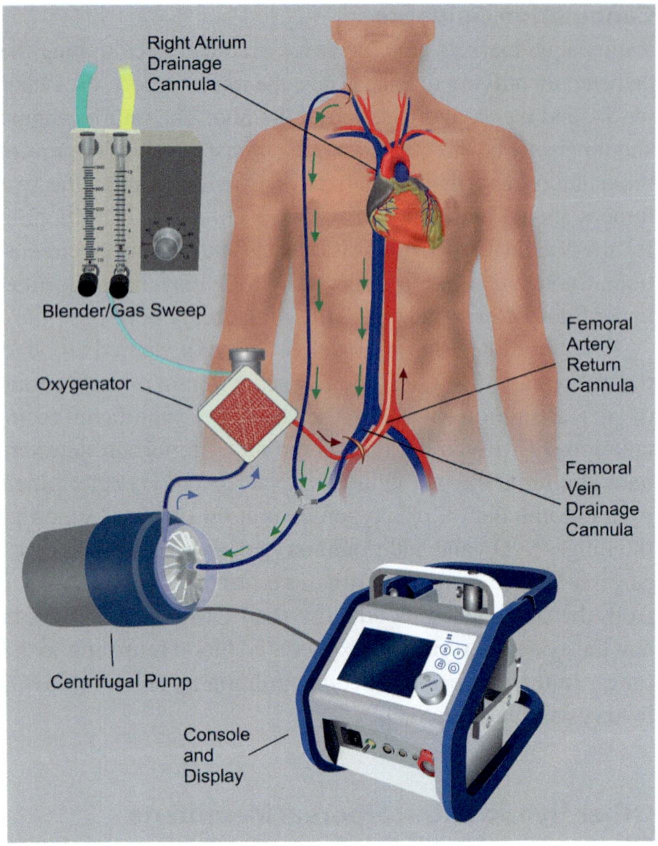

Fig. 34.8 VV-A ECMO configuration. This diagram illustrates a V-AV ECMO setup, utilizing two drainage cannulae and one return cannula to address inadequate venous drainage and blood shunting. One drainage cannula is inserted into the right common femoral vein and the other in the right internal jugular vein toward the RA. The return cannula is positioned in the femoral artery to direct flow toward the aorta

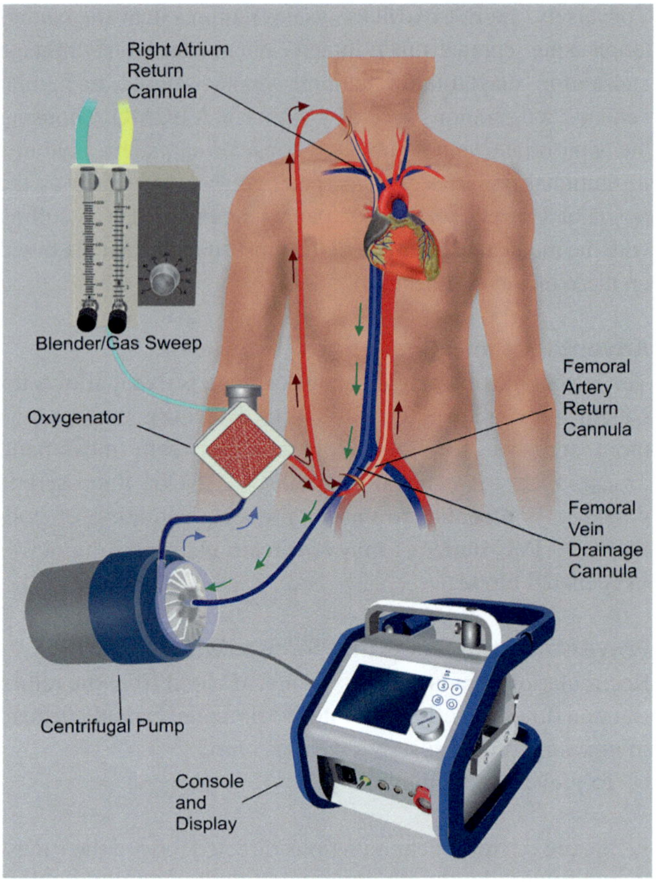

Fig. 34.9 V-AV ECMO configuration. This diagram illustrates a V-AV ECMO setup, which involves one drainage cannula and two return cannulae for optimal therapy. The drainage cannula is placed in the right common femoral vein, while one return cannula is positioned in the right internal jugular vein and the second in the femoral artery, directing flow toward the aorta. This configuration ensures comprehensive ECMO support

artery (toward the aorta) This triple cannula configuration can help augment cardiac output (Fig. 34.8).

- *Veno-arterio-venous (V-AV) ECMO*: A combination of both V-V and V-A ECMO that provides respiratory and cardiac support. It utilizes one drainage cannula (typically in the IVC) and two return cannulae. Venous blood is oxygenated and CO_2 is removed, before being divided into balanced volumes for returns to both the femoral artery (toward the aorta) and the RA (toward the lungs). The ECMO outflow is divided by a Y-connector. (Fig. 34.9) Flow through the returning cannulae is controlled using an adjustable clamp and monitored with a separate flow sensor on the upper return cannula. (ELSO Registry).

ECMO Circuit and Management

ECMO Circuit Components and Design

The core ECMO circuit includes a centrifugal blood pump, a membrane oxygenator, a gas blender to control oxygen concentration, and conduit tubing to connect these components. Additionally, circuits often feature a heat exchanger to regulate blood temperature, along with essential monitors and alarms for patient safety. Newer-generation centrifugal pumps are designed with features like non-occlusive technology and coated surfaces to minimize blood trauma (hemolysis) and reduce the risk of thrombus formation. The cannulae and tubing are also coated with biocompatible surface coatings like heparin or phosphorylcholine to further reduce thrombosis. These pumps utilize a spinning impeller, operating at about 3000 revolutions/min, creating a negative pressure of up to 100 mm Hg to draw blood through the circuit.

Flow Rate and Cannula Size

Adequate circuit flow is achieved by using appropriate cannula sizes.

For adults:

- Arterial cannula for peripheral insertion usually ranges from 15 to 21 French.
- Venous cannula ranges from 21 to 29 French, depending upon the body surface area of the patient.

Tubing for adult ECMO is typically 3/8-inch in diameter and is constructed from polyvinylchloride, which makes it highly resistant to kinking and rupture.

Perfusion Management in ECMO

Blood Flow and Oxygenation

The desired ECMO blood flow is influenced by vascular access, drainage tubing resistance, and pump properties. Systemic perfusion is effectively monitored by SvO_2 levels, where SvO_2 above 65% indicates adequate perfusion. The goal is to maintain systemic oxygen delivery (DO_2) at least three times higher than oxygen consumption (VO_2), typically maintaining a (DO_2:VO_2) ratio around five. In shock states, the ratio drops below three.

Adjustments for Optimal Perfusion

Adjusting hemoglobin levels and ECMO flow can help maintain SVO_2 above 65% and DO_2/VO_2 above three. For effective gas exchange in respiratory failure, the membrane oxygenator should match the patient's metabolic demands, ideally providing a DO_2 of 3 ml/kg/min, which equates to a flow rate of 60–80 ml/kg/min. Flows above 5 L/min are manageable without a significant increase in in-line pressures. DO_2 is determined by blood flow, hemoglobin concentration, inlet hemoglobin saturation, and membrane lung properties.

CO_2 Removal and Acid–Base Balance

CO_2 removal is determined by blood flow, sweep gas rate, the inlet PCO_2, and membrane oxygenator properties. Targeting a normal arterial pH of 7.35 to 7.45, adjustments to the sweep gas flow may be required to achieve this balance.

Hemodynamic Monitoring

Continuous monitoring of hemodynamics and oxygen saturations is crucial. In V-A ECMO, targeting a mean arterial pressure (MAP) between 65 and 80 mm Hg may be targeted for most V-A ECMO can help sustain end-organ perfusion.

Circuit Monitoring and Troubleshooting

ECMO circuits include various in-line monitors, such as bubble detectors, to identify large bubbles that can cause airlocks on the venous side. If a low circuit blood flow alarm occurs, inspect the ECMO circuit tubing and cannulae for kinks and chattering—the latter often caused by excessive negative suction on the venous drainage cannula and potentially aggravated by hypovolemia. Address hypovolemia by reducing pump speed and administering a fluid bolus.

Ventilator Settings for V-V ECMO

For patients on V-V ECMO, ventilation should be managed using the following parameters:

- Protective lung ventilation with tidal volume ≤6 mL/kg of predicted body weight.
- Plateau pressure ≤25 cmH_2O.
- Driving pressure ≤10 cmH_2O.
- PEEP ~10 cmH_2O, titrated to optimize pulmonary compliance and/or minimize driving pressure. PEEP helps maintain alveolar recruitment.

Role of TEE in ECMO Management

TEE is a valuable tool for ECMO management, facilitating the insertion and correct positioning of guidewires and cannulae while also detecting any misplacement. It helps confirm proper RA cannula position, ensuring it is not obstructed by the interatrial septum or RA walls. For V-V ECMO, TEE assesses tricuspid valve pathology, excluding tricuspid stenosis or previous tricuspid valve replacement. It guides the correct positioning of the dual-lumen single cannula in the RA and IVC, can detect recirculation of blood in the ECMO circuit by identifying cannula malposition, and in diagnosing causes of low flow. TEE also helps in evaluating biventricular function in response to ECMO and in monitoring RV and LV function during ECMO weaning. RA involution on echocardiography is a sign of hypovolemia. In centrally placed V-A ECMO, TEE can help visualize the return cannula in the aorta.

Indications and Contraindications for ECMO

V-A ECMO is used to support patients with cardiac failure from various etiologies. Cardiac arrest or cardiogenic shock occurs in approximately 5% to 10% of all patients experiencing acute myocardial infarction and is associated with an in-hospital mortality rate of 30% to 50%. This scenario is one of the most common reasons for V-A ECMO.

V-V ECMO is used to assist patients with respiratory failure resulting from hypoxic or hypercarbic conditions or from ARDS. Patients with severe hypoxia and/or hypercapnia unresponsive to optimal medical management, including protective ventilation with low-tidal volumes, plateau pressure less than 28–30 cmH_2O, high levels of PEEP, prone positioning, neuromuscular blockers, and/or other adjunctive therapies, including nitrous oxide or almitrine, qualify for V-V ECMO. A PaO_2/FIO_2 ratio of 70–80 mmHg, Murray score >3, and pH <7.2 provides a reasonable threshold for considering VV-ECMO in adults. V-V ECMO facilitates gas exchange but does not provide circulatory support. ARDS stemming from multiple etiologies is the most common indication for V-V ECMO (as referenced in Table 34.2).

Table 34.2 The indications and contraindications for both V-A and V-V ECMO. This format organizes the data clearly, highlighting the differences and similarities in the applications of each type of ECMO

Feature	V-A ECMO	V-V ECMO
Indications		
Cardiac support	Acute myocardial infarction Cardiogenic shock Refractory ventricular arrhythmias Acute fulminant myocarditis Post-cardiotomy with failure to wean off CPB Primary graft failure after lung transplantation Hyperacute rejection following organ transplantation Congenital heart disease with acute decompensated heart failure Peripartum cardiomyopathy Acute RV failure secondary to massive pulmonary embolism Post-myocardial infarct VSD Amniotic fluid embolus ECPR for reversible etiology	Acute pulmonary edema due to cardiac dysfunction Severe respiratory failure (ARDS, pneumonia, etc.) with right ventricular dysfunction Severe hypercapnic respiratory failure affecting cardiac function by normalizing CO_2, thus improving cardiac function
Pulmonary support	Acute RV failure secondary to massive pulmonary embolism Hyperacute rejection of lung graft post-transplantation	ARDS Severe bacterial or viral pneumonia, including COVID-19 Aspiration syndrome Alveolar proteinosis Pulmonary contusion Inhalational injury Pulmonary hemorrhage or massive hemoptysis Meconium aspiration syndrome Difficulty with single-lung ventilation Managing mediastinal masses
Surgical/procedural support	Post-cardiotomy with failure to wean off CPB Periprocedural for high-risk percutaneous coronary or valvular interventions	Conduct of complex thoracic procedures Airway surgery Advanced pulmonary and esophageal resections Intra-operative stabilization
Transplantation support	Primary graft failure after heart transplantation	As a bridge to lung transplant Primary graft dysfunction after lung transplant
Contraindications		
Cardiovascular issues	Aortic dissection Severe aortic insufficiency	Severe left ventricular dysfunction with low cardiac output Irreversible cardiac failure
Patient condition limitations	Irreversible etiology for cardiogenic shock Unwitnessed cardiac arrest Prolonged CPR without adequate tissue perfusion Advanced age > 80 Immunosuppression Irreversible multi-organ failure Life-limiting disseminated malignancy	Advanced age with significant comorbidities Severe neurological injury Uncontrolled sepsis
Medical suitability	SOFA score greater than 11 Not a candidate for transplant or VAD support	Bleeding diatheses Terminal illnesses with limited prognosis Morbid obesity
Treatment compatibility	Contraindications to anticoagulation Morbid obesity	Lack of vascular access Contraindication to anticoagulation Chronic conditions unlikely to benefit from temporary support

Perioperative Indications of ECMO

Encouraged by successful outcomes with ECMO in complex surgeries, the rapid expansion of its pre- and peri-procedural use has occurred, offering life-saving support for previously inoperable patients.

V-A ECMO Indications

V-A ECMO, providing both circulatory and respiratory support, is increasingly used for:

- *Cardiac Surgery*: Post-cardiotomy shock, primary graft failure after heart or lung transplant, hyperacute rejection, ECPR.
- *High-Risk Interventions*: Support during complex percutaneous procedures for coronary artery intervention (PCI), valvular disease, and structural heart disease.
- *Other*: Acute RV failure due to massive pulmonary embolism, peripartum cardiomyopathy, myocardial infarction with shock, severe pulmonary hemorrhage, and Takotsubo cardiomyopathy. Another emergent indication for V-A ECMO is the rupture of aortic annulus or ventricular septal defect following transcatheter aortic valve replacement (TAVR). Utilizing ECMO in cases of life-threatening complications related to structural heart disease can significantly restore end-organ function and improves patient survival rates.

V-V ECMO Indications

V-V ECMO, primarily for respiratory support, is beneficial in:

- *Thoracic Surgery*: Complex cases involving infiltrative masses, critical airway compromise, and airway reconstruction following traumatic injuries.

V-V ECMO can temporarily support gas exchange in traumatic lung injury or massive alveolar hemorrhage.

The use of extracorporeal life support (ECLS) has also expanded to include a unique population of peripartum women. Cardiovascular disease is currently the leading cause of pregnancy- related mortality in the United States, contributing to more than 25% of maternal deaths and maternal morbidity. The most common indications for ECLS in pregnancy include ARDS, post-partum cardiomyopathy, bleeding, and cardiac arrest.

Key Considerations

- ECMO is NOT a cure, but a bridge to recovery, decision-making, or transplant.
- Thorough patient selection and careful consideration of risks/benefits are crucial.
- Multidisciplinary collaboration is essential for optimal management.

(See Table 34.2 for a comprehensive list of V-V and V-A ECMO indications and contraindications)

Anesthetic Considerations for ECMO

Successful ECMO management in the operating room demands a comprehensive understanding of ECMO physiology, adept troubleshooting skills, and meticulous hemodynamics management. An in-depth knowledge of how ECMO influences anesthetic drug behavior and potential sequestration is crucial.

Total Intravenous Anesthesia (TIVA) is the recommended, although higher doses might be necessary because of the larger volume of drug distribution (for lipophilic anesthetic drugs) and drug loss from adsorption within the membranous oxygenator of the ECMO circuit. This adsorption causes sequestration of protein bound intravenous anesthetic drugs.

Volatile anesthetics are not effective in patients with significantly impaired gas exchange (due to pulmonary parenchymal disease or low pulmonary blood flow with low-tidal volumes).

Transporting ECMO patients requires careful planning and a multidisciplinary team (perfusionist, respiratory therapist, and anesthesiologist) to prevent complications like tubing kinks or dislodgement. Transport should be done with the patient on a portable ventilator.

As perioperative ECMO use grows, anesthesiologists will play an increasingly important role. If an emergent procedure is needed for patients on ECMO, it is generally safe to temporarily halt anticoagulation for a few hours, provided that ECMO flow exceeds 3.5 Liters.

Anticoagulation

Interaction of blood with a non-endothelial surface of the ECMO circuit leads to a hypercoagulable pro-thrombotic state. Initially, there is adsorption of proteins like fibrinogen, fibronectin, and von Willebrand factor (vWF) onto the surface of the tubing, which further mediates platelet adhesion of its surface Glycoprotein IIb/IIIa (GPIIb/IIIa). The most utilized anticoagulant for ECMO is unfractionated heparin due to its rapid onset and reversibility. ELSO recommends heparin be administered continuously after an initial bolus of 50–100 units per kilogram body weight, followed by an infusion dose between 7.5 and 20 units/kg/hr. to maintain an activated partial thromboplastin time (aPTT) of 50–60. Heparin's anticoagulant effects may be monitored using activated clotting time (ACT) and anti-factor Xa assay. Disadvantages of heparin include anti-thrombin III deficiency and heparin-induced thrombocytopenia (HIT) from platelet factor 4 (PF4) being bound to exogenous heparin, triggering the formation of antibodies (HIT antibodies) to the heparin-PF4 complex. Other anticoagulants used for ECMO include bivalirudin, argatroban, and desirudin, three direct thrombin (IIa) inhibitors. Direct thrombin inhibitors offer the advantage of more consistent anticoagulation effects at the cost of not having a reversible agent like protamine sulfate. Bivalirudin has a 20% renal clearance percentage, and thus, renal function must be monitored. Monitoring of direct thrombin inhibitors can be performed using the activated partial thromboplastin time (aPTT). The oxygenator status should be monitored for thrombotic events, which will require changing the entire circuit.

ECMO Complications

While ECMO provides critical life support, it also introduces significant risks that can substantially increase morbidity and mortality. Each case requires careful management to balance these factors effectively.

Bleeding

Bleeding around the cannulation sites is a common and potentially life-threatening complication in ECMO. This is often due to systemic heparinization, fibrinolysis, hemodilution of clotting factors, and platelet dysfunction. To mitigate bleeding risk, the following is recommended:

- Platelet count >150,000 mm^3.
- Fibrinogen >200 mg/L.
- Prothrombin ratio (PT/INR) <1.5.
- Lower ACT.

HIT is an uncommon complication, more often seen with long-term ECMO usage.

Thrombosis: Blood clots can form within the ECMO circuit, potentially leading to pulmonary embolism. Arterial thromboembolism in the arterial system can also occur, resulting in stroke.

Limb ischemia: Occurs when the femoral artery is partially occluded by the cannula, reducing blood flow to the lower extremity.

North-South Syndrome (in peripheral VA-ECMO): Refers to differential hypoxia, where the lower body receives oxygenated blood from ECMO, while the upper extremities (including the brain) receive deoxygenated blood from the LV. This can increase LV afterload, distension, and wall stress due to retrograde flow of blood to the aorta, potentially leading to pulmonary edema.

Recirculation: Cannula malposition can cause oxygenated blood to flow back into the ECMO circuit instead of the patient, leading to severe hypoxemia and end-organ damage.

Air embolism: The negative pressure up to 100 mmHg generated in the circuit between the pump and drainage cannula can entrain air, leading to gas embolism.

Hemolysis: Mechanical stress applied to red blood cells from flow or pressure gradient can cause hemolysis, measured by free hemoglobin levels.

Other Complications: Ventilator-associated pneumonia and acute kidney injury (AKI) due to acute tubular necrosis may occur. Sepsis is another serious, well-known complication.

ECMO Weaning

Successful weaning off VA-ECMO involves gradually decreasing support while simultaneously monitoring of patient's pulmonary and cardiac function. Echocardiographic assessment of LV function is crucial as flows are reduced to 1–2 L/min.

Predictors of Successful Weaning from V-A ECMO:

- LV ejection fraction ≥20%.
- Aortic velocity-time integral ≥12 cm per contraction.
- Lateral mitral annular peak systolic velocity ≥6 cm per second.
- Minimal ECMO support.

Discontinuation Criteria

Patients can be discontinued from ECMO if they can tolerate a flow less than 2.5 L/min with the following parameters:

- Central venous pressure <18 mm Hg.
- Pulmonary artery wedge pressure <20 mm Hg.
- Cardiac index >2.4 L/min.
- MAP >60 mm Hg.
- LV ejection fraction >30%.

After reducing the sweep gas flow rate, monitor the lungs' ventilation capacity and cardiac output. If cardiac output is adequate, the sweep gas flow rate can be further decreased. MAP ≥65 mmHg should be maintained with minimal inotropic support.

Weaning from V-V ECMO

The weaning process from V-V ECMO begins following successful treatment of the underlying disease and improvement of lung function. Tidal volumes begin to return to normal values, and the fraction of inspired oxygen (FiO_2) is <0.45, PEEP <10 cmH_2O, and peak inspiratory pressure (PIP) <27 cmH_2O. Blood gas values are checked every 30 minutes. The perfusionist adjusts the sweep gas flow to maintain the pre-set goals for pH and pCO_2. Gas flow is tapered in parallel with the blood flow and finally switched off for 30–60 minutes. If blood gases remain stable and the patient does not develop dyspnea or tachypnea, the decision to wean the patient from V-V ECMO is made.

Additional Considerations

During the ECMO weaning process, if there are signs of LV failure, the patient should immediately return to full ECMO support. When ECMO support level are lows, unfractionated heparin may be discontinued, and the pump rate increased to prevent clot formation. Decannulation can proceed if the patient's cardiac and pulmonary functions are stable. However, the weaning process can pose both technical and ethical challenges, particularly if complications arise, necessitating changes in care goals. Involvement of palliative care is essential to support the patient and family. Ideally, patients should be weaned from ECMO within 5–7 days; if not possible by day 25–30, alternative strategies should be considered. (Fig. 34.10).

Long-Term Survival and Quality of Life After ECMO

The COVID-19 pandemic significantly increased the need for ECMO. It has provided an opportunity to evaluate the long-term survival of patients supported by ECMO. Patients' quality of life after ECMO is significantly reduced temporarily, but most patients did not experience permanent disability.

Key Pearls

- ECMO provides advanced life support in acute respiratory failure and circulatory collapse.
- ECMO is indicated for use in right heart failure, as a bridge to recovery or heart and lung transplantation.
- ECMO provides hemodynamic support for primary graft failure after heart or lung transplantation.
- There is an emerging role for ECMO use in complex tracheobronchial surgery and thoracic mass excisions where ECMO-related risks may be justified.
- Periprocedural support for high-risk percutaneous cardiothoracic procedures in advanced structural heart disease reduces the risk score.
- The use of ECMO is resource-intensive, posing new institutional challenges.

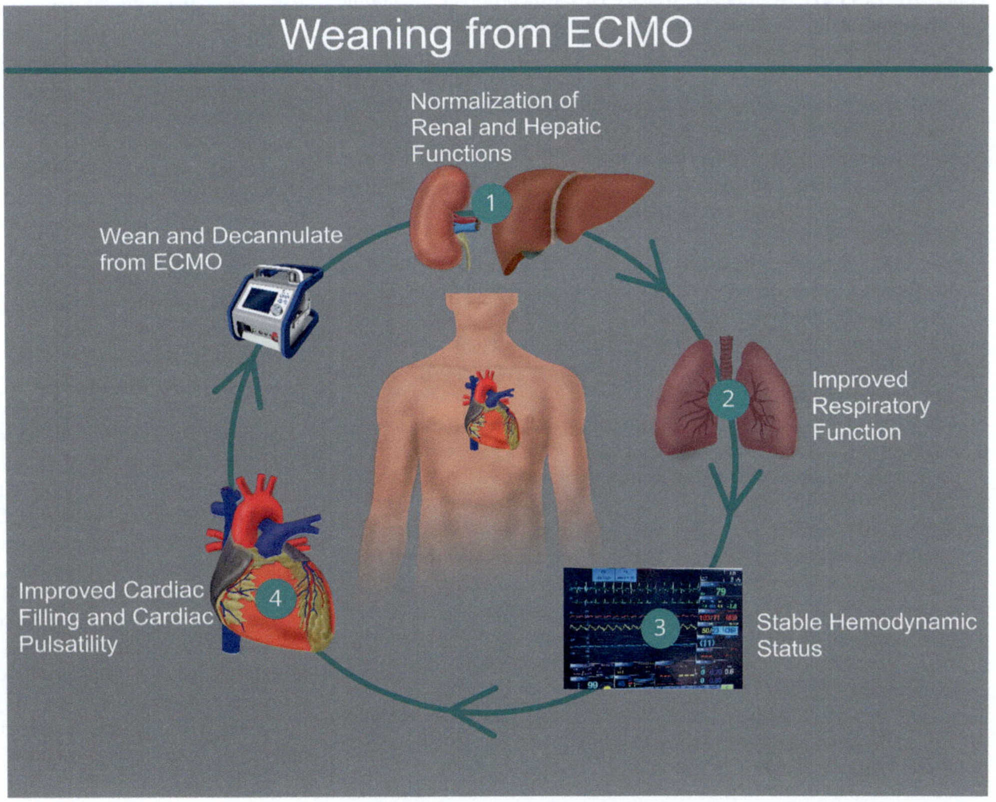

Fig. 34.10 ECMO weaning **process.** This diagram illustrates the weaning process from Extracorporeal Membrane Oxygenation, highlighting the critical parameters needed to assess a patient's readiness to discontinue mechanical support

Further Reading

Allen S, Holena D, McCunn M, et al. A review of the fundamental principles and evidence base in the use of extracorporeal membrane oxygenation (ECMO) in critically ill adult patients. J Intensive Care Med. 2011;26(1):13–26.

Amarelli C, Musumeci F, Loforte A, Montalto A, Di Franco S, Hernandez-Monfort J. Flow optimization, management and prevention of left ventricular distension during VA ECMO. In: Advances in extracorporeal perfusion therapies [Internet]. IntechOpen Limited; 2018.

Arif R, Eichhorn F, Kallenbach K, et al. Resection of thoracic malignancies infiltrating cardiac structures with use of cardiopulmonary bypass. J Cardiothorac Surg. 2015;10:87.

Bartlett RH, Roloff DW, Custer JR, Younger JG, Hirschl RB. Extracorporeal life support: the University of Michigan experience. JAMA. 2000;283(7):904–8.

Bartlett R, Arachichilage DJ, Chitlur M, et al. The history of extracorporeal membrane oxygenation and the development of extracorporeal membrane oxygenation anticoagulation [published online ahead of print, 2023 Feb 7]. Semin Thromb Hemost. 2023;50:10.1055/s-0043-1761488.

Bowles C, Hiesinger W. Postcardiotomy shock extracorporeal membrane oxygenation: peripheral or central? JTCVS Open. 2021;8:66–9.

Brogan T, Lequier L, Lorusso R, McLaren G, Peek G. Extracoporeal life support ELSO Red book. 5th ed. ELSO; 2017.

DeFilippis EM, Clerkin K, Truby LK, et al. ECMO as a bridge to left ventricular assist device or heart transplantation. JACC Heart Fail. 2021;9(4):281–9.

ELSO. General guidelines for all ECLS cases ELSO. Version 1.4. August 2017. Accessed June 23, 2023.

ELSO Registry. International summary and reports [internet]. ELSO; [cited 2023 July 11]. https://www.elso.org/registry/international-summaryandreports/internationalsummary.aspx

Esper SA, Levy JH, Waters JH, Welsby IJ. Extracorporeal membrane oxygenation in the adult: a review of anticoagulation monitoring and transfusion. Anesth Analg. 2014;118(4):731–43.

Genzor S, Pobeha P, Šimek M, et al. Long-term follow-up of patients needing extracorporeal membrane oxygenation following a critical course of COVID-19. Life (Basel). 2023;13(4):1054.

George B, Parazino M, Omar HR, et al. A retrospective comparison of survivors and non-survivors of massive pulmonary embolism receiving veno-arterial extracorporeal membrane oxygenation support. Resuscitation. 2018;122:1–5.

Hoyler MM, Flynn B, Iannacone EM, et al. Clinical management of venoarterial extracorporeal membrane oxygenation. J Cardiothorac Vasc Anesth. 2020;34(10):2776–92.

https://www.elso.org/ecmo-resources/elso-ecmo-guidelines.aspx

https://www.elso.org/registry/internationalsummaryandreports/internationalsummary.aspx

Huang W, Ye H, Cheng Z, et al. Outcomes from the use of perioperative extracorporeal membrane oxygenation in patients undergoing thoracic surgery: an 8-year single-center experience. Med Sci Monit. 2021;27:e931842.

Intraoperative Management of Adult Patients on Extracorporeal Membrane. Oxygenation: An Expert Consensus Statement from the Society of Cardiovascular Anesthesiologists—Part I, Technical Aspects of Extracorporeal Membrane Oxygenation.

Javidfar J, Bacchetta M. Bridge to lung transplantation with extracorporeal membrane oxygenation support. Curr Opin Organ Transplant. 2012;17(5):496–502.

Javidfar J, Brodie D, Wang D, et al. Use of bicaval dual-lumen catheter for adult venovenous extracorporeal membrane oxygenation. Ann Thorac Surg. 2011;91:1763–8.

Khorsandi M, Dougherty S, Bouamra O, et al. Extra-corporeal membrane oxygenation for refractory cardiogenic shock after adult cardiac surgery: a systematic review and meta-analysis. J Cardiothorac Surg. 2017;12(1):55.

Khoshbin E, Roberts N, Harvey C, et al. Poly-methyl pentene oxygenators have improved gas exchange capability and reduced transfusion requirements in adult extracorporeal membrane oxygenation. ASAIO J. 2005;51:281–7.

King CS, Roy A, Ryan L, Singh R. Cardiac support: emphasis on Venoarterial ECMO. Crit Care Clin. 2017;33(4):777–94.

Kittleson MM, Patel J, Moriguchi J, Kawano MA, Davis SD, Hage A, et al. Heart transplant recipients supported with extracorporeal membrane oxygenation: outcomes from a single-center experience. J Heart Lung Transplant. 2011;30(11):1250–6.

Ko M, dos Santos PR, Machuca TN, et al. Use of single-cannula venous-venous extracorporeal life support in the management of life-threatening airway obstruction. Ann Thorac Surg. 2015;99:e63–5.

Kumar G, Maskey A. Anticoagulation in ECMO patients: an overview. Indian J Thorac Cardiovasc Surg. 2021 Apr;37(Suppl 2):241–7.

Kwak J, Majewski MB, Jellish WS. Extracorporeal membrane oxygenation: the new Jack-of-all-trades? J Cardiothorac Vasc Anesth. 2020;34(1):192–207.

Lüsebrink E, Orban M, Kupka D, et al. Prevention and treatment of pulmonary congestion in patients undergoing venoarterial extracorporeal membrane oxygenation for cardiogenic shock. Eur Heart J. 2020;41(38):3753–61.

Mazzeffi MA, Rao VK, Dodd-o J, et al. Intraoperative management of adult patients on extracorporeal membrane oxygenation: an expert consensus statement from the society of cardiovascular anesthesiologists—Part I, technical aspects of extracorporeal membrane oxygenation. Anesth Analg. 2021a;133(6):1459–77.

Mazzeffi MA, Rao VK, Dodd-o J, et al. Intraoperative management of adult patients on extracorporeal membrane oxygenation: an expert consensus statement from the society of cardiovascular anesthesiologists—Part II, intraoperative management and troubleshooting. Anesth Analg. 2021b;133(6):1478–93.

Mehta T, Sallehuddin A, John J. The journey of pediatric ECMO. Qatar Med J. 2017;2017(1):4.

Meneveau N, Guillon B, Planquette B, et al. Outcomes after extracorporeal membrane oxygenation for the treatment of high-risk pulmonary embolism: a multicenter series of 52 cases. Eur Heart J. 2018;39:4196–204.

Naoum EE, Chalupka A, Haft J, et al. Extracorporeal life support in pregnancy: a systematic review. J Am Heart Assoc. 2020;9:e016072.

Nicoara A, Fitzsimons M, Maisonave Y. UpToDate [Internet]. Mark J, editor. www.uptodate.com. 2021 [cited 2023 Jun 12]. Available from: https://www.uptodate.com/contents/extracorporeal-life-support-in-adults-in-the-intensive-care-unit-the-role-of-transesophageal-echocardiography-tee

Pappalardo F, Schulte C, Pieri M, Schrage B, Contri R, Soeffker G, et al. Concomitant implantation of Impella((R)) on top of veno-arterial extracorporeal membrane oxygenation may improve survival of patients with cardiogenic shock. Eur J Heart Fail. 2017;19:404–12.

Pavlushkov E, Berman M, Valchanov K. Cannulation techniques for extracorporeal life support. Ann Transl Med. 2017;5(4):70.

Peek GJ, Clemens F, Elbourne D, et al. CESAR: conventional ventilatory support vs extracorporeal membrane oxygenation for severe adult respiratory failure. BMC Health Serv Res. 2006;6:163.

Rao P, Khalpey Z, Smith R, Burkhoff D, Kociol RD. Venoarterial extracorporeal membrane oxygenation for cardiogenic shock and cardiac arrest. Circ Heart Fail. 2018;11(9):e004905.

Ratnani I, Tuazon D, Zainab A, Uddin F. The role and impact of extracorporeal membrane oxygenation in critical care. Methodist Debakey Cardiovasc J. 2018;14(2):110–9.

Sangalli F, Patroniti N, Pesenti A. ECMO-extracorporeal life support in adults. 1st ed. Springer; 2014.

Scherer M, Sirat AS, Moritz A, Martens S. Extracorporeal membrane oxygenation as perioperative right ventricular support in patients with biventricular failure undergoing left ventricular assist device implantation. Eur J Cardiothorac Surg. 2011;39(6):939–44.

Sertic F, Bermudez C, Rame JE. Venoarterial extracorporeal membrane oxygenation as a bridge to recovery or bridge to heart replacement therapy in refractory cardiogenic shock. Curr Heart Fail Rep. 2020;17(6):341–9.

Shekar K, Roberts JA, Mullany DV, et al. Increased sedation requirements in patients receiving extracorporeal membrane oxygenation for respiratory and cardiorespiratory failure. Anaesth Intensive Care. 2012a;40:648–55.

Shekar K, Roberts JA, Mcdonald CI, et al. Sequestration of drugs in the circuit may lead to therapeutic failure during extracorporeal membrane oxygenation. Crit Care. 2012b;16:R194.

Sidebotham D, McGeorge A, McGuinness S, Edwards M, Willcox T, Beca J. Extracorporeal membrane oxygenation for treating severe cardiac and respiratory failure in adults: part 2-technical considerations. J Cardiothorac Vasc Anesth. 2010;24(1):164–72.

Sidebotham D, Allen SJ, McGeorge A, et al. Venovenous extracorporeal membrane oxygenation in adults: practical aspects of circuits, cannulae, and procedures. J Cardiothorac Vasc Anesth. 2012;26:893–909.

Singhvi A, Punnen J. Acute mechanical circulatory support for cardiogenic shock in India. Indian J Thorac Cardiovasc Surg. 2023;39:47. https://doi.org/10.1007/s12055-023-01530-7.

St-Arnaud C, Thériault MM, Mayette M. North-south syndrome in venoarterial extra-corporeal membrane oxygenator: the other Harlequin syndrome. Can J Anesth/J Can Anesth. 2022;69(2):262–3.

Sun W, Wang S, Chen Z, Zhang J, Li T, Arias K, et al. Impact of high mechanical shear stress and oxygenator membrane surface on blood damage relevant to thrombosis and bleeding in a pediatric ECMO circuit. Artif Organs. 2020;44(7):717–26.

Toomasian JM, Bartlett RH. Hemolysis and ECMO pumps in the twenty-first century. Perfusion. 2011;26:5–6.

Tsao N-W, Shih C-M, Yeh J-S, et al. Extracorporeal membrane oxygenation-assisted primary percutaneous coronary intervention improved 30-day clinical outcomes in patients with ST-segment elevation myocardial infarction complicated with profound cardiogenic shock. Crit Care Med. 2010;38:1810–7.

Tsao N-W, Shih C-M, Yeh J-S, et al. Extracorporeal membrane oxygenation-assisted primary percutaneous coronary intervention may improve survival of patients with acute myocardial infarction complicated by profound cardiogenic shock. J Crit Care. 2012;27(530):e1–e11.

Vallabhajosyula S, Patlolla SH, Sandhyavenu H, et al. Periprocedural cardiopulmonary bypass or Venoarterial extracorporeal membrane oxygenation during Transcatheter aortic valve replacement: a systematic review. J Am Heart Assoc. 2018;7(14):e009608.

Vyas A, Bishop MA. Extracorporeal membrane oxygenation in adults. In: StatPearls. Treasure Island: StatPearls Publishing; 2022.

Watkins AC, Maassel NL, Ghoreishi M, et al. Preoperative venoarterial extracorporeal membrane oxygenation slashes risk score in advanced structural heart disease. Ann Thorac Surg. 2018;106:1709–15.

Wendel HP, Ziemer G. Coating-techniques to improve the hemocompatibility of artificial devices used for extracorporeal circulation. Eur J Cardio-Thoracic Surg. 2011;16:342–50.

Zhang Y, Luo M, Wang B, Qin Z, Zhou R. Perioperative, protective use of extracorporeal membrane oxygenation in complex thoracic surgery. Perfusion. 2022;37(6):590–7.

Part XI

Cardiopulmonary Bypass in Unique Circumstances

35 Deep Hypothermic Circulatory Arrest

Kunal Panda, Rahul S. Thandla, Nishank P. Nooli, and Ahmed Zaky

Introduction

Deep hypothermic circulatory arrest (DHCA) is a sophisticated surgical technique used predominantly in cardiac and major vascular surgeries where conventional methods of cardiopulmonary bypass (CPB) are insufficient. DHCA involves cooling the patient to very low body temperatures (18–20 °C) to enable the temporary cessation of CPB. The concept of DHCA emerged in the mid-twentieth century but gained prominence in the 1970s, due to advancements in cooling techniques and cardiopulmonary equipment. With its successful inception, the technique has been substantially refined. It was initially proposed as a method to create a bloodless surgical field for complex cardiac repairs, particularly those requiring extensive aortic arch reconstruction. The deep hypothermic component of circulatory arrest is designed to mitigate the ischemic sequelae associated with cessation of flow to vital organs, especially the brain. Despite its benefits, DHCA is not without risks. The process requires meticulous planning and precise execution to balance the protective hypothermic effects against potential complications such as coagulopathy, arrhythmias, and renal dysfunction. Furthermore, the method's success heavily relies on the careful management of the patient's temperature, the timing of cooling and rewarming phases, and the integration of multimodal monitoring techniques to guide the perioperative management. In the current era, DHCA is used selectively and for short intervals.

K. Panda (✉) · R. S. Thandla
Department of Anesthesiology & Perioperative Medicine, University of Rochester, Rochester, NY, USA
e-mail: Kunal_Panda@urmc.rochester.edu; Rahul_Thandla@urmc.rochester.edu

N. P. Nooli · A. Zaky
Department of Anesthesiology and Perioperative Medicine, University of Alabama at Birmingham, Birmingham, AL, USA
e-mail: nnooli@uabmc.edu; azaky@uabmc.edu

Target Temperatures for DHCA

Various definitions of the levels of hypothermia exist in the surgical literature. A consensus statement defined four categories of hypothermia based on the expected degree of global metabolic and neuronal activity suppression in each temperature range. These categories are summarized in Table 6.1. For a comprehensive review of hypothermia, refer to Chap. 6, "Physiologic Changes and Inflammatory Response to Cardiopulmonary Bypass."

The target temperature for initiating DHCA varies by institutional practice and surgeon preference, heavily influenced by the anticipated duration of arrest needed to complete the procedure. Nasopharyngeal (NP) temperature is considered the most reliable surrogate for brain temperature.

Some institutions employ continuous Electroencephalography (EEG) monitoring during cooling, targeting electrocortical silence (isoelectric EEG) to indicate maximum suppression of cerebral metabolic rate ($CMRO_2$). EEG monitoring allows surgery to proceed at a higher temperature if the EEG is isoelectric. In the absence of EEG monitoring, understanding the relationship between NP temperature and the $CMRO_2$ as determined by EEG activity is crucial. While the average temperature for electrocortical silence is 18 °C in adults, this varies, with 12.5 °C necessary in over 95% of patients, whereas an average of 24 °C is needed for burst suppression.

Regardless of the target NP temperature, the arterial outflow temperature should maintain a <10 °C gradient with the venous inflow to prevent gas emboli. Cooling an adult to the target DHCA temperature typically takes at least 30 minutes, utilizing the CPB heat exchanger and discontinuing all external patient heating devices. Neuromuscular blockade should be maintained to prevent shivering.

A. S. Awad, J. DiNardo (eds.), *Clinical Perfusion for Cardiac Surgery*, https://doi.org/10.1007/978-3-031-91163-7_35

Table 35.1 Estimated safe durations for brain circulatory arrest at various hypothermic levels

Hypothermia level	Temperature (°C) (nasopharyngeal)	$CMRO_2$ (% of baseline)	Calculated maximum duration of circulatory arrest (min)
Mild	28.1 °C–34 °C	50–70%	7–10
Moderate	20.1 °C–28 °C	25–40%	10–20
Deep	14.1 °C–20 °C	15–25%	20–30
Profound	≤14 °C	10–15%	30–45

Physiological Principles of DHCA

Mechanism of Action

Hypothermia's Effects on Metabolism

Hypothermia reduces $CMRO_2$, slowing the depletion of high-energy phosphates and the development of acidosis, thereby delaying or preventing energy failure and subsequent neuronal injury. The Q_{10} concept, which is the ratio of O_2 consumption at two temperatures differing by 10°C, quantifies this effect. Children have a higher brain Q10 (~3.65) compared to adults (~2.3), indicating their metabolism slows more dramatically with cooling. However, even at 15 °C, the brain still needs about 10–15% of its normal oxygen supply.

Impact on Cerebral and Organ Protection

To estimate safe ischemic times during hypothermia, a simplified Q10 of 3.0 is used, meaning that for every 10 °C drop, the safe ischemic time triples. Thus, if 3–5 minutes is tolerated at normal body temperature (37 °C), cooling to 27 °C might allow 9–15 minutes, and at 17 °C, it could be 27–45 minutes (see Table 35.1). Additionally, Fig. 28.4 illustrates the relationship between temperature and $CMRO_2$. This topic is covered in greater detail in Chaps. 6 and 28.

Beyond reducing $CMRO_2$, pre-ischemic hypothermia mitigates the effects of ischemia by markedly decreasing the release of the excitatory neurotransmitters (glutamate, aspartate, and glycine) during ischemia and subsequent reperfusion. In energy-deprived cells, glutamate can induce neurotoxicity partly through its role in inducing massive calcium influx via NMDA receptors. Hypothermia may also help attenuate neutrophil migration into ischemic tissue. For more detailed information, please refer to Chap. 6. Additionally, a decrease in regional oxygen saturation (rSO_2) in one hemisphere indicates reduced cerebral blood flow in that area of the brain. However, this does not necessarily imply cerebral ischemia or hypoperfusion, as it does not directly measure neuronal function.

Benefits of Circulatory Arrest

DHCA creates a still, bloodless surgical field, essential for complex procedures like aortic arch repairs and congenital heart defect corrections. This allows for precise surgical manipulation and reduces the risk of air embolism and bleeding.

Risks and Physiological Challenges

While DHCA offers significant benefits, it also carries inherent risks. The rewarming phase can be particularly challenging, as rapid temperature changes can induce physiological stress and potential complications. Moreover, hypothermia can alter acid–base balance, impacting cerebral blood flow. The choice of pH management strategy (α-stat vs. pH-stat) can significantly influence outcomes. Although monitoring cerebral oxygenation using Near-Infrared Spectroscopy (NIRS) can provide insights into blood flow, it doesn't directly assess neuronal function.

Indications and Considerations for DHCA

Types of Surgeries Requiring DHCA

DHCA is a specialized technique employed in adult cardiac surgery when temporarily reducing or stopping blood flow to the upper body and arch vessels is necessary to create a motionless, bloodless surgical field. This is especially crucial for complex cardiovascular procedures where standard techniques are insufficient, such as:

1. *Aortic Arch Surgery*: Repairs of aneurysms, dissections, and other complex anomalies involving the ascending and transverse aorta, particularly when head vessels are involved.
2. *Complex Congenital Heart Repairs*: Certain congenital heart defects, particularly those involving the aortic arch or requiring intricate intracardiac repairs, may necessitate the use of DHCA.
3. *Other Cardiovascular Procedures*: DHCA may be employed in selected cases of tumor resection (renal cell carcinoma), trauma repair, pulmonary thromboendarterectomy, or complex reoperative procedures where conventional techniques are insufficient.

During DHCA, alternative methods, such as selective cerebral perfusion, are used to maintain blood flow to the brain while lower-body perfusion is reduced or halted.

Patient Selection Criteria

The candidacy for DHCA is determined by a careful evaluation of the patient's overall health and surgical needs:

- *Surgical Necessity*: The procedure must require a bloodless field and temporary circulatory arrest for technical feasibility or improved safety.
- *Medical Stability*: The patient should be optimized preoperatively, ensuring adequate organ function and minimal comorbidities that could increase the risks associated with DHCA.
- *Age and Neurological Status*: While DHCA can be used in both children and adults, factors such as age and baseline neurological function are considered in risk assessment.

Preoperative Considerations

Thorough preoperative planning is crucial for the safe and successful implementation of DHCA:

- *Multidisciplinary Team*: Effective collaboration between cardiac surgeons, anesthesiologists, perfusionists, and other specialists is essential.
- *Neuroprotection*: Strategies to minimize the risk of neurological injury during DHCA, such as selective cerebral perfusion and the use of neuroprotective agents, should be carefully considered.
- *Cardioprotection*: Optimizing myocardial preservation techniques to ensure adequate cardiac function before and after DHCA is critical.
- *Informed Consent*: A thorough discussion with the patient and their family regarding the risks and benefits of DHCA is essential for informed decision-making.

Techniques of DHCA

Preparatory Steps for DHCA

Patient Cooling Methods

DHCA involves cooling the patient to a nasopharyngeal temperature of 15–22 °C through a combination of core and surface cooling methods, before initiating circulatory arrest and disconnecting from the CPB machine to create a bloodless surgical field.

- *Core Cooling*:

Core cooling is achieved by cooling the blood as it circulates through the heat exchanger on the CPB circuit.

- *Surface Cooling*:

Surface cooling, employed during anesthesia induction, surgical exposure, and cannulation for CPB, complements core cooling and includes several steps:

1. Lowering the room temperature to below 20 °C.
2. Positioning the patient on a cooling blanket set to about 10 °C.
3. Using systems that circulate cold air or water around blankets or pads.
4. Ice-filled bags are placed around the patient's head and neck to enhance the cooling effect.

Surface cooling offers uniform and effective head cooling by reducing heat transfer from the environment. This cost-effective method is generally safe, with only theoretical risks of thermal, pressure, or eye injuries associated with ice packs; yet no such injuries have been described. One limitation of surface cooling is the potential for disruption or displacement of sensors placed on the forehead, which are used for monitoring modalities, such as BIS (Bispectral Index) or NIRS. Although the skull's poor thermal conductivity may restrict the amount of heat transfer between the brain and the ice packs, the blood flow in the carotid arteries provides an excellent mechanism for distributing thermal energy, potentially enhancing the effectiveness of cooling the brain.

This integrated approach of core and surface cooling prepares the patient optimally for DHCA, ensuring both safety and effectiveness during complex cardiovascular procedures.

Monitoring Techniques

- *NIRS*: NIRS technology, covered in detail in Chap. 14 (see Figs. 14.1, 14.2, and 14.3), can continuously monitor cerebral regional oxygen saturation (rSO_2) in the frontal cortex in patients undergoing operations with CPB and DHCA or Antegrade Cerebral Perfusion (ACP) / Retrograde Cerebral Perfusion (RCP), but its limitations must be acknowledged. During cooling on CPB prior to DHCA, rSO_2 values often increase to reach maximum levels, especially when the pH-stat strategy for acid–base management is employed, which promotes abundant cerebral blood flow. Upon initiating circulatory arrest, values begin to decline, with the rate of this decline determined by the rate of tissue oxygen desaturation as shown in Fig. 35.1. Also demonstrated in Fig. 35.1 are represen-

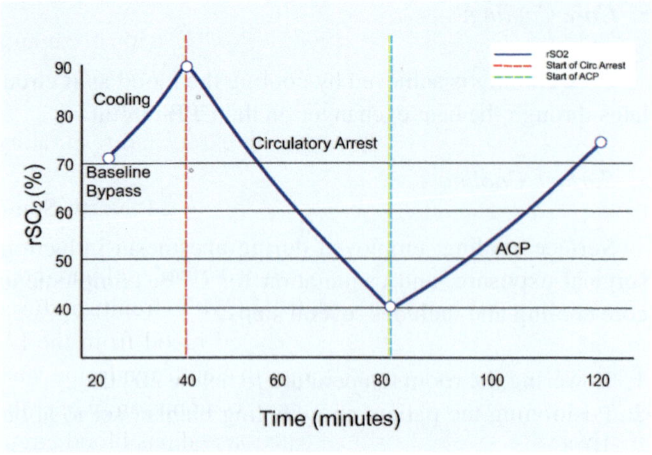

Fig. 35.1 The graph illustrates the expected trend of rSO_2 values during deep hypothermic cooling on CPB, using the pH-stat acid-base management strategy. Initially, rSO_2 values increase to their maximum during the cooling phase. Upon initiating circulatory arrest, there's a notable decline in rSO_2, reflecting tissue oxygen desaturation. The graph also shows how increased ACP flow subsequently restores rSO_2 levels

tative NIRS values, which increase toward baseline with the initiation of ACP as ACP flows are increased.

- A sudden unilateral decrease in rSO_2 likely indicates a reduction in regional cerebral blood flow and should be communicated to the surgeon and perfusionist as soon as possible. Potential causes of this could include temporary clamping of the common carotid or innominate artery, cerebral embolization, or an extension of aortic dissection, causing a unilateral decrease in cerebral perfusion.
- Bilateral decreases in rSO_2 are likely indicators of reduced cerebral blood flow, although it is important to note that this is not necessarily indicative of cerebral ischemia, as NIRS does not assess neuronal activity. Additionally, since the critical NIRS threshold values for identifying inadequate cerebral blood flow have never been clearly defined, NIRS data must be interpreted in the context of all other available data relevant to cerebral perfusion. Please refer to the algorithms in Chap. 14 (see Fig. 14.4) for managing unilateral and bilateral cerebral desaturation. These provide detailed strategies to optimize cerebral oximetry values during CPB.
- *EEG*: EEG can be used as a surveillance tool to assess neuronal function before and during hypothermic arrest. Monitoring somatosensory or motor evoked potentials helps protect the spinal cord and provides valuable information about brainstem, cortical, and subcortical regions. Cerebral hypoperfusion is typically manifested by a decrease in EEG amplitude and frequency. EEG neuromonitoring requires cumbersome equipment and trained personnel for data interpretation, making its use less common than cerebral oximetry. As a result, many institutions have transitioned from traditional raw EEG monitoring to more user-friendly processed EEG systems such as BIS (Medtronic, Minneapolis, MN, USA) or SedLine (Masimo, Irvine, CA, USA). These systems feature intuitive interfaces and provide simpler interpretation through proprietary algorithms that analyze brain activity and output a numerical value (0–100) that can assist in timing circulatory arrest. However, both raw EEG and pEEG are affected by anesthetic drugs. To ensure accurate interpretation, it's crucial to establish baseline readings at multiple key stages: before and after anesthesia induction, throughout CPB, and before the onset of hypothermia.
- *Transesophageal echocardiography (TEE)*: TEE aids in assessing cardiac function, guiding cannula placement, and detecting air embolism during cooling.

Cannulation Strategies for DHCA

Several arterial cannulation strategies can initiate CPB and achieve cooling prior to DHCA. The choice of cannulation site depends on the surgical procedure, patient anatomy, and the desired direction of blood flow during CPB. Common options include central aortic, axillary, subclavian, and femoral artery cannulation, each with distinct advantages and disadvantages.

Central Aortic Cannulation

Central aortic cannulation offers the advantage of maintaining antegrade flow during CPB while avoiding the need for additional incisions and tissue dissection. However, direct manipulation of the proximal aorta increases the risk of dislodging calcified plaque or debris, potentially leading to embolic events.

Furthermore, in cases of proximal aortic dissection, there is a higher risk of inadvertently cannulating the false lumen. This can result in partial or complete loss of perfusion to major arterial branches supplying the brain and other major organs. To mitigate this risk, the Seldinger technique, combined with TEE guidance, can confirm guidewire placement within the true lumen of both the proximal and descending aorta before cannula insertion over the wire.

Axillary or Subclavian Cannulation

Right axillary or subclavian artery cannulation can be achieved by either placing an end-to-side chimney graft or through direct cannulation (Figs. 35.2 and 35.3). This approach offers the advantage of antegrade perfusion to the brain and body, reducing the risk of dislodging proximal aortic debris and subsequent cerebral embolization. However, this technique may prolong surgical time and carries risks such as brachial plexus injury, impaired right arm perfusion, and localized vessel injury or dissection.

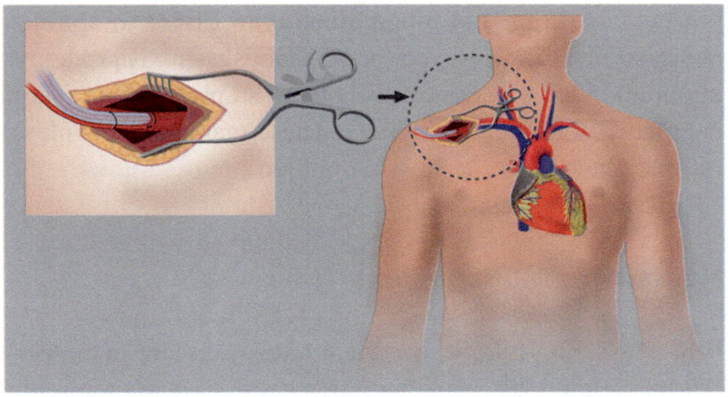

Fig. 35.2 Diagram of right axillary artery cannulation for ACP. This illustration demonstrates how the right axillary artery can be utilized to provide arterial inflow. It is directly cannulated using a purse-string suture technique

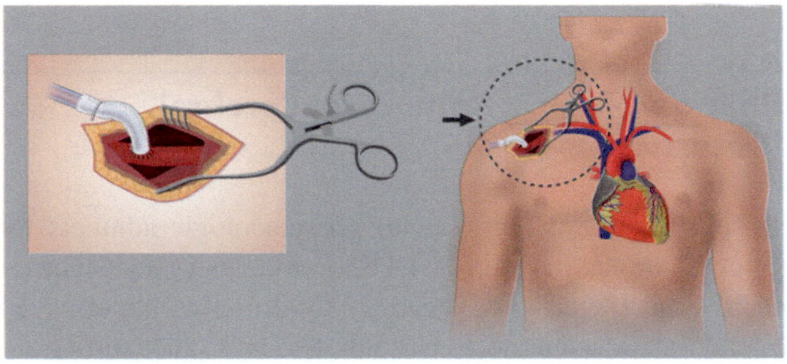

Fig. 35.3 Diagram of right axillary artery cannulation for ACP. This illustration demonstrates the surgical technique of using a Dacron graft to establish arterial inflow through the right axillary artery for ACP during DHCA

The European Society of Cardiology weakly recommends (Class IIa, Level C) the axillary artery as the first choice for cannulation in aortic arch surgery and dissection. However, studies comparing central and axillary cannulation techniques have not demonstrated significant outcomes differences.

During CPB with axillary artery cannulation, a key consideration is that invasively measured right radial artery pressure will be higher than pressures measured in the left radial or femoral arteries due to preferential flow down the right arm. This must be factored into decisions about mean arterial pressure (MAP) during CPB. On the other hand, right radial artery pressure accurately reflects cerebral perfusion pressure during ACP (discussed in the section below) via the axillary cannula.

Innominate Artery Cannulation

This method establishes an arterial line for CPB through the innominate artery, which can be accessed by direct cannulation or via an end-to-side Dacron graft anastomosis (Fig. 35.4). This approach eliminates the necessity of a second incision that would be required for exposing the axillary artery, however, it does involve more dissection. Following the administration of heparin (5000 units), a side-biting clamp is applied to partially occlude the innominate artery, thus permitting some antegrade blood flow while performing the graft anastomosis. However, if the artery is deemed too small, clamps are applied proximal and distal to the arterial incision to facilitate the anastomosis. Precise blood pressure management is critical to ensure sufficient cerebral perfusion through the left carotid artery. Monitoring techniques, such as cerebral oximetry or EEG, are invaluable in providing guidance to ensure sufficient cerebral perfusion. Notably, this technique enables a precise assessment of cerebral perfusion pressure by monitoring the pressure in the right radial artery during ACP.

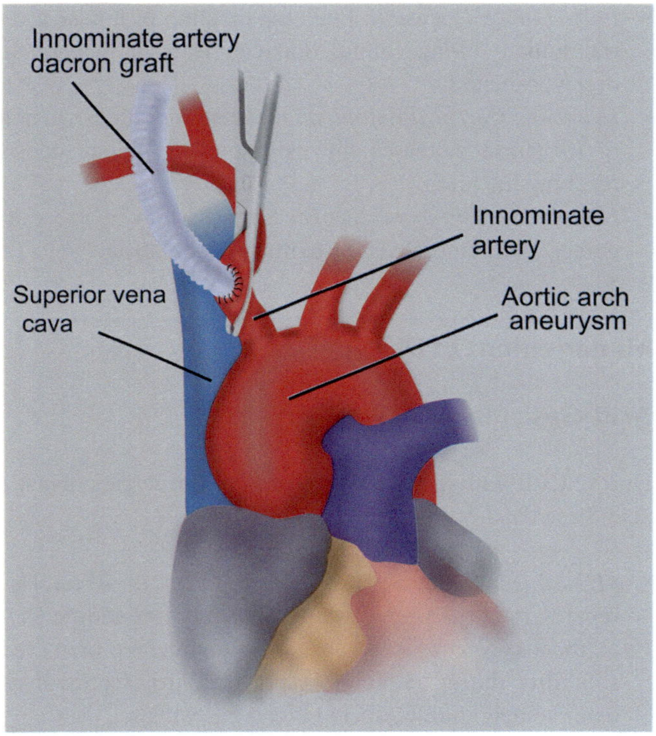

Fig. 35.4 Diagram of innominate artery cannulation with Dacron graft. This illustration shows the process of achieving proximal and distal control of the innominate artery using a side-biting clamp, followed by the end-to-side anastomosis of a Dacron graft. This graft not only provides access for CPB but also enables selective ACP during circulatory arrest by allowing occlusion of the proximal innominate segment

Femoral Cannulation

Femoral artery cannulation offers rapid access for CPB, making it valuable in complex dissections, contained aneurysm rupture, or unstable patients. While conventionally used to resume total body perfusion after distal anastomosis is complete, it carries notable risks:

- *False Lumen Perfusion*: Potential creation of a false arterial lumen during cannulation can lead to inadequate organ perfusion.
- *Increased Cerebral Embolism Risk*: Retrograde perfusion of the aorta increases the likelihood of plague debris reaching the brain.
- *Higher Mortality and Stroke*: Studies show worse outcomes with femoral versus axillary cannulation.

Management of DHCA

Acid–Base Management

During CPB with hypothermia, two main strategies manage acid–base balance: pH-stat and alpha-stat.

- *pH-stat*: Maintains a pH of 7.4 and $PaCO_2$ of 40 mmHg, regardless of body temperature. This requires adding CO_2 to the oxygenator's sweep gas to counteract increased solubility during cooling. In practice, pH-stat involves using temperature-corrected blood gas values.
- *Alpha-stat*: Maintains a progressively alkalotic pH and $PaCO_2$ as blood cools, mimicking the body's natural response to hypothermia. This approach uses uncorrected blood gas values (warmed to 37 °C).

Key Differences and Considerations

- *Cerebral Autoregulation*: Alpha-stat preserves cerebral autoregulation, the brain's ability to adjust blood flow based on its needs. pH-stat disrupts this mechanism, potentially leading to excessive blood flow and an increased risk of embolization.
- *Brain Cooling*: The increased cerebral blood flow caused by pH-stat can enhance brain cooling, but this may also increase the risk of delivering emboli to the brain.

Current Practice

In adults, alpha-stat is predominantly used during both cooling and rewarming phases of CPB. However, research indicates that the pH-stat method may offer advantages in pediatric surgeries. For a more detailed discussion of acid–base management and its implications, please refer to Chap. 6.

Blood Glucose Management

DHCA often induces hyperglycemia, which is exacerbated by glucocorticoids commonly administered in this setting to mitigate the systemic inflammatory response. Although the precise target range of blood glucose necessary to optimize neuronal protection has not been established, it is prudent to maintain blood glucose levels below 180 mg/dL. For a more detailed discussion of blood glucose management, please refer to Chap. 6.

Hematocrit Management

While a hemodilution-associated decrease in hematocrit (Hct) to around 20% can theoretically improve microcirculation during deep hypothermia, a target Hct of about 30% is generally aimed for to optimize systemic oxygen delivery. This topic is explored in more detail in Chap. 16 "Hematocrit and Transfusion Management During Cardiopulmonary Bypass."

Pharmacological Adjunct for Cerebral Protection

Despite routine use of various pharmacologic adjuncts for cerebral protection during DHCA, conclusive evidence of their efficacy remains elusive. Commonly administered agents include mannitol, barbiturates, and glucocorticoids, often cited for their low risk despite limited evidence supporting their neuroprotective role.

In the setting of DHCA and ischemia-reperfusion injury, steroid pretreatment may mitigate end-organ damage by dampening the activation and release of pro-inflammatory cytokines. Mannitol can reduce cerebral edema after ischemia, and scavenges free radicals, thus reducing tissue damage. Barbiturates such as thiopental reduce $CMRO_2$, enhancing EEG suppression and potentially enabling circulatory arrest at a higher temperature, as EEG suppression will not be dependent on temperature alone. However, thiopental's significant myocardial depressant effect may necessitate inotropic support following termination of CPB.

Hypothermic Circulatory Arrest: Techniques and Applications

Basic Steps for DHCA

1. *Cannulation*: It begins with cannulation to initiate CPB using the chosen arterial and venous access points.
2. *Cooling*: Cooling of the patient then starts, aiming for a target temperature of 18–20 °C or until EEG silence is achieved.
3. *Proximal Procedure*: During this cooling phase, the initial part of the operation involving the proximal part is performed.

4. *DHCA Initiation*:
   - Once the target temperature is reached, DHCA is initiated by stopping CPB.
   - To prevent air trapping in the brain, the patient is positioned in a steep Trendelenburg position.
   - Allow 1 liter of blood to remain in the patient to prevent air emboli.
   - Then clamping the venous cannula follow.
5. *Distal Procedure*: The surgery then proceeds in the now bloodless field.
6. *Resume CPB*: Following this, CPB is resumed by either cannulating the graft directly or via a sidearm, or by resuming flow through the axillary artery.
7. *Complete Proximal Procedure*: The operation concludes with the completion of the remaining steps of the proximal procedure.

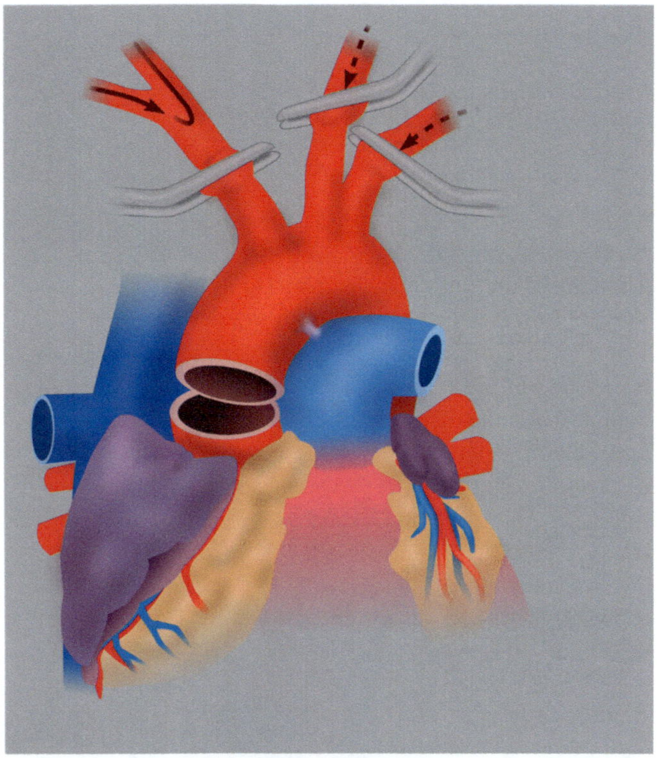

Fig. 35.5 Diagram of oxygenated blood flow during circulatory arrest. This illustration depicts how, during DHCA, selective ACP is achieved by delivering oxygenated blood from the CPB circuit to the right axillary artery at a rate of approximately 10 ml/kg/min. The aortic arch vessels remain clamped during this process. Solid arrows in the diagram show the intended flow of oxygenated blood towards the brain via the right carotid artery, while dotted arrows represent potential backflow originating from the left carotid and subclavian arteries, a result of collateral brain circulation

Adjuncts to DHCA: Selective Cerebral Perfusion

Selective cerebral perfusion techniques offer an alternative to complete circulatory arrest during DHCA, allowing for continuous or near-continuous cerebral blood flow while maintaining a bloodless operative field. These techniques enable warmer perfusion temperatures, as complete suppression of $CMRO_2$ is not required when adequate oxygen delivery matches $CMRO_2$.

Antegrade Cerebral Perfusion

ACP, typically achieved through unilateral cannulation, or via a Dacron graft, of the innominate, axillary, or common carotid arteries using the CPB arterial cannula (Fig. 35.5). If the expected duration of ACP is to exceed 40 to 50 minutes, bilateral ACP may be employed with additional cannulation of the left common carotid artery.

Advantages of ACP

- ACP allows for a higher target core temperature, which reduces the total CPB time needed for cooling and rewarming.
- Decreased complications associated with deep hypothermia, such as vasoplegia, enhanced inflammatory response, endothelial dysfunction, and coagulation abnormalities.

Typical ACP Parameters

- Adults: Cerebral perfusion pressures of 40–60 mmHg with flow rates between 6 and 10 ml/kg/min at a target temperature of 24–28 °C.
- Infants: Flow rates of 40–60 mL/kg/min.

Ideally, the ACP flow rate should be sufficient to match $CMRO_2$ at the target temperature. However, optimal perfusion pressure and flow rates for a given degree of hypothermia remain unclear, and the risks of hypoperfusion (leading to CNS ischemia) and hyperperfusion (leading to cerebral edema) must be carefully considered.

Retrograde Cerebral perfusion (RCP)

RCP is achieved via superior vena cava (SVC) cannulation, with the cannula directed cranially and ensnared between the right atrium and the azygous vein. Cold, oxygenated blood is perfused into the SVC retrogradely at a rate of 100–500 mL/minute (Fig. 35.6). To minimize the risk of cerebral air embolism, the patient is positioned in a 10° Trendelenburg.

A central venous pressure (CVP) line is transduced, and retrograde flow is adjusted to maintain CVP <25 mmHg, preventing cerebral edema. While RCP likely provides some cerebral microvascular flow, it does not, unlike ACP, deliver

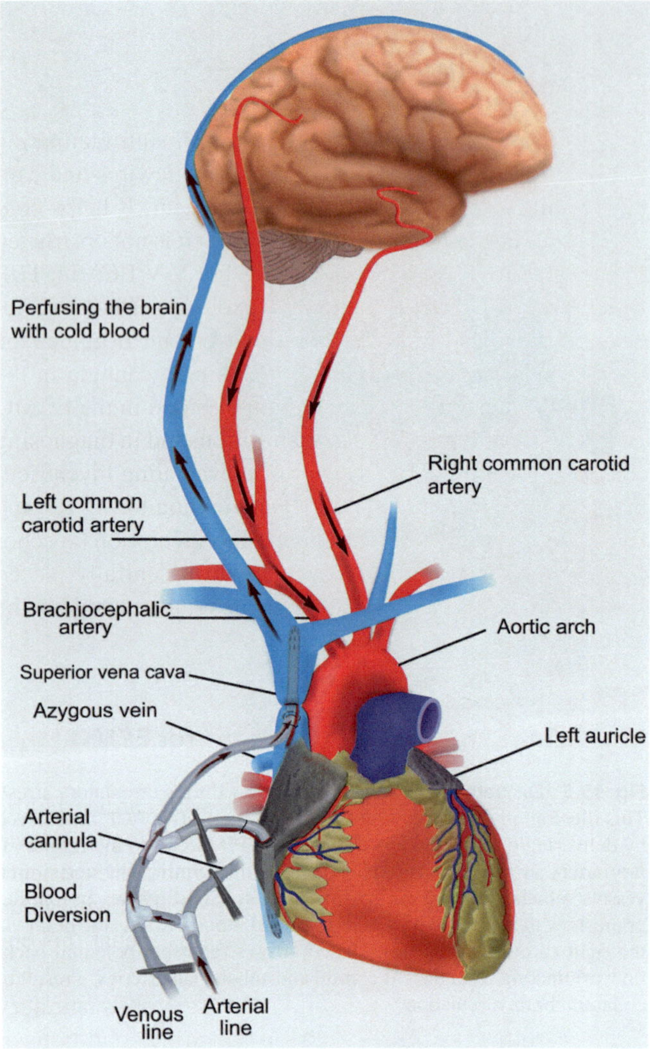

Fig. 35.6 Diagram of retrograde cerebral perfusion. This illustration depicts the precise placement of a cannula in the SVC, avoiding the azygous vein, for the delivery of cold, oxygenated blood to the brain during deep hypothermic circulatory arrest. A shunt between the arterial and venous lines is opened, allowing blood to be diverted into the SVC cannula. This retrograde flow is clearly indicated by the arrows

sufficient flow to meet the brain's $CMRO_2$. The primary advantages of RCP include the maintenance of regional hypothermia and the effective flushing of air and debris out of the cerebral circulation. These benefits contribute to extending the allowable period of DHCA, enhancing the safety and effectiveness of the procedure.

There is no clear consensus on the best cerebral protection strategy during circulatory arrest. No single technique has been proven superior, leading to wide variation in practice among aortic centers.

Rewarming Following Hypothermic Cardiac Arrest

Once the surgical phase requiring DHCA is completed, rewarming begins by reinstituting CPB at the initial cold target temperature for 10 minutes. Subsequently, rewarming proceeds slowly, typically not exceeding 0.5 ° C per minute, with the temperature gradient between the venous inflow and arterial outlet on the oxygenator is maintained at ≤4 °C. This gradual approach can take 60 to 90 minutes or longer following moderate or deep hypothermia.

Crucially, the arterial outlet temperature should never exceed 37 °C. Cerebral hyperthermia can cause severe complications like cognitive dysfunction and increased intracranial pressure, particularly after cerebral thromboembolic events during aortic surgery.

Management of Coagulopathy Following DHCA

Managing bleeding after aortic surgery with DHCA can be challenging due to multiple factors. Surgical bleeding is worsened by coagulopathy, which is a consequence of the anti-hemostatic effects of deep hypothermia, fibrinolysis, and platelet activation associated with prolonged CPB and ischemia-reperfusion injury. Employing retrograde autologous priming of the CPB circuit, cell salvage, and routine use of antifibrinolytics can help reduce transfusion requirements.

Another beneficial strategy is autologous whole blood collection. This involves withdrawing blood from the patient into citrated collection bags early in the procedure and replacing it with crystalloid or colloidal solutions, a technique known as acute normovolemic hemodilution. The collected autologous whole blood is typically reinfused after protamine administration but can also be given during CPB if needed. This strategy has been shown to significantly reduce intraoperative transfusion rates of red blood cells, platelets, plasma, and cryoprecipitate in cases involving circulatory arrest.

Further Reading

Arnaoutakis GJ, Ogami T, Bobba CM, Serna-Gallegos D, Brown JA, Jeng EI, Martin TD, Beaver TM, Yousef S, Navid F, Sultan I. Cerebral protection using deep hypothermic circulatory arrest versus retrograde cerebral perfusion for aortic hemiarch reconstruction. J Card Surg. 2022;37(10):3279–86. https://doi.org/10.1111/jocs.16809.

Engelman R, Baker RA, Likosky DS, Grigore A, Dickinson TA, Shore-Lesserson L, Hammon JW. The Society of Thoracic Surgeons, The Society of Cardiovascular Anesthesiologists, and The American Society of ExtraCorporeal Technology: clinical practice guidelines for cardiopulmonary bypass—temperature management during cardiopulmonary bypass. Ann Thorac Surg. 2015;100(2):748–57., ISSN 0003-4975. https://doi.org/10.1016/j.athoracsur.2015.03.126.

Hage A, Stevens LM, Ouzounian M, Chung J, El-Hamamsy I, Chauvette V, Dagenais F, Cartier A, Peterson MD, Boodhwani M, Guo M, Bozinovski J, Moon MC, White A, Kumar K, Lodewyks C, Bittira B, Payne D, Chu MWA. Impact of brain protection strategies on mortality and stroke in patients undergoing aortic arch repair with hypothermic circulatory arrest: evidence from the Canadian Thoracic Aortic Collaborative. Eur J Cardiothorac Surg. 2020;58(1):95–103. https://doi.org/10.1093/ejcts/ezaa023.

Peterss S, Pichlmaier M, Curtis A, Luehr M, Born F, Hagl C. Patient management in aortic arch surgery†. Eur J Cardiothorac Surg. 2017;51(suppl 1):i4–14. https://doi.org/10.1093/ejcts/ezw337.

Stecker MM, Cheung AT, Pochettino A, Kent GP, Patterson T, Weiss SJ, Bavaria JE. Deep hypothermic circulatory arrest: I. Effects of cooling on electroencephalogram and evoked potentials. Ann Thorac Surg. 2001;71(1):14–21. https://doi.org/10.1016/s0003-4975(00)01592-7.

Cardiopulmonary Bypass and the Jehovah's Witness Patient

36

Patrick Hussey and Ahmed Zaky

Introduction

The undertaking of cardiopulmonary bypass (CPB) during cardiac surgery for Jehovah's Witness (JW) patients presents unique challenges due to their religious convictions, which strictly preclude the acceptance of blood products. This chapter focuses on the key considerations and strategies for successful cardiac surgery under CPB on these patients. Despite the relatively high likelihood of the need for blood transfusion in cardiac open-heart surgery, the over 8.5 million JWs worldwide generally decline the transfusion of allogeneic primary blood components. This rejection stems from their interpretation of Acts 15:19–20 in the Bible. Blood components usually declined by a JW include red blood cells (RBCs), platelets, and fresh-frozen plasma (FFP). Conducting surgery without blood transfusion poses a unique challenge for the entire surgical team. However, recent reviews on various bloodless protocols for JW's patients have demonstrated comparable outcomes in JW patients and non-JW patients, where the latter group has the option to receive blood products.

Undertaking cardiac surgery on a JW patient necessitates meticulous preoperative discussion and optimization involving the surgeon, anesthesiologist, and perfusionist. These discussions should aim to review acceptable blood components and expanders, if any, strategize for blood management during surgery, and prepare for suitable contingency plans as needed. The 2021 Society of Thoracic Surgeons Blood Conservation Guidelines (STS/SCA/AmSECT/SABM) provide recommendations for reducing blood loss during cardiac surgery and improving patient outcomes based on evidence-based blood conservation strategies. These guidelines encompass 19 Class I recommendations, 14 Class II recommendations, and 11 Class III recommendations. In this chapter, we will delve into those recommendations pertinent to the management of JW patients.

P. Hussey · A. Zaky (✉)
Department of Anesthesiology and Perioperative Medicine, University of Alabama at Birmingham, Birmingham, AL, USA
e-mail: phussey@uabmc.edu; azaky@uabmc.edu

Demographics

JW is a global religious group with a broad reach and a diverse membership. In 2022, the official statistics indicated that approximately 19.7 million people worldwide attended the JW's observance of the Memorial of Christ's death. The JW community reported a monthly average membership of roughly 8.5 million individuals actively engaged in preaching during the same year.

In terms of racial and ethnic distribution, particularly in the United States, JW stands out as one of the most diverse religious groups. No single racial or ethnic background comprises more than 40% of the membership. The composition of the JW community includes 36% White, 32% Hispanic, 27% Black, and 6% from other or mixed races.

A noteworthy characteristic of the JW demographic profile is the gender distribution. The majority of JW are women, accounting for about two-thirds or 65% of the total membership, while men represent the remaining 35%. This distribution speaks to the inclusive nature of the community and its wide-ranging appeal across different demographics.

The Comprehensive Strategy for Managing JW Patients in the Surgical Setting

- Integrates the utilization of potential blood substitutes when acceptable. Blood substitutes fall into two main categories: oxygen carriers, like bovine hemoglobin and perfluorocarbons, which emulate RBCs' oxygen-carrying role but face approval limitations due to potential side effects; and volume expanders, such as hydroxyethyl starches, dextrans, and saline solutions, that maintain blood volume and pressure during surgical procedures,

A. S. Awad, J. DiNardo (eds.), *Clinical Perfusion for Cardiac Surgery*, https://doi.org/10.1007/978-3-031-91163-7_36

without replicating the oxygen-carrying capacity of blood.

- Proactive measures to elevate the patient's red blood cell count prior to the procedure. It involves specific, personalized strategies, which will be explored further in the preoperative considerations for bloodless cardiac surgery section.
- The meticulous implementation of techniques to minimize blood loss during surgery. These strategies involve specific techniques and approaches that will be further discussed in the intraoperative considerations for bloodless cardiac surgery section.
- Recover any lost blood during the procedure.

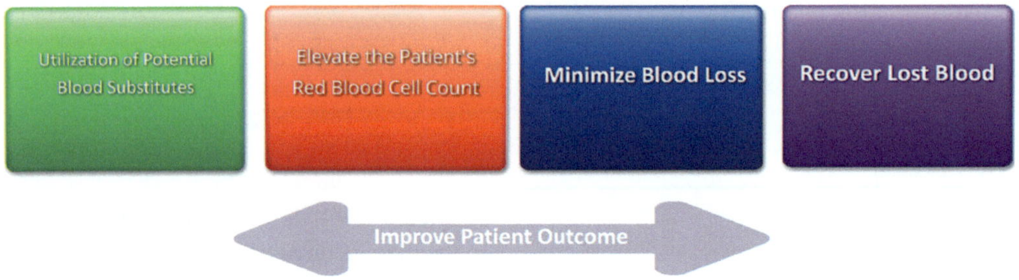

Preoperative Considerations for Bloodless Cardiac Surgery in JW Patients

1. *Preoperative Informed Consent and Comprehensive Documentation:*

The initiation of discussion about bloodless cardiac surgery should involve a broad spectrum of participants, including the patient, their family, a bloodless medicine specialist, a social worker, and the surgeon. It is not uncommon for the patient's church pastor to also partake in these discussions as well. To foster an understanding of the process, institutional guidelines, or protocols—established jointly by surgeons, anesthesiologists, perfusionists, and the blood bank—should be shared with the patient.

It is of paramount importance to determine and comprehensively document the patient's preferences concerning blood components, the extent of their refusal of blood transfusions (which may include erythrocyte concentrates, FFP, and platelets), and alternative measures to be taken in case of severe intraoperative blood loss.

Most significantly, it is imperative that JW patients are fully informed about the potential risks and benefits of the proposed surgery and associated blood conservation strategies. This includes discussing the possible risks associated with refusing blood transfusions and discussing the alternative treatment options available. This dialogue can and should be repeated multiple times throughout the preoperative process.

Furthermore, considerations of intra-operative use of hemostatic agents and the adoption of autologous retransfusion (using systems like Cell Saver®) should be consistently reviewed, documented, and validated during the pre-surgical process at the preoperative assessment clinics.

Checklists, such as the one listed below, serve as a valuable aid in understanding and corroborating patient preferences regarding the variety of blood components.

UAB PERIOPERATIVE BLOOD OPTIONS AND SELECTION GUIDE	
WHOLE BLOOD COMPONENTS *(some people call these Major Fractions)* Blood carries oxygen and nutrients through the body. The four main parts (or components) can be separated and used for treatment.	
RED BLOOD CELLS (Other Names: Erythrocytes, RBCs) take oxygen from your lungs to your organs and tissues. They also take carbon dioxide back to your lungs to breathe out. We give RBCs if your blood count is too low.	❑ Accept ❑ Decline
WHITE BLOOD CELLS (Other Names: Leukocytes, WBCs) are one of your body's defenses against bacteria, viruses, and diseases the body produces. We give WBCs to help you fight certain diseases.	❑ Accept ❑ Decline
PLATELETS (Other Name: Thrombocytes) are small pieces of cells. They help your blood make clots that prevent or stop bleeding. We give platelets if your bleeding is hard to stop or if your platelet count is very low.	❑ Accept ❑ Decline
PLASMA is the liquid part of blood. It is made of water, albumin, clotting factors, salts, sugars, fats, vitamins, and hormones. We give this if you need more plasma or clotting factors.	❑ Accept ❑ Decline
TYPES OF PLASMA ▶ Frozen (or thawed) plasma (FFP) is plasma removed from whole blood. It is frozen so it can be used later. ▶ Solvent detergent-treated plasma is plasma that is cleaned to reduce the chance of infection or allergic reaction.	
FRACTIONATED BLOOD COMPONENTS are separated from whole blood components *(some people call these Minor Fractions).*	
*– – **Clotting Factors** are proteins in plasma. They help your blood make clots that stop bleeding. – –*	
CRYOSUPERNATANT is plasma that has most of the solid parts taken out. The leftover liquid is called cryosupernatant. We give cryosupernatant to replace plasma.	❑ Accept ❑ Decline
CRYOPRECIPITATE is plasma that has the liquid part taken out. The leftover clotting factors are called cryoprecipitate. We give cryoprecipitate to help stop bleeding.	❑ Accept ❑ Decline
PROTHROMBIN COMPLEX CONCENTRATE is a mix of many clotting factors. We give this mix to help stop bleeding or to reverse the effects of blood thinning medicine.	❑ Accept ❑ Decline
CONCENTRATED CLOTTING FACTORS are single clotting factors. We give them to help stop bleeding.	❑ Accept ❑ Decline
ALBUMIN is the main protein in plasma. We give albumin to increase blood volume.	❑ Accept ❑ Decline
ANTIBODIES (Other Name: Immune Globulins) are proteins your body makes to fight disease. We can also give you antibodies to help your body fight some types of infections.	❑ Accept ❑ Decline
YOUR OWN BLOOD can be used in the procedures below in a closed system. Your blood is not mixed with any other blood.	
APHERESIS (Other Names: Plasma exchange, Plasmapheresis) is when a closed-system machine replaces bad plasma with a good plasma substitute. It is used if your plasma has antibodies that are attacking your body.	❑ Accept ❑ Decline
AUTOTRANSFUSION (Other Names: Cell Saver, Cell Salvage, Salvaged Autologous Blood) is when your blood is collected during surgery, washed and filtered, and then given back to you in a closed system.	❑ Accept ❑ Decline
HEMODILUTION is when your blood is replaced with IV fluids during surgery. After surgery, we give your blood back to you in a closed system.	❑ Accept ❑ Decline
HEART AND LUNG MACHINE is when your blood flows into a machine that adds oxygen to it. Your blood then flows back into your body in a closed system primed with nonblood fluid. It is used during some surgeries.	❑ Accept ❑ Decline
DIALYSIS (Other Names: Renal Dialysis, Hemodialysis) is when your blood flows into a machine that filters and cleans it, then flows back into your body in a closed system. It is used if your kidneys are not working well or harmful substances need to be taken out of your blood.	❑ Accept ❑ Decline
EPIDURAL BLOOD PATCH is when your blood is injected around your spinal cord to stop a spinal fluid leak.	❑ Accept ❑ Decline
PLATELET GEL is made of your platelets and white blood cells. We use it to cover wounds and help stop bleeding.	❑ Accept ❑ Decline
RECOMBINANT PRODUCTS are like whole blood components, but they are made with protein technology and do not come from blood.	
RECOMBINANT CLOTTING FACTORS* are like the clotting factors that come from whole blood components that are listed above. We give them to help stop bleeding.	❑ Accept ❑ Decline
RECOMBINANT ERYTHROPOIETIN* (Other Names: EPO, ESA, Hematopoietin) is like your body's erythropoietin. It is a hormone that tells bone marrow to make more red blood cells. We give it if your blood count is too low.	❑ Accept ❑ Decline
OTHER TREATMENT (Please Specify):	❑ Accept ❑ Decline

**Some formulations may contain a small amount of albumin.*

Adapted From American Society Of Anesthesiologists Transfusion Consent Form, Committee For Patient Blood Management

PERIOPERATIVE BLOOD OPTIONS AND SELECTION GUIDE VERSION 1, 06/01/2018

Adapted from the American Society of Anesthesiologists, Transfusion Consent Form, Committee for Patient Blood Management

2. *Preoperative Assessment Clinics*

Before surgery, a comprehensive review of the patient's medical history and a detailed physical examination should be conducted. Any existing medical conditions that could potentially increase bleeding risk or necessitate transfusions, such as anemia or bleeding disorders, should be identified and effectively managed to optimize their overall medical status.

3. *Strategies for Preoperative Blood Management Optimization*

Several approaches are essential to consider. These may encompass a thorough and proactive plan, emphasizing the aggressive optimization of hemoglobin levels. This is accomplished by administering iron and folic acid supplements or erythropoietin therapy, tailored to each patient's specific condition. Through careful monitoring, this approach aims to elevate preoperative hemoglobin levels, with a potential target of 14.

1. *Surgical Planning*

This process requires meticulous customization to the individual patient's needs with the goal of minimizing the risk of bleeding and the requirement for transfusions. This planning stage may involve the careful selection of an appropriate surgical technique and equipment to ensure optimal patient care.

Intraoperative Considerations for Bloodless Cardiac Surgery in JW Patients

Intraoperative management of JW patients undergoing cardiac surgery requires meticulous planning and execution to honor their refusal of blood transfusions. Adhering to this requirement involves a comprehensive strategy that integrates various blood conservation techniques and careful monitoring procedures. Anesthesiologists, surgeons, and perfusionists collaborate closely to tailor medical interventions with patient beliefs, employing advanced techniques to minimize blood loss and enhance anemia tolerance. Surgeons use meticulous and minimally invasive methods to reduce bleeding, while perfusionists optimize hemodynamics and oxygen delivery during CPB with strategies like lower hemodilution, biocompatible circuits, and normothermia. This multidisciplinary approach effectively minimizes transfusions and ensures successful surgical outcomes for patients with religious objections to blood products. For a comprehensive review of overall blood conservation strategies during cardiac surgery, please refer to Chap. 18.

Anesthetic Approach for Blood Conservation in JW

On the day of surgery, the anesthesia provider is responsible for delineating blood conservation strategies and acceptable products.

1. *Acute Normovolemic Hemodilution (ANH)*

The anesthesia providers can employ ANH, a blood conservation technique in which a portion of the patient's own blood is drawn prior to surgery and stored in citrate phosphate dextrose adenine-containing (CPDA) bags. These bags are placed either in a cooler or on rockers, or mixers to maintain gentle agitation and to facilitate mixing the blood with CPDA solution, helping to prevent clot formation. The bags remain attached to the infusion line throughout the procedure. The stored autologous blood is later reinfused post-CPB and after protamine administration. JW patients often request that the blood remains "in continuity," meaning it stays connected to them via stopcocks and intravenous tubing.

- *Benefits of ANH in JW:*
  - *Reduced Blood Loss:* ANH can help reduce blood loss during surgery by diluting the concentration of RBCs and plasma proteins, including clotting factors. With a lower hematocrit, the patient experiences less blood loss during surgery, as this process decreases the loss of these active components during bleeding.
  - *Optimal Hemostasis:* Unlike stored blood, freshly harvested blood contains functional platelets and normal levels of coagulation factors, enhancing clotting and reducing bleeding after reinfusion.
  - *Preservation of 2,3-DPG:* ANH maintains normal levels of 2,3-diphosphoglycerate (2,3-DPG) in RBCs, unlike stored blood. This molecule is crucial for efficient oxygen delivery to tissues, as it helps hemoglobin release oxygen more readily.

Determining Blood Withdrawal for ANH: A Stepwise Approach

The amount of blood withdrawn during ANH is personalized based on the patient's weight and desired hemoglobin (Hb) target. Here is a step-by-step approach:

1. *Calculate Ideal Body Weight (IBW):*
   - IBW (kg) = Height (cm)—105 (males) or 108 (females). This simplified formula is derived from Dr. B.J. Devine formula.
   - Alternatively: IBW (kg) = Height (m)^2 × 22.
2. *Estimate Blood Volume (BV):*
   - BV (mL) = IBW (kg) x Average Blood Volume (mL/kg).
   - Average Blood Volume varies by age and sex:
     - Adult male: 75 mL/kg.
     - Adult female: 65 mL/kg.
     - Infants: 80 mL/kg.
     - Neonates: 85 mL/kg.
     - Premature neonates: 95 mL/kg.
3. *Estimate Hb After Priming:*
   - Hb after priming (HbCPB) = (Patient's blood volume x Initial Hb) / (Patient's blood volume + Priming volume).
4. *Calculate Target Withdrawal Volume:*
   - Volume to Withdraw (L) = Estimated Blood Volume (L) x [(Initial Hb - Target Hb) / Average Hb].

   Initial Hb here is equal to Hb After Priming HbCPB.

Example: Calculating Blood Withdrawal for ANH

Scenario:

- Estimated Blood Volume (EBV): 5 liters.
- Initial Hemoglobin (Hb): 13 g/dL.
- Priming Volume: 1.4 liters (Plasmalyte + heparin 10 cc, solumedrol 4 cc, albumin 50 cc, MgSO4 50 cc).
- Target Hb: 8 g/dL.

Calculations:

1. *Hemoglobin After Priming (HbCPB):*
   - HbCPB = (Patient's blood volume * Initial Hb) / (Patient's blood volume + Priming volume).
   - HbCPB = (5 L * 13 g/dL) / (5 L + 1.4 L).
   - HbCPB ≈ **10.16 g/dL.**
2. *Average Hemoglobin Concentration:*
   - Average Hb = (HbCPB + Target Hb) / 2.
   - Average Hb = (10.16 g/dL + 8.0 g/dL) / 2.
   - Average Hb ≈ **9.08 g/dL.**
3. *Volume to Withdraw (L):*
   - Volume to Withdraw (L) = EBV (L) x [(HbCPB - Target Hb) / Average Hb].
   - Volume to Withdraw (L) = 5 L x [(10.16 g/dL - 8.0 g/dL) / 9.08 g/dL].
   - Volume to Withdraw (L) ≈ **1.19 L.**

Theoretical Withdrawal: Up to 1.19 liters could be removed during ANH. However, this does not account for retrograde autologous prime (RAP), which would further necessitate adjusting the withdrawal volume accordingly.

Important Note This is a theoretical calculation. In cardiac surgery, factors like additional CPB dilution and surgical blood loss should be considered. The actual withdrawal volume should be determined by the clinical team, balancing the desired Hb reduction with the patient's individual risks and needs.

2. *Antifibrinolytic Therapy:*
   Antifibrinolytics, such as tranexamic acid or aminocaproic acid, can be administered by anesthesia providers before or after bypass to prevent fibrinolysis.
3. *Minimized Blood Draws:*

Anesthesia and perfusion teams should minimize lab draws, given the absence of a transfusion target. Necessary lab tests, such as those for determining heparin and protamine dosing or correcting electrolyte imbalances, should only be conducted when required.

Surgical Techniques for Blood Conservation

Surgical procedures should be performed quickly and efficiently to minimize both operating room time and the duration of CPB. Increased surgical trauma, extensive dissection, and prolonged CPB can lead to significant consumption of coagulation factors. Whenever possible, minimally invasive approaches should be employed to lessen tissue disruption and blood loss. Additionally, using fewer or smaller surgical laps and sponges, and reinfusing blood collected from these using cell salvage, can help conserve blood volume. Furthermore, hemostatic agents such as fibrin glue, thrombin, or sealants are effective in controlling intraoperative bleeding.

Perfusion Techniques for Blood Conservation in JW Patients

- *Intraoperative Cell Salvage:*
  Intraoperative cell salvage, which involves using a cell saver to collect, clean, and re-infuse the patient's own blood, is commonly used in JW undergoing cardiac surgery (Figs. 18.6 and 18.7). All salvaged blood should be continuously reinfused through the cell saver in a closed circuit (Fig. 36.1). For more details, please refer to Chap. 18 titled "Blood Conservation Techniques."
- *Perfusion Pump Flow Considerations:*
  When managing perfusion pump flows, it is essential to balance minimizing blood loss while ensuring adequate oxygen delivery to the tissues. Generally, the perfusion pump flow should be set at a level that maintains adequate tissue perfusion without causing excessive blood loss. Hypotensive perfusion techniques, which involve lowering the blood pressure during surgery, can be effective in reducing blood loss. However, it's crucial to maintain appropriate perfusion levels, especially given that these patients are undergoing cardiac surgery and may have underlying cardiac conditions. Systemic vascular resistance (SVR) should be maintained at greater than 1000 in an attempt to decrease overall circulating volume. Centrifugal pumps are preferred over roller pumps due to their lower associated rates of blood trauma and hemolysis to the patient's blood.
- *Hemoconcentration Techniques:*
  During CPB, several strategies can be employed to maintain optimal hemoglobin concentration and blood viscosity. The priming volume for the bypass should be kept to a minimum. After cannulation, but before initiating bypass, the perfusionist can perform RAP of the bypass circuit via either or both the arterial and venous cannulae, clearing the circuit of crystalloid prime. RAP has been shown to benefit JW patients by maintaining blood viscosity, which can reduce microvascular injury, thrombotic events, and inflammatory response. This inflammatory response can also be reduced by minimizing bypass tubing length, keeping the circuit as close to the patient as possible. During bypass, diuretics and hemoconcentration should be used aggressively to maintain a high hemoglobin concentration and blood viscosity.
- *Modified Ultrafiltration (MUF):*
  After completion of the surgical procedure, MUF can be utilized to remove excess fluid and potentially

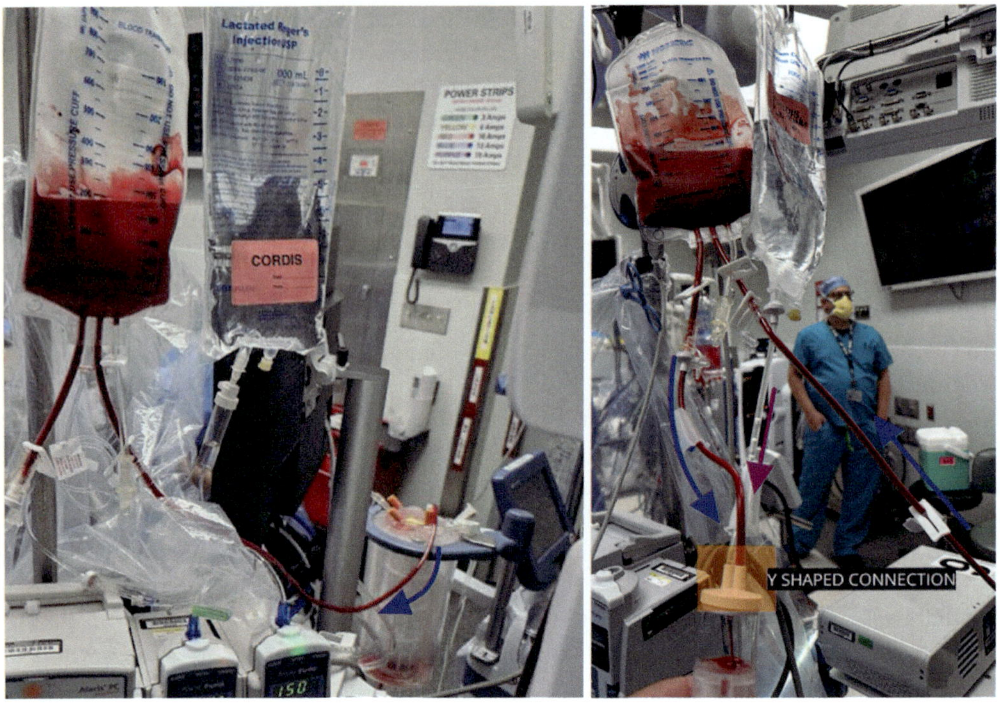

Fig. 36.1 Intraoperative cell salvage for JW patients in cardiac surgery. These two images illustrate intra-operative cell salvage, a process in which a cell saver is used to collect, clean, and re-infuse a patient's own blood during surgery. This technique is commonly employed in surgeries involving JW, who typically object to blood transfusions. *The left image*, indicated by a blue arrow, shows the connection between the cell saver machine and the collection bag. *In the right image*, blue arrows highlight the path of blood entering and exiting the collection bag. The purple arrow indicates fluid from the crystalloid bag merging with the blood through a Y-connector before entering the patient's venous system. This closed-circuit setup ensures the patient's blood remains in continuity, aligning with the beliefs of JW and avoiding external blood storage

harmful substances from the blood. This technique involves passing the patient's blood through a specialized membrane filter, which removes fluid and small molecules while retaining red and white blood cells, platelets, and larger proteins (Fig. 19.6). Studies suggest MUF may reduce edema, inflammation, blood transfusions, and postoperative complications while improving cardiac function. (Please refer to Chap. 19, "Ultrafiltration and Leukofiltration," for more information.)

- *Laboratory Monitoring and Recombinant Factors:* Lab draws should be minimized, with careful monitoring to ensure adequate anticoagulation with heparin and its reversal with protamine. JW patients often consent to the use of synthetic recombinant factors such as activated factor seven, prothrombin complex concentrate, and fibrinogen concentrates, which may be administered prophylactically to minimize blood loss. However, the potential prothrombotic risks associated with these treatments must be carefully weighed by the patient's care team.

Postoperative

In the postoperative period, it is advisable to minimize lab draws, focusing only on treatable concern such as electrolytes and anticoagulation levels. Activated clotting time (ACT) should be monitored if coagulopathy is suspected, as heparin rebound may require additional protamine administration. Chest tube output can be monitored and reinfused directly or processed via cell salvage using a closed circuit.

Future Research in Blood Substitutes: Implications for JW

Research into synthetic or artificial blood has a long history, dating back to the discovery of circulation in 1616. Once these products are approved, or in cases of last resort, it will be crucial to discuss with JW patients which synthetic options they deem acceptable.

Two promising categories for synthetic blood have emerged:

- *Hemoglobin-Based Oxygen Carriers (HBOCs)*: These products utilize modified bovine hemoglobin, formulated in a modified lactated Ringer's solution, to carry oxygen. One such product, Hemopure, has not yet received FDA approval but is currently permitted for compassionate use, with case reports of successful utilization in JW patients.
- *Perfluorocarbons (PFCs):* PFCs are entirely synthetic compounds capable of carrying both oxygen and carbon dioxide. However, various trials of PFCs have been suspended due to the lack of demonstrated beneficial outcomes.

Beyond HBOCs and PFCs, research is underway to explore innovative alternatives for blood transfusion:

- *Lab-Grown Blood from Stem Cells:* Scientists are investigating methods to generate RBCs from stem cells in the laboratory. This approach could offer a potentially unlimited source of blood for transfusion, free from disease transmission risks and compatibility issues. However, challenges remain in scaling up production and ensuring the functionality and longevity of lab-grown cells.
- *Reconstituted Freeze-Dried Blood Components:* This method involves freeze-drying blood components for long-term storage and later reconstitution with fluids for transfusion. This could improve blood availability in remote areas and disaster scenarios. However, ongoing research aims to address potential damage to blood components during the freeze-drying process and ensure functionality after reconstitution.

Conclusion

A multidisciplinary approach, encompassing preoperative optimization, intraoperative management, and postoperative care, is crucial for JW patients undergoing cardiac surgery. This approach focuses on blood conservation strategies, preoperative evaluation and optimization, surgical planning, anesthetic management, and informed consent. The objective is to minimize the risk of bleeding while ensuring the best possible outcomes for the patient.

Overall, multiple techniques and opportunities exist for JW patients to achieve the best possible bloodless outcome. Many of these techniques have shown promising results, but further research is needed to determine the most effective approaches for these patients.

Further Reading

Chambault AL, Brown LJ, Mellor S, Harky A. Outcomes of cardiac surgery in Jehovah's witness patients: a review. Perfusion. 2021;36(7):661–71. https://doi.org/10.1177/0267659120980375.

Jubouri M, Hedayat F, Abrar S, Mellor SL, Brown LJ, Harky A. Optimising bloodless cardiovascular surgery for Jehovah's witnesses and beyond. Coron Artery Dis. 2022;31(1):52–60. https://doi.org/10.1097/MCA.0000000000001050.

Marinakis S, Van der Linden P, Tortora R, Massaut J, Pierrakos C, Wauthy P. Outcomes from cardiac surgery in Jehovah's witness patients: experience over twenty-one years. J Cardiothorac Surg. 2016;11:67. https://doi.org/10.1186/s13019-016-0455-6.

Stamou SC, White T, Barnett S, Boyce SW, Corso PJ, Lefrak EA. Comparisons of cardiac surgery outcomes in Jehovah's versus non-Jehovah's witnesses. Am J Cardiol. 2006;98(9):1223–5. https://doi.org/10.1016/j.amjcard.2006.05.055.

Tanaka A, Ota T, Uriel N, Asfaw Z, Onsager D, Lonchyna VA, Jeevanandam V. Cardiovascular surgery in Jehovah's witness patients: the role of preoperative optimization. J Thorac Cardiovasc Surg. 2015;150(4):976–83.e1-3. https://doi.org/10.1016/j.jtcvs.2015.06.059.

Vasques F, Kinnunen EM, Pol M, Mariscalco G, Onorati F, Biancari F. Outcome of Jehovah's witnesses after adult cardiac surgery: systematic review and meta-analysis of comparative studies. Transfusion. 2016;56(8):2146–53. https://doi.org/10.1111/trf.13657.

37 Cardiopulmonary Bypass and Perfusion Management in Distal Aortic Repairs

Juan C. Restrepo Cardenas and Ahmed Zaky

Introduction

Distal aortic repairs are complex surgical procedures aimed at addressing life-threatening conditions such as aortic aneurysms and dissections. These procedures require meticulous surgical precision and an understanding of the aorta's critical role in systemic circulation. The success of such surgeries often hinges on effective management of blood flow during the operation, primarily achieved through various bypass techniques. Despite the development and evolution of transcatheter endovascular repair approaches for thoracoabdominal aortic aneurysms (TAAA) and type B aortic dissection, open surgical repair remains the gold standard. The use of extracorporeal circulation has become routine in the repair of these conditions. This chapter delves into the critical role of perfusion management in distal aortic surgery.

We will examine various bypass techniques, equipment, and decision-making strategies impacting patient outcomes. The challenges, complications, and future of perfusion technology in this context will also be explored. This introduction provides a foundation for understanding the processes vital to successful distal aortic repairs.

Classification and Management Approaches

The DTA, extending from the distal aortic arch to the diaphragm, can develop conditions requiring open surgical repair. These are broadly categorized as:

1. *Aortic aneurysms*
2. *Aortic dissections*
3. *Aortic Transection*
4. *Developmental Anomalies*: Such as coarctation or vascular rings

J. C. Restrepo Cardenas · A. Zaky (✉)
Department of Anesthesiology and Perioperative Medicine, University of Alabama at Birmingham, Birmingham, AL, USA
e-mail: jrestrepocardenas@uabmc.edu; azaky@uabmc.edu

Note: "Aortic syndrome" is a term that encompasses a range of aortic pathologies such as aneurysms, dissections, penetrating aortic ulcers, and intramural hematomas.

Understanding Aortic Aneurysms and Dissections

While both aortic dissections and aortic aneurysms have their classifications and clinical presentations, there can be overlap. Familiarity with the nomenclature is crucial for understanding a patient's specific situation and facilitating communication between surgical, anesthesia, and perfusion teams.

Aortic Dissection

Aortic dissections are categorized using the Stanford and Debakey classifications (Fig. 37.1), which are essential for determining the appropriate surgical approach.

DeBakey Classification

This classification is divided into three different types:

Type I: Intimal tear occurs in the ascending aorta; involves all portions of the thoracic aorta.

Type II: Intimal tear occurs in the ascending aorta only; it terminates before the origin of the innominate artery.

Type III: Intimal tear is located in the descending segment; almost always involves the descending thoracic aorta only, starting distal to the origin of the left subclavian artery; can propagate proximally into the arch.

Stanford Classification

This classification is divided into two types:

Type A: Any involvement of the ascending aorta, regardless of intimal tear location or extent of dissection.

Type B: Involves the aorta distal to the origin of the left subclavian artery.

A. S. Awad, J. DiNardo (eds.), *Clinical Perfusion for Cardiac Surgery*, https://doi.org/10.1007/978-3-031-91163-7_37

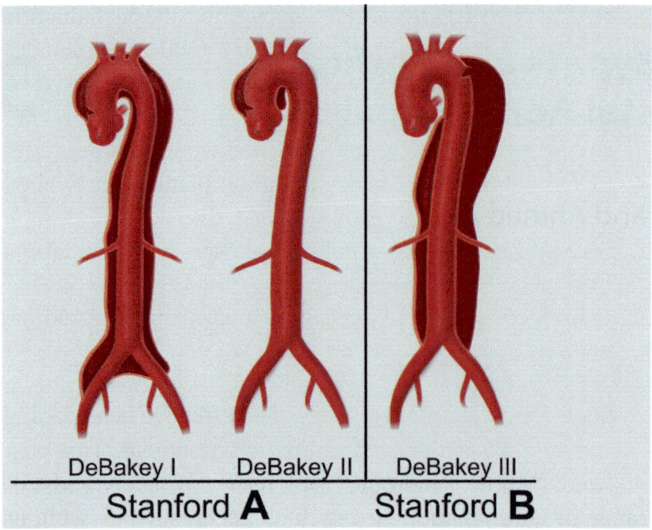

Fig. 37.1 Anatomical overview and classification according to DeBakey and Stanford systems for aortic dissection. This illustration offers a detailed visual overview of aortic dissection, pinpointing key anatomical landmarks. It clearly delineates the distinctions between the DeBakey (Types I, II, and III) and Stanford (Types A and B) classifications, providing a comparative view that enhances comprehension of this complex cardiovascular disorder

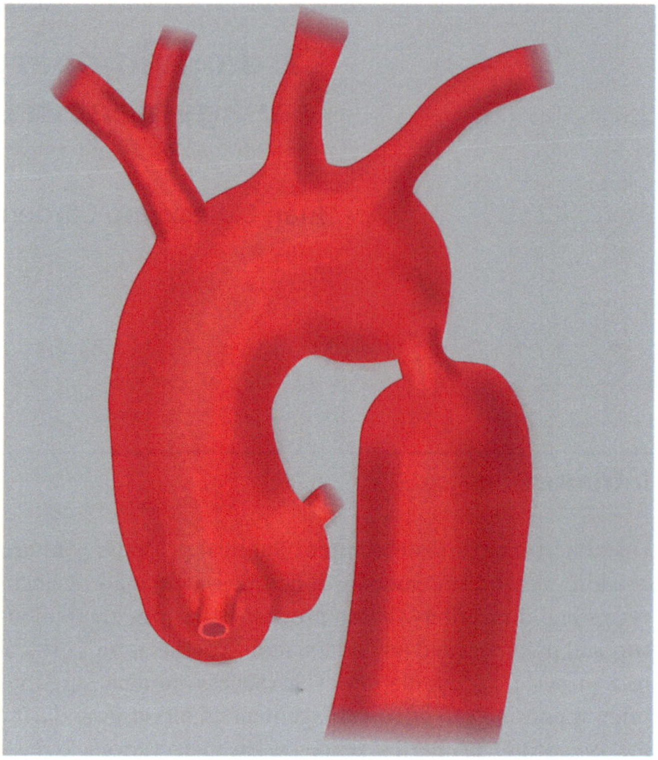

Fig. 37.2 CoA. This illustration depicts CoA, a congenital condition characterized by the narrowing of the aorta, typically occurring between the left subclavian artery and the ligamentum arteriosum. Often not evident until adulthood, this diagram highlights the typical location

Management of Descending Aortic Dissections

Descending aortic dissections, such as Stanford Type B or DeBakey Type III, are primarily managed through medical interventions, with surgery considered under specific conditions. Medical management typically targets maintaining systolic blood pressure within the range of 90–120 mmHg, aiming to stabilize the patient and prevent further complications.

Indications for Surgical Intervention: Surgery is typically reserved for severe cases characterized by:

- *Aortic Rupture*: Immediate surgical intervention is necessary to prevent fatal outcomes.
- *Persistent Pain*: Ongoing discomfort suggesting the progression of the dissection.
- *Aneurysm Expansion*: Surgical repair is considered when the aneurysm's diameter exceeds 5.5 cm or shows rapid expansion, indicating an increased risk of rupture.
- *End-Organ Ischemia*: Signs of impaired blood flow to vital organs necessitate corrective surgery to restore proper circulation.

Acute Intervention with TEVAR: Thoracic Endovascular Aortic Repair (TEVAR) is the preferred acute surgical approach. It involves the placement of an endograft via the femoral artery to seal off the intimal tear, effectively excluding the aneurysm from blood circulation. This technique aims to minimize the risks of severe complications such as paraplegia and renal failure.

Long-Term Management and Elective Repair

In patients without acute malperfusion, an initial approach of medical management accompanied by periodic re-imaging is common. Elective surgical interventions, either via TEVAR or an open thoracoabdominal approach, may be planned for aneurysms that exceed 6.0 cm in diameter, or 5.5 cm in cases involving connective tissue disorders, or those exhibiting a rapid growth rate of more than 0.5 cm per year.

Coarctation of the Aorta (CoA)

CoA, a congenital condition characterized by narrowing of the aorta typically occurring between the left subclavian artery and the ligamentum arteriosum (Fig. 37.2), often manifests in adulthood. It is marked by hypertension in the upper extremities, a delayed pulse between the radial and femoral arteries, and weak or absent pulses in the lower extremities.

(For more detailed information on pediatric CoA, please refer to Chap. 24.)

Historically, open surgical repair via left thoracotomy was the conventional treatment for CoA. This involved various techniques, including simple resection with end-to-end anastomosis, or more complex reconstructions such as prosthetic patch aortoplasty. Initially, Dacron grafts were used to expand the narrowed aorta, but due to high rates of aneurysm formation, their use was discontinued. Subsequently, polytetrafluoroethylene (PTFE) patches were introduced to reduce aneurysm risk, but their adoption has been limited due to increased re-coarctation rates. Another method, subclavian flap aortoplasty, utilizes the patient's own subclavian artery for reconstruction.

However, advancements in minimally invasive techniques have led to the growing use of endovascular approaches, particularly for isolated coarctation cases where additional open-heart procedures are not required. Transcatheter procedures such as balloon angioplasty and stent implantation are increasingly utilized for treating both native and recurrent CoA. Stent implantation has replaced balloon angioplasty due to concerns about long-term re-coarctation and aneurysm formation. Stents provide better outcomes by preventing recoil, minimizing pressure gradients, and reducing the risk of aortic wall abnormalities, making them the preferred treatment for CoA.

Aortic Transection

Aortic rupture, commonly caused by sudden deceleration or traumatic injuries, is associated with a high mortality rate. These ruptures typically happen just distal to the left subclavian artery, a location vulnerable to shearing forces due to its fixed position. Diagnosis is based on a combination of:

- *Clinical Suspicion*: Especially in the context of high-risk mechanisms of injury.
- *Hemodynamic Imbalance*: Increased upper extremity blood pressure and decreased lower extremity pressure.
- *Imaging*: Chest X-ray may reveal mediastinal widening and loss of aortic arch contour.

While symptoms are often nonspecific, early recognition is crucial for prompt intervention.

Surgical Repair Options

There are two primary approaches to surgical repair: open and endovascular.

Open surgery typically involves the excision of the damaged segment followed by anastomosis, patching, or the placement of an interposition graft. Common techniques include the clamp and sew method, although shunting or partial cardiopulmonary bypass (CPB) may also be utilized depending on the specific case (see below for more details).

On the other hand, endovascular repair, particularly TEVAR, has become increasingly preferred due to studies indicating that it results in lower mortality and fewer complications, such as spinal cord ischemia and renal failure.

Aortic Aneurysms

Aortic aneurysms occur when there is a localized dilatation of the aorta that exceeds 50% of its typical diameter. The most common types in the descending thoracic aorta are as follows:

- *Fusiform Aneurysms*: These manifest as symmetrical expansions and are the most prevalent.
- *Saccular Aneurysms*: These appear as localized bulges, which may be associated with infections. Although less common than fusiform aneurysms, saccular aneurysms tend to grow more rapidly.

The Crawford Classification (Fig. 37.3), first described in 1986, is widely used for categorizing aortic aneurysms based on the extent of aortic involvement:

Type I: Originates above the sixth intercostal space, usually near the left subclavian artery, and extends to include the origins of the celiac axis and superior mesenteric arteries. While the aneurysm may involve the renal arteries, it does not extend into the infrarenal aortic.

Type II: Begins above the sixth intercostal space, may include the ascending aorta, and extends distally to include the infrarenal aortic segment, often reaching the level of the aortic bifurcation.

Type III: Starts in the distal half of the descending thoracic aorta (below the sixth intercostal space) and extends into the abdominal aorta.

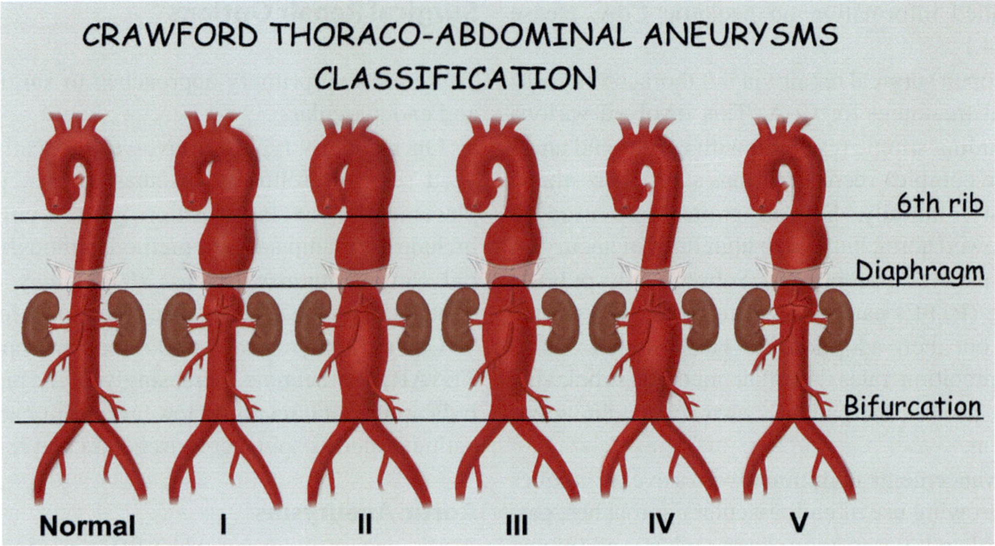

Fig. 37.3 This illustration contrasts a normal thoraco-abdominal aorta with the five Crawford types of aneurysms. Type I involves the descending thoracic aorta extending to the renal arteries. Type II originates from the descending thoracic aorta at the sixth intercostal space, possibly including the ascending aorta, and extends distally to include the infrarenal aortic segment, often reaching the aortic bifurcation. Type III begins below the distal half of the descending thoracic aorta, below the sixth intercostal space, and extends into the abdominal aorta. Type IV encompasses the entire abdominal aorta. Type V is limited to the visceral segment

Type IV: Involves the entire abdominal aorta, from the level of the diaphragm to the aortic bifurcation.

Type V: *Similar to Type III, originating* below the sixth intercostal space, and extending into the abdominal aorta, but limited to the visceral segment.

Management of Descending Thoracic Aortic Aneurysms (DTAA)

Endovascular Approaches of DTAA Repair

TEVAR has emerged as the preferred treatment for DTAA. It offers a minimally invasive approach, employing cylindrical endografts to create a new lumen within the aorta, effectively excluding the aneurysm sac. This approach is advantageous for patients with specific anatomical conditions and significant comorbidities as it involves inserting the endograft through catheters in the femoral artery, minimizing the invasiveness of the procedure. TEVAR allows for targeted treatment of the affected aortic segment while reducing overall recovery time and associated surgical risks compared to open surgery.

Open Surgical Repair

Open surgical repair remains the gold standard for certain cases of DTAA and TAAA. This approach necessitates a left thoracotomy (for DTAA) or a left thoracoabdominal incision (for TAAA) to access the aneurysm. The diseased aortic segment is then replaced with a synthetic graft. In cases of infection, cryopreserved allografts or pericardial tubes are utilized instead of synthetic grafts. If major aortic branches are involved, they are carefully detached and reimplanted onto the new graft. While open repair allows for more extensive reconstruction and direct visualization of the surgical field, it is associated with greater surgical risk, longer recovery times, and higher complication rates compared to endovascular approaches (Fig. 37.4).

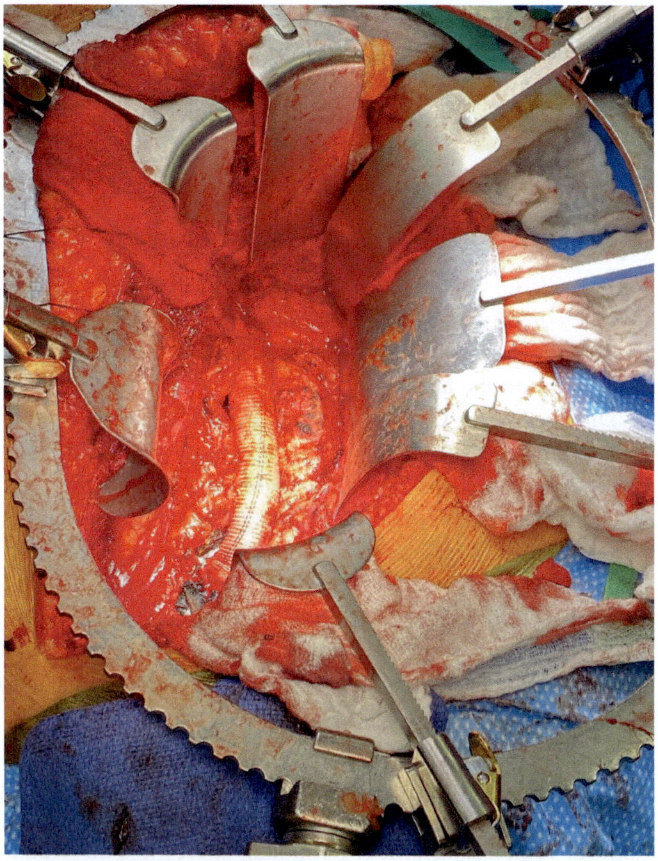

Fig. 37.4 Open surgical repair of TAAA. This image displays the extensive surgical exposure and long graft required for open repair of a TAAA. The diseased aortic segment is replaced with a meticulously positioned graft, secured by clamps above and below the aneurysm. This visualization emphasizes the technical complexity and precision necessary during this high-risk procedure

Perfusion Techniques in Distal Aortic Repair

Fundamentals of Perfusion

During distal aortic repair, managing perfusion is crucial for sustaining blood flow and oxygen delivery to tissues when normal circulation is disrupted. The aim is to closely replicate physiological conditions by controlling blood flow, pressure, and composition—including temperature, hemoglobin levels, and electrolytes—to reduce cellular stress and prevent tissue damage. A deep understanding of the circulatory system, particularly the aorta and its branches, is vital for effective perfusion management in these surgeries.

Bypass Techniques in Distal Aortic Repair

Various bypass techniques are employed during distal aortic repairs, each with its own advantages and limitations. The choice of technique depends on the specific pathology, the segments of the aorta involved, and the patient's overall condition. The common surgical techniques are summarized as follows:

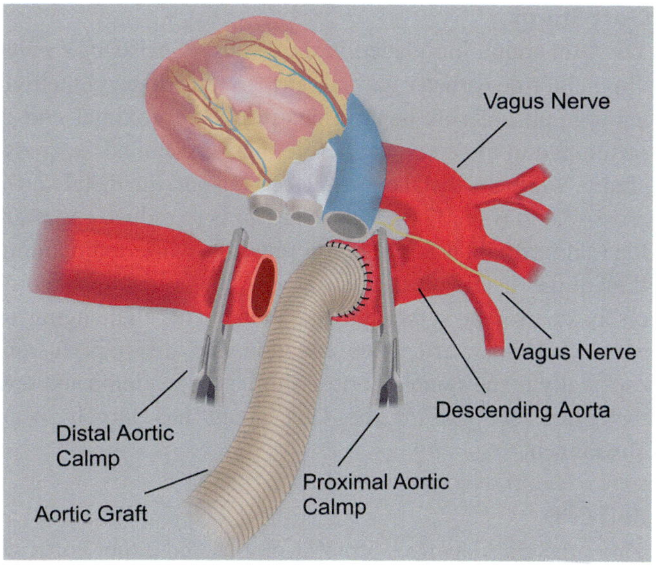

Fig. 37.5 Clamp and sew technique. This illustration demonstrates the "clamp and sew" technique, which does not utilize CPB and is performed on a beating heart. The technique involves placing two aortic cross-clamps, one proximal and one distal to the area requiring resection and repair, without providing perfusion to the distal aorta

Clamp and Sew Technique

Clamp and sew was the original technique used for TAAA repairs; it does not employ any component of CPB and is performed with a beating heart. This technique involves placement of two aortic cross-clamps; one proximal and one distal to the area to be resected and repaired with no provision for perfusion to the distal aorta (Fig. 37.5). Placement of the proximal clamp causes an enormous increase in afterload to the left ventricular (LV) with potential for myocardial supply-demand imbalance and ischemia as well as afterload mismatch and LV dilation. The cerebral circulation is exposed to high arterial pressures, which increases the risk of cerebral edema and intracranial hemorrhage. There is severe hypoperfusion and potential for ischemia in end-organs distal to the distal aortic clamp. The swift completion of the repair is critical to mitigate these risks. Additionally, the lack of opportunity for reimplantation of intercostal arteries cuts off collateral blood supply to the spinal cord, heightening the risk of paraplegia.

Due to advancements in techniques that better manage blood pressure above the proximal cross-clamp and ensure aortic perfusion below the distal clamp, the clamp and sew technique has been largely abandoned.

Gott Shunt

The Gott shunt, introduced in the 1960s, consists of a polyvinyl chloride catheter with a transparent tridodecyl methylammonium chloride heparin coating. The proximal end is positioned in the aorta just before the proximal aortic cross-clamp, while the distal end is placed beyond the distal aortic cross-clamp (Fig. 37.6). This setup aims to reduce LV afterload and proximal aortic blood pressure while maintaining flow to the distal aorta. However, due to the inability to precisely control flow through the shunt, it is challenging to ensure adequate afterload reduction and distal perfusion, especially to the spinal arteries. Similar to the clamp and sew technique, the use of the Gott shunt has largely been abandoned.

Full CPB

This procedure involves femoral venous and either aortic or femoral arterial cannulation, conducted without the use of deep hypothermic circulatory arrest.

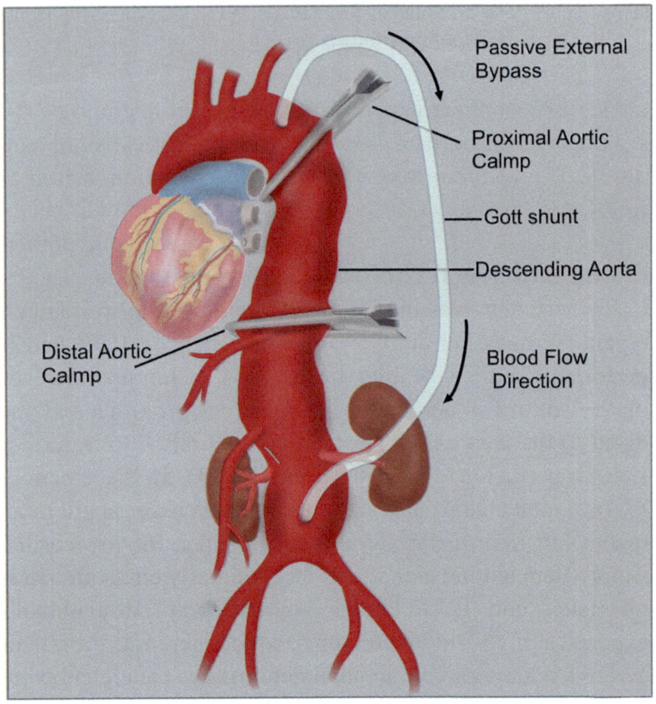

Fig. 37.6 Gott shunt technique. This illustration showcases the "Gott shunt" technique, performed without the use of CPB. It involves placing two aortic cross-clamps: one proximal and one distal to the section needing resection and repair. The Gott shunt, a polyvinyl chloride tube-like structure, is strategically inserted with one end above the proximal clamp and the other below the distal clamp. This setup facilitates passive external bypass, ensuring continued perfusion to the distal aorta throughout the procedure

Full CPB with Deep Hypothermic Circulatory Arrest

This technique can be applied to thoracoabdominal aortic repair and is described in detail in Chap. 35.

Partial Cardiopulmonary Bypass

Overview

Partial CPB is a technique used in cardiac surgery that involves diverting a portion of the venous blood returning to the heart into an external CPB circuit for oxygenation before returning it to the arterial system.

During partial CPB, the remainder of systemic venous return flows into the right atrium, continues to the pulmonary bed for gas exchange, and then returns to the left atrium and left ventricle to be pumped into the systemic circulation. For partial CPB to function effectively, the heart must continue beating and ejecting blood, and the lungs must be ventilated. Without ventilation, the systemic venous blood entering the right atrium will proceed to the systemic circulation without undergoing gas exchange, leading to hypercarbia and hypoxemia.

Mechanism

In partial CPB, venous blood is drawn from a source like the femoral vein, left atrium, or pulmonary artery and directed to the CPB circuit. The circuit comprises a venous reservoir, a heat exchanger, and optionally, an oxygenator. The oxygenator is unnecessary when the left atrium is the venous source. Oxygenated blood is returned to the arterial system, usually at the distal aorta or femoral artery.

Advantages

- *Active Rewarming*: The patient can be actively warmed. This is a major advantage if hypothermia becomes a problem.
- *Fluid and Blood Management*: Blood and fluid can be added easily to the system via the venous reservoir.
- *Efficient Blood Salvage*: All shed blood can be scavenged by the cardiotomy suction and returned to the venous reservoir without the need for a cell-saver system.
- *Precise Flow Control*: Precise control of the amount of blood diverted from the heart to the distal aorta is possible. The perfusionist partially occludes the venous drainage line with a clamp and controls arterial outflow with the pump head to balance proximal and distal blood flow. Close communication with the surgeon, anesthesiologist, and perfusionist is essential.

Disadvantages

- *Systemic Anticoagulation*: Full systemic anticoagulation with heparin is necessary.

Optimizing Hemodynamic Management

The use of partial CPB necessitates rigorous monitoring of hemodynamics, which demands close attention from both the anesthesiologist and the perfusionist due to the shared circulation in place. There is a risk that the perfusionist may divert too much blood from the heart, potentially compromising blood supply to the heart, head, and upper extremities. To manage and assess these risks effectively, the team utilizes both upper and lower arterial lines along with intraoperative transesophageal echocardiography (TEE). These tools are crucial for evaluating LV filling and function, ensuring optimal patient outcomes.

Management Strategy for Partial CPB

A prudent management strategy involves the team collaboratively establishing specific flow and pressure targets for the distal aorta. The perfusionist is responsible for adjusting the CPB circuit to achieve these targets. Concurrently, the anesthesia team manages the proximal aortic pressure, employing volume expansion along with inotropic and vasoactive agents as necessary to maintain hemodynamic stability. This coordinated approach ensures optimal management of both circulatory systems throughout the repair.

Left Heart Bypass (LHB)

Operative Technique and Setup

LHB is a specialized technique employed in aortic surgery to decompress and bypass the left side of the heart by diverting a portion of oxygenated blood from either the left atrium or the pulmonary vein for delivery to the distal aorta or femoral artery using a centrifugal pump. Notably, no oxygenator is required since the blood used is already oxygenated (Figs. 37.7 and 37.8).

LHB: Circuit Configuration and Step-by-Step Guide

1. *Administer Anticoagulation*: Initiate the procedure by administering heparin to achieve systemic anticoagulation, preventing clot formation within the bypass circuit.
2. *Establish Arterial Cannula*: Insert an arterial cannula into the descending thoracic aorta to facilitate the reinfusion of oxygenated blood.

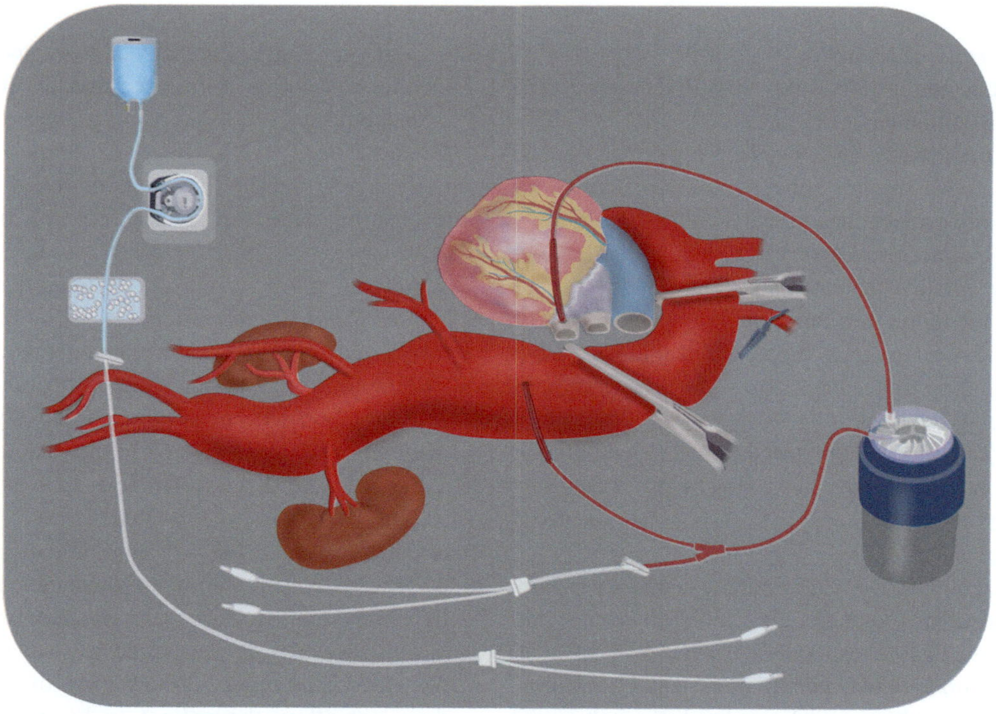

Fig. 37.7 Diagram of LHB circuit setup. This illustration displays the setup for a LHB. The procedure begins by establishing an arterial cannula for reinfusion to the descending thoracic aorta and a draining cannula to the left atrium or pulmonary vein. As depicted, a proximal aortic clamp is positioned just proximal to the left subclavian artery, with a bulldog occluding the left subclavian to control blood flow. Another clamp is applied to the descending thoracic aorta to secure the surgical area. A centrifugal pump maintains continuous flow, decompressing the left side of the heart and pumping blood back into the distal descending thoracic aorta. This targeted approach facilitates the surgical repair or replacement of the descending thoracic aorta while ensuring continuous perfusion to the lower body and vital organs

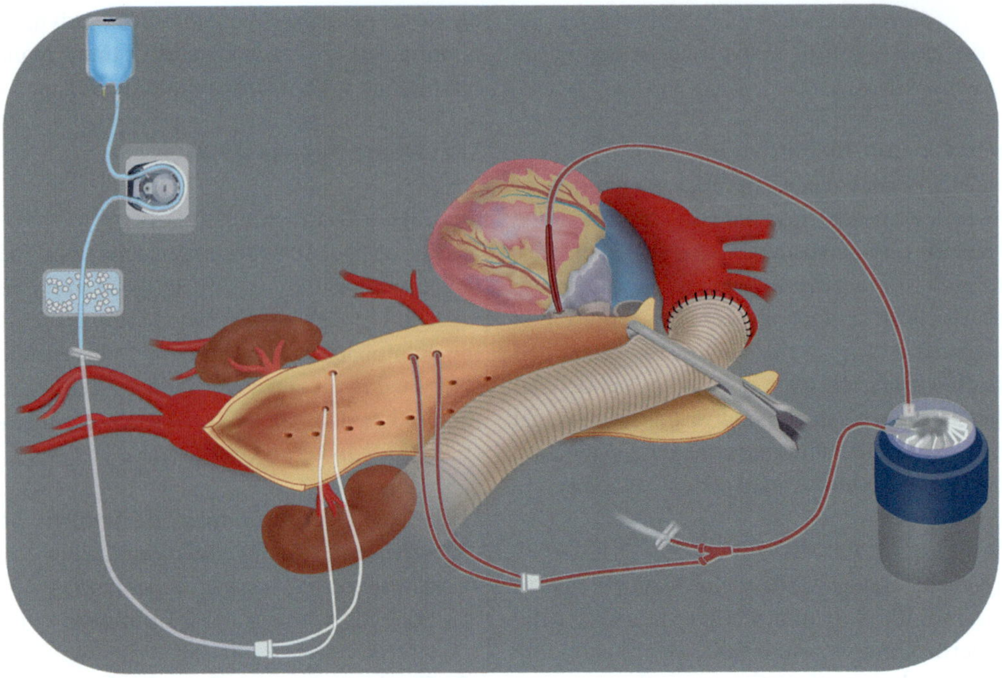

Fig. 37.8 Diagram of LHB circuit setup. This illustration displays the setup for an LHB. The procedure begins by establishing an arterial cannula for reinfusion to the descending thoracic aorta and a draining cannula to the left atrium or pulmonary vein. As depicted, a proximal aortic clamp is positioned just proximal to the left subclavian artery, with a bulldog occluding the left subclavian to control blood flow. Another clamp is applied to the descending thoracic aorta to secure the surgical area. A centrifugal pump maintains continuous flow, decompressing the left side of the heart and pumping blood back into the distal descending thoracic aorta. This targeted approach facilitates the surgical repair or replacement of the descending thoracic aorta while ensuring continuous perfusion to the lower body and vital organs

3. *Establish Draining Cannula*: Place a draining cannula into the left atrium or pulmonary vein to divert oxygenated blood from the heart.
4. *Apply Proximal Aortic Clamp*: Place a proximal aortic clamp just above the left subclavian artery to control blood flow and protect the surgical area.
5. *Occlude Left Subclavian Artery*: Use a bulldog clamp to temporarily occlude the left subclavian artery, further controlling the blood flow during the procedure.
6. *Apply Distal Aortic Clamp*: Apply a distal aortic clamp to the descending thoracic aorta to isolate the section of the aorta being repaired.
7. *Activate Centrifugal Pump*: Start the centrifugal pump to maintain continuous blood flow. This helps decompress the left heart and ensures adequate perfusion to the distal descending thoracic aorta.
8. *Perform Surgical Repair*: Carry out the necessary repairs or replacement of the descending thoracic aorta while monitoring the heart's response.
9. *Monitor and Adjust*: Continuously monitor and adjust flow rates, pressures, and anticoagulation levels throughout the procedure to ensure optimal perfusion and patient stability.
10. *Wean and Remove Cannulas*: Gradually wean the patient off the bypass and reverse anticoagulation, typically using protamine. Carefully remove the cannulas once stable circulation is restored and the repair is deemed successful.

By meticulously following these steps, the surgical team can effectively manage the complexities of the LHB procedure, ensuring patient safety and favorable outcomes.

Advantages

- *Precise Control*: The amount of blood diverted from the left atrium to distal aorta can be precisely controlled. Communication with the perfusionist is essential.
- *Ease of Insertion*: The system is relatively easy to insert.
- *Minimal Heparinization*: Only a moderate level of anticoagulation is needed (ACT = 150–200 sec).

Disadvantages

- *No Reservoir*: No blood or fluid can be added to the bypass system because there is no reservoir. Large-bore peripheral or central venous access is a necessity.
- *No Heat Exchanger*: The absence of a heat exchanger does not allow the patient to be actively warmed or cooled.

Hemodynamic Considerations

Like partial CPB, LHB requires vigilant monitoring of hemodynamics by both the anesthesiologist and the perfusionist due to the shared circulation. The perfusionist must ensure not to divert excessive blood, which can compromise perfusion to the heart, head, and upper extremities. The use of both upper and lower arterial lines, along with intraoperative TEE, helps assess LV filling, function, and blood flow distribution.

Management Strategy

It is vital for the team to establish target flow and pressure in the distal aorta, allowing the perfusionist to adjust the pump flow accordingly. Meanwhile, the anesthesia team manages the proximal aortic pressure using volume expansion and administers inotropic and vasoactive agents as necessary.

Anesthetic Considerations for DTAA and TAAA Repairs

Preoperative Assessment

Patients undergoing DTAA/TAAA repair often present with multiple comorbidities, including hypertension, coronary artery disease, chronic obstructive pulmonary disease (COPD), and diabetes. Comprehensive preoperative evaluation is essential to address these conditions and optimize patient outcomes.

Cardiac Assessment

Given the potential impact of the placement of a proximal aortic cross-clamp on myocardial function, a comprehensive cardiac evaluation is necessary prior to repair. This typically includes an echocardiogram, detailed history, and physical examination, and in certain cases, pharmacologic stress testing or coronary angiography. Coronary revascularization may be considered based on individual patient needs.

Pulmonary Assessment

The incidence of postoperative pulmonary complications, such as atelectasis, pneumonia, and lung injury, is elevated in this patient population. Therefore, a detailed pulmonary evaluation is necessary. This typically includes pulmonary function tests, chest radiography, and computerized tomography. Additionally, it is crucial to determine the patient's tolerance for one-lung ventilation, which is often required during the procedure.

Airway Management

Airway management can be challenging due to the mediastinal deviation caused by the aneurysmal aorta. A thorough review of all imaging, including computed tomography and chest radiography, is essential to anticipate potential difficulties with airway access and endotracheal tube placement. Similar considerations apply to TEE probe placement.

Neurological Assessment

A comprehensive neurological examination and evaluation of any existing deficits are vital. Meticulous documentation of baseline neurological status is crucial for postoperative comparison and detection of potential complications.

Vascular Access and Blood Product Availability

TAA repairs, particularly in the case of aortic rupture, are prone to significant bleeding. Therefore, securing adequate intravenous access is paramount. A common practice is to "double stick" the left internal jugular vein, cannulating it with two large-bore catheters. One of these catheters should be connected to a rapid infuser system to facilitate the quick infusion of fluid and blood products. The left-sided internal jugular cannulation site is preferred by some to avoid the potential kinking associated with right-sided cannulas when the patient is in a modified right lateral decubitus position. Availability of sufficient blood products is crucial and should be ordered well in advance and ready for use prior to surgical incision.

Intraoperative Considerations

Careful consideration and attention to the physiology of mechanical one-lung ventilation as well as to lateral decubitus positioning, are warranted.

Organ Protection in TAAA Repair

Monitors and their Importance

The risk of organ malperfusion during TAAA repair necessitates a comprehensive monitoring strategy that extends beyond standard ASA monitoring. Various monitors are employed to detect early signs of organ ischemia and guide prompt interventions. Table 37.1 summarizes these monitoring techniques and their roles in ensuring patient safety during surgery.

Neurological Monitoring

- *MEP*: Decreases in MEP amplitudes are strong predictors of immediate spinal cord injury. This allows for timely interventions to optimize spinal cord perfusion and restore blood flow to the lower extremities.
- *Somatosensory Evoked Potentials (SSEP)*: While SSEP monitoring is also used, it is less predictive of paraplegia compared to MEP. However, loss of the SSEP signal may indicate a potential for permanent neurological deficit.

The Role of Neuromonitoring

Although neuromonitoring has gained popularity, there is no consensus regarding whether MEP or SSEP offers greater benefits. However, current evidence suggests that MEP is more effective than SSEP at predicting paraplegia, whereas loss of SSEP is weakly associated with permanent neurologic deficit.

Table 37.1 Monitoring for organ protection during TAAA repair

Monitoring and organ protection strategies during TAAA repairs		
Monitor	Function	Relevance to TAAA repair
Arterial line (upper)	Continuous blood pressure monitoring (upper body)	Assess perfusion to the head, and upper extremities during cross-clamping and distal perfusion. Blood sampling
Arterial line (lower)	Continuous blood pressure monitoring (lower body)	Assess perfusion to the lower extremities and organs supplied by the distal aorta during repair
Central venous catheter	Assess central venous pressure (CVP) and guide fluid resuscitation	Maintain adequate preload and cardiac output, especially during periods of blood loss
Pulmonary artery catheter (PAC)	Monitor pulmonary artery pressure, cardiac output (CO), and mixed venous oxygen saturation (SvO_2)	Assess cardiac function, pulmonary vascular resistance, and tissue oxygenation
TEE	Assess cardiac function, valvular function, and regional wall motion abnormalities, volume status, cannula placement	Detect myocardial ischemia or dysfunction during cross-clamping and guide inotropic/vasopressor therapy
Cerebral oximetry	Monitor cerebral oxygen saturation (rSO_2)	Detect cerebral hypoperfusion and guide interventions to maintain adequate oxygen delivery to the brain
Neuromonitoring	Spinal cord perfusion, motor evoked potentials (MEP) more reliable as the anterior column is more susceptible to ischemia	Detect early signs of spinal cord ischemia and guide interventions to prevent neurological injury
Intrathecal pressure monitoring via lumbar drain	Monitor cerebrospinal fluid (CSF) pressure	Detect increased CSF pressure, which can indicate spinal cord ischemia, and guide CSF drainage
Urine output	Assess renal perfusion, volume status, and kidney function	Detect renal hypoperfusion and guide interventions to maintain adequate renal blood flow
Temperature	Monitor core body temperature	Maintain normothermia or mild hypothermia to reduce metabolic demand and protect organs

Additional Considerations

Beyond neuromonitoring, other strategies for organ protection during TAAA repair include maintaining optimal perfusion pressure, utilizing adjuncts like cerebrospinal fluid drainage and distal aortic perfusion, and employing hypothermia to reduce metabolic demand.

Spinal Cord Protection in TAAA Repair

Spinal Perfusion

The spinal cord is primarily supplied by three major arteries originating from the two vertebral arteries in the neck: one anterior artery covering the anterior two-thirds and two posterior arteries supplying the posterior one-third. Additional blood flow comes from collateral segmental arteries, which branch off the descending aorta in the thoracolumbar region. This includes nine pairs of posterior intercostal arteries, one pair of subcostal arteries in the thoracic area, and four pairs of lumbar arteries. These segmental arteries divide at the intervertebral foramina into anterior and posterior radicular arteries. The largest of these, the artery of Adamkiewicz, typically originates from the left side of the aorta between T8 and L2. Spinal cord perfusion also benefits from collateral blood flow from the lumbar and pelvic systems. Spinal cord perfusion pressure (SCPP) is determined by the mean arterial pressure minus the higher of either lumbar cerebrospinal fluid (CSF) pressure or CVP.

Paraplegia Risk and Intercostal Artery Reimplantation

Paraplegia remains a significant risk in the surgical repair of TAAA, with incidence rates ranging from 2.7% to 20%, depending on the volume and surgical experience of the center. During surgery, the interruption of blood flow through intercostal arteries due to exclusion by cross-clamp placement of the diseased portion of the thoracoabdominal aorta directly impacts the segmental spinal arteries and the crucial artery of Adamkiewicz. Given the significant role of these arteries in spinal cord blood supply, their flow disruption poses a high risk of spinal cord ischemia. To effectively reduce this risk, standard practice includes reimplanting intercostal arteries, particularly at the level of T8 to T12, which is a useful adjunct in reducing the rates of paraplegia following TAAA repair. This technique, which extends the operative time by only about 1–2 minutes per vessel, is pivotal in significantly lowering the chances of both early and delayed paraplegia post-operation.

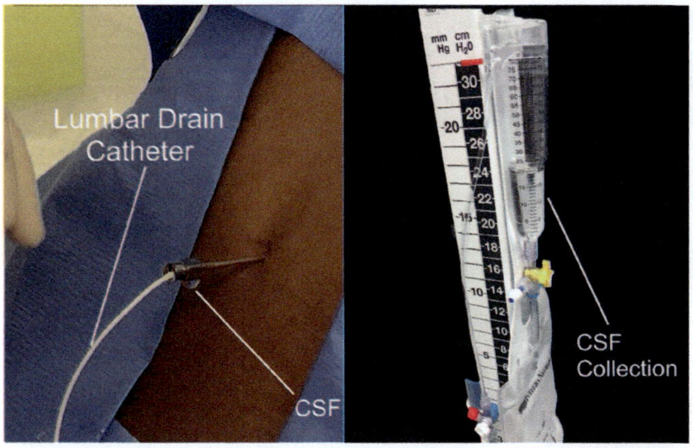

Fig. 37.9 Lumbar drain insertion and CSF collection system. The left image illustrates the insertion of a lumbar drain, while the right image showcases the CSF collection system. Note that the yellow stopcock is closed to the patient after each hour of CSF collection to ensure controlled drainage and accurate measurement, which is crucial to avoid complications such as subdural hematoma or herniation

SCPP and CSF Drainage

SCPP is defined as the difference between mean arterial pressure and spinal cerebrospinal pressure which is normally >60 mmHg. Spinal lumbar drains are placed to provide continuous CSF pressure monitoring and to provide a method to reduce spinal CSF pressure and hence increase spinal cord perfusion. Once the drainage catheter is placed, the target rate of CSF drainage is set between 10 and 15 ml per hour as the normal physiologic CSF replacement rate is believed to be 20 ml/hr. (Fig. 37.9).

SPINAL CORD PERFUSION PRESSURE

$$SCPP = MAP - CSFP$$

Where SCPP = Spinal Cord Perfusion Pressure
MAP= Mean Aortic Pressure
CSFP= Cerebrospinal Fluid Pressure

Acute CSF Pressure Elevation and Cautious Drainage

If acute increases in CSF pressure occur or evidence of cord ischemia becomes evident by neuromonitoring, CSF can be withdrawn to reduce spinal CSF pressure with the caveat that a judicious approach is necessary to avoid creating a subdural intracranial hematoma when excessive CSF drainage leads to stretching and tearing of bridging veins. Because the placement of a lumbar drain may cause trauma and bleeding, some centers elect to place this catheter the day before the scheduled surgery to allow time for hemostasis before heparinization or the occurrence of a coagulopathy associated with the surgical procedure.

Additional Protective Measures

Center-specific protocols also utilize regional epidural hypothermia and the administration of naloxone and/or glucocorticoids as adjuvants for cord protection. Figure 37.10 illustrates the multifaceted approach to neuroprotection during TAAA repair, aimed at preventing spinal cord ischemia and subsequent complications.

Mesenteric and Renal Protection

Protection against mesenteric ischemia involving the liver, gut, and kidneys during aortic surgery is associated with increased perioperative complications. Liver ischemia may exacerbate any coagulopathic state due to the compromise of factor production by the liver. Gut ischemia is associated with bacterial translocation and an alteration of the gut microbiome. The incidence of acute kidney failure has been reported to be as high as 5–13% after TAAA repair, with clamp time as the strongest predictor of injury.

Surgical techniques for mesenteric protection focus on intraprocedural perfusion and reduction of ischemic time. Selective renal perfusion with catheters connected to side arms of the aortic graft or directly to the CPB circuit to perfuse the kidneys can help decrease the renal ischemia time. Furthermore, these catheters can also be used to provide antegrade regional hypothermia using infused ice-cold saline or to deliver adjuvant medications such as steroids.

Prevention and Management of Coagulopathy

TAAA repairs are associated with coagulopathy and increased risk of bleeding. This may be due to the complexity of the procedure itself, as well as other contributing factors such as coagulopathy resulting from liver and kidney injuries, hypothermia, systemic inflammatory response, and a consumption-type coagulopathy resulting from sequestration of blood elements on the aortic graft.

Blood conservation strategies such as cell-saver transfusion and acute normovolemic hemodilution protocols are frequently employed depending on institutional protocols. Massive transfusion protocols that transfuse various proportions and amounts of blood products also vary by institution. Some institutions have protocolized the use of the antifibrinolytics epsilon aminocaproic acid or tranexamic acid based on data extrapolated from cardiac surgery.

Point of care testing, such as thromboelastography (TEG) or rotational elastography (ROTEM), is often used in conjunction with point of care testing of traditional coagulation

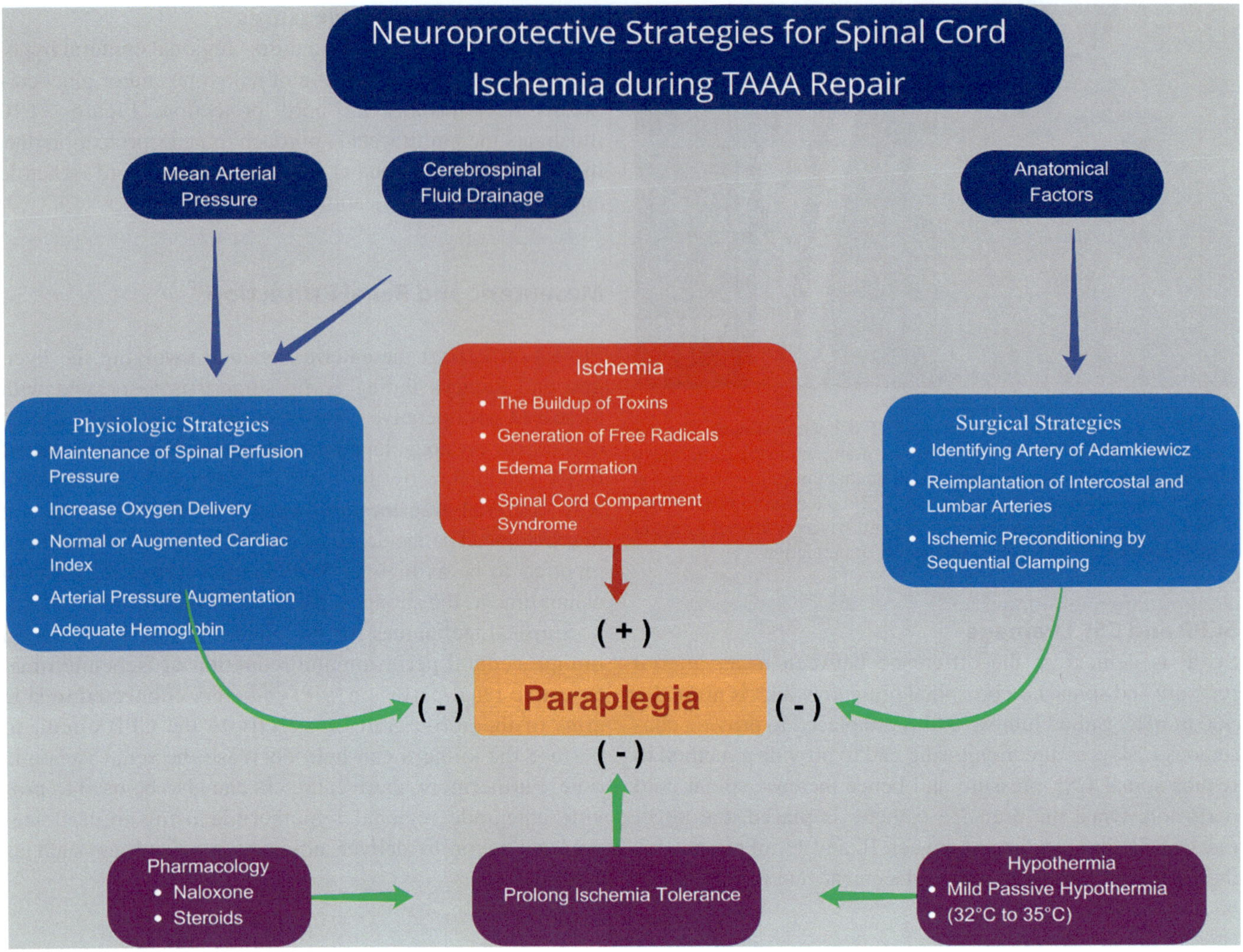

Fig. 37.10 Diagram of neuroprotective strategies for spinal cord ischemia during TAAA repair. This illustration displays key interventions, including maintaining adequate blood pressure and spinal perfusion, optimizing oxygen delivery and cardiac function, and strategically identifying and reconnecting vital arteries. Additionally, managing factors that exacerbate ischemia—such as toxin buildup, free radical generation, and edema formation—is essential. The use of medications like naloxone and steroids is crucial for neuroprotection. Employing mild hypothermia to reduce spinal cord metabolic demand further aids in protecting the spinal cord during the repair process

assays. Transfusion prediction models and component therapy administration decision trees vary among institutions.

Further Reading

Agasthi P, Pujari SH, Tseng A, Graziano JN, Marcotte F, Majdalany D, Mookadam F, Hagler DJ, Arsanjani R. Management of adults with coarctation of aorta. World J Cardiol. 2020;12(5):167–91. https://doi.org/10.4330/wjc.v12.i5.167. PMID: 32547712; PMCID: PMC7284000

Atkins AD, Atkins MD. Branched and fenestrated aortic endovascular grafts. Methodist Debakey Cardiovasc J. 2023;19(2):15–23. https://doi.org/10.14797/mdcvj.1200. PMID: 36910555; PMCID: PMC10000330

Cheung AT, Weiss SJ, McGarvey ML, Stecker MM, Hogan MS, Escherich A, Bavaria JE. Interventions for reversing delayed-onset postoperative paraplegia after thoracic aortic reconstruction. Ann Thorac Surg. 2002;74(2):413–9.; discussion 420–1. PMID: 12173822. https://doi.org/10.1016/s0003-4975(02)03714-1.

Fedorow CA, Moon MC, Mutch WA, Grocott HP. Lumbar cerebrospinal fluid drainage for thoracoabdominal aortic surgery: rationale and practical considerations for management. Anesth Analg. 2010;111(1):46–58. https://doi.org/10.1213/ANE.0b013e3181ddddd6. Epub 2010 Jun 3. PMID: 20522706

Gedney R, Wooster M. Thoracic aortic aneurysms and arch disease. Surg Clin North Am. 2023;103(4):615–27. https://doi.org/10.1016/j.suc.2023.04.013. Epub 2023 May 21. PMID: 37455028

Lester LC, Kostibas MP. Anesthetic management for open thoracoabdominal and abdominal aortic aneurysm repair. Anesthesiol Clin. 2022;40(4):705–18. https://doi.org/10.1016/j.anclin.2022.08.013. PMID: 36328624

Rocha RV, Lindsay TF, Friedrich JO, Shan S, Sinha S, Yanagawa B, Al-Omran M, Forbes TL, Ouzounian M. Systematic review of contemporary outcomes of endovascular and open thoracoabdominal aortic aneurysm repair. J Vasc Surg. 2020;71(4):1396–1412.e12. https://doi.org/10.1016/j.jvs.2019.06.216. Epub 2019 Nov 2. PMID: 31690525

Tanaka A, Smith HN, Safi HJ, Estrera AL. Open treatments for Thoracoabdominal aortic aneurysm repair. Methodist Debakey Cardiovasc J. 2023;19(2):49–58. https://doi.org/10.14797/mdcvj.1178. PMID: 36910546; PMCID: PMC10000325

Cardiopulmonary Bypass During Pregnancy

38

Melinda Eshelman and Eugene A. Hessel II

Introduction

Cardiovascular disease during pregnancy is a pressing health concern, representing a significant cause of morbidity and mortality among expectant mothers. The increasing prevalence of these conditions can be attributed to several factors, including the rising average age of pregnant women and a higher incidence of women with congenital heart disease reaching childbearing age. These demographic shifts have catalyzed the development of a specialized interdisciplinary field known as "Cardio-obstetrics," which integrates cardiology and obstetrics to manage heart disease in pregnancy more effectively.

Recent trends in the management of cardiovascular conditions during pregnancy emphasize minimizing invasive procedures such as cardiac surgery employing cardiopulmonary bypass (CPB). Instead, there is a preference for interventional cardiology procedures such a balloon valvuloplasty, endovascular valve replacement, percutaneous coronary intervention (PCI), and Off-pump coronary artery bypass grafting (CABG). These approaches align with the 2018 recommendations from the European Society of Cardiology, which advise reserving cardiac surgery for situations where non-surgical interventions fail and the mother's life is threatened.

Despite these guidelines, the necessity for cardiac surgery employing CPB during pregnancy remains a reality for certain severe cases, underscoring the need for ongoing research and refined clinical strategies. This chapter delves into the physiological challenges, treatment modalities, and both maternal and fetal outcomes associated with managing cardiovascular disease in pregnant patients, guided by the latest research and clinical practices.

Physiological Changes of Pregnancy

Pregnancy induces profound physiologic changes to meet the increased metabolic demands of both the mother and fetus. Notably, by the end of pregnancy, uterine blood flow may increase tenfold and renal blood flow by 50%. To support this increased flow, plasma volume and cardiac output (CO) typically rise by 40–50% above baseline levels by the 32nd week, with 75% of this increase occurring by the end of the first trimester. Initially, this rise in CO is achieved by an increase in stroke volume, with the heart rate gradually increasing in the second half.

The structural changes in the heart include enlarged atrial and ventricular diameters and an increase in left ventricular end diastolic volume, while the end systolic volume remains unchanged, thereby enhancing the ejection fraction. By term, the left ventricular mass has typically increased by 50%, attributed to the growth in size of pre-existing cardiomyocytes, leading to eccentric hypertrophy.

Additionally, elevated levels of the hormone progesterone and signaling molecules such as nitrous oxide and prostaglandins contribute to significant peripheral vasodilation. This hormonal and molecular activity leads to a decrease in systemic and pulmonary vascular resistance, with blood pressure reaching its lowest between the 20th and 24th weeks of gestation. Despite these changes, central venous, pulmonary artery diastolic, and pulmonary capillary wedge pressures generally remain within the normal range for non-pregnant individuals.

Table 38.1 summarizes these normal physiological changes during pregnancy and their potential implications for preexisting cardiovascular conditions.

M. Eshelman · E. A. Hessel II (✉)
Department of Anesthesiology & Perioperative Medicine, University of Kentucky, Lexington, KY, USA
e-mail: Melinda.Eshelman@uky.edu; ehessel@uky.edu

A. S. Awad, J. DiNardo (eds.), *Clinical Perfusion for Cardiac Surgery*, https://doi.org/10.1007/978-3-031-91163-7_38

Table 38.1 Normal physiological changes during pregnancy and their potential implications for pre-existing cardiovascular conditions

Physiological change	Effect	Implications for CVD
Cardiovascular		
Increased blood volume (up to 50%)	Higher CO, decreased systemic vascular resistance	Can exacerbate heart failure, valvular disease
Increased heart rate (10–15 bpm)	Shorter diastolic filling time	May worsen mitral stenosis, diastolic dysfunction
Mild left ventricular hypertrophy	Increased cardiac workload	Can exacerbate cardiomyopathy
Decreased blood pressure (initially)	Lowered systemic resistance	May mask hypertension initially
Respiratory		
Increased oxygen consumption	Increased demand on the heart	Can exacerbate heart failure, pulmonary hypertension
Hematologic		
Dilutional anemia	Reduced oxygen-carrying capacity	Can exacerbate existing anemia or ischemia
Hypercoagulability	Increased risk of blood clot formation	Increased risk of thromboembolism with prosthetic valves, existing hypercoagulable states

Impact on Preexisting Heart Conditions

These cardiovascular adaptations, while necessary for supporting fetal development, can exacerbate existing heart conditions or unveil previously undiagnosed issues. Women with conditions like hypertrophic cardiomyopathy or valvular heart diseases may experience worsened symptoms due to increased blood volume and CO. These physiological stresses can lead to complications, making pre-pregnancy cardiac assessment and careful monitoring throughout pregnancy crucial for maternal and fetal health.

Cardio-Obstetrics: A Growing New Field

Maternal morbidity and mortality rates are rising in the United States, owing mostly to cardiovascular disease (CVD), the primary and often preventable cause of death. Pregnancy-related hemodynamic and physiologic alterations can worsen existing or latent CVD, resulting in complications such as heart failure, arrhythmias, hypertension, and myocardial ischemia events. Additionally, negative pregnancy outcomes can increase the long-term susceptibility to CVD.

Cardio-obstetrics has emerged to manage the complex relationship between heart health and pregnancy. This multidisciplinary field provides comprehensive care for women with CVD, aiming to optimize outcomes for both mother and child. Its growth is driven by more women having children later in life and an increasing number of women with congenital heart disease reaching childbearing age, along with rising cases of acquired heart disease.

Effective management requires a collaborative approach with a diverse team of experts, such as obstetricians, cardiologists, maternal-fetal medicine specialists, anesthesiologists, and other specialists. This collaborative approach involves using risk assessment tools, conducting appropriate testing and imaging, safely administering medications during pregnancy and lactation, and providing specialized care for conditions like arrhythmias, congenital heart disease, and peripartum cardiomyopathy. By understanding the causes and developing comprehensive care programs, Cardio-obstetrics aims to improve maternal outcomes and address disparities in cardiovascular care during pregnancy.

Conditions Requiring Cardiac Surgery During Pregnancy

Maternal mortality during cardiac surgery with CPB is similar to that of non-pregnant women; however, fetal mortality remains high. Therefore, as previously mentioned, cardiac surgery is recommended only when medical or interventional procedures fail and the mother's life is at risk. The latest data suggest the optimal period for cardiac surgery with CPB for fetal safety is the third trimester, while no specific trimester has been identified as preferable for maternal outcome.

The physiologic changes of pregnancy can exacerbate pre-existing cardiac conditions. With close monitoring by a cardiologist and a high-risk obstetrician, the goal should be to carry the pregnancy to term and then address the maternal cardiovascular disease 6 weeks or more post-partum. For women without heart disease, induction of labor at 40 weeks has been shown to decrease the risk of emergency cesarean section by 12% and reduce the risk of stillbirth by 50%. Consequently, induction of labor at 40 weeks of gestation should be considered in all women with cardiac disease.

Conditions in which cardiac surgery is commonly performed during pregnancy are listed in Table 38.2.

Table 38.2 Common conditions requiring cardiac surgery during pregnancy

Condition	Type	Subtypes/examples	Potential complications in pregnancy
Congenital heart disease	Structural	Atrial/ventricular septal defects, tetralogy of Fallot, coarctation of the aorta	Heart failure, arrhythmias, cyanosis, fetal growth restriction
Valvular heart disease	Rheumatic	Mitral stenosis, aortic stenosis	Heart failure, pulmonary edema, fetal distress
	Acquired	Bicuspid aortic valve disease, myxomatous degeneration	Aortic dissection, worsening regurgitation, arrhythmias
Prosthetic valve dysfunction	Mechanical or bio-prosthetic		Thromboembolism, bleeding (anticoagulation complications), structural failure
Infective endocarditis	Infection		Heart failure, sepsis, embolic events, fetal infection
Ischemic heart disease	Vascular	Spontaneous coronary artery dissection (SCAD), CAD	Increase flow, manage anemia, consider packed RBCs (with caution)
Aortic dissection	Vascular	Type A (ascending), type B (descending)	Aortic rupture, organ ischemia, maternal and fetal death
Pulmonary embolism	Thromboembolic		Respiratory failure, right heart failure, maternal and fetal death
Cardiac tumors	Neoplastic	Myxoma (most common)	Obstruction of blood flow, embolic events, arrhythmias

Stenotic Valve Lesions

Increased CO during pregnancy can cause an increase in trans-valvular gradient by approximately 50% between the first and second trimesters.

Mitral Stenosis (MS)

Pregnancy often exacerbates the symptoms of MS. The risk of heart failure exacerbation increases as valve area decreases, with 50% of patients whose valve area ≤ 1.0 cm^2 requiring admission for heart failure during pregnancy. The physiologic increase in CO leads to a heightened gradient across the mitral valve, resulting in increased pressure in the left atrium, dyspnea, and pulmonary edema. Pregnant women with MS frequently present in the third trimester with decreased functional status and atrial arrhythmias. For this reason, patients with MS should be counseled to consider intervention pre-pregnancy, even if asymptomatic. If a parturient with MS experiences worsening condition and/or systolic pulmonary artery pressure greater than 50 mmHg despite optimal medical treatment, percutaneous mitral commissurotomy may be performed, preferably after 20 weeks of gestation. The goal of percutaneous mitral commissurotomy in these patients is not for complete resolution, but to improve the hemodynamic status of the patient, with a high reported success rate of 95–97%. Open heart surgery should only be performed if all other measures have failed and a mother's life is at risk.

Aortic Stenosis (AS)

AS in pregnancy is most commonly due to a bicuspid aortic valve, followed by rheumatic heart disease. Heart failure during pregnancy is rare in patients who were asymptomatic before pregnancy but occurs in 25% of symptomatic patients. Estimated trans-valvular gradients increase during pregnancy due to the physiologic increase in CO, yet both the calculated valve area and dimensionless index remain unchanged. Symptomatic patients with severe AS or asymptomatic patients with impaired LV function should have surgery performed pre-pregnancy. Patients who are severely symptomatic during pregnancy may require percutaneous valvuloplasty. Although highly successful for MS, valvuloplasty for AS carries a high risk of aortic regurgitation post-valvuloplasty, and restenosis commonly occurs within 1 year. If valvuloplasty is not feasible, valve replacement should be considered after early delivery. There are a few case reports of transcatheter aortic valve replacement (TAVR) in pregnancy to bridge patients to a healthy delivery. Both vaginal delivery and cesarean section can be safe in patients with AS.

Regurgitant Valvular Lesions

Mitral and Aortic Regurgitation

Generally, mitral and aortic insufficiency is well-tolerated in pregnancy; however, parturients with severe regurgitation and symptoms or reduced ejection fraction (EF) are at high risk of developing heart failure. Approximately 25% of patients with moderate or severe rheumatic mitral regurgitation (MR) develop heart failure. Like in non-pregnant patients, the acute onset of mitral or aortic regurgitation is poorly tolerated. If these patients develop heart failure refractory to medical therapy, surgery may become unavoidable.

Prosthetic Valve Dysfunction and Thrombosis

Pregnant women with mechanical valves have a higher risk of death compared to patients with an uncomplicated pregnancy. Death in these patients usually occurs due to thromboembolism of the prosthetic valve, exacerbated by the hypercoagulable state of pregnancy. The risk of thromboembolism for a mechanical valve during pregnancy ranges from 3–14%, and anticoagulation should be closely monitored. Asymptomatic prosthetic valve thrombosis has been successfully treated with careful infusion of tissue-type plasminogen activator. Occasionally, surgery is required, but it carries considerable risk. Acute malfunctioning valves may also require surgery, which also presents considerable risk. An interventional transvenous valve-in-valve procedure is an option for some patients.

Aortic Dissection During Pregnancy

The exact effects of pregnancy on changes in aortic wall structure are not fully understood; however, pregnancy-induced cardiovascular changes, such as increased arterial wall tension and intimal shear stress, may contribute to aortic dissection. Notably, approximately half of aortic dissections and ruptures in women younger than 40 occur during pregnancy, most often in the third trimester. Conditions like Marfan syndrome, Ehlers-Danlos syndrome, bicuspid aortic valves, and Turner syndrome increase the risk of aortic dissections in pregnant women. Dissections are also associated with pre-eclampsia and chronic hypertension, with an average aortic diameter of 4.8 cm at the time of dissection.

Management of Acute Dissection in Pregnancy

Type B dissections may be managed by thoracic endovascular aortic repair (TEVAR), but type A dissections (ascending aortic dissections, see Fig. 37.2) are surgical emergencies requiring immediate repair. If the fetus is viable, cesarean section should be performed before aortic repair. If the baby is not viable, aortic surgery should be performed with the fetus in utero.

Endocarditis During Pregnancy

While endocarditis is uncommon during pregnancy, it carries high mortality rates for both mother (15%) and fetus (22%). Risk factors include intravenous drug use, congenital heart disease, and rheumatic heart disease. Diagnosis and antibiotic treatment follow the same principles as in non-pregnant patients, using the modified Duke criteria and considering potential fetal toxicity of certain antibiotics. However, surgical treatment is ideally delayed until the infection is eradicated.

Cardiac Myxoma

Cardiac myxomas are rare tumors in pregnant patients. The clinical presentation of a cardiac myxoma is influenced by its size, mobility, and location within the heart. They are most frequently found in the left atrium. Symptoms are nonspecific and include constitutional, embolic, and obstructive cardiac symptoms. These symptoms can include dyspnea, palpitations, and fatigue, which may be misinterpreted as asthma or typical fatigue associated with pregnancy. Diagnosis is initially made by transthoracic echocardiography (TTE), while cardiovascular magnetic resonance imaging (MRI) provides further tumor characterization. Atrial thrombi with stalk may be mistaken for myxomas and can lead to unnecessary and potentially harmful surgery. Indications for surgical resection are embolic events, frequent syncope episodes, or sudden cardiac arrest caused by the myxoma obstructing the mitral valve orifice. The literature on maternal mortality is promising, reporting 100% maternal survival and 85% fetal survival in 61 pregnant women.

Pulmonary Embolism (PE)

Deep vein thrombosis (DVT) and PE are unfortunately not uncommon in pregnancy. Martillotti, et al., provided a systematic review of the management of severe PE during pregnancy. Therapeutic options include thrombolysis, percutaneous catheter thrombectomy, and ECMO, and if required, surgical thrombectomy with CPB. An earlier summary of seven case reports and five subsequent reports of pulmonary embolectomy during pregnancy reported a maternal survival of 100% and fetal survival of 67%.

Acute Coronary Syndrome

Acute coronary syndrome (ACS), which encompasses unstable angina, non-ST-segment elevation myocardial infarction (NSTEMI), and ST-segment elevation myocardial infarction (STEMI), can occur during pregnancy. Only 40% of pregnant patients with MI have evidence of coronary artery atherosclerosis. Spontaneous coronary artery dissection (SCAD) is seen in up to 27% of patients. Angiographically, normal coronary arteries are observed in 13% of cases; in these instances, MI is most likely due to a coronary artery spasm or an embolic event.

Atherosclerosis is more commonly the cause of MI during the antepartum period, whereas SCAD resulting in MI is most often observed in the postpartum period. The high rate of SCAD in postpartum patients is likely related to hormonal changes occurring during pregnancy. Approximately 75% of SCAD cases during pregnancy present with STEMI, and EF is often reduced, with a mean EF of 40%. The left anterior descending coronary artery is frequently the culprit vessel; however, 40% of patients experience multivessel SCADs. While most patients with SCAD who are managed conservatively demonstrate angiographic healing, revascularization should be considered for those exhibiting active myocardial ischemia, hemodynamic instability, or a left main dissection. CABG should be reserved for patients with left main or multivessel proximal large-vessel dissection.

Percutaneous Interventions During Pregnancy

Depending on the type of cardiovascular disease, alternatives to CPB can be considered during pregnancy. For example, STEMIs during pregnancy should be treated with primary PCI, preferentially accessed through the radial artery due to the increased bleeding risk associated with femoral access. Anticoagulation is typically achieved with heparin, with larger doses often required in pregnant patients to achieve the desired effect compared to non-pregnant patients.

Percutaneous interventions include balloon angioplasty and stent placement. While balloon angioplasty does not require dual antiplatelet therapy (DAPT), stent placement offers a lower risk of vessel closure in the short term and a lower long-term risk of restenosis. DAPT with aspirin and clopidogrel is mandatory after stent placement to prevent in-stent thrombosis. However, drug-eluting stents require 6 months of DAPT, whereas bare metal stents only require 1 month, making them more suitable during pregnancy. Polymer-Free Biolimus A9 stents, currently in US clinical trials, allow for 1 month of DAPT and offer some of the same long-term advantages as drug-eluting stents.

Mechanical Circulatory Support (MCS) and TAVR

Peripartum cardiomyopathy, the most common cause of cardiogenic shock in pregnancy, may have improved outcomes with early initiation of MCS. Intra-aortic balloon pumps (IABP), temporary ventricular assist devices (VADs), and extracorporeal membrane oxygenation (ECMO) have all been utilized in treatment. These interventions are discussed in more detail subsequently.

TAVRs have been highly successful in non-pregnant patients. However, since the valves used in TAVR are bioprosthetic with a lifespan of approximately 10 years, patients undergoing TAVR during pregnancy are likely to need another valve replacement within their lifetime. Gestational age, severity of AS, and patient symptoms must all be considered when considering TAVR. While only a few case reports exist, TAVR in pregnancy has shown promising results. Valve-in-valve procedures have also been reported during pregnancy.

Maternal and Fetal Outcomes

Cardiac surgery requiring CPB poses risks for both the mother and the fetus. While maternal mortality is estimated at 3–15%, fetal mortality is significantly higher, ranging from 16 to 35%. A recent meta-analysis reported a 7.3% maternal mortality rate, which was not influenced by trimester or prior C-section. Fetal mortality was 26.5%, with the lowest rate occurring in the third trimester (29.4%, compared to 33.9% in the second trimester and 44.8% in the first trimester). Significantly, it was lower when preceded by C-section (6.7% vs 35.7%).

Maternal risk factors for mortality include severe symptoms (NYHA Class III/IV), while fetal mortality is associated with maternal age over 35 years, emergency surgery, and severe maternal symptoms.

Timing of Cardiac Surgery During Pregnancy

In non-emergent situations, the timing of cardiac surgery during pregnancy requires balancing the risks to both the maternal and fetal risks. Fetal mortality decreases as pregnancy progresses, with survival rates below 50% at 20–23 weeks and as high as 94% at 28–31 weeks. Conversely, the mother's risk increases with advancing gestation, as the physiologic changes of pregnancy can worsen underlying heart conditions.

Ideally, cardiac surgery is postponed until 6 weeks postpartum. However, if immediate intervention is necessary, preterm delivery combined with simultaneous cardiac repair should be considered when the fetus has reached at least 28 weeks of gestation.

Intraoperative Management of Cardiac Surgery During Pregnancy with or Without CPB

Optimal care for parturients undergoing cardiac surgery, with or without CPB, aims to minimize maternal and fetal risk. Current recommendations, primarily based on expert opinion, are summarized in Table 38.3. Because of advances in neonatal care and the persistent risks to the fetus during CPB, many experts suggest elective delivery of the fetus, often with standby CPB, around 28-week gestation. In these cases, completing a full course of preoperative maternal corticosteroids is recommended, if possible.

Anesthesia and Hemodynamic Management

- *Preoxygenation:* The patient should be pre-oxygenated for at least 5 min, as oxygen consumption is increased in the pregnant patient and functional residual capacity is decreased.
- *Induction:* Rapid sequence induction is recommended due to decreased tone of the lower esophageal sphincter and increased risk for aspiration.
- *Agents:* Propofol, morphine, fentanyl, succinylcholine, and nondepolarizing muscle relaxants have all been used safely in pregnancy.
- *Volatile Anesthetics:* Although volatile anesthetic gases cross the placenta, they have been safely used during pregnancy and, as an added benefit, inhibit uterine contractility. Minimal alveolar concentration (MAC) requirement is decreased by 30–40% in pregnant patients, so less volatile agent is required to achieve the same depth of anesthesia.

Table 38.3 Recommended management of CPB during pregnancy

Category	Maternal considerations	Fetal considerations	Recommendations and management strategies
Anesthesia	Primarily based on maternal needs	Safety for the fetus is paramount	Volatile agents (may lower uterine tone) Avoid teratogens Adjust doses for placental transfer Consider regional if feasible
CPB management			
Heparin and protamine			Routine management of heparin and protamine
CPB flow	High flow is essential due to increased CO (2.5–3.5 L/min/m^2)	Maintain adequate placental perfusion	Aim for flow rate > 2.5 L/min/m^2 or < 3 L/min/m^2
Perfusion pressure	Normal to slightly elevated for adequate organ perfusion (>70 mmHg or > 60–70 mmHg)		Use phenylephrine or norepinephrine as needed, maintain MAP above 60–70 mmHg
Pulsatile flow	Unproven benefit, but some advocate for it to reduce placental vasoconstriction	May improve fetal oxygenation and heart rate	Consider IABP or a pulsatile arterial pump
Acid-base & oxygenation	Alpha-stat pH management, prevent acidosis, maintain normal SaO_2	Fetal Well-being depends on maternal acid-base balance	Maintain maternal $PaCO_2$ ~ 30 mmHg, PaO_2 ~ 150 mmHg, avoid hyperventilation
Hematocrit	Maintain >25–27% or > 28%		Avoid excessive hemodilution
Temperature	Normothermia or mild hypothermia (32–34 °C)	Fetal heart rate correlates with maternal temperature; avoid hypothermia	Gradual rewarming to avoid uterine contractions and fetal distress
Positioning	15° left lateral tilt to prevent aortocaval compression	Ensure adequate placental blood flow	Avoid supine position
Venous drainage	Prevent obstruction by IVC cannula	Can impact placental circulation	Ensure proper cannula placement and monitor venous return
Cardioplegia		Unknown impact on fetus	Limited data, individualized approach
Tocolytic therapy	Prevent or treat uterine contractions	Ensure fetal Well-being	Use beta-mimetics, magnesium sulfate, calcium channel blockers, or indomethacin with caution
Fetal monitoring		Continuous monitoring of FHR and uterine tone before, during, and after CPB. Doppler assessment if >20–24 weeks	Obstetrician and neonatologist on standby for emergency cesarean section

- *Hypotension:* Address promptly with left lateral tilt positioning and fluid administration. Position the patient in a left lateral tilt to prevent aortocaval compression and maintain uretero-placental blood flow. If hypotension persists, administer vasopressors. Both phenylephrine and ephedrine can effectively treat hypotension; however, phenylephrine is preferred due to its more favorable fetal blood gas results and has become the most frequently used pressor in pregnancy. Norepinephrine and vasopressin are also increasingly recommended.

CPB Considerations

- *Off-pump:* Off-pump approach is recommended for coronary artery surgery.
- *Bypass Time:* Bypass duration should be minimized.
- *Antifibrinolytics:* Antifibrinolytic agents such as tranexamic acid are not recommended as pregnancy is a hypercoagulable state.
- *Heparin Resistance:* Anticipate heparin resistance due to decreased antithrombin III concentrations during pregnancy. Protamine, while not well-studied in pregnancy, has been used occasionally to reverse the effects of heparin.
- *Cannulation:* Ensure careful positioning of venous cannulae, as obstruction of venous drainage may lead to adverse effects on the fetus.
- *Pump Flow and MAP:* While on bypass, it is advisable to use a higher pump flow rate of 2.5–3.5 $l/min/m^2$ to match the increased CO of the pregnant patient. Maintaining a mean arterial pressure higher than 60–70 mmHg is recommended.
- *Pulsatile Flow:* The benefit of providing pulsatile flow during CPB in pregnant patients is controversial and unproven. However, many experts advocate for its use to prevent placental vasoconstriction, based on studies in fetal lambs that indicated pulsatile flow promoted nitric oxide-mediated placental vasodilation. Clinical case reports also suggest improved fetal bradycardia with the use of pulsatile flow. Pulsatile arterial pressure can be most effectively provided by using an IAPB, although pulsatile arterial pumps may also be employed. An example of its apparent benefits was well demonstrated in a case report by K. Masada, et al., in 2018 (Fig. 38.1).
- *Fetal Monitoring:* Fetal heart rate and uterine tone monitoring should be performed during CPB and continued in the postoperative period. During CPB, Doppler indices in the umbilical and middle cerebral arteries are measured and flows adjusted for optimization of placental blood flow.
- *Maternal Hematocrit:* It should be maintained at 28% or greater.
- *Maternal Acid-Base Management:* Maternal $PaCO_2$ should be maintained at 30 mmHg and arterial PO_2 around 150 mmHg. Care must be taken not to hyperventilate as hypocarbia due to hyperventilation leads to a significant decrease in uterine blood flow.
- *Temperature Management*: Optimal temperature management during CPB in pregnant patients remains controversial. Fetal heart rate is directly influenced by maternal temperature, and hypothermic perfusion has been linked to fetal complications such as asystole, uterine contractions, and decreased placental blood flow. Additionally, both cooling and rewarming phases can induce sustained uterine contractions, leading to fetal distress. While earlier literature suggested that normothermic CPB was associated with lower fetal mortality, recent reports indicate successful fetal outcomes following the use of mild hypothermia (32–34 °C), which is now used in the majority of cases. Notably, even deep hypothermia with circulatory arrest (DHCA) has been reported with 68% fetal survival in a series of 22 cases.

Uterine Contractions and Fetal Heart Rate

- *CPB and Uterine Contractions:* CPB may induce sustained uterine contractions, which should be treated promptly with tocolytics. Tocolytic therapies include beta-mimetic agents (such as terbutaline), magnesium sulfate, calcium channel blockers, and cyclooxygenase inhibitors (like indomethacin).
  - Beta-mimetic agents can induce pulmonary edema in a small percentage of patients (typically around 0.5–1%, though some reports suggest up to 5%). They may also cause sinus tachycardia, atrial fibrillation, supraventricular tachycardia, and hypotension. Therefore, these agents should be used with caution, especially in patients with pre-existing cardiac conditions.
  - Magnesium offers the added benefit of fetal cerebral protection, has a negligible effect on hemodynamics, and does not affect fetal blood flow. It is typically administered as a bolus followed by a continuous infusion, and magnesium levels should be monitored regularly, especially in anesthetized patients.
  - Calcium channel blockers relax myometrial smooth muscle; nifedipine, for instance, decreases pulmonary and systemic vascular resistance, which may lead to hypotension.
- *Fetal Heart Rate Changes During CPB:* Initiation of CPB almost always results in fetal bradycardia, and fetal tachycardia is commonly observed at the end of CPB. Fetal bradycardia often manifests as a response to fetal hypoxia and acidosis.

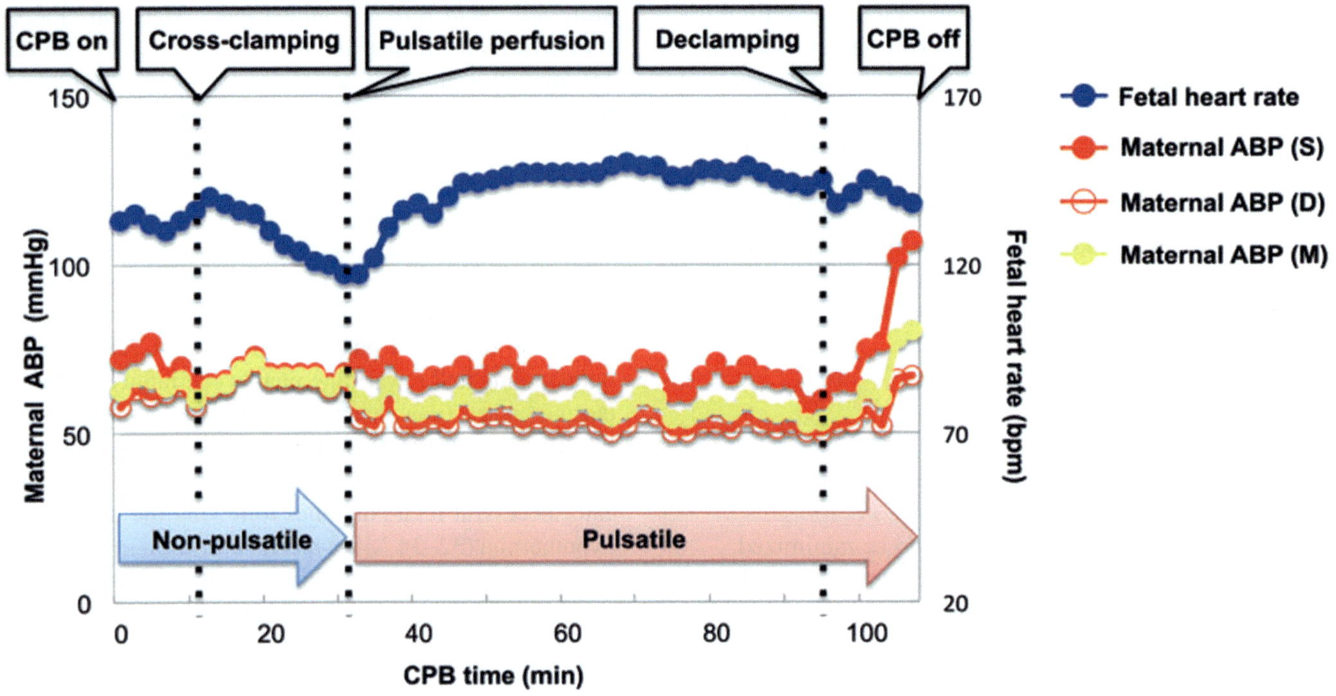

Fig. 38.1 This graph illustrates the monitoring of fetal heart rate and maternal hemodynamics during CPB with transitions between non-pulsatile and pulsatile flow. Key phases of the procedure are marked, including CPB initiation, cross-clamping, the start of pulsatile perfusion, declamping, and CPB termination. Notably, maternal arterial blood pressure (ABP) is shown in three traces: systolic (S), diastolic (D), and mean (M), highlighting the impact of pulsatile flow on these parameters and on fetal heart rate (bpm)

Mechanical Circulatory Assistance and ECMO During Pregnancy

ECMO, primarily veno-arterial (V-A), but also veno-venous (V-V), is increasingly used during pregnancy and offers insights into the use of CPB considerations in this context. Common indications for ECMO include acute respiratory distress syndrome (ARDS), PE, peripartum cardiomyopathy, pulmonary hypertension, postpartum hemorrhage, and Eisenmenger syndrome. Four systematic reviews covering 257 pregnant women on ECMO report a 19% maternal mortality rate (range: 9–23%) and 29% fetal mortality (range: 22–35%). Notably, fetal mortality with ECMO appears lower than with CPB, a finding warranting further research.

Additional reports highlight the use of IABP, Impella devices, and chronic implanted VADs in pregnant patients. For critically ill pregnant women, C-section with CPB on standby, or immediate post-delivery cardiac surgery often results in positive outcomes for both mother and fetus.

Recommended management of CPB during pregnancy is summarized in Table 38.3, which organizes the complex protocols into clear categories for ease of reference in clinical settings. The table encompasses anesthesia choices, specific procedures, and key parameters to monitor for both maternal and fetal well-being during CPB. Remember that these are guidelines, and individualized approaches, based on the patient's specific condition and expert consultation, may be necessary.

Further Reading

Alameh A, Jabri A, Aleyadeh W, et al. Pregnancy-associated myocardial infarction: a review of current practices and guidelines. Curr Cardiol Rep. 2021 Aug 19;23(10):142.

Balough JB, Kickinson KJ, Mhlyre JM. ECMO for obstetric patients: a new era. A&A. 2022;135(2):64–7.

Barrus A, Afshar S, Sani S, et al. Acute type A aortic dissection and successful surgical repair in a woman at 21 weeks gestational pregnancy with maternal and fetal survival: a case report. J Cardiothorac Vasc Anesth. 2018 Jun;32(3):1487–93.

Bauchat JR, Van de Velde M. Nonobstetric surgery during pregnancy. Chapter 17. In: Chestnut DH, Wong CA, Tsen LC, et al., editors. Obstetric anesthesia, principles and practice. 6th ed; 2020. p. 369–91.

Braverman AC, Mittauer E, Harris KM, et al. Clinical features and outcomes of pregnancy-related acute aortic dissection. JAMA Cardiol. 2021 Jan 1;6(1):58–66.

Brízido C, Madeira S, Silva C, et al. Spontaneous coronary artery dissection: a review for clinical and interventional cardiologists. Rev. Port Cardiol. 2023 Mar;42(3):269–76.

Carlier L, Devroe S, Budts W, et al. Cardiac interventions in pregnancy and peripartum—a narrative review of the literature. J Cardiothorac Vasc Anesth. 2020;34(12):3409–19.

Cauldwell M, Johnson M, Jahangiri M, Roos-Hesselink J. Cardiac interventions and cardiac surgery and pregnancy. Int J Cardiol. 2019;276:43–7.

Chen SW, Zhong YL, Ge YP, et al. Successful repair of acute type A aortic dissection during pregnancy at 16th gestational week with maternal and fetal survival: a case report and review of the literature. World J Clin Cases. 2019;7(18):2843–285.

Countouris ME, Marino AL, Raymond M, et al. Infective endocarditis in pregnancy: a contemporary cohort. Am J Perinatol. 2022 Aug 22; https://doi.org/10.1055/a-1877-5763.

Dayanand S, Martinez JM, Figueredo VM, Gupta S. Mechanical circulatory support in women. J Cardiol. 2021;77(3):209–16.

Elkayam U, Schäfer A, Chieffo A, et al. Use of Impella heart pump for management of women with peripartum cardiogenic shock. Clin Cardiol. 2019 Oct;42(10):974–81.

Elsayed AAA, Abdelaal KM, Abdelghaffar AMM, et al. Poor outcome of surgical management of acute malfunctioning mechanical mitral valve during pregnancy. Should centers with limited resources find different options? Heart Surg Forum. 2019;26:E405–10.

Escolà-Vergé L, Rello P, Declerck C, et al. Infective endocarditis in pregnant women without intravenous drug use: a multicentre retrospective case series. J Antimicrob Chemother. 2022 Sep 30;77(10):2701–5.

Foolchand S, Ramnarain H. Prosthetic heart valve thrombosis in pregnancy: a case series on acute management. Cardiovasc J Afr. 2021 Jul-Aug 23;32(4):228–32.

Fukuda W, Chiyoya M, Taniguchi S, et al. Management of deep vein thrombosis and pulmonary embolism (venous thromboembolism) during pregnancy. Gen Thorac Cardiovasc Surg. 2016 Jun;64(6):309–14.

Gayam S, Staab J, Shih G, Stoops S. Cesarean delivery in a parturient with a left ventricular assist device. Int J Obstet Anesth. 2020 Nov;44:53–5.

Gevaert S, Van Belleghem Y, Bouchez S, et al. Acute and critically ill peripartum cardiomyopathy and 'bridge to' therapeutic options: a single center experience with intra-aortic balloon pump, extra corporeal membrane oxygenation and continuous-flow left ventricular assist devices. Crit Care. 2011;15(2):R93.

Ginwalla M, Pillai D, Gandhi S. Use of intra-aortic balloon counterpulsation during emergent cesarean section in a pregnant patient with myocardial infarction. J Invasive Cardiol. 2010 Jun;22(6):E104–6.

Girnius A, Meng ML. Cardio-obstetrics: a review for the cardiac anesthesiologist. J Cardiothorac Vasc Anesth. 2021 Dec;35(12):3483–8.

Grocott H, Smith MS, Shore-Lesserson L. CPB Management and organ protection. Chapter 31. In: Kaplan JA, et al., editors. Kaplan's cardiac anesthesia. 7th ed; 2017. p. 1111–61.

Jha N, Jha AK, Chand Chauhan R, Chauhan NS. Maternal and fetal outcome after cardiac operations during pregnancy: a meta-analysis. Ann Thorac Surg. 2018;106(2):618–26.

John AS, Connolly HM, Schaff HV, Klarich K. Management of cardiac myxoma during pregnancy: a case series and review of the literature. Int J Cardiol. 2012 Mar 8;155(2):177–80.

Johnson MZ, Damianopoulos NJ, Lee F, Yong G. Mitral valve-in-valve implantation during pregnancy. BMJ Case Rep. 2021 Nov 23;14(11):e244270.

Kacmar RM, Gaiser R. Physiologic changes of pregnancy. Chapter 2. In: Chestnut DH, Wong CA, Tsen LC, et al., editors. Obstetric anesthesia, principles and practice. 6th ed; 2020. p. 13–31.

LaRue S, Shanks A, Wang IW, et al. Left ventricular assist device in pregnancy. Obstet Gynecol. 2011 Aug;118(2 Pt 2):426–8.

Liu Y, Han F, Zhuang J, et al. Cardiac operation under cardiopulmonary bypass during pregnancy. J Cardiothorac Surg. 2020;15(1):92.

Makdisi G, Jan MY, Dungy-Poythress L, et al. Successful delivery in a patient with left ventricular assist device and unplanned pregnancy. Ann Thorac Surg. 2017 Jul;104(1):e31–3.

Masada K, Shimamura K, Kuratani T, Sawa Y. Management of foetal circulation by switching to pulsatile perfusion during cardiovascular surgery in pregnancy. Eur J Cardiothorac Surg. 2018;53(3):680–1.

Meng ML, Smiley R. The cardio-obstetrics patient and the cardiothoracic anesthesiologist. J Cardiothoracic Vasc Anesth. 2022 Feb;36(2):546–8.

Meng ML, Arendt KW, Banayan JM, et al. Anesthetic care of the pregnant patient with cardiovascular disease: a scientific statement from the american heart association. Circulation. 2023 Mar 14;147(11):e657–73.

Merlo AC, Rosa GM, Porto I. Pregnancy-related acute myocardial infarction: a review of the recent literature. Clin Res Cardiol. 2022 Jul;111(7):723–31.

Moore SA, Dietl CA, Coleman DM. Extracorporeal life support during pregnancy. J Thorac Cardiovasc Surg. 2016;151:1154–60.

Nallapati C, Park K. Ischemic heart disease in pregnancy. Cardiol Clin. 2021 Feb;39(1):91–108.

Nguyen A, Schaff HV. Cardiac surgery during pregnancy. In: Elkayam U, editor. Cardiac problems in pregnancy; 2019. https://doi.org/10.1002/9781119409861.ch26.

O'Kelly AC, Ludmir J, Wood MJ. Acute coronary syndrome in pregnancy and the post-partum period. J Cardiovasc Dev Dis. 2022 Jun 23;9(7):198.

Ong J, Zhang JJY, Lorusso R, et al. Extracorporeal membrane oxygenation in pregnancy and the postpartum period: a systematic review of case reports. Int J Obstet Anesth. 2020;43:106–13.

Pitfield AF, Annie Bedard A, Jamil BJ. Anesthetic management for cardiac surgery during pregnancy complicated by postoperative threatened abortion. J Cardiothorac Vasc Anesth. 2023 Jan;37(1):158–66.

Pomini F, Mercogliano D, Cavalletti C, Caruso A, Pomini P. Cardiopulmonary bypass in pregnancy. Ann Thorac Surg. 1996;61(1):259–68.

Regitz-Zagrosek V, Lundqvist CB, Borghi C, et al. Guidelines on the management of cardiovascular diseases during pregnancy. Eur Heart J. 32(24):3147–97.

Rimmer L, Heyward-Chaplin J, South M, Gouda M, Bashir M. Acute aortic dissection during pregnancy: trials and tribulations. J Card Surg. 2021;36(5):1799–805.

Samalavicius RS, Puodziukaite L, Radaviciute I, et al. Prophylactic use of an intra-aortic balloon pump in a high-risk patient with peripartum cardiomyopathy requiring cesarean delivery. Int J Obstet Anesth. 2018;33:67–71.

Sebah MB, Mengistu AD, Tadesse KD, Tekleab AM. Immediate maternal and fetal outcome following percutaneous mitral valve balloon commissurotomy: a 6-year single-center experience from sub-Saharan Africa. Cardiol Young. 2022 Oct;32(10):1616–20.

Sebastian NA, et al. Extracorporeal membrane oxygenation in pregnant and postpartum patients: a systematic review. J Matern Fetal Neonatal Med. 35(24):4663–73.

Sharma JB, Yadav V, Mishra S, et al. Comparative study on maternal and fetal outcome in pregnant women with rheumatic heart disease and severe mitral stenosis undergoing percutaneous balloon mitral valvotomy before or during pregnancy. Indian Heart J. 2018 Sep-Oct;70(5):685–9.

Shook LL, Barth WH Jr. Cardiac surgery during pregnancy. Clin Obstet Gynecol. 2020;63(2):429–46.

Song S, Lu L, Li L, et al. Antepartum acute stanford type A aortic dissection: a case report and literature review. J Cardiothorac Surg. 2022 Apr 12;17(1):73.

Srichawla BS, Sekhon M. Biventricular impella (BiPella) utilization in fulminant COVID-19 myopericarditis-mediated cardiogenic shock during pregnancy. Clin Res Cardiol. 2023 Feb;112:1475–8.

Taha B, Guglielminotti J, Li G, Landau R. Utilization and outcomes of extracorporeal membrane oxygenation in obstetric patients in the United States, 1999–2014: a retrospective cross-sectional study. Anesth Analg. 2022;135(2):268–76.

Tran TQ. Successful emergency management for aortic arch rupture in pregnancy at first trimesters: a case report. Int J Surg Case Rep. 2019;64:28–30.

van Hagen IM, Thorne SA, Taha N, et al. Pregnancy outcomes in women with rheumatic mitral valve disease: results from the registry of pregnancy and cardiac disease. Circulation. 137(8):806–16.

van Steenbergen GJ, Tsang QHY, van der Heijden OWH, et al. Timing of cardiac surgery during pregnancy: a patient-level meta-analysis. Eur Heart J. 2022 Aug 1;43(29):2801–11.

Vidovich MI. Cardiovascular disease. Chapter 41. In: Chestnut DH, Wong CA, Tsen LC, et al., editors. Obstetric anesthesia, principles and practice. 6th ed; 2020. p. 987–1024.

Weiner MM, Hamburger J, Beilin Y. The pregnant patient with cardiac disease. Chapter 50. In: Kaplan JA, et al., editors. Kaplan's cardiac anesthesia: for cardiac and noncardiac surgery. 7th ed; 2017. p. 1582–99.

Wong MJ, Bharadwaj S, Galey JL, Lankford AS, Galvagno S, Kodali BS. Extracorporeal membrane oxygenation for pregnant and postpartum patients. Anesth Analg. 2022;135(2):277–89.

Würdinger M, Cammann VL, Ghadri JR, Templin C. Spontaneous coronary artery dissection: a rare event? Heart Fail Clin. 2022 Jan;18(1):189–99.

You Y, Liu S, Wu Z, et al. Cardiac surgery under cardiopulmonary bypass in pregnancy: report of four cases. J Cardiothorac Surg. 2021;16(1):268.

Yuan SM. Cardiac myxoma in pregnancy: a comprehensive review. Rev. Bras Cir Cardiovasc. 2015 Jul-Sep;30(3):386–94.

Zhang JJY, Ong JA, Syn NL, et al. Extracorporeal membrane oxygenation in pregnant and postpartum women: a systematic review and meta-regression analysis. J Intensive Care Med. 2021;36(2):220–8.

Zhu JM, Ma WG, Peterss S, et al. Aortic dissection in pregnancy: management strategy and outcomes. Ann Thorac Surg. 2017 Apr;103(4):1199–206.

Part XII

Charting and Record Documentation

Paper and Electronic Record Charting in Perfusion

39

Kayla You

Introduction

In the rapidly evolving medical landscape, documentation has become a cornerstone of patient care, ensuring transparency, continuity, and accountability. This is particularly true in the field of perfusion, where data recording is of paramount importance. According to the American Society of Extracorporeal Technology (AmSECT) Standards and Guidelines for Perfusion Practice, documentation not only fulfills an obligatory requirement but also establishes a pivotal connection between clinical practice and patient outcomes. Each perfusion record is more than just a transcript of numbers and notes; it is a vital component of the patient's overall medical story.

This inclusion in the permanent medical records serves multiple purposes. It not only provides a chronological account of the patient's treatment but also aids in the streamlined transition of care from the operating room to postoperative teams. The mandate to maintain and store these records according to institutional policies further emphasizes their enduring value. It ensures that they remain accessible, unaltered, and intact for future reference, legal requirements, or other clinical needs.

In this chapter, we will discuss the different ways of charting in perfusion: traditional paper charting and modern electronic record charting. We will explore the advantages and disadvantages of each method and how they are used in clinical practice today. The objective is to shed light on the significance of meticulous documentation and how it has evolved over time to improve patient care.

Importance of Documentation

Accurate and detailed charting in perfusion is not simply a protocol but a fundamental requirement. Highlighted by the AmSECT Standards and Guidelines, the information meticulously captured on the perfusion chart serves purposes beyond its immediate application (Fig. 39.1). Here are the reasons emphasizing its paramount importance:

1. *Foundation for Postoperative Care*: A comprehensive perfusion record serves as a reference point for the postoperative care team. It provides insight into the patient's physiological responses and the interventions made during the surgical procedure, ensuring continuity of care.
2. *Legal Implications*: The perfusion chart, when viewed as a part of the patient's permanent medical record, can serve as evidence in medical-legal cases. A detailed and timestamped documentation can validate the actions taken by the perfusionist and the medical team.
3. *Quality Assurance and Continuous Improvement*: Regularly maintained and detailed records can be analyzed for patterns and trends. This can highlight potential areas of improvement in the surgical and perfusion processes, leading to enhanced patient outcomes in future.
4. *Communication Among Medical Team*: Often, surgical procedures involve multiple specialists and medical professionals. A well-documented perfusion record can act as a medium of communication, ensuring that everyone is in agreement regarding the patient's condition and the interventions made.
5. *Patient Safety*: In scenarios where immediate decisions need to be made, having an exhaustive perfusion record can be invaluable. It ensures that the medical team is equipped with all the necessary information, minimizing the chances of oversight and enhancing patient safety.

K. You (✉)
Department of Clinical Perfusion, Keystone Perfusion Services, PC., Headquartered in Mountain Top, Mountain Top, PA, USA

A. S. Awad, J. DiNardo (eds.), *Clinical Perfusion for Cardiac Surgery*, https://doi.org/10.1007/978-3-031-91163-7_39

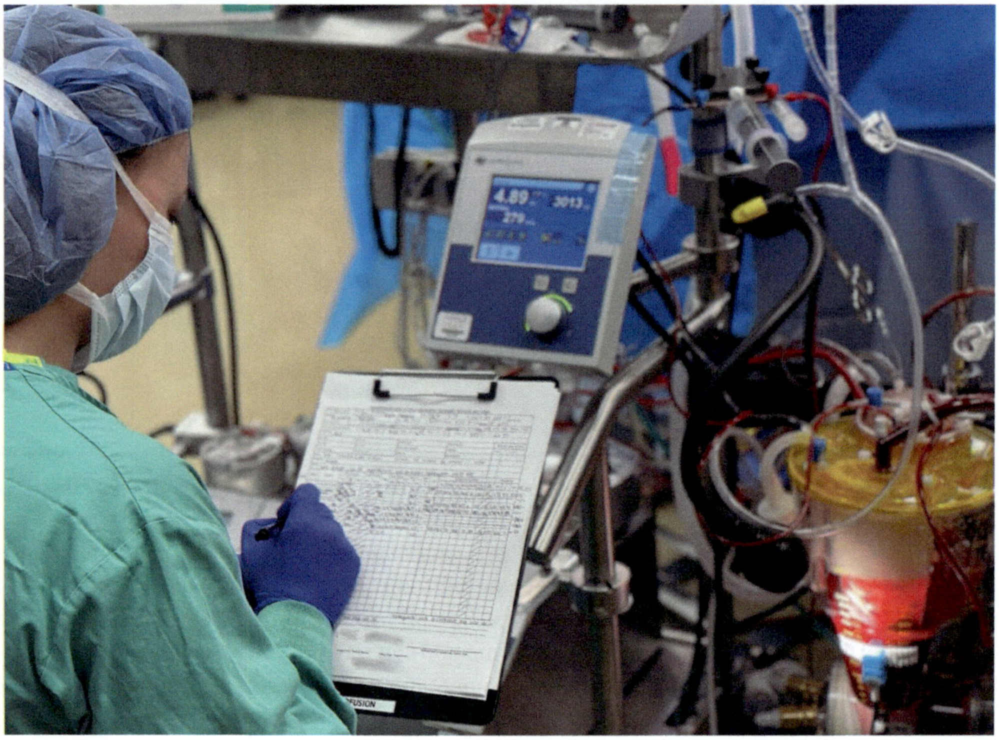

Fig. 39.1 A focused clinical perfusionist diligently records patient data on a paper record during a cardiopulmonary bypass run, ensuring precision and attention to detail amidst the critical environment of a cardiac surgery operating room

What to Include in a Perfusion Record:

- Patient demographics and preoperative risk factors.
- Description of the procedure, equipment used, and involved personnel.
- Physiological parameters, such as blood flow rates, arterial pressures, and temperatures [of both the patient and the cardiopulmonary bypass machine blood (CPB)].
- Results of blood gas, anticoagulation monitoring, and oxygen saturations.
- Other specific values such as cardioplegia and oxygen flow rate.
- Signatures of all involved perfusionists.

Frequency of Documentation

During CPB charting, frequent documentation is essential for accurate and continuous patient care. Throughout the procedure, perfusionists are responsible for the diligent recording of various critical parameters. These recordings are typically carried out at intervals of 15 minutes, or more often if significant events or changes occur. These parameters include, but are not limited to, patient vitals, pump speed, oxygenator performance, temperature, blood gas levels, and administered medications and blood products.

Immediate documentation is required for critical incidents or interventions, such as flow rate adjustments or reactions to medications, to accurately capture the details and timing of these events.

The perfusionist must also document any communication with the surgical team, particularly the surgeon and anesthesiologist, regarding changes in the patient's status or the procedure. This real-time documentation is essential for postoperative review and quality assurance, ensuring that every aspect of the CPB run is recorded and can be analyzed for future reference, whether for educational purposes, quality improvement, or regulatory compliance.

Types of Record Charting in Perfusion

Traditional Paper Charting

Traditionally, perfusion has relied on paper charting to document patient data during cardiac surgeries (Fig. 39.2). This method requires perfusionists to manually record a variety of details, including the patient's medical history, the surgical intervention, and physiological parameters. Ensuring the accuracy and completeness of these paper records is essential during cardiac surgeries. While paper charting has been a tried-and-true method for many years, it has multifaceted challenges. Not only is the process tedious, demanding undivided attention for real-time manual documentation, but the physical nature of paper charts also exposes them to risks of misplacement or damage—both of which could jeopardize the integrity of a patient's medical record. Additionally, an often-overlooked pitfall of paper charting during the conduct

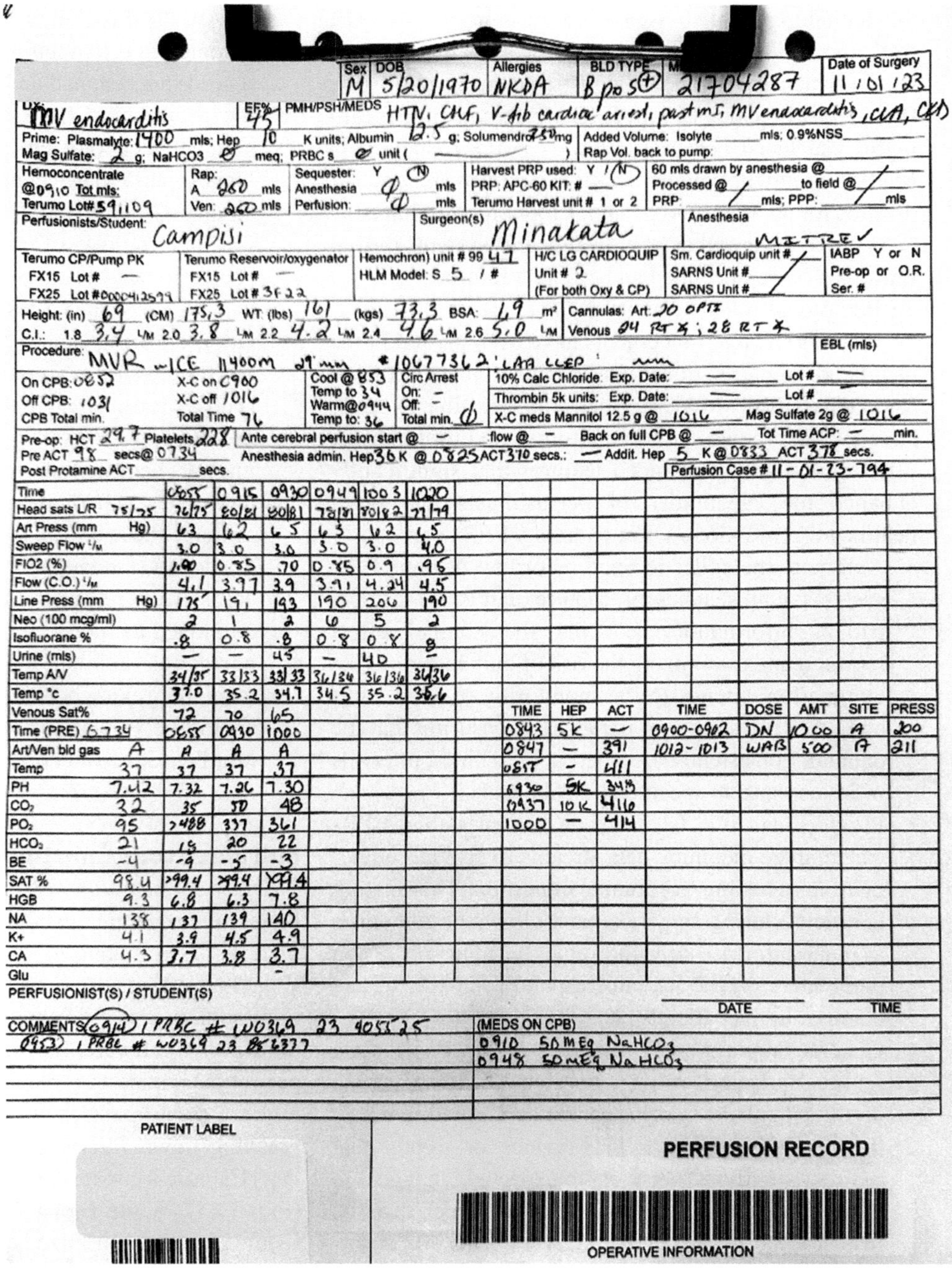

Sex: M | DOB: 5/20/1970 | Allergies: NKDA | BLD TYPE: B pos ⊕ | 21704287 | Date of Surgery: 11/01/23

DX: MV endocarditis | EF%: 45 | PMH/PSH/MEDS: HTN, CHF, V-fib cardiac arrest, past MI, MV endocarditis, CVA, CKD

Prime: Plasmalyte: 1400 mls; Hep 10 K units; Albumin 12.5 g; Solumendrol 250 mg | Added Volume: Isolyte ____ mls; 0.9%NSS ____
Mag Sulfate: 2 g; NaHCO3 Ø meq; PRBC s Ø unit ( ) | Rap Vol. back to pump:

Hemoconcentrate @0910 Tot mls: Terumo Lot# 59,109 | Rap: A 260 mls Ven: 260 mls | Sequester: Y / (N) Anesthesia Ø mls Perfusion: Ø mls | Harvest PRP used: Y / (N) PRP: APC-60 KIT: # — Terumo Harvest unit # 1 or 2 | 60 mls drawn by anesthesia @ / Processed @ / to field @ / PRP: / mls; PPP: / mls

Perfusionists/Student: Campisi | Surgeon(s): Minakata | Anesthesia: Mitrev

Terumo CP/Pump PK FX15 Lot # — FX25 Lot #0000412599 | Terumo Reservoir/oxygenator FX15 Lot # — FX25 Lot # 3F22 | Hemochron) unit # 9947 HLM Model: S 5 / # | H/C LG CARDIOQUIP Unit # 2 (For both Oxy & CP) | Sm. Cardioquip unit # / SARNS Unit # / SARNS Unit # / | IABP Y or N Pre-op or O.R. Ser. #

Height: (in) 69 (CM) 175.3 WT (lbs) 161 (kgs) 73.3 BSA: 1.9 m² | Cannulas: Art: 20 OPTI
C.I.: 1.8 3.4 L/M 2.0 3.8 L/M 2.2 4.2 L/M 2.4 4.6 L/M 2.6 5.0 L/M | Venous 24 RT ∡; 28 RT ∡

Procedure: MVR w/ ICE 11400M 29 mm #10677362; LAA clip | EBL (mls)

On CPB: 0852 Off CPB: 1031 CPB Total min. | X-C on 0900 X-C off 1016 Total Time 76 | Cool @ 853 Temp to 34 Warm @ 0944 Temp to: 36 | Circ Arrest On: – Off: – Total min. Ø | 10% Calc Chloride Exp. Date: — Lot # — | Thrombin 5k units: Exp. Date: — Lot # | X-C meds Mannitol 12.5 g @ 1016 Mag Sulfate 2g @ 1016

Pre-op: HCT 29.7 Platelets 228 | Ante cerebral perfusion start @ – flow @ – Back on full CPB @ – Tot Time ACP: – min.
Pre ACT 98 secs @ 0734 | Anesthesia admin. Hep 36 K @ 0825 ACT 370 secs.: — Addit. Hep 5 K @ 0833 ACT 378 secs.
Post Protamine ACT ____ secs. | Perfusion Case # 11-01-23-794

Time		0855	0915	0930	0949	1003	1020
Head sats L/R	75/75	76/75	80/81	80/81	78/81	80/82	77/79
Art Press (mm Hg)		63	62	65	63	62	65
Sweep Flow L/M		3.0	3.0	3.0	3.0	3.0	4.0
FIO2 (%)		1.00	0.85	.70	0.85	0.9	.95
Flow (C.O.) L/M		4.1	3.97	3.9	3.91	4.24	4.5
Line Press (mm Hg)		175	191	193	190	206	190
Neo (100 mcg/ml)		2	1	2	6	5	2
Isofluorane %		.8	0.8	.8	0.8	0.8	.8
Urine (mls)		–	–	45	–	40	–
Temp A/V		34/35	33/33	33/33	36/34	36/36	36/36
Temp °c		37.0	35.2	34.7	34.5	35.2	35.6

	Pre (0734)			
Venous Sat%		72	70	65
Time (PRE)	0734	0855	0930	1000
Art/Ven bld gas	A	A	A	A
Temp	37	37	37	37
PH	7.42	7.32	7.26	7.30
CO_2	32	35	50	48
PO_2	95	>488	337	361
HCO_3	21	18	20	22
BE	-4	-9	-5	-3
SAT %	98.4	>99.4	>99.4	>99.4
HGB	9.3	6.8	6.3	7.8
NA	138	137	139	140
K+	4.1	3.9	4.5	4.9
CA	4.3	3.7	3.8	3.7
Glu				–

TIME	HEP	ACT
0843	5K	–
0847	–	391
0857	–	411
0930	5K	343
0937	10K	416
1000	–	414

TIME	DOSE	AMT	SITE	PRESS
0900-0902	DN	1000	A	200
1012-1013	WAB	500	A	211

PERFUSIONIST(S) / STUDENT(S)

DATE TIME

COMMENTS (0914) 1 PRBC # W0369 23 405525
(0953) 1 PRBC # W0369 23 862377

(MEDS ON CPB)
0910 50 mEq $NaHCO_3$
0948 50 mEq $NaHCO_3$

PATIENT LABEL

PERFUSION RECORD

OPERATIVE INFORMATION

Fig. 39.2 A meticulously maintained paper chart captures real-time data and critical observations of a patient's physiological status during a CPB run, ensuring precise monitoring and immediate responsiveness from the medical team

of CPB is the potential distraction it can pose. As perfusionists engage in manual logging, their primary focus can inadvertently shift from the patient's immediate care, potentially compromising safety and efficacy.

Transition from Paper to Digital

The transition from paper to digital records in healthcare represents a significant transformation driven by government regulations and technological advancements.

Drivers of Change:

(a) Government Regulations

The evolution of electronic charting in medicine, spurred by the American Recovery and Reinvestment Act of 2009, marked a pivotal shift from paper records to electronic medical records (EMRs). The Act championed the "meaningful use" of Electronic Health Records (EHRs)—digital tools designed to enhance healthcare quality, safety, and efficiency. Furthermore, EHRs promote better patient and family engagement, streamline care coordination, and safeguard health data. To accelerate the adoption of EHRs, the Act provided financial incentives for healthcare providers who embraced this technology and showcased its meaningful use. The Act offered financial incentives to healthcare providers who adopted EHRs and demonstrated meaningful use. Providers who did not adopt EHRs or demonstrate meaningful use faced penalties, such as a 1% reduction in Medicare reimbursements. This two-pronged approach—rewards for adoption and penalties for non-compliance—helped to ensure that the healthcare system moved towards a more integrated and efficient future.

(b) Technological Advancements

Technological advancements have been pivotal in the healthcare sector's transition to Electronic Perfusion Records (EPRs). Modern electronic charting systems have evolved to become more intuitive and user-centric, offering a suite of advanced features that significantly enhance the capabilities of perfusionists and other healthcare professionals. For example, EPRs can:

- Automate the collection and recording of data. EPR systems can seamlessly capture and store critical patient information, reducing the manual effort required and minimizing the risk of human error. This automation extends to the monitoring of vital signs and other physiological parameters, ensuring that the data are consistently recorded at predefined intervals or in response to specific clinical events.
- Provide real-time feedback on patient status. EPRs can analyze incoming data streams to provide immediate insights into a patient's condition. This feature is crucial during surgeries, as it allows perfusionists to make informed decisions quickly, adjust perfusion parameters on the fly, and respond promptly to any changes in the patient's physiological state.
- Generate reports and alerts. The ability to generate reports and alerts is an extension of this real-time monitoring. EPR systems can be configured to notify the perfusionists of critical values or trends that require attention, such as unexpected changes in blood flow or oxygenation levels. These alerts can be instrumental in preventing adverse events and ensuring patient safety.
- Integrate with other clinical systems. The ability of EPRs to integrate with other clinical systems is one of their most transformative aspects. This feature consolidates all patient information into a single, comprehensive profile. This holistic approach provides healthcare professionals with an in-depth and complete picture of the patient's medical status. For example, clinicians anywhere can instantly view the operative note and CPB run chart, enabling them to thoroughly examine the full scope of patient records, including the detailed documentation of the CPB run, regardless of their physical location.

Amidst this shift, some hospitals have adopted a transitional, hybrid methodology, where traditional paper records are scanned and digitized to be incorporated into the overarching EMR. While this strategy bridges the gap between old and new methods, it presents challenges, particularly concerning data accuracy and accessibility. Other hospitals adopt post-procedure data entry. For this, the role of clinical perfusionists or data entry professionals becomes crucial in transcribing historical paper charts into EPR systems. Prioritizing data for entry, ensuring quality control, and providing continuous training are essential steps in this process. Challenges such as missing or illegible information, inconsistency in data formats, and potential misinterpretation due to unclear handwriting may arise. Clear procedures for data entry and quality control must be established to mitigate these issues. For efficient data entry, it is crucial to adopt a standardized template that ensures uniformity across all records. Keyboard shortcuts should be employed to speed up the process, allowing for quicker navigation and data input. Additionally, a rigorous protocol for reviewing data before finalizing submissions should be in place, involving a thorough double-check of all entries to catch and correct any errors.

Full Electronic Charting (E-Charting)

Numerous academic establishments are undergoing a complete shift from hybrid record-keeping to full E-charting (Fig. 39.3), driven by the compelling reasons outlined in the section "Drivers of Change." This shift, often facilitated by third-party software, ensures seamless access to crucial patient data, making it readily available in real-time to every relevant department. E-charting streamlines patient care by breaking down interdepartmental barriers and automating Data Capture from devices like anesthesia and CPB Machines (Fig. 39.4). While E-charting offers clear benefits, such as secure data and minimized errors, it also presents challenges, such as training and initial costs. A primary challenge is the need for comprehensive training for clinical perfusionists, as the shift from paper to digital requires a certain level of tech-savviness and familiarity with new systems. This can be a steep learning curve for some staff members. Additionally, the upfront costs of purchasing and setting up E-charting systems can be substantial, posing a financial challenge, especially for smaller healthcare facilities. Lastly, in this post-modern era of easily accessible data, there is always a risk that electronic medical records can be compromised by unauthorized individuals or groups. Therefore, it is of utmost important that a hospital and hospital system maintain thorough security of their EMR.

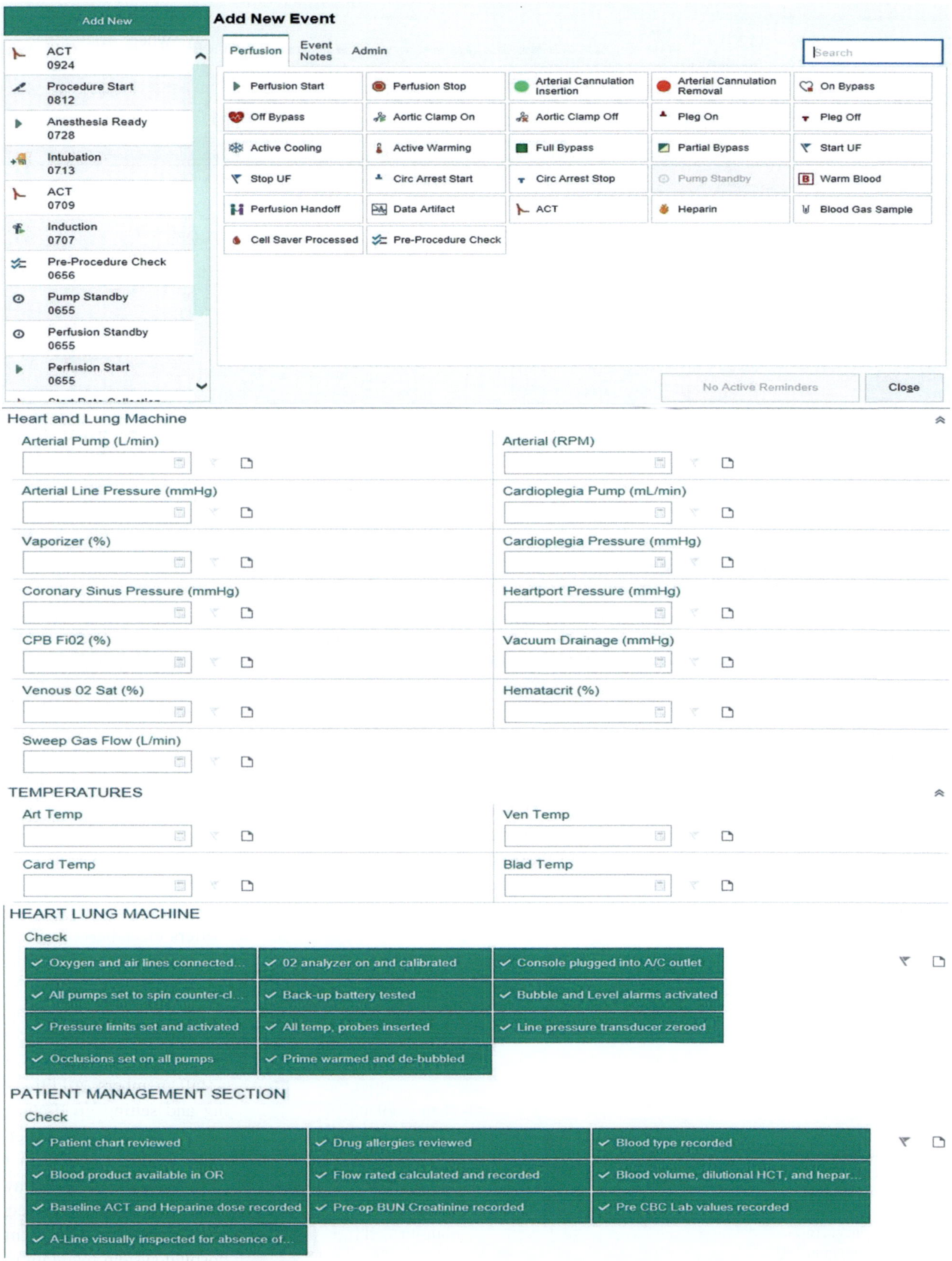

Fig. 39.3 Seamless digital integration: the future of perfusion charting in action. This series of screenshots demonstrates the advanced features of third-party software, highlighting its role in revolutionizing perfusion charting. With seamless digital integration and user-friendly interfaces, such as simple checkbox selections, it offers a glimpse into the future of medical record-keeping in perfusion practices

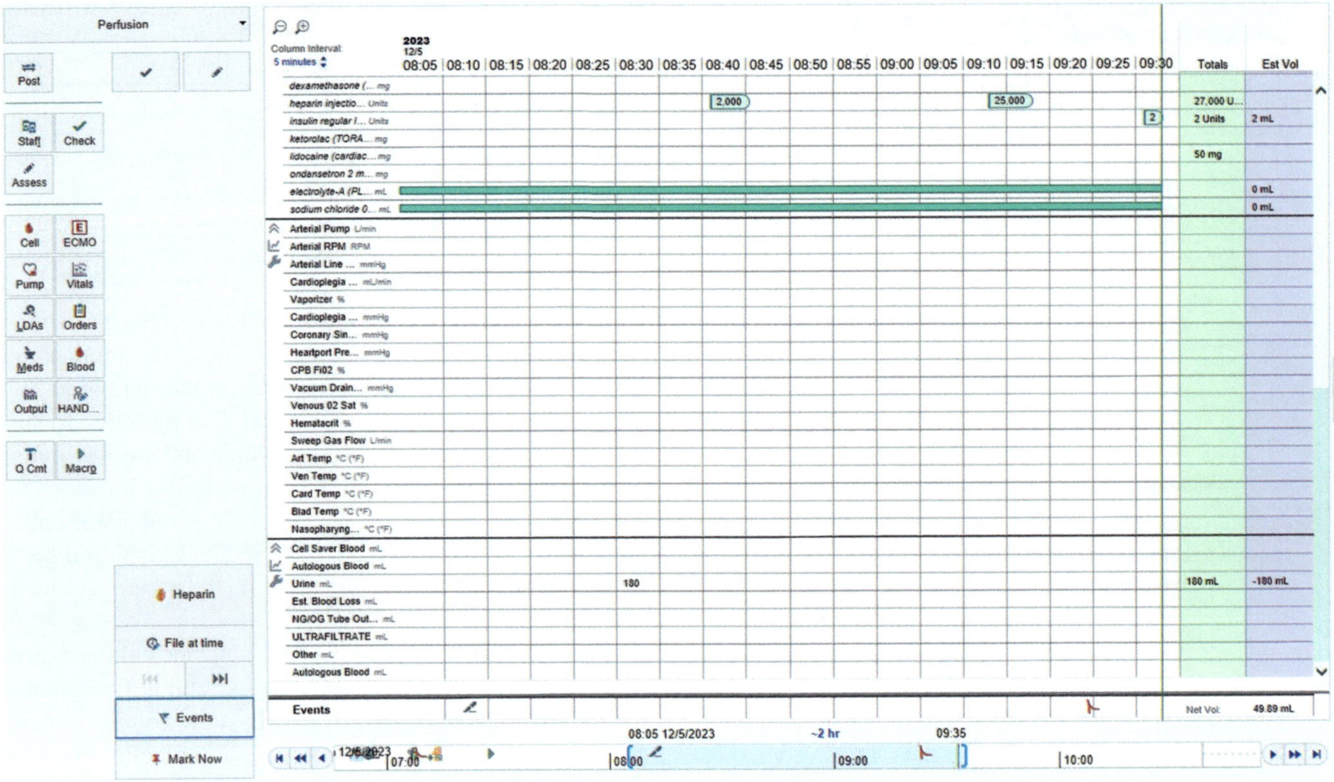

Fig. 39.4 Screenshot of Epic software: automating Data Capture from CPB Machines. This image showcases the Epic software interface, highlighting its capability to automate Data Capture directly from the CPB machine, streamlining the process of recording and managing critical patient information during surgical procedures

Artificial Intelligence (AI) and Machine Learning

The integration of cutting-edge technologies, like AI and machine learning, indicates a promising future for E-charting. These technologies promise to take E-charting to the next level by enabling more sophisticated analysis of patient data for faster, more accurate, and tailored interventions, enhancing patient care.

Further Reading

American Society of ExtraCorporeal Technology Standards and Guidelines for Perfusion Practice. Standard 4: Perfusion Record. 2023. https://www.amsect.org/Policy-Practice/AmSECTs-Standards-and-Guidelines

CMS finalizes definition of meaningful use of certified electronic health records (EHR) technology. https://www.cms.gov

Index

A. S. Awad, J. DiNardo (eds.), *Clinical Perfusion for Cardiac Surgery*, https://doi.org/10.1007/978-3-031-91163-7

D

E

F

I

O

P

GPSR Compliance

The European Union's (EU) General Product Safety Regulation (GPSR) is a set of rules that requires consumer products to be safe and our obligations to ensure this.

If you have any concerns about our products, you can contact us on ProductSafety@springernature.com

In case Publisher is established outside the EU, the EU authorized representative is:

Springer Nature Customer Service Center GmbH
Europaplatz 3
69115 Heidelberg, Germany

Batch number: 10105642

Printed by Printforce, the Netherlands